# Reference Ranges (continued)

## Endocrinology (continued)

### Thyroid

| | CONVENTIONAL UNITS | SI UNITS |
|---|---|---|
| FT$_3$ | 1.4–4.4 pg/mL | |
| FT$_3$I | 85–205 | |
| FT$_4$ | 0.8–1.8 ng/dL | 10.3–23.2 pmol/L |
| FT$_4$I | 4.2–13.0 | |
| rT$_3$ | 10–28 ng/dL | 0.15–0.43 nmol/L |
| RT$_3$U | 25–35% | |
| sTSH | 0.4–4.2 μU/mL | 0.4–4.2 mIU/L |
| T$_3$ | 80–180 ng/dL | 1.232–2.772 nmol/L |
| T$_4$ | 5.0–12.0 μg/dL | 64.5–154.8 nmol/L |
| Tg | 3–42 ng/mL | 3–42 μg/L |
| THBR | 0.72–1.24 | |

### Parathyroid & Calcium–Phosphorus

| | CONVENTIONAL UNITS | SI UNITS |
|---|---|---|
| Calcium (s) | 8.5–10.5 mg/dL | 2.25–2.60 mmol/L |
| (u) | 100–400 mg/d | 2.5–10.0 mmol/d |
| Calcium, ionized | 4.48–4.92 mg/dL | 0.11–1.23 mmol/L |
| Inorganic phosphorus | 2.8–4.0 mg/dL | 0.90–1.29 mmol/L |
| PTH | 10–65 pg/mL | 1.05–6.84 pmol/L |

### Adrenal

| | CONVENTIONAL UNITS | SI UNITS |
|---|---|---|
| Aldosterone (upright) | 5–30 ng/dL | 0.14–0.83 nmol/L |
| (supine) | 3–10 ng/dL | 0.08–0.28 nmol/L |
| Cortisol (0800 h) | 5–23 μg/dL | 138–635 nmol/L |
| (1600 h) | 3–15 μg/dL | 83–414 nmol/L |
| Dopamine | 0–83 pg/dL | |
| Epinephrine (u) | 0.5–20 μg/24 h (HPLC) | |
| HVA (u) | <15 mg/24 h | <82.4 μmol/d |
| Metanephrines, Total (u) | 0.3–0.9 mg/24 h | |
| Norepinephrine (u) | 14–80 μg/24 h (HPLC) | |
| VMA (u) | 2–7 mg/24 h | 10.1–35.4 μmol/d |

### Reproductive

| | CONVENTIONAL UNITS | SI UNITS |
|---|---|---|
| Androstenedione | | |
| (m) (adult) | 75–205 ng/dL | 2.62–7.16 nmol/L |
| (f) (adult) | 85–275 ng/dL | 2.97–9.60 nmol/L |
| Estradiol | | |
| (f) | | |
| Prepubertal | 4–12 pg/mL | 14.68–44.04 pmol/L |
| Early follicular phase | 30–100 pg/mL | 110.1–367 pmol/L |
| Late follicular phase | 100–400 pg/mL | 367–1468 pmol/L |
| Luteal phase | 50–150 pg/mL | 183.5–550.5 pmol/L |
| Postmenopausal | 5–18 pg/mL | 18.35–66.06 pmol/L |
| (m) | | |
| Prepubertal | 2–8 pg/mL | 7.34–29.36 pmol/L |
| Adult | 10–60 pg/mL | 36.7–220.2 pmol/L |
| DHEA | | |
| (m) | 3.6–6.3 ng/mL | 12.5–21.9 nmol/L |
| (f) | 4.4–6.0 ng/mL | 15.3–20.8 nmol/L |
| DHEA-S | | |
| (m) (adult) | 151–446 μg/dL | 3.9–11.4 μmol/L |
| (f) (premenopausal) | 84–433 μg/dL | 2.2–11.1 μmol/L |
| (postmenopausal) | 1.7–177 μg/dL | 0.04–4.5 μmol/L |
| Free Testosterone | | |
| (m) (adult) | 50–210 pg/mL | 174–729 pmol/L |
| (f) (adult) | 1.0–8.5 pg/mL | 3.47–29.5 pmol/L |
| FSH | | |
| (m) | 2–10 mIU/mL | 2–10 IU/L |
| (f) | | |
| Follicular phase | 2–10 mIU/mL | |
| Mid-cycle peak | 9–18 mIU/mL | |
| Luteal phase | 0–9 mIU/mL | |
| Postmenopause | 20–100 mIU/mL | |
| LH | | |
| (m) | 0–9 mIU/mL | |
| (f) | | |
| Follicular phase | 0–14 mIU/mL | |
| Mid-cycle peak | 20–70 mIU/mL | |
| Luteal phase | 0–16 mIU/mL | |
| Postmenopause | 20–70 mIU/mL | |

## Endocrinology (continued)

### Reproductive (continued)

| | CONVENTIONAL UNITS | SI UNITS |
|---|---|---|
| Progesterone | | |
| (m) | 0.12–0.3 ng/mL | 0.38–0.95 nmol/L |
| (f) | | |
| Menstrual cycle | | |
| Follicular phase | <1 ng/mL | <3.18 nmol/L |
| Luteal phase | 5–20 ng/mL | 15.9–63.6 nmol/L |
| Testosterone | | |
| (m) | | |
| Prepubertal | 10–20 ng/dL | 0.35–0.69 nmol/L |
| Adult | 300–1000 ng/dL | 10.41–36.44 nmol/L |
| (f) | | |
| Prepubertal | 10–20 ng/dL | 0.35–0.69 nmol/L |
| Adult | 20–75 ng/dL | 0.69–2.60 nmol/L |
| Postmenopausal | 8–35 ng/dL | 0.28–1.21 nmol/L |

### GI & Pancreatic Function

| | CONVENTIONAL UNITS | SI UNITS |
|---|---|---|
| Basal Acid Output (m) | 2.2–2.7 mmol/h | |
| (f) | 1.0–1.5 mmol/h | |
| Bile Acids (s) | 200–2000 ng/mL | |
| (u) | 180–400 μg/24 h | |
| Fecal Fat | <6 g/24 H | |
| Gastrin | 0–100 pg/mL | 0–100 ng/L |
| d-Xylose (s) 2 h | >25 mg/dL | >1.65 mmol/L |
| (u) | >4 g/5 h | >26.64 mmol/5 h |

### Nutrition

| | CONVENTIONAL UNITS | SI UNITS |
|---|---|---|
| Creatinine height index | >90% | |
| Hydroxyproline, Total (u) | 15–50 mg/d | |
| Hydroxyproline, Free (u) | <1.3 mg/d | |
| 3-methyl histidine | 3.0–9.0 mg/d | |
| Nitrogen balance (u) | 2–4 g/d | |
| Vitamin C | 0.4–0.6 mg/dL | 22.71–34.07 μmol/L |
| Vitamin B$_{12}$ | 110–800 pg/mL | 81.18–590.4 pmol/L |
| Folate | 3–16 ng/mL | 6.80–36.24 nmol/L |
| Vitamin A | 300–800 μg/L | 1.05–2.79 μmol/L |
| 25(OH)D$_3$ | 14–42 ng/mL | 35–104.83 nmol/L |
| 1,25(OH)$_2$D$_3$ | 15–45 pg/mL | 36–108 pmol/L |
| Vitamin E | 5–18 mg/L | 11.6–59.8 μmol/L |
| Vitamin B$_1$ | 0.21–0.43 μg/dL | |
| Vitamin B$_2$ | 4–24 μg/dL | |
| Vitamin B$_6$ | 5–30 ng/mL | 20.23–121.38 nmol/L |
| Selenium | 50–140 μg/L | 6.35–17.78 μmol/L |
| Zinc | 70–150 μg/dL | 10.71–22.95 μmol/L |
| Copper (m) | 71–140 μg/dL | 11.15–21.98 μmol/L |
| (f) | 80–155 μg/dL | 12.56–24.34 μmol/L |
| Fluoride (u) | 0.2–3.2 mg/L | 10.5–168.3 μmol/L |

### Pregnancy

| | CONVENTIONAL UNITS | SI UNITS |
|---|---|---|
| DHEA-S (term) | 0.23–1.17 μg/mL | 0.6–3.0 μmol/L |
| Estradiol (term) | 5–25 μg/mL | 466–1031 pmol/L |
| Estriol, Total (term) (s) | 48–350 ng/mL | 167–1215 nmol/L |
| (u) | 5,000–50,000 μg/mL | 17,350–173,500 nmol/d |
| FSH (s) | undetectable | |
| hPL (term) (s) | 3.6–8.2 μg/mL | 3.6–8.2 mg/L |
| Progesterone | | |
| 1st trimester | 20–50 ng/mL | |
| 2nd trimester | 50–100 ng/mL | |
| 3rd trimester | 70–250 ng/mL | |
| Testosterone | 3–4 × adult level | |

f = female, m = male, s = serum, u = urine.

# Clinical Chemistry
## Concepts and Applications

# Clinical Chemistry
## Concepts and Applications

**Shauna C. Anderson, PhD**

*Professor, Department of Microbiology*
*Brigham Young University*
*Provo, Utah*

**Susan Cockayne, PhD**

*Associate Professor, Department of Microbiology*
*Brigham Young University*
*Provo, Utah*

**McGraw-Hill**
Medical Publishing Division

*New York / Chicago / San Francisco / Lisbon*
*London / Madrid / Mexico City / Milan / New Delhi*
*San Juan / Seoul / Singapore / Sydney / Toronto*

## Clinical Chemistry: Concepts and Applications

1234567890  PBT PBT  098765432

ISBN 0-07-136047-6

This book was set in Adobe Garamond by Matrix Publishing Services.
The editors were Julie Scardiglia, Michael Brown, Kitty McCullough, and Karen Davis.
The production supervisor was Lisa T. Mendez.
The cover designer was Aimée Nordin.
The index was prepared by Editorial Services, Maria Coughlin.
RR Donnelley was printer and binder.

This book is printed on acid-free paper.

## Library of Congress Cataloging-in-Publication Data

Clinical chemistry : concepts and applications / [edited by] Shauna C. Anderson, Susan Cockayne.
    p. ; cm.
  Includes bibliographical references and index.
  ISBN 0-07-136047-6
  1. Clinical chemistry.  I. Anderson, Shauna Christine, 1945–  II. Cockayne, Susan.
  [DNLM: 1. Chemistry, Clinical. QY 90 C64105 2003]
RB40.C573 2003
616.07'56—dc21
                                                 2002030946

# CONTENTS

# CONTRIBUTORS

**Jane Adrian, EdM, MT(ASCP)**

Director, Clinical Laboratory
Lincoln Developmental Center
Department of Human Services, State of Illinois
Lincoln, Illinois

*Inherited Metabolic Disorders*
*Laboratory Assessment of Psychiatric Disorders*

**Joan E. Aldrich, PhD**

Associate Professor, Department of Medical
  Laboratory Sciences
University of Texas Southwestern Medical Center
Dallas, Texas

*Spectrophotometry*
*Clinical Enzymology*

**Shauna C. Anderson, PhD**

Professor, Department of Microbiology
Brigham Young University
Provo, Utah

*The Parathyroid Glands and Calcium-Phosphate*
  *Metabolism*

**Nancy A. Brunzel, MS**

Clinical Chemistry Teaching Specialist
University of Minnesota
Minneapolis, Minnesota

*Renal Anatomy and Physiology*
*Renal Function: Nonprotein Nitrogen Compounds,*
  *Function Tests, and Renal Disease*

**Eileen Carreiro-Lewandowski, MS, CLS (NCA)**

Professor, Department of Medical Laboratory
  Science
University of Massachusetts Dartmouth
North Dartmouth, Massachusetts

*Neonatal and Pediatric Laboratory Assessment*

**Susan Cockayne, PhD**

Associate Professor, Department of Microbiology
Brigham Young University
Provo, Utah

*Laboratory Reagents and Calculations*
*Porphyrins*
*Therapeutic Drug Monitoring*
*The Parathyroid Glands and Calcium-Phosphate*
  *Metabolism*

**Mary Coleman, MS, CLS(NCA), CLSp(CG), CLSp(H)**

Instructor, Department of Pathology
University of North Dakota
Grand Forks, North Dakota

*Laboratory Resources*
*Method Evaluation and Preanalytical Variables*

**Margot Hall, PhD, FAIC, CChem MRSC**

Professor, Department of Medical Technology
University of Southern Mississippi
Hattiesburg, Mississippi

*Carbohydrates*
*Tumor Markers*

**Audrey E. Hentzen, PhD, MT(ASCP)**

Director, Clinical Laboratory Science Program, and
  Assistant Professor
Illinois State University
Normal, Illinois

*Principles of Molecular and Immunoassays*
*Immunologic Disorders*

**Marcia H. Hicks, MAEd, MT(ASCP)**

Teaching Coordinator, Clinical Chemistry
Department of Pathology and Laboratory Medicine
Evanston Northwestern Healthcare/Evanston
  Hospital
Clinical Instructor, Clinical Chemistry
Medical Technology Program, Division of Allied
  Health
National–Louis University
Evanston, Illinois

*Thyroid Endocrinology*

**Jean D. Holter, EdD**

Professor and Medical Technology Program
  Director
West Virginia University
Morgantown, West Virginia

*Laboratory Safety*
*Laboratory Automation*
*Point-of-Care Testing*

## Jocelyn J. Hulsebus, PhD, MT(ASCP)

Assistant Department Chair
Department of Clinical Laboratory Sciences
University of Kansas Medical Center
Kansas City, Kansas

*Introduction to Hormones and Endocrinology*
*Hypothalamus and Pituitary Endocrinology*
*Adrenocortical Endocrinology*
*Adrenal Medullary Endocrinology*

## Lynn R. Ingram, MS

Associate Professor
University of Tennessee Center for Health Sciences
Memphis, Tennessee

*Liver Function*

## Lisa J. Johnson, MHS, MT(ASCP)SC

Manager of Scientific Research and Development
Endocrine Society
Bethesda, Maryland

*Acid-Base and Blood Gas Physiology*

## Mark D. Kellogg, PhD, MT(ASCP)

Captain, U.S. Army Medical Service CorpResearch
Biochemist, U.S. Army Research Institute of
    Environmental Medicine
Natick Massachusetts

*Quality Assurance*
*Computers in the Clinical Laboratory*

## George B. Kudolo, PhD, FAIC CPC

Associate Professor of Clinical Chemistry
Coordinator, Graduate Toxicology
Department of Clinical Laboratory Science
University of Texas Health Science Center at
    San Antonio
San Antonio, Texas

*Reproductive Endocrinology*
*Biochemical Assessment During Pregnancy*

## Elia Mears, MS, MT(ASCP)SM

Director of Laboratory Services
Leonard J. Chabert Medical Center
Houma, Louisiana

*Nutritional Status Assessment*

## Claudia E. Miller, PhD, MT(ASCP), CLS

Professor, Health Studies Department
National–Louis University
Evanston, Illinois

*Gastrointestinal and Pancreatic Function*

## Sharon M. Miller, PhC, CLS(NCA), MT(ASCP)

Interim Dean and Professor
College of Health and Human Sciences
Northern Illinois University
DeKalb, Illinois

*Nutritional Status Assessment*
*Geriatric Laboratory Assessment*

## Richard C. Mroz, Jr., DA, MT(ASCP)

Department of Clinical Laboratory Sciences
University of South Alabama
Mobile, Alabama

*Lipids*
*Electrolytes*

## Joan Radtke, MS, MT(ASCP)SC, CLS(NCA)

Clinical Assistant Professor, SBHIS Education
    Coordinator
College of Health and Human Development
    Sciences
University of Illinois at Chicago
Chicago, Illinois

*Proteins*
*Toxicology*

# FOREWORD

In preparing for careers in laboratory medicine, students continually face the difficult challenge of deciding what is most important within the vast knowledge base available on each topic. Too frequently, important principles may be hidden in a deluge of correct but relatively unimportant material. The editors and authors of this textbook have focused on key topics in each subject area. This book is a practical aid for students preparing for careers in laboratory medicine. It brings together the basics in chemistry, physiology, and pathology that are relevant to the practice of laboratory medicine. The design will help students understand the role of laboratory testing in health care. Experienced laboratorians, who change disciplinary focus during their career, may also find the book to be a valuable reference. The organization within each chapter is reader friendly and includes a summary of concepts deemed to be most important.

The scope of the subject matter is necessarily broad, extending the traditional boundaries of clinical chemistry to include immunology and endocrinology. Contributors have been selected from educational centers throughout the United States. Traditional analyte groupings include nitrogenous compounds, electrolytes, proteins, carbohydrates, enzymes, porphyrins, lipids, and drugs. Others chapters focus on liver, GI, pancreatic, renal, thyroid, immunologic disorders, and nutrition. Chapters on quality assurance, laboratory safety, laboratory calculations, automation, spectrophotometry, and laboratory resources will help students' transition to the clinical laboratory work environment. Specific patient populations are emphasized in the chapters on neonatal/pediatric and geriatric patients. The reader-friendly design will find wide acceptance among students, as well as experienced clinical laboratory scientists who want to review basics in a new area of interest.

*K. Owen Ash, PhD*
Professor of Pathology
The University of Utah School of Medicine
Salt Lake City, Utah

# PREFACE

*Clinical Chemistry: Concepts and Applications* was designed primarily for the clinical laboratory science student. It would also be of interest to anyone involved in laboratory medicine or clinical chemistry. The emphasis is on the concepts of clinical chemistry, the mechanisms of diseases, and the correlation of laboratory data with those diseases. Although laboratory procedures are important, the principle of the procedure is more important than the actual step-by-step process. For that reason, and because procedures vary among institutions, we have not included procedures but have discussed the principles.

This textbook was designed and formatted with educational principles in mind. Numerous tables, figures, and examples have been included in the chapters for further clarification of the instructional material. Where applicable, each chapter discusses physiologic concepts and specific analytes. Laboratory data are also applied and correlated with the disease process. The analyte section includes a discussion of specimen collection, sources of error, and reference ranges. Each chapter concludes with a brief summary.

Each chapter in *Clinical Chemistry* has been updated to include the most recent information and technological advances in clinical chemistry at the time of publication. While addressing the common areas of clinical chemistry, the book also includes a discussion of molecular techniques in the chapters on Principles of Molecular and Immunoassays (Chapter 7), Method Evaluation and Preanalytical Variables (Chapter 5), Nutritional Status Assessment (Chapter 33), Laboratory Assessment of Psychiatric Disorders (Chapter 35), Neonatal and Pediatric Laboratory Assessment (Chapter 37), Geriatric Laboratory Assessment (Chapter 38), and, finally, Point-of-Care Testing (Chapter 34).

It is our hope and intention that *Clinical Chemistry: Concepts and Applications* with its inclusion of pedagogical principles, fundamental information, updates, and additions will better prepare the students for their role in the clinical laboratory.

*Shauna C. Anderson*
*Susan Cockayne*

# ACKNOWLEDGMENTS

Every edition of a textbook represents a tremendous undertaking and journey for many people. The authors of this edition would like to extend their heartfelt thanks to their families and special friends for their unwavering support of this project. Many times they have assumed duties that have allowed us the time to devote to this project.

We are also grateful to our colleagues in the clinical laboratory science profession who have contributed so diligently to this edition. Their expertise will help make this an outstanding textbook.

We are indebted to those people at The McGraw-Hill Companies for their professionalism in seeing this project to completion. We are especially grateful to Steve Zollo for his enthusiasm and direction in initiating this project and to Martin Wonsiewicz and Julie Scardiglia for guiding and overseeing the final manuscript preparation.

We would like to acknowledge the authors of the first edition of the textbook who have not participated in this edition. Their work was much appreciated. Thanks to Donald N. Wright, Suzanne W. Connor, Rosemary C. Bakes-Martin, Prabhaker Khazanie, Maria J. Steinbeck, Lauri R. Wyner, Kathleen Doty, J. Helen Cronenberger, John E. Hammond, Naomi Q. Hanson, Leslie I. Onaka, Sonia E. Christensen, Keila B. Poulsen, Kory M. Ward, Robert F. Labbe, Christine King, Carole Ann Allston, Kathleen McEnerney, Beverly A. Lyman, Andrew Maturen, Allen J. Nice, Marcia K. Leise, Ruth A. Sibilia, Steven C. Kazmierczak, Rebecca Rettmer, Lois Hill Berg, Paul M. Urie, and Gregory C. Critchfield.

*Shauna C. Anderson*
*Susan Cockayne*

# CHAPTER 1

# Laboratory Resources

*Mary Coleman*

Clinical laboratorians should be familiar with the basic supplies and equipment used in clinical chemistry laboratories for preparing reagents and specimen handling. Many of the manual techniques used in clinical laboratories of the past have become automated but knowledge and skills utilized in operating basic equipment are still needed in a variety of clinical laboratories. Laboratories dealing with research and esoteric testing may use these basic skills more so than the automated chemistry laboratories.

Basic supplies and equipment to be discussed include pipets, other types of glassware and plasticware, chemicals, purified water, standards, calibrators, controls, analytical balances, centrifuges, desiccators, and thermometers.

## PIPETS

Manual pipets are used to transfer or measure aliquots of a liquid. A number of different pipets are available to choose from and have different features that the clinical laboratorian should be aware of when selecting a type of pipet to use (Figure 1–1). Always consult manufacturer's guidelines about the use, accuracy, and tolerance (inaccuracy limits) of the types of pipets used in the laboratory.

Pipets used to measure accurate amounts of a liquid should have information available as to the tolerances of the pipet. The National Institute of Standards and Technology (NIST), known as the National Bureau of Standards (NBS) before 1988, has established standard tolerances for different volumetric glassware used in the clinical chemistry laboratory. NIST was established by the U.S. Congress in 1901 and charged with the responsibility of establishing a measurement foundation to facilitate both U.S. and international commerce. NIST provides a calibration service for manufacturers of volumetric labware that directly links the glassware standards to national and international standards.[1]

Another organization, the American Society for Testing and Materials (ASTM), is a membership organization that writes voluntary consensus standards. Class A volumetric glassware is defined in ASTM standards. The letter A stamped on the side of volumetric glassware indicates that it complies with class A requirements for accuracy. See Table 1–1 for some example class A inaccuracy tolerance limits.[2] Manufacturers of pipets and glassware should have the information available about the NIST and ASTM standards met by their labware.

Providing a certificate of traceability with a serialized class A pipet is one example of how a manufacturer complies with NIST and ASTM. It indicates that a serial number has been fused in the pipet to indicate that the pipet was individually calibrated and certified against equipment whose calibration is traceable to the NIST. Certificates list the weight set used, the test number, and the date of testing. Each pipet is also calibrated in accordance with ASTM E542 and meets accuracy requirements of ASTM E969. The glass meets the requirements of ASTM E438 for type 1, class A. Not all pipets sold meet this certification or will be serialized. A variety of quality grades of pipets are sold by manufacturers. Therefore, one must check with the manufacturer for this information.

## Serological and Mohr Pipets

Graduated pipets that can measure different amounts of liquid include the serological (Figure 1–1**a.**) and Mohr pipet (Figure 1–1**b.**). They are also called measuring pipets. These pipets come in various sizes, usually ranging from 1, 5, and 10 mL, and can be purchased as reusable glass pipets or disposable pipets.

To use a serological pipet, the liquid must be aspirated into the pipet (Figure 1–2**a.**). Mouth pipetting should not be done. A pipetting aid or bulb should be used (Figure 1–1**e.,f.**). The pipet aid will automatically sample and dispense a desired volume at a touch of a button. The bulb must be squeezed and placed over the pipet, creating suction as the bulb is released, then the bulb is removed and the index finger is placed over the pipet (Figure 1–2**b.,c.**). When the liquid has been aspirated into the pipet, the sides of the pipet, but not the tip, are wiped off with a tissue to remove excess liquid (Figure 1–2**d.**). It is important to remember that when pipetting a solution, the lower level of the meniscus of the liquid should be level with the calibration line (Figure 1–2**e.**) as the pipet is held vertical and at eye level. The amount of liquid to be measured in a serological pipet can be determined by the amount measured between gradations on the pipet. If the clinical laboratorian wishes to measure the entire volume, the lower level of the meniscus of the liquid is level with the first calibration/gradation mark and the contents are allowed to drain to the tip and then the last few drops are blown out with a safety bulb. The pipet should be held vertical during this process (Figure 1–2**f.**). The serological pipet is known as a "to deliver (TD)/blowout" pipet. The volume has been determined by the

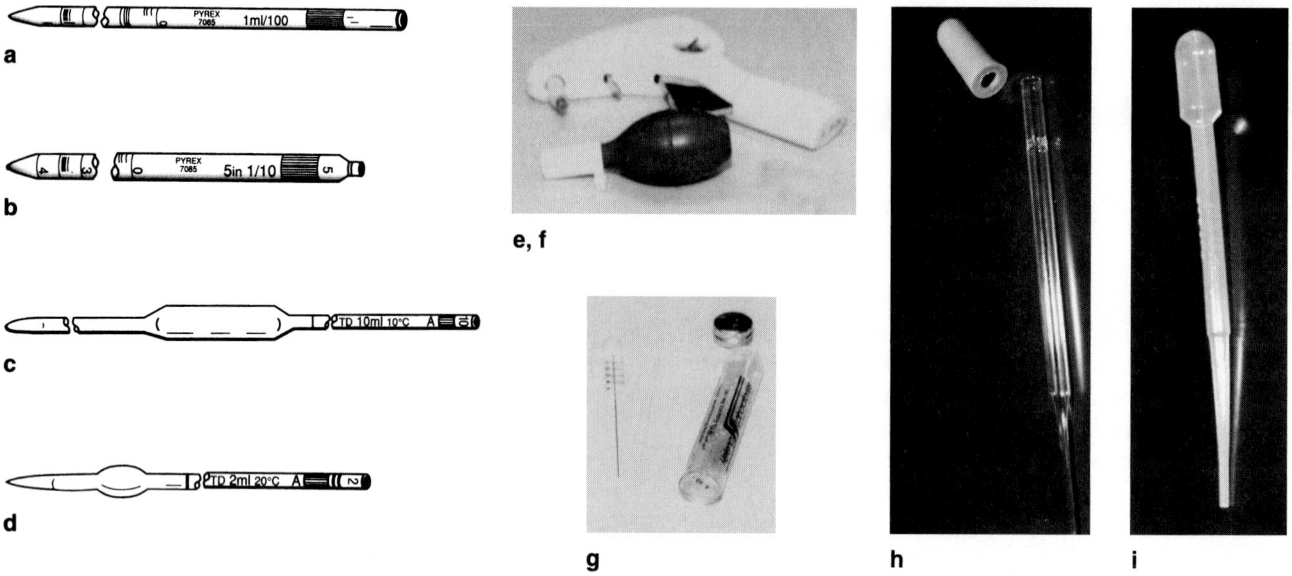

**F I G U R E    1 – 1**

Types of manual pipets. **a.** Mohr pipet. **b.** Serological pipet. **c.** Volumetric pipet.
**d.** Ostwald-Folin pipet. **e.** Pipet aid. **f.** Pipet bulb. **g.** Micropipet. **h.** Glass Pasteur
pipet and bulb. **i.** Plastic transfer pipet.

manufacturer to be the "to deliver" volume and the calibration for the full amount contained in the pipet has been calibrated to the tip of the pipet. Traditionally an etched ring or double ring markings toward the top of the pipet indicates that it is a "blowout" pipet (Figure 1–3). The technique of manual pipetting is best learned in the laboratory by observing and practicing the correct technique.

Use of the Mohr pipet (Figure 1–1**b.**) requires the same techniques as with the serological pipet, except that the Mohr pipet is a TD/ "no blowout" pipet. The end-calibration line for measuring the full volume of the pipet is before the tip of the pipet. The pipet is held vertical and the liquid is allowed to drain from the beginning calibration line to the end cali-

bration line to measure the full volume. The receiving receptacle is tilted so that the pipet tip touches the inside wall of the container. The rest of the liquid in the tip is discarded.

The Mohr pipet is more accurate than the serological pipet, but both are used for measuring reagents. They are not used to measure calibrators or controls.

## Volumetric Pipets

The volumetric pipet (Figure 1–1**c.**) has a bulb in the middle of the pipet and two slender pieces of glass on either side. To use the pipet, the same technique is used to fill the pipet as with the serological and Mohr pipet. The volumetric pipet is

**T A B L E    1 – 1**

**Class A Tolerances (± mL) for Volumetric Glassware**

| CAPACITY (mL) | MEASURING PIPETS (SEROLOGICAL AND MOHR) | TRANSFER PIPETS (VOLUMETRIC) | VOLUMETRIC FLASKS (TOLERANCE) | GRADUATED CYLINDERS |
|---|---|---|---|---|
| 1 | 0.01 | 0.006 | 0.01 | |
| 5 | 0.02 | 0.01 | 0.02 | 0.05 |
| 10 | 0.03 | 0.02 | 0.02 | 0.10 |
| 50 | | 0.05 | 0.05 | 0.25 |
| 100 | | 0.08 | 0.08 | 0.50 |
| 250 | | | 0.12 | 1.00 |
| 500 | | | 0.20 | 2.00 |
| 1000 | | | 0.30 | 3.00 |
| 2000 | | | 0.50 | 6.00 |

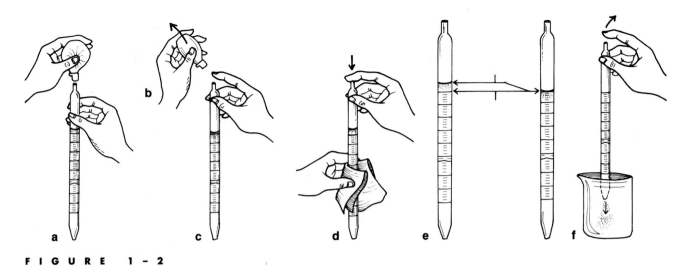

**FIGURE 1-2**

Steps in pipetting. **a.** Compressed pipet bulb is placed over the serological pipet.
**b.** The pipet bulb is removed. **c.** The index finger is placed over the pipet. **d.** The
sides of the pipet are wiped off. **e.** The level of the meniscus of the liquid should be
at the calibration line. **f.** The pipet is held vertical as it is drained.

a TD/"no blowout" pipet. Its liquid is allowed to drain to the tip as the pipet is held vertical and touches the side of the receiving receptacle. The volumetric pipet is not graduated; it only measures one volume. Volumetric pipets come in varying sizes, including 1 to 10 mL and 25 mL. The volumetric pipet has one half the inaccuracy tolerance limits of the serological pipet, and is therefore more accurate. Volumetric pipets have been used to add the diluent to a lyophilized control or to measure standards and reagents.

## Ostwald-Folin Pipet

The Ostwald-Folin pipet (Figure 1–1**d.**) is a "TD/blowout" pipet. Its use is for measuring viscous solutions such as whole

blood, but it is not used much in the laboratory anymore. The same technique is used to fill the pipet as discussed above. To empty the pipet, the pipet is held vertical while the fluid is allowed to drain slowly and the final drop is blown out. The Ostwald-Folin and volumetric pipets are sometimes referred to as transfer pipets.

## Micropipets

Micropipets (Figure 1–1**g.**) measure small amounts of a liquid. They come in a variety of sizes including 1 to 200 $\mu$L. They may be used to measure serum or plasma samples or small reagent volumes. Micropipets are usually "to contain" (TC) pipets, which means the measured volume is contained

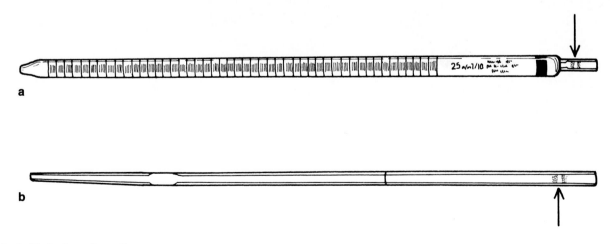

**FIGURE 1-3**

Two deliver/blowout pipets. **a.** Serological pipet with a double-etched ring at the arrow. **b.** Ostwald-Folin pipet with a double-etched ring at the arrow.

in the pipet but will not be the delivered volume. To deliver the contained volume, the pipet contents are usually pushed out by a small pipetting bulb and the pipet inner walls are rinsed out with the diluent in the receiving receptacle using an aspiration technique and a small pipetting bulb.

## Pasteur and Disposable Transfer Pipets

Pasteur (Figure 1–1**h.**) and disposable transfer pipets (Figure 1–1**i.**) are used for transferring liquid from one receptacle to another. They may be used to remove serum from a clot tube or plasma from an anticoagulated tube. Disposable transfer pipets are made of plastic, and Pasteur pipets usually have a reusable suction top and a disposable glass pipet bottom.

## Semiautomated Pipets

Semiautomated pipets offer more convenience and efficiency to pipetting. They may be single channel (Figure 1–4**a.**) or multichannel (Figure 1–4**b.**). Multichannel pipets can pipet a multiple number of samples, usually 8 or 12, at the same time. No pipetting bulb is required for pipetting, nor do pipets have to be washed. A plunger or trigger, versus the pipetting bulb, is used to aspirate the liquid into the pipet. Some semiautomated pipets use air displacement to draw up the fluid and others use positive displacement. The air-displacement technique uses suction to draw up the fluid. Positive displacement uses a mechanical device such as a piston to displace the liq-

uid to be drawn up. It operates much like the movement of the barrel in a hypodermic syringe. Semiautomated pipets use plastic tips, usually polypropylene, which are disposable and autoclavable. The pipet tips tend to retain less inner surface film than does glass. Such pipets, if used properly, improve the precision of measurements. For information on the proper technique, use, accuracy, and precision of a semiautomated pipet, always consult the manufacturer's directions. Semiautomated versions of pipets are available in a variety of sizes including the range from 0.2 $\mu$L to 10.0 mL.

Electronic pipetters are also available. They provide a variety of programmable application parameters. The applications may include the pipetting mode, the fixed-volume mode, and the dispensing mode. The pipetting mode allows the user to create programs for reverse pipetting, a method that is used with highly viscous liquids. The pipetting modes include: (1) blowout, which provides manual control when dispensing residual liquid, (2) manual pipetting for manual-like control of aspiration and dispensing, and (3) rinsing, which is used for mixing applications. The fixed-volume mode allows the user to program a number of the most commonly used volumes for quick recall and the dispensing mode provides repetitive dispensing of a constant volume. The electronic pipetter may be able to program sequences too, such as sequential pipetting, dispensing, and sequential dispensing, automatic dispensing and dilutions, and serial dilutions.

Some solutions (e.g., serum, protein-containing solutions, and organic solvents) can leave a film on the inside tip wall, resulting in an error larger than the tolerance specified. Since

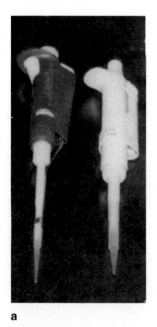
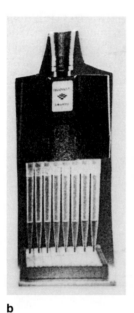
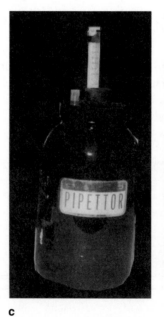
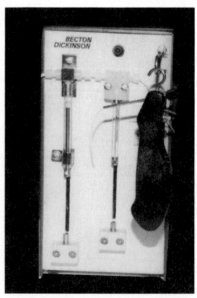

a                    b                    c                    d

### F I G U R E   1 - 4

Semiautomated pipets and dispensers. **a.** Single-channel semiautomated pipet. **b.** Multichanneled semiautomated pipet. **c.** Manual dispenser. **d.** Automated dispenser.

this film remains relatively constant in successive pipettings with the same tip, excellent precision may be obtained by refilling the tip and using the refilled volume as the sample. Successive samples from the same tip will exhibit good reproducibility (low variance). Very dense liquids may not be suitable for air-displacement pipetting. Positive displacement pipets are recommended for those liquids. Saline, water, and phosphate buffers do not need prewetting, although manufacturers may recommend it for some liquids. When measuring with a semiautomated pipet, hold the pipet vertically and do not lay the pipet down with liquid in the tip. Use a consistent immersion depth when measuring a substance. See manufacturer's guide for each size pipet. If a pipet is dropped or damaged by liquid being accidentally drawn into the body of the pipet, a leak may develop. Pipets may fail to work if small leaks develop in the pipet.[3]

A reverse mode of pipetting, which is opposite the reference method for semiautomated pipets, is when the plunger is depressed all the way beyond the first stop of the pipet to aspirate the sample and depressed only to the first stop to deliver the aliquot. This method may be used with viscous samples but it is more difficult to obtain accurate and precise results. Techniques among pipet users may vary because of their training and use. These differences can cause variances in accuracy and consistency in the laboratory. Lab managers should adopt standard operating procedures for pipetting techniques to ensure that all operators are trained to an adequate level of proficiency. It has also been suggested that semiautomated pipets be assigned to an operator or workstation so that errors are located and isolated to one area.[3]

## DISPENSERS

Manual and automated dispensers (Figure 1–4c. and 1–4d., respectively) may be used in the laboratory to add repeated volumes of reagent or diluent to serial solutions or receptacles. They usually consist of a reagent bottle to which a plunger with a valve system is attached. The volume to be delivered is adjusted on the pipetter-dispensing device, which generally is attached by tubing to a reagent bottle containing the reagent to be dispensed. The dispenser is fitted with a tube that reaches to the bottom of the bottle. The device must be primed with liquid to ensure removal of any air bubbles. Once primed, depression of the plunger delivers a selected amount of liquid. Return of the plunger to the raised position refills the dispenser chamber. Manual dispensers may require frequent cleaning to remove material that can hamper piston action.

Automated dilutor dispensers may be used to prepare samples for analysis. Usually the dispenser pipets a preset volume of sample and diluent into a receiving vessel or instrument. Check with the manufacturer as to the use, accuracy, precision, and care of the automated and manual dispensers.

## Pipet Quality Control

Three activities should be performed in pipet quality control (QC): performance verification, maintenance, and calibration. First, performance verification should be checked under working conditions. Mechanical pipets should be considered as instruments in the laboratory and the same QC should apply to them as to other instruments in the laboratory. The QC should be set up to identify pipet malfunctions in a timely manner. Second, maintenance should include the disassembly, cleaning, replacement of worn, corroded, or suspect parts, and relubrication and reassembly. Third, calibration should include measurement of the pipet by a trained technician under controlled conditions.[3] According to the College of American Pathologists (CAP) guidelines, pipet calibration checks should be carried out on a routine schedule, at least monthly.[4] A pipet QC procedure should be included in the appropriate laboratory manual and results and dates should be recorded in a designated log.

Two other steps are added to the pipet quality control program to detect and prevent errors: Fourth, assign all pipets to an operator or a workstation, to localize your problem pipets. If a pipet is malfunctioning, the data affected can be identified. Fifth, train and certify all operators. All operators should check their pipets on a regular basis.

Pipets may be calibrated commercially or in one's own laboratory. There are three methods that can be used to calibrate pipets: gravimetric method, spectrophotometric methods, and gravimetric/spectrophotometric comparison verification. Techniques that use radioisotopic analyzers, enzymatic analysis, and acid-base filtration are not recommended.

The National Committee for Clinical Laboratory Standards (NCCLS) has recommended the gravimetric method as the primary method of calibration. It is based on determining the weight of water dispensed by the pipet and should be limited for use of pipetters that dispense volumes greater than 2 $\mu$L. This method will discriminate between imprecision of at least 0.02 mg standard deviation. It must be done under controlled conditions that include: a proper analytical balance environment, temperature reading with a calibrated thermometer, proper barometric air pressure, and a proper weighing vessel.[5] See the NCCLS and CAP document for details.[4,5]

The spectrophotometric method may include measuring a solution at two different wavelengths. The recommended chemical is a potassium dichromate. It is a primary standard that is readily available and has a sharp peak at 350 nm. It is soluble in water and stable for one year. CAP considers this procedure a secondary method for calibration of pipetters.

A gravimetric/spectrophotometric comparison verification method is done by carrying out the gravimetric procedure on a solution and then transferring the solution from a balance to a spectrophotometer instrument. This method permits direct point-by-point comparison between the gravimetric and photometric methods.

## Cleaning Pipets

See the cleaning labware section for a discussion of cleaning pipets.

---

## GLASSWARE AND PLASTICWARE

Besides pipets, other types of glassware and plasticware may be used in the clinical chemistry laboratory for measuring, transferring, and reagent preparation. Always contact the manufacturer for the proper use and accuracy of the glassware and plasticware. An understanding of the quality and use of a variety of glass and plastic is helpful before purchasing these products. Glassware and plastic supplies found in the chemistry laboratory may include beakers, reagent bottles, volumetric and Erlenmeyer flasks, graduated cylinders, funnels, centrifuge and test tubes, tubing, and pipets.

## Glassware Characteristics

Different grades of glass may be available in the laboratory. Types of glass used include borosilicate, high thermal, soda-lime, boron-free, high silica, high alkali resistant, and low actinic. Some glassware is more resistant to breakage and heat, and may therefore be preferred for most uses in the laboratory. Preferred glassware should consist of high thermal borosilicate or alumina silicate glass and should meet class A tolerances prescribed by NIST (see Table 1–1). This information should be available from the manufacturer when ordering glassware.

Borosilicate glass contains the addition of boron oxide ($B_2O_3$) and is more resistant to heat and breakage. Exax™ is a brand of low-grade borosilicate glass. Pyrex™ and Kimax™ are brand names for high thermal resistant borosilicate glass. Corex™ is a brand name for a glass that is six times stronger than borosilicate glass. It is made of alumina silicate and has been strengthened chemically. It is used in higher temperatures, thermometers, graduated cylinders, and centrifuge tubes.

Soda-lime glass or standard flint glass is composed of a mixture of oxides of silicon, calcium, and sodium. It has poor resistance to high temperatures and sudden changes of temperature. Its resistance to attack by chemicals is only fair. Soda-lime glass materials should be used only for glassware that does not need to be heated or centrifuged. Caution should also be taken when using it for analytical procedures. Minerals may leach from the glass and cause interference problems with some assay procedures.

Other types of specialty glass include boron-free glass, high silica glass, and low actinic glass. Boron-free glassware has high resistance to alkali and was developed particularly for use with strongly alkaline solutions. Its thermal resistance is much less than that of borosilicate glass, and therefore it must be heated and cooled carefully. Its primary use should be with solutions or digestion involving strong alkali.

High silica glass is 96% silica content. This glass is made by removing almost all elements except silica from borosilicate glass. It has good optical qualities and temperature capabilities. It is good for optical reflectors and mirrors. Low actinic glass is used to reduce light exposure to its contents. This amber-colored glass was developed to protect compounds, such as carotenes, vitamin A or bilirubin, that are sensitive to light in the 300 to 500 nm range.

## Plasticware Characteristics

Types of plastic include polyethylene, polypropylene, polycarbonate, Teflon, polycarbonate, polymethylpentene, polystyrene, polyvinyl chloride, and styrene acrylonitrile. Plasticware has advantages in the laboratory because it is unbreakable, may be disposable, tends to be cheaper, and does not release ions into solution as glass does. However, before purchasing plasticware, the manufacturer should be contacted as to its physical properties. When a new plastic material is substituted for glass in the lab setting, comparison studies should be done.

Polyethylene and polypropylene are used in making many types of labware. Polyethylene is less expensive and is used for a lot of disposable labware. However, reagents stored in polyethylene may lose water to the air, resulting in higher concentration of standards and reagents. Polypropylene can withstand higher temperatures and can be sterilized. Polycarbonate is twice as strong as polypropylene and may be used for centrifuge tubes. Teflon has high corrosive resistance at extreme temperatures. Linear polyethylene, polypropylene, polymethylpentene, and Teflon may be autoclaved. Polycarbonate can be autoclaved for limited amounts of time and temperature. Polystyrene, polyvinyl chloride, and styrene acrylonitrile are not autoclavable. They may be gas sterilized with ethylene oxide or chemically sterilized by rinsing with benzalkonium chloride.

## Volumetric Flasks

Volumetric flasks are used in the diluting of a sample or a solution to a certain volume. Flasks come in a variety of sizes, usually from 1 mL to 4 L (Figure 1–5a.). The most accurate flasks are certified to meet standards set by NIST, and designated as class A. They are designated to contain an accurate volume at the specified temperature (20 to 25°C) when the bottom of the meniscus just touches the etched filled line across the neck of the glass. The flask should be held vertical and at eye level when the flask is being filled to the bottom of the meniscus. When a nonacid solution or sample is to be diluted, the solution or sample is added first and then the diluent is added in a stepwise process. The solution is swirled before more diluent is added. The diluent is added until it is level with the bottom of the meniscus. A dropper may be needed for final additions of the solvent. The flask is then stoppered and inverted to ensure complete mixing of the specimen. When an acid solution is made, the acid must be added to the diluent; otherwise excess heat is generated when the diluent is added to acid.

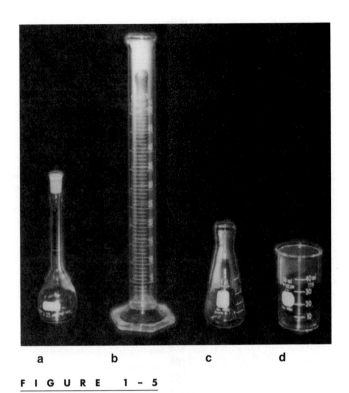

a          b          c          d

**FIGURE     1 - 5**

Laboratory glassware. **a.** Volumetric flask.
**b.** Graduated cylinder. **c.** Erlenmeyer flask. **d.** Beaker.

## Graduated Cylinders

A graduated measuring cylinder is a long straight-sided cylindrical piece of glassware (Figure 1–5**b.**) with calibrated markings on it. It can be made from polyethylene or other types of plastic as well as from glass. Cylinders come in a variety of sizes usually from 10 mL to 1 L. Graduated cylinders are used to measure volumes of liquid when a high degree of accuracy is not essential.

## Erlenmeyer Flasks

Erlenmeyer flasks are used in the laboratory for general mixing and preparing reagents. Their sizes range from 10 mL to several liters (Figure 1–5**c.**).

## Beakers

Beakers are wide-mouthed cylindrical vessels available in both glass and plastic. Beaker volumes usually range from 5 mL to several liters (Figure 1–5**d.**). They are used for general mixing and reagent preparation.

## Labware Quality Control

Volumetric labware that is utilized in the testing process must be calibrated. Manufacturers of volumetric labware calibrate the item before it is sold but this calibration must be checked

by the laboratory using the labware. Gravimetric calibration, similar to pipet gravimetric calibration, can be done. See the NCCLS and CAP documents for details.[4,5] Calibration procedures must be included in the appropriate lab manuals and documentation of calibration dates and results should be done.

## CLEANING LABWARE

In clinical laboratories today, most labware is disposable, which is preferable because cleaning labware properly can be difficult and expensive. Unclean labware can result in an inaccurate lab test result and cleaning labware containing blood or other body fluids must be handled with proper precautions.

Labware that must be reused should be immediately rinsed after use and immersed in a detergent solution. A 10% dilution of a commercial bleach solution (5% sodium hypochlorite solution) should be added if blood or body fluids are present in the labware and soaked for a sufficient time to allow potentially present infectious agents to be killed. Most labware can be washed in an automatic washer. Consult the manufacturer's directions as to the proper use of the washer and the proper detergent to use. Pipets are usually washed in a specifically designed pipet washer. They also should be put into a detergent solution immediately after use and be allowed to soak for a few hours. Consult the manufacturer's directions for the proper use of the pipet washer and the proper detergent to use. Pipets may be allowed to air dry or dry in a pipet dryer.

If labware is washed manually, it too should be rinsed immediately after use and soaked in a detergent solution. Generally a metallic-free, nonionic detergent is used. The labware may be scrubbed with a brush and then rinsed with tap water a few times and then rinsed with a reagent grade water that is the same as that used in the labware. For example, if a solution is to be made in the labware using reagent grade II water, reagent grade II water should be the last rinse water used to rinse the labware.

When glassware is clean, reagent grade rinse water will drain as a continuous film. Unclean vessels will have small drops of water clinging to the surface. Spots on the labware may also indicate unclean glassware. This procedure cannot be used with nonwettable plastics.

If acid washing is necessary for labware cleaning, a 1 molar HCl or 1 molar $HNO_3$ solution may be used. A chromic acid solution is no longer recommended due to residual contamination and hazards of handling or preparing the solution.[6]

A quality assurance plan should be established to check for the effectiveness of the cleaning process. A selected piece of glassware should be filled with reagent grade water and emptied to see if it wets uniformly. The presence of droplets of water or imperfect wetting indicates that the glassware is not clean. Further evaluation of clean glassware can be made by rinsing a selected vessel with reagent grade water and measuring the pH of the reagent grade water before and after it was used to rinse the vessel. If alkaline or acid detergents are still present, they will alter the pH of the water. Another method to use is to rinse the vessel with dilute (20 mg/L) aqueous solution of sulfobromophthalein (bromsulphalein) dye or some other acid-base indicator.[6]

Linear polyethylene, polypropylene, Teflon, polymethylpentene, and polycarbonate plastics are cleaned in ordinary glassware washing machines. Detergents specially made for cleaning plastics can be purchased. The use of abrasive cleaners and strong oxidizing agents should be avoided. Contact the manufacturer for specific instructions.

## CHEMICAL REAGENTS AND HANDLING

### Chemical Purity Grades

Most reagents used in the clinical chemistry laboratory today are prepared ready to use by the manufacturer. Occasionally, especially in clinical laboratories involved in research, new methodology development, or esoteric tests, there may be a need for a laboratorian to do a reagent preparation. To prepare reagents, a knowledge of chemicals, standards, solutions, water requirements, and lab calculations is necessary.

Chemicals are graded for purity by their manufacturer and certificates of analysis should be available on request. Examples of chemical grades are listed in Table 1–2. The American Chemical Society (ACS) has established specifications for analytical reagent grade chemicals. Labels on these reagents either state the actual impurities for each chemical lot or list the maximum allowable impurities. The label should have either the initials AR or ACS or the term "for laboratory use" clearly printed on it. Chemicals of this category are suitable for use in most analytical laboratory procedures. United States Pharmacopeia (USP) and National Formulary (NF) grade chemicals have met specifications established by these agencies. The limitations established for this group of chemicals are based only on the criterion of not being injurious to individuals. Chemicals in this group are used in the production of drugs and may not be pure enough for some chemical procedures. Ultrapure chemicals, such as HPLC and chromatographic grade, have been put through additional purification steps for use in specific procedures such as chromatography, atomic absorption, fluorometry, standardization, or other techniques that require extremely pure chemicals. Other brand name terms may be used for chemical grades by the manufacturer. Contact the manufacturer for information on the purity and the application of the chemical.

### Chemical Handling Precautions

Manufacturers should provide Material Safety Data Sheets (MSDS) with each chemical. The MSDS sheet will provide information on how to handle, store, and dispose of the chem-

T A B L E   1 – 2

**Purity Grades of Chemicals**

| GRADE | DEFINITION |
|---|---|
| Certified American Chemical Society (ACS) plus | Acids, which in addition to meeting or exceeding the latest specifications of the ACS, are analyzed for more than 16 metals |
| Certified American Chemical Society (ACS)/ also called reagent grade (AR) | Reagents that meet or exceed the latest ACS specifications, actual lot analysis on label |
| USP/NF/FCC/EP/BP | Reagent chemicals that meet or surpass specifications of the United States Pharmacopeia (USP), the National Formulary (NF), the Food Chemicals Codex (FCC), the European Pharmacopoeia, and/or the British Pharmacopeia |
| Chromatographic grade | Minimum purity of greater than 99% as determined by gas chromatography; no single impurity exceeding 0.2% |
| HPLC | Solvents manufactured specifically for use with HPLC instruments, meets all ACS specifications. Submicron filtered |
| Spectroscopic grade | Spectrally pure in the visible, ultraviolet, and near- and mid-infrared ranges |
| Chemically pure (CP) | Almost as pure as reagent grade chemicals |
| Laboratory and technical | Chemicals of reasonable purity for situations where no official standards for quality or impurity exist |
| Practical grade | Contains some impurities but usually adequate for most organic preparations, it should not be used in clinical chemical analysis without prior purification. |

ical. It will also provide information on health, flammability, and reactivity hazards or other special warnings associated with the chemical.

## Desiccants and Desiccators

A **desiccant** is a compound used to absorb and remove water from the air or from another substance. In the chemistry laboratory, desiccants are primarily used to prevent moisture absorption by chemicals or other compounds. If a desiccant absorbs enough water from the atmosphere to cause it to become a liquid, it is called a **deliquescent** substance. Some desiccants are deliquescent and lose their efficiency after they have absorbed a certain amount of water. Desiccants with indicators for moisture absorption added, such as cobaltous chloride, can indicate when the desiccant has lost its efficiency. Usually the indicator will change from a blue to pale pink with moisture absorption. The blue color can be regenerated by heating the drying agent. It is best to check with the manufacturer as to the use and regeneration time and temperature needed for the drying agent. The regeneration type of desiccants are probably more cost effective than nonregeneration desiccants. It has been recommended to avoid desiccants that are granular, such as calcium chloride, since they produce dust.

A desiccator is an air-tight container that holds the desiccant and substances requiring storage under such conditions (Figure 1–6). In the laboratory, various chemicals may need to be stored, dried, or cooled down in a desiccator. Desiccators come in various sizes and shapes and may be made of glass, plastic, or stainless steel. It is best to contact the manufacturer about the proper use and care of the desiccator.

## REFERENCE MATERIALS AND CONTROLS

Clinical laboratory testing requires that the testing process must be run in a quality manner and that the materials and equipment used in the testing process conform to known standards. Reference materials (RMs) are materials assigned a known value because of their purity and/or their assigned values have been determined by a technically valid procedure. RMs are used in the clinical laboratories as the calibrator of a method (i.e., to verify or assign values to a lab method). Reference materials include standard reference materials, certified reference materials, and primary and secondary reference materials. Temperature and time in the laboratory can be critical and must be compared to standards.

## Standard Reference and Certified Reference Materials

Increased requirements for quality systems documentation for trade and effective decision making regarding the health and safety of the U.S. population have increased the need for demonstrating "traceability-to NIST" and establishing a more formal means for documenting measurement comparability with standards laboratories of other nations and regions. Standard reference materials (SRMs) are certified reference materials (CRMs) issued under NIST trademark that are well characterized using state-of-the-art measurement methods for the determination of chemical composition and physical properties. NIST assigns values to SRMs and reference materials (RM), which in turn are used for calibrating and validating instrumentation and methods and procedures used for chemical measurements. SRMs are used to ensure the accuracy, traceability, and comparability of measurement results in many diverse fields of science, industry and technology, both within the United States and throughout the world.[1]

## Primary Reference Material and Calibrators

A primary reference material, also called primary standard, is a material prepared from reagent grade chemicals that are directly weighed or measured to produce a standard solution with an exact known concentration. Calibrators are solutions that contain a known amount of an analyte and are used to calibrate an assay method.

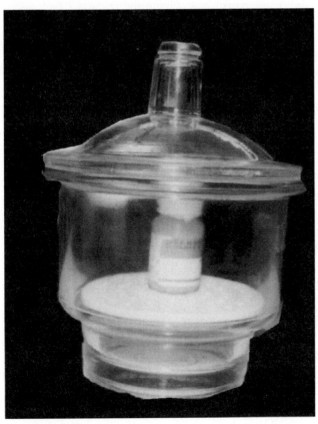

**FIGURE  1 - 6**

Desiccator.

## Secondary Reference Material

A secondary reference material or secondary standard is a solution whose exact concentration cannot be determined by measuring the solute. It is compared to a primary standard to assign its value.

## Controls

Once a method has been calibrated, precision and accuracy must be monitored. Controls, which are patient-like substances, are run alongside patient samples to assess accuracy and precision of lab tests.

## Time and Temperature

NIST certifies the correct time, which can be used to check stopwatches and timers used in the laboratory. One can call the NIST number 1–303-499-7111, or access the web site for the correct time.[1]

Two types of thermometers may be found in the laboratory. They include the thermometer that usually consists of a sealed glass tube containing a liquid such as mercury. A thermistor is a thermally sensitive resistor, usually used for detecting minute changes in temperature.

All thermometers used in the clinical chemistry laboratory for quality control purposes must be verified against a NIST certified thermometer. SRM 934 is a laboratory thermometer, mercury in glass, available from NIST, and has calibration points at 0 °C, 25 °C, 30 °C, and 37 °C. A NCCLS document provides details of thermometer's calibration.[7] Calibration procedures must be included in the appropriate lab manuals and documentation of calibration must be recorded.

## WATER PURIFICATION

Water can contain four types of impurities that can cause significant errors in chemistry lab tests. Those impurities include: inorganics, organics, bacteria, and particles. Dissolved inorganics include calcium, magnesium, zinc, iron, and other salts and heavy metals. Organics include contaminants from soil and rain runoff. Examples include detergents, tannins, and humic acid. Bacteria or byproducts of bacteria, pyrogens, or endotoxins may contaminate water. Colloids and suspended particles may also contaminate water. To prevent introduction of an interference from water impurities into the testing process, purified water is used in the laboratory.

## Water Purity Specifications

There are different levels of water purity that can be prepared and used in the laboratory. The NCCLS has published standards for three types of reagent grade water: grades I, II, and III (Table 1–3).[8] To ascertain reagent grade I to III water purity, manufacturers of water purity systems should test the water for microbiological content, pH, resistivity, and soluble silica.

Reagent grade I water is the most pure water used in the laboratory. No single process of purification can produce water that meets the specifications of reagent grade I water; therefore, manufacturers of water purification systems have devised a series of purification processes to produce reagent grade I water. In general, water from a municipal feed source is put through a purification system. The manufacturer of the water purification system may require the municipal feed source water to be tested to ascertain the initial purity of the water. Some manufacturers require the source water be pretreated by either distillation, deionization, or reverse osmosis. The purification system may include use of a dual-filtration cartridge to remove organic compounds and particulate matter. A mixed bed ion exchange resin will remove unwanted ions and a 0.2-$\mu$m membrane filter removes microorganisms and particulate matter >0.2 $\mu$m. The final product must have a resistivity of 10 M$\Omega \cdot$ cm. The higher the resistivity of the water, the fewer ions present, and the more pure the water. Type I water must be used immediately after production. The high resistivity of the water cannot be maintained during storage.

TABLE   1 – 3

### The National Committee for Clinical Laboratory Standards Specifications for Reagent Grade Water

|  | TYPE I | TYPE II | TYPE III |
|---|---|---|---|
| Bacterial content (maximum CFU/mL) | 10 | $10^3$ | N.S. |
| pH | N.S. | N.S. | N.S. |
| Resistivity (minimum $\Omega$-cm 25°C) | 10 | 2.0 | 0.1 |
| Silicate mg/L (max) | 0.05 | 0.1 | 1.0 |
| Particulate matter | 0.20-$\mu$m filter | N.S. | N.S. |
| Organic contaminants | Activated carbon | N.S. | N.S. |

CFU = colony-forming unit.

N.S. = not specified.

## Water Purification Methods

Four processes of purifying water may be used prior to or in the process of making reagent grade I water. Those processes are distillation, deionization, reverse osmosis, and filtration. Used by themselves they do not meet the requirements of reagent grade I water.

## Distillation

Distillation is the process of vaporization of a liquid followed by condensation in a separate part of the system. The purpose of distillation is to purify or concentrate a substance or separate a volatile substance from less volatile substances. Distillations will remove bacteria, pyrogens, particulate matter, dissolved ionized solids, and some organic contaminants. A problem with the distillation process is that there is a carryover of impurities into the distilled water. This carryover results in contamination of the distilled water with dissolved ionized gases such as ammonia, carbon dioxide, and chlorine, and low boiling point organic compounds. As a result, water treated with distillation alone does not meet the specific conductivity requirement of type I water.

## Deionization

In water, dissolved mineral salts separate into positively charged cations and negatively charged anions. Deionization can reduce the amounts of these ions to very low levels through the process of ion exchange. Water is passed through columns of insoluble resin polymers that exchange $H^+$ and $OH^-$ for other cations and anions. The columns may contain cation exchangers, anion exchangers, or a mixture of cation and anion exchange resins in the same container known as a mixed-bed resin exchanger. Cations are removed by a cation exchange resin. Sodium, calcium, magnesium, and other cations are replaced with hydrogen ions ($H^+$). This exchange produces acids that must be removed or neutralized by an anion exchange resin. Two general types of anion resins are used for deionization: weak-base resin and strong-base resin. Weak-base resins adsorb strong acids, whereas strong-base resins exchange chloride, sulfate, and alkaline anions for hydroxide ions ($OH^-$). The hydrogen ions from the cation exchange process combine with the hydroxide ions from the anion exchange process to form water.

## Reverse Osmosis

Reverse osmosis is a process by which water is forced through a semipermeable membrane from a concentrated solution into a more dilute solution. The membrane removes almost all organic compounds, bacteria, other particulate matter, and ionized and dissolved minerals. It does not remove dissolved gases effectively.

## Filtration

Different types of filtration systems exist. Microporous membrane filtration, depending on the type filter, may filter out suspended solids or colloidal particles and microorganisms. Ultrafilters remove impurities based on the size of the filter, i.e., a .22-$\mu$m filter removes particles larger than 0.22 $\mu$m.

## Reagent Grade Water Uses

Reagent grade I water is used for lab tests requiring minimal interference. This includes lab tests for enzymes, electrolytes, trace metals, and preparation for calibrators and reference material solutions. Reagent grade II water can be used for laboratory tests that do not require reagent grade I water. Reagent grade II water can be stored for a while but bacterial and chemical contamination is always a possibility the longer it is stored. Reagent grade III water can be used for glassware washing but the final rinse should be done with the water grade that will be used in the glassware.

## Reagent Water Quality Control

Reagent water should be monitored for bacterial content, pH, resistivity, silicate content, particulate, and organic matter. A reagent water preparation and testing quality control procedure should be included in the laboratory manual and dates and results should be recorded in a designated log.

## BASIC CHEMISTRY EQUIPMENT

The clinical chemistry laboratory of today is highly automated, but may include some less automated equipment such as weighing balances and centrifuges.

## Weighing and Balances

In the highly automated chemistry laboratory, weighing substances may be done infrequently, to be used only in gravimetric calibration of volumetric measuring devices or to make up a rare solution or reagent.

Weighing is done by making a comparison of an unknown with a known mass. Weight is a function of mass under the influence of gravity: weight = mass × gravity. When the gravitational force for two masses is the same, the weights should be equivalent to the masses; hence, in practice, the terms *mass* and *weight* are used interchangeably.

## Types of Balances

The process of weighing small quantities in the laboratory is done by using a balance. There are two general types of balances found in the clinical laboratory: electronic and mechanical. Mechanical balances include the torsion, double pan, single pan, and analytical varieties. Electronic balances may be either top loading or analytical balances. Balances can also be differentiated or described by their weighing capability. An analytical balance may be defined by some as an instrument capable of weighing to 0.01 mg and possessing a draft shield.

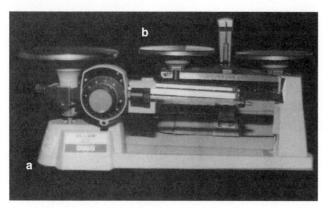

**FIGURE    1 - 7**

**a.** One-pan triple balance (front). **b.** Two-pan triple balance (back).

Other types of balances may be described as precision and microbalance. A precision balance may be capable of weighing to 1 mg and a microbalance may be capable of weighing to 0.1 $\mu$g. Laboratories purchasing a balance can choose from a number of designs, features, and functions.

When weighing to 0.1 g is satisfactory, a nonanalytical balance may be used. Nonanalytical balances include torsion, double-pan, single-pan, and double- and triple-beam balances.

A torsion balance is often found in a pharmacy and is different from other balances in that it uses metal bands to support the weight of the beam instead of a knife-edge fulcrum. Having no knife edges, the torsion balance requires little maintenance from misaligned or damaged knife edges.

A double-pan balance has two weighing pans dangling from the ends of a beam. A knife-edge fulcrum supports the beam at the beam's center. The substance to be weighed is placed on the left pan. Standard weights are usually added to the right pan and fine adjustments are made with a dial or vernier.

A single-pan balance has arms with unequal length. Double beam or triple beam balances are forms of the unequal arm balance (Figure 1–7**a.**). The knife-edge fulcrum is located close to the weighing pan and the long arm has two or three parallel beams to which different size weights are attached. Some models of the triple-beam balance have two pans (Figure 1–7**b.**). Two-pan triple balances have been used when two objects were balanced against each other, as in balancing tubes for use in a centrifuge.

When weighing more precise measurements an analytical balance can be used. A type of analytical mechanical balance, also called a type of substitution balance, is a single-pan balance enclosed by sliding transparent doors, which minimize the environmental influences on pan movement. The operator places the substance to be measured within a tared (a deduction from gross weight made to allow for the weight of the paper or container) weighing vessel on the sample pan. The pan is attached to a series of calibrated weights that are counterbalanced by a single weight at the opposite end of the beam

and pivoted on a knife's edge. When a substance is placed on the pan, individual weights are removed from the pan end of the beam to restore equilibrium. This is accomplished by means of knobs on the front of the balance that lift weights or combinations of weights from the beam. Weights less than 100 mg are read from an optical scale attached to the end of the beam opposite the pan. A light source coupled with appropriate lenses and mirrors projects the optical scale (0 to 100 mg) on a screen located in the front of the balance. Weights to the nearest 0.1 to 0.01 mg are read by a vernier. A beam arrest knob should be in place while substances are being placed on or removed from the measuring pan. Otherwise, the knife edges could become damaged.

An electronic analytical balance (Figure 1–8**a.**) has a single-pan balance. It utilizes magnetic force restoration cells instead of weights. The pan sits on the arm of a movable hanger. The position of the hanger is monitored by an electrical position-scanning device. When a load is placed on the pan, the electrical position-scanning device changes position and transmits a current to an amplifier that increases the current flow through the coil and restores the pan to its original position. The compensation current is proportional to the weight placed on the pan. This is sent in digital form to a microprocessor that converts it into the corresponding weight value, which appears as a digital display.

A single-pan top-loading electronic balance (Figure 1–8**b.**) is most often self-balancing and can be coupled to a computer or recording device. When a substance is placed on the pan, the beam tilts downward. A null detector senses when the beam has deviated from the equilibrium point.

## Use and Care of Balances

The location of the balance should be in an area free of drafts, extreme vibrations, static electricity, and aggressive chemical

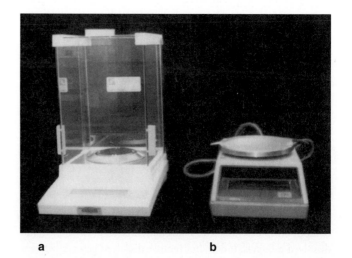

**FIGURE    1 - 8**

Electronic balances. **a.** Electronic analytical balance. **b.** Single-pan top loading electronic balance.

vapors. The balance should be set on a stable, even surface away from extreme heat or direct sunlight. These requirements are more critical, the more sensitive the balance. All weighing on a pan should be performed using a weighing paper or vessel. The pan and surrounding area should be kept clean and free of loose chemical crystals. Before a balance is used, consult the manufacturer's directions for leveling, zeroing, calibration procedures, and proper care of the balance.

Balances should be serviced at least on an annual basis, more frequently if heavily used. Service should be performed by the manufacturer or its representative. Analytical balances should be calibrated at least annually by trained professionals to verify weight accuracies and records must be kept documenting quality control and maintenance procedures.

## CENTRIFUGES

A centrifuge is an instrument used to separate fractions of a mixture by spinning the mixture at a high speed in a circular motion. Centrifuges are used often in chemistry to separate serum or plasma from blood cells. The serum or plasma can then be analyzed for chemical analytes. Centrifuges may also be used in urinalysis procedures to concentrate the sediment at the bottom of the tube. The precipitate is discarded and sediment can then be analyzed for cellular components. Sometimes a special type of centrifuge, called an ultracentrifuge, is used to separate lipid components such as chylomicrons from other components of plasma or serum. Other various uses for component separation will not be discussed here, but exist in the chemistry laboratory as well.

Centrifuges usually have three basic components: a rotor, a drive shaft, and a motor. The rotor holds the containers of mixture to be centrifuged. The rotor can be mounted on a drive shaft that connects to the motor. The motor will generate the power to turn the rotor. Usually the centrifuge is enclosed in a housing case that protects the operator in the event that a tube in the centrifuge should break. Operation controls and indicators may be located on the outer wall of the housing case. Centrifuges vary in their features, including refrigeration, minimum and maximum speed, tachometer readings, breaking capacities, automatic balancing, or balancing alarms. Consult with the manufacturer about the proper use and features of their centrifuges.

Centrifugation is the process used by a centrifuge to separate components. Centrifugal force is the natural force that occurs when objects undergo circular motion. Relative centrifugal force (RCF) is the term used to describe the force required to separate two phases in a centrifuge and is the product of the radial acceleration and the mass of the mixture. It is measured in number of times greater than gravity, $\times$ g. The RCF can be calculated by the following formula:

$$RCF = 1.12 \times 10^{-5} \times r \times rpm^2$$

r = radius in centimeters from the center of rotation to the bottom of the tube in the rotor cavity or bucket during centrifugation and the speed of rotation of the rotor in revolutions per minute (rpms).

The RCF of a centrifuge also can be determined from a nomogram distributed by manufacturers of centrifuges (Figure 1–9). A tachometer device can determine the rpms of an instrument and the radius can be determined by measuring the appropriate distance in the centrifuge. If the rpm and radius measurement are known, the $\times$ g are obtained by drawing a straight line between the radius and rpm points on the nomogram, and reading where it intercepts with the $\times$ g.

## Types of Centrifuges

Three types of centrifuges are usually used in the clinical chemistry laboratory: swinging bucket or horizontal head, fixed angle or angle head, and ultracentrifuges.

A horizontal head or swing-bucket centrifuge rotor (Figure 1–10) enables the containers of mixture to be centrifuged in a horizontal position when the rotor is centrifuging and in a vertical position at rest. During the centrifugation process, particles move along to the end of the tube and are evenly distributed at the bottom of the tube. When the rotor is at rest, the tube resumes its vertical position and the sediment is flat with the supernatant above it. Horizontal head or swinging bucket centrifuges may generate RCFs up to 3,200 $\times$ g and attain speeds of 4,000 rpms. The fixed-angle or angle-head centrifuge rotor (Figure 1–11) holds the tubes at a specified angle, usually 25 to 50 degrees to the vertical axis of rotation. During the centrifugation process, particles move along the side of the tubes to form a sediment that packs against the side and bottom of the tube. Fixed-angle centrifuges produce less heat and friction than horizontal head or swinging bucket centrifuges and may generate RCFs up to 5,600 $\times$ g and attain speeds of 7,000 rpms.

Ultracentrifuges are high-speed centrifuges that are used in the clinical chemistry laboratory to separate lipoproteins from the serum or plasma sample. Ultracentrifuges attain rpms in the 100,000 range and generate RCFs of 175,000 $\times$ g and higher.

### USE AND CARE OF THE CENTRIFUGE

All types of centrifuges can vary in size, speed, and other features. The manufacturer should be contacted for the exact specifications of each centrifuge. Only tubes recommended by the manufacturer should be used in the centrifuge. Tubes must be balanced in the centrifuge for smooth operation. Some centrifuges have automatic balancing features; others must have the operator provide proper balances for each tube to be centrifuged. Blood specimens should be centrifuged with their stoppers on to reduce the generation of aerosols. Blood specimens should also be centrifuged at an appropriate RCF. NCCLS provides guidelines to the proper handling and cen-

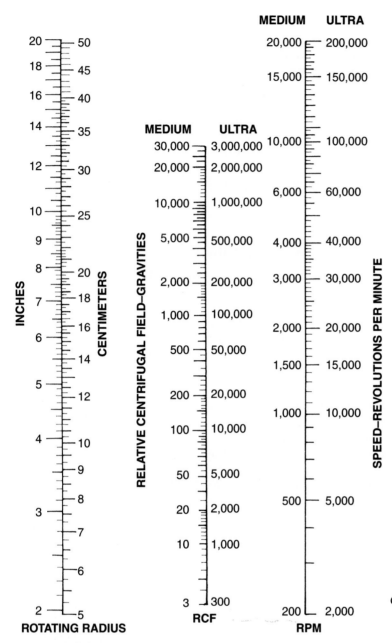

Using the RCF Nomograph

To determine the relative centrifugal field (RCF), place a straightedge on the nomograph connecting the known speed (RPM) and the known rotating radius. The point at which the straightedge intersects the RCF axis is the field.

For example, if the rotating radius is 10 cm and the speed is 3,000 rpm, the relative centrifugal field is 1,000 • g (gravity).

If the field and the radius are known, the corresponding speed can be determined.

To Calculate RCF

| | | |
|---|---|---|
| RCF | = | $0.00001118 \cdot r \cdot N^2$ |
| RCF | = | relative centrifugal field (gravities) |
| $r$ | = | rotating radius (centimeters) |
| N | = | rotating speed (revolutions per min) |

**ROTATING TIP RADIUS**

The distance measured from the rotor axis to the tip of the liquid inside the tubes at the greatest horizontal distance from the rotor axis is the rotating tip radius. The radius is listed for your convenience in the speed and force tables.

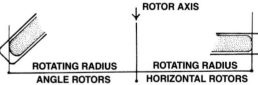

**F I G U R E     1 – 9**

Relative centrifugal force nomograph. Because models and sizes of centrifuges vary considerably, the use of gravity (g) forces instead of revolutions per minute (rpm) is suggested. A nomograph for calculating centrifugal speed is provided. The rotating radius of the centrifuge head is the basis for the calculation and it must be carefully determined. (Reprinted with permission from International Equipment Co., Needham Heights, MA)

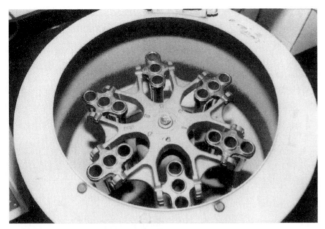

**FIGURE  1 - 1 0**

Horizontal head or swing-bucket centrifuge rotor.

trifuging of blood specimens.[9] Centrifuges should be kept clean and should be disinfected properly if a body fluid spillage occurs.

The speed of a centrifuge should be checked periodically using a photoelectric or strobe tachometer. The centrifuge timer and temperature should be checked periodically against reference standards. Centrifuges should be checked and cleaned regularly to ensure proper operation. Centrifuges may have brushes or other items listed in the manufacturer's manual that need to be checked on a routine basis, although many centrifuges made today do not have brushes. Quality control and maintenance procedures must be included in the appropriate lab manuals and documented when performed.

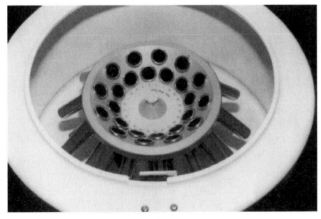

**FIGURE  1 - 1 1**

Fixed-angle or angle-head centrifuge rotor.

## SUMMARY

Basic laboratory resources for the chemistry laboratory include pipets, beakers, flasks, graduated cylinders, analytical balances, centrifuges, chemicals, desiccators, standards, calibrators, controls, and water purification systems.

A knowledge of the above resources is necessary for working in or managing a clinical chemistry laboratory. Quality control and assurance procedures must be in place to ensure that the basic resources used in the laboratory are calibrated, handled, and stored in the proper manner.

## REFERENCES

1.  National Institute of Standards and Technology (NIST). Standard Reference Materials Program. Available at: http://ts.nist.gov/srm. Accessed Dec 29, 2000.
2.  American Standards and Testing Materials (ASTM). Available at: http://www.astm.org. Accessed Dec 29, 2000.
3.  Curtis R: Controlling pipette performance in the real world. Cal Lab 7:32-36, 2000.
4.  College of American Pathologists: *Evaluation, Verification, & Maintenance Manual.* 5th ed. Northfield, IL, College of American Pathologists, 1999.
5.  National Committee for Clinical Laboratory Standards: *Determining Performance of Volumetric Equipment: Proposed Guideline.* NCCLS publication no. 18-P. Wayne, PA, National Committee for Clinical Laboratory Standards, 1984.
6.  Seamonds B, Byrne EA: Basic laboratory principles and techniques. In Kaplan LA, Pesce AJ (eds.): *Clinical Chemistry: Theory, Analysis, Correlation.* 3rd ed. St Louis, Mosby, 1996; pp 3–44.
7.  National Committee for Clinical Laboratory Standards: *Temperature Calibration of Waterbath Instruments, and Temperature Sensors. Approved Guideline.* NCCLS document I2-A2. Wayne, PA, National Committee for Clinical Laboratory Standards, 1990.
8.  National Committee for Clinical Laboratory Standards: *Preparation and Testing of Reagent Water in the Clinical Laboratory. Approved Guideline.* 3rd ed. NCCLS document C3-A3. Wayne, PA, National Committee for Clinical Laboratory Standards, 1997.
9.  National Committee for Clinical Laboratory Standards: *Procedures for the Handling and Processing of Blood Specimens: Approved Guideline.* 2nd ed. NCCLS document H18-A2. Wayne, PA, National Committee for Clinical Laboratory Standards, 1999.

# C H A P T E R  2

# Laboratory Reagents and Calculations

*Susan Cockayne*

The performance of accurate and precise chemical analyses is a function of many variables in addition to the technical skill and expertise of the laboratorian. One of these variables is the use of chemical reagents, including water, of sufficient purity to exclude interfering substances that would invalidate analytical results. A **reagent** denotes any chemical compound or solution used in clinical analyses. The need to prepare reagents in the laboratory is not as prevalent as it once was because of the availability of prepackaged reagents in kits. However, when necessary, certain reagents must be prepared from chemicals of recommended purity.

## REAGENTS

Different designations of chemical purity exist. Chemicals that are designated as **reagent grade** or **analytical reagent grade** are those that meet the specifications of the American Chemical Society (ACS). These chemicals are recommended for analytical use because of their high degree of purity. Ultra pure reagents have an even higher degree of purity and are indicated for use in those instruments or techniques that require this higher specification.

The designation **USP** and **NF** grade denote chemicals that meet specifications of the United States Pharmacopeia or the National Formulary, respectively. Impurity tolerances that are not injurious to health are indicated by these designations, thus they are of interest to the pharmaceutical chemist but may not be of sufficient purity for chemical analysis.

Those chemicals not considered of sufficient purity for use as reagents are designated **chemically pure** (CP). Other designations indicating insufficient purity for clinical analyses include **purified, practical, technical,** and **commercial.** Since there is no standard for such labeling, the quality of the reagent may vary from one manufacturer to another.

## STANDARDS

Standards are solutions of a known concentration used to calculate the concentrations of controls and patient specimens when performing clinical analyses. Standards for use in the clinical laboratory are usually designated as primary or secondary or as reference standards. **Primary** standards are pre-

pared from reagent grade or better chemicals that are directly weighed or measured to produce a standard solution with an exact known concentration. The degree of purity of primary standards is 99.98% as proposed by the International Union of Pure and Applied Chemistry. This degree of purity usually exceeds the limits achievable or necessary for standards used in the clinical laboratory. **Secondary** standards are standard solutions whose exact concentration cannot be determined by measuring the solute but is determined by assaying an aliquot of the solution using a primary standard for calibration. The secondary standard is suitable for clinical analyses and is the most commonly utilized standard. **Reference** standards were initially developed by the National Bureau of Standards and include substances that are difficult to purify, such as cholesterol and bilirubin. They are issued with a certificate listing their chemical and physical properties. Although they do not attain the percent purity specified by primary standards, they may be used in clinical analyses to determine the concentration of other specimens or to determine the concentration of a secondary standard.

## LABORATORY CALCULATIONS

### Metric System

Scientific measurements are most commonly reported in terms of the metric system. The metric system is a decimal-based system and thus is compatible with mathematics using decimals. It has the advantage that fractional parts of standard units of measurement can be made according to decimal fractions. The standard units for the expression of weight, length, volume, and time are the gram, meter, liter, and second, respectively. Fractional parts of the standard units are derived by multiplying the standard by some power of 10. Each fractional part has a designated symbol and prefix. Table 2–1 lists the basic units of the metric system with their corresponding symbols and prefixes.

Clinical laboratory scientists performing quantitative analyses must be familiar with the use of the metric system and the relationships between fractional units. It is oftentimes necessary to convert from one unit to another. A familiarity with the common prefixes and their corresponding decimal fractions will facilitate such conversion.

TABLE    2-1

**Metric System**

| PREFIX | SYMBOL | POWER OF 10 | DECIMAL |
|--------|--------|-------------|---------|
| Tera | T | $10^{12}$ | 1 000 000 000 000.0 |
| Giga | G | $10^{9}$ | 1 000 000 000.0 |
| Mega | M | $10^{6}$ | 1 000 000.0 |
| Kilo | k | $10^{3}$ | 1 000.0 |
| Hecto | h | $10^{2}$ | 100.0 |
| Deca | da | $10^{1}$ | 10.0 |
| Deci | d | $10^{-1}$ | 0.1 |
| Centi | c | $10^{-2}$ | 0.01 |
| Milli | m | $10^{-3}$ | 0.001 |
| Micro | $\mu$ | $10^{-6}$ | 0.000001 |
| Nano | n | $10^{-9}$ | 0.000000001 |
| Pico | p | $10^{-12}$ | 0.000000000001 |
| Femto | f | $10^{-15}$ | 0.000000000000001 |
| Atto | a | $10^{-18}$ | 0.000000000000000001 |

*Example 2–1*

Perform the indicated conversions

$50\ \mu L = \underline{\quad}\ mL$

$mL = 50\ \mu L \times \dfrac{1\ mL}{1000\ \mu L}$

$mL = 5 \times 10^{-2}$

$0.5\ mg = \underline{\quad}\ \mu g$

$\mu g = 0.5\ mg \times \dfrac{10^{3}\ \mu g}{1\ mg}$

$\mu g = 500$

$250\ mL = \underline{\quad}\ L$

$L = 250\ mL \times \dfrac{1\ L}{1000\ mL}$

$L = 0.25$

$0.05\ mg = \underline{\quad}\ ng$

$ng = 0.05\ mg \times \dfrac{10^{6}\ ng}{1\ mg}$

$ng = 5 \times 10^{4}$

$10\ cm = \underline{\quad}\ mm$

$mm = 10\ cm \times \dfrac{10\ mm}{1\ cm}$

$mm = 100$

## Temperature

Currently, three different temperature scales are in use. The **Fahrenheit** (F) and **Celsius** (C) scales are used most commonly. On both scales the fixed points are the freezing and boiling points of water at sea level. The Fahrenheit scale designates 32° as the freezing point and 212° as the boiling point of water, whereas the Celsius scale designates 0° and 100° as the freezing and boiling points of water, respectively. The Celsius scale is divided into 100 units and the Fahrenheit scale is divided into 180 units. The **Kelvin** (K) scale has the same size divisions as the Celsius scale but its zero point corresponds to absolute zero, which is equal to −273° on the Celsius scale. It is used particularly when dealing with very high or very low temperatures. Although the Celsius scale is most commonly used in the clinical laboratory, there may be occasions when it is necessary to convert among scales. The following formulas can be used for temperature conversions.

$$°F = (°C \times \tfrac{9}{5}) + 32$$

$$°C = (°F - 32) \times \tfrac{5}{9}$$

$$°C = °K - 273$$

$$°K = °C + 273$$

## Concentration

A **solution** can be defined as a homogeneous mixture of two or more substances. The substance is termed a **solute** when it is dissolved in a solution; and the dissolving matrix is known as the **solvent**. Although a solution may be either gaseous, liquid, or solid, this discussion will center on the preparation of liquid solutions.

*Example 2–2*

What weight of glucose is needed to prepare 100 mL of a 10% w/v solution?

% w/v solution problems can easily be solved by using the following general formula:

$$grams = \frac{X\ g}{100\ mL} \times X\ mL\ desired\ solution$$

Using this formula the problem can be solved by:

$$grams = \frac{10\ g}{100\ mL} \times 100\ mL\ desired\ solution$$

$$= 10\ g$$

Add 10 g of glucose to a 100 mL volumetric flask and bring up to a total volume of 100 mL

*Example 2–3*

Make 300 g of a 20% w/w aqueous solution of NaCl.

To solve this problem, the weight of the solute (NaCl) must first be calculated. Then, the weight of the solvent must be determined so that when added to the weight of the solute, it will equal the weight of the final solution.

$$grams\ NaCl = \frac{20\ g\ NaCl}{100\ g} \times 300\ g\ desired\ solution$$

$$= 60\ g\ NaCl$$

Since water is the solvent, simply subtract the weight of the solute from the weight of the final solution to determine the weight of solvent:

$$\begin{array}{r} 300\ g\ desired\ solution \\ -\ \ 60\ g\ NaCl \\ \hline 240\ g\ solvent\ (H_2O) \end{array}$$

Mix 60 g NaCl with 240 g $H_2O$

## PERCENT SOLUTIONS

The concentration of solutions may be expressed in different ways. One common expression is percent concentration. Three means of expressing percent concentration are:

1. % w/v (weight/volume)
2. % w/w (weight/weight)
3. % v/v (volume/volume)

**% W/V** is used as a unit of measurement when the solute is a solid substance and the solvent is a liquid. % w/v concentrations are usually written in a form such as 5% w/v. When written in this manner, it is understood that the units of measurement of the concentration are **grams/100 mL** solution. Thus, a 5% w/v solution is equal to 5 g of solute per 100 mL of solution. When calculating % w/v problems, determine how many grams of solute are needed per 100 mL of solution.

**% W/W** Percentage solutions expressed as % w/w are calculated using the weight of the final solution rather than the volume. The weight is usually expressed in grams.

**% V/V** Percentage solutions involving volume per unit volume are used when both solute and solvent are liquids. The typical unit of measurement is milliliters of solute in 100 mL of solution.

*Example 2–4*

How much ethanol is needed to prepare 150 mL of a 15% v/v solution?

$$mL = \frac{15\ mL}{100\ mL}\ ethanol \times 150\ mL\ desired\ solution$$

$$= 22.5\ mL\ ethanol$$

Combine 22.5 mL ethanol with 127.5 mL $H_2O$

## MOLARITY

Another means of expressing the concentration of a solution is **molarity.** Molarity designates the number of moles of solute in one liter of solution. The units of measurement of molarity, then, are **moles/liter.** A 1 molar solution contains 1 mole of solute per liter of solution and is commonly expressed as mol/L or M.

One mole of a particular compound is equal to the gram molecular weight of that compound and can be obtained by adding the atomic weights of the atoms comprising the compound. For example, the molecular weight of NaCl is

$$\begin{array}{r} Na = 23 \\ Cl = 35.5 \\ \hline 58.5 \end{array}$$

A 1 molar solution of NaCl contains 58.5 g of NaCl per liter of solution.

A simplified approach to the calculation of molarity and other problems of this type that does not require the memorization of formulas is to use the process of unit cancellation. A three-step approach can be used to perform these calculations.

1. Identify the units of the desired answer and write them on the left side of the equation.

2. Write all given numbers and units in ratio form on the right side of the equation. Add any additional units in ratio form to enable cancellation of all units except those desired in the answer.
3. Perform the calculations.

Another important concept to understand when dealing with molarity problems is the unit of millimole. A millimole is 1/1000 of a mole and, conversely, 1 mole equals 1000 millimoles. Thus,

$$\frac{moles}{liter} = \frac{millimoles}{milliliter}$$

### Example 2–5

Calculate the molarity of a solution of NaCl containing 87 g/L of solution.

1. Express desired units on the left side of equation

$$\frac{moles}{liter} =$$

2. Write all given units in ratio form so that all but desired units will cancel.

$$= \frac{87 \text{ g}}{1 \text{ L}} \times \frac{1 \text{ mole}}{58.5 \text{ g}}$$

3. Perform the calculation

$$\frac{moles}{liter} = \frac{87 \text{ g}}{1 \text{ liter}} \times \frac{1 \text{ mole}}{58.5 \text{ g}}$$

$$= \frac{1.49 \text{ moles}}{liter} = 1.49 \text{ mol/L} = 1.49 \text{ M}$$

### Example 2–6

How many grams of NaOH (MW = 40) are contained in 500 mL of a 4 M solution?

$$grams = \frac{4 \text{ moles}}{1 \text{ L}} \times \frac{40 \text{ g}}{1 \text{ mole}} \times 500 \text{ mL} \times \frac{1 \text{ L}}{1000 \text{ mL}}$$

$$= 80 \text{ g}$$

### Example 2–7

A solution contains 3.5 g of HCl in 1 L. How many millimoles does it contain?

$$\frac{mmole}{L} = \frac{3.5 \text{ g}}{1 \text{ L}} \times \frac{1 \text{ mole}}{36.5 \text{ g}} \times \frac{1000 \text{ mmole}}{1 \text{ mole}}$$

$$= 95.9 \frac{mmole}{L}$$

## MOLALITY

Molality is an expression of concentration that differs from molarity in that **molality** designates the amount of solute per 1000 g (kilogram) of solvent rather than final solution as used in molarity. The units of molality are **moles/1000 g** of solvent. Molality is a weight/weight measurement rather than weight/volume and is thus independent of temperature variation, making it a more accurate concentration measurement than molarity. However, it is less convenient to work with and is not commonly used in the clinical laboratory. Since most solutions used in the clinical laboratory are aqueous solutions, there is very little difference between molality and molarity.

### Example 2–8

What is the molality of a solution if 127 g of NaCl (MW = 58.5) were dissolved in 1000 g of distilled water?

$$\frac{moles}{1000 \text{ g}} = \frac{127 \text{ g}}{1000 \text{ g}} \times \frac{1 \text{ mole}}{58.5 \text{ g NaCl}}$$

$$= \frac{2.17 \text{ mole}}{1000 \text{ g } H_2O}$$

## NORMALITY

The normality of a solution is another expression of the concentration of a solution. Normality is similar to molarity except that concentration is based on equivalent weight instead of molecular weight. An **equivalent weight** can be defined as the mass of an element or compound that will combine with or replace 1 mole of hydrogen. The equivalent weight is dependent on the total charge of the positive ion, or the valence, of the element. The valence can be determined by inspection of the formula of the chemical compound or by reference to a periodic chart of the elements. As a general rule, the equivalent weight of a compound is equal to the molecular weight divided (MW) by the valence:

$$equivalent \text{ weight} = \frac{molecular \text{ weight}}{valence}$$

If the compound is an acid, an equivalent is the quantity of substance that contains one replaceable hydrogen. For example, in the case of a monovalent compound such as HCl, the valence of $H^+$ is 1 so that the equivalent weight = molecular weight. However, any element with a valence greater than 1 will have an equivalent weight less than the molecular weight. Sulfuric acid, $H_2SO_4$, contains two replaceable hydrogens that can be determined by inspection of the formula. Thus, the valence of $H_2SO_4$ is 2 and the equivalent weight is 49 g (98 g/2).

The relationship between equivalents and moles in this example is:

$$1 \text{ equivalent} = 0.5 \text{ moles}$$

or

$$1 \text{ mole} = 2 \text{ equivalents}$$

If one is dealing with a base or a salt, an equivalent weight is the quantity of a substance that will react with one replaceable hydrogen. NaOH will dissociate into $Na^+$ and $OH^-$. The valence, or total positive charge, is 1. Hence, with one replaceable hydrogen the equivalent weight equals the molecular weight. For $Al(OH)_3$, there are 3 replaceable hydrogens. The valence, or total positive charge, is 3. The equivalent weight is 78 g = 26 g/3.

Since normality is equal to the number of equivalent weights (or equivalents) of solute per liter of solution, the units of measurement of normality are **equivalents/liter.** A 1 normal solution is expressed as 1 N.

*Example 2–9*

What is the normality of a solution that contains 150 g of NaCl per liter? (MW = 58.5)

$$\frac{eq}{L} = \frac{150 \text{ g}}{1 \text{ L}} \times \frac{1 \text{ eq}}{1 \text{ mole}} \times \frac{1 \text{ mole}}{58.5 \text{ g}}$$

$$= 2.56 \frac{eq}{L} = 2.56 \text{ N}$$

*Example 2–10*

Calculate the normality of a solution containing 75 g of $Ba(OH)_2$ in 850 mL $H_2O$. (MW = 171)

$$\frac{eq}{L} = \frac{75 \text{ g}}{850 \text{ mL}} \times \frac{1000 \text{ mL}}{1 \text{ L}} \times \frac{1 \text{ mole}}{171 \text{ g}} \times \frac{2 \text{ eq}}{1 \text{ mole}}$$

$$= 1.03 \frac{eq}{L} = 1.03 \text{ N}$$

The calculation of normality problems requires the inclusion of the proportional relationship of equivalents and moles. The number of equivalents per mole or moles per equivalent must be determined in order to calculate the desired answer.

Another important expression in laboratory calculations is the **milliequivalent** (mEq). A milliequivalent is 1/1000 of an equivalent, and just as 1000 mg = 1 g, 1000 mEq = 1 eq.

*Example 2–11*

Calculate the chloride concentration in mEq/L of a solution prepared by diluting 25 g of $BaCl_2$ to 2 L (MW = 208)

$$\frac{mEq}{L} = \frac{25 \text{ g}}{2 \text{ L}} \times \frac{1 \text{ mole}}{208 \text{ g}} \times \frac{2 \text{ eq}}{1 \text{ mole}} \times \frac{1000 \text{ mEq}}{1 \text{ eq}}$$

$$= 120 \frac{mEq}{L}$$

## Conversions

There are many occasions in the clinical laboratory when a solution will be encountered where the concentration is not expressed in the desired form. For example, it may be necessary to convert from molarity to normality. The conversion between units of concentration can easily be performed using the method of unit cancellation.

*Example 2–12*

Convert 5 M $H_2SO_4$ to normality.

$$\frac{eq}{L} = \frac{5 \text{ moles}}{1 \text{ L}} \times \frac{2 \text{ eq}}{1 \text{ mole}}$$

$$= 10 \frac{eq}{L} = 10 \text{ N}$$

*Example 2–13*

Convert 12 N $H_3PO_4$ to molarity.

$$\frac{moles}{L} = \frac{12 \text{ eq}}{1 \text{ L}} \times \frac{1 \text{ mole}}{3 \text{ eq}}$$

$$= 4 \frac{moles}{L} = 4 \text{ M}$$

*Example 2–14*

Convert 0.4 M NaOH to % w/v. (MW = 40)

$$\frac{g}{100 \text{ mL}} = \frac{0.4 \text{ moles}}{1 \text{ L}} \times \frac{40 \text{ g}}{1 \text{ mole}} \times \frac{.1 \text{ L}}{100 \text{ mL}}$$

$$= \frac{1.6 \text{ g}}{100 \text{ mL}} = 16\% \text{ w/v}$$

Notice that one does not use 100 as a divisor even though it is present in the denominator of the last unit. The reason for not dividing by 100 is that the desired unit in the denominator on the left side of the equation is **100 mL**—not just **mL.**

Laboratory calculations frequently involve problems requiring the conversion of mg/dL to mEq/L. These conversions can also be solved by this same approach.

*Example 2–15*

A sodium concentration is reported as 250 mg/dL. What is its concentration in mEq/L? (MW = 23)

$$\frac{mEq}{L} = \frac{250 \ mg}{100 \ mL} \times \frac{1 \ eq}{1 \ mole} \times \frac{1000 \ mEq}{1 \ eq}$$

$$\times \frac{1 \ mole}{23 \ g} \times \frac{1 \ g}{1000 \ mg} \times \frac{1000 \ mL}{1 \ L}$$

$$= 109 \ \frac{mEq}{L}$$

*Example 2–16*

A calcium concentration is reported as 10 mg/dL. What is its concentration in mmol/L? (MW = 40)

$$\frac{mmole}{L} = \frac{10 \ mg}{100 \ mL} \times \frac{1 \ mmole}{40 \ mg} \times \frac{1000 \ mL}{1 \ L}$$

$$= 2.5 \ \frac{mmole}{L}$$

## Hydrates

Often, when a chemical compound is manufactured, it contains varying amounts of water molecules attached to each molecule of salt. These water molecules are called the **water of hydration.** Some salts are available in the anhydrous (no water) form and in the form of one or more hydrates. The molecules of this water must be included in calculations.

Often a prescribed hydrate of salt is not readily available but some other form is. For example, copper sulfate comes in an anhydrous form ($CuSO_4$), as a monohydrate ($CuSO_4 \cdot H_2O$), or as a pentahydrate ($CuSO_4 \cdot 5 \ H_2O$). One liter of a 1 molar solution of copper sulfate would require:

160 g $CuSO_4$
178 g $CuSO_4 \cdot H_2O$
250 g $CuSO_4 \cdot 5 \ H_2O$

The most straightforward approach to hydrate calculations is to use a ratio-proportion setup to complete the problem.

*Example 2–17*

A procedure states to make a 10% solution of $CuSO_4$. Only $CuSO_4 \cdot H_2O$ is available. We know from the definition of % w/v that:

$$10\% = \frac{10 \ g}{100 \ mL}$$

But we need to know how much of the monohydrate would be equivalent to 10 gm of the anhydrous form. A ratio-proportion approach compares the molecular weights of both compounds to calculate the number of grams of hydrate to use.

$$\frac{160 \ g \ anhydrous \ form}{178 \ g \ monohydrate} = \frac{10 \ g \ anhydrous \ form}{X \ g \ monohydrate}$$

$$160X = 178 \times 10$$

$$X = 11.13 \ g$$

In 100 mL of solution, 11.13 g of the monohydrate would be equivalent to 10 g of the anhydrous form. Note that the difference in the molecular weights (178 − 160 = 18) represents the molecular weight of one molecule of water.

*Example 2–18*

Calculate the number of grams required to prepare 400 mL of a 0.5 N solution of $CaCl_2$ using $CaCl_2 \cdot 2H_2O$.

First determine the number of g in 400 mL of 0.5 N $CaCl_2$. (MW = 111)

$$g = \frac{0.5 \ eq}{L} \times \frac{111 \ g}{2 \ eq} \times \frac{1 \ L}{1000 \ mL} \times 400 \ mL$$

$$= 11.1 \ g$$

Once the number of grams of the anhydrous form is known, the ratio-proportion comparison of the molecular weights of anhydrous and hydrous forms can be used to determine the number of grams of hydrate.

$$\frac{111 \ g \ anhydrous \ form}{147 \ g \ hydrate} = \frac{11.1 \ g \ anhydrous \ form}{X \ g \ hydrate}$$

$$111X = 147 \times 11.1$$

$$X = 14.7 \ g \ of \ CaCl_2 \cdot 2 \ H_2O$$

## Dilutions

When a dilution is performed, a weaker solution is made from a stronger solution. A diluent, such as water, is added to an aliquot of the stronger solution, resulting in a solution of lesser concentration. Dilutions are commonly expressed in the clinical laboratory as one part of the original solution to the total parts of final solution, which includes both solute and solvent.

A 1:10 dilution calls for 1 part of the concentrated solution to be diluted to a total volume of 10 parts. A 1:10 dilution can be expressed as 1:10, 1 to 10, or 1/10. If a 1:10 dilution of serum was being made, the appropriate proportions would be:

$$\begin{array}{r} 1 \text{ part serum} \\ +9 \text{ parts diluent} \\ \hline 10 \text{ parts final solution} \end{array}$$

### Example 2–19

Calculate the dilution if 5 mL of serum are diluted with 15 mL of saline.

$$\begin{array}{r} 5 \text{ mL serum} \\ +15 \text{ mL saline} \\ \hline 20 \text{ mL final solution} \end{array}$$

The dilution of this solution would be 5:20. However, dilutions are usually stated as 1 to some number. To convert a 5:20 dilution to a 1 to something dilution, set up a ratio-proportion problem:

$$\frac{5}{20} = \frac{1}{X}$$

$$5X = 20$$

$$X = 4$$

The dilution is 1:4. There is 1 part of serum to 4 parts of total solution.

### Example 2–20

Make 250 mL of a 1:5 dilution of serum in saline.

$$\frac{1 \text{ part serum}}{5 \text{ parts total}} = \frac{X \text{ mL serum}}{250 \text{ mL total solution}}$$

$$5X = 250$$

$$X = 50 \text{ mL}$$

To produce 250 mL of a 1:5 dilution of serum in saline, place 50 mL of serum in a flask and add enough saline to bring the total volume to 250 mL.

Another type of dilution problem that involves changing the concentration of a given solution can be performed with the use of a simple formula:

$$V_1 \times C_1 = V_2 \times C_2$$

The general use of this formula involves changing a solution of known volume and concentration ($V_1C_1$) to one of weaker concentration ($V_2C_2$). Three of the four values must be known to solve the equation. The units can be any units of volume and concentration as long as they are the same for both sides of the equation.

This same formula can also be applied to acid-base problems where it is desirous to know what volume or what concentration of one substance will neutralize a known volume and concentration of another substance. (See Example 2–23.)

### Example 2–21

How much 20% alcohol is required to make 1 L of 10% alcohol?

$$V_1 \times C_1 = V_2 \times C_2$$

$$1 \text{ L} \times 10\% = X \text{ L} \times 20\%$$

$$20X = 10$$

$$X = .5 \text{ L}$$

500 mL of 20% alcohol when diluted to 1 L with $H_2O$ will make a 10% solution of alcohol.

### Example 2–22

What is the concentration of a solution if 25 mL of a 1.5 M solution is diluted to 250 mL?

$$V_1 \times C_1 = V_2 \times C_2$$

$$250 \text{ mL} \times X = 25 \text{ mL} \times 1.5 \text{ M}$$

$$250X = 37.5$$

$$X = 0.15 \text{ M}$$

The resulting solution will have a concentration of 0.15 M.

*Example 2–23*

How much 5 N $H_2SO_4$ is needed to neutralize 100 mL of 4 N NaOH?

$V_1 \times C_1 = V_2 \times C_2$

$100 \text{ mL} \times 4 \text{ N} = X \text{ mL} \times 5 \text{ N}$

$400 = 5X$

$X = 80 \text{ mL}$

80 mL of 5 N $H_2SO_4$ will neutralize 100 mL of 4 N NaOH.

*Example 2–24*

What is the dilution fold of the following serial dilution system consisting of 5 tubes? The following amounts of diluent have been added to the tubes: 0.5 mL is added to tube 1 and 0.5 mL to tubes 2 to 5. Next, 0.5 mL of patient serum is added to tube 1 and 0.5 mL is serially transferred through tube 5. Finally, 0.5 mL is discarded from tube 5.

$\dfrac{1}{X} = \dfrac{0.5}{1.0}$

$0.5X = 1.0$

$X = 2$

## Serial Dilutions

In some assays performed in the clinical laboratory, a semi-quantitative technique known as titering is done. These types of procedures are particularly useful in serologic tests when estimates of the volume of antibody in a clinical specimen are necessary. The technique involves preparing serial dilutions of the serum. A serial dilution constitutes a series of dilutions of progressive, regular increments in which each subsequent dilution is less concentrated than the preceding dilution by a constant amount, "N". In an N-fold serial dilution system, the solute concentration in each successive dilution is 1/N of the preceding dilution. Often, serial dilutions are "twofold," where each dilution is ½ as concentrated as the one immediately preceding it.

The dilution fold of a system can be determined by the following formula:

$$\frac{1}{\text{dilution fold}} = \frac{\text{volume transferred}}{\text{total volume}}$$

The volume transferred is equal to the constant volume transferred to each successive tube in the serial dilution system. Total volume is equal to the volume being transferred plus the volume of diluent already in the tube.

*Example 2–25*

What is the dilution of tube #3 in the above example?

$X = \dfrac{1}{2} \times \dfrac{1}{2}^{(3-1)}$

$X = \dfrac{1}{2} \times \dfrac{1}{2}^{2}$

$X = \dfrac{1}{2} \times \dfrac{1}{2} \times \dfrac{1}{2}$

$X = \dfrac{1}{8}$

The dilution of serum in tube 3 is $\dfrac{1}{8}$.

It is often desirable to determine the dilution of a given tube (X) in a serial dilution system. This dilution may be calculated by:

$$\text{Solution of tube 1} = \text{dilution of X} \left[ \frac{1}{\text{dilution fold}} \right]^{(X-1)}$$

## Specific Gravity

The most frequent use of specific gravity in the laboratory is when working with concentrated commercial liquids, such as acids or bases. When working with liquids, it is rather awkward to measure the volume in grams. It is much more convenient to measure the volume in milliliters. Grams must be converted to milliliters when only grams is given.

We can determine how much 1 mL of any liquid weighs by knowing the specific gravity. Specific gravity is a method of measuring density. It is a ratio of mass/volume. Thus, specific gravity can be expressed as:

$$\frac{g}{mL} \text{ or } \frac{mL}{g}$$

When working with concentrated commercial liquids, the bottle label will often indicate the specific gravity and another value called assay or percent purity. For example,

$HNO_3$ – specific gravity 1.42

assay 70%

These values indicate that 1 mL of the solution has a mass of 1.42 g and that 70% of this mass is a pure $HNO_3$. To find out how many grams of $HNO_3$ are in 1 mL of concentrated solution, we must multiply the specific gravity by the assay, or percent purity.

$$\frac{1.42\text{ g}}{1\text{ mL}} \times .70 = \frac{0.994\text{ g}}{1\text{ mL}} \text{ (pure } HNO_3)$$

*Example 2–26*

Prepare 2 liters of a 1.5 N HCl solution. The supply of concentrated HCl has a specific gravity of 1.19 and an assay of 38%.

$$\text{mL} = \frac{1.5\text{ eq}}{L} \times \frac{36.5\text{ g}}{\text{eq}} \times \frac{1\text{ mL}}{1.19\text{ g} \times 0.38} \times 2\ L$$

$$= 242.1\text{ mL}$$

To a flask add some water, then add 242.1 mL of concentrated HCl and dilute up to a total volume of 2 L.

*Example 2–27*

Calculate the molarity of concentrated HCl (specific gravity = 1.19, assay = 38%)

$$\frac{\text{mole}}{L} = \frac{1\text{ mole}}{36.5\text{ g}} \times \frac{1.19\text{ g} \times .38}{1\text{ mL}} \times \frac{1000\text{ mL}}{1\text{ L}}$$

$$= 12.3\ \frac{\text{mole}}{L} = 12.3\text{ M}$$

## International System of Units

Despite the general use of the metric system, discrepancies have occurred in reporting units from one laboratory to another. In an attempt to establish a system whereby all quantitative measurements could be expressed in clearly defined and standardized units, the Système International d'Unités (SI) was adopted in 1960. Most international scientific organizations have adopted the system. Some modifications of the original SI system have been accepted to make it more adaptable for the reporting of clinical laboratory data. Although it is difficult to incorporate changes of this dimension, the trend in clinical laboratories is to report all quantitative analyses in SI units. Conventional metric system units are still frequently used, however. A basic understanding of the SI system and its units will enable the laboratorian to interconvert units when both systems are not reported.

**TABLE 2–2**

**SI System**

| BASE PROPERTY | BASE UNIT | UNIT SYMBOL |
|---|---|---|
| Length | meter | m |
| Mass | kilogram | kg |
| Time | second | s |
| Electric current | ampere | A |
| Thermodynamic temperature | Kelvin | K |
| Luminous intensity | candela | cd |
| Amount of substance | mole | mol |

*Example 2–28*

Convert 90 mg/dL glucose to mmol/L. (MW = 180)

$$\frac{\text{mmole}}{L} = \frac{90\text{ mg}}{dL} \times \frac{10\text{ dL}}{1\text{ L}} \times \frac{1\text{ mole}}{180\text{ g}}$$

$$\times \frac{1\text{ g}}{1000\text{ mg}} \times \frac{1000\text{ mmole}}{1\text{ mole}}$$

$$= 5\ \frac{\text{mmole}}{L}$$

*Example 2–29*

Convert 140 mEq/L of sodium to mmole/L. (MW = 23)

$$\frac{\text{mmole}}{L} = \frac{140\text{ mEq}}{L} \times \frac{1\text{ eq}}{1000\text{ mEq}}$$

$$\times \frac{1\text{ mole}}{1\text{ eq}} \times \frac{1000\text{ mmole}}{1\text{ mole}}$$

$$= 140\ \frac{\text{mmole}}{L}$$

The SI system is developed around seven basic properties. Table 2–2 lists the basic SI properties and units.

Many of the clinical laboratory SI units are based on mmol/L or its various subunits and g/L as the only acceptable mass/volume designations. Conversion from conventional units to these SI units requires knowledge of the molecular weight of the substance. The mathematical calculations can then be easily performed by the unit cancellation method as shown above and in Example 2–30.

*Example 2–30*

Convert 4.5 g/dL albumin to g/L. (MW = 65,000)

$$\frac{g}{L} = \frac{4.5\ g}{100\ mL} \times \frac{1000\ mL}{L}$$

$$= 45\ g/L$$

## SUMMARY

Many calculations are performed in the clinical laboratory. Clinical laboratory scientists must become proficient in these basic calculations to minimize errors, to facilitate efficient work flow and to perform mental checks of various parameters. The method of unit cancellation allows many different types of calculations to be performed without the need to memorize formulas.

# CHAPTER 3
# Laboratory Safety

*Jean D. Holter*

## REGULATIONS

Laboratory safety is a legal responsibility of the employer as well as a moral obligation to the employee. Many federal, state, and local laws regulate safe practices to protect employees, the community, and the environment. An overview of these regulations is presented in this section.

Congress enacted the Occupational Safety and Health Act (PL 91-596) in 1970 and established the Occupational Safety and Health Administration (OSHA) (website: www.OSHA. gov) within the Department of Labor. OSHA has the authority to establish regulations, conduct on-site inspections of workplaces to determine compliance with mandatory safety standards and assess fines if it finds noncompliance with the regulations. The National Institute of Occupational Safety and Health (NIOSH) serves as OSHA's research and advisory arm.

OSHA has drafted or promulgated regulations that specifically affect clinical laboratories. The details in each regulation are too voluminous to present in this chapter but may be obtained by contacting an area OSHA office. The regulations most specific to clinical laboratories are:

- Occupational Exposure to Formaldehyde Standard— 29CFR 1910.1048
- Hazard Communication Standard—29CFR 1910.1200
- Occupational Exposure to Bloodborne Pathogens— Federal Register, May 30, 1989, pp 23134–23139; Updated November 5, 1999
- Occupational Exposure to Hazardous Chemicals in Laboratories—29CFR:1910.1450

OSHA Bloodborne Pathogen Compliance Directive, published November 5, 1999, establishes the responsibilities of personnel service firms to provide hepatitis B vaccinations, postexposure evaluation and follow-up, and record keeping on their employees. There must be an annual update of the exposure control plan to reflect technology changes.[1]

Agencies other than OSHA also have regulations that affect laboratories:

- Resource Conservation and Recovery Act (RCRA)— Environmental Protection Agency (EPA)—40CFR, parts 260–265.
- Department of Transportation (DOT)—49CFR, parts 171–179

- Medical Waste Tracking Act—EPA, 1989—40CFR, parts 22 and 259
- Nuclear Regulatory Commission (NRC)—Title 10 CFR, sections 19, 20, 35

In addition, there are local and state laws that regulate sewer disposal, fire and building codes, and hazardous waste disposal.

Laws and regulations administered by federal, state, and local agencies are mandatory. However, there are government and private agencies that provide guidance by adopting safety standards, codes, and guidelines that are voluntary but are often adopted by regulatory agencies and become mandatory. Some of these organizations are the National Fire Protection Association, National Committee on Clinical Laboratory Standards (NCCLS), Centers for Disease Control and Prevention (CDC), NIOSH, National Institutes of Health, and American Conference of Governmental Industrial Hygienists.

Voluntary accrediting agencies such as the Commission on Laboratory Accreditation of the College of American Pathologists (website: www.cap.org) and Joint Commission for Accreditation of Healthcare Organizations (website: www. jcaho.org) adopt standards for inspection and accreditation based on both mandatory regulations and standards adopted by the aforementioned voluntary organizations.

## SAFETY PRACTICES

Safe practices in the clinical laboratory need to be followed by all personnel who work in or enter the laboratory. Mandatory regulations and accrediting agency standards address most of the following safe work practices.

### General Practices

Smoking, eating, and application of cosmetics are prohibited to prevent the spread of hand to mouth infectious agents or toxic chemicals. To prevent contact with or spread of infectious agents, a protective garment such as a fluid-resistant lab coat or gown should be worn over clothing. These same protective outer garments should not be worn outside the laboratory. Shoes should be made of a nonporous material with closed toes and heels. Contact lenses should be discouraged because of fumes and splashes that might occur. Contact lenses inhibit tearing and allow substances to remain on the cornea longer. Goggles or face shields are recommended if contact lenses are worn, especially if there is a high risk of fumes, aerosols, or splashes. Dangling jewelry, long hair, and beards may pose a safety hazard by coming in contact with specimens or other surfaces or by becoming entangled or caught in moving instruments such as rotators or centrifuges. Sampling specimens, reagents, water, or any substance through a pipet by mouth should be strictly prohibited.

## Spills

A written policy and procedure should be developed to instruct employees in how to handle chemical and biological spills. Spill kits for both types of spills are available commercially. The laboratory should develop a procedure for handling spills and ensure a safe work environment. More specific information on spill cleanup can be found in the sections on chemical and biological safety in this chapter.

## Hoods

### FUME HOODS

Fume hoods are used when chemical reagents may produce a hazardous fume. The sash or window should be lowered when working in the hood. Air flow should be checked to assure proper ventilation. Controls such as power, gas, and vacuum should be located externally to prevent a spark that may cause a fire when using volatiles.

### BIOLOGICAL HOODS

Biological hoods remove particles that may infect the person working with the biologically infected specimen. These hoods contain a HEPA (high-efficiency particulate air) filter and are used typically in a microbiology laboratory.

## Hand Washing

Hand washing is one of the major ways of preventing the spread of infectious agents. Even if gloves are worn, hand washing is necessary because of microscopic holes in gloves that may occur. When dealing with patients, hand washing should be done between each patient even if gloves are worn.

## Housekeeping

Trash, infectious waste, and dirty glassware should not be allowed to accumulate in large quantities in the laboratory. Containers of discarded specimens and causative agents should be covered when not in use. Work surfaces should be frequently cleaned with a disinfectant and at the beginning and end of each shift. The disinfectant should be a 10% bleach solution, which is made fresh every 24 hours.[1] The time to disinfect an area is the time for the disinfected surface to air dry.[1] Laboratory personnel should be responsible for maintaining a clean sanitary work area even if there is an institutional janitorial service.

## Labels and Signs

All chemical containers should be clearly labeled with the name of the chemical and any precautions for handling. Areas where flammables, hazardous or toxic chemicals, and carcinogens are stored or being used must be clearly marked. Areas where blood and body fluids are being stored or analyzed should be clearly marked with a biohazard sign (Figure 3–1).

## Waste Disposal

There are EPA regulations regarding the disposal of chemicals. For further information, consult the section in this chapter on chemical safety. Disposal of biological materials such as infectious waste is coming under greater scrutiny and is regulated by federal, state, and local laws. See the section on biological safety in this chapter for more information.

## Needles and Sharps

Needles and other sharps pose a physical hazard and a potential infectious hazard to laboratory and support personnel. All disposable needles and other sharps should be discarded into puncture-resistant and leakproof containers marked with a biohazard symbol. These containers should be discarded according to institutional policy when they are one-half to three-fourths full. Most institutions incinerate sharp containers. Needles should not be recapped unless a recapping device is used that is designed to prevent accidental skin puncture. Needles should never be cut because cutting may splatter blood or other fluids into the environment.

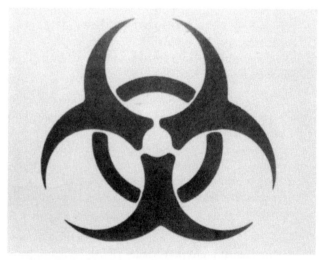

**F I G U R E   3 - 1**

The international biohazard symbol. (Courtesy of Lab Safety Supply, Inc., Janesville, WI)

## Employee Training

Each new laboratory employee should be instructed in safe work practices before exposure to hazardous substances or situations. Annual training in chemical safety and in exposure control is required by OSHA regulations and must be documented.[2] The laboratory should appoint a person to be responsible for laboratory safety training.

## FIRE SAFETY

### Classes of Fire

Flammable and combustible liquids are necessary in the clinical laboratory for some procedures. There is also the potential danger of electrical fires in the laboratory. The clinical laboratory scientist must understand these dangers and how to deal with them in an emergency. Fires are classified as class A through class D. Class A fires are ordinary combustibles, such as wood or paper; class B are flammable liquids; class C involve energized electrical circuits regardless of fuel; class D are combustible metals such as sodium and magnesium. Each class of fire requires the appropriate type of fire extinguisher for efficient fire fighting and prevention of the spread of fire.

### Extinguishers

Fire extinguishers contain different substances and are labeled according to the class of fire on which they should be used. Class A extinguishers are filled with water and should never be used on an electrical fire because the water can conduct electricity back to the person holding the extinguisher. Class B extinguishers are filled with dry chemicals, aqueous film-forming foam (AFFF), or carbon dioxide. Class C extinguishers are filled with carbon dioxide or Halon. Class D extinguishers are filled with a special dry powder containing a thermoplastic binder that allows the agent to form a solid crust on heating. Extinguishers also are available that are rated for class A to C fires. They contain a dry powder and may be used effectively and safely on all three classes of fire. However, if this type is used on electrical equipment in the laboratory, the powder will be difficult or impossible to clean from the internal workings of an instrument. Therefore, carbon dioxide or Halon is recommended for fires in electrical equipment.[3] Fire extinguisher types are compared in Table 3–1.

### Causes and Prevention

Basic causes of fires in laboratories are carelessness, lack of knowledge regarding chemicals being used, unattended operations, and circuit overload. Safety in-service education should

TABLE  3 – 1

**Comparison of Fire Extinguisher Types**

| TYPE | ADVANTAGES | DISADVANTAGES | NOTES |
|---|---|---|---|
| Halon—class A, B, C or B, C | Quick fire knockdown<br>Will reach hidden fires<br>No damage to equipment<br>Good visibility<br>Good discharge range<br>Heat absorber | Requires rapid discharge<br>More expensive<br>Personnel hazard (Halon 1211)<br>Not for deep-seated fires | Most common system for electrical and electronic fires<br>Maximum effectiveness requires rapid detection |
| Dry chemical—class A, B, C | Good on oil or grease<br>Good knockdown<br>Low cost | Limited personnel hazard<br>Equipment damage likely<br>Cleanup required<br>Not suitable for hidden fires | Compatible with other agents<br>Subject to equipment interference |
| Carbon dioxide—class B, C | Good fire suppression capability<br>Will reach hidden fire<br>Good visibility<br>No equipment damage<br>No cleanup<br>Quickest way to cool a fire | May be toxic to personnel<br>May cause thermal static (shock) damage<br>Heavy vapor settles out limiting total discharge range | Second choice to Halon when fighting class B and C fires |

(Courtesy of Lab Safety Supply, Inc., Janesville, WI)

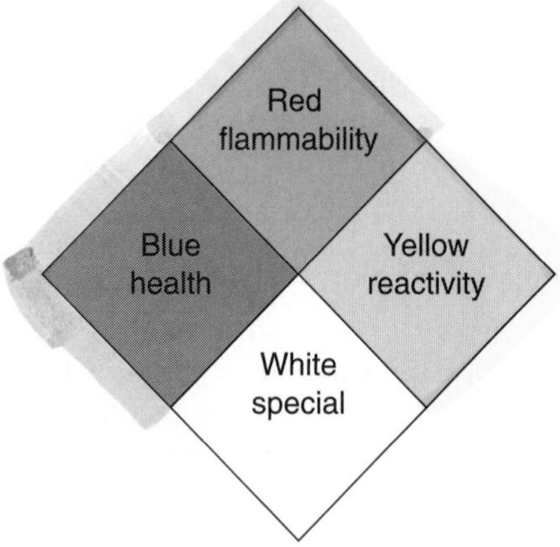

**FIGURE 3-2**

NFPA Chemical Hazard Label. This warning system is intended to be interpreted and applied only by properly trained individuals to identify fire, health, and reactivity hazards of chemicals. The user is referred to certain limited numbers of chemicals with recommended classifications in NFPA 49 and NFPA 325M, which would be used as a guideline only. Whether the chemicals are classified by NFPA or not, anyone using the 704 system to classify chemicals does so at his or her own risk. (Used with permission. Copyright © 1996, National Fire Protection Association, Quincy, MA)

be held annually to remind employees about safe work practices to prevent fire and other accidents.

If a fire does occur, the fire department or other assistance must be summoned first before attempting to extinguish the fire. The steps to take in the event of a fire are:

1. Rescue anyone in danger.
2. Isolate the fire by closing a door.
3. Call for help.
4. Try to extinguish fire.
5. Evacuate if the fire cannot be extinguished.

If several people are available, these steps can be carried out simultaneously in a team effort. Laboratory personnel should be trained in the use of fire extinguishers. The local fire department or institutional safety committee can usually provide this training.

The National Fire Protection Agency (NFPA) has a system for identifying laboratory hazard for fighting fires. It is a diamond-shaped symbol divided into four parts: blue represents health hazards; yellow represents safety hazards; red represents fire or flammable hazards; and white represents specific information such as no water or radiation (Figure 3–2). These labels should be displayed on the door of all laboratories and chemical storage areas so that the firefighters are aware of the types of hazards that may be present.

# CHEMICAL SAFETY

## Material Safety Data Sheets

In August 1987, OSHA amended the federal Hazard Communication Standard—29 CFR 1919.1200 (Right to Know/HCS Standard) to expand the standard to all industries, including health care facilities. This standard requires that employers determine if hazardous chemicals are present, make material safety data sheets (MSDSs) available to employees, label chemical containers with the hazard, maintain a chemical inventory and hazardous chemical list, provide employee information and training, and develop a written hazard communication program.

Manufacturers are required to provide a MSDS with any chemical manufactured. MSDSs are technical documents containing detailed information about the chemicals. The information that is included on a MSDS is shown in Table 3–2. An example of a MSDS is shown in Figure 3–3.

These sheets must be available to laboratory employees at all times. The employer is responsible for providing adequate training and providing employees with the necessary protective equipment.

## Chemical Hygiene Plan

In early 1990, OSHA published a final rule on occupational exposure to hazardous chemicals in laboratories (29CFR:1910.1450). This regulation became effective May 1, 1990, and laboratories were required to have a written chemical hygiene plan (CHP) as of January 31, 1991. Clinical and research laboratories in hospitals as well as private clinical laboratories are included.

The written CHP must include:

- Criteria for and methods of monitoring chemical exposure
- Standard operating procedures for handling hazardous chemicals

TABLE 3-2

**Information contained on a Material Safety Data Sheet**

1. Identification of chemical (e.g., CAS no. synonyms)
2. Hazardous ingredients
3. Physical data
4. Fire and explosion data
5. Health hazard information
6. Reactivity data
7. Spill, leak, and disposal procedures
8. Personal protection information
9. Special precautions and comments

## Material Safety Data Sheet

May be used to comply with OSHA's Hazard Communication Standard
29CFR1910.1200 Standard must be consulted for specific requirements

Quick Identifier
Common Name used on label and test

### SECTION 1

Manufacturer's Name

Address                          Emergency Telephone No.

City, State and Zip              Other Information Calls

Signature of Person
Responsible for Preparation (Optional)          Date Prepared

### SECTION 2 - Hazardous Ingredients/Identity

| Hazardous Components (chemical and common name) | OSHA/PEL | ACGIH/TLV | Other Exposure | CAS NO |
|---|---|---|---|---|
|  |  |  |  |  |
|  |  |  |  |  |

### SECTION 3 - Physical & Chemical Characteristics

| Boiling Point | Specific Gravity (g/ml) | Vapor Pressure (mmHg) |
|---|---|---|
| Vapor Pressure |  |  |
| Solubility in Water | Reactivity in Water | |
| Appearance and Odor | Melting Point | |

### SECTION 4 - Fire & Explosive Data

| Flash Point  F   C | Flammable Limits in Air & by Volume | LEL Lower | UEL Upper |
|---|---|---|---|

Auto Ignition       Extinguisher
Temperature         Media
Special Fire
Fighting Procedures

Unusual Fire and
Explosion Hazards

### SECTION 5 - Physical Hazards (Reactivity Data)

Stability   Unstable/Stable   Conditions to Avoid

Incompatibility
(Materials to Avoid)

Hazardous
Decomposition Products

Medical Conditions Generally
Aggravated by Exposure

Chemical Listed as Carcinogen
or Potential Carcinogen

National Toxicology      IARC             OSHA  Yes/No
Program  Yes/No          Monographs  Yes/No

Emergency and
First Aid Procedures

**Routes of Entry**  1. Inhalation  2. Eyes  3. Skin  4. Ingestion

### SECTION 7 - Special Precautions and Spill/Leak Procedures

Precautions to Be Taken
in Handling and Storage

Other
Precautions

Steps to Be Taken in Case
Material Is Released or Spilled

Waste Disposal
Methods (Consult federal, state and local regulations)

### SECTION 8 - Special Protection Information/Control Measures

Respiratory Protection
(Specify Type)

| Ventilation | Local Exhaust | Mechanical (General) | Special | Other |
|---|---|---|---|---|

Protective
Gloves              Eye Protection

Other Protective
Clothing or Equipment

Work Hygiene Practices

**IMPORTANT**
Do not leave any blank spaces. If required information is unavailable, unknown, or does not apply, so indicate.

**F I G U R E   3 - 3**

Material safety data sheet. (Courtesy of Labelmaster Division, American Labelmart Co., Chicago, IL)

- Criteria for implementing engineering controls (fume hoods)
- Use of personal protective equipment and other hygiene practices
- Special precautions for extremely hazardous chemicals
- Specific measures to ensure that fume hoods and other protective equipment are working properly
- Provision for employee information and training
- Provision for medical consultation and examination
- Designation of a chemical hygiene officer responsible for implementation of the CHP

This regulation basically directs laboratory employers to comply with existing OSHA exposure limits and right to know requirements (HCS) and to provide medical surveillance programs.

## Categories of Chemicals

Since the laboratory deals with a wide variety of chemicals, clinical laboratory scientists must understand the potential hazards involved in their use. Chemicals may have health hazards or physical hazards. The hazard categories of chemicals are:

- **Corrosives**—chemicals with a pH of $\leq 2$ or $\geq 12.5$.
- **Toxic substances**—poisons, irritants, and asphyxiants.
- **Carcinogens**—capable of causing cancer.
- **Mutagens and teratogens**—capable of causing chromosomal aberrations or congenital malformations.
- **Ignitable**—flammable and combustibles.
- **Reactive**—explosive and oxidizers.

Corrosive chemicals cause visible destruction of human tissue on contact. Some commonly used corrosives in laboratories are concentrated acids such as hydrochloric acid or acetic acid and alkalies such as sodium hydroxide. Corrosives can produce injury upon inhalation or contact.

Toxic substances include poisons, irritants, and asphyxiants. They do not act directly with human tissue but interfere with the metabolic processes of the body. They may enter the body by ingestion, inhalation, or skin absorption. Studies in humans and animals form the basis for guidelines that set limits for exposure to toxic chemicals in the workplace. These limits are called threshold limit values (TLVs) and may be found on the MSDS. The TLV indicates the amount an individual can have exposure to without any adverse effect. There are three different TLVs[3]:

1. Time-weighted average (TLV-TWA)—represents the maximum allowable exposure over an 8-hour work day.
2. Short-term exposure limit (TLV-STEL)—represents the maximum amount of allowable exposure for a short period such as 15 minutes.
3. Ceiling value form (TLV-C)—represents the concentration of an agent that must never be exceeded.

Carcinogens are chemicals that have been shown to cause cancer in animals or humans. Occupational exposure to carcinogens directly accounts for about 4 % of the cancer incidence in the United States.[4] Chemicals labeled or noted on the MSDS as being carcinogenic, cancer causing, potential carcinogen, or cancer suspect should be clearly labeled and handled in a specific area of the laboratory with appropriate personal protective equipment. The carcinogenic chemicals regulated by OSHA are listed in Table 3–3.[5]

Many other chemicals are classified as cancer suspect agents or select carcinogens. Lists of these chemicals can be obtained from the National Toxicology Program (NTP) and from the International Agency for Research on Cancer (IARC). Formaldehyde is considered a potential carcinogen and is regulated by OSHA.[6]

Mutagenic and teratogenic chemicals are reproductive hazards that have the potential to cause irreversible damage or death to future generations. Before conception, mutagens can produce chromosomal mutations and genetically induce congenital problems. Maternal exposure after conception may result in fetal death or abnormalities. The MSDS identifies chemicals that have been shown to be mutagenic or teratogenic. Pregnant laboratory workers should be aware of the chemicals with which they are working.

Flammable and combustible chemicals may also have associated health hazards, but the primary immediate hazard is risk of fire. Examples are xylene, diethyl ether, acetone, and alcohols. Flammable liquids have a flashpoint below 140 °F and combustible liquids have a flashpoint at or above 140 °F.[7] The flashpoint is the lowest temperature that produces sufficient vapor to form an ignitable mixture at the surface of the liquid. A heat source must be present to ignite the vapor. This heat source may be an electrical spark or static spark. The greatest risk of fire from flammable or combustible liquids in the laboratory is from improper storage. OSHA and NFPA have published specifications for storage of flammable liquids.[7]

TABLE  3 – 3

**OSHA Regulated Carcinogenic Chemicals**

Chloromethyl methyl ether—vinyl chloride
N-Nitrosodimethylamine
N-2-Fluorenylacetamide (2-AAF)
Benz[a]pyrene
4-Aminobiphenyl
Benzidine
1-Naphthylamine
2-Naphthylamine
4-Nitrobiphenyl
Benzene
Ethylenimine
p-Dimethylaminoazobenzene
beta-Propiolactone
bis Chloromethyl ether

Flammable and combustible liquids should be limited to one pint quantities if stored in glass containers and the rest stored in a flammable safety cabinet (Figure 3–4) or in an approved flammable safety can (Figure 3–5). Flammables should never be stored in a refrigerator unless it is designated by the manufacturer as an explosion-proof refrigerator with all electrical switches outside the refrigeration compartment.

When flammables are used, there should be no nearby heat sources or sources of ignition from electrical equipment. When the contents of one metal container are transferred to another, the two containers should be connected by a metal conductor to prevent static electricity buildup. Flammable liquids should not be poured into another container because the turbulence of the liquid can generate static electricity. The liquid should be poured through a funnel that has its tip immersed in the receiving container.

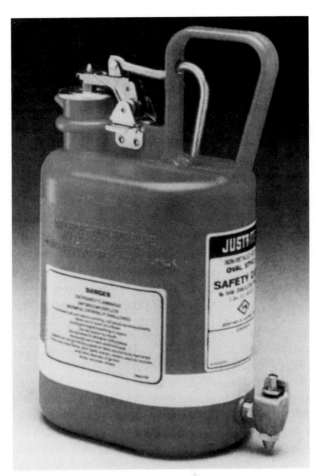

**FIGURE 3 - 5**

Flammable safety can. (Courtesy of Lab Safety Supply, Inc., Janesville, WI)

An explosive chemical is one that rapidly decomposes and produces energy that creates an explosion. Picric acid in its crystalline form is know to be explosive upon impact. The MSDS for each chemical received by the laboratory should be consulted for potential hazards.

Reactive compounds have molecular structures of high reactivity. They may be oxidizers with high oxygen content or compounds with redox groups (hydrazine, hydroxylamine), compounds that react violently with water or moist air (anhydrous metal oxides), pyrophoric compounds that react spontaneously with air, or compounds that can form peroxides over time and become explosive, such as diethyl ether.[3]

## Handling and Labeling

It is important to wear personal protective equipment when handling chemicals. A coat or rubber apron, eye protection, and gloves will greatly reduce the chances of severe injury when handling chemicals. The use of a fume hood or appropriate respirator is necessary when handling toxic volatile liquids.

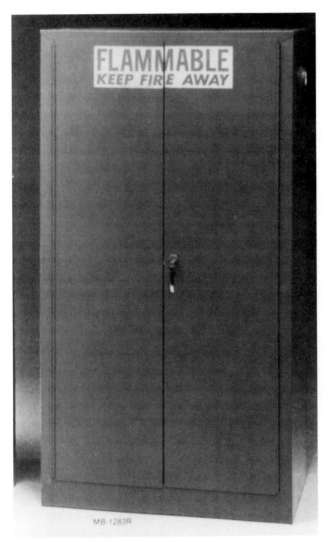

**FIGURE 3 - 4**

Flammable safety cabinet. (Courtesy of Lab Safety Supply, Inc., Janesville, WI)

Chemicals or other equipment should not be stored in fume hoods because these stored objects may interfere with the airflow. If anything must be stored in the hood, install narrow shelves on the back or side walls.

All chemicals in primary and secondary containers must be labeled with the name of the chemical and any known hazard. OSHA requires that the label be legible, in English, contain the necessary information, and be prominently displayed. It can be written, printed, or in graphic form (pictogram). Many labeling systems are available to relay hazards to employees:

- National Fire Protection Association, NFPA 704, Standard System for the Identification of the Fire Hazards of Materials
- Hazardous Materials Identification System (HMIS), of the National Paint and Coating Association
- American National Standards Institute, ANSI, Z129.1-1988
- Department of Transportation (DOT)

Because the NFPA numerical rating for hazards was developed primarily for short-term exposures created by fires, it may differ from HMIS, which is a numerical system designed for situations where the chemical is actually being used. The DOT and ANSI systems use pictograms (Figure 3–6) and/or signal words to relay the hazard information and do not require looking at a reference for the meaning of the number and color. For example, a skull and crossbones denotes poison and a flame denotes flammable materials with the DOT and ANSI systems. It is important to use a system that is simple and readily understood by all personnel coming into contact with the chemical.

## Storage

Chemicals should be stored in an uncluttered area that is properly ventilated and away from a heat source. They should not be stored above eye level. It is not a good idea to store chemicals alphabetically because reactive groups of the chemicals may be incompatible. As a rule, inorganics should be stored separately from organics. Inorganic acids should be stored together with the exception of nitric acid. Nitric acid should be isolated from the other acids. Acetic acid can be stored with inorganic acids.[3]

Flammables should be stored in an approved flammable safety cabinet. These cabinets may be vented or unvented. The primary purpose of a flammable safety cabinet is to keep fire away from flammable liquids.

Toxic chemicals should be handled with great care in a well-ventilated area. The containers should be clearly marked with the hazard. They should be stored separately from acids and oxidizing agents. A secondary container should be used to contain the chemical in event of breakage or leakage if the substance is highly toxic or carcinogenic.

Water-reactive chemicals such as sodium, potassium, and metal hydrides should be segregated from the other chemicals and stored in a dry environment. These areas should not be equipped with automatic sprinkler systems.

## Spills

A written plan for containing and cleaning up chemical spills should be developed. The MSDS should be consulted for information on personal protective equipment and spill cleanup procedures. Spill pillows or other absorbent materials should

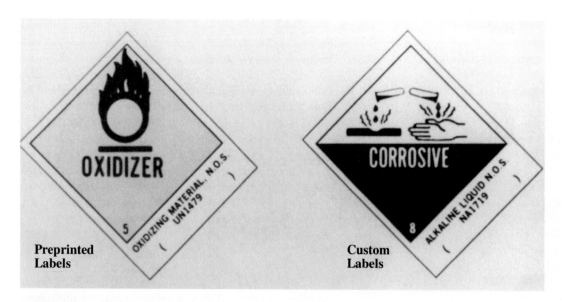

**FIGURE 3-6**

Hazard information pictograms. (Courtesy of Lab Safety Supply, Inc., Janesville, WI)

be available. Concentrated acid spills or base spills should be diluted with water before cleanup is attempted. The spill should then be covered with a neutralizer such as sodium bicarbonate for acids or boric acid for bases. The spill should then be absorbed with a spill pillow or other absorbent material and disposed of according to the institutional policy on chemical waste disposal. The surface should be cleansed with soap and water after the chemical is cleaned up. If a solvent is spilled, no water or diluent should be added and the solvent should not be allowed to flow down a drain. Since solvents may present a fume problem, respiratory protective equipment needs to be available. After absorption with absorbent material or a spill pillow, the material should be placed in a closed container to prevent fumes from escaping. All containers should be labeled with the chemical name and any hazard and disposed as chemical waste. Commercially available spill control kits that contain neutralizing and absorbing materials are available.

## Disposal

Specific EPA (website: www.epa.gov) regulations as well as state and local laws regulate the disposal of chemicals. Clinical laboratories can be classified as **small quantity generators** by EPA if they generate between 100 and 1000 kg of hazardous chemicals per month. They are classified as **conditionally exempt small quantity generators** if they generate less than 100 kg/month.[8] EPA regulates the disposal of hazardous chemicals (chemicals that have ignitability, corrosivity, reactivity, or toxicity).

In general, only small amounts (100 mL or less) of water-soluble chemical waste may be put into the sewer drains. Flammable liquids such as xylene, ether, azides, peroxides, mercury, and other heavy-metal–containing compounds should not be flushed down drains. The drain should flow to a wastewater treatment plant and not into a storm sewer system. The drain should be flushed with at least 100-fold excess of water to dilute the chemical.[9] The local sanitary sewer district should be contacted to determine specifically what is acceptable to put into the sanitary sewer.

Most laboratory chemicals will need to be disposed by an EPA-licensed chemical hauler or disposal company. This company must comply with the RCRA regulations, which are enforced by EPA and DOT regulations for transporting chemicals. The laboratory is responsible for the chemicals from "cradle to grave" and is liable for their ultimate disposal. According to RCRA, the generator of the chemical, the transporter and disposal facility must be registered with EPA. The movement and disposal of the chemicals is monitored by a multicopy manifest that lists the materials being shipped. Completion of the manifest assures the generator of arrival and acceptance of the chemicals at the disposal site. The generator must keep copies of the manifest for 3 years.[8] Chemicals should never be mixed when discarded but should be kept

in their individual containers. Extremely reactive chemicals should be segregated from other chemicals. An inventory of the stored waste chemicals should be kept and the list given to the transporter.

Time limits on waste chemical storage are based on the generator's classification. The NCCLS document GP5-T is an excellent source of information on EPA waste chemical compliances. Many transporters prefer to pack the waste chemicals to their own specifications based on chemical class and disposal methods. The materials management department of the institution can assist with arrangements for chemical transport, disposal, and compliance with EPA regulations.

## COMPRESSED GASES

Compressed gas cylinders of varying sizes can be found in laboratories and especially in research laboratories. Since the cylinders are pressurized, they can become "torpedoes" that can even penetrate block walls if the main valve stem is sheared by falling over.

A good working practice when using a flammable gas is to allow only one cylinder of gas to be in use at a time and to use the smallest size possible. Gas cylinders, both flammable and nonflammable, should never be stored in flammable safety cabinets with flammable and combustible liquids. They should be grouped by type and stored in a ventilated room reserved exclusively for cylinder storage. The room should have a fire resistance rating of at least 2 hours.[10]

Cylinders should always be secured by a chain or other device to prevent them from falling over and shearing the valve stem. When cylinders are transported, valve protective caps should be used. When cylinders are not in use, the valves should be tightly closed.

## ELECTRICAL SAFETY

Laboratories have a great deal of electrical equipment in proximity to sinks, liquids, and other grounded surfaces. Burns, shock, electrocution, ignition, and explosion are hazards associated with electricity. Burns, shock, and electrocution are avoided by preventing electrical potentials from developing across personnel. Fire and explosion hazards are avoided by preventing the occurrence of high temperatures. Circuit breakers, fuses, and ground fault interrupters (GFI) are designed to detect overloaded circuits that could cause ignition and explosion.

Grounding provides protection against a possible short between one side of the power line and the chassis of the instrument or the person touching the instrument. Three-pronged grounded plugs provide this grounding and should never be plugged into a two-wire extension cord. The use of three-prong adaptors is discouraged because the internal ground wire may be broken or the grounding "pigtail" wire may not be properly connected to a good ground source. A GFI is sensitive to current leaks or "faults" between the instrument and the ground and rapidly interrupts the circuit if current is detected.

Equipment should be checked annually for current leakage and ground integrity. All equipment should have a grounded plug or polarized plug, which has one prong larger than the other so current is directed to the switch first. Multiple outlet strips should be avoided because they may overload the circuit.

Daily use of extension cords is not in compliance with most local or state electrical codes. If extension cords must be used for emergency power, only properly grounded heavy-duty cords that have been checked by the facility's maintenance department should be used.

If equipment is damaged, malfunctions, smells strong, makes unusual noise, or gets wet, it should be immediately turned off and inspected by a qualified person. If anyone gets a shock (even a small tingle) or a frayed wire or loose connection is noticed, the instrument should be disconnected immediately from the power supply and the problem reported to maintenance or other qualified personnel. Electrical equipment merely needs to be plugged in to be dangerous, it does not need to be turned on.

## BIOLOGICAL SAFETY

### Personal Protection

The epidemic spread of acquired immunodeficiency syndrome (AIDS) has created concern about bloodborne pathogens in the laboratory community. Clinical laboratory workers are recognized as a high-risk group for job-related infection with hepatitis B (HBV) and human immunodeficiency virus (HIV). In 1987, the Centers for Disease Control and Prevention (CDC) (website: www.cdc.gov) published recommendations to protect health care workers and others from acquiring HIV infection[11] and updated them in 1988.[12] Among the recommendations was "blood and body fluid precautions should be consistently used for **all** patients and patient specimens." This has become known as **Universal Precautions.** These recommendations include the use of personal protective equipment such as fluid-resistant gowns or lab coats, gloves, and eye protection when handling blood and body fluids in the laboratory. The 1988 CDC revision removed nonbloody urine, feces, saliva, sputum, and vomitus from the list of body substances requiring Universal Precautions. Since this created some confusion, many institutions started to use **Body Substance Isolation** (BSI), which requires the use of personal protective equipment to handle **all body substances**. It is good practice to treat all body secretions and excretions as potentially infectious because diseases other than HBV and HIV may be transmitted via body substances.

In 1991, OSHA issued a final rule for Occupational Exposure to Bloodborne Pathogens[13] and a Compliance Directive in 1999.[1] This rule requires the employer to supply personal protective equipment that does not permit potentially infectious materials to reach the employee's clothes, skin, eyes, and mouth under normal conditions of use. The rule also requires the safe disposal of sharps and other biohazardous waste, and requires that HBV vaccine and postexposure treatment be made available free of charge to all employees at risk of exposure. Annual training is required that provides information regarding the risks of exposure and transmission and necessary precautions to avoid exposure.

In addition to personal protective equipment, the proposed rule also addresses hand washing, specimen transport, use of pipetting devices, spill cleanup, waste disposal, and decontamination of equipment.

### Spills

During biological spill cleanup, always wear gloves and a gown or lab coat. Disposable towels should be placed over the spill and disinfectant poured on the towel. After standing a few minutes, the biological material and disinfectant can be absorbed with absorbent material (spill pillow). The contaminated material is then placed in a biohazard container. After most of the spill is absorbed, the area is cleaned with an intermediate- to high-level disinfectant, such as a 1:10 dilution of bleach. The bleach solution must be fresh and prepared every 24 hours for the disinfectant to be effective. The disinfectant should be absorbed with disposable material. The spill site is rinsed with water and the area dried.[14] The hepatitis B virus can survive for at least a week in dried blood on environmental surfaces or contaminated needles and instruments.[1] These surface areas should be cleansed with a 10% fresh bleach solution. A biohazard spill kit that contains all the necessary materials for spill cleanup can be prepared so that it is readily available in the laboratory.

### Disposal

Infectious waste is defined as any solid or liquid waste that is known to contain or suspected of containing pathogens. EPA divides infectious waste into 6 categories.[15]

Infectious waste should be segregated from the regular trash and placed in infectious waste containers clearly marked with a biohazard label. Needles and sharps should be placed in rigid, puncture-proof containers that can be sealed with a tight-fitting lid. These containers should be disposed in a manner consistent with the institutional policy on infectious waste disposal.

Infectious waste can be treated by incineration, autoclaving, or discharge into the sanitary sewer system. It is common practice to dispose of suctioned fluids, urine, and small amounts of unclotted blood into the sanitary sewer system with copious amounts of water. The local water treatment plant should be contacted for specific guidelines.

Autoclaving can be used to decontaminate or sterilize infectious waste; culture plates are often decontaminated using this method. In some localities, sanitary landfills will accept autoclaved infectious waste. Where autoclaved waste is not acceptable to landfill, the only alternative is to incinerate the waste.

Incinerators can be used to dispose of all types of infectious waste. There are strict EPA standards for incinerators and they must meet federal, state, and local regulations. It is possible to contract with an off-site incineration company to pick up and incinerate infectious waste for a fee. Some states have adopted laws that require tracking the ultimate disposal of the infectious waste through a manifest system similar to the chemical disposal manifest system.[16]

## RADIATION SAFETY

### General Information

There are four types of ionizing radiation hazards:

- Alpha particles
- Beta particles
- Electromagnetic radiation (gamma rays and x-rays)
- Neutrons

Alpha particles are large and can travel only a very short range in air. They may be stopped by skin or a sheet of paper. They may, however, cause serious tissue damage if ingested or inhaled. It is not common to find alpha emitters in the clinical laboratory. Plutonium is an alpha emitter. Beta particles they are smaller than alpha particles and are negatively charged electrons. They have limited penetrating power, but like alpha particles they are a significant health hazard if inhaled or ingested. Beta particles are emitted by $^3$H, $^{14}$C, $^{32}$P. Gamma radiation and X rays are composed of electromagnetic energy and not composed of atomic particles. Gamma radiation has no mass or charge but does have great penetrating power and poses a significant internal and external hazard if in high enough concentration. Gamma radiation is produced by both $^{125}$I and $^{131}$I. X rays differ from gamma rays only in the origin of the radiation. Neutron emitters are rarely used in the clinical laboratory. Neutrons arise from spontaneous fission of some isotopes and are produced by atomic reactors and accelerators.

The biological effect of all types of ionizing radiation is damage to DNA in the cell nucleus. This damage can lead to mutation, cancer, or cell death. The clinical diagnostic laboratory does not usually use radioisotopes in concentrations high enough to cause cell damage, but exposure should be controlled because exposure may be cumulative.

### Handling

Someone knowledgeable of or willing to learn about radiation and the handling of radioisotopes should be appointed as laboratory radiation safety officer. Many institutions have an institutional radiation safety officer and a committee with representation from all the departments that handle radioisotopes in the institution (e.g., radiology, nuclear medicine, laboratory). All personnel working with radioisotopes must be instructed in proper handling techniques and safety precautions. Pregnant women should be advised of the potential hazard to the fetus. There should be written procedures for receiving shipments and using, storing, and disposing of the material. There should also be written spill procedures for spill cleanup and monitoring protocols.

Receipt of radioisotopes should be documented and broken packages monitored for significant leakage. If monitoring exceeds 200 millirads per hour at the surface, the Nuclear Regulatory Commission (NRC) mandates that the laboratory supervisor, courier, supplier, and RNRC be notified and proper decontamination be carried out. Radioisotopes should be stored in clearly labeled refrigerators or cabinets.

Procedures using radioisotopes should be performed in a separate room. The door to the room should be labeled "Radioactive Material—Authorized Personnel Only." Waste containers should also be clearly labeled. The areas in which radioisotopes are used should be monitored with a survey meter and a series of wipe tests. A record of all survey results must be kept as well as a record of any corrective action.

When personnel are using radioisotopes, all precautions against eating, drinking, and smoking must be strictly followed. Most clinical in vitro radioimmunoassay (RIA) kits contain $^{125}$I. If $^{125}$I is ingested, it may be concentrated by the thyroid gland and accumulate into a harmful dose. All personnel should wear an exposure-monitoring device such as a film badge or use a dosimeter when working with radioactive material. Gloves and laboratory coats are required. Hands should be thoroughly washed after working with radioisotopes, even if gloves are worn. For easy containment and proper disposal of spills or drips, it is recommended that procedures be performed over an absorbent pad or contained area. Report accidental inhalation, ingestion, injury or spills to the supervisor or radiation safety officer immediately.

### Spills

If a spill occurs on a surface, it may be cleaned up with soap and water or a commercial cleaning agent. Begin cleaning at the outer edge of the spill and work inward. Cleaning should be continued until monitoring shows acceptable radiation levels. If the spill involves skin contact, use soap and water for cleaning and take care not to abrade the skin or get material into open wounds or onto mucous membranes. The area of contact should be monitored for radioactivity after cleaning.

## Waste Disposal

A general license by the NRC is required for use of radioimmunoassay (RIA) kits in the clinical laboratory even when exempt material is used. Under these guidelines, effluents from RIA in vitro tests may be flushed into the sanitary sewer and diluted with large amounts of water.[17] However, many states also have regulations regarding disposal of radioisotopes, so local and state regulations should be consulted. When disposing of radioisotopes into the sanitary sewer, designate one sink for this purpose. This sink should be clearly labeled and routinely monitored with a wipe test for residual radioactivity. Liquid waste disposed in this manner must be material that is readily soluble or dispersible in water. Other material such as disposable tubes and pipets that have been in contact with the radioisotopes may be safely discarded in the routine trash after all radioactive labels are removed. If the waste also contains biohazardous material, it may be autoclaved before disposal into the routine trash. The laboratory's NRC license should be consulted for disposal guidelines.

## LABORATORY SAFETY PROGRAM

Safety in a laboratory cannot be accomplished by training alone. Hazards should be removed wherever possible, such as substituting a less toxic chemical for a more toxic one. If a hazard exists, the personnel should be guarded from the hazard by engineering practices, such as installation of a fume hood. If personnel must handle hazardous substances, protective clothing and equipment must be provided.

Emergency plans should be established for fire, spills, and evacuation. There should be periodic drills to test these plans. Drills should be documented with the dates, nature of drill, outcome, and names of personnel participating. This is a requirement of some accrediting agencies such as the College of American Pathologists.

There should be a reporting system for accidents involving personal injury and incidents not involving injury. Such incidents suggest unsafe conditions or actions and can be useful for investigating the cause of and ways to prevent future incidents and possible personal injury. It should be made clear in actions and policies that the reporting of incidents is to improve safety practices and provide a safe working environment. Employees should be encouraged to recommend changes to avoid future occurrence.

An individual who is willing to learn about OSHA standards and other federal, state, and local regulations that affect laboratory safety should be appointed as a laboratory safety manager. This individual should be knowledgeable of good laboratory safety practices. It is also recommended that a safety committee, composed of staff technologists, be appointed. Under the leadership of the safety manager, this committee should recommend safety polices, write and update the safety manual, conduct safety training programs, investigate accidents and

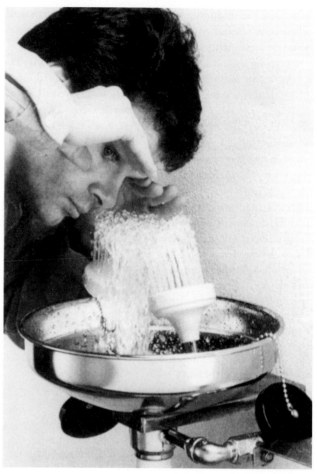

**F I G U R E   3 – 7**

Eyewash fountain. (Courtesy of Lab Safety Supply, Inc., Janesville, WI)

incidents, conduct periodic safety inspections and drills, recommend changes in work practices, and disseminate safety information to the rest of the laboratory staff.

Safety equipment that should be available in any laboratory handling chemicals includes showers, eyewash fountains (Figure 3–7), fire extinguishers, fume hoods, and fire alarms. These items should be tested periodically to ensure they are working correctly. Employees should be trained in the use of this equipment. Other items that should be available include a first-aid kit, a chemical spill control kit, fire blankets, respirators, safety goggles or face shields, masks, gloves, fluid-resistant lab coats or gowns, and plastic or rubber aprons.

## SUMMARY

The clinical laboratory contains a variety of potential biological, chemical, and mechanical hazards. Laboratory personnel with an awareness and understanding of safe work practices will find it to be a safe environment in which to work. To maintain a safe environment, all levels of laboratory personnel should be educated in safe work practices and emergency preparedness at job entry and periodically thereafter.

## RESOURCES FOR SAFETY INFORMATION

American National Standards Institute (ANSI)
11 W 42nd St. FL 13
New York, NY 10018
(212) 642-4900

Centers for Disease Control and Prevention (CDC)
Division of Biosafety
1600 Clifton Rd., NE
Atlanta, GA 30333
(404) 639-3311
www.cdc.gov

Code of Federal Regulations (CFR) and Federal Register
Superintendent of Documents
U.S. Government Printing Office
732 N Capitol St., NW #808
Washington, DC 20402
202/512-0000

College of American Pathologists (CAP)
325 Waukegan Rd.
Northfield, IL 60093
(847) 832-7000
www.cap.org

Compressed Gas Association
1725 Jefferson David Hwy.
Arlington, VA 22202-4102
(703) 412-0900

Department of Transportation (DOT)
Materials Transportation Bureau, Information Services
   Division
400 7th St., SW
Washington, DC 20590
(202) 366-4000

Environmental Protection Agency (EPA)
401 M St., SW
Washington, DC 20460
202/382-4700
www.epa.gov

Joint Commission on Accreditation of Healthcare
   Organizations (JCAHO)
One Renaissance Blvd.
Oakbrook Terrace, IL 60181
(630) 792-5000
www.jcaho.org

National Committee for Clinical Laboratory Standards
   (NCCLS)
940 W Valley Rd.
Ste 1400
Wayne, PA 19087-1898
(610) 688-1100
www.nccls.org

National Fire Protection Association (NFPA)
One Battery March Park
Quincy, MA 02169
(800) 344-3555
www.nfpa.org

National Institute for Occupational Safety and Health
   (NIOSH)
Office of Technical Publications, Robert A. Taft Laboratories
4676 Columbia Pkwy.
Cincinnati, OH 45226
(513) 533-8377
www.cdc.gov/niosh

Occupational Safety and Health Administration (OSHA)
U.S. Department of Labor
200 Constitution Ave., NW
Washington, DC 20210
(202) 693-1999
www.cdc.gov

U.S. Nuclear Regulatory Commission (NRC)
Washington, DC 20555
(301) 415-7000
www.nrc.gov

## REFERENCES

1. OSHA: Bloodborne Pathogen Compliance Directive. *Vantage Point* 33 (22), 1999.
2. OSHA: Hazard Communication Standard. 29CFR 1910.1200, 1986.
3. Rayburn SR: *The Foundations of Laboratory Safety.* New York, Springer-Verlag, 1990.
4. Doll R, Petro R: *The Causes of Cancer: Qualitative Estimates of Avoidable Risk of Cancer in the US.* Oxford, England, Oxford University Press, 1981.
5. OSHA: 29CFR 1910.1001–1047, 1989.
6. OSHA: Occupational Exposure to Formaldehyde. 29CFR 1910.1048, 1988.
7. National Academy of Sciences, National Research Council: *Prudent Practices for Handling Hazardous Chemicals in Laboratories.* Washington, DC, National Academy Press, 1981.
8. Phifer RW, McTigue WR: *Hazardous Waste Management for Small Quantity Generators.* Chelsea, MI, Lewis Publications, 1988.

9.  National Academy of Sciences, National Research Council: *Prudent Practices for Disposal of Chemicals from Laboratories.* Washington, DC, National Academy Press, 1983.

10. Standard P-1. Arlington, VA, Compressed Gas Association, 1984.

11. CDC: Recommendations for prevention of HIV transmission in health care settings. MMWR 36 (Suppl 25), 35–185, 1987.

12. CDC: Update: Universal precautions for prevention of transmission of HIV, HBV, and other blood-borne pathogens in health care settings. MMWR 37, 337–392, 1988.

13. OSHA: Occupational Exposure to Bloodborne Pathogens (proposed rule). Federal Register, May 30, 1989, 23134–23139, 1989.

14. National Committee for Clinical Laboratory Standards: Protection of laboratory workers for disease transmitted by blood, body fluids and tissue. NCCLS Document M29-T, Villanova, PA, NCCLS, 1989.

15. EPA: Guide for Infectious Waste Management. Washington, DC, U.S. Government Printing Office, 1986.

16. EPA: Medical Waste Tracking Act. 40CFR, parts 22 and 259, 1989.

17. Nuclear Regulatory Commission: 10CFR, parts 19, 20, 34, 2000.

# C H A P T E R 4
# Quality Assurance

*Mark D. Kellogg*

Quality assurance is often used to refer to all of the processes a laboratory takes to ensure quality in test results. However, assurance is more properly defined as a pledge, or guaranty, a self-confidence. Thus, using this definition quality assurance is the *result* of the processes focused on achieving quality. That is, by using planning, assessment, and monitoring tools, we can pledge, guaranty, and assure the quality of the products laboratories produce.

The first part of this chapter will address the quality management framework that is integral to the implementation of an effective quality control program. This will be followed by a more detailed description of the quality control monitoring process and the statistics used in this process. This chapter will utilize the terms and concepts proposed by Westgard, Burnett, and Bowers as part of their framework for managing the quality of laboratory tests.[1]

## THE QUALITY MANAGEMENT FRAMEWORK

The first step in achieving quality laboratory processes requires a definition of the goals and objectives and the establishment of quality requirements to satisfy the customer. Without these definitions, there is no way to measure whether acceptable quality is being achieved. Imagine having your clinical chemistry instructor start a lecture stating, "Today you will learn" and then describing the process of changing tires on semi-trailers. By the end of class, you will have learned something, but does it satisfy your need as a student in clinical chemistry? Was there any relevant quality in the instruction? This example shows the importance of having well-defined goals and objectives.

The next step in the framework is **quality planning.** This encompasses the creation, selection, and validation of the methods and processes used in the laboratory. What are the best available methods? Do they meet the quality requirements? The selection of quality control procedures is an example of quality planning and will be addressed later in this chapter. Remember, the plan is what gets you to the desired quality. As

an example, imagine preparing for a long journey. You will need to decide how you will get there. Will you use a plane, car, train? What routes will you travel to get there? It is very difficult to accomplish the goal without a plan.

**Quality laboratory processes** (QLP) result from the quality planning and describe the means by which work is conducted in the laboratory. Personnel policies, standard operating procedures (SOPs), specimen-collection guidelines all belong to the QLP domain. These should represent the best way for your laboratory to get the work done. But no process is perfect and the remaining components of the management framework serve to monitor these processes and provide correction if they deviate from the established quality requirements.

**Quality assessment** (QA) in the clinical laboratory includes all actions a laboratory takes to measure and monitor performance of the laboratory processes. QA includes verification of the quality of sample collection, sample processing, reporting of results, and interpretation of the final report by the physician. In addition, quality assessment should address the prompt reporting and better use of test results as well as the competency and adequacy of laboratory staff.

If QA activities determine that quality requirements are not being achieved, then **quality improvement** (QI) processes must determine the cause of the problem and provide input to further quality planning to eliminate the problem. A good example would be the monitoring of hemolyzed blood samples arriving in the laboratory. A QA program may keep track of these and create a warning if more than X specimens arrive in a defined period. If this warning is given, an investigation (a QI process) might find that the specimens all came from a specific lot of evacuated tubes or resulted from incomplete training of specimen-collection personnel. Once the problem is identified, then quality planning can be used to create measures for assuring evacuated tube quality or additional training can be designed for specimen-collection personnel.

Quality improvement is more than just simply changing something to fix a problem, but a thorough assessment of what the problem is and then the use of quality planning to modify or create quality laboratory processes to eliminate the problem. Dr. Westgard provides an excellent example from his essay on total quality management.[2] In his example he describes how a physician who has ordered a stat or emergency test calls for the answer before the specimen has arrived in the laboratory. The physician insists that the laboratory needs to do testing faster. However, performing the test faster does not solve

The views, opinions, and/or findings contained in this chapter are those of the author and should not be construed as an official Department of the Army position, policy, or decision unless so designated by other documentation.

the problem, which most likely is due to problems in the collection and transport of specimen to the laboratory. Listening to the customer (physician) does not mean doing what the customer says. It is important to use your knowledge of the testing process to analyze where problems might exist and investigate to determine the root cause.

Quality control (QC) provides the tools to detect problems early and prevent errors from exceeding established quality requirements. QC is somewhat narrowly defined as the monitoring of work processes, detecting problems and making corrections prior to delivery of products or services.[1] This contrasts to the broader measures of QA described earlier that detect errors after they have occurred but before they reach a defined "critical" level. Typically, QC is applied to the analytical process (the actual measurement of analytes in a specimen) and not the pre-analytical or post-analytical phases. Statistical process control, or statistical quality control, is the major procedure for monitoring the analytical performance of laboratory methods.

QC will be the focus of the remainder of this chapter. Readers are highly encouraged to learn more about the total quality management approach to laboratory testing and to read the works of Westgard and others on quality control. The World Wide Web (WWW) provides an amazing abundance of resources, and in particular Dr. Westgard has an excellent web site at www.westgard.com.

## QUALITY CONTROL MONITORING

### Selection of Quality Control Materials

Before discussing the criteria for selection of control material, it is appropriate to make a distinction between a standard and a control. A **standard** is a solution that contains a known amount of an analyte and is used to calibrate an assay method. A standard has one assigned value; for example, it contains 100 mg/dL of glucose. Not 100 mg/dL ± X amount, but exactly 100 mg/dL. If we know that we are putting 100 mg/dL of glucose into the instrument, the result should be 100 mg/dL. If the result is not 100 mg/dL, then the system is adjusted (calibrated) to produce the desired 100 mg/dL value. This adjustment may be performed by you or automatically by the microprocessors controlling the instrument. Assay results are then calculated from calibration settings. **Controls,** on the other hand, are used to monitor the performance of an assay method once it has been calibrated. Controls are run alongside patient samples and results are calculated from calibration data in the same manner that patient results are calculated. The controls are used to make sure that the measurement process is stable (the same as it was when calibrated) and if the results produced are acceptable.

A control should have the same **matrix** or closely mimic the characteristics of the patient sample that is being tested.

Matrix refers to all of the characteristics of the sample. In broad terms the matrix can be defined as serum, plasma, or urine. However, controls usually have additional material added as preservatives, or may be entirely synthetic. When these additional materials or components of synthetic controls do not act like a biological sample when tested, we call this **matrix interference.** Because of this interference, it is important that a test designed to be performed on serum have control material that is as similar to serum as possible. This can be accomplished by pooling actual samples of human serum or animal serum, lyophilizing or dehydrating serum samples, or using an artificial protein-based solution that has the same physical characteristics as serum. These control samples are usually purchased from commercial vendors, often from the manufacturer of the instrument or reagents that you are using.

Every QC system should include at least two levels of controls with analyte concentrations focused at medical-decision levels. The importance of this is illustrated in the following example.

A physician receiving an abnormal creatinine result on a patient may make two very different medical decisions based on the magnitude of the abnormal value:

1. For some patients, the physician may decide the value is elevated enough from normal to diagnose kidney dysfunction.
2. For other patients, the physician may decide the result is so elevated that aggressive medical intervention such as dialysis is necessary.

The laboratory that has this physician as a client could have one control focused at or near the value that distinguishes normal from abnormal and the other control focused at a value that would indicate a need for extensive medical intervention.

Many chemistry laboratories use three levels of controls with values focused at low normal, high normal, or very abnormal concentrations. An example that illustrates the benefit of using three levels of controls is shown by the physician who treats diabetic patients.

This physician might make three levels of medical decisions based on abnormal glucose values. The physician may decide that:

1. a patient has a value elevated enough to have his or her condition diagnosed as diabetes.
2. a patient with a previously diagnosed condition of diabetes has a value so elevated that the patient requires immediate insulin therapy.
3. the diabetic patient has a value low enough to be near insulin shock.

Thus, a laboratory with three levels of controls could adequately ensure quality results at all three decision points.

It is advantageous to have sufficient amounts of the same lot number of control material to last at least a year. This is because whenever a new lot of control is put into place, a laboratory must reestablish target ranges for the control pool. This process, if performed correctly, takes approximately a month and would be inconvenient to perform more than once a year. In addition to the sufficient amounts to last at least a year, it is important that the control material remain stable for that period of time.

Controls should also be available in aliquots convenient for daily use. Once a control vial is opened, it is subject to evaporation and thus a change in concentration could easily occur. Commercial controls are usually available in 1-mL, 5-mL, or 10-mL aliquot vials.

## Statistical Procedures

Quality control samples can be used to monitor both quantitative (produces a numerical result) and qualitative (produces a nonnumerical or positive or negative result) tests. Since most chemistry procedures are quantitative, the focus of this section will be on the statistical procedures for evaluating QC results that are numerical or quantitative.

Once controls have been selected, the next step is to assay the selected controls for a period of time so that sufficient data points are generated to establish the target range. When a control is put into operation and run alongside patient samples, the value of the control is monitored against the target range. This monitoring process is the basis for determining acceptance or rejection of patient sample results.

The usual procedure for establishing a target range is to assay each control at least once per day or once per shift for a full month. A good rule of thumb is that data sets should contain at least 20 points if the statistics calculated on the data are to be considered valid. Therefore, the time allowed to collect data to establish a control's target range should be sufficient to produce at least 20 data points. In addition, the control should be assayed over an extended period to ensure that it is subjected to changes in the laboratory environment that may occur with different operators or at different times of day.

In an ideal world, repeated sampling of a control should produce the same result each time. However, the world is not perfect and unfortunately neither is the laboratory. There will always be a certain amount of variability in repeated measurements. This variability is affected by operator technique, the laboratorian, and by the inherent variability in the assay method (the instrument or procedure used to run the test). By measuring the control sample over 20 different time points, we hope to measure this inherent variation and use this information to decide if the process changes later.

Data from repeated measurements will have a distribution or spread in the values that reflect how easy it is to repeat the measurement and obtain the same value. We can visually represent this variability in repeat measurements with frequency plots. To design a frequency plot from repeat measurements of controls, the values obtained are plotted on the x-axis, and the number of times a value is obtained is plotted on the y-axis. The resulting plot takes the shape of a curve, with the area

*Example 4–1*

Laboratory A assays a control for glucose 2 to 3 times per day for 30 days. The laboratory then lists all assay values in descending order and counts the number of times each value was obtained. The following table lists the laboratory values for the control and the frequency each value was obtained during the 30 day period.

| Value (mg/dL) | Frequency |
|---------------|-----------|
| 106 | 1 |
| 105 | 1 |
| 104 | 1 |
| 103 | 2 |
| 102 | 3 |
| 101 | 4 |
| 100 | 3 |
| 99 | 2 |
| 98 | 1 |
| 97 | 1 |
| 96 | 1 |

The laboratory labels the x-axis of a frequency plot with the range of values obtained on the control (96 to 106) and the y-axis of the plot with the minimum to maximum number of times the values were obtained (1 to 4). As seen in Figure 4–1, once the points were plotted and the curve drawn, the area under the curve gave a visual representation of the frequency of data points at each value.

under the curve representing the number of data points at each control value.

As can be seen from the curve in Figure 4–1, the value that is in the middle of the range of values is also the value that is repeated most often. Therefore, the peak of the curve is at this value. Conversely, the values that have only one data point or are rarely repeated are also the values that are the lowest and the highest numbers in the data set. Thus, these values are found in the tails of the curve.

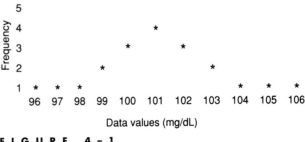

**F I G U R E　4 – 1**

A frequency plot.

## CENTRAL TENDENCY AND NORMAL DISTRIBUTION

Although it is impossible to obtain the same value for repeated measurements of a control, it is desirable that the majority of data points be nearly the same. This concept of clustering of data points about one value is referred to as central tendency. The frequency plot that results from data that exhibit central tendency has a peak that represents the value that is repeated most often. If the data points to the right of the peak (positive direction) are about equal to the data points to the left of the peak (negative direction), the data are said to have a normal distribution about the point of central tendency. The curve that results from plotting data that have a normal distribution is bell-shaped, with most values having frequencies in the top portion of the curve and few values having frequencies in the tails of the curve. These characteristics give the curve its spreading symmetrical or bell shape as shown in Figure 4–2.

Although plotting the data and observing the shape of the curve will indicate whether the data display central tendency and normal distribution, the interpretation of the curve is left to the observer. Statistical analysis of the curve will produce a mathematical picture of its shape that is less open to interpretation.

The statistical parameters used to measure central tendency are the mean, median, and mode. The **mean** is defined as the average of all the data points or values. The formula for calculating the mean is:

$$\bar{x} = \frac{\sum x_i}{n}$$

where    $\bar{x}$ = statistical designation for the mean
$\sum$ = symbol for "sum of"
$x_i$ = each data point or value
$n$ = the number of data points or values

The **median** is defined as the middle data point observed once the data are arranged in descending or ascending order. It is calculated by listing the data points in numerical order (including repeat data points) and selecting the middle value. For example, in a data set of 19 data points arranged in numerical order from 1 to 19, the value listed at position 10 is the median. Nine numbers are below this value (positions 1 to 9) and 9 numbers are above this value (positions 11 to 19). If the data set contains an even number of data points, the values at the two middle positions are averaged to obtain the median. For example, in a data set containing 20 values, the value at position 10 and the value at position 11 are averaged and that average becomes the median.

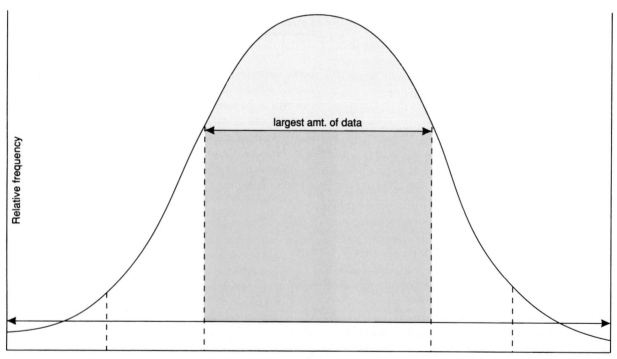

**FIGURE 4-2**

Normal distribution curve.

The **mode** is the value that occurs with the greatest frequency. In Example 4–1, the mode was 101 because it was the value repeated most often.

When data have a normal distribution, the mean, median, and mode are about the same. In other words, the central tendency about which the data are clustered is not only the value repeated most often but is also the middle value of the data set as well as the average of all values. This mathematically confirms that the data are clustered about the point of central tendency, the values above the peak are about equal to those below and the majority of values have frequencies near the peak.

In the example below, the calculated mean, median, and mode are essentially the same, and thus the data are normally

*Example 4–2*

The first two columns in the table below list the data from Example 4–1 by date in the order in which the control was sampled. The last two columns of the table list each data point, including all repeats, by its position in descending order.

| Date | Value | Position | Descending Order |
|------|-------|----------|------------------|
| 6-1  | 103   | 1        | 106              |
| 6-2  | 99    | 2        | 105              |
| 6-3  | 100   | 3        | 104              |
| 6-4  | 101   | 4        | 103              |
| 6-5  | 98    | 5        | 103              |
| 6-8  | 105   | 6        | 102              |
| 6-9  | 102   | 7        | 102              |
| 6-10 | 101   | 8        | 102              |
| 6-11 | 103   | 9        | 101              |
| 6-12 | 99    | 10       | 101}middle       |
| 6-15 | 102   | 11       | 101}middle       |
| 6-16 | 97    | 12       | 101              |
| 6-17 | 101   | 13       | 100              |
| 6-18 | 96    | 14       | 100              |
| 6-19 | 102   | 15       | 100              |
| 6-22 | 104   | 16       | 99               |
| 6-23 | 106   | 17       | 99               |
| 6-24 | 100   | 18       | 98               |
| 6-25 | 101   | 19       | 97               |
| 6-26 | 100   | 20       | 96               |

SUM = 2020

The mean, median, and mode for the data in Example 4–2 are as follows:

Mean = 101 (2020 divided by 20 data points)
Median = 101 (indicated in last column of example 4–2)
Mode = 101

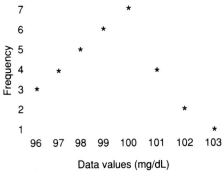

**F I G U R E   4 - 3**

This frequency plot is from data that are skewed towards the left side of the peak.

distributed. Some data sets will have central tendency but not normal distribution because the spread of points about the center is not symmetrical. The curve from this type of data set is said to have a skewed distribution and is asymmetrical because there are more data points on one side of the peak than on the other.

The calculated mean, median, and mode for the data represented by the frequency plot in Figure 4–3 are as follows:

Mean = 98.9
Mode = 100
Median = 99

Since the three measures of central tendency are not close enough to be considered equal, mathematical calculations indicate that the data are not normally distributed.

There are some instances in which data sets may have two points of central tendency. As shown in Figure 4–4, the curve resulting from these data has two peaks and is thus termed bimodal. The calculated mean, median, and the mode for these data are as follows:

Mean = 101.2
Median = 101
Mode = 99

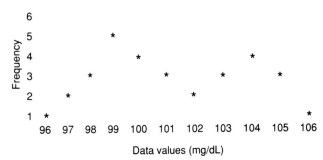

**F I G U R E   4 - 4**

Curve resulting from data set with a bimodal distribution.

These calculations are not the same and therefore the curve is not normally distributed.

Since the goal for repeat measurements of controls is that all values be about the same, it is critical that their frequency plots exhibit true central tendency with very little bias on either side of the peak. Therefore, the mean, median, and mode should always be calculated to confirm that the data are normally distributed before attempting to establish a target range.

## MEASURES OF DISPERSION

Once it has been determined that the data for repeat control measurements are normally distributed, it is important to consider the dispersion or the spread of the data within the distribution about the mean. The spread of data around a central tendency can be tight or broad, depending on the ability of a method or an operator to repeat the same value for a control each time it is sampled.

Both the curves in Figure 4–5 and Figure 4–6 have central tendency. The mean, median, and mode for each are about the same and thus the curves are normally distributed. However, the curve in Figure 4–5 has more points at or about the mean than the curve in Figure 4–6, and thus the data from Figure 4–5 are closer to that "perfect world" of obtaining the same value for each repeat sampling of the control. Since our goal is to have repeat control values that are as close to one value as possible, it is desirable that control data have a slim distribution about the mean. We assume that if we are successful at repeating the value for a control, we will be just as successful at repeating a value for a patient sample. Thus the ability to successfully repeat measurements and obtain the same value gives credibility to lab results.

As with determining central tendency of data, it is possible to draw a frequency plot and observe the curve for tight or broad distribution of points about the mean. Since this depends on interpretation by the observer, which can be subjective, there are statistical parameters that will give us a mathematical picture of the spread of the data about the mean. Those parameters are the range, variance, standard deviation, and coefficient of variation.

**Range** is defined as the difference between the highest and lowest value in a data set. To calculate the range, arrange the data set in order and subtract the lowest value from the

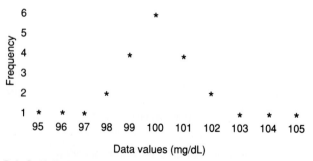

**F I G U R E   4 - 5**

Curve for tight distribution of points about the mean.

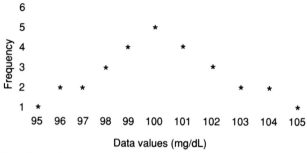

**F I G U R E   4 - 6**

Curve for broad distribution of points about the mean.

highest value. Looking at the data in Example 4–1, the highest value in the data set is 106 and the lowest value is 96. Therefore the range of the data is 10. If we add the units of mg/dL to the data, we can now say that repeated measurements of the control pool covered a range of 10 mg/dL.

Although the range gives an indication of the dispersion of data points, it is not clear how the data within the range vary about the mean. **Variance** is defined as the measure of the average squared distance of data points from the mean.

The formula for calculating variance is:

$$S^2 = \frac{\sum(x_i - \bar{x})^2}{n - 1}$$

where

$S^2$ = statistical symbol for variance

$\sum$ = symbol for "the sum of"

$(x_i - \bar{x})^2$ = (each data point minus the mean), squared

$n - 1$ = number of data points minus one degree of freedom

As you can see from the formula, the calculation of the variance is actually the calculation of an average. The data set that is averaged is the squared differences of data points from the mean. As with any average, the variance is calculated by summing members of a data set and dividing by the number of data points. In the variance formula, the total number of data points are adjusted for a loss in degrees of freedom.

**Degrees of freedom** are defined as the number of independent data points that are contained in a data set. Suppose you are told to select any 5 numbers and calculate their average. You have complete freedom in the selection of numbers since no restriction has been placed on the data set. You, therefore, have 5 independent numbers in the set. However, if you are told to take the average of any 5 numbers whose sum is 20, there is now a restriction placed on the data set and you have only 4 independent numbers. Once you select 4 numbers, the fifth number is set. For example, if you select 2, 3, 5, and 6 for the first 4 numbers, the last number must be 4 to obtain the sum of 20. Therefore, you have lost one degree of freedom.

*Example 4-3*

In the following example, the variance is calculated on the data from Example 4–1. The mean of the data was calculated previously as 101.

| $x$ | $x - \bar{x}$ | $(x - \bar{x})^2$ |
|---|---|---|
| | $(\bar{x} - 101)$ | |
| 103 | 2 | 4 |
| 99 | −2 | 4 |
| 100 | −1 | 1 |
| 101 | 0 | 0 |
| 98 | −3 | 9 |
| 105 | 4 | 16 |
| 102 | 1 | 1 |
| 101 | 0 | 0 |
| 103 | 2 | 4 |
| 99 | −2 | 4 |
| 102 | 1 | 1 |
| 97 | −4 | 16 |
| 101 | 0 | 0 |
| 96 | −5 | 25 |
| 102 | 1 | 1 |
| 104 | 3 | 9 |
| 106 | 5 | 25 |
| 100 | −1 | 1 |
| 101 | 0 | 0 |
| 100 | −1 | 1 |
| SUM = 2023 | | SUM = 122 |

n = 20

When we calculate the variance of a data set, we have previously calculated the mean and will use this in the variance formula. Therefore, we have lost one degree of freedom in the data and the sum of the squared differences must be divided by "n − 1" instead of "n".

The calculations for variance in Example 4–3 are as follows:

Sum of squared differences = 122

n − 1 = 19

Variance = 6.4 (122 divided by 19)

For the purpose of ease in demonstration, the mean and the differences from the mean have been expressed as whole numbers. The mean for these data is actually a decimal that should make the differences decimals. Also, actual statistical calculations, such as those performed on calculators, will retain at least 2 decimal places beyond the original number throughout all steps in the calculation. Therefore, this data set should have 3 decimal places in the numbers listed under the

squared differences column. Consequently, if these data are subjected to calculator manipulations, the final standard deviation (SD) will be slightly different.

If the original units in the data were mg/dL, the unit for the final variance calculation would be $mg^2/dL^2$. Although we have used a calculation that should give us valuable information about the spread of data, the final answer is of little use because the units are difficult to interpret. However, it is necessary to use the squared differences instead of the actual differences to compensate for the positive and negative variability about the mean. By squaring the differences, the resulting numbers are positive integers and represent the distance from the mean without taking direction into account.

**Standard deviation** is defined as the square root of the variance. The SD is merely a mathematical manipulation of the variance that converts it to a more usable statistic.

The formula to calculate SD is:

$$SD = \sqrt{\frac{(x_i - \bar{x})^2}{n - 1}}$$

As you can see, the formula for SD is merely the square root of the formula for variance. The advantage to this calculation is that the units for SD are the same as the units in the original data set.

From Example 4–3:

Variance = 6.4
SD = 2.5 (the square root of 6.25)

The SD is a measurement statistic that describes the average distance each data point in a normal distribution is from the mean. The SD unit of measure covers about one sixth the total distance of the x-axis on a normal distribution curve. If the mean of the data is the middle point on the x-axis, then 3 SD units lie on the right side of the mean and 3 SD units lie on the left side of the mean.

As shown in Figure 4–7, specific areas under a normal distribution curve are bound by the SD units on the x-axis. As you will recall, most of the data in a normal distribution lie close to the mean. Therefore, the area of the curve cut by the SD units immediately to the right and left of the mean would contain the largest number of data points. In fact, the SD unit immediately to the right and the SD unit immediately to the left of the mean each contain about 34.1% of the data. As we progress down the x-axis in both directions, the next SD unit takes in about 13.65% of the data on each side of the mean. The final SD units on each end of the x-axis contain 2.1% of the data. The remaining 0.3% of the data theoretically spreads out to infinity.

**Confidence intervals** are defined as the limits between which we expect a specified proportion of a population to lie. In statistical analysis of repeat measurements that follow a normal distribution, confidence limits refer to the percentage of data contained within intervals that includes the mean and

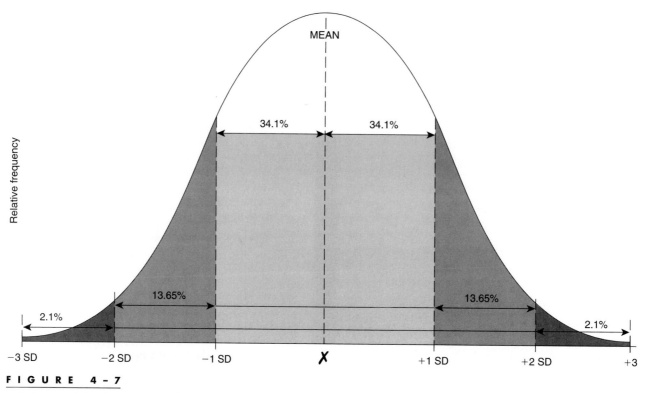

A normal distribution curve showing specific SD units.

specified SD units about the mean. The usual confidence limits used in the clinical laboratory are as follows:

68.2% confidence limits — the mean ± 1 SD.
68.2% equals the sum of 34.1% of the data on the left side of the mean and 34.1% on the right side.
95.5% confidence limits — the mean ± 2 SD.
95.5% is the total of 68.2% ($\bar{x} \pm 1$ SD) of the data plus two additional units of 13.65% from both sides of the mean.
99.7% confidence limits — the mean ± 3 SD.
99.7% is the sum of 95.5% of the data ($\bar{x} \pm 2$ SD) and two units of 2.1% from the final SD sections on the x-axis.

As you can see from Figure 4–8, the confidence limits combine equal areas from both sides of the mean that are bound by equal SD units. Even though the length of the SD units will change if the distribution changes from tight to broad, the area of the distribution curve defined by an SD unit will not change. Therefore, the percentage of data points contained within an area will not change with distribution changes.

If the data from repeat measurements do not exhibit a normal distribution, the SD and the mean ± SD confidence intervals cannot be used to describe the dispersion of data about the mean. This is because the SD is merely a mathematical description of a normal distribution. This is best illustrated in the following example:

If you were to calculate dispersion statistics for the data

that produced the bimodal distribution curve in Figure 4–4, you would obtain the following results:

range = 96 − 106    mean = 99
variance = 7.7    3 ± SD = 8.4
SD = 2.8    mean ± 3 SD = 91 − 107

The calculated SD for these data is invalid because the confidence interval that should represent 99.7% of the data ($\bar{x} \pm 3$ SD) defines a range that is larger than the actual data range, an impossibility. Therefore, data must be determined to follow a normal distribution before the SD can be used to describe its dispersion about the mean.

Although the standard deviation gives an accurate mathematical picture of the spread of the data about the mean, it is often difficult to determine if the value for the SD is acceptable. Acceptability is judged by obtaining a relatively small number for the SD, which indicates that the data have a tight distribution about the mean.

**Coefficient of variation** (CV) is the standard deviation expressed as a percentage of the mean. The CV is calculated by dividing the standard deviation by the mean and multiplying by 100.

The formula for calculating the CV is:

$$\frac{SD}{\bar{x}} \times 100$$

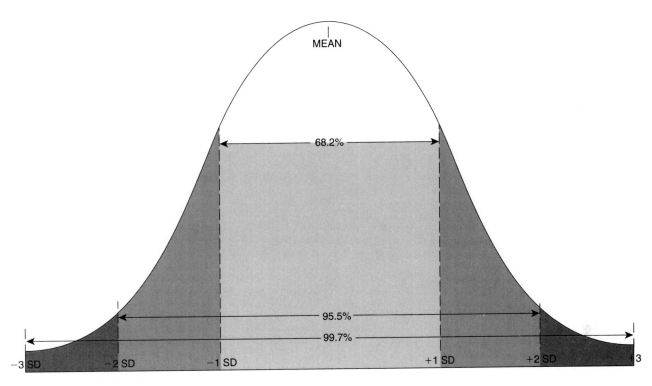

Confidence limits and SD units in a normal distribution curve.

Since the coefficient of variation is a percentage rather than a statistic with units as is the case with SD, it is easier to set criteria for acceptability. The usual limits for acceptability are that the CV on repeat laboratory measurements should be less than 5%.

The coefficient of variation for the data from Example 4–1 is 2.3% (2.3/99 × 100). This indicates that the size of the SD in relationship to the mean is acceptable and therefore the distribution is tight rather than broad about the mean.

## Internal Quality Control Procedures

Once data from repeat measurements of a control are shown to have a normal distribution and the distribution is confirmed to be tight rather than broad about the mean, the control is ready to be put into use in the laboratory. The control is then assayed along with patient samples at intervals within the assay procedure that are defined by the method and by protocols within the laboratory. Control assay values are monitored against preestablished confidence intervals to verify accuracy and precision in measurement. **Accuracy** is the ability to obtain the established or "true" value for a sample, whereas **precision** is the ability to obtain the same value for repeat measurements of a sample.

These two definitions seem similar and, in fact, the terms are often used incorrectly. Accuracy and precision are very dif-ferent concepts. Accuracy in measurement describes the correctness of a result, whereas precision in measurement describes the ability of the method to maintain the same value on repeat measurements and over time. Laboratory methods must be monitored for both accuracy and precision since it cannot be assumed that a method has both if only one or the other is confirmed. For example, a method may be precise in that repeat measurements are nearly the same, but the repeated value is not the true value, which therefore makes the method inaccurate.

In theory, it would be possible to have a method that is accurate but imprecise in that measurements do not repeat well but the overall average of the repeat values is near the true value. In practice, however, this rarely occurs. If a method is imprecise, it is usually also inaccurate.

A control monitoring system must give immediate information to the test operator (bench tech) who makes decisions about the quality of patient results. The system must also give periodic information to the laboratory supervisor who makes decisions about the overall performance of a method (precision and long-term accuracy of measurement).

### LEVEY-JENNINGS CHARTS

One of the oldest methods for monitoring control values is a Levey-Jennings chart. A Levey-Jennings chart is a normal distribution curve (also referred to as a Gaussian distribution

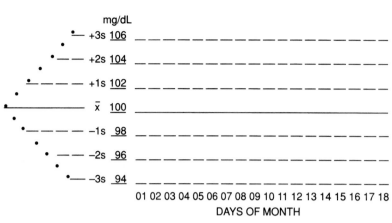

**F I G U R E   4 - 9**

Levey-Jennings chart.

curve) lying on its side with specific points on the curve extended into a chart format designed for plotting values. This is shown graphically in Figure 4–9.

*Example 4–4*

A small laboratory is using a Levey-Jennings chart to record and monitor values for a midrange glucose control. The method being monitored is an automated glucose oxidase method that is run about 2 to 3 times per day. The laboratory assayed the control for 30 days to establish the target range. The mean for the data was 100 mg/dL and the SD was 2 mg/dL. The 95.5% confidence limit ($\bar{x} \pm 2$ SD) was 96 mg/dL to 104 mg/dL. The laboratory labels the chart and puts the control into regular use. Each control value is plotted at the time of assay and the values are monitored daily by the supervisor. The first 10 values obtained for the control after it was put into use are listed below. The resulting Levey-Jennings chart for these values is shown in Figure 4–10. Notice that the bottom of the chart in Figure 4–10 is designed to be labeled sequentially in the order that controls are run each day and over a number of days.

| Date | Assay No. | Value |
| --- | --- | --- |
| 7-14 | 1 | 101 mg/dL |
|  | 2 | 100 mg/dL |
|  | 3 | 98 mg/dL |
| 7-15 | 1 | 99 mg/dL |
|  | 2 | 102 mg/dL |
| 7-16 | 1 | 103 mg/dL |
|  | 2 | 98 mg/dL |
| 7-17 | 1 | 100 mg/dL |
|  | 2 | 101 mg/dL |
|  | 3 | 100 mg/dL |

On a Levey-Jennings chart, the point that defines the mean on the Gaussian curve becomes a solid line located in the middle of the chart. Points on the curve corresponding to SD intervals become dashed lines located equidistant from the mean both above and below the midline. The left side of the chart is labeled with the mean and appropriate SD values at line intersection points. The base of the chart is labeled from left to right in time units that reflect the sequence of control measurements. The time units could be days, number of sequential values over several days, or numbers of values within one day, but should cover a period sufficient to display at least 30 sequential assay results.

The values on the left side of a Levey-Jennings chart are the values obtained from the repeat control measurements that were performed for the purpose of establishing target ranges. Once data from these measurements are collected and shown to be normally distributed, confidence intervals are calculated and mean and SD points of intersection are labeled on the chart. Once the chart is labeled, it is then used to monitor control values.

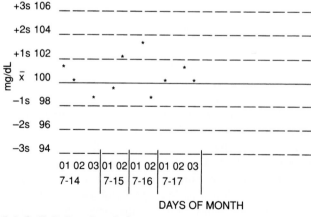

**F I G U R E   4 - 1 0**

A Levey-Jennings chart using a midrange control serum with an automated glucose oxidase procedure.

In the simplest Levey-Jennings QC monitoring system, immediate decisions about the quality of patient results are based on the degree to which control values remain within a preestablished limit. If a control value is within this limit, the assumption is made that results on patient samples run concurrent with the control are correct. For example, a common acceptable limit for a control might be that all values must be within the 95.5% confidence interval, which is shown on a Levey-Jennings chart as the area covered by the mean ± 2 SD. In other words, current assay values for the control must be essentially the same as 95.5% of the data obtained on the control during the period that the target range was established. Using this control rule criteria, a control value is considered acceptable if it lies within the shaded area shown in Figure 4–11.

Precision and long-term accuracy of a method are confirmed on a Levey-Jennings chart by control values remaining clustered about the mean with little variation in the upward or the downward direction as shown in Figure 4–12. Note also in Figure 4–12 that approximately the same number of points lie above the mean as below the mean.

Imprecision in measurement is indicated by a large amount of scatter about the mean and usually an uneven distribution above and below the mean. The Levey-Jennings chart in Figure 4–13 shows control values that demonstrate imprecision in measurement.

Imprecision is most often caused by technique errors such as variability in pipetting or inattention to detail by the oper-ator. Imprecision results in an increase in the SD or a broadening of the distribution about the mean.

Inaccuracy that occurs over time is also detected by a Levey-Jennings chart. Changes in long-term accuracy are subtle changes that occur in a method and often go unnoticed by the operator who is making immediate decisions about patient results. This type of inaccuracy occurs because there has been a change in the measurement process that is not large enough to be noticed immediately but that can affect patient results. Long-term inaccuracy is indicated on a Levey-Jennings chart by either a trend or a shift.

A **trend** is a gradual change in the mean that proceeds in one direction.

Figure 4–14 shows a Levey-Jennings chart of control values that demonstrate a trend occurring from value 9 through value 20. A trend is usually caused by gradual changes in the method of assay such as deterioration of reagents and standards or deterioration in instrument performance. Values may still be clustered about the mean but the mean itself is gradually trending toward either higher or lower values.

A **shift** is an abrupt change in the mean that becomes continuous.

The Levey-Jennings chart in Figure 4–15 shows a shift in control values that occurred at value 9. A shift is caused by the introduction of something new into the assay procedure. The usual causes of shifts are new lots of standards and reagents or a slight malfunction in an instrument that results in an

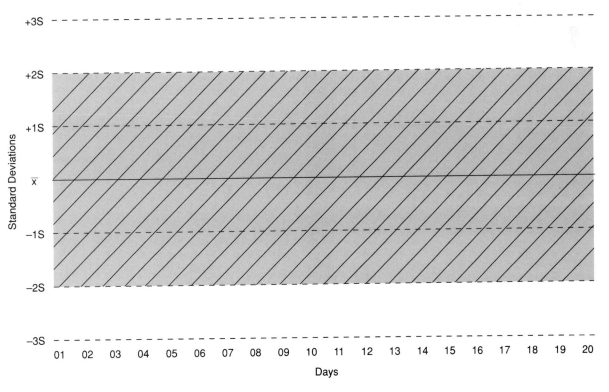

**FIGURE 4-11**

Levey-Jennings chart.

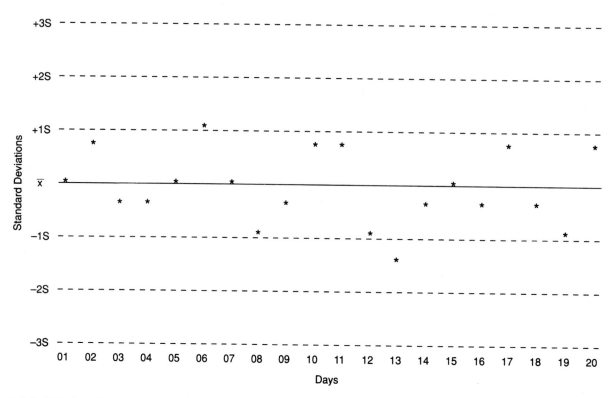

**FIGURE 4-12**

Levey-Jennings chart demonstrating precision.

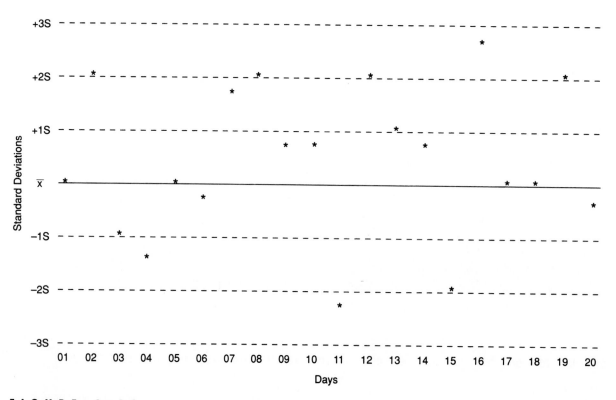

**FIGURE 4-13**

Levey-Jennings chart that demonstrates imprecision.

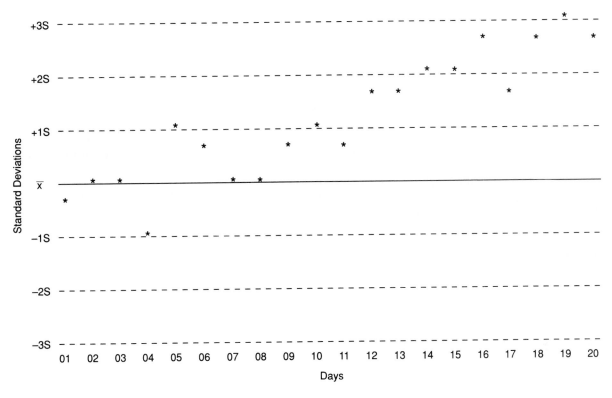

**FIGURE 4-14**

Levey-Jennings chart that demonstrates a trend.

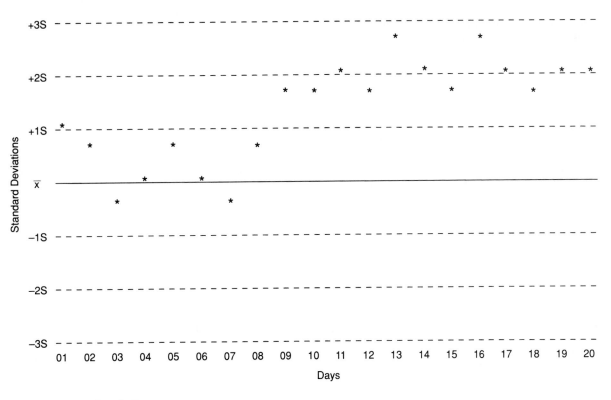

**FIGURE 4-15**

Levey-Jennings chart that demonstrates a shift.

immediate and somewhat permanent change in performance. The exact time the new solution was introduced or the change occurred can be pinpointed on a Levey-Jennings chart as the point at which the mean shifted to either a higher or a lower value.

The most obvious advantage of a Levey-Jennings chart is that it gives a good visual representation of precision and long-term accuracy and is easy to interpret. The disadvantage of a Levey-Jennings chart is the amount of time required to maintain chart data. For effective use, control values must be plotted at the time of assay and in the order of measurement. In addition, separate charts are required for each assay and each level of control. Computers can be very useful tools in maintaining and analyzing the large of amount of data generated.

## Error Detection

Since the goal of QC is to monitor processes and detect problems, it may be useful to think of the QC process as an alarm system. The system collects data (control values) about the process, and if these values exceed some preestablished value, an alarm is sounded. Similar to the temperature monitors on many laboratory refrigerators or freezers, they measure temperature and sound an audible alarm if the temperature goes too high or too low. The values for these "too high" and "too low" temperatures are usually set by the user. But how high is too high? Is it okay for the 4°C refrigerator to reach +10°C? Or to go down to −20°C and freeze the items inside? Someone had to do some research, create a plan, and implement the high and low temperature limits for the alarm system. Quality control is just the same. To have a good QC alarm, one has to define what is the acceptable range of error and then select tools that will be capable of detecting that error.

Control monitoring and error detection can be characterized by two key factors: (1) the probability of error detection ($P_{ed}$), and (2) the probability of false rejection ($P_{fr}$).

The probability of error detection describes the ability (probability, since this is a statistical analysis) of the detector to detect an error that is beyond the stable imprecision of the instrument. Ideally, our detector would detect 100% of the errors ($P_{ed} = 1.00$). In the clinical laboratory, a practical objective is 90% detection of errors.[3]

The probability of false rejection describes the probability of an alarm when no error exists. Ideally, the detector would not sound an alarm if nothing is wrong ($P_{fr} = 0.00$). However, think of your home smoke detector. How many times has it sounded when no dangerous fire existed? This is an example of a false rejection. Detectors can be designed to differentiate the smoke from your burned toast and that of your burning draperies, but it is practically difficult in terms of cost. Thus, smoke-detector manufacturers have to balance the sensitivity of their device to detect any smoke with the possible severity of the outcome (your death in a real fire). The device needs to have a very high probability of error detection. Manufacturers thus have to accept a number of false rejection alarms (burned toast sets off the alarm) to improve the ability to detect all fires

(a 100% probability of error detection). Laboratory quality control faces a similar situation. The QC process needs to be able to detect errors before they cause harm to patients but a laboratory cannot afford (financially or in terms of time spent) to have a process that is so sensitive to changes that there are large numbers of false rejection and results in continually trying to find a problem when none exists. Careful planning (quality planning) is required for proper selection of control processes and rules that are sensitive enough to prevent harm but avoid large numbers of false rejections.

## QUALITY PLANNING FOR QUALITY CONTROL

As stated previously, the first step in quality is the definition of quality goals, objectives, and the establishment of quality requirements. Analytical quality results from a complex relationship between the imprecision and inaccuracy of the method, normal physiologic variation in the analyte, changes in the specimen after it is collected, or even differences in the sample that result from collection procedures. Each analyte has a different set of the listed characteristics and, as such, the quality of measurement cannot be measured with the same rule system for each. If you haphazardly select rules, you may have a high false-rejection rate or have a low error-detection rate and, more important, you will not have any valid assurance that you are getting quality results.

Fortunately, the laboratory technologist does not need to be an expert in the establishment of quality goals and requirements. There are a number of tools available from professional organizations, websites, and other resources. Guidelines created by regulatory agencies, standards creating organizations (e.g., National Committee for Clinical Laboratory Standards, NCCLS) can be found in publications, texts, and on the WWW.[4,5] Essentially, the process requires three steps. The laboratory (1) defines the quality required by the test, (2) measures the imprecision and inaccuracy of the method, (3) selects rules based on their probability of error detection and false rejection.

Resources for defining quality requirements include the allowable error as defined by the Proficiency Testing limits under the Clinical Laboratory Improvement Act (CLIA), medically relevant limits found in the literature, or in consultation with physicians.[4-8] These limits describe how far apart the measures on the same specimen can be before the difference changes clinical decisions. For example, under CLIA, acceptable variation in sodium is the target value ± 4 mmol/L. Thus, if you run a sodium analysis and get 140 mmol/L, then rerun that same sample and get 142 mmol/L, that is acceptable quality. If you got 148 mmol/L on the repeat test, that would not be acceptable quality because the clinician would see that as a significant change and think something has changed in the patient.

The measures of imprecision and inaccuracy are conducted as part of the method evaluation when a test is being installed. After a test has been in use, the bias (inaccuracy) can be determined from peer comparison programs or proficiency testing survey results. The imprecision can be determined from the daily QC values. If the measures of imprecision and inaccuracy fall outside what you determined to be acceptable quality, your method is not acceptable and needs to be improved or another method selected.

Once you have determined the quality required and the performance (inaccuracy, imprecision) of your method, then you need to select control rules and determine the frequency that they need to be run so you will know when the quality of results is declining. There are a number of ways to select these rules to maximize error detection and minimize false rejections. Readers are referred to the multitude of resources for rule selection found in journals, quality control texts, and on the WWW. The Westgard QC website provides numerous tools to assist with this process (www.westgard.com).

## Multirule Systems

Although simple control rules may provide the required error detection and avoid significant false rejection (as determined during the quality planning process), it is more common to see a multirule system in place. These systems use multiple rules that define specific limits for control values. If a control value violates a rule by exceeding the limits, an error in measurement has been detected and the results on patient samples assayed concurrently with the control cannot be released to the

physician. A common set of laboratory QC multirules is Westgard's multirule system.[9] Control rules are usually described using abbreviations such as 1-2S or 4-1x, where the first number represents the number of control values that have been observed and the second and third characters describe the control limit. For example, 1-2S means that one control value was more than two standard deviations away from the mean value. The 4-1x notation indicates that four control values were more than one standard deviation away from the mean. Other texts and papers may use slightly different notations (e.g., $1_{2s}$ or 1:2s). The original Westgard rules and the definitions for each are presented below. Levey-Jennings charts giving visual representations of the violations for each rule are presented in the accompanying figures.

1-2S—One control value exceeds the mean by more than 2 SD but less than 3 SD. The control can exceed the mean in either the upward or the downward direction. This rule is demonstrated in Figure 4–16.

1-3S—One control value exceeds the mean by more than 3 SD in either the upward or the downward direction. The violation of this rule is shown in Figure 4–17.

2-2S—Two consecutive control values exceed the mean by more than 2 SD but less than 3 SD. These two control values must be consecutive and they must lie in the same

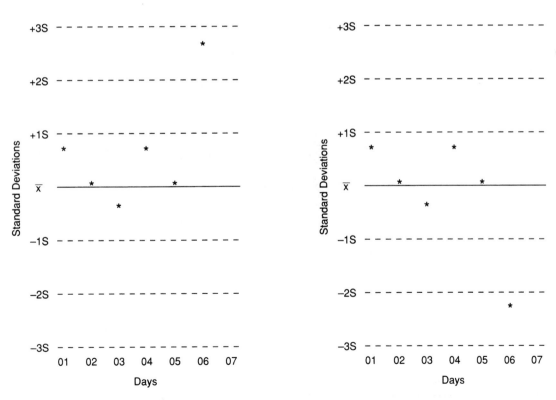

**FIGURE 4-16**

Levey-Jennings chart representing the 1-2S multirule system. *Left,* a control value exceeds 1-2S in the upward direction on day 6. *Right,* a control value exceeds 1-2S in the downward direction on day 6.

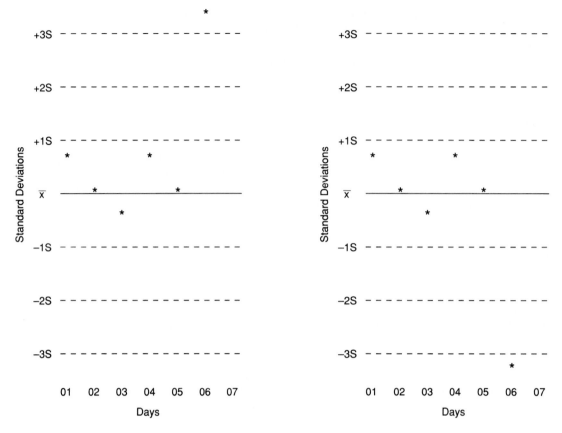

**FIGURE 4-17**

Levey-Jennings chart representing the 1-3S multirule system. *Left*, a control value exceeds 1-3S in the upward direction on day 6. *Right*, a control value exceeds 1-3S in the downward direction on day 6.

direction from the mean. This rule violation is shown in Figure 4–18.

R-4S—The difference between two consecutive controls is greater than 4 SD. These two consecutive control measurements have assay values in opposite directions from each other and the difference between the two spans at least 4 SD. The violation of this rule is shown in Figure 4–19.

4-1S—Four consecutive control values exceed the mean by more than 1 SD. These four controls must be consecutive and lie in the same direction from the mean. The violation of this rule is shown in Figure 4–20.

10x—Ten consecutive control values exceed the mean in the same direction. This rule violation is shown in Figure 4–21.

In the original Westgard multirule system, the 1-2S rule is a flag that indicates a possible change in long-term accuracy or precision. If a control value exceeds 2 SD in either direction but is less than 3 SD, the remaining rules are applied to the data. If there are no violations of the remaining rules, the control values are considered acceptable and patient assay results are released to the physician. Thus the 1-2S flag does not always indicate error in measurement.

The justification for using the 1-2S rule as a flag and not

a violation is based on the definition for the 95.5% confidence limit of a control's target range data. By definition, the 95.5% confidence limit ($\bar{x} \pm 2$ SD) contains 95.5% of the data points obtained while establishing the target range for the control. Conversely, 4.5% of the control data, although representing very real values, are outside these limits. There is no requirement to use rules as flags (or warning rules). The use of the 1-2S rule as a flag is often designed to save time and effort when interpreting control data manually. When computers are used to interpret control data a flag or warning rule may not be utilized.[10]

When a control is put into use and run alongside patient samples, it is expected that assay values will duplicate those obtained on the control during the target range period. As mentioned previously, a common rule for acceptance of control data is that all control values must be within the 95.5% confidence limit. This criteria would mean that 1 in every 20, or 4.5%, of the values would be out of this range due to chance alone even though the control may be duplicating values from the target period. In fact, if the control is rerun, chances are the assay value will now be within the 95.5% confidence limits. NOTE: It is not appropriate to simply rerun a control that exceeds the 1-2S limit. You must follow the defined control rules and base your decision on that result. If you exceed the

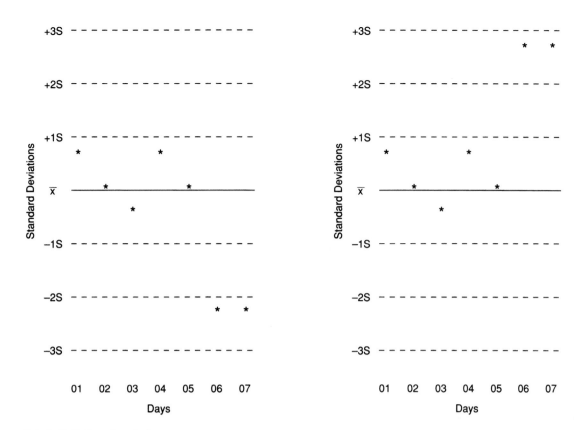

FIGURE 4-18

Levey-Jennings chart representing the 2-2S multirule system. *Left*, two consecutive control values on day 6 and on day 7 violate the 2-2S rule in the downward direction. *Right*, two consecutive control values on day 6 and on day 7 violate the 2-2S rule in the upward direction.

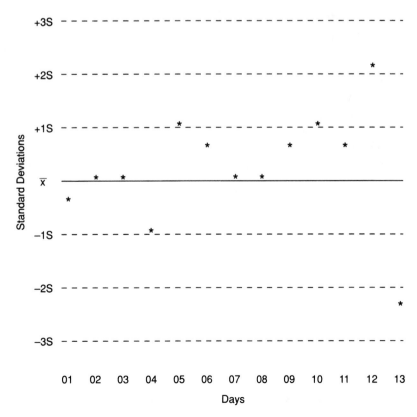

FIGURE 4-19

Levey-Jennings chart representing the R-4S multirule system. The difference between two consecutive control values (days 12 and 13) exceeds 4 SD.

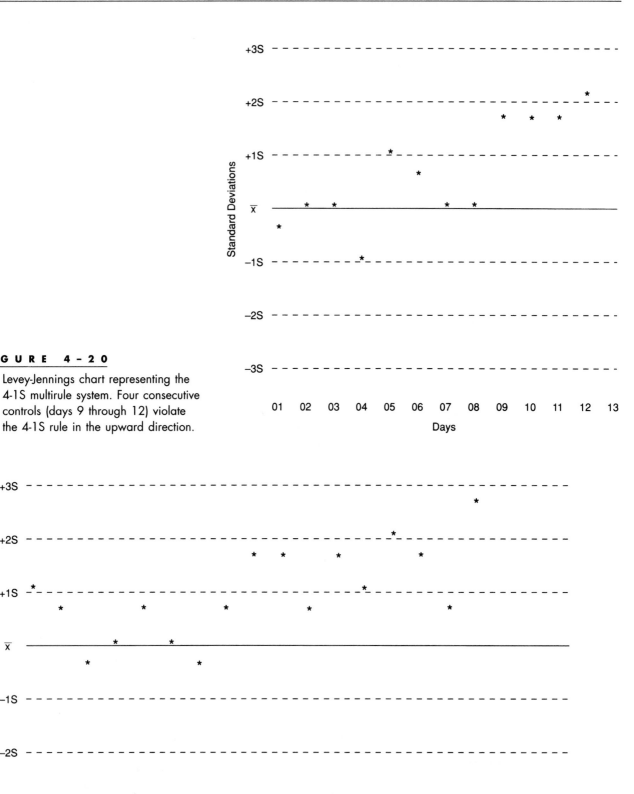

**FIGURE  4-20**

Levey-Jennings chart representing the
4-1S multirule system. Four consecutive
controls (days 9 through 12) violate
the 4-1S rule in the upward direction.

**FIGURE  4-21**

Levey-Jennings chart representing the 10x multirule system. Ten consecutive control
values (days 8 through 17) violate the 10x rule in the upward direction.

*Example 4–5*

A laboratory is using the Westgard multirule system to monitor control values on an automated instrument. The following results are twelve consecutive assay values for the calcium control and are in units of mmol/L. Values flagged by the 1-2S rule are indicated and any rule violations are listed after the flag.

Target values for control: mean = 3.3 mmol/L
and                                  SD = 0.1 mmol/L

Mean ± 1 SD range = 3.2 to 3.4 mmol/L
Mean ± 2 SD range = 3.1 to 3.5 mmol/L

| Consecutive Order of Controls | Value | Flag | Westgard Rule Violated |
|---|---|---|---|
| 1 | 3.2 | | |
| 2 | 3.3 | | |
| 3 | 3.4 | | |
| 4 | 3.2 | | |
| 5 | 3.1 | 1-2S | none |
| 6 | 3.3 | | |
| 7 | 3.4 | | |
| 8 | 3.5 | | |
| 9 | 3.6 | 1-2S | none |
| 10 | 3.6 | 1-2S | 2-2S |

*Example 4–6*

The following data are from a laboratory that assays two levels of controls for potassium. The values for the two levels are given in the order in which they were assayed.

Target values (high control)

Mean = 6.6 mmol/L
$\bar{x}$ ± 1 SD = 6.5 to 6.7 mmol/L
$\bar{x}$ ± 2 SD = 6.4 to 6.8 mmol/L

Target values (low control)

Mean = 3.5 mmol/L
$\bar{x}$ ± 1 SD = 3.4 to 3.6 mmol/L
$\bar{x}$ ± 2 SD = 3.3 to 3.7 mmol/L

| Consecutive Order of Controls | Value | Flag | Westgard Rule Violated |
|---|---|---|---|
| 1 low | 3.6 | | |
| 2 high | 6.7 | | |
| 3 low | 3.3 | | |
| 4 high | 6.4 | | |
| 5 low | 3.7 | | |
| 6 high | 6.3 | 1-2S | none |
| 7 low | 3.5 | | |
| 8 high | 6.6 | | |
| 9 low | 3.4 | | |
| 10 high | 6.5 | | |
| 11 low | 3.7 | | |
| 12 high | 6.8 | | |
| 13 low | 3.7 | | |
| 14 high | 6.9 | 1-2S | 4-1S across controls |

1-2S limit (a warning in the Westgard multirule system) but no other control rules are violated, you have valid assurance that nothing is wrong and patient results can be reported. If you rerun the control material, you are wasting reagent, time, and control material.

The original Westgard system attempts to beat those 1 in 20 odds by using the 1-2S rule as a flag and not as a violation. If, in addition to being outside the 95.5% confidence limit, a control value also violates a second rule, we can be more confident that there has been a change in assay performance since the establishment of the target range.

Before presenting a few exercises on the use of multirules, it is necessary to review a few points about the application of control rules:

1. Control values must exceed the limits to be considered a violation. For example, if the 95.5% confidence limits for a glucose control were 95 to 100 mg/dL and one control assay value was 100 mg/dL, it would not exceed the $\bar{x}$ ± 2 SD limit. A value of 101, on the other hand, would exceed the limit.

2. The value of the control that was the 1-2S trigger is included in the count of consecutive controls for applying rules. This is most easily demonstrated by the 2-2S rule. As can be seen from Figure 4–18, the value on day 6 was

a flag that triggered the other rules but none were violated; therefore, patient values were accepted and results were sent to the physician. The value on day 7 was again a flag, but now two flags have occurred consecutively. The flag on day 7 is included in the count when applying the 2-2S rule and the rule has now been violated.

3. The R-4S, 4-1S, and 10x rules are not applied unless a 1-2S flag has occurred to initiate their application (the 2-2S rule contains the flag as a part of the violation and the 1-3S rule is always a violation even without a flag). In Figure 4–21, the values on days 12, 13, 14, and 15 all exceed $\bar{x}$ ± 1 SD. However, the 4-1S rule has not been violated because a 1-2S flag did not occur to initiate the application of the other rules. On day 17, a 1-2S flag did occur and when the rules were applied, the 10x rule was violated. The 4-1S rule was not violated because on day 16, the value of the control did not exceed the mean plus 1 SD.

Example 4–5 demonstrates the use of the Westgard system for monitoring control data.

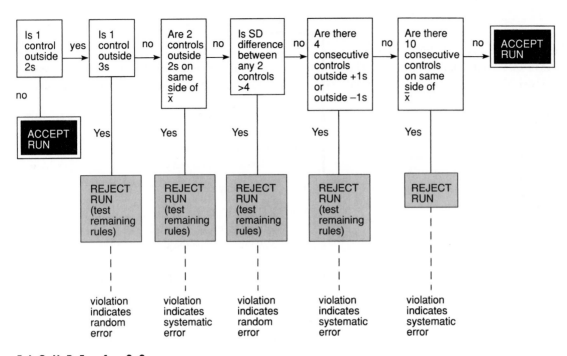

**FIGURE 4-22**

The Westgard multirule system.[11]

The greatest advantage to any multirule system is the power of the rules for distinguishing between random and systematic error. **Random error** is the error that occurs without any real pattern and **systematic error** is the error that is continuous and affects all results equally.

On a Levey-Jennings chart, random error is indicated by a control value that is significantly different from the other values. Systematic error on a Levey-Jennings chart is indicated by a trend or a shift. Systematic errors are errors that require investigation to identify their causes. Random errors can usually be considered a one-time event and patient samples and controls can be rerun with success. The exception to this is that a consistent random error problem requires investigation because it could indicate a change in precision.

In the Westgard system, specific rules indicate random error and other rules indicate systematic error. As shown in Figure 4–22, the 1-3S rule and R-4S rule are rules whose violation indicates the presence of a random error. The 2-2S, 4-1S, and 10x rules are rules whose violation indicates a systematic error.

In addition to distinguishing between random and systematic error, the Westgard system also indicated the direction that the investigation of a systematic error should take. This ability to indicate the direction for investigation of error is realized when a specific process for applying the rules is followed:

1.  The rules are applied across controls. This is illustrated for a two-control system in Example 4–6. In this example, the value on day 14 exceeded the mean plus 2 SD and was thus a flag that initiated the application of the rules to previous control data. Values on days 14, 13, 12, and 11 are all above the mean plus 1 SD. The values are consecutive and lie in the same direction from the mean. Therefore, Westgard rules indicate a systematic error has occurred. The rules can be applied across control pools for systems containing three or more control pools in a similar manner.

2.  The rules are applied across runs. This may require a system for retrieving data such as a computer monitoring system. The 4-1S rule and the 10x rule are the most powerful rules for application across consecutive runs or days.

3.  Once a rejection is identified, the operator continues to apply the rules until all have been tested. This is illustrated in Example 4–7. In this example, the operator did not stop after the first rule rejection and ultimately identified three rule rejections. If the process had been terminated after the 4-1S rejection within control II, the full extent of the error would not have been realized. In this example, the systematic error extended throughout the range represented by both controls. A violation within a single control, on the other hand, might be due merely to a loss of calibration at that end of the linear range as opposed to a complete instrument malfunction.

*Example 4–7*

The following data are from a laboratory which assays two levels of controls for an analyte. The values for the two levels are given in the order in which they were assayed.

Target Values (control I)

Mean = 16.1 mmol/L
$\bar{x} \pm 1$ SD = 15.8 to 16.4 mmol/L
$\bar{x} \pm 2$ SD = 15.5 to 16.7 mmol/L

Target Values (control II)

Mean = 25.6 mmol/L
$\bar{x} \pm 1$ SD = 25.2 to 26.0 mmol/L
$\bar{x} \pm 2$ SD = 24.8 to 26.4 mmol/L

| Consecutive Order of Controls | Value | Flag | Westgard Rule Violated |
|---|---|---|---|
| 1 I | 16.2 | | |
| 2 II | 25.8 | | |
| 3 I | 16.0 | | |
| 4 II | 25.4 | | |
| 5 I | 16.2 | | |
| 6 II | 26.1 | | |
| 7 I | 16.5 | | |
| 8 II | 26.2 | | |
| 9 I | 16.3 | | |
| 10 II | 26.3 | | |
| 11 I | 16.6 | | |
| 12 II | 26.3 | | |
| 13 I | 16.7 | | |
| 14 II | 26.5 | 1-2S | 4-1S within control II |
| | | | 4-1S across controls |
| | | | 10 x across controls |

## External Quality Control

The QC procedures addressed previously in this chapter are referred to as internal quality control. A laboratory QC program is not complete unless it also includes an external component. External quality control is a process by which a laboratory uses an outside unbiased source to verify the quality of patient results.

The most common type of external quality control involves testing biological samples submitted to a laboratory by an outside agency. The laboratory assays the unknown samples "blind" just as though they were actual patient samples and sends the results back to the agency. The laboratory's accuracy of measurement is also compared with other laboratories using similar methods. This method of external QC is

called *proficiency testing* and is often tied to requirements for laboratory accreditation.

Proficiency testing is administered by a number of companies including the American Proficiency Institute, American Association of Bioanalysts, and the College of American Pathologists. These companies must be approved by the Health Care Financing Administration (HCFA) and successful participation in a recognized proficiency testing program is required for proper compliance with CLIA '88. In addition to meeting HCFA requirements, some accrediting agencies will have more stringent or additional proficiency testing requirements to maintain accreditation.

The acceptable limits for passing proficiency events are defined by HCFA.[4] Qualitative tests are graded using the result that 90% of participants provided. For example, if 100 laboratories participate in a pregnancy testing survey and 92 report the sample as positive, then the correct answer is positive (and the 8 laboratories reporting negative will not pass). Immunohematology results are an exception to this rule and are based on a 95% consensus.

Quantitative results are graded against a target value $\pm$ a fixed amount. The fixed amount can be expressed as a percentage, a number of standard deviations, or a quantity. For example, HCFA requires that chloride results be target value $\pm$ 5%, whereas total calcium is graded against target value $\pm$ 1.0 mg/dL and TSH is graded against target value $\pm$ 3 SD. The target value is the mean value obtained by a peer group using the same instrument or reagent as your laboratory. A peer group must have at least 10 laboratories participating to be valid. Additionally, like qualitative results, only those analytes having a 90% consensus are graded.

The statistical term standard deviation interval (SDI) quantitates the number of SD units a single result differs from the group mean. The SDI is used by proficiency organizations to define the amount a lab result may differ from the average of the results from a group of peers. This difference is then adjusted for the average difference (standard deviation) of the group. The calculation of an SDI is as follows:

$$SDI = \frac{\text{Lab result} - \text{Peer group mean}}{\text{Peer group SD}}$$

Example 4–8 shows proficiency survey results using both fixed criteria and standard deviation intervals to report results. As can be seen in Example 4–8, laboratory A's potassium result on the proficiency sample is outside the acceptable limits. The SDI for their result on the BUN proficiency sample is acceptable, though it is close to the limit.

Since proficiency testing is closely tied to accreditation, the original intent of verifying accuracy in measurement by testing unknown samples blind is often overshadowed by the concern that a wrong answer may affect accreditation. For that reason, in addition to proficiency testing, many laboratories also subscribe to a method for external QC that does not carry penalties for incorrect answers. As an example, some lab groups have established their own regional proficiency testing programs in which samples are sent to participating laboratories by one of the larger laboratories in the group. The results and comparisons are reported in the same manner as the agencies involved in proficiency testing. This regional approach attaches no penalty to wrong answers and the original concept of self-evaluation by peers is retained.

*Example 4–8*

On a proficiency survey, fixed criteria of $\pm$ 0.2 mmol/L were used for potassium evaluation. For BUN, limits of acceptability were $\pm$ 2 SDI from peer group results. Laboratory A's proficiency report is as follows:

|  | Lab A Result | Target Value | Peer Group Mean | Peer Group SD |
|---|---|---|---|---|
| Potassium | 4.0 | 4.3 | | |
| BUN | 24 | | 21 | 1.5 |

The acceptability limits for potassium are calculated as follows:

Target value $\pm$ allowable concentration deviation
$(4.3 + 0.2 = 4.5; 4.3 - 0.2 = 4.1) = 4.1$ to $4.5$

The SDI interval for Laboratory A's BUN result is as follows:

$$SDI = \frac{Lab\ result - peer\ group\ mean}{Peer\ group\ SD}$$

$$\frac{24 - 21}{1.5} = 2\ SDI$$

Some laboratories subscribe to external QC programs provided by companies who supply daily control materials to laboratories. The laboratory uses the control materials for daily internal QC procedures and sends statistical or raw data on the daily control values to the company at the end of each month. The company provides the laboratory with information on the amount of long-term inaccuracy and imprecision that may be occurring within the laboratory. The company also provides the laboratory with information on the closeness of their results on the control pools to peer laboratories using the same control materials. This information is provided in much the same format as provided by the proficiency testing groups.

## SUMMARY

Quality assurance is the result of processes by which a laboratory defines, measures, and improves quality in laboratory

results by closely monitoring the preanalytical, analytical, and postanalytical stages of laboratory testing. The process can be defined with a total quality management approach to quality that includes quality planning, processes, assessment, control, and improvement.

Quality control is a section of the analytical stage of quality assurance and is the process of monitoring results from control samples to verify quality in results from patient samples run alongside the controls. QC processes have both an internal and an external component.

The first step in an internal QC process is to establish the target range for the control sample. The target range is set by assaying the control repeatedly and verifying the existence of a point of central tendency and a tight distribution in the resulting data set. Once the range has been established, control results are monitored over time to detect any significant change in values that might indicate variability in method performance and a possible imprecision or inaccuracy in patient results. Imprecision in results is known as random error, and inaccuracy is termed systematic error. The monitoring of control results to detect random and systematic error is done by visual methods such as Levey-Jennings charts or by control rule methods that rely on rule violations to indicate that an error has occurred. The selection of rules to achieve error detection while reducing false rejection requires a thorough planning process that determines the quality required and is based on the known characteristics (bias, imprecision) of the method.

External QC is the process of assaying unknown samples from an outside agency and thus verifying accuracy of testing by comparison to an established value for the outside sample or comparison to the average result obtained on the sample by laboratories within a peer group. The most common external quality control systems are proficiency testing programs.

## REFERENCES

1.  Westgard JL, Burnett RW, Bowers GN: Quality management science in clinical chemistry: A dynamic framework for continuous improvement of quality. *Clin Chem* 36:1712–1716, 1990.
2.  Westgard JO: Assuring quality through total quality management. Available at: http://www.westgard.com/essay4.htm
3.  Westgard JO: QC—The chances of rejection. Available at: http://www.westgard.com/lesson15.htm#alarm
4.  U.S. Department of Health and Human Services: Clinical laboratory improvement amendments of 1988; final rules and notice. 42CFR Part 493. Federal Register 57:7188–7288, 1992.
5.  Guideline: Internal quality control testing: Principles and definitions. Villanova, PA, National Committee for Clinical Laboratory Standards (C24-T), 1987.
6.  Skendzel LP, Barnett RN, Platt R: Medically useful cri-

teria for analytic performance of laboratory tests. Am J Clin Pathol 83:200–205, 1985.

7.  Fraser CG: Biological variation in clinical chemistry. An update: collated data, 1988–1991. Arch Pathol Lab Med 116:916–23, 1992.

8.  Westgard JO, Seehafer JJ, Barry PL: Allowable imprecision for laboratory tests based on clinical and analytical test outcome criteria. Clin Chem 40;1909–1914, 1994.

9.  Westgard JO, Barry PL, Hunt MR, Groth T: A multi-rule shewhart chart for quality control in clinical chemistry. Clin Chem 27:493–501, 1981.

10.  Westgard JO: QC—The multirule interpretation. Available at: http://www.westgard.com/lesson18.htm

11.  Bakes-Martin R, Romph P, Myers K: Quality control pool evaluation. *Basic Quality Assurance for the Medical Laboratory, LAP LM-5—A Self Study Course.* Denver, CO Association for Continuing Medical Laboratory Education, March 1988.

# CHAPTER 5

# Method Evaluation and Preanalytical Variables

*Mary Coleman*

Internal and external quality control (QC) programs are processes performed daily or at other intervals to ensure the quality of an analytical procedure and are integral parts of analytical quality assurance. Preanalytical continuous quality improvement (CQI) and quality assurance (QA) refer to procedures designed to ensure quality and improvement in quality in all processes that precede the analytical testing procedure. Ensuring quality in the selection of a new method is a QA process that is performed before the introduction of a new procedure into a laboratory and before the establishment of internal and external QC programs. If a change in analytical performance is detected by QC programs after a new method is established, many of the original method evaluation procedures may be repeated to reverify optimal performance. Therefore, method evaluation is an important part of both preanalytical and analytical QA.

## METHOD EVALUATION

All personnel within a laboratory who will be performing or managing the performance of a new test method should be involved in the process of method selection and evaluation. Some may have direct involvement by performing the evaluation experiments or making selection decisions. Others may have indirect involvement in that their ability to correctly perform the new procedure in their particular laboratory environment will be evaluated by someone else. It is of no benefit for a new method to be evaluated for its ability to perform in the hands of a few well-skilled individuals who are not pressured by daily workload commitments.

A new method must be evaluated for both precision and accuracy as well as for its ability to correctly diagnose disease. Although package inserts and instrument manuals list manufacturer claims for these parameters, individual laboratories must verify that the claims can be met within the laboratory's own environment, using its own equipment and its own personnel.

### Linearity

The first manufacturing claim that is often verified within a laboratory is linearity. Linearity checks are preliminary checks on the accuracy of the new method. An evaluation of linearity is also a method of familiarizing laboratory staff with the nuances and special requirements. Traditionally, linearity studies have been performed by assaying a set of standards of known purity that span the desired range of linearity and have concentrations focused at specific points. Protocols from the National Committee on Clinical Laboratory Standards (NCCLS) have defined a method for checking linearity that uses patient samples having values at specific levels or that have been diluted to obtain specific concentrations.[1] Regardless of the type of material used, a few factors should be considered when checking the linearity of a new method. Just as it is important to have control values focused at medical decision points, it is advisable to check for linearity and accuracy of measurements at major medical decision points. Therefore, when evaluating a new method for glucose, a laboratory may want standards or linearity patient samples focused at 50, 120, and 250 mg/dL. The linearity protocol should include concentrations at approximately 20 and 500 mg/dL, even if these are beyond medical decision points. A laboratory cannot in good conscience report patient results that exceed the limits of linearity established within the laboratory's own environment.

Once the standards or linear patient samples have been selected and assayed, usually in triplicate, the laboratory graphs the expected concentrations of each sample on the x-axis against the mean of the results obtained for each sample on the y-axis. Linearity is confirmed by a line drawn through the data points that has a 45-degree angle and does not deviate at either end before the expected range of linearity is achieved. This method of evaluation depends on the judgment of the observer to determine if the resulting line is truly linear. A mathematical method for determining linearity is to calculate the percent recovery of each standard or linear patient sample. If the results for all samples recover within 5% of the expected value, linearity is confirmed.

Determining linearity by calculating percent recovery of linear samples is presented in Example 5–1. The limits for acceptable recovery are defined as 95% to 105% (within 5%). Although the standards in Example 5–1 all recovered within acceptable limits, the laboratory will subject the method to rigorous evaluation protocols since all standards recovered are lower than expected. This type of recovery could indicate a potential accuracy problem. Depending on the manufacturer's analysis of a method, laboratories may perform less extensive studies to validate method performance which is referred to as method validation.

*Example 5–1*

A laboratory purchases a set of linear standards for glucose and assays each level in triplicate using a new glucose method. The laboratory then takes the average of each triplicate value and calculates the % recovery for each standard.

| Standard No. | Expected Glucose Values (mg/dL) | Mean Value of Triplicate Observed Glucose Values (mg/dL) |
|---|---|---|
| 1 | 25 | 24 |
| 2 | 60 | 57 |
| 3 | 100 | 96 |
| 4 | 120 | 115 |
| 5 | 250 | 241 |
| 6 | 400 | 390 |

$$\% \text{ Recovery} = \frac{\text{Value recovered}}{\text{Value expected}} \times 100$$

|  | Recovery |
|---|---|
| Standard 1: | 96.0% |
| Standard 2: | 95.0% |
| Standard 3: | 96.0% |
| Standard 4: | 95.8% |
| Standard 5: | 96.4% |
| Standard 6: | 97.5% |

## Precision

The first true experiments on method evaluation performed within a laboratory should be verifications of the precision of a new method. You may recall that if a method is not precise, it probably will not be accurate. Therefore, if method evaluation experiments show a method to be imprecise, it is of no value to continue with the evaluation process. Two types of precision must be confirmed: within-run precision and between-run precision.

## Within-run

Within-run precision checks the ability of a method to repeat a value for a sample regardless of where that sample is placed within a run. To validate within-run precision, either aliquots of a patient sample or a control are placed at selected points throughout a run or an entire instrument sample tray is filled with the aliquots. The standard deviation (SD) and coefficient of variation (CV) for the resulting values are calculated. The CV must be less than or essentially the same as the manufacturer's or within previously defined limits. Most analytical methods in the chemistry laboratory should be able to demonstrate CVs of less than 5%.

*Example 5–2*

Laboratory B is evaluating a method for glucose. The following results are obtained: low pool mean 60 mg/dL, SD 2.5 mg/dL; normal range pool mean 100 mg/dL, SD 2.5 mg/dL; high pool mean 200 mg/dL, SD 2.5 mg/dL. What are their CVs?

$$\text{Coefficient of variation (\%CV)} = \frac{\text{Standard deviation}}{\text{Mean}} \times 100$$

$$CV = \frac{2.5}{60 \text{ mg/dL}} \times 100\% = 4.2\%$$

$$CV = \frac{2.5}{100 \text{ mg/dL}} \times 100\% = 2.5\%$$

$$CV = \frac{2.5}{200 \text{ mg/dL}} \times 100\% = 1.2\%$$

## Between-run

Between-run precision evaluates the ability of a method to repeat measurements when aliquots are placed on different runs. This is often referred to as day-to-day precision. Assuming that no medical intervention or change in health status has occurred between the time of sampling, this type of precision verifies that a laboratory will obtain essentially the same value for an analyte on a particular patient even if the samples are drawn days apart.

As can be seen from Example 5–2, precision is related to concentration. The same SD at different concentrations can give very different CVs. Therefore, precision should be verified at more than one level of concentration. These concentration levels normally represent low, middle, and high points within the established linear range that correspond to values found in the laboratory's own patient population. These levels are usually related to medical decision points.

### F TEST

Another statistic that can be used to evaluate precision is the F test. The F test is used when a new method's precision appears to be either about the same or slightly higher than a reference method or manufacturer's claims and there are no defined limits of acceptability for precision for the method or analyte. The formula for the F test is as follows:

$$F \text{ test} = \frac{\text{Larger variance}}{\text{Smaller variance}}$$

The F test merely compares the variances of two methods and judges whether the two variances are essentially the same. If the F test confirms the variances to be essentially the same, the assumption is made that the new method is performing as well as the reference method or the manufacturer's claims.

Before the use of the F test is demonstrated, two statistical terms must be defined:

**Null hypothesis**—A scientific hypothesis that states there is no significant difference between two sets of data.
**P value**—The probability of being wrong when a test statistic proves the null hypothesis.

When the F test is used for comparing variances, the goal is to prove the null hypothesis or to prove there is no significant difference between the variances of the two methods. If the calculated F value is smaller than a predetermined cutoff, we assume there is no difference between the variances; i.e., they are statistically the same. This cutoff point is related to the degrees of freedom in the data and is dependent on the probability level at which we are testing.

The degrees of freedom for each data set are n − 1 or the degrees of freedom from the calculation for the SD and the variance of each data set. When the F test is used to evaluate a new method that has a variance higher than expected, the numerator contains n − 1 degrees of freedom from the new method data set and the denominator contains n − 1 degrees of freedom from the reference method data set.

If the calculated F test value is larger than the cutoff point at the appropriate degrees of freedom in the numerator and the denominator, the statement is made that the difference in the variances of the two sets of data is significant and the new method

*Example 5–3*

Laboratory B ran between-run precision experiments on a new method for PTH using a low, mid, and high control for 1 month. The mid and high controls produced coefficients of variation that were less than those listed by the manufacturer. The low control produced a standard deviation and a coefficient of variation that was larger than that listed by the manufacturer. The laboratory decided to use the F test to determine if their precision data were significantly different from that of the manufacturer.

| Manufacturer's Data | Laboratory B's Data |
|---|---|
| Mean = 23.4 | Mean = 23.8 |
| SD = 2.0 | SD = 2.2 |
| CV = 8.6 | CV = 9.2 |
| N = 12 | N = 21 |

Manufacturer's variance: $(2.0)^2 = 4.00$

Laboratory B's variance: $(2.2)^2 = 4.84$

$$F \text{ test} = \frac{\text{Larger variance}}{\text{Smaller variance}}$$

$$F \text{ test} = \frac{4.84}{4.00} = 1.21$$

**TABLE 5–1**

**Table for Significance of F Test***

| DEGREES OF FREEDOM (DENOMINATOR) | DEGREES OF FREEDOM (NUMERATOR) | | | | |
|---|---|---|---|---|---|
| | 10 | 12 | 14 | 16 | 20 |
| 10 | 2.97 | 2.91 | 2.86 | 2.82 | 2.77 |
| | **4.85** | **4.71** | **4.60** | **4.52** | **4.41** |
| 11 | 2.86 | 2.79 | 2.74 | 2.70 | 2.65 |
| | **4.54** | **4.40** | **4.29** | **4.21** | **4.10** |
| 12 | 2.76 | 2.69 | 2.64 | 2.60 | 2.54 |
| | **4.30** | **4.16** | **4.05** | **3.98** | **3.86** |
| 13 | 2.67 | 2.60 | 2.55 | 2.51 | 2.46 |
| | **4.10** | **3.96** | **3.85** | **3.78** | **3.67** |
| 14 | 2.60 | 2.53 | 2.48 | 2.44 | 2.39 |
| | **3.94** | **3.80** | **3.70** | **3.62** | **3.51** |
| 15 | 2.55 | 2.48 | 2.43 | 2.39 | 2.33 |
| | **3.80** | **3.67** | **3.56** | **3.48** | **3.36** |
| 16 | 2.49 | 2.42 | 2.37 | 2.33 | 2.28 |
| | **.69** | **3.55** | **3.45** | **3.37** | **3.25** |
| 17 | 2.45 | 2.38 | 2.33 | 2.29 | 2.23 |
| | **3.59** | **3.45** | **3.35** | **3.27** | **3.16** |
| 18 | 2.41 | 2.34 | 2.29 | 2.25 | 2.19 |
| | **3.51** | **3.37** | **3.27** | **3.19** | **3.07** |
| 19 | 2.38 | 2.31 | 2.26 | 2.21 | 2.15 |
| | **3.43** | **3.30** | **3.19** | **3.12** | **3.00** |
| 20 | 2.35 | 2.28 | 2.23 | 2.18 | 2.12 |
| | **3.37** | **3.23** | **3.13** | **3.05** | **2.94** |

*Values for 0.05 probability level are in regular type and values for 0.01 probability level are in boldface type.

is more imprecise than the reference method. The correctness of that statement is related to the probability level at which the statistic is tested. In the clinical laboratory, significance statistics are usually tested at a 0.05 probability level. If a test statistic is larger than the cutoff value at the 0.05 level, the statement that there is a difference between the two sets of data would be incorrect 5% of the time. In other words, 5% of the time there could be a value for the statistic this large when there is no difference in the variances or in the precision between the two methods.

Example 5–3 demonstrates the use of the F test to verify precision in evaluation of a new method. Cutoff points for the F test are listed in tables of significance. A portion of a table of significance for the F test is shown in Table 5–1. In the example, Laboratory B had 20 (n − 1) degrees of freedom in the numerator (new method) and 11 (n − 1) degrees of freedom in the denominator (reference method). The cutoff or critical value for F at these degrees of freedom tested at the 0.05 level is 2.65. Since the F value calculated by Laboratory B is less than the critical value, the laboratory can assume that the variance in its data is essentially the same as the manufacturer's.

## Accuracy

Most method evaluations performed in clinical chemistry laboratories are for replacement methods. A replacement method is a new method or instrument purchased to replace an existing method or instrument, usually because the new method has advantages in price, speed, or ease of use. Verification of accuracy for replacement methods is done by patient comparison studies. Several patient samples are split, and one split is assayed on the new method while the other split is assayed on the existing method. A comparison is then made between the assay values on the new method and the assay values on the existing method. The purpose of this type of evaluation is to verify that the new method will perform as well as or better than the existing method. Patient comparison studies can also be used to verify the accuracy of a new method for an analyte that is being introduced into the laboratory but these comparisons require the cooperation of a neighboring facility that has an acceptable method for the analyte being tested. Ideally, comparisons should be made to a recognized reference method—a method that has been determined to be the most accurate one available for the analyte.

Patient comparison studies require a minimum of 40 patient samples. The samples should represent a wide range of concentrations with at least 50% being outside the analyte reference range. The percentage of samples selected with concentrations in the high and low ranges should reflect the percentage of high and low concentrations normally seen in the laboratory's patient population. The analyses should be performed in duplicate on each method and analysis on one method should be followed within 2 to 4 hours by analysis on the other method. If duplicates do not match on one method because of random error and there is not a sufficient amount of sample to repeat both duplicates, all values for that sample should be eliminated from the study. The usual criterion for acceptance is that duplicates should agree within 5% of each other.

Once samples have been assayed on both methods, the bias is calculated by subtracting the mean of the results on the reference method from the mean of the results on the new method. If the bias is positive, results on the new method, in general, will be higher than those on the reference method. If the bias is negative, the new method will have values lower than those on the reference method. In an ideal situation, every patient sample should assay the same on both methods, which would produce a bias of zero.

### PAIRED t-TEST

A paired t-test may be used to determine if there is a statistical difference (bias) between a new method and an old method and may be an indicator of accuracy of a new method. One method is considered the reference method and the other method is considered the test method. The data are considered paired because the evaluation protocol calls for split samples, each data point on the new method is coupled to a data point on the existing method.

Evaluating the significance of the difference in the means (bias) of paired data requires a bit more mathematical manipulation than was required to evaluate a difference in variances. This is because the bias can deviate in either a positive or negative direction from the ideal value of zero. The first step in the calculation of the paired t-test is to calculate the difference for each split and then calculate the average deviation of the differences from the bias or the overall difference. These deviations should follow a normal distribution with most deviations being close to the bias or the deviation from the bias being close to zero. The formula for the SD of the differences (SDd) is as follows:

$$SDd = \sqrt{\frac{[\sum(Y - X) - Bias]^2}{n - 1}}$$

where Y-X is the difference between each pair value on the Y method (new method) minus the value on the X method (reference method); bias is the mean of the Y method minus the mean of the X method; $n - 1$ is $n - 1$ pairs (loss of one degree of freedom because bias was calculated previously).

This formula is similar to the formula for the SD of unpaired data. The formula for the SD of unpaired data calculated the average deviation of each data point from the overall mean of the data. The formula for unpaired data is presented as follows for comparison:

$$SD = \sqrt{\frac{\sum(Y - X)^2}{n - 1}}$$

Example 5–4 lists data for a comparison study and calculations for SDd.

In this example, the analyte is not defined and the number of pairs presented is below the recommended amount. This was done to facilitate the mathematical manipulation required for the example. The steps in the calculation for data pair 1 are presented as follows to assist in the manipulation of the formula:

1. $Y - X = 99 - 100 = -1$
2. $(Y - X) - Bias = (-1) - (0.4) = -1.4$
3. $[(Y - X) - Bias]^2 = [-1.4]^2 = 1.96$

The last calculation needed for the paired t-test is the standard error of the mean (SEM). Whenever an average is calculated, a certain amount of error is inherent in the calculation that is related to the number of data points on which the average is calculated. The SD of the differences is actually an average of the deviations from the bias and is subject to the same calculation errors as any other average. The calculation of the standard error of the mean for the SDd is as follows:

$$SEM = \frac{SDd}{\sqrt{n}}$$

*Example 5–4*

The bias for the following patient comparison data is 0.4.

| Pair No. | Result X | Result Y | Y − X | [(Y − X) − Bias] | [(Y − X) − Bias]$^2$ |
|---|---|---|---|---|---|
| 1 | 100 | 99 | −1 | −1.4 | 1.96 |
| 2 | 99 | 100 | 1 | 0.6 | 0.36 |
| 3 | 98 | 97 | −1 | −1.4 | 1.96 |
| 4 | 97 | 100 | 3 | 2.6 | 6.76 |
| 5 | 105 | 104 | −1 | −1.4 | 1.96 |
| 6 | 100 | 101 | 1 | 0.6 | 0.36 |
| 7 | 87 | 88 | 1 | 0.6 | 0.36 |
| 8 | 100 | 101 | 1 | 0.6 | 0.36 |
| 9 | 82 | 83 | 1 | 0.6 | 0.36 |
| 10 | 97 | 100 | 3 | 2.6 | 6.76 |
| 11 | 99 | 100 | 1 | 0.6 | 0.36 |
| 12 | 82 | 83 | 1 | 0.6 | 0.36 |
| 13 | 85 | 84 | −1 | −1.4 | 1.96 |
| 14 | 87 | 88 | 1 | 0.6 | 0.36 |
| 15 | 83 | 81 | −2 | −2.4 | 5.76 |
| 16 | 114 | 113 | −1 | −1.4 | 1.96 |
| 17 | 82 | 83 | 1 | 0.6 | 0.36 |
| 18 | 91 | 91 | 0 | −0.4 | 0.16 |
| 19 | 57 | 58 | 1 | 0.6 | 0.36 |
| 20 | 85 | 84 | −1 | −1.4 | 1.96 |
| | | | | | $\Sigma$ = 34.8 |

$$SDd = \sqrt{\frac{\Sigma[(Y - X) - Bias]^2}{n - 1}} = \sqrt{\frac{34.8}{19}} = \sqrt{1.83} = 1.35$$

The calculation of the standard error for the SDd of the data given in Example 5–4 is as follows:

$$SEM = \frac{1.35}{\sqrt{20}} = \frac{1.35}{4.47} = 0.30$$

We are now ready to calculate the paired *t*-test. The formula for the paired *t*-test is as follows:

$$t = \frac{Bias}{SEM}$$

The value for the paired t test for the data from Example 5–4 is as follows:

$$t = \frac{0.4}{0.30} = 1.33$$

Just as tables of significance are available for the F test, tables are available to aid in making a judgment about ac-

cepting or rejecting the null hypothesis for the *t*-test. A portion of a two-tailed table of significance for the paired *t*-test is presented in Table 5–2.

Tables for *t* are related to the degrees of freedom in the data and probability levels. As with all laboratory data, the *t*-test is evaluated at the 0.05 probability level. The degrees of freedom are n-1 data pairs (the same degrees of freedom used to calculate the SDd). All laboratory data are evaluated using a two-tailed *t*-test because laboratory data can deviate from a mean in either the negative or the positive direction. The one-tailed *t*-test is used only for data that would deviated from a baseline in one direction such as data from a patient study in which participants who were given an experimental drug would experience one of two effects (no change or either a decrease or an increase in a physiologic parameter but not both). An example of this might be a trial study for a new blood pressure medication in which the control (placebo) group would show no effect and the drug group would show a decrease in blood pressure.

The critical *t* value for the data from the laboratory in Example 5–4 is 2.093 at 19 degrees of freedom tested at the 0.05 probability level. Since calculated *t* values can be either positive or negative, the allowable limits for the calculated *t* for these laboratory data are −2.093 to +2.093. The calculated value for *t* for the data from Example 5–4 is 1.33, which is within these limits. Therefore, the laboratory can accept the null hypothesis and conclude there is no difference between the means of the two methods. In other words, the bias between the two methods is essentially zero.

TABLE 5–2

**Two-Tailed Table for Significance of Paired *t*-Test**

| DEGREES OF FREEDOM | PROBABILITY FOR GREATER VALUE, P | | |
|---|---|---|---|
| | 0.10 | 0.05 | 0.01 |
| 10 | 1.812 | 2.228 | 3.169 |
| 11 | 1.796 | 2.201 | 3.106 |
| 12 | 1.782 | 2.179 | 3.055 |
| 13 | 1.771 | 2.160 | 3.012 |
| 14 | 1.761 | 2.145 | 2.977 |
| 15 | 1.753 | 2.131 | 2.947 |
| 16 | 1.746 | 2.120 | 2.921 |
| 17 | 1.740 | 2.110 | 2.898 |
| 18 | 1.734 | 2.101 | 2.878 |
| 19 | 1.729 | 2.093 | 2.861 |
| 20 | 1.725 | 2.086 | 2.845 |
| 21 | 1.721 | 2.080 | 2.831 |
| 22 | 1.717 | 2.074 | 2.819 |
| 23 | 1.714 | 2.069 | 2.807 |
| 24 | 1.711 | 2.064 | 2.797 |
| 25 | 1.708 | 2.060 | 2.787 |

## LINEAR REGRESSION BY LEAST SQUARES

An evaluation of the correlation between two methods can be done by plotting the current or reference method values on the x-axis against values for the new method on the y-axis. Perfect correlation would be achieved when the splits assayed are exactly the same on both methods and would be indicated on the graph by a line through the data points that has a 45-degree angle and passes through zero. A statistical method to calculate the best-fit line, normally referred to as the regression line, uses the least-squares concept.

### Slope

The first parameter of the best-fit regression line to be calculated by least-squares statistics is the slope. The slope indicates the angle of the line. The slope selects a specific length of the line and defines the ratio of values on the y-axis to values on the x-axis contained within the length of the line. The basic formula for the slope is:

$$\text{Slope} = \frac{\Delta Y}{\Delta X}$$

The calculation of the slope for linear regression takes into account the concept of least squares but is still a ratio of

*Example 5–5*

| Pair No. | Result X | Result Y | $X^2$ | XY |
|---|---|---|---|---|
| 1 | 100 | 99 | 10000 | 9900 |
| 2 | 99 | 100 | 9801 | 9900 |
| 3 | 98 | 97 | 9604 | 9506 |
| 4 | 97 | 100 | 9409 | 9700 |
| 5 | 105 | 104 | 11025 | 10920 |
| 6 | 100 | 101 | 10000 | 10100 |
| 7 | 87 | 88 | 7569 | 7656 |
| 8 | 100 | 101 | 10000 | 10100 |
| 9 | 82 | 83 | 6724 | 6806 |
| 10 | 97 | 100 | 9409 | 9700 |
| 11 | 99 | 100 | 9801 | 9900 |
| 12 | 82 | 83 | 6724 | 6806 |
| 13 | 85 | 84 | 7225 | 7140 |
| 14 | 87 | 88 | 7569 | 7656 |
| 15 | 83 | 81 | 6889 | 6723 |
| 16 | 114 | 113 | 12996 | 12882 |
| 17 | 82 | 83 | 6724 | 6806 |
| 18 | 91 | 91 | 8281 | 8281 |
| 19 | 57 | 58 | 3249 | 3306 |
| 20 | 85 | 84 | 7225 | 7140 |
| n = 20 | $\sum 1830$ | $\sum 1838$ | $\sum 107224$ | $\sum 170928$ |

$$b = \frac{(20)(170928) - (1830)(1838)}{20(170224) - (1830)^2} = 0.990$$

*Y* values to *X* values. The formula for calculating the slope for the least-squares regression line is:

$$b = \frac{(n)(\sum XY) - (\sum X)(\sum Y)}{(n)(\sum X^2) - (\sum X)^2}$$

where *b* is the mathematical symbol for slope; $\sum XY$ is the sum of each X value multiplied by each Y value; $\sum X$ is the sum of all the X values; $\sum Y$ is the sum of all the Y values; $\sum X^2$ is the sum of all the squared X values; $(\sum X)^2 = $ The squared sum of all the X values and *n* is the number of data pairs.

Example 5–5 contains a list of data and calculations from a laboratory that performed a patient comparison study and calculated the best-fit line using least-squares statistics. The slope calculated in the example was 0.990. In the clinical laboratory, a slope of 0.95 to 1.05 is considered acceptable. A new method that has a positive slope will assay above the current method and a new method that has a negative slope will assay below the reference method. In both cases, this deviation from the current method usually becomes larger as concentration increases.

### Y Intercept

The Y intercept is the point at which the best fit line intersects the y-axis. The Y intercept is actually the bias corrected for the slope of the line. The Y intercept is calculated as follows:

$$a = \overline{Y} - b\overline{X}$$

where *a* is the mathematical symbol for Y intercept; $\overline{Y}$ is the mean of values on the Y method (new method); $b = $ slope of the line and $\overline{X}$ is the mean of values on the X method (current or reference method). The data in Example 5–5 had a slope of 0.990, the mean of the values on the *X* method was 91.5, and the mean of the values on the Y method was 91.9. The calculation of the Y intercept for these data is as follows:

$$a = 91.9 - (0.990)91.5$$

$$a = 91.9 - 90.585$$

$$a = 1.315$$

If you refer to Example 5–4, you will see that these are the same data on which we used the paired *t*-test to evaluate the bias of 0.4 that was not adjusted for the slope. The calculation of the Y intercept has given us a more correct bias. This bias intersects the Y axis at a value of 1.315 above the origin. This means that, in general, the new method will assay 1.315 units above the new method. The Y intercept for a new method should be close to zero. If the *t*-test has shown the bias to be acceptable and the slope is within limits, it can usually be assumed that the Y intercept is acceptable. A new method that has a significant Y intercept will assay either above or below the reference method, depending on the sign of the Y intercept. This deviation from the reference method will remain the same throughout the concentration range. We can now write the equation for the least-squares regression line:

$$\hat{Y} = a + bX$$

where $a$ is the Y intercept; $b$ is the slope; $X$ is the specified $X$ value; and $\hat{Y}$ is the value of $Y$ on the regression line (this distinguishes it from the observed value for Y). With this formula, we can calculate any value for $Y$ on the line at any specified $X$ value.

## OTHER LINEAR REGRESSION STATISTICS

### Sdy/x

The standard deviation of $Y$ about $X$ quantitates the average difference between the actual value of $Y$ at each $x$ coordinate and the value for $Y$ on the regression line. The SDy/$x$ is calculated by the following formula:

$$\text{SDy}/x = \frac{\sum(Y - \hat{Y})^2}{n\text{-}2}$$

where $Y$ is the observed value for $Y$ at each $X$ value; $\hat{Y}$ is the calculated value for $Y$ on the line at each $X$ value. This is equal to $a + bX$; and n-2 is the number of data pairs corrected for the loss of two degrees of freedom. When using $a + bX$ to calculate $\hat{Y}$, both the slope and the bias have been calculated previously.

The SDy/$x$ measures the dispersion of the data points about the regression line and is an indication of the random error inherent in the new method. Unfortunately, there are no standard criteria for acceptable values for SDy/$x$. However, precision experiments performed during the first part of method evaluation studies indicate the random error attributable to the new method.

### Correlation Coefficient

The formula for the correlation coefficient is as follows:

$$r = \frac{(n)(\sum XY) - (\sum X)(\sum Y)}{\sqrt{[(n)(\sum X^2) - (\sum X)^2][(n)(\sum Y^2) - (\sum Y)^2]}}$$

The correlation coefficient is a linear regression statistic that estimates the strength of the association between two variables and grades this strength from $-1$ to $+1$. A negative correlation is one in which both variables decrease together. A positive correlation is one in which both variables increase together. This statistic is of little value in assessing the difference between two methods. The $r$ value is affected by the range of sample values in that a wide range of values gives a value for $r$ that is close to one regardless of the scatter of data. A laboratory correlation study should include a wide range of values to be considered valid and many investigators use the $r$ value

to verify that their data set contains sufficient number and range of values. The correlation coefficient should only be used in conjunction with other statistics and should not be the sole justification for accepting a new method. Unfortunately, its misuse is more common than its correct use. The evaluator who understands the concepts of coefficient of variation, F test, paired $t$-test, slope, and intercept will have little use for the correlation coefficient.

## RECOVERY EXPERIMENTS

There are two other method evaluation studies that can be done to assess accuracy, recovery, and interference. Recovery experiments estimate the amount of proportional systematic error inherent in a method and gives the same information as the slope that is calculated from method comparison studies. Recovery experiments may be done in addition to method comparison, though they may not be indicated if method comparison studies demonstrate a minimal amount of proportional error. If patient comparisons are not done, recovery experiments should be performed to assess proportional systematic error.

To perform recovery experiments, patient samples are spiked with known amounts of an analyte. The patient sample chosen as a baseline sample should have a low concentration and should be spiked with analyte, usually as a pure standard, of high concentration. The volume of standard added should be such that addition to the patient baseline sample will result in no less than a 1:10 dilution. The formula for calculating concentration of standard added, concentration recovered, and percent recovery are presented below:

$$\text{Concentration added} = \text{Standard concentration}$$
$$\times \frac{\text{mL standard}}{\text{mL serum} + \text{mL standard}}$$

$$\text{Concentration recovered} = \text{Concentration of spiked sample}$$
$$- \text{Concentration of baseline}$$

$$\%\ \text{Recovery} = \frac{\text{Concentration recovered}}{\text{Concentration added}} \times 100$$

For most recovery studies, a percent recovery of 95% to 105% is considered acceptable.

## INTERFERENCE EXPERIMENTS

Interfering substances in the matrix of a sample are one of the causes of constant systematic error. The total amount of constant error is given by the Y intercept. Interference experiments are done to verify the cause of a significant Y intercept or in place of a calculation of the Y intercept. Interference could be caused by lipemia, hemolysis, interfering drugs, analytes, or chemicals. The manufacturer usually lists possible method interfering substances. The experimental protocol is similar to recovery except that the interfering substance, instead of the analyte spike, is added to the baseline sample. The one exception to this is interference from hemolysis. To check for interference from hemolysis, two samples are drawn from a patient and one sample is artificially hemolyzed. Differences between the sample containing the interfering substance and the baseline are not quantitated as percentages but are merely noted.

## Errors Identified by Method Evaluation Studies

Method evaluation studies identify two types of error. Random error occurs without prediction and systematic error occurs within the system and has direction. Proportional systematic error is a systematic error that grows larger as the concentration of the analyte increases. Constant systematic error is a systematic error that affects the method by a constant amount over the entire analytical range.

The following statistical parameters discussed in this section pinpoint specific types of error and are listed in Table 5–3.

## Diagnostic Method Evaluation Studies

A new method must also be evaluated for its ability to correctly diagnose disease. In this evaluation process, the results of a laboratory test are matched to the presence or absence of disease in the patient and a judgment is made about the ability of the test to reflect true patient status. This type of evaluation is impractical for most laboratories but manufacturers usually list data for these parameters for all new tests. For that reason, it is important to understand the concepts of the diagnostic value of a test so that a manufacturer's data can be interpreted correctly. The diagnostic value of a test is also an important piece of information that a laboratory can share with the physician who must interpret laboratory test data.

A laboratory test that is used to diagnose disease can have four possible outcomes:

1. **True positive (*TP*)**—A positive result for patients who have the disease.
2. **True negative (*TN*)**—A negative result for patients who do not have the disease.
3. **False positive (*FP*)**—A positive result for patients who do not have the disease.

### TABLE 5–3

**Statistical Parameters and Type of Error**

| PARAMETER | TYPE OF ERROR |
|---|---|
| Coefficient of variation | Random error |
| F test | Random error |
| Paired *t* test | Total systematic error |
| Slope | Proportional systematic error |
| Y intercept | Constant systematic error |

4. **False negative (*FN*)**—A negative result for patients who have the disease.

Ideally, all positive test results should be true positives and all negative test results should be true negatives. However, this is not always the case, and usually there is a balance between true positives and negatives and false positives and negatives that must be weighed for all new tests.

### SENSITIVITY

Diagnostic sensitivity is the probability that a test result will be positive when the disease the test is detecting is present. It compares the number of true positives with all patient tests in the study that should have given positive results.

$$\text{Sensitivity} = \frac{TP}{TN + FN} \times 100$$

where *TP* is the number of true positives and *FN* is the number of false negatives.

### SPECIFICITY

Diagnostic specificity is the probability that a test result will be negative when the disease the test is detecting is not present. It compares the number of true negatives with all the patients whose results should have been negative.

$$\text{Specificity} = \frac{TN}{TN + FP} \times 100$$

where *TN* is the number of true negatives and *FP* is the number of false positives.

*Example 5–6*

A manufacturer evaluates a new pregnancy test. The manufacturer enlists 800 study subjects, 300 pregnant women and 500 nonpregnant women. The manufacturer lists the following information in a 4 × 4 table:

| Test Results | Number of Pregnant Subjects | Number of Nonpregnant Subjects |
|---|---|---|
| Positive | 250 (TP) | 4 (FP) |
| Negative | 50 (FN) | 496 (TN) |
| Total | 300 (TP + FN) | 500 (FP + TN) |

$$\text{Sensitivity} = \frac{250}{300} \times 100\% = 83\%$$

$$\text{Specificity} = \frac{496}{500} \times 100\% = 99\%$$

Example 5–6 demonstrates the calculation of diagnostic sensitivity and specificity. The laboratory that is reviewing the diagnostic value of this test recognizes that although the test may produce some false negatives, a positive result is very specific for diagnosing pregnancy. This means that a positive result is a strong indication that a woman is pregnant. The physician and the laboratory may decide this is not an acceptable test for screening presurgical patients because of the possibility of false negatives.

## EFFICIENCY

Another statistic that can be used to assess diagnostic value for a test is the efficiency of the test. The efficiency of a test relates the total number of correct results for a test to the total number of participants in the study population. The formula for efficiency is:

$$Efficiency = \frac{TP + TN}{TP + FP + FN + TN} \times 100$$

The efficiency for the pregnancy test described in Example 5–7 is:

$$Efficiency = \frac{250 + 496}{250 + 4 + 50 + 496} \times 100 = 93.25\%$$

## PREDICTIVE VALUE

Another statistic that is used to evaluate diagnostic usefulness is the predictive value for a test. A negative and a positive predictive value can be determined for a method. The negative predictive value is the ability of a method to correctly determine the absence of a disease in patients who do not have the disease. The positive predictive value is the ability of the method to correctly determine the presence of a disease in those patients who have the disease. The following formulas are used to calculate the predictive values:

$$\frac{Negative}{predictive\ value} = \frac{True\ negative}{True\ negative + false\ negatives} \times 100$$

$$\frac{Positive}{predictive\ value} = \frac{True\ positive}{True\ positive + false\ positive} \times 100$$

As an example, a laboratory checks the predictive value of a troponin I method. Of 1000 positives, 980 had a myocardial infarction. Of the 2000 negatives, 20 had a myocardial infarction. The predictive values are calculated as follows:

$$Negative\ predictive\ value = \frac{1980}{1980 + 20} \times 100\% = 99\%$$

$$Positive\ predictive\ value = \frac{980}{980 + 20} \times 100\% = 98\%$$

## REFERENCE INTERVALS

Another part of the analytical process that can directly affect the quality of laboratory results is the reference interval or range of normal values used to interpret test results. Using incorrect reference intervals can compromise the quality of the test even when all aspects of the preanalytical and analytical processes conform to standards. The use of correct reference intervals is part of postanalytical QA. The main purpose of postanalytical QA is to correctly initiate or monitor patient care as a result of quality laboratory data.

It is theoretically desirable that each laboratory establish its own reference ranges for all analytes. A facility's patient or client population could be quite different from the patient population of a neighboring facility. For example, a laboratory that serves a facility specializing in treating women of childbearing age has a very different population from a laboratory serving a children's hospital. Reference values for many analytes can change with increasing age, differences in ethnic origin, and geographic location. Additionally, reference values are often quite different for men and women.

Unfortunately, it is often impractical for laboratories to establish their own reference ranges. Laboratory managers and physicians usually rely on previously published values that appear to fit the population of interest to interpret laboratory test results. Many of these published values, however, have been retained through the years with very little modification. Whenever possible, establishing laboratory reference ranges should be considered as part of an overall QA program. This is especially true for tests resulting from new technology.

When reference range studies cannot be done, reference interval transference can be done. This is a way to establish reference intervals with considerably less effort and less data than used for the establishment of reference intervals discussed below. Reference ranges obtained in one study may be transferred to a laboratory's reference range. The laboratory should review information from the study including the patient selection process demographics, analytical system used, and statistical analysis used. The medical director of the laboratory should be responsible for making the decision as to transfer of reference ranges. Reference ranges can also be validated by sampling a small population of patients. A 20-individual study can be done when documentation of a reference range study is available from the manufacturer. Specimens should be collected and analyzed from 20 individuals who represent the reference sample population. The reference range is validated if two or fewer test results fall outside the published reference range. When information from the manufacturer is not adequate, an experimental validation may be done using a 60-sample approach. The reference interval is determined and statistically compared to the reported reference interval.[2,3]

## Selection of Population

When establishing a new reference range, data should contain 100 to 150 values. If the test is applicable to both male and female subjects, there should be equal representation of both genders. The participants should also demonstrate a wide range of age and activity level. Other factors such as smoking, obesity, and use of medications (including oral contraceptives) that could influence health status should be recorded for each subject. In some cases it may be best to form subsets of groups to determine if a subset factor has a direct influence on the reference range. A participant who has a chronic disease, even though he or she may appear healthy, should be excluded from the study population.

## Calculation of Reference Range

Once data have been collected, the 95% confidence interval of the data is calculated and this interval becomes the reference range. Quite often reference range data do not follow a normal distribution. If this occurs, the usual method of calculating the confidence interval based on the calculation of the SD is not applicable. The 95% confidence limits for reference ranges are usually calculated by nonparametric statistics as opposed to parametric statistics. Nonparametric statistics do not assume that the underlying data have a normal distribution.

*Example 5–7*

A laboratory collects 150 data points for a reference range. The laboratory determines that the data do not follow a normal distribution. A partial list of the data by its position in ascending order is listed below:

| Position No. | Data Value | Position No. | Data Value |
|---|---|---|---|
| 1 | 27 | . | — |
| 2 | 28 | . | — |
| 3 | 29 | 145 | 52 |
| 4 | 29 | 146 | 52 |
| 5 | 30 | 147 | 52 |
| 6 | 31 | 148 | 53 |
| . | — | 149 | 53 |
| . | — | 150 | 54 |

The laboratory calculated the position of the 2.5 percentile by multiplying the number of data points by 2.5%

$(n)0.025 = (150)0.025 = 3.8$ or position 4

The laboratory calculated the position of the 97.5% percentile in the same manner

$(n)0.975 = (150)0.975 = 146.25$ or position 146

The most common method of calculating a reference range using nonparametric statistics is by percentile ranking. With percentile ranking, data are arranged in sequential order and the data points that occupy the 2.5% position at the low end and the 97.5% position at the high end define the range for the 95% confidence interval. Example 5–7 illustrates the use of percentile ranking to calculate a reference range. The reference range for this analyte is determined to be 29 to 52 (the value at position 4 is 29 and the value at position 146 is 52).

## PREANALYTICAL VARIABLES

Laboratory quality assurance can be divided into preanalytical, analytical, and postanalytical areas. Traditionally, only the analytical phase was of concern to the laboratorian. However, modern advances in the practice of laboratory medicine that include an increase in the number of tests and their complexity as well as their effect on patient care demand that QA activities extend outside the laboratory. To reduce errors, we must identify where they occur and to be successful in this process, the preanalytical and postanalytical phases of QA must involve individuals and departments outside the laboratory.

Two studies in the 1990s identified that the largest percent of errors were not in the analytical testing phase but were in the preanalytical and postanalytical phases.[4,5] There has been a concern that not all errors in health care are reported because health care institutions are reluctant to draw attention to these mistakes. This reluctance is unfortunate since systematic analysis of errors and their causes is a good way for organizations to improve their operation. To be able to prevent these errors from occurring, one must have a good understanding of these preanalytical variables.

Preanalytical variables can be grouped into categories. One example of preanalytical variable categories includes: physiologic, specimen collection, handling, and interference variables. Examples in each category are discussed in this chapter (Table 5–4). A brief review of variables will be discussed below. For a more complete discussion, refer to references cited.[6–8]

## Physiologic Variables

### AGE, GENDER, AND RACE

One must always look at the age of the patient when evaluating laboratory results. Pediatric values vary in many lab tests and are too numerous to commit to memory. Gender can be a factor because of hormonal variations that occur with each gender. Limited studies have been done on the variations of lab results with race, but some are available.[6]

### DIURNAL VARIATION

Test values may vary depending on the time of day collected. Aldosterone, bilirubin, BUN, catecholamines, cortisol, therapeutic

**Preanalytical Variables**

| PHYSIOLOGIC | SPECIMEN COLLECTION | HANDLING | INTERFERING SUBSTANCES |
|---|---|---|---|
| Age | Requisition errors | Light | Lipemia |
| Gender | Patient identification | Temperature | Hemolysis |
| Race | Tourniquet time | Evaporation | Bilirubin |
| Time of day | Timing of collection | Aliquoting/labeling | Fibrin strands |
| Season | IVs | Processing time | Clots |
| Altitude | Capillary vs. venous | Centrifugation | |
| Menstruation | Serum vs plasma | Separation time | |
| Pregnancy | Anticoagulants | | |
| Exercise | Gel vs nongel | | |
| Fasting, nonfasting | Order of draw | | |
| Diet | Short draws | | |
| Dehydration, clinical state | Mixing | | |
| Tobacco use | Labeling | | |
| Drug use | | | |
| Posture—standing, sitting, lying | | | |

drugs, testosterone, luteinizing and follicle-stimulating hormone, iron, potassium, thyroxine-stimulating hormone, triglycerides, and uric acid all are affected by diurnal variation.

## EXERCISE

Strenuous exercise can increase the bilirubin, creatine kinase (CK), aspartate aminotransferase (AST), high-density lipoprotein (HDL) cholesterol, lactate, lactate dehydrogenase (LD), and uric acid.

## LIFESTYLE

Diet, caffeine, smoking, and alcohol intake can have an effect on some chemical analytes. High protein diets increase levels of uric acid, urea, and ammonia in blood compared with vegetarians. Caffeine can decrease pH, increase ionic calcium and catecholamine levels. Smoking can increase glucose, triglycerides, cholesterol, and LDL cholesterol. Short-term effects of ethanol include a decrease in glucose, increase in plasma lactate, and an increase in uric acid and triglyceride. Moderate intake of alcohol increases the HDL cholesterol. Long-term effects of alcohol include an increase in gamma glutamyltransferase (GGT), AST, and alanine aminotransferase (ALT).

## NONFASTING SPECIMENS

Certain specimens are required to be fasting. They include fasting glucoses and lipid profiles. A nonfasting glucose will be increased compared to a fasting sample. The triglycerides and low-density lipoprotein (LDL) cholesterol will be increased in a nonfasting sample compared to a fasting sample.

## PROLONGED FASTING

Prolonged fasting can decrease transthyretin (prealbumin), glucose, albumin, LD, HDL cholesterol, and insulin. Transthyretin has a shorter half life than albumin, and is therefore a better indicator of malnutrition in hospitalized patients.

## DEHYDRATION

Dehydration causes hemoconcentration, which can result in the false elevation of some chemical analytes including iron, calcium, sodium, and enzymes. An elevated hematocrit or protein can be an indication of dehydration and the patient should be rehydrated before reassessing the chemical analytes.

## PATIENT POSITION

Patients who change from a standing position to a reclining (supine) position may see a change in the analytes measured. A decrease in aldosterone, antidiuretic hormone, catecholamines, renin, albumin, alkaline phosphatase, ALT, bilirubin, calcium, cholesterol, total protein, and triglycerides is noted when going from a standing position to a supine position. The laboratory standardization panel on blood cholesterol measurement of the National Institutes of Health recommends that patients sit for 5 minutes before collection of specimens for cholesterol and other lipoprotein measurements to minimize this posture related change.[8]

# Specimen Collection Variables

Specimen collection variables include requisition errors, patient identification errors, tourniquet time variability, improper cleaning agents, improper collection time, and intravenous or drug medication interference with the sample.

## TOURNIQUET APPLICATION TIME

A tourniquet that is kept on too long (>3 minutes) will increase the total protein, iron, AST, bilirubin and total lipids. A total cholesterol level may increase 5% at 2 minutes and 15% at 5 minutes. Repeated fist clenching can increase the potassium 1 to 2 mmol/L.

## INTRAVENOUS INFUSION SITE

Drawing from above an intravenous infusion (IV) site should be avoided if at all possible. Drawing from below the IV site after turning off the IV for 2 to 5 minutes and discarding the first 5 mL seems to be preferable. Some laboratories may draw from above the IV as a last resort if the IV has been shut off for 10 minutes.

## CLEANSING AGENTS

Povidone-iodine (Betadine) used as a cleansing agent falsely elevates phosphorus, uric acid, and potassium. Isopropyl (70%) alcohol should not be used for medical or legal ethanol levels.

The type of collection sample, capillary or venous serum, or serum versus plasma sample can cause variances in the analyte measurement. Glucose capillary values are 1.4% higher than venous serum samples and potassium capillary samples are 0.9% higher than venous samples. Capillary samples of bilirubin, calcium, chloride, sodium, and total protein are lower than venous serum samples. Plasma values of potassium, phosphorus, and glucose are lower than serum values. Plasma values of total protein, LD, and calcium are higher then serum values. A cholesterol, triglyceride, and HDL cholesterol measured with EDTA plasma should be multiplied by 1.03 to be equivalent to a serum sample.

## ANTICOAGULANTS

Most chemistry analytes are run on serum or heparinized plasma samples depending on the analyte and methodology used to analyze it. Each laboratory should have documentation in their procedure manuals as to what type samples they require. Some anticoagulants cannot be used for certain tests. Anticoagulants containing fluoride may be used for glucose testing but will interfere with electrolyte studies by altering blood cell membrane permeability. Plasma samples for prostate specific antigen and iron are unacceptable.

## GEL VERSUS NONGEL TUBES

Serum or plasma separator tubes may be unacceptable for some analytes, for example, therapeutic drugs. The manufacturer of the separator tube should provide documentation of analytes that have been shown to give comparable results in serum or plasma obtained from tubes containing gels versus nongel tubes.

## GLASS VERSUS PLASTIC TUBES

If a laboratory is switching from glass to plastic tubes, the manufacturer of the plastic tube should provide documentation of analytes that have been shown to give comparable results in serum or plasma from plastic tubes compared to serum or plasma obtained from glass tubes.

## ORDER OF DRAW

NCCLS recommendations for vacutainer or syringe order of the draw of filling tubes is the following: blood culture tubes, nonadditive or serum tubes, citrate or coagulation tubes, gel separator tubes, heparin, EDTA, and fluoride tubes. Filling the tubes out of this order may cause some cross contamination in the tubes leading to interference in testing the analytes.

## Handling

### LIGHT AND TEMPERATURE

Bilirubin, vitamin $B_{12}$, vitamin A, and carotene are affected by light. Collection devices for these substances that are light-restricting are available. Precautions can also be taken by covering the container with a light-restricting material. Temperature labile analytes include ammonia, blood gases, lactate, pyruvate, gastrin, renin, and parathyroid hormone. Specimens can be chilled by placing in ice water. If blood gases are collected in plastic syringes and run within 20 minutes, they do not need to be iced.

### SPECIMEN PROCESSING

A laboratory should have documentation of specimen-handling information, including the time of specimen delivery to the laboratory, time and date drawn, type of specimen, phlebotomist obtaining specimen, and the reason for rejection, if the specimen was not acceptable.

A procedure should be in place regarding specimen processing. If the plasma needs to be separated from an anticoagulated specimen, it should be separated from cells within 1 hour of collection. A clot-tube specimen should be allowed to clot for 30 to 60 minutes and no longer than 2 hours before it is centrifuged and the serum separated from the clot. Clot tubes that contain clot activators can be processed sooner. The manufacturer should be contacted regarding the recommended clotting time. Clot tubes should be spun at 1200 × g for 10 to 15 minutes.[9] Analytes that increase on standing include CK, lactate, LD, phosphate, and ammonia. Analytes that may decrease on standing include glucose and bicarbonate.[8] Glycolysis will decrease serum glucose by ~5% to 7% in 1 hour. The rate is higher in the presence of leukocytosis. In separated nonhemolyzed sterile serum, the glucose concentration is generally stable for as long as 8 hours at 25°C. Glycolysis can be inhibited and glucose stabilized for as long as 3 days at room temperature by collecting the specimen in a sodium iodoacetate or sodium fluoride additive tube.

## Interfering Substances

The presence of lipemia, hemolysis, and fibrin strands can be evaluated in the specimens before the analytical run. Lipemia representing an increase in lipid material produces turbidity in plasma and serum. Lipemia may cause interference with some chemistry methodologies. Methods exist to remove the lipids by ultracentrifugation or by taking bichromatic readings of an analyte in order to eliminate interference from the turbidity.

Hemolysis, which is red cell lysis, causes the release of chemical analytes present in the red cells such as potassium and enzymes. If this occurs due to an in vitro phenomenon such as a traumatic phlebotomy collection, a false increase in the reported results of serum or plasma analytes occurs. To eliminate in vitro hemolysis, specimens need to be recollected.

Fibrin strands can be caused by partial clotting in an anticoagulated specimen. The strands can cause interference in analysis of analytes by plugging up the probes in the automated analyzers, interfering with the analyte reaction, or interfering with the reading of the analyte. To correct for fibrin strands, the sample would have to be recollected and mixed properly to avoid partial clotting of the sample.

## Detecting Preanalytical Errors

Error detection for preanalytical errors includes visually checking for lipemia, hemolysis, fibrin threads, and short draws in anticoagulated tubes. It may also include delta checks (comparing a patient's lab result with a previous lab result) and evaluating timeliness of the specimen.

## Error Prevention

When there are few ways to detect errors, more devices must be in place for error prevention. Strict guidelines on patient identification and collection processes must be followed.

# COMPONENTS OF AN EFFECTIVE CQI/QA PROGRAM

## Preanalytical

Some components of an effective preanalytical CQI/QA program include:

1. Correct ordering of tests—This implies that the laboratory must consult with physicians on the laboratory tests that are available to fit their diagnostic and monitoring needs. The physician, in turn, should look to the laboratory to give the best advice on proper ordering and sequencing of tests. This communication is particularly important when the laboratory is considering implementing a new test.
2. Preparing of the patient—The patient should have enough information about test orders so that he or she is not anxious about the collection of a test sample. The patient must also be informed of any pretest preparations such as fasting or medical restrictions.
3. Correct identification of the patient by the phlebotomist—The name and identification on the collection sample and the request form must match each other and must also match the correct patient.
4. Proper collection of the sample—The sample must be collected in the correct container and under conditions specified by the test procedure.
5. Timely transportation of the sample to the laboratory—The time between collection and point of assay should be within limits defined by the laboratory.
6. Proper handling of the sample from time of transportation to time of analysis—This may include avoiding exposure or keeping the sample on ice. All samples should be handled as though they are infectious.
7. Proper handling of the sample within the lab—This includes correct documentation of sample identification within the lab, correct centrifugation techniques, and, if necessary, timely separation of the cells from the serum or plasma.

These procedures cannot be verified or monitored by traditional statistical procedures. The indication that there has been a lapse in quality in this area usually reaches the laboratory in the form of a complaint or a report of a quality-compromising event. The possible compromise in quality is then evaluated by a formalized process that defines the indicator of the possible lapse in quality, standards of performance for the indicator, and mechanisms for monitoring the performance.

The following is an example of the process:

*Indicator*
Phlebotomist reports an inpatient does not have an armband, which makes identification difficult.

*Standard*
All hospital inpatients should have armbands to verify identification.

*Monitor*
The number of patients without armbands will be counted for the next 30 days.

If the laboratory discovers after 30 days that the report from the phlebotomist was not an isolated incident, a compromise in quality has been identified and must be corrected. The correction requires the cooperation and involvement of hospital personnel responsible for admission of patients to the hospital and assurance that armbands remain on patients. It may be discovered, when this problem is reported to the nursing staff, that some admitting personnel were not aware of the importance of the policy or that one nursing floor did not realize their patients needed armbands. Once a tentative solution to the problem has been reached, the laboratory monitors the identification process for another 30 days to ensure compliance. Most preanalytical QA monitoring procedures take this problem-oriented approach to ensure quality.

## Analytical

In addition to internal and external QC programs, analytical CQI/QA includes:

1. Proper labeling and use of reagents. Reagents must be labeled with concentration, lot number, date of preparation or time put into use, expiration date, and initials of preparer.
2. Periodic calibration of pipetting devices.
3. Preventive maintenance of instruments.
4. Periodic checking of the temperatures of refrigeration units.
5. Periodic checking of the accuracy of all analytical balances and thermometers.
6. Periodic verification of the accuracy of centrifuge speeds and timing devices.
7. Periodic checking that procedure manuals are complete and up-to-date.
8. Constant assurance that safety procedures are followed.

These processes are usually monitored by function sheets or periodic written verification that these procedures are followed on a regular basis. These written verifications may be in the form of checklists that the laboratorian must initial as the functions are performed. These sheets are then verified at periodic intervals by the supervisor for completeness and compliance.

## Postanalytical

Postanalytical CQI/QA is the process of verifying quality in all procedures that occur once the report leaves the laboratory and is in the hands of the physician or care provider. In addition to the use of correct reference intervals, areas of postanalytical CQI/QA include:

1. Verification of calculations on final reports.
2. Review of test results for possible transcription errors.
3. Reports that are easy to read and interpret.
4. Procedures for informing the physician of results that require immediate attention.
5. Timeliness of reporting values to patient chart.
6. Verification of correct interpretation of lab tests by physicians.
7. Constant interaction with the institution to ensure quality in direct patient care as a result of lab tests.

The monitoring of this section of CQI/QA usually takes two forms. One is the process described for preanalytical QA in that a possible lapse in quality may be identified by a complaint from a physician or other care provider. These complaints are usually related to incorrect lab reports or an excessive time lapse between the ordering of a lab test and the receipt of final results. These potential lapses in quality would be handled in the same manner as that described for the preanalytical process. The other type of monitoring for quality in this area by an ongoing assessment of the impact of laboratory results and procedures in the institution that the laboratory serves. The purpose of these ongoing assessments is to promote excellence in patient care by interfacing with all departments of an institution. Institutional CQI/QA programs usually take the form of QA committees, continuous quality improvement committees, or review committees. The focus of these groups is not to solve problems but to prevent them from occurring.

In addition, the laboratory must have its own form of ongoing CQI/QA in which the laboratory is periodically evaluated for its ability to function as a quality department. This may include an evaluation of laboratory space to ensure efficiency in services, review of qualifications of laboratory staff, and encouragement of staff to participate in continuing education activities.

CQI/QA within the clinical laboratory is the responsibility of every member of the laboratory staff. CQI/QA must become a way of life, an attitude that is apparent in every level of practice within the laboratory. This quality must extend beyond the physical confines of the laboratory and include a responsibility to every physician who orders a test and a concern for every patient who receives treatment as a result of laboratory data.

## SUMMARY

Method evaluation is a part of preanalytical QA. Evaluation studies verify that a method is accurate and precise before it is incorporated into a laboratory's testing menus. Linearity and precision studies are done to verify manufacturer's claims. Accuracy is verified by patient comparison studies. Diagnostic evaluation studies are sometimes performed to test the ability of a new method to correctly diagnose disease.

Quality in the final lab result depends heavily on using the correct reference range. Verification of this range is considered part of postanalytical QA. Subjects for reference interval studies must represent the population of interest, and since data often do not follow a normal distribution, nonparametric statistics are often used to calculate the interval.

A complete and effective CQI/QA program verifies quality at every step in the testing process: preanalytical, analytical, and postanalytical.

### REFERENCES

1. National Committee for Clinical Laboratory Standards: *Evaluation of the Linearity of Quantitative Analytical Methods: Proposed Guideline.* NCCLS publication no. EP6-P2-2001. Wayne, PA, National Committee for Clinical Laboratory Standards, 2001.

2. National Committee for Clinical Laboratory Standards: *How to Define and Determine Reference Intervals in the Clinical Laboratory: Approved Guideline.* NCCLS publication no. C28-A-2000. Wayne, PA, National Committee for Clinical Laboratory Standards, 2000.

3. Barry PL, Westgard JO: Method Validation: Reference interval transference. In Westgard JO (ed.): *Basic Method Validation: Training in Analytical Quality Management for Healthcare Laboratories.* Madison, WI, Westgard Quality Corporation, 1999.

4. Boone DJ: Comment on Houwen B: Random errors in haematology tests: A process control approach. Clin Lab Haematol 12(Suppl 1):169–170, 1990.

5. Nutting PA, Main DS, Fischer PM, et al: Problems in laboratory testing in primary care. JAMA 275:635–639, 1996.

6. Young DS, Bermes EW: Specimen collection and processing: Sources of biological variation. In Burtis CA, Ashwood ER (eds.): *Tietz Textbook of Clinical Chemistry*, 3rd ed. Philadelphia, W. B. Saunders, 1999, pp 42–72.

7. Narayanan S: The preanalytic phase: An important component of laboratory medicine. Am J Clin Pathol 113: 429–452, 2000.

8. Dale J C: Preanalytical variables in laboratory testing. Lab Med 29(9):540–545, 1999.

9. National Committee for Clinical Laboratory Standards: *Procedures for the Handling and Processing of Blood Specimens: Approved Guideline*, 2nd ed. NCCLS publication no. H18-A2. Wayne, PA, National Committee for Clinical Laboratory Standards, 1999.

## Additional Reading

National Committee for Clinical Laboratory Standards: *Testing in the Clinical Laboratory.* NCCLS publication no. EP7-P. Wayne, PA, National Committee for Clinical Laboratory Standards, 1986.

# C H A P T E R   6

# Spectrophotometry

*Joan E. Aldrich*

## SPECTROPHOTOMETRIC PRINCIPLES

### Characteristics of Light

Spectrophotometry is an analytical method that uses properties of light for qualitative and quantitative measurements. The measurements depend on both the wave and particle properties of light.

#### WAVELENGTH

The wavelength of light equals the distance between identical sites on consecutive waves; for example, the distance between two crests (Figure 6–1). The closer two crests are, the shorter the wavelength and the greater the energy contained in the light. The shorter the wavelength, the larger the number of photons of light that will be contained in a given distance. More photons represents more energy; hence, short wavelength represents higher energy than long wavelength light.

#### ELECTROMAGNETIC SPECTRUM

Wavelengths of light are expressed in units of nanometers (nm, $10^{-9}$ m) with wavelengths from 190 to approximately 390 nm being invisible **ultraviolet** light (UV) and from 390 to approximately 750 nm being **visible** light (able to excite retinal cells). Although color identification is somewhat subjective, each visible color corresponds to a range of wavelengths (Table 6–1). A convenient mnemonic for remembering the sequence of visible colors is ROY G BIV, which stands for red, orange, yellow, green, blue, indigo, and violet (from longest to shortest wavelength).

Wavelengths of light longer than 800 nm correspond to the **infrared** portion of the electromagnetic spectrum. Its wave-

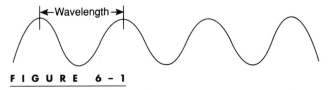

**FIGURE   6 – 1**

Wavelength: distance between two successive peaks.

### TABLE   6 – 1

**Characteristics of Visible Light**

| APPROXIMATE WAVELENGTH (nm) | COLOR OF LIGHT ABSORBED | COLOR OF LIGHT TRANSMITTED |
|---|---|---|
| 390–435 | Violet (V) | Yellow-green |
| 435–490 | Blue (B) | Yellow |
| 490–580 | Green (G) | Red |
| 580–595 | Yellow (Y) | Blue |
| 595–650 | Orange (O) | Green-blue |
| 650–750 | Red (R) | Blue-green |

lengths are expressed in $\mu$m ($10^{-6}$ m) and are perceived as heat instead of light. In a molecule, these wavelengths correspond to the energy associated with vibrating, bending, and twisting covalent bonds. Wavelengths of electromagnetic energy that are even longer (cm) are radio waves used for radar and radio.

Wavelengths shorter than 190 nm include **X rays** and **gamma radiation.** These photons have such high energy that they can penetrate flesh. Their energies are sufficient to break covalent bonds and to strip electrons from atoms (Figure 6–2).

### Spectral Absorption Curves

Each colored solute absorbs a unique pattern of wavelengths whose energies correspond to the energy levels of the electrons in its chemical bonds. In general, the perceived color of a solution will be dominated by the wavelengths that are transmitted (not absorbed) by the solute. The transmitted and absorbed wavelengths are complementary to each other (Table 6–1). Thus, the visible color of a solution will be the complement of the wavelengths that are absorbed; for example, a solution of red hemoglobin absorbs green light at 540 nm and a solution of yellow bilirubin absorbs blue light at 450 nm. Often, the pattern of absorbances at different wavelengths is so distinctive that a solute can be identified by its absorption spectrum. A spectral absorption curve is a graph that shows the pattern of absorbances by a solute at different wavelengths (Figure 6–3).

| wavelength (nm) | 0.1 | 1.0 | 200 | 400 | 1000 | $2.5 \times 10^7$ |
|---|---|---|---|---|---|---|
| EM radiation | gamma | X ray | ultraviolet | visible | infrared | radio |

**FIGURE   6 - 2**

Nomenclature for different wavelengths of electromagnetic energy.

Another use of an absorption spectrum is using it to de-cide which wavelength of light to use for quantitative analy-sis. Quantitative spectrophotometry compares the absorbance of an unknown concentration of solute to the absorbance of a known concentration (see Beer's law later in this chapter). In general, the wavelength where absorbance is greatest would be selected because even a small amount of solute would cause a measurable amount of absorbance. In the examples above, hemoglobin is measured by its absorbance at 540 nm and bilirubin by its absorbance at 450 nm.

Technical considerations sometimes modify the decision of which wavelength to use for analysis. In Figure 6–3, for ex-ample, the solute has three distinct absorption peaks. The peak at 300 nm ("B") is not suitable as the analytical wavelength because its absorbance is small compared to the other two peaks. The peak at 255 nm ("A") is not suitable for quantita-tive analysis because it is very narrow; thus a very small change or error in wavelength would cause a large change in ab-sorbance that was not due to change in concentration of solute. In addition, peak A is at 255 nm, an ultraviolet wavelength of light, which requires special optical components (see Spec-trophotometer Components later in this chapter). The peak at 480 nm ("C") has high absorbance and has a rounded top, making it suitable among the three peaks available for analy-sis of this solute.

## Transmission and Absorption of Light

The physical principle behind all forms of spectrophotometry is that visible and ultraviolet wavelengths of light correspond to the range of energy levels associated with valence electrons. The electron bonds between the atoms of a colored solute can absorb limited energy without disrupting the chemical bond. An electron can be raised to its next energy level by absorbing the energy of a photon if the photon carries the appropriate amount of energy for that electron in that compound. A spec-trophotometer detects the presence of and measures the num-ber of those bonds by measuring the number of photons ab-sorbed by the solute.

In practice, a spectrophotometer uses a high-intensity lamp and measures the amount of light that penetrates the col-ored solution (Figure 6–4). The proportion of light that pen-etrates the solution is called transmittance (abbreviated T). It is usually expressed as a percent of the maximum light trans-mitted when the colored solute is absent ($I_o$). As the concen-tration of photon-absorbing solute is increased, less light (I) is transmitted through the solution.

$$\%T = \frac{I \times 100}{I_o}$$

The relationship between the amount of light transmit-ted and the concentration of solute is inversely proportional and logarithmic (Figure 6–5).

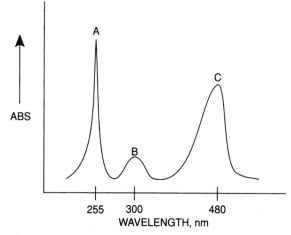

**FIGURE   6 - 3**

Spectral absorption curve.

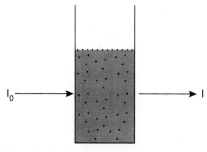

**FIGURE   6 - 4**

Transmittance of monochromatic light through a cuvette. $I_o$ is the incident radiation; $I$ is the transmitted radiation.

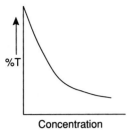

**FIGURE   6 - 5**

Percent transmittance (%*T*) is a function of concentration.

## ABSORBANCE

For ease of calculation, a new term is defined that is directly proportional to the concentration of solute. This term, absorbance, is defined as the negative logarithm of *T*. Algebraic manipulation and the common definition that $I_0$ is set at 100 leads to the following simplification: $A = 2 - \log \%T$ (Figure 6–6). Since $-\log \%T$ is proportional to concentration of the photon-absorbing solute, absorbance is directly proportional to its concentration. Thus using absorbance (instead of %*T*) removes both the negative sign and the logarithm from the relationship with concentration and permits straight lines for calibration (Figure 6–7).

In the experiment that produced Figure 6–7, four calibrators of known concentration and a solution of unknown concentration were measured in a spectrophotometer. The instrument meter was set to read 100 %*T* when there was no colored solute present and the %*T*s of both an unknown solution and known calibrators were measured. After converting %*T* readings to absorbances, the calibration line was plotted (Figure 6–7). Interpolation determines that the concentration of the unknown is 8.8.

## BEER'S LAW

Beer's law is the formal expression of the relationship between absorbance and concentration of solute. In its commonly used form, the contributions of Beer and Bernard and Bouguer and Lambert are combined into one equation: $A = \varepsilon lc$.

Since absorbance measures the number of molecules of solute in the path of the photons, absorbance depends on both

$$A = -\log T = -\log I/I_0 = +\log I_0/I = \log I_0 - \log I$$

When $I_0 = 100$, then *I* is %*T*.

$$A = \log 100 - \log \%T = 2 - \log \%T$$

**FIGURE   6 - 6**

Derivation of absorbance (*A*).

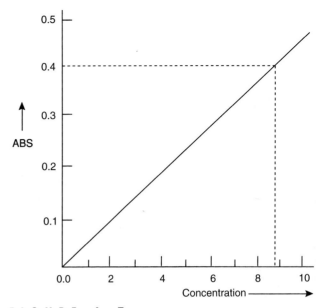

**FIGURE   6 - 7**

Relationship of absorbance to concentration.

the concentration of solute and the depth of the solution. In other words, $A \propto lc$, where *l* = depth of the solution and *c* = concentration of solute. Substituting a proportionality constant produces the equation commonly referred to as Beer's law: $A = \varepsilon lc$. Absorbance has no units; thus the proportionality constant takes on whatever units are necessary to cancel the units associated with *l* and *c*. $\varepsilon$ is referred to as molar absorptivity when the depth of solution (*l*) is expressed in centimeters and the concentration of solute (*c*) is expressed in moles/liter.

Molar absorptivity is the conversion factor between absorbance and concentration. One of its uses occurs when a stable calibrator is not available, for example, when measuring the concentration of an NADH solution. The molar absorptivity of NADH at 340 nm is $6.22 \times 10^3$; in other words, a 1 cm depth of a 1 mol/L solution of NADH has an absorbance of 6220 or, in more practical terms, a 100 $\mu$mol/L solution of NADH has an absorbance of 0.622. Thus, measuring the absorbance of an unknown solution of NADH at 340 nm in a 1-cm cuvette allows for the calculation of NADH concentration (Example 6–1).

Molar absorptivity also has a use as an indicator of purity. The expected value for $\varepsilon$ can be obtained from reference tables, and compared to the measured absorbance of a prepared solution. If the solution was made using analytical-grade equipment (balance, glassware), its concentration will depend only on the purity of the material that was used to make the solution. Deviation from the expected absorbance indicates the degree of impurity (Example 6–2).

*Example 6–1*

The molar absorptivity of NADH at 340 nm is $6.22 \times 10^3$ L $\cdot$ mole$^{-1}$ cm$^{-1}$. The absorbance of NADH in a 1-cm cuvette at 340 nm is 0.38. Calculate the concentration of NADH.

$$A = \varepsilon c l$$

$$c = \frac{A}{\varepsilon l} = \frac{0.38}{6.22 \times 10^3 \text{ L} \cdot \text{mole}^{-1} \times \text{cm}^{-1} \times 1 \text{ cm}}$$

$$= \frac{0.38}{6.22 \times 10^3 \text{ L} \cdot \text{mole}^{-1}}$$

$$= 6.11 \times 10^{-2} \times 10^{-3} \text{ mole/L}$$

$$= 6.11 \times 10^{-5} \text{ mole/L}$$

*Example 6–2*

Method:

175.4 mg of bilirubin (molecular weight 584.65) was weighed on an analytical balance, and quantitatively transferred to a class A volumetric flask for dilution to 1000 mL total volume. After mixing, 1 mL of the solution was diluted to 100 mL in another volumetric flask. The absorbance of the second solution at 453 nm, read in a 1-cm cuvette, was 0.175. The molar absorptivity of pure bilirubin using these conditions is 60,700. Calculate the purity of the bilirubin.

Concentration of bilirubin (if pure):

175.4 mg/1000 mL $\times$ 1/100 $\div$ 584.65
$$= 3.0 \times 10^{-6} \text{ mol/L}$$

Absorbance of the solution (if pure):

$3.0 \times 10^{-6}$ mol/L $\times$ 60,700 A/mol/L = 0.182 A

% purity:

$0.175 \div 0.182 \times 100 = 96\%$ pure

Beer's law has three important assumptions:

• the light striking the solute is monochromatic (only one wavelength),
• the solute being analyzed is the only colored solute (chromophore) present in the solution,
• the only light being measured comes from the analytical beam of light.

Strict adherence to all of these conditions is difficult. In addition, there are inherent limitations to the accuracy of measuring the amount of light transmitted. Since %$T$ is a logarithmic function, readings between 95 and 100 %$T$ and between 0 and 10 %$T$ are suspect and should be avoided.

## CALIBRATION

If all conditions were optimal, the absorbance of a solution would be proportional to the concentration of its colored solute and one calibrating solution would be sufficient. If that condition were met, it would only be necessary to (1) anchor the scale of the spectrophotometer by setting complete darkness to read 0 %$T$ (= infinite absorbance), and (2) set pure solvent (complete lack of colored solute) to read 100 %$T$ (= 0 absorbance). Then, when the detector responded to transmitted light, $A = 2 - \log \%T$ would be true and thus $A = \varepsilon l c$ would also be true. Calibration could then be simplified to:

$$\frac{A_{unknown}}{A_{calibrator}} = \frac{\text{Concentration}_{unknown}}{\text{Concentration}_{calibrator}}$$

The two absorbances would be measured in the procedure and the concentration of the calibrator is known. Thus, concentration of the unknown solution could be calculated.

In Figure 6–7, any one of the calibrators could have been used to determine the relationship between absorbance and concentration, allowing calculation of the concentration of the unknown solution. In practice, at least two calibrators are usually used to verify that the relationship is consistent over the whole range of analyte concentrations that will be found in the patients' samples (Example 6–3).

*Example 6–3*

Two standard solutions of urea and a patient's serum are analyzed, and the following absorbances are obtained:

| | |
|---|---|
| 15 mg/dL urea standard | A = 0.150 |
| 50 mg/dL urea standard | A = 0.400 |
| Patient's serum | A = 0.250 |

If only the 15 mg/dL standard had been used, the patient's serum would appear to contain 25 mg/dL urea:

$$\frac{0.250}{0.150} = \frac{x}{15 \text{ mg/dL}} \qquad x = 25 \text{ mg/dL}$$

Whereas, if only the 50 mg/dL standard had been used, the patient's serum would appear to contain 31 mg/dL urea:

$$\frac{0.250}{0.400} = \frac{x}{50 \text{ mg/dL}} \qquad x = 31 \text{ mg/dL}$$

Clearly, in this example an error or uncontrolled variable has occurred. Failure to use two standards would overlook the error and cause an erroneous result for the patient's serum.

## SPECTROPHOTOMETRIC INSTRUMENTS

### Spectrophotometer Components

Since spectrophotometry measures the amount of light transmitted through a solution, provision must be made for generating the light, selecting the desired wavelength, holding a known depth of solution in the pathway of the light, and measuring the amount of light that is transmitted through the solution. These requirements outline the basic components of a spectrophotometer (Figure 6–8).

#### LIGHT SOURCE

The light source must be a stable lamp that provides the desired wavelength and provides enough light to penetrate the solution. No single type of lamp can provide all the wavelengths that might be needed for all applications.

An incandescent lamp with a **tungsten** filament heated to 3000° K is the most common source of visible wavelengths. At this temperature, the filament emits continuous wavelengths of light from 350 nm through infrared, although most of the emitted energy is in the infrared range (heat), less is in the visible range, and very little is emitted in the violet and near-ultraviolet range. The amount of light emitted at each wavelength depends on the temperature of the filament. Therefore, the lamp must warm up to a stable operating temperature before use. Often, the heat that is generated may have to be dispersed or blocked to prevent error. For example, the amount of light emitted by fluorescent solutes decreases when they are warmed. Nevertheless, a tungsten lamp provides a cheap, reliable source of light across the whole range of visible wavelengths.

Commonly, the glass envelope surrounding the tungsten filament is filled with a halogen gas. These tungsten-halogen lamps do not darken with use because the halogen reacts with tungsten atoms that are boiled off the filament and prevents depositing a film of tungsten on the inside of the envelope. Since the envelope remains clear, these lamps are able to emit sufficient energy even during extended use.

**Ultraviolet** wavelengths of light are most commonly provided by high-voltage discharge arcs. In these, a high-voltage power supply ionizes the gas (hydrogen, deuterium, xenon, or mercury) contained in a glass envelope. As the excited ions return to ground state, a continuum of wavelengths in the ultraviolet range is emitted. Some visible wavelengths are also emitted but that spectrum is not a smooth continuum. Discharge arc lamps emit more short-wavelength UV light than long-wavelength UV light. Since the spectrum of emitted light shifts with change in voltage supplied to the lamp, the power supply must be tightly regulated. In addition, the glass envelope containing the ionized gas must be transparent to UV wavelengths. Generally, a window of special silica glass or quartz glass is fused into the envelope to accommodate this requirement.

The amount of light emitted by a xenon discharge arc is greater than that emitted by a deuterium discharge arc, which in turn is greater than that emitted by a hydrogen discharge arc. Selecting which type of discharge arc to purchase depends largely on how much energy is required to penetrate the solutions to be measured.

A mercury vapor lamp is also available as a discharge arc. It is less useful as a general-purpose source of UV wavelengths because the discrete electron orbits in mercury atoms result in sharply defined wavelength peaks instead of a continuous spectrum of wavelengths. These peaks are so sharp that they can be used to calibrate the monochromator that selects the desired wavelength from the continuum (see Blanking and Checking a Spectrophotometer later in this chapter).

A few instruments use a laser as the light source. This provides a very intense beam of light of very specific wavelength. Lasers are most often found in instruments used for immunoassay, where the indicator label is a fluorescent compound that becomes excited by the wavelength of the laser.

#### MONOCHROMATOR

The function of a monochromator is to select a narrow range of wavelengths of light from the continuous spectrum that is provided by the light source. Except when using a monochromatic light source (e.g., a laser), there is a trade-off between the intensity of the light beam selected and the range

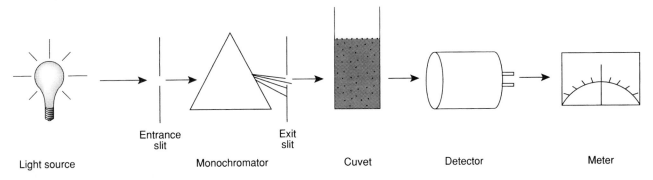

Entrance slit       Exit slit

Light source          Monochromator          Cuvet          Detector          Meter

**FIGURE 6-8**

Basic components of a spectrophotometer.

of wavelengths in that light beam. If a larger variety of wavelengths is permitted, then more photons of those wavelengths are available from the light source. However, if only a very narrow range of wavelengths is permitted, the light source will have to be more intense because only a few photons will meet the criterion.

In its simplest form, a filter of colored glass or colored plastic could act as a monochromator. Since a spectrophotometer measures a solute by the amount of complementary light that is absorbed, selecting a colored glass or colored plastic filter that is the complementary color would provide an appropriate range of wavelengths. For example, hemoglobin is red and the complement of red is blue-green (Table 6–1); therefore, it would be appropriate to use a blue-green filter to measure hemoglobin. However, recall that Beer's law assumes that there is only a single colored solute and one wavelength of light. In practice, a very narrow band of wavelengths is desirable for absorbance and concentration to be proportional over the widest range possible and to avoid interference from other similarly colored interfering solutes in the sample.

The actual range of wavelengths transmitted by a monochromator is called the **bandpass**. It is determined by measuring the spectrum of wavelengths transmitted by the monochromator (Figure 6–9). All wavelengths are counted that pass greater than 50% of the maximum light. In Figure 6–9, the bandpass is 10 nm because all wavelengths between 445 and 455 nm transmit more than half of the maximum transmission. The biggest limitation of the colored glass and colored plastic filters described above is that the bandpass is usually 30 to 50 nm. In other words, a piece of green glass may actually transmit all wavelengths from 500 to 550 nm and the resulting absorbance of a red solute may deviate from Beer's law at all but an impractical narrow range of concentrations.

A popular type of monochromator is an **interference filter.** It is composed of two parallel sheets of half-silvered glass

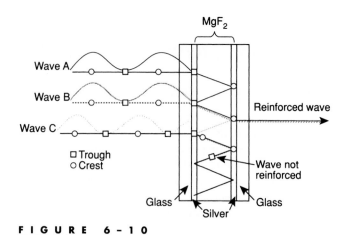

**FIGURE 6-10**

Passage of light waves through an interference filter. Wave A reinforced by wave B breaks through. Wave C is not reinforced by any wave and does not break through.

surrounding a core of dielectric, for example, $MgF_2$ (Figure 6–10). The distance between the parallel sheets determines the wavelength of light that is transmitted through the filter. Photons of light that enter the filter are reflected between the two silvered surfaces. Photons whose wavelengths are an integer fraction of the distance between the surfaces are synchronous and their amplitudes add together (constructive interference), whereas those wavelengths that are not an integer fraction are out of phase when they meet other photons of the same wavelength and they are destroyed (destructive interference). Only the constructively reinforced wavelengths of light remain to emerge from an interference filter. This includes the desired wavelength as well as harmonic wavelengths that are one half and twice as long as the desired wavelength. Considering the range of ultraviolet and visible wavelengths, those harmonic wavelengths usually are not significant sources of interference but a **cutoff filter** (also called sharp-cut filter) can be used if desired. A cutoff filter absorbs all light below a specified wavelength and transmits all light above that limit. Thus, it can be inserted between the monochromator and the sample to remove unwanted harmonic wavelengths.

With modern engineering methods to produce planar parallel surfaces, interference filters are available in a wide variety of wavelengths and they characteristically have a narrow bandpass (usually 5 to 15 nm). They are very stable and provide a convenient method for selecting filters with a variety of wavelengths.

When a continuous spectrum of wavelengths is required, the monochromator of choice is a **diffraction grating.** It is composed of a polished reflective surface onto which sharply defined, parallel grooves have been etched (Figure 6–11). When light hits a sharp edge, it is diffracted into a spectrum of its component wavelengths. When many rays of light diffract off many parallel sharp edges, the multitude of spectra overlap each other, constructive and destructive interference

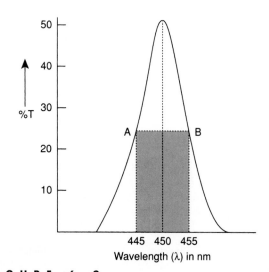

**FIGURE 6-9**

Bandpass of a spectrophotometer (isolated by a filter).

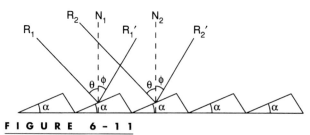

**FIGURE 6-11**

Reflectance grating showing two incident rays, $R_1$ and $R_2$, which are in phase, emerging as $R_1'$ and $R_2'$. Those rays not in phase will be destroyed by interference. $\alpha$ = blade angle; $\theta$ = angle of light striking; $\phi$ = reflectance angle.

occurs between overlapping spectra and a single linear spectrum of all the impinging wavelengths results. This is similar to the way a single rainbow is produced when sunlight diffracts off of myriad water droplets. Diffraction gratings can be made of material that reflects (or transmits) both visible and UV wavelengths.

For the overlapping spectra to produce a single spectrum, the incoming light must be collimated (in parallel light rays). This is accomplished by passing the light from the lamp through a lens (also called an entrance slit) before it hits the diffraction grating. The lens is often made of heat-absorbing material, which also protects subsequent parts from the heat of the lamp.

The desired wavelength is selected from the final spectrum by aligning a pinhole (also called an exit slit) between the correct area of the spectrum and the cuvette (Figure 6–8). The bandpass of the diffraction grating monochromator is determined by the width of the final spectrum and the size of the pinhole. The spacing of the grooves etched on the surface of the diffraction grating determines the width of the final spectrum: the more grooves, the wider the spectrum; the wider the spectrum, the smaller the bandpass transmitted through a pinhole. Typical diffraction gratings have several hundred to several thousand grooves per millimeter. Some instruments allow the user to adjust the size of the pinhole: a wider pinhole (exit slit) lets through more light and causes a wider bandpass.

## SAMPLE HOLDER

A typical sample holder is a glass cuvette with a square cross section. The walls of the cuvette must be transparent to the wavelength of light used. For visible and near-UV wavelengths, both ordinary flint glass and certain plastics are sufficient; for wavelengths below 340 nm, quartz glass or fused silica cuvettes are required. The cuvette must meet optical quality standards.

Recalling the assumptions of Beer's law, the distance that the light passes through the solute must be constant for absorbance to be proportional to concentration. Thus, the distance between the walls of a cuvette must be constant. The molar absorptivity coefficient in Beer's law assumes that a 1-cm depth of solution is measured, which implies use of

a 1-cm deep square cuvette. Round cuvettes can also be used provided they have been matched for equal absorbing properties and the absorbances of calibrators are measured in the same cuvettes. The molar absorptivity cannot be used for calculations when round cuvettes are employed because the depth of solution is not constant.

Most automated instruments either have built-in cuvettes that are automatically washed between samples or use disposable cuvettes that are automatically advanced into position and then discarded after use. In either case, the quality of the optical path is an important aspect of monitoring the quality of spectrophotometric results. Whether automated or manual, cuvettes must be optically matched, clean and not scratched in order to produce accurate absorbances.

In special circumstances, solutes are measured by burning them in a flame instead of being dissolved in a solvent. These conditions are found in flame emission spectrophotometry and atomic absorption spectrophotometry. However, neither of these instruments is in common use in clinical laboratories.

## DETECTOR

The function of the detector in a spectrophotometer is to produce electrical energy (current or voltage) in response to light energy. The detector is placed in line with the light beam that is transmitted through the solution being analyzed. The amount of light hitting the detector is converted to current or voltage, which then can be converted to absorbance. Thus, Beer's law relates detector response to solute concentration.

Detectors rely on the fact that when certain materials are exposed to visible or ultraviolet light, their valence electrons become excited and may even be ejected from the surface of the metal. Examples of these materials include selenium and cadmium as well as certain semiconductors made from silicon or germanium that is doped with gallium salts.

In a solid-state **photodiode,** light enables electrons to flow in one direction across the diode junction, which causes a change in voltage across the semiconductor. The magnitude of the change in voltage is proportional to the amount of light that reaches the detector. Photodiodes have a significant advantage because they can be closely spaced in an array. Then several wavelengths of light, passing through a single cuvette, can be directed to adjacent photodiodes and measurements of several chromophores can be made simultaneously. This is the arrangement used for bichromatic analysis in many instruments in the clinical laboratory (see Bichromatic Analysis later in this chapter).

In **photomultiplier tubes** and **photocells,** a photosensitive metal (e.g., selenium or cadmium) is used as a cathode and photons striking the cathode cause electrons to be released from its surface. The current flow created by the free electrons is proportional to the intensity of the light transmitted through the solution and hitting the detector.

Photocells directly measure the very small current; a very strong light source is required that restricts their use to very few applications. Photomultiplier tubes (PMTs) amplify the

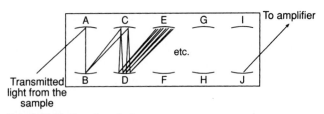

## FIGURE   6 - 1 2

Schematic of photomultiplier tube. A = cathode;
B → J = dynodes represented by crescent shape.

*Example 6–4*

|                               | Cuvette A        | Cuvette B      | Cuvette C          |
|-------------------------------|------------------|----------------|--------------------|
| Absorbance due to:            | Reagent Blank    | Serum Blank    | Analytical Cuvette |
| Cuvette                       | yes              | yes            | yes                |
| Color or turbidity of reagent | yes              | most           | yes                |
| Color or turbidity of sample  | no               | yes            | yes                |

current from the photosensitive cathode many-fold. This allows the PMT to be very sensitive to small amounts of light or to small changes in the amount of light striking the cathode. PMTs also have very fast response time, which makes them suitable for measuring rapid changes in absorbance. The electrons ejected from the cathode are attracted to an adjacent dynode whose voltage is slightly lower than the cathode (Figure 6–12). As each electron strikes the next dynode it causes ejection of several more electrons. Thus, by careful alignment of 10 to 20 dynodes with progressively lower voltages, a few electrons ejected from the cathode can be multiplied into a larger, easily measured current.

PMTs are so sensitive that they must be protected from excessive light that could burn out the circuit with the large current generated. They are also temperature sensitive since the photoemissive cathode may emit a small number of electrons even at room temperature (dark current). PMTs also require a regulated power supply to set the voltages of the dynodes. They are used in instruments where their sensitivity to small variations of light is needed.

## BLANKING AND CHECKING A SPECTROPHOTOMETER

Using Beer's law to quantitate an analyte is based on the assumption that the absorbance reading of the spectrophotometer is an accurate reflection of the amount of chromophore in the light path. This requires (1) proper blanking to eliminate extraneous sources of absorbance, (2) checking the components to be certain they are performing their functions within acceptable limits, and (3) calibrating the variables that will affect absorbance readings.

**Blanking** refers to reading the absorbance of a solution that includes all light absorption not due to the desired chromophore. Possible sources of extraneous absorption include absorption or reflectance of light by the cuvette, absorption or scattering of light by the solvent or the reagents, and absorption or scattering of light by color or turbidity in the sample.

A **reagent blank** contains all the components of the chromogenic reaction except the sample with its analyte. The absorbance of the reagent blank includes absorbances due to the cuvette and all reagents. Alternatively, a **serum blank** contains the sample and all reactants except one reagent that is required for the chromogenic reaction. Therefore, the absorbance of a serum blank includes absorbances due to the cuvette, the sam-

ple's color and turbidity, and most reagents' absorbances. When one of these blanks is set to 100 % *T* (0 absorbance), all of its absorbances are effectively subtracted from the absorbance of the analytical cuvette. This compensates for absorbance due to the analytical cuvette and other extraneous absorbances (Example 6–4). Setting cuvette A at 100% *T* (0 absorbance) before reading absorbance of cuvette C will subtract all interfering absorbances except background color or turbidity of the sample. Setting cuvette B at 100 % *T* (0 absorbance) before reading absorbance of cuvette C will subtract all interfering absorbances except for color or turbidity in the one reactant that was omitted.

**Checking** the performance of spectrophotometer components generally includes monitoring the responses to known situations. The intensity of the **lamp** can be checked by selecting a wavelength where only minimal photons are emitted (e.g., 400 nm for a tungsten-halogen lamp) and testing whether a cuvette containing deionized water can be set to read 100 % *T* (0 absorbance). If it cannot, then the lamp is too weak and may require replacement. Checking the **monochromator** means making sure that the light that it emits is the same as the wavelength indicated on the control dial. Wavelength calibrating filters and solutions are commercially available. Holmium oxide and didymium filters are frequently used since they have a variety of known, sharp absorption peaks across the visible and ultraviolet wavelengths (Figure 6–13). With a calibrating filter or solution in the cuvette, the wavelength knob is adjusted through the region of wavelengths where the greatest absorbance is expected. If the observed maximum absorbance does not occur at the expected wavelength, then the wavelength dial must be adjusted to reflect the true wavelength going through the cuvette. Often this simply requires loosening a setscrew on the wavelength knob.

The width of the **bandpass** of the spectrophotometer can be checked using the same holmium oxide or didymium filters from above. Two absorption peaks are chosen that differ in wavelength by one bandpass. When the wavelength knob is adjusted through that range of wavelengths, the two distinct peaks should be apparent on the absorbance meter (Figure 6–14). A wide bandpass is indicated if the two absorbance peaks merge

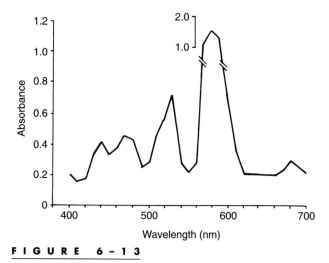

**FIGURE 6-13**

Absorption spectrum of a didymium filter.

into one peak of lesser absorbance. If the bandpass has become wider than specified by the instrument manufacturer, the most common causes are dirt or warping of the exit slit or the surface of the monochromator.

**Cuvettes** are checked by reading the absorbance of a colored solution in every cuvette using an absorbed wavelength. Clean, unscratched cuvettes are considered a matched set if they all give the same (±0.005) absorbance reading.

The **detector** is checked for the absence of stray light and for response that is proportional to the light transmitted through the cuvette. **Stray light** is any light that reaches the detector but is not part of the analytical light beam. Stray light may enter through a misplaced cover, a crack in the instrument chassis or a reflecting surface between an ambient light source and the detector. When a colored solution is placed in

a cuvette and a wavelength is selected that is completely absorbed by the solution, the absorbance reading should be near infinity (0 %$T$). Any significant detector response indicates the presence of stray light, which must be minimized in order to obtain accurate absorbance readings.

Commercially available neutral density filters are used to check the linearity of detector response. These filters have known absorbance and known relationship between the absorbances of different filters. If their absorbance readings fall outside specification, the most common detector malfunction is loss of linearity at very high or very low readings. Fatigue may cause loss of linearity when the detector has been exposed to intense light that exhausted the readily available electrons on the photosensitive cathode. Allowing the detector to "rest" by protecting it from all light for a period of minutes to hours will allow the cathode to replenish its electrons and may restore linearity. If linearity is not restored, replacement or intervention by an electronics technician is indicated.

## Basic Spectrophotometer

The components of a basic spectrophotometer are usually arranged as shown in Figure 6–8. Absorbances of solutions are measured in either consecutive cuvettes or consecutively in one cuvette. In many instruments, the electrical output of the detector is sent to a central processor that stores the readings from calibrators and calculates absorbances and quantitative results for unknown samples.

### BICHROMATIC ANALYSIS

An alternative arrangement found in many high-output instruments places the monochromator between the cuvette and the detector (Figure 6–15). The advantage of this arrangement is that it allows use of several fiberoptic cables to direct light transmitted through the cuvette to several different interference filters and then to an array of photodiodes. Thus a single spectrophotometer can be used to measure a variety of analytes at a variety of wavelengths. This is the arrangement used in bichromatic analyzers.

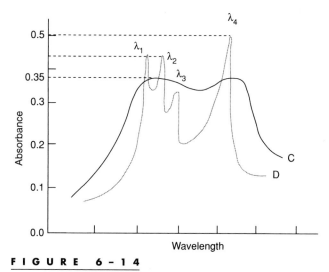

**FIGURE 6-14**

Comparison of the spectral scan using a wide bandpass width (curve C) and a narrow bandpass width (curve D).

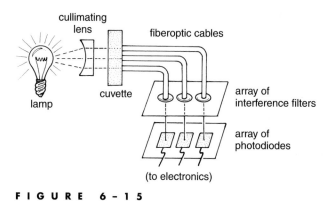

**FIGURE 6-15**

Components of a multiwavelength spectrophotometer.

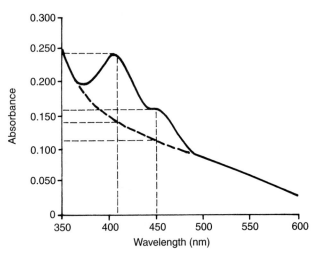

**FIGURE    6-16**

Absorption spectrum of a hemolyzed amniotic fluid.

In bichromatic analyzers, the primary filter selects the wavelength where the desired chromophore has maximum absorbance. The secondary filter is chosen because, at its wavelength, the desired chromophore has zero absorbance but common interfering substances do have absorbance. The interfering substances have a known relationship between their absorbances at the two wavelengths. The true absorbance that is due only to the desired chromophore can then be calculated.

*Example 6–5*

You are analyzing an amniotic fluid sample for bilirubin by measuring $\Delta A_{450}$, i.e., the difference between measured absorbance at 450 nm and the interpolated absorbance at 450 nm if bilirubin were not present. However, the sample also contains hemoglobin, which has an absorption peak at 410 nm but also absorbs at 450 nm. Bichromatic analysis can be used to correct for this overlapping absorbance because the absorbance of hemoglobin at 410 nm is known to be 20 times its absorbance at 450 nm. Bilirubin does not absorb at 410 nm.

The absorption spectrum of the amniotic fluid is scanned between 350 and 600 nm (Figure 6–16) and these data are obtained:

| | |
|---|---|
| Absorbance at 450 nm | 0.162 |
| Absorbance at 410 nm | 0.248 |
| Interpolated absorbance at 450 nm without bilirubin | 0.118 |

Calculate the $\Delta A450$ for this sample:

Absorbance at 450 nm corrected
for hemoglobin = 0.162 − (0.248/20) = 0.150
$$\Delta A450 = 0.150 - 0.118 = 0.032$$

Bichromatic analysis is used to correct for interference when a color-producing reaction is performed on a patient's sample that is hemolyzed, icteric, or lipemic. Here the absorbance measured at the analytical wavelength may be a composite of the absorbance due to the desired chromophore plus absorbance due to the background color or turbidity of the sample (Example 6–5 and Figure 6–16).

The processing unit of many laboratory instruments automatically calculates the bichromatic correction for common interfering substances. For naturally occurring colored or turbid interfering substances, bichromatic analysis is an effective method for obtaining accurate (corrected) absorbance readings that does not require additional sample or additional analysis time.

### DOUBLE-BEAM SPECTROPHOTOMETER

Another method of correcting for inherent color or turbidity in samples uses a double-beam spectrophotometer (Figure 6–17). This instrument splits the light beam into two paths, sending one through the analytical solution and the other through a serum blank in which the sample was not allowed to produce chromophore (See Blanking and Checking a Spectrophotometer earlier in this chapter). The absorbances of both solutions are read at the analytical wavelength. The absorbance of the solution in the analytical cuvette is the sum of absorbance owing to the desired chromophore plus absorbance from interfering substances contributed by the sample; the absorbance in the blank cuvette is the result of interfering substances only. The true absorbance due to the desired chromophore equals the difference between the two readings.

All components of the instrument contribute to both light beams. Therefore, small deviations in lamp intensity or detector sensitivity affect both light beams equally and do not affect the net absorbance reading. The major advantage of double-beam spectrophotometry compared to bichromatic analysis is that it does not rely on any assumptions regarding relative absorbances of different interfering substances at different wavelengths. Its disadvantages are that it requires twice as much sample as well as a separate reagent. Modern automated analyzers do not use double-beam spectrophotometry to correct for interfering substances.

### Fluorometer and Fluorescence Polarization Spectrophotometer

Fluorescent compounds are uncommon; they are most often compounds with conjugated (alternating) double bonds. The valence electrons of fluorescent compounds are able to temporarily achieve higher level orbits by absorbing the energy of photons just as other chromophores do. However, in fluorescent compounds, those excited electrons lose a small amount of energy by kinetic motion or bond vibration and emit the remaining amount of energy as a photon (Figure 6–18). Nonfluorescent chromophores dissipate all of the excitation energy kinetically. The energy of the photon emitted by a fluorescent

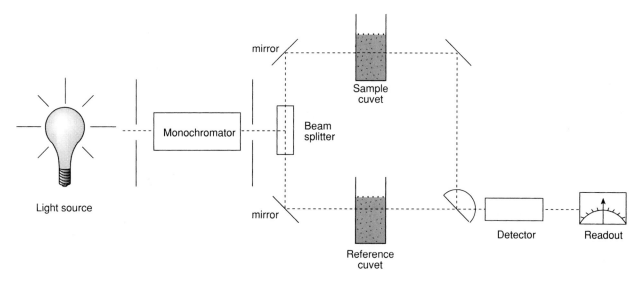

**F I G U R E   6 - 1 7**

Main components of a double-beam spectrophotometer.

molecule is less than the energy of the exciting photon; therefore, the wavelength emitted by a fluorescent molecule is always longer than the excitation wavelength. The time delay between excitation and emission is $10^{-8}$ to $10^{-4}$ seconds.

## FLUOROMETRY

A **fluorometer** is similar to a basic spectrophotometer in its light source, cuvette, and detector. It differs from a spectrophotometer in two basic ways: (1) it has two monochromators to select the excitation wavelength and the emission wavelength, and (2) the detector is at right angles to the excitation light beam in order to avoid measuring transmitted light (Figure 6–19).

Simple fluorometers use interference filters for both the primary and secondary monochromators, whereas scanning

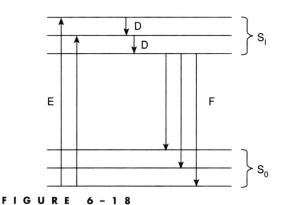

**F I G U R E   6 - 1 8**

Representation of fluorescence emission. $S_0$ = ground state with three vibrational energy levels; $S_1$ = first excited state with three vibrational energy levels; $E$ = excitation process; $D$ = radiationless vibrational deactivation; $F$ = fluorescence emission.

fluorometers require the continuous wavelengths from diffraction gratings. The excitation wavelength of many fluorescent compounds is in the ultraviolet range, which requires that the lamp provide ultraviolet wavelengths; xenon lamps are commonly used. Quartz cuvettes must be used because they are transparent to ultraviolet wavelengths of light. In addition, fluorometry cuvettes must meet optical quality standards in two dimensions: the axis of the incoming excitation light beam and the axis of the exiting emitted light beam.

Fluorometry has three major advantages compared to absorption spectrophotometry.[1] Fluorometric methods are often more specific than chromogenic methods. In both methods, the analyte only absorbs certain wavelength(s) and few (if any) other compounds in the solution will absorb that wavelength. Fluorometry has greater specificity because the secondary monochromator selects only the emitted wavelength of light. Positive interference could only occur from another compound that was fluorescent, absorbed the same wavelength, and emitted the same wavelength.[2] The amount of emitted light is directly proportional to the concentration of the fluorophore. Thus, no mathematical treatment of the data is required before calculating concentrations and, like absorbance, the relative amount of fluorescence does not have a unit associated with it. The proportionality also implies another contrast with absorption spectrophotometry, namely, there is only one anchor for calibrating the instrument scale of a fluorometer. A black cuvette is placed in the sample holder and the meter reading is adjusted to zero fluorescence similar to the method of setting 0 % $T$ (infinite absorbance) on a spectrophotometer. In fluorometry, there is no meter setting comparable to setting a blank at 100 % $T$ (0 absorbance) in a spectrophotometer; the fluorometer scale is open-ended.[3] Fluorometry is much more sensitive than absorption spectrophotometry. In both methods, the amount of incident (exciting) light that is absorbed

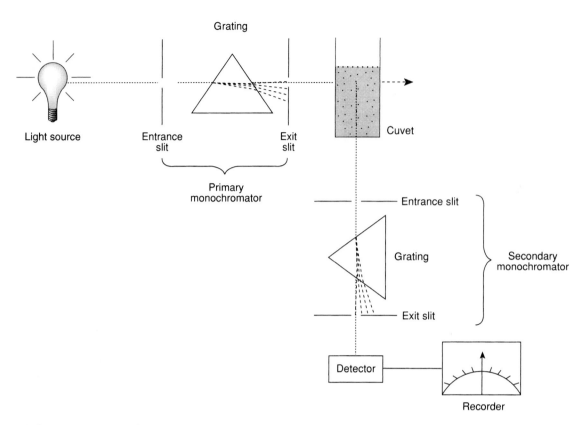

**FIGURE  6-19**

Components of a spectrofluorometer.

in the cuvette is directly proportional to the concentration of the analyte. But in fluorometry, when the emitted light is measured, it is compared to darkness, and in absorption spectrophotometry, it is compared to maximum transmitted light ($100\%\,T$). Thus, fluorescence emission has no theoretical upper limit. As long as there is sufficient excitation light to react with all the molecules of fluorophore, increased concentration will cause more emitted light to reach the detector. However, there is a practical upper limit to fluorescence readings because at very high concentrations of fluorophore, self-absorption of emitted light can occur. This reduces the amount of light reaching the detector and causes falsely low fluorescence readings.

There are several analytical disadvantages to fluorometry in addition to self-absorption at high concentration. Quenching is the term for decreased fluorescence readings due to absorption of emitted light by other solutes in the cuvette, e.g., solvents and reagents used in the fluorogenic reaction or contaminants from insufficient washing. Also, the amount of light emitted is sensitive to pH due to the effect on resonance stabilization of the molecule. Increased temperature causes decreased fluorescence (although the emitted wavelength is not changed) because heat increases the amount of energy that is dissipated by intermolecular collisions. Increased viscosity decreases the frequency of intermolecular collisions and causes increased fluorescence readings.

**Flow cytometry** is a modern technique for distinguishing different cell types by their surface antigens. Different fluorochromes are attached to antibodies that are specific for the surface antigens that identify different cell types. As the cells flow through a narrow tube in the flow cytometer, a xenon lamp or laser excites the different fluorophores and their emitted photons are detected by an array of interference filters and photomultiplier tubes. Flow cytometers also utilize nephelometric principles to count cells (See Nephelometer and Turbidimeter later in this chapter).

## FLUORESCENCE POLARIZATION

**Fluorescence polarization** is a modification of fluorometry that is specifically designed to measure homogeneous immunoassays. The instrument has all the components of a fluorometer plus two polarizing filters, one in front of each monochromator. A polarizing filter has the function of passing light waves that are in one plane and blocking all other light; it does not alter the wavelength of the light. The movement of the two polarizers is coordinated so that they alternate between being parallel and perpendicular to each other. When they are parallel, emitted light that is in the same plane as excitation light is passed to the detector; when they are perpendicular, emitted light that is in the same plane as excitation light is blocked from the detector.

The immunoassays that use this principle measure the amount of fluorescently labeled antigen that is bound to antibody in the cuvette. The fluorescent label on the antigen absorbs and emits light as usual for a fluorophore whether it is antibody-bound or unbound. However, during the $10^{-8}$ to $10^{-4}$ seconds between absorption and emission, the small, unbound fluorophore-antigen molecules rotate rapidly and thus emit light in a random plane instead of the plane of the excitation light. In contrast, the much greater molecular mass of the antibody-bound fluorophore-antigen molecules damps their movement so that their emitted light is in the same plane as the excitation light.

When the two polarizers of the instrument are parallel to each other, the emitted light striking the detector is mostly due to antibody-bound fluorophore-antigen and includes only a small random amount of light emitted by the unbound fluorophore-antigen. But when the two polarizers are perpendicular to each other, the light striking the detector is only the result of the same small random amount of light emitted by the unbound fluorophore-antigen. Subtracting the two fluorescence readings leaves only the emitted light resulting from the antibody-bound fluorophore-antigen, which is related to the concentration of antigen in the patient's sample.

## Nephelometer and Turbidimeter

When a photon in the light beam of a spectrophotometer strikes a solid particle in the cuvette, the photon is scattered. This is the principle of both nephelometry and turbidimetry. A **turbidimeter** measures the amount of light transmitted to the detector through a suspension of particles, that is, the amount of unscattered light. Like spectrophotometry, the amount of light transmitted in a turbidimeter is related to the concentration of suspended particles by a negative logarithm. Since absorbance is simply a mathematical concept, it is legitimate to say that absorbance (calculated from the transmitted light) is directly proportional to concentration of particles in a turbid solution.

**Nephelometry** measures the light that is scattered by suspended particles instead of the light that is transmitted through the suspension. The direction of maximum scatter depends on the relationship between particle size and the wavelength of light but in clinical practice most suspensions contain particles that are much larger than the wavelength of visible light. Under these circumstances, most of the scattered light is directed forward in a cone that surrounds the transmitted light beam (called Mie scatter).

The simplest form of a nephelometer is a fluorometer in which the secondary monochromator has been removed. The secondary monochromator is not needed because scattering does not alter the wavelength of the photons. Like fluorometry, the detector reading is directly proportional to the concentration of suspended particles. As in the comparison between fluorometry and spectrophotometry, nephelometry is more sensitive than turbidimetry for the same reason.

Two major disadvantages of turbidimetry and nephelometry are the problem of maintaining a homogeneous suspension in the path of the light beam and the assumption that all of the suspended particles are the same size. These are important considerations when measuring precipitated particles to determining the concentration of a soluble compound (e.g., measuring a protein by an antigen-antibody precipitin reaction). Nevertheless, over a fairly narrow range of concentrations and using very consistent techniques, turbidimetry and nephelometry can be used for quantitative analysis.

## Chemiluminometer

A recently developed method for immunoassay uses chemiluminescent compounds that are conjugated to antigens or antibodies to act as a label. Chemiluminescent compounds resemble fluorophores because they emit excess energy as photons. However, in contrast to fluorescence, the excitation is produced by a chemical reaction instead of absorbing a particular wavelength of light. Furthermore, self-quenching is not seen in chemiluminescence. A **chemiluminometer** resembles a spectrophotometer with a PMT detector. The PMT output is fed to an analogue-to-digital converter that counts the pulses of light emitted by the chemiluminescent reaction product. The number of pulses is used to calculate the concentration of labeled reagent, which is subsequently used to measure the unknown analyte concentration.

## Reflectance Spectrophotometer

Major examples of instruments that use reflectance spectrophotometry in clinical laboratories are urine dipstick readers and dry-slide technology instruments. As in spectrophotometry, a lamp and monochromator provide a suitable incident light beam that is directed to a colored reaction product. The chromophore of the reaction product absorbs an amount of light that is dependent on its concentration and the remaining light is reflected to a photodiode or PMT. Like multichannel spectrophotometers, fiberoptic cables may be used to direct the reflected light to several interference filters and several photodiodes.

Unfortunately, the relationship between reflected light and concentration of chromophore is not linear. Although a single calibrator is sufficient when reflectance is used for qualitative results, quantitative results require multiple calibrators and a complex algorithm (called a spline) that is built into the microprocessor.

## SUMMARY

The wavelength of light and its energy level are inversely proportional to each other. Thus, short wavelength light can damage cells (ultraviolet, X rays, gamma radiation). Visible light, which includes wavelengths 350 through 750 nm, and ultraviolet light, which includes wavelengths from 190 through 350 nm, are used in clinical spectrophotometry. These wavelengths have energy in the same range as chemical bonds and the electrons in the bonds can absorb light of corresponding energy level.

The exact pattern of wavelengths that is absorbed by chemical bonds in a compound determines the color of the compound and its absorption spectrum. When white light (containing all visible wavelengths) shines on a colored solution, the solute molecules absorb certain wavelengths leaving the remaining wavelengths to be transmitted through the solution. Those wavelengths that are transmitted determine the perceived color of the solution and are complementary to the wavelengths that were absorbed.

Spectrophotometry (also called transmission spectrophotometry) measures the concentration of a dissolved solute by measuring the amount of light of specific wavelength that is transmitted through a solution. The percent of light that is transmitted (%$T$) is proportional to the negative logarithm of the number of light-absorbing solute molecules in the light path. By making the depth of the solution constant, the %$T$ depends only on the concentration of the solute.

Absorbance, defined as the negative logarithm of the fraction of light transmitted, is a convenient simplification for converting light measurement into concentration. When solvent alone ("blank solution") is used to calibrate the spectrophotometer at 100 %$T$, then Beer's law can be used to estimate the concentration of solute by using proportions:

$$\frac{A_{unknown}}{A_{calibrator}} = \frac{Concentration_{unknown}}{Concentration_{calibrator}}$$

The broad term spectrophotometry encompasses several variations that use the light-absorbing properties of chemical bonds to detect solutes and measure their concentrations. All variations require the same basic components, though they are arranged in different orientations for specific applications.

The light source in any spectrophotometer must provide the desired wavelength. Tungsten-halogen lamps are most commonly used for visible wavelengths, and deuterium or xenon lamps are used for ultraviolet wavelengths. An interference filter is a convenient method for selecting a narrow band of wavelengths from the spectrum provided by the lamp, whereas a diffraction grating separates the light into its complete spectrum of wavelengths and uses an exit slit to select the desired band of wavelengths. Both of these monochromators provide

acceptably narrow bandpass of wavelengths for accurate analyses. The solution being analyzed is held in a cuvette made of optical quality glass or plastic that must be transparent to the wavelength of light being used. Photomultiplier tubes are often used as the detector in spectrophotometry because of their high sensitivity and rapid response. Photodiodes are a common alternative since they can be manufactured in an array that allows simultaneous absorbance readings at multiple wavelengths of light. Bichromatic analyzers and double-beam spectrophotometers utilize multiple absorbance readings to correct for absorbance by extraneous colored solutes found in patients' samples.

Fluorescence spectrophotometry is applicable to those compounds that fluorescently re-emit light energy that was absorbed by their chemical bonds. The emitted wavelength of light is always longer than the absorbed wavelength because of energy lost kinetically. Fluorometry is more sensitive than absorption spectrophotometry, but it is also subject to more interferences such as self-absorption and quenching. Fluorescence polarization spectrophotometry is an adaptation of fluorometry that allows distinction between fluorophores that are bound to small molecular weight compounds and those that are bound to large molecular weight compounds. Nephelometry and turbidimetry are variations of spectrophotometry that are used to measure insoluble particles in suspension. The amount of light transmitted through the suspension (turbidimetry) or scattered by the insoluble particles (nephelometry) can be related to the concentration of particles in a manner analogous to transmission spectrophotometry or fluorometry. Chemiluminometry resembles fluorometry by measuring emitted light, though the manner of producing the light is chemical instead of physical. Reflectance spectrophotometry is analogous to ordinary transmission spectrophotometry in that it measures the light that is not absorbed by the colored analyte. However, in this case, the light is reflected from the material that is supporting the analyte.

## REFERENCES

1.  Burtis CA, Ashwood ER: *Tietz Textbook of Clinical Chemistry*, 3rd ed. Philadelphia, W. B. Saunders, 1998.
2.  Karselis TC: *The Pocket Guide to Clinical Laboratory Instrumentation*. Philadelphia, F. A. Davis, 1994.
3.  Lehmann CA, Leiken AM, Ward KM: *Clinical Laboratory Instrumentation and Automation*, 2nd ed. Philadelphia, W. B. Saunders, 1997.

# CHAPTER 7
# Principles of Molecular and Immunoassays

*Audrey E. Hentzen*

## INTRODUCTION

### Target Molecules

Target molecules for molecular and immunoassays are biological substances that are specifically found in disease conditions or made by an infectious agent. These molecules are unique to those infectious agents or disease states and are not normally present in healthy individuals. Antibodies or molecular probes can be synthesized to bind to protein structures (antigens) or nucleic acid target molecules so that they can be detected for clinical diagnosis. Whether the target molecule is nucleic acid, protein, or a modification of either of these, they can serve as targets for molecular and immunoassays that are rapid, sensitive, and specific. Target molecules can be obtained from infected or diseased tissue or tumor cells and used in the development of assays for clinical testing. Nucleic acids can be isolated, cloned, and their sequence characterized by molecular techniques. Proteins can be purified, sequenced, and antibody made through traditional and new molecular methods. The GenBank is a depository of nucleic acid and protein sequences that are accessible by anyone.[1] Scientists contribute nucleic acid and protein sequences as they become known so that others may utilize this information in their research. The Human Genome Project has provided complete mapping and sequencing of all genes and will correlate genes with protein products and functions.

### Types of Nucleic Acids

Nucleic acid can be found free in the cytoplasm of prokaryotic cells or within the nucleus organelle of eukaryotic cells. Viruses also contain nucleic acid, usually bound to protein within their viral capsid. Nucleic acid is of two types, **deoxyribonucleic acid (DNA)** or **ribonucleic acid (RNA);** both are composed of nucleotides and sugar-phosphate backbones (Figure 7–1**a.** and 7–1**b.**). DNA is a double-stranded molecule (dsDNA) that forms a double helix through its hydrogen bonding. The **nucleotide** bases found in each strand of DNA are adenine (A), guanine (G), cytosine (C), and thymine (T), each of which is attached to a sugar molecule (deoxyribose) bound to a phosphate group. The base with the sugar group forms a nucleoside. RNA contains A, G, C as well, but uracil (U) is used instead of T in forming polymers of RNA (Figure 7–1**b.**). A and G are purines, whereas C, T, and U are pyrimidines and due to the nature of their hydrogen bonding, A can only bind T or U and G can only bind C (Figure 7–1**c.**). This principle is essential and naturally inherent in DNA and is extremely useful in molecular probe assays.

### Nucleic Acid Synthesis

DNA is the molecule that carries within its structure the genetic code or gene information for all of the cell processes needed to maintain life. Genes determine the structure and function of all molecules within an organism and this is encrypted in the nucleic acid sequence (one gene, one protein concept). A gene is a hereditary unit or sequence of ACGT nucleotides, occupying a fixed location or locus in the chromosome. DNA is replicated during the cell cycle and passed to future generations of the organism. DNA is rewritten or transcribed into three types of RNA, **messenger RNA (mRNA),** which carries the message of the protein to the cytoplasm for protein synthesis (translation), **transfer RNA (tRNA),** which is part of the translation machinery and functions primarily in transporting appropriate amino acids to the translational apparatus, and **ribosomal RNA (rRNA),** which combines with ribosomal proteins to form ribosomes, which are the physical translational apparatus where protein synthesis occurs.

DNA is located within the nucleus, a membrane-bound organelle in eukaryotic cells or as a circular strand in the cytoplasm of prokaryotic organisms, which do not contain organelles. DNA must be replicated prior to cell division and a finely orchestrated series of events utilizing enzymes accomplishes this task of copying it exactly.[2] DNA replication is a semiconservative process, that is, each parent strand of dsDNA is a template to direct the synthesis of a new DNA or daughter strand. Each new cell will contain a parent strand and a newly synthesized complementary strand.

For DNA to be copied, it must first be unwound or opened up. To do this, the enzyme helicase nicks one strand of DNA and allows it to rotate about the other strand of DNA and then reconnects it forming the double strand again (Figure 7–2). This forms a fork in the double helix that allows a short segment of the single-stranded DNA to be exposed. DNA is only synthesized in the 5′ to 3′ direction, by the enzyme DNA polymerase. DNA polymerase reads the parent

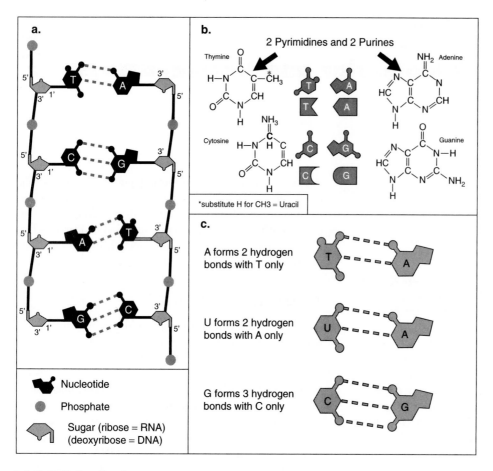

**F I G U R E   7 - 1**

Nucleic acid structure. **a.** Double-stranded nucleic acid showing sugar-phosphate backbone, nucleotides, and hydrogen bonding. The backbone of the DNA is a sugar molecule with the base attached to the first carbon of each sugar. The phosphate group is attached to the fifth carbon of ribose (RNA) and deoxyribose (DNA). There are four possible bases in DNA, adenine (A), guanine (G), cytosine (C), and thymine (T). RNA is single stranded and may form secondary structures through complementary binding to itself. RNA is similar to DNA in that it is made up of a sugar phosphate backbone except the sugar is not missing a hydroxyl group on the second carbon. Additionally, uracil (U) base is used instead of T in RNA molecules. **b.** Nucleotide structure of ACGT and uracil substitution. **c.** A · T, A · U, and G · C specific base pairing due to the nature of the hydrogen bond formation.

strand of DNA in the 3′ to 5′ direction, matching A to T and G to C, connecting nucleotides into a polymer of DNA complementary to the parent strand. When the parent strand of DNA is unwound, one new strand can be synthesized continuously since the parent template sequence can be read 3′ to 5′ (moving away from the replication fork) while synthesizing DNA 5′ to 3′. However, the other parent strand is 5′ to 3′ and cannot be read in the 3′ to 5′ orientation to make a new DNA polymer. Instead, RNA primers (short polymers or oligonucleotides of RNA) bind as the DNA is exposed and offer a starting site for DNA polymerase to synthesize the new

DNA in the 5′ to 3′ direction. This forms many short pieces of DNA called Okazaki fragments. These must be connected to one another by the enzyme DNA ligase to form a continuous strand.

## Protein Synthesis

The flow of information encoded in the DNA sequence is through protein molecules, which can be structural, regulatory, or functional (enzymes). Genes within the DNA are activated through transcription factors, small proteins that bind

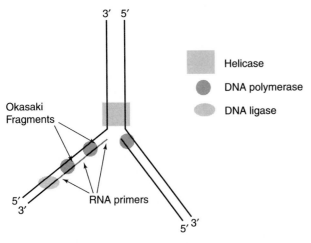

## FIGURE 7 - 2

DNA replication fork with enzymes and orientation. Helicase enzyme unwinds the DNA for replication. DNA is read 3′ to 5′ and synthesized by DNA polymerase in the 5′ to 3′ direction. The leading arm is continuous, whereas the lagging arm is made up of discontinuous Okazaki fragments. Okazaki fragments are synthesized by binding DNA polymerase to RNA primers and extension of those primers. Fragments are then joined together by the enzyme DNA ligase to make the strand continuous.

DNA promoter sites.[3] Promoter sites are special sequences of DNA that signal the initiation of RNA transcription. Once the transcription factors have bound, the enzyme RNA polymerase can associate with the promoter site to synthesize RNA. DNA is read 3′ to 5′, whereas the new complementary strand of RNA is made 5′ to 3′. There are three types of RNA made from DNA: messenger RNA (mRNA), transfer RNA (tRNA), and ribosomal RNA (rRNA). In eukaryotic organisms there are three RNA polymerases that carry out the production of these RNAs. RNA polymerase I transcribes preribosomal RNA, RNA polymerase II synthesizes mRNAs, and RNA polymerase III synthesizes tRNA (Figure 7–3**a.**).[4] mRNA carries the genetic information to the cytoplasm where it associates with ribosomes and is translated into an amino acid sequence (7–3**b.**). rRNA associates with proteins to form ribosomes, the synthetic machinery for the translational process. tRNAs are adapter molecules that read the mRNA information, one codon at a time, binding the codon sequence in a complementary manner. A codon is a triplet of bases in the mRNA that specifies a single amino acid. The tRNA will transfer the appropriate amino acid to the growing polypeptide chain during protein synthesis. Some amino acids have more than one codon to direct the recruitment and placement of that amino acid in the primary amino acid sequence; this is called degeneracy. Primary amino acid sequence may be made freely in the cytoplasm or protected from the cytoplasmic environment by

**a.**

| RNA Polymerase | Product |
|---|---|
| RNA Pol I | Ribosomal RNA |
| RNA Pol II | messenger RNA |
| RNA Polymerase III | transfer RNA |

**b.**

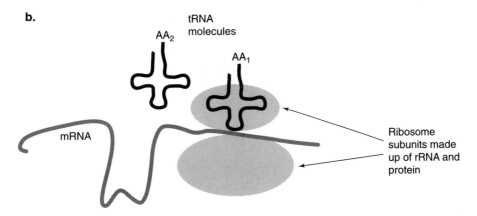

## FIGURE 7 - 3

**a.** The three types of RNA polymerase (RNA Pol) and their products. **b.** Diagram of the translational apparatus where proteins are formed. mRNA associates with the ribosome, then tRNA brings in the appropriate amino acid by complementary binding of the tRNA anti-codon to the mRNA codon. An amino acid polymer is created by the formation of a peptide bond between adjacent amino acids brought to the translational apparatus by tRNA.

synthesis into the endoplasmic reticulum. Either way, the primary amino acid sequence may form secondary, tertiary, and quaternary structures that are further modified by post-translational enzymes. Proteins may be retained within the cell's cytoplasm or internal membranes or placed on the plasma membrane or even secreted. Control or trafficking of proteins within the cell is a complex, highly regulated process.[4]

## SPECIMEN COLLECTION AND HANDLING

### Immunoassays

Immunoassays are designed to detect antigens or antibodies present in patient samples. Serum or plasma should be collected using the normal venipuncture procedures and precautions. Serum should be separated from the clot and can be refrigerated at 2 to 8°C for up to 2 days following collection. If there is a longer delay in running the test, the specimen should be frozen. For accurate results, the specimen should not be hemolyzed or grossly lipemic. Icteric specimens with high porphyrin content may also cause problems in some of the assays. If the serum or plasma does contain particulate matter, it should be centrifuged at 1000 × g for 15 minutes before testing. Each manufacturer package insert indicates the proper sample collection method and storage for that assay procedure.

For fluorescent immunoassays, if possible, blood specimens should be collected from fasting subjects, as lipids tend to stick to the glass and produce a green halo of nonspecific fluorescence. It is important to prevent hemolysis, since fluorescing porphyrins can interfere with the reading of a test.

Urine samples for hormone and drug testing may be collected in plastic or glass containers. Freshly voided urine specimens should be used. If not tested within 1 day, samples may be stored at 2 to 8°C for up to 3 days to avoid drug degradation. To store samples longer than 3 days, keep them frozen and thaw just prior to testing. Samples should be at room temperature for testing. The effect of urine preservatives has not been established and their use is not recommended. Drug analysis results of samples that are known to be drug free have not been observed to test positive due to storage conditions or pH changes.

### Molecular Assays

Molecular assays examine patient samples for the presence of specific nucleotide sequences in nucleic acids (DNA or RNA) by specialized techniques. In certain human disease states (genetic, hematologic disorders, and cancer), base sequence may be altered, deleted, or rearranged and can be detected by molecular techniques. Additionally, assays are designed to detect and identify foreign DNA or RNA, which correlates with nucleic acid belonging to pathogenic microorganisms, viruses, fungi, and parasites.

A number of different technologies have been developed, and in some cases multiple methods are available to detect the same abnormality. The selection of one methodology over another is dependent on an individual laboratory's clinical use, sensitivity, specificity, cost, turnaround time, technical expertise, and knowledge requirements for personnel.

DNA is relatively stable at room temperature and it can be recovered from organisms that are not viable. The nucleic acid remains chemically intact enough to be manipulated by bioengineering techniques even after centuries of dormancy, inactivity, or cold storage. mRNA on the other hand is extremely labile and sensitive to RNAse digestive enzymes that are found in cellular extracts and secreted on your fingertips. RNAse inhibitors may be added to sample lysates to protect mRNA until it can be reverse transcribed into complementary DNA (cDNA), which is more stable and useful for further testing. Gloves must be worn at all times when working with mRNA to reduce exposure to RNAse. rRNA is considerably more stable than mRNA due to its association with ribosomal proteins to form ribosomes. rRNA can be stored at room temperature until the sample is lysed but once cellular enzymes are released on cell lysis, the rRNA should be processed. rRNA can also be reverse transcribed or in some cases measured directly.

Universal precautions should be observed when handling any patient samples, tissues, or infectious agents. Blood should be drawn into yellow top (ACD solution A) tubes, filled completely, and stored at room temperature or refrigerated if RNA is the target molecule. Amniocytes and chorionic villi for cell culture and cytogenetics are collected and placed in media containing culture flasks and stored or shipped at room temperature. Additionally, amniotic fluid, fixed tissue, and cheek swabs are also processed, stored, or shipped at room temperature. Vaginal swabs for direct nucleic acid testing for *Candida albicans, Gardnerella vaginalis, Trichomonas vaginalis* (VP AFFIRM, Becton Dickinson, Franklin Lanes, NY), *Neisseria gonorrhoeae, Chlamydia trachomatis,* and *Mycobacterium tuberculosis* (Gen-Probe, San Diego, CA) testing are stored and processed at room temperature. *N. gonorrhoeae* and *Chlamydia* samples used for testing by molecular probes are stable for up to 7 days, compared to fastidious culture requirements, and thus remove the urgency for culture setup and viable growth.

## IMMUNOASSAYS

### Immunogenicity and Antigen-Antibody Interactions

Several terms used throughout this chapter may need to be defined to aid in the overall understanding of immunoassay principle. In particular, **antigen** is often misused as a synonym for immunogen. An **immunogen** is a substance that when introduced into a particular species stimulates an immune response and the production of immunoglobulins or **antibodies** that recognize and bind to the immunogen. An immunogen stimulates the production of antibodies in contrast to an antigen that only combines with an antibody. The part of the antibody molecule that makes contact with the antigen during an antigen-antibody reaction is called the **antibody-binding site.** The portion of the antigen that combines with the binding site of the antibody is called an **antigenic determinant.** This is a three-dimensional chemical structure present on an antigen that determines the specificity of the antigen-antibody reaction. **Specificity** of an antigen-antibody reaction is the degree to which an antibody binds to a particular antigen (e.g., homologous antigen) while not binding structurally similar molecules. A heterologous antigen is a molecule with a similar structure that participates in a weaker, nonspecific antigen-antibody reaction referred to as a cross-reaction. A high-molecular-mass antigen can have more than a single antigenic determinant, such as human chorionic gonadotropin hormone, allowing it to react with several different antibody molecules. A **hapten** is a low-molecular-mass molecule (<20,000 daltons) such as a drug that acts as a single antigenic determinant. It is incapable of eliciting an antibody response when injected into an animal unless it is coupled to a macromolecular carrier.

## Monoclonal Antibodies

Each B cell produces an antibody that binds only to a specific part or antigenic determinant of an immunogen. The serum of an animal immunized with an immunogen contains polyclonal antibodies, a mixture of antibodies that recognize different antigenic determinants. Monoclonal antibodies are synthesized by a single population of B cells (a clone) and the antibody that results from the clonal expansion is homogeneous in structure and specificity for the stimulating antigen.

This natural phenomenon has been harnessed by bioengineers to develop techniques for the production of monoclonal antibodies that are specific for single antigenic determinants. These techniques include genetically engineered chimeric monoclonal antibodies or grafting mouse complementarity-determining regions into human variable regions of an Ig molecule for expression by bacterial cultures and the formation of B lymphocyte–hybridoma cell lines that are eternal and produce monoclonal antibodies.[5] These antibodies are chemically, physically, and immunologically homogeneous since each antibody is made from cells originating from a single cell. Production of the monoclonal antibody has allowed the development of immunoassays that are highly specific for antigens associated with infectious agents, certain disease states, or even therapeutic drug monitoring.

## Antigen-Antibody Reactions

Immunoassays are procedures that rely on the use of antibodies as "specific" binding reagents. These assays are used in most

clinical laboratories to quantitate or determine the presence of therapeutic and nontherapeutic drugs, numerous biological substances, infectious agents, or host-response antibodies in serum, urine, and cerebrospinal fluid. The principle of these assays is that a specific, reversible binding between an antigen and its corresponding antibody will take place and that this interaction will form a complex that can be differentiated from bound or "free" ligand. A **ligand** is any molecule that forms a specific complex with another molecule. To measure this interaction or complex formation, various labels have been covalently coupled to ligands that allow for the detection and quantitation of the molecule of interest. For many years the label of choice has been radionuclides, with the measurement of radioactivity used for the quantitation of these labels. These assays are referred to as radioimmunoassays and they provide accurate, sensitive, specific, and reproducible results. However, the use of radioisotopes poses a problem concerning special safety measures in the handling and disposal of these reagents. Increasing public awareness and concern about the dangers of radioisotopes has led to more stringent regulations that limit their use in the clinical setting. Enzyme immunoassays have essentially replaced radioimmunoassays, since these procedures use enzymes as labels and enzyme-substrate reactions to quantitate the molecule of interest. Recent use of fluorescent compounds as labels or the use of fluorogenic substrates in enzyme immunoassays have become more common as well.

The strength of the bond between an antigenic determinant of an antigen or hapten and the binding site of a single antibody is termed antibody **affinity.** The affinity is the summation of the attractive and repulsive forces between an antibody and its corresponding antigen. The binding affinity of an antibody can be expressed in terms of an equilibrium constant K, since the noncovalent bonding between an antibody and an antigen is reversible. K represents the approximate amount of antibody and antigen that will be in the form of a complex at any given time after the initial mixture and incubation of known concentrations of antigen and antibody. According to the law of mass action, $K =$ [Ab-Ag complex]/[Ab][Ag]. $K$ is also equal to the forward reaction rate $k_1$ (association due to attractive forces) divided by the reverse reaction rate $k_2$ (disassociation due to repulsive forces). $K = k_1/k_2 =$ [Ab-Ag]/[Ab][Ag].

$$\text{Antibody} + \text{Antigen} \underset{k_2}{\overset{k_1}{\rightleftharpoons}} \text{Antibody-antigen complex}$$

## Competitive-Binding Reactions

Competitive-binding reactions are frequently used in the various immunoassay procedures. The principle of these reactions is that binding of an antigen to an antibody (specific for that antigen) takes place in proportion to antigen concentration contained in a standard, control, or test sample. Not all of the antigen will be bound since it is competing with a fixed amount of labeled antigen, also present in the reagent mix, for a limited number of antibody-binding sites. In competitive assays, there are several idealized assumptions: (1) the antigens and antibodies are homogeneous and that their reversible interaction will reach equilibrium, (2) the label on an antigen in no way interferes with the antigen-antibody interaction, (3) the antibody and antigen can only form bimolecular complexes (i.e., both the antigen and the antibody are univalent), and (4) antigen-antibody complexes can be separated completely from free labeled-antigen. Deviations from these ideal conditions change only the details without changing the general properties of competitive reaction immunoassays.

Competitive assays, also utilized in molecular test systems, are under similar assumptions but they apply to the unique interaction between oligonucleotide probes (or primers in amplification methods) with target sequences and unlabeled synthetic nucleic acid sequence that is also complementary to the oligonucleotide. These unlabeled synthetic nucleic acid sequences are added to the reagent mix to compete with patient (target) nucleic acid for labeled probe during the hybridization reaction. Oftentimes, this competitive assay is used as a confirmatory test for direct or amplified assays.

## Radioactive Labels

### RADIOIMMUNOASSAY

**Radioimmunoassay** (RIA) is an immunologic technique that uses radioisotopes to detect antigens or antibodies in biological fluids. RIA was developed by Yalow and Berson[6] in 1959 based on the observation that the reaction between soluble antibodies and antigens will form an antigen-antibody **precipitate** or insoluble aggregate under optimal conditions. The RIA method incorporates a competitive-binding reaction in which a fixed amount of radiolabeled-antigen and antigen in the samples compete for a limited number of specific antibody binding sites. Both unlabeled and radiolabeled antigen are bound by the antibody and form precipitable complexes. Bound and free radiolabeled antigens must then be separated before the radioactivity of the bound radioisotope can be measured. The percentage of precipitated radiolabeled antigen decreases as the concentration of unlabeled antigen in the test sample increases. The concentration of the antigen in the test sample is therefore inversely related to the amount of radioactivity in the bound fraction.[7]

### Reagents

The antibody reagents used in RIAs are frequently attached to solid supports such as plastic tubes or polystyrene beads. The antibodies specifically recognize an antigen or hapten, i.e., a drug or a low-molecular-mass steroid hormone of interest. The antibody reagents can be characterized as either polyclonal (a mixture of purified antibodies recognizing different antigenic determinants of an antigen or the same portion of the antigen with differing affinities) or monoclonal (a solution containing identical antibody molecules recognizing a single antigenic determinant).[8]

The radiolabeled antigen or **hapten** is a purified molecule covalently labeled with a radioisotope. The radioisotope most frequently used is sodium iodide I 125 ($^{125}$I) which, for safety reasons, cannot be above 0.5 $\mu$Ci/tube.

Buffers are used in commercial RIA kits as diluents and generally contain EDTA, bovine serum albumin (BSA) to reduce nonspecific bindings and a preservative.

Standards and controls consist of human source material, sodium azide, and a stated concentration of antigen, hapten, or antigenic antibody of interest. Many of the RIAs and other immunoassay kits contain human source components that should be considered potentially infectious material and no known test can offer complete assurance that products derived from human sources will not transmit infection. It is recommended that these reagents and human specimens be handled and disposed of using good laboratory practices. Some reagents also contain sodium azide, which may react with lead and copper plumbing to form highly explosive metal azides. If waste is discarded down the drain, flush it with a large volume of water to prevent azide buildup.

### Assay Protocols and Separation Methods

RIAs are **heterogeneous immunoassays** that require the physical separation of free labeled antigen from antibody-bound radiolabeled antigen before the radioactivity of the bound label can be measured. The fundamental difference between heterogeneous immunoassays and homogeneous immunoassays is whether there are separation steps or washes before detection of the signal from the labeled substance. In **homogeneous immunoassays,** there are no separation or wash steps prior to detecting immunocomplex formation. Three commonly used heterogeneous immunoassay protocols and separation techniques are described below.

**Solid-phase attachment** is the simplest of the separation assay techniques and the most frequently used. Originally, Catt and associates[9] in 1966 observed that antibodies could be covalently coupled to polystyrene or polypropylene beads[10] and later reported, along with another group, that antibodies could be adsorbed to tubes consisting of these materials.[9,11] The present immunoassay techniques use antibodies adsorbed in a limited number to the inner wall of an assay tube. The samples containing the unlabeled antigen and radiolabeled antigen are added directly to the coated assay tubes. During an incubation period the antigens compete with each other for binding to a limited number of immobilized antibodies. Following incubation, the liquid is aspirated or decanted to remove free radiolabeled antigen in solution. The radioactivity of the labeled-antigen-antibody complex bound to the wall of the tube can then be quantitated using a gamma counter (Figure 7–4). Antibody can also be adsorbed onto polystyrene beads, which can be pelleted by centrifugation or polymer-coated iron oxide particles and are separated using a magnetic separation unit. This

**a.**

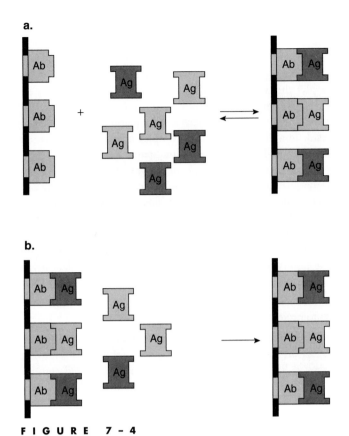

**b.**

**FIGURE 7-4**

Solid-phase attachment RIA. **a.** Radiolabeled antigen (shaded) and standards, controls, and samples containing antigen (Ag) are added to antibody (Ab) coated tubes. Labeled and unlabeled Ags compete for a limited number of Ab binding sites and form complexes. **b.** The free radiolabeled Ags are removed and the radioactivity of the bound fraction is measured.

unit retains the magnetic particles in a thin layer on the side of the assay tube so that the tube can be easily decanted.

The **"activated" charcoal** method of separation uses the adsorbent properties of activated or dextran-coated charcoal. Activated charcoal will adsorb low-molecular-mass antigens without binding antibody or antigen-antibody complexes. Using the adsorbent properties of activated charcoal, free radiolabeled antigens can be separated from bound by using centrifugation to pellet the charcoal. The radioactivity of the pellet containing the free label is then determined. The activated charcoal method has the advantage of reducing nonspecific binding or trapping of small molecules within the antigen-antibody complexes, although contact time with the charcoal is critical to achieve reproducible results. This technique cannot be used for high-molecular-mass antigen detection, since large molecules cannot be adsorbed by the charcoal. A more recent method using polystyrene beads coated with activated charcoal has made it even easier to separate the bound and free

fractions. Tubes containing the beads can easily be covered with a screen and decanted.

The **precipitation technique** is also based on an initial competitive reaction between radiolabeled antigen and unlabeled antigen for binding to a limited number of antibodies. However, the antigen-antibody complexes that are formed are separated from free label by precipitating them out of solution with saturated ammonium sulfate (Farr technique). A second precipitation technique uses a **double antibody** method to aid in the separation of the antigen-antibody complexes. To separate the bound and free labeled antigen, a second antibody, recognizing the primary antibody, is added, producing a large complex made up of radiolabeled antigen, primary antibody, and secondary antibody. The precipitates from either method can be pelleted by centrifugation. The radioactivity of the labeled antigen contained within the precipitate is then determined and used to quantitate the amount of antigen present in the test sample. A double antibody technique that does not require precipitation is one that uses a second antibody, e.g., recognizing the primary antibody adsorbed to polystyrene beads to aid in the separation of bound from free labeled antigen.

**Detection**

A gamma counter or scintillation counter is used to measure gamma rays or electromagnetic radiation emitted by very high energy isotopes. A **radioisotope** is an atom of an element possessing an increased number of neutrons in the nucleus. This increase creates an unstable nucleus that will spontaneously transform into more stable nuclear species with the emission of radiation. The unstable radioisotope nuclei are called **radionuclides** and are capable of emitting three kinds of radiation: alpha particles, positively or negatively charged electrons, and gamma rays. The gamma counter is used to measure emitted gamma rays, often referred to as radioactivity. A tube containing the radioisotope $^{125}I$ is placed into the gamma counter. The $^{125}I$ emits gamma rays, which strike the detector, a sodium iodide crystal activated by trace amounts of thallium and protected by lead to prevent background radiation. When gamma rays are adsorbed by the crystal, a brief flash of light is given off called **scintillation.** This in turn will be detected and amplified by a photomultiplier (PM) tube. By selecting the size of the pulse to be counted, it is possible to count the gamma emissions from one type of atom and exclude others. The pulse threshold is also selected so that pulses coming from the PM tube that are less than the preselected threshold will not be conducted. Many of the current scintillation counters have levels preset for commonly used radionuclides. The pulses are received and counted by a timing mechanism connected to a counting device. The final component is the readout, displayed in preset intervals of counts per minute (cpm).

**Standard Curve**

The data obtained in RIAs are plotted and the concentration of the antigen is determined from a dose-response curve. To plot a dose-response curve, one must know the amount of radiolabeled antigen that is bound to the antibody (cpm) and the amount of unlabeled antigen contained in each standard reagent. The percentage of radiolabeled antigen bound to antibody expressed as a percentage of the total amount of label added to each tube (% B) is plotted as a function of the log concentration of the unlabeled antigen contained in each standard creating a sigmoidal curve (Figure 7–5**a.**). The curvature

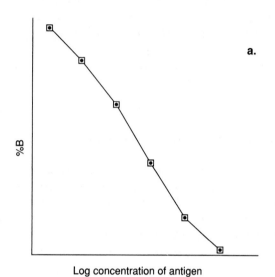

Log concentration of antigen

**a.**

%B

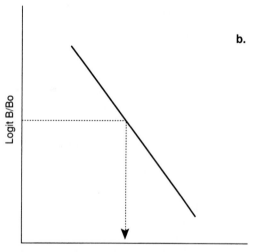

Log concentration of antigen

**b.**

Logit B/Bo

**FIGURE  7 – 5**

**a.** Representative schematic of a dose-response curve. The percentage of labeled antigen bound to antibody (%B) is plotted on the y-axis as a function of the corresponding log concentration of unlabeled antigen in each standard on the x-axis. **b.** Schematic of logit-log transformation. This is a plot of logit of bound cpm per total cpm (B/Bo) versus the log of the concentration of the unlabeled antigen in each standard.

represents the percentage of the labeled antigen that is bound when the concentration of the unlabeled antigen or dose is increased.

Although nonlinear curves can be plotted and used to interpret the data, linear plots are more advantageous if an error is present because an obvious variation in the linear pattern will be observed. There is no equation that will always result in a linear curve but a complex mathematical equation using **logit-log transformation** can approximate a linear curve. This is a plot of logit of the fraction of bound radioactivity (B/Bo) versus the log of the concentration of the unlabeled antigen in each standard (Figure 7–5**b.**). Bo represents the total amount of radioactivity added (cpm) or the zero standard. The disadvantage to the logit-log method of curve fitting is the frequent bias the system implies in the plotting of the results owing to the natural curvature of the data being plotted.

## Automation

RIAs are amenable to automation for large-scale processing. Automated approaches can be used to perform the following steps in RIA: (1) the addition of the sample, a fixed amount of the specific antibody, and a fixed amount of a labeled antigen, (2) incubation and performance of the actual separation of the bound and free antigens, (3) measurement of radioactivity, and (4) calculation of the test sample antigen concentration from a plotted standard curve. Most automated instruments, although they differ greatly in design, are capable of performing these tasks without the need of an operator. This eliminates the risks of working with radioactive materials. Other important aspects of RIA automation include the precision and reproducibility that cannot be attained manually.[12]

## Advantages and Disadvantages

One of the advantages of RIA is the use of a high-gamma-emitting radioisotope label, [125]I, which creates an assay that is sensitive enough to detect antigen at the picomolar concentration or lower. **Sensitivity** is the degree of response to a change in the ligand concentration represented by a dose-response curve. Sensitivity is dependent on the label used in the assay and the affinity of the antibody for an antigen. This term is synonymous with the specific detection and the limit of that detection within an assay. Chemiluminescence detection systems have been developed and are rapidly replacing many RIAs because of their limit of detection and ease of use without the inherent risk. RIA is easily automated as mentioned above and practical if large batches are to be tested. Disadvantages are that radioisotope labels have a short shelf life of 1 to 2 months, which causes inefficiency, high cost, and waste. These substances can also be inconvenient and expensive to dispose of and store. Finally, unless dealing with a fully automated system, the dangers of human exposure to radioisotopes must also be considered. In laboratories that work with radioisotopes, regulations must be monitored by a licensed radiation safety committee and the instrumentation and the manner in which the isotopes are handled are subject to routine inspections.

## Laboratory Applications

Radioimmunoassays are used to quantitate high- and low-molecular-mass hormones, normal and abnormal plasma proteins, coagulation factors, antibodies directed toward viral antigens, isoenzymes, and cerebrospinal fluid myelin basic protein. They are also used to monitor therapeutic drug levels.

## IMMUNORADIOMETRIC ASSAY

The principle of the **immunoradiometric assay** (IRMA) is that a radiolabeled antibody is used to determine the presence of an antigen in biological fluids. The IRMA uses an excess of radiolabeled antibody to detect all of the antigen present, making this a noncompetitive assay. This excess eliminates the requirement for a purified antigen reagent, which is often difficult to obtain in sufficient quantities. A separation step is required to differentiate between radiolabeled antibody bound to the antigen and free label. The radioactivity of the bound label is then determined using a gamma counter. The IRMA is similar to RIA in that radiolabeled molecules are used to detect antigen-antibody reactions. However, in IRMAs the radiolabeled molecule is an antibody as opposed to a radiolabeled antigen in the RIA. In addition, all of the unlabeled antigen is bound by the presence of excess antibody, making the IRMA a more sensitive assay as compared with RIA.

There are two types of IRMAs used in the clinical laboratory, a two-site, solid-phase assay and a one-site, fluid-phase assay. **Two-site, solid-phase** immunoradiometric assay, also known as the "sandwich" technique,[13] is used to detect high-molecular-mass antigens with at least two antigenic determinants. This assay relies on the use of an immobilized antibody specific for a unique antigenic determinant on the antigen of interest and a second antibody labeled with [125]I that recognizes a second unique antigenic determinant on the same molecule. Samples containing the antigen are added to antibody-coated tubes, followed by the addition of a second antibody labeled with [125]I. During incubation, the antigen binds to the immobilized antibody, which orients the antigen so that the labeled antibody can bind to its recognition site forming a sandwich. Following incubation, any free labeled antibody is removed by decanting the tube. The radioactivity of the bound fraction is then determined (Figure 7–6). There are several variations in the above-mentioned protocol depending on the antigen to be assayed. The forward two-step method described above is the most commonly used two-site IRMA. The reverse two-step method changes the order in which the antibody reagents are added. Finally, the simplest and fastest method is when the antibody reagents are added simultaneously, although this method is not always applicable.

## Reagents

Unlabeled antibody reagents are generally adsorbed onto a solid support. The adsorbed antibody is often referred to as the primary antibody and specifically recognizes a unique anti-

**a.**

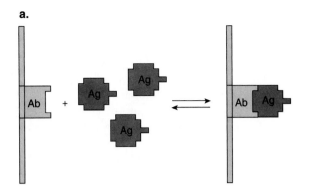

**b.**

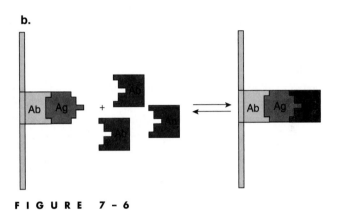

### FIGURE 7-6

Two-site, solid-phase IRMA. **a.** Samples, controls, and standards containing antigen (Ag) are added to antibody (Ab)-coated tubes and Ag-Ab complexes are formed. **b.** A radiolabeled second Ab (shaded) is added that recognizes and binds to a unique site on the same Ag, forming a larger complex. The free labeled second Ab is then removed and the radioactivity is measured.

genic determinant on the antigen of interest. The antibodies are frequently monoclonal antibodies which are rapidly replacing the use of polyclonal antiserum. Monoclonal antibodies can be produced in large quantities using the hybridoma technology developed by Kohler and Milstein[8] and are high affinity, homogeneous reagents, specific for a single antigenic determinant. A second antibody labeled with [125]I (usually monoclonal) is directed toward a second unique antigenic determinant on the same antigen. As mentioned under RIA in this chapter, the label cannot exceed $0.5\beta Ci$/tube limiting the amount of [125]I-labeled antibody that can be added.

Reference standards and high and low controls are provided in the assay kit and contain specified amounts of antigen. The reagents are run in duplicate with the test samples.

## Standard Curve

The bound radioactivity is assessed in counts per minute (cpm) and the average cpm for the background is subtracted from the average for each duplicate standard, control, and sample. Using semi-log paper or linear graph paper, the average cpm for each standard is plotted on the y-axis and the concentration of each standard is plotted on the x-axis. A smooth curve is drawn through all five standard points. The concentration of each test sample and control can be determined by finding the value of the average cpm on the standard curve and reading the x-axis for the proper concentration. A linear curve is possible if monoclonal antibody reagents are used and the concentration of antigen does not exceed the amount of antibody reagent.

The **one-site, fluid phase** IRMA depends on the selective precipitation of immunocomplexes.[9,14] Radioiodinated antibody in solution is incubated with standards, controls, or test samples containing antigen. A labeled antigen-antibody complex is formed and separated from free labeled antibody by differential precipitation using ammonium sulfate. The radioactivity in the precipitate is directly related to the concentration of the unlabeled antigen contained in the standards, controls, and test samples. The excess free labeled antibody can also be removed by adding precipitating binders, often antigen-coated beads, and radioactivity is determined in the fluid phase rather than the precipitate. The amount of radioactivity in the final step of the one-site technique is measured and expressed as a percentage of the total amount of label added to each tube. This information is plotted on a linear-logarithmic graph and used to construct a dose-response curve. This technique is not frequently used in assays developed for clinical laboratories.

### Advantages and Disadvantages

The IRMA is a faster and more sensitive assay than the RIA because the antibody is present in excess, increasing the chances of antigen-antibody interaction and all of the unknown antigen is bound. The use of radiolabeled antibody (1) eliminates the need to isolate the antigen, which is often present in very low quantities, (2) provides reagents that are more stable, and (3) decreases the problems of labeling structurally dissimilar antigens. Nonspecific binding tubes containing the labeled reagent are run concurrently with each RIA and IRMA assay to determine the amount of nonspecific binding of labeled reagent to an assay tube or to serum proteins. In general, the nonspecific binding in RIA is higher than in the IRMA, particularly when using radiolabeled-monoclonal antibody. In the two-site, solid-phase technique, two antibodies are used, increasing the specificity of the assay. However, this technique requires the production of two specific antibody reagents for the detection of one molecule, which is not always possible. As mentioned earlier under RIA, there are numerous disadvantages in the use of radioisotopes.

### Laboratory Applications

IRMAs are used for the measurement of serum proteins, coagulation factor VIII, ferritin, thyroid-binding protein, carcinoembryonic antigen, alpha-fetoprotein, IgE, prostatic acid phosphatase, prostatic-specific antigen, and hormones such as thyroid-stimulating hormone, prolactin, human growth hormone, serum, and urine human chorionic gonadotropin.

## ENYZME LABELS

The assays using enzyme labels are generally referred to as enzyme immunoassays (EIA) or enzyme-labeled molecular probes. There are many variations of immunotechniques that are enzyme-linked assays, whereas the molecular-enzyme linked assay uses an enzyme-labeled probe for the detection of the hybridization reaction. Enzymes increase the sensitivity of the assay due to their turnover rate and ability to catalyze chemical reactions.

### Enzyme-Linked Immunosorbent Assay

The **enzyme-linked immunosorbent assay** (ELISA) uses an enzyme label instead of a radioisotopic label to measure the formation of antigen-antibody complexes. Numerous variations of the ELISA method are available for the detection and quantitation of high-molecular-mass ligands ($>30,000$ daltons) but all of the methods are based on principles originally described by Engvall and Perlmann[15] and Van Weemen and Schuurs in 1971.[16] The enzyme label used in these assays is conjugated to a ligand, which can be an antigen, an antibody specific for the antigen of interest, or an antibody to the primary antibody. Most ELISAs are solid-phase assays in which an antigen or antibody is adsorbed onto a solid support. Some of the protocols rely on competitive and others noncompetitive binding reactions but all ELISAs require a separation step to remove free enzyme conjugate before the amount of bound enzyme conjugate can be determined. The determination of bound enzyme conjugate requires the addition of the enzyme substrate and the measurement of an enzyme-substrate catalytic reaction. Enzymes, because of their catalytic properties, are very sensitive and versatile labels. A single enzyme protein has the ability to convert, within minutes, a large number of substrate molecules to an equally large number of the end product, producing an amplified and easily detectable color change. In the **inhibition ELISA** method, the color change is reduced rather than enhanced because the enzyme activity is inhibited by the binding of the antibody to the enzyme conjugate.

The principle of the ELISA is based on several assumptions: (1) the antigen or antibody can be linked to an insoluble carrier surface and will retain immunologic reactivity, (2) the enzymes have a high specific activity, converting a relatively large amount of substrate to detectable product (related to signal amplification), allowing for the detection of very low concentrations of ligand, (3) enzymatic activity or immunologic reactivity of the conjugates is preserved and remains stable during assay and storage, and (4) the enzymes are not present in the biological fluid that is to be analyzed.

## Reagents

Antibodies used in the ELISA can be monoclonal in origin[8] or polyclonal supplied as unfractionated antiserum or purified immunoglobulin fractions. The antibodies may be soluble or immobilized onto a solid support. They can be used as unlabeled or enzyme-conjugates, and finally, they can react with either a specific antigenic determinant on an antigen or to a ligand-specific antibody (primary antibody), depending on the assay protocol.

Antigens are purified or produced using recombinant technology, used as labeled or enzyme conjugates and immobilized or soluble, depending on the assay protocol.

Standards and controls consist of lyophilized human source material, sodium azide, and a stated concentration of antigen.

Enzyme conjugates are either antigens or antibodies covalently coupled to the enzyme of choice. A reagent, formed by covalently coupling two molecules together, is called a **conjugate.** It is also possible to noncovalently label antibodies or enzymes with biotin and then add avidin. Avidin possesses four binding sites for biotin, not all of which are engaged in the interaction with biotin-labeled antibody. The remaining free binding sites can then function as acceptors for the biotin-labeled enzyme. This procedure can be shortened by using biotin-labeled antibody and enzyme-labeled avidin.

Buffers are used to maintain reaction pH and ion concentration, for sample dilutions or as diluents in reconstituting the lyophilized assay reagents.

Enzymes and substrate combinations include the enzyme horseradish peroxidase, its substrate hydrogen peroxide, and chromogen o-phenylenediamine. The product of this reaction produces a strong yellow-orange color. Other enzymes include β-galactosidase and its substrate o-nitrophenyl-β-D-galactopyranoside, which is converted to a yellow nitrophenolate ion, and alkaline phosphatase and its substrate p-nitrophenyl phosphate, which is converted to nitrophenolate ion.

Stopping reagent 1-N sulfuric acid is used to inhibit enzyme activity and stabilize the final colored reaction product.

## Competitive-Binding Assays

A solid-phase competitive-binding reaction ELISA is frequently used for the detection of antigen or hapten. In this type of assay, unlabeled ligand (patient sample) competes with enzyme-conjugated ligand for a limited number of immobilized antibody-binding sites. After a brief incubation, separation of bound and free enzyme-conjugated ligand is accomplished using the solid-phase separation technique described under RIA in this chapter. Substrate is added and enzyme present in the bound fraction converts substrate to a colored product. The amount of product formed is inversely related to the concentration of the unlabeled ligand in the test sample. The absorbances of the standards, controls, and test samples are determined using a spectrophotometer set at the appropriate wavelength within 2 hours after the addition of the stopping reagent. The reference wells containing only enzyme-conjugated

ligand show the greatest coloration. Decreased color changes in the wells is proportional to the amount of antigen present in the standards, controls, and test samples (Figure 7–7).

A standard curve is obtained by plotting the average absorbance value of each set of duplicate standards on the y-axis versus the antigen concentration contained in each standard on the x-axis of linear graph paper. A straight-line graph is obtained. The antigen concentration in the controls and test samples run concurrently with the standards can be determined from the standard curve using the average absorbance values of duplicate samples. To obtain the control and test sample concentrations, the value of the average absorbance is located on the y-axis of the standard curve and the corresponding concentration is read on the x-axis.

A competitive "inhibition ELISA" method is most frequently used for the detection of antibody. In this type of assay, unlabeled antibody in the test sample competes with a fixed concentration of enzyme-conjugated antibody for binding to a limited amount of antigen immobilized onto a solid support. After incubation, the unbound material is removed by washing. The enzyme substrate is added and, following incubation and color development, the enzyme reaction is stopped by the addition of the stopping reagent. Enzyme activity is decreased in the presence of antibody in the test sample so that within the detectable range of the assay, the greater the concentration of the antibody, the less the absorbance of the sample.

## Immunoenzymetric Assays

### NONCOMPETITIVE ASSAYS

**Immunoenzymetric assays** (IEMA), also referred to as the sandwich technique, are the most commonly used ELISA methods for the detection of antigens bearing at least two antigenic determinants. An excess of antibody, specific for the antigen, frequently monoclonal, is adsorbed onto polystyrene beads. These antibodies are specific for a unique antigenic determinant on the antigen of interest. Sample solutions are incubated with the antibody-coated beads so that all of the antigen present in the test sample will be bound by the immobilized antibody. After removal of unbound material, the amount of antigen bound to the antibody is quantitated by adding an enzyme-conjugated antibody that recognizes a second antigenic determinant on the same antigen. Following a second incubation and separation step, the enzyme activity remaining associated with the sandwich is determined by the addition of the substrate. Product formation is directly related to the amount of antigen in the standards, controls, and test samples. If the second antibody is monoclonal, the antibody reagents can be added simultaneously and only one wash step is required.

The color change is proportional to the amount of antigen in the test solution. A standard curve is obtained by plotting the average absorbance value of each set of duplicate standards versus the antigen concentration contained in each

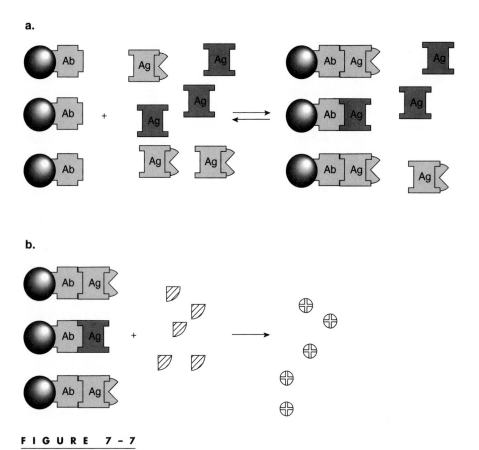

ELISA. **a.** A limited number of antibody (Ab) molecules attached to polystyrene beads are reacted with antigen (Ag) and enzyme-conjugated antigen. These antigens compete for binding and complexes are formed. **b.** The beads are washed to remove unbound antigen, enzyme substrate is added, and the bound enzyme-conjugate antigen converts the substrate to measurable colored product.

standard on linear graph paper. This produces a straight line. Concentrations of antigen in control and test sample duplicates run concurrently with the standards can be determined from the curve using the average absorbance values. Alkaline phosphatase is the enzyme of choice since it catalyzes a single hydrolysis step and a linear enzymatic response curve is obtained.

## Advantages and Disadvantages

The advantages of using enzyme-conjugated antigens and antibodies are that they can be stored under sterile conditions and used for years without any appreciable loss of their enzymatic and immunologic activities. The use of enzymes as labels entails minimal risk of contamination or pollution and the procedures are relatively easy to perform. There is no need for costly equipment and the assay can be performed in laboratories equipped with simple spectrophotometers. The specificity of the assay depends, as does that of RIA, on the specificity of the antibodies used. Similar to the IRMA, the IEMA uses an excess of labeled antibody. Because the label is an enzyme and not a radioisotope, the IEMA is not limited by how much labeled antibody can be added to each assay tube. Therefore, the IEMA can be used to detect antigen over a wider

range of concentration. The competitive and noncompetitive methods are highly sensitive, detecting picogram quantities of hormones and other substances. Disadvantages are that most of the assays require multiple incubation and separation steps and take longer to perform than either RIA or IRMA, increasing the chance of error. Automation has helped to alleviate these problems, reducing carryover errors, increasing precision though robotics and reducing turnaround times.

## Laboratory Applications

ELISAs are available for the measurement of factor VIII–related antigen, tumor markers such as carcinoembryonic antigen, alpha-fetoprotein, human chorionic gonadotropin, and antibodies (IgG and IgM) produced by the host in response to various viral infections. During the last decade, ELISA solid-phase assays have become the standard method of screening for hepatitis (hepatitis A, B, C, D, and E (HAV, HBV, HCV, HDV, HEV, respectively), antibodies and B surface or core antigens) and the human immunodeficiency virus (HIV). ELISAs for HIV antibodies (Electronucleonics, Inc., or Biotech Laboratories, Rockville, MD) are confirmed by Western blot. In addition to HIV antigens, other viral antigens, cytomegalovirus

(CMV) and Epstein-Barr virus (EBV) can be detected using an ELISA technique. The recent trend in antigen detection has been the use of monoclonal antibodies to identify specific viral antigens, since these antibodies are generated more easily to low-molecular-mass viral proteins. IEMAs, many using monoclonal antibodies, are available for the detection of carcinoembryonic antigen, alpha-fetoprotein, creatine kinase isoenzyme (CK-MB), ferritin, follicle-stimulating hormone, human chorionic gonadotrophin, IgE, luteinizing hormone, prolactin, prostatic acid phosphatase, prostate-specific antigen, and thyroid-stimulating hormones.

## Enzyme-Multiplied Immunoassay Technique

The **enzyme-multiplied immunoassay technique** (EMIT) is a separation-free, competitive binding assay that uses an enzyme as a label, conjugated to the hapten of interest, and an enzyme-substrate reaction as a detection system. This type of assay was originally described by Rubenstein and colleagues[17] in 1972. This is a homogeneous assay where the antibody-antigen reaction does not require a separation step to separate the free from the bound before detection of the immuno-complex.

The principle of enzyme-multiplied immunoassays is that the amount of hapten-antibody interaction can be determined by use of an enzyme label. It is based on a competitive-binding reaction between the hapten in the patient samples, controls, and standards and the enzyme-conjugated hapten for a limited number of antibody binding sites. Binding of the antibody to the enzyme-conjugated hapten results in the inhibition of the enzyme activity. This inhibition is due to the antibody sterically interfering with the binding of substrate to the catalytic site of the enzyme or binding of the antibody conformationally changing the enzyme. The amount of the unlabeled hapten in the test sample determines the number of antibody sites that will be available to bind and inactivate the enzyme-conjugated hapten. The more unlabeled hapten present, the less antibody available to inhibit enzymatic activity. The observable color change is therefore directly proportional to the amount of hapten in the test sample (Figure 7–8).

## REAGENTS

Antibody-coated tubes are solid supports coated with antibodies specific for the hapten (a drug, a drug metabolite, or a peptide hormone). It is more common to use monoclonal antibodies since the generation of a monoclonal antibody to a low-molecular-mass hapten is considerably easier than to a high-molecular-mass antigen.

Enzyme-conjugated reagents are hapten derivatives commonly covalently coupled to the enzyme glucose-6-phosphate dehydrogenase label.

Enzyme substrate and coenzyme are the substrate glucose-6-phosphate and the coenzyme nicotinamide adenine dinucleotide. The enzyme reaction results in the reduction of the coenzyme to a measurable product.

a.

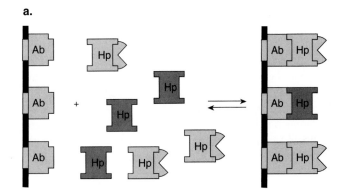

b.

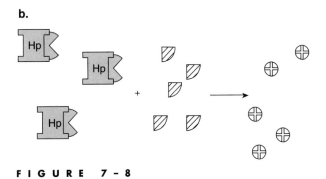

**FIGURE 7-8**

EMIT. **a.** Hapten (Hp) and enzyme-conjugated hapten compete for binding to a limited number of antibody binding sites (Ab) on a coated tube and hapten-antibody complexes are formed. **b.** Substrate is added and the enzyme on the free conjugate hapten converts the substrate to a measurable product.

Calibrator and controls consist of lyophilized human urine or serum, sodium azide, and a stated concentration of drug or hapten. These reagents have to be reconstituted with distilled or deionized water to the appropriate volume, allowed to dissolve an appropriate amount of time, and must be at the correct temperature before use.

Buffers are used to maintain reaction pH and ion concentrations or are used to increase the assay volume.

## CALCULATIONS

The conversion of a substrate or coenzyme to a measurable end product produces a change in the absorbance at a given wavelength and that end product is measured using a spectrophotometer. The calculation of test sample antigen concentrations is based on concurrent testing of the calibrator, controls, and zero diluent. Two absorbance values are recorded, the initial absorbance after a timed reagent reaction process, and a subsequent recording after a given interval of time, showing an absorbance shift that represents a measure of the reaction rate. It is this value that is used to quantitate the amount of hapten present in the sample. The higher the sample concentration of hapten, the greater the absorbance change.

The EMIT urine drug assays are designed to be qualitative and are not meant to be used to measure the concentration of drug present in the sample. The absorbance change in the sample mixture is compared to that in the calibrator mixture and the result is reported as positive or negative. The concentration of the drug or metabolite can be estimated from the results obtained from the EMIT assays, although there is some question as to its significance since highly individualized metabolic and excretory patterns create extreme variables in the amount of detectable drug present at any given period of time. High-pressure liquid chromatography or gas chromatography/mass spectrometry are the preferred methods for confirmation of a positive urine drug test.

### Laboratory Applications

EMIT systems by Syva Company (Palo Alto, CA) have been used as screening tests for therapeutic drugs and drugs of abuse or their metabolites including: acetaminophen, amphetamines, barbiturates, benzodiazepines, cannabinoids, cocaine metabolite, methadone (a synthetic narcotic/analgesic drug), methaqualone (a sedative-hypnotic drug), opiates, phencyclidine (PCP, a hallucinogenic drug), propoxyphene, tricyclic antidepressants, and others. By using the enzyme malate dehydrogenase, an EMIT has recently been developed that is sensitive enough to detect nanogram quantities of the hormone $T_4$. This development has expanded and should continue to expand the capabilities of the EMIT system beyond its present use in drug monitoring.

### ADVANTAGES AND DISADVANTAGES

The advantages of this type of assay are that no separation step is needed. It is very suitable for automation on many existing enzyme analyzers and it is a relatively easy assay to perform. The reagents have a relatively long shelf life as compared with radioisotopic reagents. EMIT urine drug tests have proved to be among the most sensitive as well as accurate testing methods in current use. Literature is available as to which medications with very similar chemical structures cross react with the test antibody and affect the assay specificity, producing false-positive results. Interference by endogenous enzymes or substances that affect enzyme activity may occur and the user should be aware of this possibility. Disadvantages are that some of the assays are less sensitive than heterogeneous enzyme immunoassays and the advantage of no separation step is sometimes offset by a required pretreatment of the samples.

### FLUORESCENT LABELS

### Substrate-Labeled Fluorescent Immunoassay

The **substrate-labeled fluorescent immunoassay** (SLFIA) is a homogeneous enzyme immunoassay developed by Burd and associates[18] in 1977. This assay uses a fluorogenic enzyme substrate as a label and an enzyme-substrate reaction for the detection of antibody-antigen complexes. Although the original assays were developed for determination of low-molecular-mass ligands,[19] Ngo and co-workers[20] in 1979 developed the first separation-free assay for high-molecular-mass ligands, thereby allowing for the detection of serum IgG and IgM. SLFIA relies on a competitive-binding reaction between a **fluorogenic ligand** and unlabeled ligand for a limited number of specific antibody-binding sites and the corresponding complexes are formed. When antibodies bind to the ligand portion of the fluorogenic-ligand, it is no longer a substrate for the enzyme; hence the free form of the label can produce fluorescence, whereas the antibody-bound label cannot. Enzyme is added after the corresponding complexes are formed. No separation steps are required to distinguish the free and antibody-bound label because only the free label can serve as an enzyme substrate and generate a fluorescent product. The fluorescent product is measured using a fluorometer. **Fluorescence** is the emission of light at a longer wavelength following the excitation of the fluorescent molecule with a light of a shorter wavelength. Excitation refers to the transition of an electron to a higher energy level when the molecule is excited. Emission occurs when the electron returns to a lower ground state energy level with some of the energy transferred to the chemical bonds of the excited molecule. Fluorometric measurement is more sensitive than colorimetric spectrophotometry.

The fluorogenic ligand in this assay plays a dual role; it competes with the unlabeled ligand for binding to a limited number of antibody-binding sites and it serves as a substrate for the enzyme. The enzyme in this assay, usually *Escherichia coli* β-D-galactosidase and its fluorogenic substrate, galactosylumbelliferone, are used merely to distinguish and to quantitate the proportion of free fluorogenic ligand rather than to provide an amplified signal. The fluorescence product, umbelliferone, is present in proportion to the level of the unlabeled ligand in the reaction mixture.

A standard curve is obtained by plotting the average fluorescence emission readings of each set of duplicate standards on the y-axis of linear graph paper. A straight-line graph is obtained. The ligand concentration of the controls and test samples run concurrently with the standards can be determined from the standard curve using the average fluorescence emission readings. To obtain the control and test sample concentrations, the value of the average fluorescence emission readings is found on the y-axis of the standard curve and the corresponding concentration is read on the x-axis.

### LABORATORY APPLICATIONS

The SLFIA has been used to quantitate a number of therapeutic drugs as well as specific serum IgG and IgM antibodies produced by the host in response to viral infections. SLFIA has been automated: the Stratus® analyzer (DADE-Behring, Deerfield, IL) uses an interesting solid-support system consisting of glass fiber paper onto which the antibody reagent is complexed; it has been successfully used to quantitate therapeutic drugs and hormones.

## ADVANTAGES AND DISADVANTAGES

The sensitivity of the SLFIA is in the micromolar range for most assays, which limits its use to therapeutic drugs present in relatively high concentrations. The precision and accuracy of this method is comparable to that of RIA and other EIA methods.[21] The advantages are that the reagents are stable for greater than a year if stored properly, no separation is required, and it is a rapid method to perform.

## Fluorescence Polarization Immunoassay

The **fluorescence polarization immunoassay** (FPIA) is a homogeneous, competitive assay developed by Colbert and others[22] in 1984 for the detection of low-molecular-mass haptens of less than 20,000 daltons. This method monitors the reaction between hapten and antibody using a fluorescent label conjugated to a hapten. In the assay, test sample is added to the **fluorescent-conjugated hapten** and an initial fluorescent reading is made using a fluorometer equipped with a polarized light source to compensate for sample quenching or background variation. To the extent that the test sample contains the substance of interest, competition occurs between unlabeled and labeled hapten for a limited number of antibody-binding sites. Following incubation, the polarized-fluorescence is measured again to determine the amount of hapten present.

Polarized fluorescence is measured using a polarized light source. The excitation of the fluorescent conjugates by the polarized light source results in the transition of its electrons to a higher energy level and the orientation of these electrons in the same direction as the polarized light. The emission of polarized fluorescence occurs when the oriented electrons return to a lower ground state energy level. The free fluorescent conjugates rotate rapidly in solution so that the oriented electrons do not remain in line with the light source and those molecules emit little detectable polarized fluorescence. The rate of rotation of the antibody-bound fluorescent conjugates (due to an increase in molecular volume) becomes much slower relative to the free fluorescent conjugate. Therefore, the bound fluorescent conjugate emits an increased amount of polarized fluorescence. This method gives a direct measure of the bound to free ratio instead of simply measuring the amount of label present so no separation of bound and free is required. The quantity of polarized fluorescence measured is the intensity of the light or the difference between the oriented and the unoriented light. The fluorometer can be standardized by using a series of calibrators containing known concentrations of the substance of interest. The fluorescence polarization is measured for the calibrators and test samples and the concentration of antigen in the test samples is calculated from a 6-point curve.

## LABORATORY APPLICATIONS

The Abbot TDx™ and AxSYM® automated analyzers (Abbott Diagnostics, North Chicago, IL) for FPIA have been

successfully used to quantitate many therapeutic drugs, drugs of abuse, and some hormones.[23]

## ADVANTAGES AND DISADVANTAGES

Fluorescence polarization measurements can be made very accurately and they are less affected by variations in fluorescence intensity than are standard fluorescence measurements. Thus, precision on the order of 1% or greater of measurement is readily achieved, which translates into more precise assay measurements. Another advantage of fluorescence polarization is that this technique does not require the separation of bound and free label. Disadvantages include the fact that FPIA is limited to measurements that can be performed with fluorescent compounds. The instrumentation required for performing fluorescence polarization measurements is very specialized and may only measure fluorescence intensity or polarization. The system is also less flexible than absorption spectroscopy. In addition, when performing fluorescence polarization measurements, it is crucial to control temperature and viscosity, and to use nonhemolyzed and nonlipemic samples that produce interfering fluorescence. Finally, the blood samples may require a pretreatment step before testing.

## Microparticle Enzyme Immunoassay

Microparticle enzyme immunoassay (MEIA) technology uses a solution of suspended, submicron-sized latex particles to measure analytes in a heterogeneous assay (Figure 7–9). This is a noncompetitive assay with resulting fluorescence being directly proportional to the analyte being measured. The particles are coated with a capture molecule (antigen, antibody, or viral particle) specific for the analyte being measured. The surface area of the microparticles increases assay kinetics and decreases assay incubation time.

In the sampling center, reactants and sample for an assay are transferred to a reaction vessel and then onto the processing center where reagents and sample are incubated to reaction temperature. The sample and reagents are mixed and then transferred to an inert glass matrix. Microparticles and any immune complexes are retained by the glass fibers while reactants pass through the matrix pores. A second antibody labeled with an alkaline phosphatase conjugate is added to the glass matrix and binds the immune complex: 4-methylumbelliferyl phosphate (MUP) substrate is added and the conjugate enzyme catalyzes the hydrolysis of MUP to methylumbelliferone (MU), which is fluorescent. The fluorescence is proportional to the concentration of the analyte tested.

## LABORATORY APPLICATIONS

The Abbot AxSYM® automated analyzer (Abbott Diagnostics, North Chicago, IL) for FPIA and MEIA has been used to quantitate hormones, some therapeutic drugs, and drugs of abuse.[23]

## ADVANTAGES AND DISADVANTAGES

The use of submicron particles coated with capture probe increases the effective surface of the immune complex reaction.

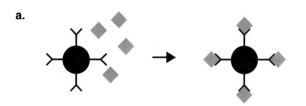

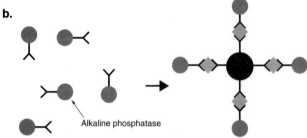

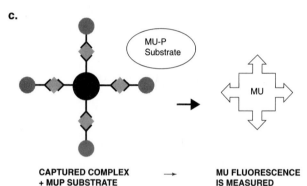

**FIGURE 7-9**

Microparticle enzyme immunoassay (MEIA) **a.** Microparticles coated with a capture molecule (antigen, antibody of analyte specific binding substance) bind and capture the analyte. **b.** Anti-analyte specific alkaline phosphatase conjugate binds elsewhere on the analyte. Antibody-antigen-antibody conjugate complex is captured by MEIA reaction cell glass fiber matrix. **c.** Fluorogenic substrate (4-methylumbelliferyl phosphate, MUP) is added to the reaction cell and MUP is catalyzed to methylumbelliferone (MU), which is fluorescent. Rate of MU production is measured. Analyte is determined from a standard curve.

This increases the diffusion distance between analyte and solid phase, resulting in increased assay kinetics and decreased assay incubation times with significantly decreased turnaround times.

Another adaptation similar to the MEIA system described above is the ion-capture technology. Polyanion anti-analytes bind analyte to increase the size of the formed immune complex. These polyanions then bind the positive surface of the glass fiber matrix while reactants pass through. A second antibody conjugate labeled with alkaline phosphatase and MUP

substrate are added as above and rate of MU formation is again measured. The increased size of the immune complex is essential for increased assay kinetics.

## Radiative Energy Attenuation

Radiative energy attenuation (REA) assays involve color development during a fluorogenic reaction process. In the presence of the analyte being tested, a chromogen (unreacted dye) is converted to a chromophore (colored dye) capable of absorbing (quenching) fluorescent light (radiant energy). The absorbance spectrum of the chromophore overlaps the excitation or emission spectrum of the fluorophores generated by the reaction process. The light-absorbing properties of the chromophore produced absorb the fluorescence and reduce the measured fluorescence (attenuates radiative energy). Changes in radiant energy intensity follow the principles of Beer's law and can be used to calculate concentration of analyte in patient samples using standards or standard curves. REA is used to quantitatively measure specific analytes based on the principle that the logarithm of measured fluorescent light intensity is inversely proportional to the amount of chromophore present.

### LABORATORY APPLICATIONS

The Abbot AxSYM® automated analyzer (Abbott Diagnostics, North Chicago, IL) has incorporated the REA to quantitate hormones, therapeutic drugs, and drugs of abuse.

### ADVANTAGES AND DISADVANTAGES

REA is a homogeneous assay that has similar advantages and disadvantages to FPIA. Homogeneous reactions have increased precision but can be plagued by interfering substances that are not removed by separation or washing steps.

## MOLECULAR ASSAYS

## Nucleic Acid Hybridization Reactions

The principle of **nucleic acid hybridization** is that a labeled complementary, single-stranded DNA (ssDNA), is used as a probe. The probe specifically interacts with single-stranded DNA or RNA target molecules in a test sample or control to form a stable double-stranded hybrid (DNA-DNA or DNA-RNA). Similar to the previously described immunoassays, a specific binding reagent (in this assay, labeled-DNA probe) is used to detect a particular DNA or RNA strand of interest. To detect hybrid formation, the DNA probes are conjugated to labels similar to those used in immunoassays including radioisotopes, enzymes, fluorescent molecules, biotin, and chemiluminescent esters.

Target sequences, regions of specific ACGT sequence within genes that are unique for a protein, organism, or dis-

| **Unique Target Sequence** | **ACTGCTAGTGTCGATTCGCGTAATGCTGATGGCCGATAA** |
| Oligonucleotide (probe) | GCTAAGCGCATTACGACTACCGG |

**FIGURE 7-10**

Probe synthesis. The oligonucleotide probe is complementary to a region within the target sequence for a specific organism, protein, or disease state. The probe is designed and synthesized to correspond to target sequence and bind specifically.

ease state, have been isolated, cloned, and characterized. Oligonucleotides (short polymers of DNA or RNA) are designed to correspond to those unique regions and then probes are synthesized for use in hybridization reactions for the identification or detection of target sequences (Figure 7–10). Hybridization is the binding of complementary oligonucleotide probes to form double-stranded molecules over that region. DNA probes hybridize to a complementary sequence of the specific target molecule sequence and hybridization events are detected by the label or detector molecule (enzyme, fluorophore, or chemiluminescent molecule) attached to the probe.

Hybridization is based on the inherent characteristics of dsDNA and nucleotide hydrogen bonding. dsDNA can be denatured or melted apart (break hydrogen bonds) by high temperature or alkaline pH and it will reanneal or reassociate specifically when the temperature is reduced or the pH neutralized (Figure 7–11). The reassociation of DNA strands will be directed by the complementary alignment of nucleotide bases, A to T or U, and G to C by the reforming of hydrogen bonds. Clinical specimens are complex environments with many different nucleic acids and proteins being present. The presence of noncomplementary strands of nucleic acid do not affect the reassociation of the complementary strands of nucleic acid but environmental conditions greatly influence the

annealing process and its specificity. Base pairing can occur between DNA and DNA, DNA and RNA, and between RNA and RNA to form duplex structures.

Factors that affect hybridization include: temperature, pH, salt concentration, G $\cdot$ C content in the probe and target sequence, probe length, and the presence of nonaqueous substances. The equation for calculating the proper environmental $T_m$ (temperature for melting dsDNA) for probe hybridization to occur shows how each factor influences the $T_m$ (Figure 7–12). $T_m$ is the temperature at which a hybridization reaction should occur, such that 50% of the probe will be bound to the target sequence and 50% will be free in solution. This provides an environment for specific interaction between the probe and target sequence only. Increased temperature "melts" DNA apart, whereas reduced temperatures can force DNA together (Figure 7–13). If the environment is cold enough, it can even force noncomplementary strands of DNA together and form nonspecific hybridization events.

Most hybridization reactions are adjusted to a pH near neutral (pH 6 to 8). Increased pH (alkaline) causes an absence of environmental hydrogen ions, disrupting the nucleotide hydrogen bonds that hold the two strands of nucleic acid together. Alkaline pH can melt the probe away from a target sequence and acidic environments can force the probe to bind nonspecifically. Likewise, high-salt conditions neutralize the negativity of the sugar-phosphate backbone of the nucleic acid, forcing nucleic acids (oligonucleotides and target sequence) to form double-stranded molecules even when regions are noncomplementary. In low-salt environments, the negativity of nucleic acid causes repulsion of the strands and reduced hydrogen bonding between complementary strands and subsequently no hybridization or false negatives can occur.

G $\cdot$ C content and overall probe length also affect the hybridization temperature through the nucleotide base hydrogen bonding that occurs. The G $\cdot$ C bond is 3/2 times stronger that A $\cdot$ T or A $\cdot$ U pair formation, since the G $\cdot$ C pair forms three hydrogen bonds and A $\cdot$ T or A $\cdot$ U pairs only form two bonds. Thermodynamically, G $\cdot$ C pairs are stronger than A $\cdot$ T or A $\cdot$ U pairs and require more energy to melt them apart. Likewise, a probe that is longer and forms more hydrogen bonds with the target sequence overall will be more strongly associated than probes that have shorter lengths and form fewer hydrogen bonds. Probes can be designed to correspond to unique target sequences over regions that contain

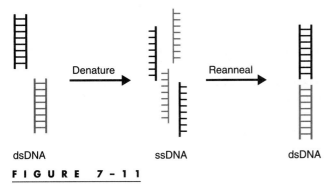

**FIGURE 7-11**

dsDNA denaturation and complementary reannealing. dsDNA can be denatured to single strands by high temperature or alkaline conditions. When the temperature is reduced or pH neutralized, complementary strands reanneal forming hydrogen bonds between the complementary nucleotide pairs (A $\cdot$ T and G $\cdot$ C).

$T_m$ is the temperature at which a hybridization reaction should occur such that 50% of the probe will be bound to the target sequence and 50% will be free in solution. This provides the environment for the specific interaction between the probe and target sequence only. To calculate $T_m$ for the hybridization reaction:

$$T_m = 81.5°C + 16.6(\log [Na]) + 0.41(\%GC \text{ content}) - 0.63[\% \text{ formamide (v/v)} - 600/\text{probe size}]$$

C = Temperature in Celsius, [Na] = salt concentration in M, %5GC content = percent of G-C pairs that are formed by the oligonucleotide binding the target sequence, % formamide = percent formamide solution in total hybridization solution, probe size = number of nucleosides making up the oligonucleotide.

**FIGURE   7 - 1 2**

Environmental factors affect temperature of hybridization. $T_m$ is the temperature at which a hybridization reaction should occur such that 50% of the probe will be bound to the target sequence and 50% will be free in solution. This provides the environment for the specific interaction between the probe and target sequence only.

many G · C pairs to keep overall probe length to manageable lengths and to increase the temperature of hybridization and specificity.

Lastly, nonaqueous substances, such as formamide, destabilize mismatches or misalignments between probes and target sequence to reduce nonspecific hybridization reactions. Because of their destabilizing affect, nonaqueous substances reduce the temperature required to melt nucleic acid strands apart so they must be considered when calculating the temperature at which hybridization is going to occur.

In the clinical setting, these conditions have all been worked out prior to the kits' approval by the Food and Drug Administration (FDA) for the use in the clinical laboratory. However, it is essential for laboratorians, who assure quality control and perform molecular testing, to understand the principles and process of each assay. When troubleshooting molecular probe assays, these factors of hybridization may need to be considered.

## Probe Design and Synthesis

Nucleic acid probes are designed to correlate to unique target sequences found within infectious agents or disease states. Unique target sequences can be identified through isolation, cloning, and sequencing of nucleic acids (DNA or RNA) from infected or diseased tissue directly or they can be made to correspond to characterized proteins made by the infectious agent or during the disease state. If proteins are initially isolated, they must first be separated (often by high-pressure liquid chromatography) and then sequenced by a protein sequencer. Once the primary amino acid is known, then the corresponding synthetic DNA sequence can be produced by taking into consideration all possible codons assigned for each amino acid. The best DNA sequence to synthesize corresponds to protein amino acids that are specified by only a single codon (methionine or tryptophan) or by just two codons (phenylalanine, tyrosine, histidine) to reduce the degeneracy in nucleic acid sequence. This process of rewriting primary amino acid sequence into DNA sequence is often called reverse translation, even though it is just a mental or computational process.

Full-length DNA sequence is analyzed for uniqueness and specificity for the infectious agent or disease state to identify target sequence for probe hybridization. Many computer pro-

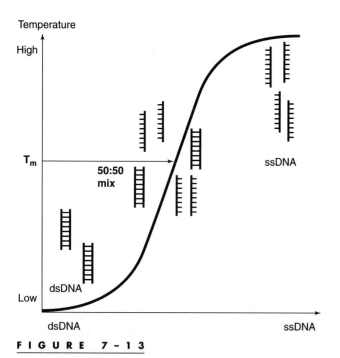

**FIGURE   7 - 1 3**

Temperature effects on dsDNA. As temperature is increased, dsDNA is "melted" apart. Hydrogen bonds are disrupted and ssDNA molecules are generated. At $T_m$, 50% of the DNA remains double stranded and 50% has formed single-stranded molecules.

grams have been developed to compare long lengths of DNA sequences and look for similarities and differences with DNA sequences deposited in GenBank.[1] GenBank sequences are available and accessible for anyone to use for this process. Additionally, as the Human Genome Project expands our DNA database, it will undoubtedly lead to the understanding and identification of many disease processes. When designing a probe, it is best to use a portion of the DNA sequence that is found only in the infectious agent or disease state or shows the least homology (likeness) to other sequences in the databases. Additionally, G · C content and overall length contribute to the probe hybridization conditions and specificity (see above).

Once the nucleic acid sequence is decided on, then a DNA probe can be produced synthetically by one of two methods: (1) a solid-phase chemical procedure adds one nucleotide on at a time to produce the oligonucleotide, or (2) by an in vitro synthesis using DNA fragments and the DNA polymerase enzyme.[24] Solid-phase synthesis is limited to synthesizing oligonucleotides up to 30 to 35 nucleotides (maximum of 100) in length due to the complex nature of the chemical reaction and the need for accurate chain elongation. Longer probes (greater than 100 nucleotides to thousands of nucleotides in length) are made by in vitro synthesis and tend to be more accurate owing to the reading and accuracy of the DNA polymerase enzyme. The reader is referred to a biotechnology or bioengineering text for discussion of the many techniques used to regenerate DNA fragments.[24]

## Nucleic Acid Detection

Molecular hybridization assays are similar to immunoassays in that they require binding specificity, in this case interaction between nucleotides. The presence of target nucleic acid sequences are detected by hybridization events that occur between probe and target sequences. The detection of these events is through the labeling of the probe nucleic acid. The label allows for quantitation or visualization of the hybridization event and many labels have been developed for this purpose.

### RADIOACTIVE LABELS

End labeling has been an extremely useful technique when labeling DNA with radioactive phosphate. Radioactive ATP [$^{32}$P-P-P-adenosine] is used to incorporate $^{32}$P onto the terminal 5' C hydroxyl group of deoxyribose at the end of the ssDNA molecule. Polynucleotide kinase enzyme specifically transfers the $^{32}$P from ATP to the free hydroxyl group of deoxyribose, covalently labeling the DNA molecule. Alternatively, [$^{32}$P$\alpha$-dATP] radionucleotide can be incorporated directly into the DNA strand through in vitro synthetic reactions (nick-translation) using DNA polymerase.[24] DNA polymerase (isolated from *E. coli*) has an exonuclease activity, that is, it nicks dsDNA and removes a nucleotide. It then repairs the nick by replacing it with a labeled nucleotide. After several cy-

cles of this the dsDNA is denatured and the ssDNA used as probes during hybridization reactions. Other labels such as fluorophores, quenchers, acridinium esters, or enzymes are similarly linked by covalent bonds to the DNA carbohydrate backbone, leaving the nucleotides free to interact with target sequences during hybridization.

Radioactive decay is detected by a scintillation counter (described above) or by autoradiography. In the autoradiography process, the radioactivity is detected by placing the sample, gel, or blot (described below) in contact with photographic film. The radioactive decay forms silver grains in the photographic film and when the photographic film is developed, hybridization can be detected by visual inspection. This technique has been used extensively in research settings, DNA fingerprinting, restriction fragment length polymorphism (RFLP) analysis, and characterization of genomic DNA.

### ENZYME OR FLUORESCENT LABELS

Enzyme- or fluorescent-linked labels involve the incorporation of modified nucleotide precursors (dTTP, dATP, dGTP, or dCTP) into synthesized probe by nick-translation. Additionally, nucleotides may be biotinylated as a label generating a generic probe. These may then be reacted with strepavidin coupled to an enzyme (horseradish peroxidase, for example) and in the presence of appropriate substrate, generate chromogenic or fluorogenic end products for detection or quantitation.[25]

### CHEMILUMINESCENT LABELS

**Chemiluminescence** is the resultant release of light energy as an end product of a chemical reaction. The most common chemiluminescent labeling reagent is an acridinium ester. When reacted with hydrogen peroxide, the acridinium ester is cleaved causing a short burst of light to be released (Figure 7–14). The light is detected by a luminometer with the amount of light proportional to the amount of hybridization that has occurred between probe and target sequence. The acridinium ester is attached to oligonucleotides through covalent bonding to the carbohydrate backbone. The acridinium ester does not interfere with the hybridization reaction between probe and target sequence.

Chemiluminescence has been used for direct and amplified nucleic acid testing. Chemiluminescence is more sensitive in its detection levels than fluorescent methodology and even surpasses isotope decay for detection of hybridization reactions without the biohazard.

## Direct Nucleic Acid Testing

Direct assays, like those described below (Southern blotting and FISH), only detect DNA or RNA already present in the sample. Nonamplified or direct probe assays have three main steps: sample preparation, probe hybridization, and detection of the hybridization reaction. Direct nucleic acid hybridization protocols, based most commonly on the Southern technique, have been developed for forensics, paternity testing, and the

**a.**

**b.**

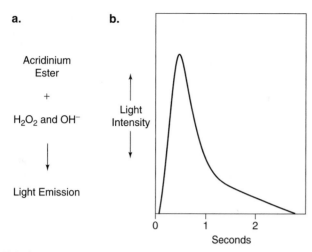

Acridinium
Ester

+

$H_2O_2$ and $OH^-$

↓

Light Emission

Light Intensity

0    1    2

Seconds

**F I G U R E   7 - 1 4**

Chemiluminescence. **a.** Chemiluminescence is the emission of light from a chemical reaction. Chemical compounds, attached to molecular probes, act as reporter molecules for hybridization events. When the acridinium ester (AE) is hydrolyzed in an alkaline environment, a burst of light is released. **b.** The energy released is a short, intense burst of light that is detected in a luminometer. The amount of light is directly proportional to the amount of AE present, which corresponds to hybridization events.

detection of infectious agents. DNA probes labeled with enzymes or biotin have been incorporated into the Southern technique to provide rapid, walk-away molecular testing with easy visualization interpretation.

## SOUTHERN AND NORTHERN HYBRIDIZATION

The **Southern hybridization** technique was developed by Edward M. Southern. This technique combines size-separating agarose-gel electrophoresis with DNA transfer and hybridization that allows for characterization of specific DNA fragments.[26]

In the Southern technique, DNA extracted from cells is digested with a bacterial **restriction endonuclease enzyme.** Bacterial restriction endonucleases differ from each other by their recognition sites and will cut the dsDNA only if their recognition site is present. These enzymes recognize short, specific dsDNA sequences to cleave adjoining, adjacent nucleotides of the dsDNA. The restriction endonuclease cleaves the covalent phosphodiester bond on the sugar-phosphate backbone to generate DNA fragments. DNA fragments are then size separated by agarose-gel-electrophoresis. Molecular weight markers are run in the gel beside the DNA fragments so DNA fragment size can be determined. Genomic DNA is very long and would not migrate by gel electrophoresis without fragmentation first.

After the DNA is size separated by agarose-gel electrophoresis, the gel is then exposed to acid and base solution to break the hydrogen bonds holding the dsDNA together, generating ssDNA molecules. The gel is then neutralized and prepared for Southern transfer (Figure 7–15). The Southern transfer is done by high-salt capillary action. A tray is prepared that has a Whatman filter paper wick that dips into a high salt solution. The gel is placed on top of the Whatman paper, then covered by a membrane (nitrocellulose is most common) followed by 2 sheets of Whatman paper, and then many paper towels to absorb and draw the high-salt solution through the gel. The salt solution carries the ssDNA to the membrane where it adheres. After 12 to 16 hours the membrane, commonly called a blot, can be removed followed by baking or ultraviolet exposure to further adhere the DNA to the membrane.

The membrane is then incubated in hybridization solution containing the labeled probe. Initially, nucleotides labeled with $[^{32}P]$ such as $[^{32}P\alpha\text{-dATP}]$ were used to make radiolabeled probes. This process has been replaced by biotin-, enzyme-, or chemiluminescent-labeled probes. Probe hybridizes to target sequence during the incubation period and then a series of washes are performed to wash away unbound labeled probe.

The DNA fragment where the probe hybridized can be visualized by phospho-imaging or by overlaying the blot with X-ray film to detect radioactive decay. The band that forms is compared to the molecular weight markers to determine the size of the DNA fragment that has hybridized with the probe. When probes are labeled with an enzyme, the membrane is simply overlaid with enzyme substrate and color develops where the hybridization has occurred, indicating the DNA fragment of interest.

## DNA FINGERPRINTING

**DNA fingerprinting** or RFLP mapping uses the Southern blotting technique in forensic testing, paternity testing, and pretransplantation HLA antigen tissue typing.[26] Genomic DNA is extracted from the patient's cells, restriction digested, and size separated by agarose-gel electrophoresis. The DNA fragments are then transferred to the membrane by capillary action or application of a vacuum. The blot is then exposed to DNA probes that encode individual HLA antigens containing a variety of labels. If hybridization occurs, then the specific marker will be visualized during the detection process. HLA antigens are determined by comparing the patient's pattern of hybridization to control patterns (known HLA antigen sequence) of hybridization. This same technique can be applied to forensic testing when tissue and blood samples are collected at crime scenes. Furthermore, RFLP mapping can be utilized in paternity testing and child custody law suits.

Direct nucleic acid hybridization is highly specific under proper hybridization conditions. Oligonucleotide probes, corresponding to unique base sequences found only in infectious agents or disease states, eliminate cross-reactivity under the

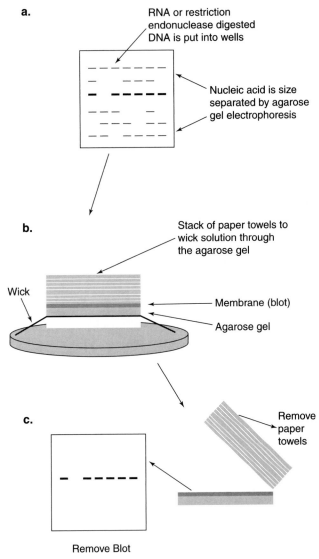

**a.**

RNA or restriction endonuclease digested DNA is put into wells

Nucleic acid is size separated by agarose gel electrophoresis

**b.**

Stack of paper towels to wick solution through the agarose gel

Wick

Membrane (blot)

Agarose gel

**c.**

Remove paper towels

Remove Blot

**F I G U R E   7 - 1 5**

Southern transfer of nucleic acid. **a.** DNA is size separated by agarose gel electrophoresis, then exposed to acid and base solution to generate ssDNA molecules. The gel is then neutralized and prepared for Southern transfer. **b.** The Southern transfer is done by high salt capillary action. A tray is prepared that has a Whatman filter paper wick (black line) that dips into a high salt solution. The gel (light grey) is placed on top of the Whatman paper, then covered by a membrane (dark grey), followed by 2 sheets of Whatman paper and many paper towels to absorb and draw the high salt solution through the gel. The salt solution carries DNA to the membrane where it adheres. **c.** After 12 to 16 hours the membrane, commonly called a blot, can be removed, then permanently affixed by baking or ultraviolet exposure. The membrane is then incubated in hybridization solution containing the labeled probe.

appropriate hybridization conditions. Unlike antibodies that exhibit a variety of affinities, oligonucleotides bind consistently and specifically every time: A always binding T or U, and G always binding C. Utilization of detection systems (labeled probes) to discern hybridization events has increased our ability to detect minute amounts of nucleic acid. Disadvantages are mainly related to small amounts of target sequence in the sample. Additionally, some detection reactions require organic chemicals that must be properly disposed of, and if radioactive labels are used, they must be disposed through regulated waste procedures and require personnel-exposure monitoring as well.

## FLUORESCENT IN SITU HYBRIDIZATION

**Fluorescent in situ hybridization (FISH)** is a highly specialized molecular procedure used to localize DNA (Southern) or RNA (Northern) target molecules in tissue sections or to diagnose structural, duplication, deletions, rearrangement, or translocation events of chromosomal abnormalities.[27] Oligonucleotide probes are designed to correspond to specific variant nucleic acid sequences in genomic DNA or to foreign nucleic acid in infectious agents. Probes detect the DNA or RNA directly, with no amplification of the initial DNA or RNA present in the sample. Probe hybridization studies provide information about genetic variation and nucleic acid subcellular location in examined tissue sections, since tissues, cells, and chromosomes may be examined without any morphologic changes in cellular structures.

Spatial and temporal localization can be investigated if one probes for mRNA. mRNA is expressed or transcribed from active genes and can be found within the cell's nucleus or cytoplasm. Additionally, it can be determined when a gene becomes actively expressed in a disease state or infection, and when the mRNA becomes detectable during the disease process. FISH requires a solid support or slide that holds the sample to be analyzed. Standard histologic methods are followed to prepare and adhere tissue, cells, or arrested chromosomes on the slide. The sample is then digested by enzymes (proteases, RNAse, and DNAse) to make the cell more porous and allow probe entry into the cellular matrix. The probe-hybridization mix is then overlaid onto the tissue, cells or chromosomes and allowed to hybridize. Unhybridized probe is washed away. Through a series of salt washes of decreasing concentration, nonspecific hybridization is removed as well. The sample may be counterstained to increase visualization of the cellular morphology. The slide is then examined by fluorescent microscopy and most commonly recorded by photography or digital imagery.

### Laboratory Applications

There are numerous cytogenetic FISH assays being performed, predominantly in special accredited molecular genetics laboratories. These laboratories are accredited by the College of American Pathologists to fulfill the mandates established by the Clinical Laboratory Improvement Amendments. Additionally, accreditation by the American Association of Blood Banks allows for parentage testing as well. Down syndrome and other chromosomal abnormalities associated with birth defects, herpes simplex, and leukemia are just a few of the tests available (Vysis Inc., Downers Grove, IL).

### Advantages and Disadvantages

Advantages include the specific information gained about the target molecule within native cellular conditions. When slides are examined for the localization of DNA or RNA within tissue sections, valuable information about pathogen host interactions and disease progression is gained. The main disadvantage to the FISH technique is the highly specialized training and technical procedures required for histologic preparation of the tissue-containing slides.

### SEMIAUTOMATED TESTING

The VP AFFIRM (Becton Dickinson, Sparks, MD) is a semi-automated, branched-direct DNA probe assay that uses three

DNA probes to detect three target rRNA sequences (*G. vaginalis, T. vaginalis,* and *C. albicans*) in the same clinical sample. By targeting rRNA, there is natural amplification because each cell has thousands of ribosomes that contain rRNA compared with the single copy of genomic DNA.

### Laboratory Applications

The VP AFFIRM branched DNA test methodology is similar to a two-site IRMA, utilizing two probes for each organism to detect regions within each of the unique target sequences. A vaginal swab is incubated with lysate to rupture all cells and release nucleic acids. The lysate is placed in the sample well and the test slide is dipped and incubated robotically. The slide contains three wells, one each for *G. vaginalis, T. vaginalis,* and *C. albicans,* to provide solid support for microparticle beads. The first organism specific probe is attached to the stationary microparticle bead localized in the well and functions to capture the target sequence and hold it on the slide (Figure 7–16). The slide is robotically washed to remove cellular debris and

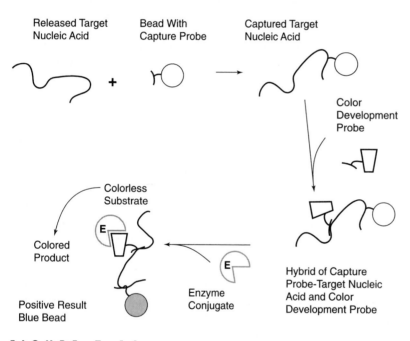

**F I G U R E   7 - 1 6**

Semiautomated direct nucleic acid detection. Scheme of the VP AFFIRM (Becton Dickinson, Franklin Lanes, NY) chemical and binding reactions that take place in each reaction well on the reagent slide. Organism-specific probe is attached to stationary microparticle beads localized to individual wells. Microparticle probes function to capture specific target sequence and bind it to the slide. The slide is robotically washed to remove cellular debris and unbound nucleic acids. The second probe, conjugated to a color development substrate, is added and binds elsewhere on the target sequence. Unbound probe is robotically washed away and hybridization is detected by adding enzyme to catalyze the color substrate reaction to a colored end product that turns the bead blue. Color development indicates that hybridization has occurred in that well and nucleic acid for that organism was present in the patient sample. (Redrawn from product insert, VP AFFIRM, Becton Dickinson, Franklin Lanes, NY) unbound nucleic acids. The second probe is added and binds elsewhere on the target sequence and is conjugated to an enzyme label. Unbound probe is washed away and hybridization is detected by adding enzyme substrate that is catalyzed to a colored end product. If color has developed in the well, then hybridization has occurred in that well. The slide is visually inspected and results reported out as positive or negative for each organism. The slide has internal positive and negative controls built into additional wells. External controls are available as well from independent manufacturers.

## Advantages and Disadvantages

Oligonucleotide probes correspond to specific unique base sequences that are found only in infectious agents or disease states. Linking this specificity with the detection of hybridization through the use of enzyme catalysis increases the sensitivity for detecting minute (picomolar) amounts of target molecules. Three easy steps of sample preparation, hybridization, and detection have allowed for automation, reduced personnel time, and shortened turnaround times. Quality control and patient results are easily visualized for qualitative interpretation and reporting. Disadvantages are related to the ability to directly detect target sequence without amplification when organisms are present in small numbers.

## HYBRIDIZATION PROTECTION ASSAY

Gen-Probe (San Diego, CA) has developed a homogeneous hybridization protection assay (HPA) that targets rRNA of infectious agents and utilizes chemiluminescence for quantitative measurement of hybridization reactions. There are three main steps: (1) sample preparation to release target rRNA from infectious agents (*N. gonorrhoeae, C. trachomatis*), (2) hybridization of DNA probe labeled with chemiluminescent molecule (acridinium ester) to target rRNA, and (3) detection of chemiluminescent label on DNA probe. There are no wash steps or solid substrate phases to be manipulated. The HPA detection of only hybridized probe is accomplished by addition of a selection reagent that degrades unprotected acridinium esters (unhybridized probe) in solution, leaving hybridized acridinium esters intact within the double-stranded duplex (Figure 7–17). Hydrogen peroxide is added to the reaction mixture and chemiluminescence is measured in a luminometer. Many Gen-Probe assays have been developed utilizing this HPA system as part of their detection process.

## Laboratory Applications

Gen-Probe direct assays have been developed and used in microbiology for confirmation or identification of isolated organisms since the early 1990s. Recent advancements include incorporating the Gen-Probe technology for testing clinical specimens directly. PACE 2 (Gen-Probe, San Diego, CA) detects both *N. gonorrhoeae* and *C. trachomatis* simultaneously as a screening procedure. A positive PACE 2 test is then reflex tested with direct assays for *N. gonorrhoeae* or *C. trachomatis* followed by a probe competition assay (PCA) for confirma-

tion. PCA is a competitive DNA probe assay distinguishing specific from nonspecific signal in the PACE 2 test. The Centers for Disease Control and Prevention have established guidelines for verification of positive chlamydial results in low-risk populations and this format meets those guidelines. Gen-Probe has developed direct assays for other bacteria, *Mycobacterium pneumoniae*, fungi, and streptococcus Group A.

## Advantages and Disadvantages

Advantages of the Gen-Probe direct assay are related to the high sensitivity and specificity of ribosomal RNA targets, probe hybridization, and the chemiluminescence detection system. Additionally, there are no wash steps and solution phase separation and detection reduce cross-contamination and personnel time required to perform the test. Application of direct-probe assay is clinically useful for detecting fastidious organisms or organisms that may be present in very low numbers. PACE 2 offers rapid screening of high-risk populations for *C. trachomatis* and *N. gonorrhoeae*. Up to 50% of patients infected with *N. gonorrhoeae* also have *C. trachomatis* infection (Gen-Probe Technical Report, 1995). These patients present with similar symptoms and need differential diagnosis since identification is important for selecting the appropriate treatment option for each organism.

## AMPLIFIED DETECTION SYSTEM

Chiron (Chiron Corp, Emeryville, CA) developed a heterogeneous direct test for blood to detect HIV target viral RNA. This procedure incorporates an amplification process for the signal or detection system. First, the patient's plasma is collected and viral RNA is extracted through cell lysis. The sample is then incubated with two DNA probes. Probe 1 is attached to a solid support (microtiter plate) and functions to capture and hold the viral RNA in the well by hybridizing to a specific region of the target RNA. Probe 2 also binds a specific region of the target RNA but elsewhere on the viral RNA, much like an IRMA. Probe 2 has additional nucleic acid sequence that is repetitive and not directed toward the viral RNA. Instead, this sequence is bioengineered to correspond to a third probe that will be added later, after the wash step. This reaction mix is incubated and then washed to remove cellular debris and unbound probes 1 and 2. Probe 3, a detector probe, is then added to the reaction well and it binds many times to the probe 2 repetitive sequence. This is called a multiple probe with multiple enzyme system since probe 3 is conjugated to alkaline phosphatase enzyme. When a chemiluminescent substrate is added (dioxetane), light is produced and measured in a luminometer. The amount of light is proportional to HIV RNA present in the sample. The third probe essentially amplifies the detection system for the hybridization reaction by binding many times to the initial hybridization reaction. This process, target capture and signal amplification, increases the sensitivity down to 50 viral particles per milliliter of patient plasma for this direct nucleic acid method without amplifying nucleic acid sequence.

**STEP ONE: HYBRIDIZATION**

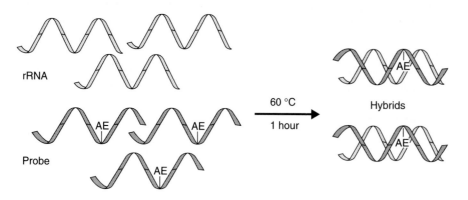

rRNA

Probe

60 °C
1 hour

Hybrids

**STEP TWO: SELECTION**

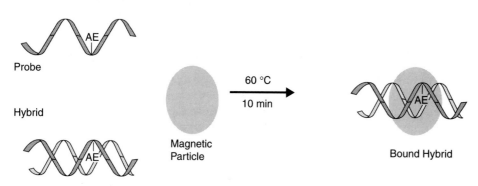

Probe

Hybrid

Magnetic
Particle

60 °C
10 min

Bound Hybrid

**STEP THREE: DETECTION**

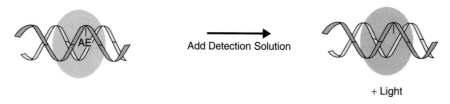

Add Detection Solution

+ Light

**F I G U R E     7 – 1 7**

Hybridization protection assay. Hybridization protection assay (HPA) developed by Gen-Probe utilizes the highly chemiluminescent acridinium ester (AE) molecule as a reporter group. In step 1, probe and target sequence are allowed to mix and form RNA:DNA hybrids. In step 2, an unhybridized probe is selectively destroyed by a chemical reaction. Alkaline hydrolysis of the ester bond of AE renders it permanently nonchemiluminescent. When covalently attached to a single-stranded oligonucleotide probe, hydrolysis of AE is rapid. In contrast, when the probe hybridizes to a complementary target nucleic acid, the hydrolysis rate of AE is greatly reduced. In step 3, hybrids are reacted with the detection solution and the acridinium ester is cleaved, releasing the burst of chemiluminescence. The chemiluminescence after hydrolysis is a direct measure of the amount of target nucleic acid present in the sample. (Courtesy of Gen-Probe, San Diego, CA)

Other signal amplification methods that have been developed to detect rare hybridization events include multiple enzymes, multiple probes, and two-tiered probes.[28] Multiple enzymes, or the attachment of many labels to a single probe, is the simplest of these methods. The use of multiple probes increases the signal as well, but it requires the development of many short probes that bind the target sequence in many areas in a specific manner. The two-tiered signal amplification method consists of a set of many secondary probes that bind a primary probe many times. These are more easily engineered because the primary probe is synthetic to begin with.

### Laboratory Applications

Assays by Chiron utilizing this same technology include HIV RNA, human papillomavirus, CMV, *C. trachomatis, N. gonorrhoeae,* and hepatitis B virus.

### Advantages and Disadvantages

The main advantage of these systems is that the sensitivity is greatly enhanced by the signal amplification detection method. In theory, a single hybridization event could be detected through the amplification of the detection system. Additionally, carryover contamination from large amounts of target sequences generated by amplification methods (DNA or RNA products) is reduced.

## Amplified Nucleic Acid Testing

Much like the culture in microbiology, the amplification of nucleic acid is performed so that it can be further characterized. In microbiology cultures, an organism is grown overnight so that one can perform biochemical and antibiotic sensitivity testing and possibly serotyping the next day. In amplification techniques, the target sequence is enzymatically amplified so it can be identified with a DNA probe that is linked with a detection system. Often, few organisms are present in a sample, especially organisms like *Mycobacterium tuberculosis,* which is fastidious and grows very slowly, if at all.

The key principle of nucleic amplification techniques is the enzymatic amplification (multiplication) of a specific nucleic acid sequence, occurring exponentially, producing billions of copies in a short time. Many amplification techniques have been developed and approved by the FDA for use in human testing. These techniques use enzymes that have been characterized in normal molecular functions (replication and transcription) and harvested through biotechnology and engineering. **DNA polymerase** is an enzyme that copies DNA from DNA during the replication process. **DNA ligase** enzyme joins together double-stranded DNA fragments (Okazaki fragments) during replication as well. **RNA polymerase** enzyme binds double-stranded DNA at promoter sites and transcribes thousands of copies of mRNA from the DNA template. **Reverse transcriptase** enzyme was identified in retroviruses and functions to rewrite RNA into DNA so that it can be inserted into the host cell genome. The genes encoding these enzymes have been isolated, cloned, and expressed through bioengineering so that they are available in pure, highly concentrated amounts.

Advantages of nucleic acid amplification assays are their higher sensitivity, faster turnaround times, and ability to detect nucleic acid from unculturable organisms, gene mutations, rearrangements, or deletions in human chromosomes. There are four basic steps for the amplification methods: (1) sample preparation, (2) amplification, (3) hybridization, and (4) detection. Currently, there are many types of nucleic acid amplification technologies. **Polymerase chain reaction** (PCR), first developed and described by Kary Mullis in the early 1980s, utilizes changes in temperature (thermocycling) to regulate enzyme activity and the amplification process. **Ligase chain reaction** is a modification of this process but still requires thermocycling. **Nucleic-acid-sequence–based amplification** (NASBA), **transcription-mediated amplification** (TMA), and **strand-displacement amplification** (SDA) have been developed and are all isothermal processes relying on a different set of enzymes and processes to regenerate copies of target molecules.

### POLYMERASE CHAIN REACTION

PCR is the reference standard in amplification techniques. PCR was made easy with the discovery and isolation of a thermal-stable DNA polymerase from the thermophilic bacterium *Thermus aquaticus.* This DNA polymerase, known as Taq polymerase, is stable up to 95°C and is unaffected by the denaturation step in PCR. However, Taq polymerase enzyme has no proofreading ability so it does make mistakes when incorporating nucleotides. Another hyperthermophilic organism, *Pyrococcus furiosus,* produces a thermal-stable DNA polymerase (up to 100°C) with proofreading activity, making it a better enzyme for reactions that require absolute accuracy.

PCR can be used with DNA or RNA starting material; however, RNA must be reverse transcribed into cDNA first before the PCR reaction begins. There are three main steps for each PCR cycle. A 92°C denaturation or melting of double-stranded DNA followed by a 37 to 45°C annealing period where oligonucleotide primers bind to target sequences, and, lastly, a 72°C period where DNA polymerase is allowed to extend the primers complementary to the target sequence (Figure 7–18). Cycles are performed (n) number of times generating $2^n$ number of amplicons at the end of the thermocycling. The amplicons are then detected by visual inspection of agarose-gel electrophoresis or labeled-probe hybridization using any one of the visualization systems.

### Laboratory Applications

PCR assays are used to detect very small (picogram) amounts of target DNA or RNA. PCR was one of the first techniques used to detect viruses (HIV, HBV, HCV, HDV, HEV, CMV, EBV, and many others) and fastidious organisms such as *M. tuberculosis, N. gonorrhoeae,* and *C. trachomatis.* Amplicor

**Polymerase Chain Reaction**
**Original Target: DNA**
**or Reverse Transcribed RNA**

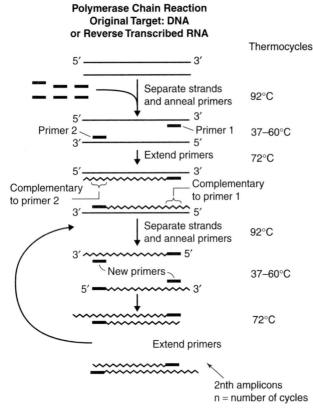

# FIGURE 7-18

Polymerase chain reaction amplification. Polymerase chain reaction (PCR) can be used with DNA or RNA starting material. However, RNA must be reverse transcribed (not shown) into cDNA prior to PCR amplification. Three temperature steps occur in a single cycle to regulate the steps of each PCR cycle. First, denaturation at 92°C "melts" or separates the double-stranded DNA. Second, a 37 to 45°C annealing period allows target-specific oligonucleotide primers to bind to target sequence. Lastly, a 72°C period of primer extension by DNA polymerase incorporates complementary nucleotides corresponding to target sequence. Cycles are performed (n) number of times generating $2^n$ number of amplicons at the end of the thermocycling. Amplicons are then detected by a visual inspection of agarose gel electrophoresis or labeled-probe hybridization using any one of the visualization systems.

HIV-1 (now owned by Chiron, Emeryville, CA) combined PCR methodology directly with the detection process. The primer involved in the amplification process is bound to a biotin molecule that is incorporated in each amplicon. The amplicons were then reacted with avidin that has been tagged with an enzyme for a colorimetric determination and the amplicon quantified spectrophotometrically.

## Advantages and Disadvantages

The main advantage to PCR is that it offers rapid amplification and identification of target nucleic acid sequences. However, the process relies on repeated specific interaction between primers and target sequences for amplification. Additionally, there is the increased risk for carryover contamination due to the large amount of amplicon generated. In many laboratories, protocols and procedures have been implemented and need strict adherence to reduce contamination and false-positive results. Most laboratories have established a clean zone or workstation just for PCR testing. Incorporating (biotin) labeled primers in the amplification process reduces the overall steps required for detection and reduces personnel time required for testing.

## LIGASE CHAIN REACTION

Ligase chain reaction (LCR) is similar to PCR in that it requires thermocycling to regulate the enzyme steps for each cycle but the process is different in that the probe is amplified instead of the target molecule. Abbott Laboratories uses this methodology on their instrumentation (LCx7, Abbott Laboratories, Abbott Park, IL). Temperature is used in the first step to denature the dsDNA apart. Much longer primers are provided in the reaction mix and they are allowed to anneal to the ssDNA target during the second step (Figure 7–19). Additionally, the primers are part of the detection systems through the incorporation of terminally placed haptens. During the last step of LCR, primers bound to the target are filled in by DNA polymerase and joined together by DNA ligase. During future cycles, the ligated primers (amplicons) become the template for the next cycle, annealing primers that are then filled in and ligated. The amplicons are then detected by an antigen-antibody reaction (microparticle enzyme immunoassay) with the hapten that has been incorporated in the amplicon (Figure 7–20). The antibody that binds the hapten is bound to a magnetic bead for easy separation of incorporated label from free. After a wash step, the second antibody labeled with a fluorophore is added and it binds to the other end of the ligated amplicon. An enzyme substrate is then added and fluorescence is generated and measured. The fluorescence is directly proportional to amplicon concentration.

## Laboratory Applications

LCR amplification has been used for the detection of *C. trachomatis, N. gonorrhoeae, M. tuberculosis* organisms, and the quantification of HIV and HCV in laboratory specimens. Additionally, Abbott laboratories have developed molecular beacon probes to increase the sensitivity of these tests. Molecular beacon probes have hairpin structures when not hybridized to target sequence. This brings fluorophore labels in close proximity to fluorescent quenchers (Figure 7–21). When the probe is unbound, there is no observable fluorescence. When the probe binds LCR products, it separates the fluorophore from the quencher and fluorescence is detectable. Furthermore, different fluorophore-labeled probes (Figure 7–21**b.**), or beacons, can be

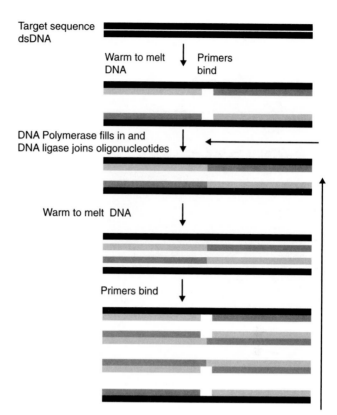

Target sequence dsDNA

Warm to melt DNA    Primers bind

DNA Polymerase fills in and DNA ligase joins oligonucleotides

Warm to melt DNA

Primers bind

## FIGURE 7-19

Ligase chain reaction. LCR is similar to PCR, requiring thermocycling to regulate the enzyme steps for each amplification cycle. First, increased temperature is used to denature dsDNA. The temperature is then reduced and long primers are allowed to bind specifically to adjacent ssDNA target sequence. Primers bound to target are then filled in by DNA polymerase and joined together by DNA ligase. In future cycles, ligated primers (amplicons) become template for the next cycle, annealing primers that are then filled in and ligated. The amplicons are then detected.

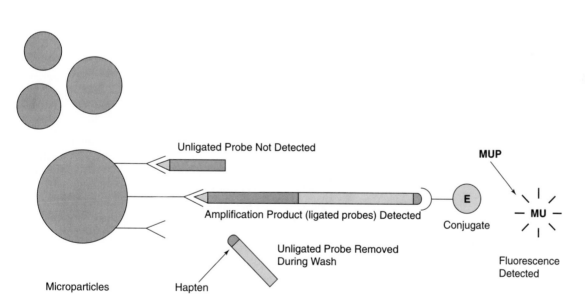

Unligated Probe Not Detected

Amplification Product (ligated probes) Detected

MUP

E
Conjugate

MU

Fluorescence Detected

Microparticles        Hapten

Unligated Probe Removed During Wash

## FIGURE 7-20

LCR combined with MEIA. Primers are incorporated into the amplicon during the LCR. The first primer (dark shade) has a hapten covalently attached to the 5′ end. This binds to the antibody-coated microparticle. The second primer (light shade) has a hapten covalently attached to the 3′ end and binds the antibody-enzyme conjugate. Unbound amplicons and unligated primers are washed away. 4-methyleneumbelliferone-phosphate is added and hydrolyzed by the antibody-enzyme conjugate to produce methyleneumbelliferone, which is fluorescent. Fluorescence is directly proportional to the amount of amplicons produced by LCR. (Courtesy of Abbott Laboratories, Waukegan, IL)

**a.**

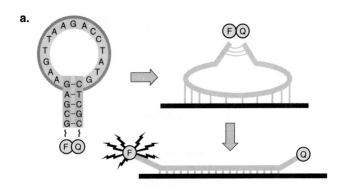

**b.**

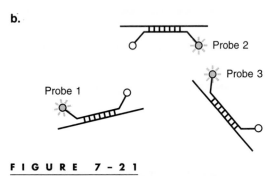

**F I G U R E    7 - 2 1**

Molecular beacons. **a.** Molecular beacon probes (Abbott Laboratories, Waukegan, IL) are designed to form hairpin structures by complementary self-binding when not hybridized to target sequence. This brings the fluorophore label (F) into close proximity to a (universal) fluorescent quencher (Q). When the probe is unbound there is no observable fluorescence during the detection process. When the probe binds LCR amplified products, it separates the fluorophore from the quencher and fluorescence is detectable. **b.** Different fluorophore labeled probes, or beacons, can be used within the same homogeneous reaction mix to detect different amplicons with simultaneous detection by a multiplex detection system. (Courtesy of Abbott Laboratories)

used within the same reaction mix to detect different target sequences with simultaneous detection at a "multiplex" detection system. Internal controls are incorporated in the LCR reaction process and monitored by the multiplex detection system.

### Advantages and Disadvantages

There are two major advantages to the LCR technique coupled with the use of molecular beacons: (1) primers themselves are much longer and extend over most of the target sequence, increasing the specificity of the interaction between target sequence and probe, and (2) primers must hybridize specifically to adjacent regions within the target sequence and be ligated together for the amplification and detection process to occur. If either primer fails to bind specifically to the target sequence,

then it is excluded from the amplification and detection system since both primers are required in both steps.

### NUCLEIC-ACID-SEQUENCE–BASED AMPLIFICATION

Nucleic-acid-sequence–based amplification (NASBA) is an isothermal amplification of target RNA. RNA is more abundant in cells because it is transcribed from a single copy of DNA. This natural amplification process increases the total number of target molecules for amplification, which reduces the number of amplification cycles required for detection of the amplicon.[29]

Nuclisens7 (Organon Teknika, Akzo Nobel, NV) utilizes the simultaneous activity of reverse transcriptase, RNAse H, and RNA polymerase to selectively amplify RNA target sequences. The RNA is first annealed to a primer that encodes an RNA polymerase promoter sequence as well as being specific for the RNA target sequence. Reverse transcriptase copies the RNA target into complementary DNA (cDNA) (Figure 7–22). This results in a RNA-DNA hybrid that is then acted on by RNAse H. RNAse H is an enzyme that digests RNA, leaving behind the single strand of cDNA. A second primer then anneals to the cDNA and is extended by reverse transcriptase, making double-stranded DNA with an intact promoter. RNA polymerase then generates multiple mRNA copies from the DNA template. The mRNA amplicons are then detected by a chemiluminescent-labeled probe and subsequent chemiluminescence.

### Laboratory Applications

Assays have been developed for the detection of CMV, HCV, and HIV, and with the use of internals controls and standards, quantitative HIV levels can be performed.

### Advantages and Disadvantages

One of the major advantages of NASBA is the targeting of RNA, which is already naturally amplified within the cells, and the use of RNA polymerase, which generates thousands of mRNA amplicons in a short time. Typical amplification is on the order of a billionfold increase in about 90 minutes. Additionally, isothermal reaction methodology removes the need to purchase expensive thermal cyclers used in PCR and LCR.

### TRANSCRIPTION-MEDIATED AMPLIFICATION

Gen Probe (San Diego, CA) developed a nucleic acid amplification method called transcription-mediated amplification (TMA) to simplify the complex, time-consuming steps initially present with early amplified nucleic acid assays. TMA is an isothermal process that can be performed in a heatblock or waterbath. The kinetics of TMA are very rapid with billions of RNA amplicons being produced from a single target molecule in less than 1 hour. TMA can be used with any type of target nucleic acid including rRNA, mRNA, or DNA, but rRNA is the most common target.

TMA system is composed of three steps: (1) sample preparation, (2) amplification, and (3) detection. Disruption of the

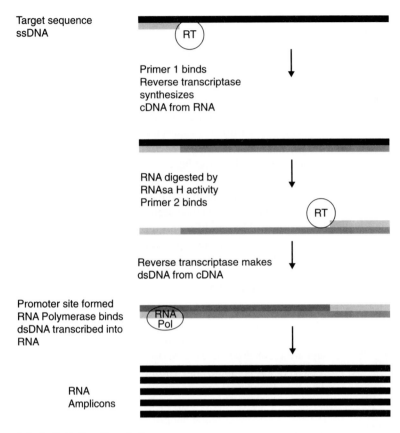

Target sequence
ssDNA

Primer 1 binds
Reverse transcriptase
synthesizes
cDNA from RNA

RNA digested by
RNAsa H activity
Primer 2 binds

Reverse transcriptase makes
dsDNA from cDNA

Promoter site formed
RNA Polymerase binds
dsDNA transcribed into
RNA

RNA
Amplicons

**F I G U R E    7 - 2 2**

Nucleic-acid-sequence–based amplification. Nucleic-acid-sequence–based
amplification (NASBA) is an isothermal amplification of target single-stranded RNA
(ssRNA). Primer 1, which encodes a RNA polymerase (RNA Pol) promoter sequence
and complementary sequence to target RNA, anneals to RNA and reverse
transcriptase (RT) enzyme transcribes the RNA into complementary DNA (cDNA).
RNAse H enzyme then digests the RNA of the RNA-DNA hybrid to leave behind the
single strand of cDNA. A second sequence specific primer anneals to the cDNA and
is extended by RT to generate double-stranded DNA (dsDNA) with an intact
promoter. RNA Pol then recognizes the promoter site and transcribes multiple mRNA
copies from the dsDNA template. The mRNA amplicons are then detected by a
labeled probe and detection system.

microorganism is necessary to release the target nucleic acid into the assay mixture. This is performed by chemical or enzymatic methods or mechanical sonication. The released nucleic acid is stabilized, denatured, and serves as a template for in vitro replication. The components of the TMA reaction mix are primers or oligonucleotides that bind to target sequence and initiate the reaction, nucleotides, and two enzymes to drive the autocatalytic reaction. T7 RNA polymerase transcribes RNA from DNA and reverse transcriptase synthesizes DNA from RNA or DNA templates. Additionally, reverse transcriptase has inherent RNAse H activity to degrade RNA in RNA-DNA hybrids after it has been copied into cDNA. In the first step of amplification, a primer encoding a promoter and complementary sequence to specific target sequence binds at a de-

fined site in the target sequence (Figure 7–23). Reverse transcriptase then extends the primer to copy target rRNA into cDNA. The DNA-RNA hybrid is then degraded by RNAse H activities of the reverse transcriptase. A second primer then binds to the cDNA copy and is extended by reverse transcriptase, creating a dsDNA molecule with an intact promoter. RNA polymerase recognizes the promoter sequence and initiates transcription. Each newly synthesized RNA reenters the TMA process (becoming autocatalytic) and serves as a template for a new round of replication, leading to an exponential expansion of RNA amplicon. Each DNA template can make 100 to 1000 copies of RNA amplicon that contribute to the autocatalytic process, resulting in billions of amplicons in less than 1 hour.

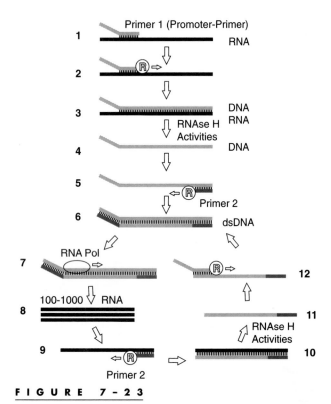

**F I G U R E   7 – 2 3**

Transcription-mediated amplification. Step 1. Promoter-primer binds to RNA target; step 2. Reverse transcriptase (RT) creates DNA copy of RNA target; step 3. RNA:DNA duplex; step 4. RNAse H activities of RT degrades the RNA; step 5. Primer 2 binds to the DNA and RT creates a new DNA copy; step 6. Double-stranded DNA template with a promoter sequence; step 7. RNA polymerase (RNA POL) initiates transcription of RNA from DNA template; step 8. 100–1000 copies of RNA amplicon are produced; step 9. Primer 2 binds to each RNA amplicon and RT creates a DNA copy; step 10. RNA:DNA duplex; step 11. RNAse H activities of RT degrades the RNA; and step 12. Promoter primer binds to the newly synthesized DNA. RT creates a double-stranded DNA (dsDNA) and the autocatalytic cycle repeats, resulting in a billion-fold amplification. (Courtesy of Gen-Probe, San Diego, CA)

Detection of the RNA amplicon produced by TMA is performed using the same hybridization-protection-assay-separation-detection process used in the Gen-Probe direct assays (Figure 7–17). Acridinium-ester–labeled DNA probes are added and allowed to hybridize to specific target sequences within the RNA amplicon produced by TMA. Separation of hybridized from unhybridized probes is done by the addition of selection reagents that hydrolyze the acridinium ester on the unhybridized probes. No light is emitted in the luminometer from the unhybridized probes; only those acridinium esters protected within the double helix are not hydrolyzed by the selection reagents and emit light during the detection process.

Dual-kinetic assays have been developed where two target rRNAs are amplified by the TMA process simultaneously. The two types of RNA amplicons are then hybridized to different, specific oligonucleotides, modified by acridinium-ester labels with different light-off kinetics (dual kinetic). Simultaneous detection is accomplished based on the light-off kinetics of the acridinium ester, one is a flasher, a short burst of light, whereas the other is a glower, a slower, less intensive burst of light (Figure 7–24). Single or combined light-off events can be detected based on the light intensity and duration of the light-off event.

A recent modification of the TMA assay includes a target capture probe to isolate target sequence away from cellular debris prior to TMA amplification (Figure 7–25). This increases enzyme activity by removing naturally inhibiting substances that are present in clinical specimens.

## Laboratory Applications

The first application of the Gen-Probe TMA system was the *M. tuberculosis* test. This assay provides same-day test results and can be performed on a routine basis. Other amplified assays are *C. trachomatis*, *N. gonorrhoeae*, HIV, HCV, *Mycobacterium avium* complex, and chronic myelogenous leukemia. The Gen-Probe dual-kinetic assay for HIV and HCV was recently adopted by the American Red Cross as the screening test for the national blood supply. Large numbers of samples (blood donor products) are first pooled and then screened by the Gen-Probe target capture dual-kinetic assay for HIV and HCV (Figure 7–26). Positive pools are then segregated, retested and individual positive samples identified. This has greatly reduced the total number of tests required to ensure a safe blood supply.

New instrumentation systems by Gen-Probe include a fully automated TMA amplification instrument (TIGRIS, Gen-Probe, San Diego, CA) and a dual-platform instrument (VIDAS, Gen-Probe, San Diego CA) that performs TMA amplification and immunoassays.

## Advantages and Disadvantages

Technological and clinical advantages provided by the TMA HPA test methodology include: RNA transcription amplification using two enzymes, RNA polymerase and reverse transcriptase, isothermal amplification of target rRNA already present in thousands of copies per cell, RNA amplicons that are more labile outside the reaction tube than a DNA product, thereby reducing laboratory contamination and false positives, rapid kinetics resulting in excess of 10 billionfold amplification within 15 to 30 minutes, and, lastly, reaction and detection occurs within a single-tube format.

## STRAND-DISPLACEMENT AMPLIFICATION

Strand-displacement amplification is a unique isothermal process for the exponential amplification of target dsDNA sequences. Target sequence can be either RNA or DNA but they must first be converted to dsDNA. Components of SDA include primers, DNA polymerase, restriction endonuclease, and

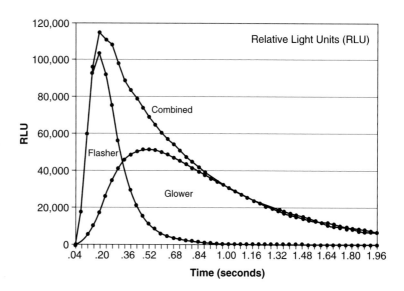

### FIGURE 7-24

Dual-kinetic chemiluminescence. Different light-off reaction kinetics allow for the use of two chemiluminescent molecules within the same reaction mixture. Flasher is a short burst of light energy, Glower is a longer, lower intensity of light, whereas combined is a unique pattern distinguishable from either the flasher or the glower. Dual-kinetic chemiluminescent probes allow for the detection of two target nucleic acid sequences. (Courtesy of Gen-Probe, San Diego, CA)

nucleotides. The target sequence is denatured to generate single-stranded DNA and two primers are then allowed to anneal to adjacent regions on the target DNA (Figure 7–27). The first primer encodes a region complementary to specific target sequence, whereas the second primer is complementary to tar-

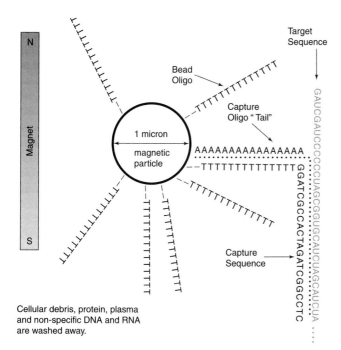

Cellular debris, protein, plasma and non-specific DNA and RNA are washed away.

### FIGURE 7-25

Target capture technology. Lysed sample is reacted with target capture beads, which bind specific RNA target sequences. Target RNA bound to the magnetic bead is held in place with a magnet, whereas cellular debris and nonspecific nucleic acids are washed away. Natural inhibiting substances present in the patient sample are also removed by this wash. The target sequence is then amplified by transcription-mediated amplification. (Courtesy of Gen-Probe, San Diego, CA)

get sequence and an additional noncomplementary sequence corresponding to a restriction endonuclease site. The second primer is also labeled with a fluorophore at the 5' end and a quencher at its 3' end. DNA polymerase extends both primers, reading DNA template and adding nucleotides to the primer. During the extension process, the extension of the first primer displaces the second primer and its extending sequence. Another set of primers binds the newly synthesized strand in a similar way and is extended by DNA polymerase to form double-stranded DNA. The restriction endonuclease site is then recognized by the restriction endonuclease and nicked. The DNA polymerase recognizes the nick and repairs the DNA by extending the sequence again while displacing the previously synthesized strand. The process is repeated generating multiple copies.

Detection is accomplished by complete cleavage of the restriction endonuclease site, releasing the fluorophore-labeled DNA fragment and freeing it from the quenching effects. Unbound primer forms a hairpin structure that brings the quencher in close proximity to the fluorophore so no fluorescence is detected. Only primer that is incorporated in the amplicon (dsDNA) is cleaved by the restriction endonuclease, releasing the fluorophor from the quenching effect.

### Laboratory Applications

SDA assays, Probe Tec ET system (BD Biosciences, Franklin Lanes, NY), have been developed for the detection of *C. trachomatis* and *N. gonorrhoeae*. Owing to the isothermal amplification process, the technology has been automated with potential to reduce cross-contamination and false positives.

### Advantages and Disadvantages

BD Probe Tec ET system is performed in a 1-hour assay with SDA generating millions of copies through a unique amplification process. The fluorescence detection system is linked directly with the primer amplification process, incorporating the label into each amplicon generated. Test methodology can be

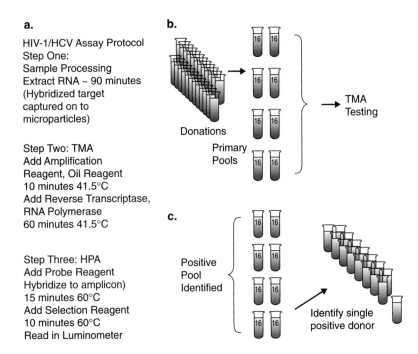

**a.**

HIV-1/HCV Assay Protocol
Step One:
Sample Processing
Extract RNA ~ 90 minutes
(Hybridized target
captured on to
microparticles)

Step Two: TMA
Add Amplification
Reagent, Oil Reagent
10 minutes 41.5°C
Add Reverse Transcriptase,
RNA Polymerase
60 minutes 41.5°C

Step Three: HPA
Add Probe Reagent
Hybridize to amplicon)
15 minutes 60°C
Add Selection Reagent
10 minutes 60°C
Read in Luminometer

**b.**

Donations

Primary
Pools

TMA
Testing

**c.**

Positive
Pool
Identified

Identify single
positive donor

**FIGURE 7-26**

Dual-kinetic TMA assay for the human immunodeficiency virus (HIV) and hepatitis C virus (HCV). **a.** The dual-kinetic assay (HIV/HCV, Gen-Probe, San Diego, CA) test and pooling scheme is used for screening the national blood donor supply. Large numbers of samples (blood donor products) are **b.** pooled into groups of 16, and then screened by target capture, TMA **(a.)** and dual-kinetic chemiluminescence with probes designed for the detection of HIV and HCV. **c.** Positive pools are then segregated, retested, and individual samples tested to determine the positive donor sample. This process greatly reduces the total number of screen tests required for blood component processing.

semi- or fully automated, reducing cross-contamination, false positives, and personnel time.

## EMERGING TECHNOLOGIES

DNA microarray or biochips based on microelectronic and semiconductor technology is under development as we gain more sequence information through the Human Genome Project and research on infectious agents. DNA fragments (probes) are anchored to glass or silicon chips and electronically act as transistors in an integrated circuit.[30] Thousands of oligonucleotide probes can be placed on a single chip, allowing for simultaneous hybridization events and detection.

DNA chips have been developed and manufactured using different methodology.[30] Affymetrix Inc. (Santa Clara, CA) utilizes a photolithographic method for the production of oligonucleotide probes (20 to 25 base pairs) coupled to glass or silicon surface. DNA microarray or spotted DNA chips are produced by robotic delivery of premanufactured oligonucleotides to a microgel on a glass slide much like an ink-jet printer. These oligonucleotides are routinely 500–5,000 base pairs.

Laser microarray technology or microelectronic circuitry may be used to detect hybridization events. Analysis may be performed on clinical samples directly or amplicons generated from an amplification procedure. Laser microarray technology requires that the clinical sample or amplicons be first coupled with a fluorescent label. The labeled sample or amplicons are then reacted with the biochip and hybridization events detected by a microarray reading device. The intensity and location of fluorescence specifies the strength or amount of hybridization and the identity of the gene or organism in the sample. Microelectronic circuitry utilizes the change in resistance due to hybridization of target sequence to oligonucleotide for detection of hybridization events. Each silicon chip consists of electrodes, independently addressable via an electron control system to detect hybridization at each oligonucleotide. Again, the location and intensity of the change is used to determine the quantity and identity of the gene or infectious agent in the sample.

A new signal amplification technology, currently under development, involves the amplified cycling of probe in a rapid, simple, isothermal method for the detection of target nucleic acid sequence.[30] VelogeneJ (ID Biomedical, Vancouver, CA) uses a unique DNA–RNA–DNA probe sequence to provide RNAse H sensitive links when the probe is hybridized

**Step One: Generation of Target Sequence**

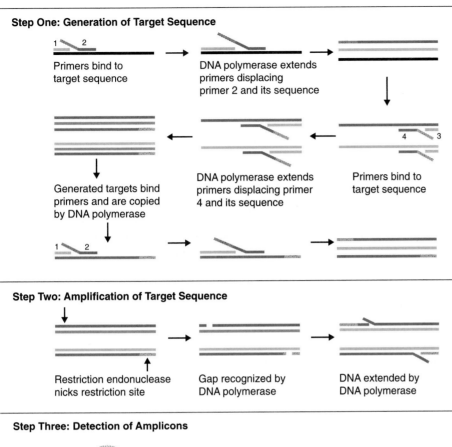

Primers bind to
target sequence

DNA polymerase extends
primers displacing
primer 2 and its sequence

Primers bind to
target sequence

DNA polymerase extends
primers displacing primer
4 and its sequence

Generated targets bind
primers and are copied
by DNA polymerase

**Step Two: Amplification of Target Sequence**

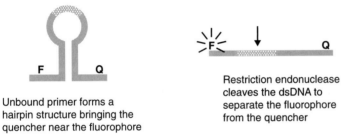

Restriction endonuclease
nicks restriction site

Gap recognized by
DNA polymerase

DNA extended by
DNA polymerase

**Step Three: Detection of Amplicons**

Unbound primer forms a
hairpin structure bringing the
quencher near the fluorophore

Restriction endonuclease
cleaves the dsDNA to
separate the fluorophore
from the quencher

# FIGURE 7-27

Strand-displacement amplification. Step 1: Generation of target sequence. Primers 1
and 2 bind specifically to target sequence. Primer 2 encodes additional sequence
that is not specific for target sequence; instead, it encodes an endonuclease restriction
site (gray patches in primer block). Both primers are recognized and extended by
DNA polymerase. As primer 1 is extended, primer 2 and its complementary
sequence are displaced. Primers 3 and 4 specifically bind to target sequence
generated by the extension of primer 1 and 2. Primer 4 encodes additional sequence
that is not specific for target sequence; instead, it encodes an endonuclease restriction
site (gray patches in primer block). Both primers are recognized by DNA polymerase
and extended, generating target that can bind primers as before. Step 2:
Amplification of target sequence. The endonuclease restriction site is recognized by
the endonuclease and partially cleaved, generating a break in a single strand of the
dsDNA. This gap is recognized by DNA polymerase, filled in and extended,
displacing the remaining complementary strand. This process is repeated many times
generating multiple copies of target sequence. Step 3: Detection of amplicons. The
primers 2 and 4 form hairpin structures when not incorporated into full-length
sequence. Primers 2 and 4 are labeled with a fluorophore (F) at the 5′ end and a
quencher (Q) on the 3′end. In the unincorporated form, the hairpin brings the
fluorophore into close proximity of the quencher so that when the sample is exposed
to incident light, no fluorescence is observed. When the primers are incorporated, the
fluorophore is cleaved free of the quencher by the endonuclease and when the
sample is exposed to incident light, fluorescence is observed.

to its target DNA sequence.[30] When the probe is bound to target sequence, the RNAse H sensitive sites are cleaved, generating multiple cleaved probe fragments that accumulate and are quantified by a detection system. The target sequence is not amplified, which greatly reduces the possibility of cross-contamination and false positives. Additionally, this probe design is generic in that it only requires the linkage of specific complementary sequence for different target sequences to the DNA–RNA–DNA hybrid complex.

## SUMMARY

In this chapter, we have discussed many molecular and immunoassays. Molecular and immunoassays use different detection systems to determine the presence or quantity of target molecules of interest. Several differences within or among the various assays include: (1) whether the molecule of interest is nucleic acid (DNA, mRNA, rRNA), antibody, antigen, or a hapten, (2) whether the reactions are competitive or noncompetitive, direct, or amplified, and (3) whether the bound and free forms of the labeled ligands or probes are separated (heterogeneous methods) or not separated (homogeneous methods) before detection.

Some of the more common molecular and immunoassay techniques were discussed. These include immunoassays that use isotopic labels, RIAs, and IRMAs; immunoassays that use enzyme labels, ELISA and EMIT; and assays that utilize fluorescent compounds as labels, such as FPIA or fluorogenic substrates in enzyme-coupled procedures, SLFIA. Molecular assays are designed to either directly detect target sequences of DNA or RNA or amplicons generated from those target sequences. rRNA target sequences are naturally amplified since they are present in the thousands of ribosomes found in each cell. Amplification methods have been developed to detect very small amounts of DNA or RNA target sequence in clinical samples. Amplification methods include PCR, LCR, NASBA, TMA, and SDA, all of which use molecular enzymes for the in vitro synthesis of amplicons that are detected by a variety of technologies (radioactivity, enzyme catalysis, fluorescence, or chemiluminescence).

RIAs were the first commonly used immunoassay methods. However, clinical laboratories have incorporated alternative, automated immunoassay methods to eliminate the storage, handling, and disposal problems associated with the use of radioisotopes. Enzyme immunoassays and fluorescent immunoassays have been developed to replace the use of RIA. Nonisotopic DNA probe hybridization procedures are also a common alternative assay for the detection of disease states or infectious agents. Our knowledge and understanding of molecular biology is ongoing and exponentially expanding as we conclude the Human Genome Project efforts and gain new technological tools. Clever manipulations of molecular enzymes and use as tools allow for the development of unique methods and protocols for the detection of disease states or infectious agents. Discussion of emerging technologies simply points out that we are only at the beginning of our capabilities.

## REFERENCES

1. GenBank: National Institutes of Health, National Center for Biotechnology Information. Accessible at: http://www.ncbi.nlm.nih.gov/GenBank/
2. Darnell J, Lodish H, Baltimore D: General features of DNA replication, repair and recombination. In Darnell J, Lodish H, Baltimore D (eds.): *Molecular Cell Biology.* 2nd ed. New York, Scientific American Books, 1990, pp 449–487.
3. Darnell J, Lodish H, Baltimore D: RNA synthesis and gene control in prokaryotes. In Darnell J, Lodish H, Baltimore D (eds.): *Molecular Cell Biology.* 2nd ed. New York, Scientific American Books, 1990, pp 229–260.
4. Lehninger AL, Nelson DL, Cox MM: RNA metabolism. In Lehninger AL, Nelson DL, Cox MM (eds.): *Principles of Biochemistry.* 2nd ed. New York, Worth Publishers, 1997, pp 856–891.
5. Darnell J, Lodish H, Baltimore D: Growing and manipulating cells. In Darnell J, Lodish H, Baltimore D (eds.): *Molecular Cell Biology.* 2nd ed. New York, Scientific American Books, 1990, pp 151–188.
6. Yalow RS, Berson SA: Assay of plasma insulin in human subjects by immunological methods. Nature 184:1648, 1959.
7. Yalow RS: Radioimmunoassay of hormones. In Williams E (ed.): *Textbook of Endocrinology.* Philadelphia, WB Saunders, 1985, pp 123–132.
8. Kohler G, Milstein C: Continuous cultures of fused cells secreting antibody of predefined specificity. Nature 256:495, 1975.
9. Catt K, Niall HD, Tregear GW: Solid-phase radioimmunoassay of human growth hormone. Biochemistry Journal 100:31C, 1966.
10. Catt K, Tregear GW: Solid-phase radioimmunoassay in antibody-coated tubes. Science 158:1570–1572, 1967.
11. Wide L, Porath J: Radioimmunoassay of proteins with the use of sephadex-coupled antibody. Biochimie Biophysica Acta 130:257–260, 1966.
12. Bowie LJ: *Automated Instrumentation for Radioimmunoassay.* Boca Raton, CRC Press, Inc., 1980.
13. Miles LEM, Hales CN: Labeled antibodies and immunological assay system. Nature 219:186–189, 1968.
14. Lazarchik J, Hoyer LW: Immunoradiometric measurement of the factor VIII procoagulant antigen. J Clin Invest 62:1048–1052, 1978.
15. Engvall E, Perlmann P: Enzyme-linked immunosorbent assay (ELISA). Quantitative assay for immunoglobulin G. Immunochemistry 8:871–874, 1971.

16.  Van Weemen BK, Schuurs A: Immunoassay using anti-gen enzyme conjugates. FEBS Letters 15:232–236, 1971.

17.  Rubenstein KE, Schneider RS, Ullman EF: Homogeneous enzyme immunoassay—a new immunochemical technique. Biochem Biophys Res Comm 47:846–851, 1972.

18.  Burd JF, Wong RC, Feeney JE, et al.: Homogeneous reactant-labeled fluorescent immunoassay for therapeutic drugs exemplified by gentamicin determination in human serum. Clin Chem 23:1402–1408, 1977.

19.  Wong RC, Burd JF, Carrico FJ, et al.: Substrate-labeled fluorescent immunoassay for phenytoin in human serum. Clin Chem 25:686–691, 1979.

20.  Ngo TT, Carrico RJ, Boguslaski RC: Homogeneous fluorescence immunoassay for protein using β-galactosyl-umbelliferone label. Paper presented at the Second International Conference on Diagnostic Immunology, New England College, Henniber, NH, 1979.

21.  Ngo TT, Wong RC: Fluorogenic enzyme substrate labeled immunoassays for haptens and macromolecules. In Ngo TT, Lenhoff HM (eds.): *Enzyme-mediated Immunoassay.* New York, Plenum Press, 1985.

22.  Colbert DL, Smith DS, Landon J, et al.: Single-reagent polarization fluoroimmunoassay for barbiturates. Clin Chem 30:1765–1769, 1984.

23.  Popelka SR, Miller DM, Holen JT, et al.: Fluorescence polarization immunoassay II. Analyzer for rapid, precise measurement of fluorescence polarization with use of disposable cuvettes. Clin Chem 27:1198–1202, 1981.

24.  Klug WS, Cummings MR: Chromosome mutations: Variations in chromosome number and arrangement. In Klug WS, Cummings MR (eds.): *Genetics.* 6th ed. Upper Saddle River, NJ, Prentice Hall, 2000, pp 251–281.

25.  Reed R, Holmes D, Weyers J, et al.: Molecular genetics I—fundamental principles. In Reed R, Holmes D, Weyers J, et al. (eds.): *Practical Skills in Biomolecular Sciences.* Harlow, England, Addison Wesley Longman Ltd, 1998, pp 228–236.

26.  Klug WS, Cummings MR: Construction and analysis of DNA clones. In Klug WS, Cummings MR (eds.): *Genetics.* 6th ed. Upper Saddle River, NJ, Prentice Hall, 2000, pp 499–529.

27.  Klug WS, Cummings MR: DNA structure and analysis. In Klug WS, Cummings MR (eds.): *Genetics.* 6th ed. Upper Saddle River, NJ, Prentice Hall, 2000, pp 282–319.

28.  Zane HD: Molecular techniques in immunology theoretical and practical concepts. In Zane HD (ed.): *Laboratory Medicine.* Philadelphia, WB Saunders, 2001, pp 314–336.

29.  Farkas DH: *DNA Simplified II: The Illustrated Hitchhiker's Guide to DNA.* Washington, DC, American Association for Clinical Chemistry, 1999, p 55.

30.  Vossler JL: Molecular diagnostics in the clinical microbiology laboratory. ADVANCE 12(17):38–42, 2000.

## BIBLIOGRAPHY

Abbas AK, Lichtman AH, Pober JS: *Cellular and Molecular Immunology.* Philadelphia, WB Saunders, 2000.

Darnell J, Lodish H, Baltimore D: *Molecular Cell Biology.* New York, Scientific American Books, 1990.

Klug WS, Cummings MR: *Genetics.* Upper Saddle River, NJ, Prentice Hall, 2000.

Reed R, Holmes D, Weyers J, et al.: *Practical Skills in Biomolecular Sciences.* Harlow, England, Addison Wesley Longman Ltd, 1998.

# CHAPTER 8

# Laboratory Automation

*Jean D. Holter*

Automation in the clinical chemistry laboratory has increased over the past 40 years. Automated instruments have become a necessity because of the volume and the variety of tests routinely performed. As medical science has improved, more patients survive illnesses and traumas that would have been fatal just a few short years ago. This advance has created a continuing need for laboratory testing to monitor these patients. In addition, more tests are now available and the results are needed by the physician in a manner that allows their timely consideration in the medical decision-making process. Along with this increasing workload has come the demand for greater productivity among laboratory workers. The result of all this has been the development of highly efficient and sophisticated automated instruments.

The first automated chemistry analyzer appeared in 1957 when the "bubble" used in the auto analyzer was patented. Early attempts at automation produced instruments that measured only one constituent at a time and simply mechanized existing manual methodology. As technology has advanced, however, more constituents can be measured by the same instrument and newer, more reliable methods have been developed. Instrument manufacturers have developed their own reagents specifically for use with their instruments.

In this chapter, the principles of automation as applied to clinical chemistry are discussed and specific examples of these principles are presented using currently available instrumentation. Before the discussion begins, however, some definitions are in order.

The term **automation** can be defined as the technique, method, or system of operating or controlling a mechanical or productive process by highly automatic means. When applied to clinical chemistry, automation means a mechanical approach to the analytical processes. Most automated analytical instruments have been designed to perform the repetitious steps in the determination of various analyte concentrations in patient samples, primarily serum, with minimal operator intervention. This has the benefit of eliminating tasks that are repetitive and monotonous, which can lead to boredom, inattention, and errors in analysis.

Automated systems do not fall into easily defined categories. A variety of approaches to automation exist, and most manufacturers use these in combination with their instruments. The following are the most common terms currently used in describing automated systems.

**Batch analysis**—Samples are processed in concert as a group or "batch" in the same analytical analysis.

**Parallel analysis**—Samples undergo a series of analytical processes, usually for one analysis at a time, concurrently, often used with batch analysis.

**Sequential analysis**—Samples are processed sequentially rather than in a batch. Samples enter the system one after another, are processed, and results are issued in the same order.

**Continuous flow**—A type of sequential analysis in which all samples pass through the same continuous stream and undergo the same analytical process at the same rate.

**Simultaneous analysis**—More than one analysis performed on a sample at the same time.

**Discrete analysis**—Each sample reaction is compartmentalized. Each sample has its own physical space in which the individual chemical reaction takes place, often used with **simultaneous analysis.**

**Selective (discretionary) analysis**—Samples can be processed by any individual method or combination of methods available on the given analyzer at the discretion of the operator.

**Test repertoire**—The tests available to be analyzed on a given instrument. The immediate test repertoire includes the tests that can be performed at any one time, and the total test repertoire includes all tests that could be performed given the appropriate instrument configuration.

**Throughput**—The maximum number of test results that can be produced by an analyzer in a given time period, usually an hour.

**Dwell time**—The minimum time from initial sampling to the production of a result.

**Closed system**—The assay parameters are set by the manufacturer and require the purchasing of reagents from the manufacturer because of a unique container or format.

**Open system**—The reagents can be purchased from a variety of sources or vendors. The assay parameters may be modified by the purchaser of the system.

**Random access analyzer**—A system where any specimen can be analyzed in any sequence with regard to the initial order of the specimens.

## ROBOTICS

Most of the instrument robotics in the clinical laboratories has involved front-end automation to move the sample. The robotics typically transfers the sample from the centrifuge and loads the sample onto the analyzer. The initial systems have used conveyor belt systems or devices for moving the sample to the instrument. Two companies, Johnson & Johnson Clinical Diagnostics and Dade International Chemistry Systems, are developing front-end conveyor systems and software for use with their own instruments.[1] Olympus at olympus.com has a laboratory automation system for sale.

The post-analytical/back-end handling phase has accomplished the most through the management of data by computerization of the reporting system. Areas that have been computerized include quality control, reviewing results to be reported, transmitting results, and reagent inventory.

Only the largest laboratories can support the high volume of samples needed for total laboratory automation (TLA). Many laboratories automate a section or a specific process rather than the complete laboratory. The advantage of this approach is the reduction of labor, which encompasses approximately 65% of the laboratory's budget.[2]

## STAGES OF AUTOMATED ANALYSIS

Each automated system involves a variety of steps that mirror the steps required in manual analysis. Figure 8–1 illustrates these steps, which are explained below.

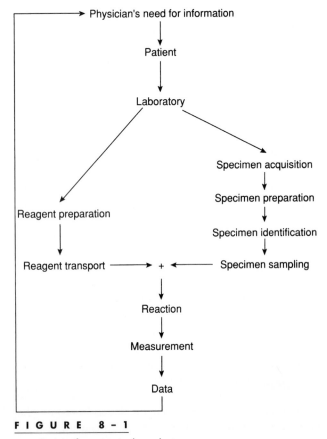

Steps of automated analysis.

## Specimen

### ACQUISITION

Although not a step in the actual analysis, acquisition is one of the most important steps in the scheme of any method of analysis, especially automated analysis. There is no substitute for a competent phlebotomist using approved venipuncture technique and appropriate collection tubes. In addition, the patient must be adequately prepared (e.g. fasting). Attention must also be paid to collection time, the time required for transport to the laboratory, and the time the results are needed by the physician. Any method of analysis can be no better than the specimen received.

### PREPARATION

Preparation is by far the most time-consuming step and is fraught with the possibility of error. Samples must be labeled, centrifuged, and split into aliquots if analysis is to be done at more than one workstation.

Some proposals have been made to expedite the specimen preparation step. These include the use of whole blood, which eliminates the need for centrifugation. Applications using ion-selective electrodes are available for measurement of such substances as sodium, potassium, and calcium in whole blood. Other proposals involve bedside testing and the use of probes to measure analytes.

Another proposal to accelerate the specimen processing step, or at least minimize human intervention, is the use of robotics. Modular robotics systems have been developed that mechanize the sample preparation steps. These systems can position tubes relative to centrifuges and racks and pipet, and pour and mix samples. The majority of the robotics systems use bar-coded specimens and sorting stations to solve many problems encountered in specimen processing.[3]

### IDENTIFICATION

Proper identification of a patient sample is one of the most critical steps in laboratory analysis. Mislabeling a patient sample can lead to the production and transmission of erroneous results, which in turn may have significant consequences for the patient. From the time of specimen procurement to the reporting of the final result, there are numerous opportunities for mismatching samples and results.

The initial connection between the patient and specimen is made at the time the specimen is collected. This is done by means of a label, which is generated manually or by computer. In many computerized laboratories, entry of a test order for a specific patient generates a label with a unique accession number, patient information, and the tests requested. It also results in the creation of a record in the computer that remains incomplete until the test results are entered. The label generated by this computer operation is affixed to the specimen when the blood is drawn. Arrival of the specimen in the laboratory is documented by log-in or checkoff procedures.

Noncomputerized laboratories rely on appropriate identification of samples by the phlebotomist at the time of collection. The phlebotomist manually prepares a label containing the patient's name and collection information. When this specimen arrives in the laboratory along with the test requisition form, it may be assigned a unique accession number.

Regardless of how a specimen is initially identified, once analysis begins there must be a way to link test results with the specimen and ultimately with the patient. At each step of the analytical process, from preparation of the specimen to reporting final results, positive specimen identification must be made. A growing number of instruments is capable of sampling from the original or primary collection tube. The use of bar-coded labels, produced by the laboratory's computer system, by hand when the specimen arrives in the laboratory, or by the instrument itself when the specimen is programmed, facilitates the identification of specimens by the instrument. The results are then matched with the patient's accession number, which is included in the bar code.

If the primary collection tube cannot be used, the specimen is usually transferred to some type of sampling device. These sample containers must be labeled with the same information as found on the original tube, including the accession number. This procedure can be done by using secondary labels or by coding the containers and correlating them to a work list or load list. Results are ultimately matched with the patient's accession number, which was assigned when the specimen was logged into the laboratory. Labels used to identify specimens while being analyzed must be readable by the operators as well as the instruments so that specimens can be readily located.

Clearly, there are many opportunities during processing and analysis for mismatching specimens and results. The risks increase with manual transcription of information during accessioning, labeling, relabeling, and preparation of load lists. If specimens must be analyzed in a specific order defined by a load list, more opportunities for error exist. The smaller number of steps requiring human intervention in identification of samples decreases the possibilities for error.

## SAMPLING AND TRANSPORT

Presentation of specimens to an instrument can occur in a variety of configurations. These configurations are divided into two general types: sampling directly from the primary collection tube or sampling from aliquots of specimen manually transferred into containers.

When the primary collection tube is used, a separator of some sort is usually present that forms a barrier between the serum and cells. One type of separator is a gel, present in the evacuated tube at the time of specimen collection, which moves into position when the blood is centrifuged. Another is a filter placed into the tube after the blood is collected but before the blood is spun. The filter also moves into position between the cells and serum when the blood is centrifuged. With a separator in place the possibility of sampling cells is minimized.

There are several observations to be made regarding the use of sample cups for presentation of the specimen to the instrument for sampling. One is that the cup should be made of an inert material so that it neither adds nor removes analytes of interest. The best materials for these container cups are glass or polyvinyl. Another consideration is that the dead volume should be at a minimum. The dead volume is that volume of specimen in excess of the sample volume that must be present to ensure that the full sample volume is aspirated. A third observation is that decreased cross-contamination and lower costs result if the sample container cups are disposable.

The specimens, whether in primary collection tubes or sample cups, are placed into a loading zone where they are moved into position for sampling by the instrument. The loading zone is an area designed to hold specimens until they are actually sampled by the instrument. Loading zones can be turntables with spaces for sample holding cups or tubes, a series of racks that hold cups or tubes or even a serpentine chain of holders for tubes.

Evaporation of the sample in the loading zone can have a serious impact on the accuracy of results. An early study claimed up to 50% analytical error over 4 hours because of evaporation.[4] A more recent study noted analytical error up to 16% after 4 hours uncovered.[5] Several factors affect the amount of evaporation, including sample size, size and shape of the cup, whether the cup is covered, and environmental factors such as temperature, relative humidity, and airflow. Many instruments have covers for the loading zone or individual caps for the cups or tubes to help minimize evaporation. A few instruments regulate the temperature of the loading zone.

Other aspects of the loading zone that may affect sample integrity require some consideration. Some analytes are temperature-labile and may be degraded at room temperature. Refrigeration of the loading zone is one solution to this problem but only a few instruments have refrigerated loading zones. Photosensitive analytes also require some consideration. Lengthy exposure to room light can destroy constituents such as bilirubin. Room light can be effectively excluded from the loading zone through the use of colored (smoke, orange, red) covers. These covers not only help prevent photodegradation but also evaporation.

Most instruments use thin, stainless-steel probes to introduce the sample. The probe enters the sample, in some cases after first piercing a protective cap, and aspirates the appropriate volume. A liquid level sensor is often associated with the sample probe so that the probe goes only a specified distance into the sample. If the same sample probe is used for all specimens, the possibility for carryover exists. Carryover is minimized on many instruments by incorporating external and internal probe flushes between sampling. It is eliminated in those systems that use disposable sample probes.

The sample, once aspirated, is transported to the reaction vessel in the instrument. Continuous flow analyzers use peristaltic pumps and plastic tubing to transport the sample and the reagents through the instruments. Most discrete analyzers use positive liquid-displacement devices such as syringes to volumetrically aspirate and dispense the sample into the reaction vessel.

Continuous flow analyzers using peristaltic pumps and plastic tubing rely on the inside diameter of the tubing and the length of time the probe is in the sample to determine sample size. Since samples are aspirated sequentially and uniformly, a precise measure of sample size is not necessary. Use of flow-rated tubing for which the volume of liquid that travels in the tubing per unit time is known and knowledge of the time the probe spends in the sample allows one to calculate the approximate sample size.

Positive displacement devices can be calibrated for accurate and precise measurement of volumes as small as 1 $\mu$L. The speed at which the motors drive these devices must be carefully controlled because sudden changes in velocity can cause imprecise and inaccurate pipetting. The accuracy of any pipetting system should be verified periodically and should not exceed $\pm$1% of the nominal volume of the system.

## Reagents

The source of the reagents depends on whether the instrument is an open or closed system. An open system is one where a variety of vendors may provide the reagents. A closed system utilizes only one vendor, typically the manufacturer of the instrument.

### PREPARATION

Many approaches to reagents and reagent preparation are available on the market. The most common approach is preprepared liquid reagents that are bulk packaged in glass or plastic bottles. In many instances the storage bottle can be placed directly on or in the instrument, attached to the delivery system, and used without any further preparation, thus minimizing any errors that could arise from improper dilution or processing.

For some systems the reagents are concentrated or in dry powder or lyophilized form and must be diluted with a specified volume of diluent before being used. Although errors could occur as a result of inept reconstitution, storage space is decreased and stability is usually increased. In some systems, human error in reconstituting reagents is avoided by having the instrument perform the reconstitution of the reagent as needed.

Stability of bulk reagents is generally very good. Expiration dates may be a year or more. Reagents that contain enzymes usually have shorter expiration dates. However, stability may be extended by packaging the enzyme components separately. The working reagent, with shorter stability, is prepared by mixing the two components.

Another approach to reagent preparation is the unit test concept. Reagents, usually in a dry form, are prepackaged in amounts sufficient for performing a single test. These premeasured reagents are reconstituted with a diluent such as water, a buffer, or, in the case of the dry slide methods, just the sample. The reconstitution is most often performed automatically by the instrument. Although unit test reagents are usually more expensive than bulk liquid or powdered reagents, they require much less storage space, avoid the possibility of reagent carryover, and are less likely to be wasted.

## TRANSPORT AND DELIVERY

The volume of reagent required for the determination of a given analyte is related directly to the volume of sample used. Most chemical reactions rely on the combination of reagents and sample in exact proportions to yield accurate results. For most instruments these proportions have been predetermined by the manufacturer. However, some manufacturers allow the instrument users to develop and use their own test applications.

In unit test systems the volume of reagent has been premeasured. The "dose" of reagent, already in the reaction vessel, needs only to be delivered to the area where the sample will be added. This is usually done mechanically by pushing the reaction container to a sampling station or loading zone.

Continuous flow systems use peristaltic pumps and plastic tubing to transport reagents through the system. The volume of reagent is determined by the inside diameter of the tubing, just as the volume of sample is determined. The streams containing the sample and reagents are mixed and continue through the system by means of the peristaltic pump action. Some discrete analyzers also use peristaltic pumps to deliver set volumes of reagents to stationary reaction vessels.

Positive displacement syringes are another method to deliver specific volumes of reagent to a reaction chamber. These syringes operate in the same manner as the positive displacement syringes used for sample aspiration and delivery. The same precautions mentioned in an earlier section are necessary: The speed of the driving motor should be controlled as closely as possible to prevent sudden changes in velocity and the accuracy should be verified periodically.

## Reaction Conditions

Discussion of reaction conditions begins with the reaction vessel. In continuous flow systems the reaction container is the tubing through which the reaction mixture flows. In discrete systems, the reaction vessel may be reusable or disposable containers that move through the system or it may be a stationary reaction chamber. In many cases, the reaction vessel is also the cuvette.

Reaction components can be mixed in several ways. In continuous flow analyzers, mixing is achieved through a combination of approaches. First, a series of inversions of the reaction mixture occurs as the stream passes through mixing coils. In addition, the action of the air bubbles that are injected into the flowing stream aids mixing by causing the fluid at the wall of the tubing to move along with the fluid in the center of the tubing resulting in turbulent rather than laminar flow.

Dry slide methods accomplish mixing of the sample with

premixed, premeasured reagents through diffusion. As the sample comes into contact with the top layer of the slide, it is drawn by capillary action into the porous layer. As the reagents hydrate, the components of interest diffuse into the reagent layers.

Discrete systems mix reaction components by means of (1) stirring paddles or sticks, (2) motion of the reaction vessel, (3) forceful addition of reagents, and (4) agitation by air bubbles or ultrasonic waves. Some systems that use stationary reaction chambers incorporate magnetic stir bars to mix components.

Incubation in automated systems involves timed delays during which the reactions proceed. The reaction vessels are usually maintained at constant temperatures to ensure the integrity of the reactions.

Continuous flow systems achieve appropriate incubation times by varying the length of tubing the components flow through; the longer the tubing, the longer the incubation. Discrete systems ensure appropriate incubation times by holding the reaction vessels in a fixed position for the specified length of time or by using microprocessors to delay measurement until the reaction is complete.

Temperature is commonly achieved by using air or water baths or heating blocks. Temperatures are characteristically monitored by thermocouples. Error conditions are flagged when temperatures exceed preset limits. Some instruments allow operator input of desired temperature. Most, however, are preset.

Mention should be made of the use of ion-selective electrodes for the measurement of sodium, potassium, chloride, and occasionally carbon dioxide. The reagent handling systems and reaction conditions for ion-selective electrodes are typically separate from those previously described that apply primarily to colorimetric or enzymatic measurements. Most ion-selective electrodes are of the flow-through variety in which the sample and reference solutions are moved via peristaltic pumps through chambers containing fixed indicator and reference electrodes. The specimen must remain in contact with the electrodes long enough to reach a steady state. The electrodes are designed to minimize response time so that a steady state can be reached rapidly, maximizing the throughput of the system.

## Reaction Measurement

Traditionally, absorbance/transmittance photometry has been used for the measurement of analytes. This method has three basic components: a light source, a method for spectral isolation, and a detector.

Many sources of radiant energy have been incorporated into automated systems. The most common include tungsten, quartz-halogen, deuterium, mercury, and xenon lamps. Each has advantages and disadvantages.

Interference filters are used most often as the method of achieving spectral isolation. These filters can be prepared quite inexpensively and can be made with relatively narrow band-

widths, 5 to 15 nm. Some instruments use monochromators such as diffraction gratings for spectral isolation. Diffraction gratings provide a continuous spectrum and therefore a greater choice of wavelengths for use. A diffraction grating also allows the use of two or more wavelengths (bichromatics) at the same time for correction purposes, to eliminate the absorbance contribution of interfering substances.

Photomultiplier tubes (PMTs) are the most prevalent detectors in automated systems. Photodiodes have adequate sensitivity for most applications but PMTs have the greater sensitivity needed for those applications that require a very rapid response time.

In recent years, methods other than absorbance/transmittance photometry have been developed for the measurement of analytes. Reflectance photometry is one of these other methods. In reflectance photometry, diffuse, reflected light rather than absorbed light is measured. The intensity of the reflected light is compared with the intensity of the light reflected from a reference surface. One drawback to reflectance photometry is that intensities are not linear with concentration of the analyte of interest; they do not follow Beer's law. To correct for this deviation, mathematical algorithms are used to linearize the relationship between the intensity of reflected light and the analyte concentration. The components of the electrooptical system used in reflectance photometry are essentially the same as for absorbance/transmittance photometry: light source, monochromator, and detector.

Turbidimetry, nephelometry, and fluorescence are other methods available for measuring analyte concentration. Turbidimetry and nephelometry have found greatest application in protein and immunochemistry measurements. Fluorescence and fluorescence polarization have been applied in immunoassays and automated immunoassay instruments.

Another aspect of reaction measurement is where the measuring is to be performed. Continuous flow systems take measurements in a stationary flow cell through which the reaction stream passes. In early models, the bubbles were removed to prevent excess noise. But in the recent systems, the number and spacing of the bubbles are controlled and the microprocessor enables the readings to be taken between the bubbles.

Most discrete analyzers take measurements in the vessel where the reaction has taken place. In the case of disposable reaction vessels, once the measurement is made the container is either automatically removed by the instrument or removed and discarded by the operator. In the case of reusable reaction vessels, the cuvettes must be thoroughly washed, checked optically, and prepared for the next reaction. Disposable reaction vessels simplify the system but often have less exacting optical properties and represent a continuing cost. Reusable vessels require elaborate washing mechanisms but can be made to more exacting optical standards and decrease the ongoing costs.

The signal produced during the measurement stage must be converted to data usable by the operators. Most systems take the analog signals from the detectors and convert them to digital form by means of analog-to-digital (A/D) converters.

These data are presented to a computer in the instrument that converts them rapidly to the readily usable results. The results are displayed either on a cathode ray tube (CRT), directly on a hard copy such as paper tape, or both. These results must then be reviewed by the technologist and transferred to report slips, if reporting is done manually, or transcribed into a laboratory computer. This step is extremely susceptible to transcription errors. Many instruments are capable of interfacing directly with a laboratory computer, thus eliminating the transcription step and its attendant errors.

## Function Verification and Preventive Maintenance

All analyzers require at least some minimal function verification even if it consists only of running control material to verify response and precision. More elaborate function verification may include checking photometer lamp intensity, verifying calibration curves, observing moving parts to ensure they are operating properly, monitoring temperatures, and performing any self-checking functions available on the analyzer.

Preventive maintenance is done to ensure the analyzer continues to function properly. Keeping an analyzer clean may be the most important maintenance procedure, regardless of the instrument. Cleaning up spilled specimens and reagents will help prevent future malfunctions. Other maintenance procedures include discarding waste, cleaning water baths, cleaning reaction vessels (if reusable), replacing reagents, replacing worn or damaged parts (e.g., filters, tubing, syringes, probes, lamps), and readjusting components to ensure proper functioning.

## EXAMPLES OF SPECIFIC SYSTEMS

The following section presents specific information for some individual instrument systems found in laboratories today. This section is not intended to be exhaustive. Some of the instruments have been included because they exemplify a type of instrument and not because they are in common use.

## Continuous Flow Analyzers

The **auto analyzer (AA)** and **sequential multiple analyzer** (both with a computer, **SMAC**, and without, **SMA**) made by Bayer (formerly Technicon Instruments Corporation) are the primary examples of continuous flow analyzers. As mentioned in the introduction, the AA was the first successful automated chemistry analyzer and was based on the continuous flow principle developed by Leonard Skeggs and patented in 1957. The first AA could process 20 samples per hour for a single test and used reagents at a rate of 5.0 mL per minute. Current versions of SMAC can process up to 150 samples per hour with up to 23 tests per sample and consume only about 0.75 mL of reagent per minute. SMAC is an example of sequential, non-

selective analysis. It uses bar codes to identify samples. Most of the reagents are in bulk form with little preparation required. Measurement is by absorption photometry using a stationary flow cell and filters for wavelength isolation. Results calculated by the computer are printed on a form that could be used as the final report form.

The Chem 1 analyzer by Bayer utilizes a single continuous flow tube with an encapsulated oil segment of sample and reagents. The use of the oil segment eliminates the carryover problem of the single continuous flow tubing.

## Parallel Analyzers

The most characteristic examples of parallel analysis are the centrifugal analyzers. Developed with federal money at the Oak Ridge National Laboratory, the principle was not patented. Several manufacturers produce centrifugal analyzers including Electro-Nucleonics GemENI, or Roche COBAS; and J.T. Baker CENTRIFICHEM.

Samples and reagents are transferred to innermost discrete compartments in a rotor using positive displacement syringes. The rotor either contains cuvettes or aligns with cuvettes on the instrument so that when the rotor is accelerated, samples and reagents are mixed together in the cuvette in the outer section by centrifugal force. Temperature is controlled by air baths or heaters mounted on the rotors. Rotors and cuvettes can be disposable or reusable, requiring a wash before they can be used again. The cuvettes rotate rapidly through an optical system consisting of a stationary light source, filters for wavelength selection, and a PMT. Readings can be taken on each cuvette each time it passes through the optical system, making it very useful for determinations in rate reactions.

Typically, centrifugal analyzers are batch instruments capable of determining only one analyte at a time. Reagents are available in bulk form with little or no preparation required. Reagents are available from a variety of distributors and in-house applications can be adapted for use on these instruments.

## Discrete Analyzers

The remaining analyzers fall into the broad category of discrete analyzers. They exemplify a multiplicity of strategies.

Johnson & Johnson manufactures and distributes the VITROS, formerly the Kodak EKTACHEM analyzer. This is the primary example of dry slide technology. Tests are requested on a CRT with a touch screen menu. Any combination of tests can be programmed. Samples are applied to slides that are automatically dispensed from test-specific cartridges. Sample application is performed by means of individual, disposable tips, thereby eliminating the carryover problem. The sample itself provides the liquid necessary to hydrate the reagent layers of the slide. The slides incubate in heated air chambers and the color that develops is measured by reflectance photometry from the bottom side of the slide. Results for each sample are collated and printed in a report form that could be suitable for use as the final chartable report. Since each slide contains reagents for a single test, the VITROS is an example of the unit test concept. The reagent slides must be stored at refrigerator or freezer temperatures depending on the test and are only available from Johnson & Johnson. This is also an example of a closed system.

Another example of the unit test concept is the Dade Behring (formerly Du Pont) ACA IV or Star. Reagents are prepackaged in plastic packs (Figure 8–2). The instrument recognizes a binary code unique to the chemistry on the header of the pack providing the test identification. The amount of sample needed for the chemistry is aspirated and then delivered to the waiting reagent pack followed by sufficient diluent to make the total volume 5.0 mL. As the chemistry pack moves through several heated air delay stations, the reagent, which was sequestered in pods, is released and mixed with the sample and diluent. The reaction is measured photometrically with filters mounted on a filter wheel as the means of wavelength isolation. The pack itself is formed into an optical cell with a path length of 1 cm. Results are printed on a report tape.

Dade Behring also makes the DIMENSION RxL (Figure 8–3), a discrete, random-access clinical chemistry system that can perform a variety of tests, including general and special chemistries, enzymes, electrolytes, and drugs. Electrolytes are measured using ion-selective electrodes. Reagents for photometric chemistries are stored in concentrated liquid or tablet form in cartridges. Cuvettes are formed as the instrument needs them from a roll of Surlyn® film and are disposable. Sample and reagent, hydrated as needed, are added to the newly formed cuvette where mixing and measurement take place. Wavelength selection is accomplished with filters mounted on a filter wheel. After readings are taken, the top of the cuvette is sealed and drops into a waste container. When all tests are completed on a given sample, a report is printed by the computer.

Beckman Instruments manufactures and distributes the SYNCHRON (formerly ASTRA) family of analyzers. The SYNCHRON CX3, designed for efficient diagnostic management of high-volume emergency and routine situations, is a multianalyte discrete analyzer that performs the eight most fre-

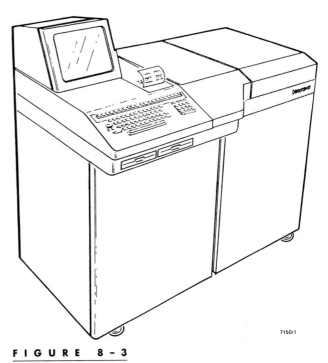

**FIGURE 8 - 3**

DIMENSION® clinical chemistry system that can perform a variety of tests, including general and special chemistry, enzyme, electrolyte, and drug tests.

quently requested tests: sodium, potassium, chloride, carbon dioxide, glucose, urea nitrogen, creatinine, and calcium. The SYNCHRON ASX (Figure 8–4) is a basic chemistry analyzer that can be configured to include up to 23 chemistries in over 300 configurations. The ASX includes the INTERLINK Systems Director, which allows the user to archive patient data, quality control data, and setup data as well as to interface with a host computer. The SYNCHRON CX4 AND CX5 analyzers can perform more than 40 different chemistries defined by Beckman with space for an additional 45 user-defined chemistries.

The larger SYNCHRON analyzers are microprocessor controlled, random-access chemistry analyzers. Samples and adequate reagent volume for the requested tests are pipetted into glass cuvettes in the reaction carousel and are thermally controlled at 30 or 37°C. These glass cuvettes rotate through the optics system, which has 10 fixed wavelengths ranging from 340 to 700 nm. When the reaction is complete and measurements taken, the cuvets are automatically washed and checked to validate the adequacy of the wash. Primary tube sampling is available for all SYNCHRON analyzers. In addition, the instruments can be connected to a host computer system for direct filing of patient results.

Boehringer Mannheim Diagnostics distributes the Hitachi analyzers. The Hitachi analyzers use positive displacement syringes to aspirate and deliver samples and reagents to cuvettes set in water baths, which maintain a stable incubation temperature, usually 37°C. Sampling can be done from the primary collection tube or from aliquot cups. Bar coding facili-

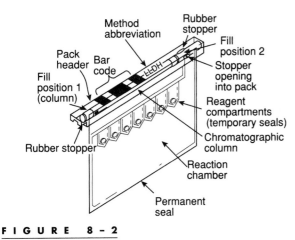

**FIGURE 8 - 2**

ACA® IV analytical test pack.

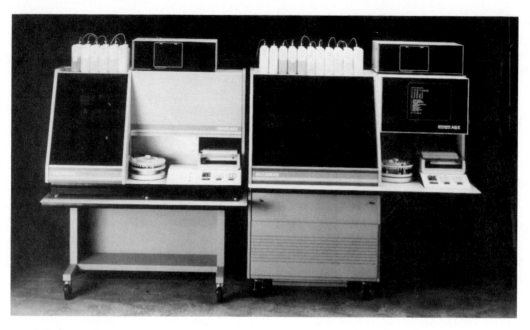

**FIGURE  8–4**

SYNCHRON ASX is a basic chemistry analyzer that can be configured to include up to 23 chemistries in over 300 configurations.

tates positive specimen identification. When the reactions are complete, the absorbance is read in the reaction cuvette using a diffraction grating spectrophotometer with detectors at fixed wavelengths. After bichromatic readings are taken, the cuvettes are washed and checked optically for the next determination. Ion-selective electrode cartridges are available for sodium, potassium, and chloride determinations. Reagents, available from Boehringer Mannheim and a growing number of other sources (open system), are packaged in bulk and require little or no preparation. In addition, in-house applications are readily adapted to these instruments since test parameters can be manually programmed. The instruments have refrigerated storage compartments for the reagents but as yet the loading zones are not temperature controlled. Hitachi analyzers offer many self-monitoring functions and real-time quality control.

## INSTRUMENT SELECTION

As the foregoing discussion indicates, many instrument systems are available. How does one choose the right system for a given laboratory situation? First, the specific laboratory needs and goals must be accurately assessed. Second, current operations must be examined to determine if there are options other than the purchase of a new instrument. And third, the analyzers available must be compared to determine which one will work best in a particular laboratory setting.[6]

Once the decision is made to purchase a new instrument, cost is not the only factor involved. The following questions should be addressed. Does the instrument perform all the tests required? Are reagents available only from one source, the maker of the instrument (proprietary reagents)? Will the instrument improve work flow? Is emergency capability required? If so, is it available? What will be the cost of operating the instrument? Are there continuing costs that are not obvious at purchase time?

Other concepts that need to be decided concerning the selection of laboratory instruments include: operator walk-away capability, minimal operator intervention, cost of consumable materials, actual cost per test (fixed or variable), performance characteristics (sample size, turnaround time), analytical characteristics, and space needed including auxiliary functions (water, drains, electrical power), and the amount of daily, weekly, and monthly maintenance required. Other decisions relate to options for purchasing, leasing, and renting. There is no one flawless instrument but, with proper attention to detail, the best instrument for a given situation can be selected.

## SUMMARY

Only 40 years ago automation was just becoming a reality in the clinical chemistry laboratory. Currently, automation has advanced far beyond the first continuous flow instruments that mechanized the steps involved in manual chemistry determinations. Improved specimen and reagent-handling options, optimized chemical reaction, improved optics and photometer systems, and the introduction of microprocessors for instrument control and data presentation have made today's instruments reliable, efficient workstations. Numerous automated instruments are available, each with something to offer in the way of enhanced laboratory operations. The difficult decision now is not finding an automated system but choosing the right one.

## REFERENCES

1. Boyd J, Felder R, Savory J: Robotics and the changing face of the clinical laboratory. Clin Chem 42:1901–1910, 1996.

2. Saineto D: Laboratory automation: Coming of age in the 21st century. Clin Lab News 26(1):1,6–7, 2000.

3. Maffetone MA, Watt SW, Whisler KE: Automated specimen handling: Bar codes and robotics. Lab Med 21: 436–443, 1990.

4. Burtis CA: Factors influencing evaporation from sample cups, and assessment of their effect on analytical error. Clin Chem 21:1907–1917, 1975.

5. Burtis CA: Sample evaporation and its impact on the operating performance of an automated selective-access analytical system. Clin Chem 36:544–546, 1990.

6. Lifshitz MS, DeCresce RP: Clinical laboratory instrument selection. Lab Med 21:367–370, 1990.

# CHAPTER 9

# Computers in the Clinical Laboratory

*Mark D. Kellogg*

The clinical laboratory was one of the first areas in medicine in which computers were utilized. In the late 1950s automated instrumentation began to appear in the clinical laboratory and using computers to manage and store the data produced only seemed natural. Eventually, computers were used to support the entire process of analysis, from collection of the sample to reporting the results. However, computers of the 1960s and 70s were large devices requiring constant attention and cost significant dollars to purchase, install, and maintain. It was not until the personal computer revolution of the early 1980s that laboratory personnel had a powerful new tool capable of markedly improving their operation. With the advent of word processing, electronic spreadsheet, and database management software, computer systems moved rapidly into routine use in the administrative offices of most clinical laboratories. Concomitant with the development of the personal computer was the addition of microprocessor systems and associated software to control a new generation of complex laboratory instruments. Microprocessor-based instrument control systems replaced the electromechanical systems. These microprocessor-controlled instruments not only supported the transfer of data directly from analyzer to computer but also provided significant new abilities. Operators could now validate results before transfer, monitor and evaluate quality control, and be alerted to problems with key operational parameters of the instrument such as temperature, reagent volume, and missing samples.

Today, laboratories use computers to manage test requests and specimen collection, control instruments, collect data from instruments, translate that data into meaningful results, collate all analyses on an individual patient, and generate reports for physician information and inclusion in patients' medical records. Because computers are part of every laboratory and because medical informatics (including clinical laboratory data) is essential to health care delivery, clinical laboratory personnel must have a basic knowledge of computers and computer communication technology. Individuals who understand how a computer operates will use computers more effectively and, when faced with decision making about computers, will not be at the mercy of those who do know. Similar to the automobile, the more you know about how it operates, the more informed decisions you can make in purchases, repairs,

and upgrades. This chapter will present general concepts of computer hardware, software, and their usage in the clinical laboratory.

## COMPUTER HARDWARE AND SOFTWARE

A computer is a machine with two key characteristics. It is designed to respond to a specific set of instructions in a defined manner and can execute programs that represent prerecorded instructions. The actual machine (wires, circuits, and transistors) is called the hardware. Software is the prerecorded set of instructions and data used to execute actions.

### Hardware

**Hardware** is the physical part of a computer system. Computer hardware includes the following five main components: (1) memory, which allows the temporary storage of data and programs, (2) mass storage, for permanent storage of large amounts of data, (3) input devices, like the mouse and keyboard, that allow a user to enter data and instructions, (4) output devices, that let you see what the computer is doing, and (5) the central processing unit (CPU), which is the component that actually executes the instructions. Additionally, all computers require a **bus** to connect all of these components for transmission of data between them during processing, calculating, and other activities. A power supply provides the necessary electrical power for components to operate. The memory, CPU, and cards connected to the input and output devices are all connected to a circuit board called the **motherboard.**

### Memory

Memory is that part of the computer where data is stored while being used and where programs or instructions for computer activities are stored. It consists of a number of physical units called chips. Memory determines the size and number of programs that can be retained by a computer and also the size of data that can be retained and processed at one time. The CPU directs the data manipulation that actually takes place in memory. There are different types of memory chips. Some retain their contents permanently after power to the computer is lost but most computer memory chips lose their contents when power is lost.

The views, opinions, and/or findings contained in this chapter are those of the author and should not be construed as an official Department of the Army position, policy, or decision unless so designated by other documentation.

**Read-only memory** (ROM) is a type of memory that remains intact when power to a computer is discontinued. ROM memory remains permanently. Memory content of ROM is programmed at the time of manufacture and thereafter the user may not alter the contents. ROM contains instructions for operations essential to basic computer functions, for example, disk drive interaction. ROM chips are used to store **BASIC Input Output System** (BIOS) instruction, which is a set of routines that activate and control peripheral devices connected to the computer. ROM BIOS greatly affects computer compatibility with software. A rewriteable form of ROM, called FLASH-ROM, allows the contents of the ROM to be changed at a later time.

The smallest piece of information that is stored within a computer is called a **bit.** A binary digit (**bit**) is a single digit in a binary code (1 or 0). Physically, it is a memory cell and is electrically either on (1) or off (0). Eight bits of memory are required to store a **byte** or an alphanumeric character, which is the common unit of computer storage. In other words, eight bits represent one letter of the alphabet (one byte).

**Random-access memory** (RAM) is the working or user accessible memory of the computer and is lost when power is discontinued. Therefore, data that are in RAM must be saved before switching off the computer power. The user may enter, change, or erase data in RAM. The number of RAM memory chips is one of the major determiners of the cost of computers. Size of RAM not only determines the amount of data that may be processed at a time but it also dictates the size and number of programs that may be held in a computer at any one time. Microcomputers today usually come with at least 32 or 64 **megabyte** (MB, $1 \times 10^6$ bytes) RAM and are expandable to 256 MB or more. Just a few years ago computers came with only 1 MB or even as little as 640 **kilobytes** (KB, $1 \times 10^3$ bytes) RAM.

Microcomputers usually have empty slots in which additional RAM may be added after purchase. When acquiring memory chips, it is important to match their speed of operation with the requirements of the computer. The unit of speed is **nanoseconds** ($1 \times 10^{-9}$ seconds). The faster the chip, the more it costs. There are many kinds of RAM. **Static RAM** (SRAM) is a faster executing and more efficient RAM chip but it is costly. **Dynamic RAM** (DRAM) chips are more common, cost less, and are slower. DRAM has been succeeded by **synchronous dynamic RAM** (SDRAM) and **extended data out RAM** (EDO RAM); both improve the execution speed and amount of memory present in a chip.[1] Typically, memory chips are physically placed on circuit boards called memory modules. Each module contains eight or nine individual memory chips each containing 16, 32, or 64 megabits of memory. **Single inline memory module** (SIMM) and **dual inline memory module** (DIMM) are common modules found in today's computers. Almost all new computers use DIMMs. Most motherboards contain slots for only one type (SIMM or DIMM) but some contain slots to accept both. It is important to ascertain which type of memory a computer can utilize before adding additional memory modules

Virtual memory is a section of the computer's hard drive that is used to augment the existing RAM. The various operating systems (UNIX, Linux, Windows) handle this differently but essentially move data from physical memory, or RAM, to the hard drive when space in the physical memory runs low. Virtual memory is also used to swap out little used portions of physical memory to free it up for other operations.

**Cache memory** or **cache RAM** is a reserved section of the fastest RAM that is used to improve computer performance. Usually, parts of a program or pieces of data that are used repeatedly are read from a disk into cache memory and stored. Thereafter, each time the computer calls for these pieces of program or parts of data, they are immediately available from high-speed RAM rather than from the slower speed disk.

## Storage Devices

As defined above, storage devices are hardware devices that hold or store data. These devices are rated according to the speed with which they react as well as to the volume of data they can accommodate. A **drive** is a peripheral device that receives data from the computer (output device), stores data (storage device), and feeds previously stored data to the computer (input device). Drives may be one of several types:

1. Floppy drives
2. Hard drives
3. Compact disc (CD) drives
4. DVD drives

Although less frequently used today, **magnetic tape** was a common form of data storage with early mini- and mainframe computers. Data that were no longer needed for daily processing were transferred to magnetic tape for archiving. Reels of tape were easier and safer to transport than large disk packs used for daily operation. Tape is linear storage and retrieval in contrast to the nonlinear or random processing of disk and hard drives. Magnetic tape may also be used to store data from microcomputers and is an economical means for backing up data on hard drives.

**Floppy disk drives** use disks that contain a disk media that is not rigid (as hard drives are) and may be removed and physically carried to different locations.[1] Earlier terminology referred to these disks as floppy diskettes or diskettes, but most people simply refer to them as floppy disks. The first floppy disks were either 8 in. or 5.25 in. in diameter and could store up to 400 kilobytes of information. Newer floppy diskettes are 3.5 in. and can store up to 1.44 MB. **Zip™** disks and **Jaz™** disks utilize a similar nonrigid disk media but can store 250 MB to 2 gigabytes (GB), respectively. The floppy disk is slowly disappearing as compact disk and DVD technology improves. Disks must be **formatted** or electronically divided into tracks and sectors before they can be used to store data. Disks must be matched with the type of drive in which they are to be used (for example, double density, high density, Zip™).

**Hard drives** store more data and store it more rapidly than do floppy drives. However, until recently, hard drives were not usually removed from the computer and carried around. A number of removable hard drives are now available, some even fitting into the palm of your hand. The disk media in the hard drive is inflexible and usually made of metal, although glass versions have been developed. The disk media is placed in a closed system (the floppy disk is open) that allows the disks to operate at greater speeds and to hold more data.

**Compact disc** (CD) drives use laser beams to read and write data. Each CD holds up to 650 MB of memory. The CD disk player is closely related to the well-known audio CD or compact audio player found in many homes. There are a number of varieties of CD drives, including CD-ROM (CD read-only memory), CD-R (CD-recordable), CD-RW (CD-rewriteable). CD-R is a type of WORM (write once, read many) type of technology that allows the user to record information onto the CD. CD-RW takes that capability one step further and allows the CD-RW disk to be erased and rewritten with new data. The CD-RW drive can write to the older CD-R disks but can rewrite only with the CD-RW disks.

**DVD drives** are the latest technology (1999–2000) and are beginning to replace CD drives. Most people call DVD either digital video or digital variable but the manufacturers state that DVD does not stand for anything.[1] The disks used in these drives are physically similar in size to CDs, but can hold between 4.7 and 18 gigabytes (GB) of information. Like the CD, these drives exist in different formats. The DVD-R (DVD-recordable) writes to a 4.7 GB disk once and then the disk can be read many times using standard DVD players. DVD+RW (DVD-rewritable) drives can read standard DVDs and also read and write to 3 GB DVD+RW media. DVD-RAM (DVD-random access memory) uses special media that cannot be used in other DVD drives, and can be written and read multiple times like RAM memory chips. The DVD-RAM uses both sides of the DVD-RAM disk, holding 2.6 GB on each side.

## Input Devices

An input device is a peripheral device that sends data to the computer, for example, a keyboard or disk drive. Because input devices are sending data to the computer, a software program (driver) must inform the receiving computer of the communications parameters with which the input device transmits. These parameters will be discussed later in the communications section of this chapter. For an input device to function, it must be physically interfaced (connected) to the computer and a program called a **driver** that instructs the computer how to interact with the device must be loaded into memory.

The **keyboard** is that input device with which most computer users are familiar. In addition to the keyboard, almost all computers today also use a **mouse** to assist communication

with the computer. There are at least three types of mice from which to choose. A **serial mouse** is connected to the serial port of the computer. A **bus mouse** connects to a special board that must be added to the computer. Therefore, a bus mouse requires inserting an extra circuit board or card into the computer motherboard. A **PS/2 mouse** plugs into the mouse port of IBM PS/2 computers.

A **bar code reader** is a device that directs a laser beam or a light beam across a series of lines of varying widths (the bar code) that code information. The reader directly enters the scanned information into an interfaced computer. Bar code devices are common to the laboratory and hospital environment. The bar code is a key element that allows automated instrumentation to identify specimen and reagent containers. **Microphones** are also used as input devices on today's computers, and as speech recognition technology improves, their use to control computer activity will be become as common as today's mouse input.

## Monitors and Video Cards

A **monitor**, cathode ray tube (CRT), or screen is a display device that is used to enable the user to view the output of a computer. A monitor receives output data from the computer and is therefore an output device. A **video card** or **video adapter** is a plug-in circuit board that generates text and graphic images for a particular kind of monitor. It is important to match the video card to the software requirements and to match the output of the video card to a monitor. Damage may occur to a monitor if it is not connected to a video card to which it is matched.

Most computer systems today use **red-green-blue** (RGB) monitors that accept separate signals for each of the colors plus an extra, individual signal for synchronization. An **interlaced** monitor denotes alternately scanning or displaying all odd lines and then all even lines. Television uses interlaced technology and generates 60 half frames or 30 full frames per second. The screen is scanned from left to right, top to bottom every odd line, and then it is scanned again every even line. A problem with this technology is that if the scan rate is too low, the picture flickers. **Noninterlaced** monitors sequentially refresh all lines top to bottom and are flicker-free.

Video cards and monitors are selected and matched in relation to video resolution modes. **Resolution** is the degree of sharpness in image or printed letters and is expressed in terms of rows and columns of **picture elements (pixels),** which are the smallest entity or dot that can be displayed on a screen. Pixel resolution is expressed in rows and columns. Thus a video card that outputs an image with a resolution of $640 \times 480$ pixels is sharper than a video card that outputs an image of $420 \times 380$ pixels. In addition to pixel resolution, the **number of displayable colors** affects resolution perceived by the human eye. A $640 \times 480$ pixel resolution with 256 displayable colors has a higher resolution or sharper image than a $640 \times$

480 pixel resolution with 16 displayable colors. Number of displayable colors is one of the video mode characteristics.

A method used to rate resolution of monitors is the dot pitch of the monitor. The **dot pitch** (dp) is a property of the monitor itself and is the width of a dot in hundredths of a millimeter. The smaller the dot, the sharper the image. Higher resolution monitors today have a 0.28 dp, which is 28/100 of a millimeter. The lower the dp, the better the resolution. A 0.28 dp monitor displays a sharper image than a 0.33 dp monitor. Displaying a 640 × 480 pixel image on a 0.28 dp monitor would produce a sharper image than displaying a 640 × 480 image on a 0.33 dp monitor.

## Printers

Printers make hard, permanent copies of computer output and are rated according to quality or sharpness of print as well as to speed of printout. Quality of print may be denoted by the terms: **draft, near-letter quality,** and **letter quality** or, more precisely, **dots per inch** (dpi). Speed of printout is assessed as **page per minute** (ppm) or **characters per second** (cps). Very roughly, 1 ppm is equivalent to 60 cps.

Interfacing or connecting printers to computers requires matching communications parameters and is covered in the communications section of this chapter. Ability to print different fonts and to print in **landscape** (horizontal) or **portrait** (vertical) is controlled by software. Ability to print graphics is also software controlled, except that the printer must be capable of performing the software instructions, e.g., daisy wheel printers can never print graphics. Printers come in many types including daisy wheel, dot matrix, ink-jet, laser, and dye sublimation.

**Daisy wheel** printers form characters by selectively impacting letters located on the end of a spoke of a revolving wagon wheel. These printers are letter quality but are not capable of printing graphics because they do not print dot by dot or pixel by pixel. Generally, daisy wheel printers are faster and of sharper quality than dot matrix printers.

**Dot matrix** printers form characters by selectively impacting tiny wires, from a group of rows and columns of wires, onto a ribbon. The formed characters are actually a series of dots. They output a draft quality or readable text, which is the most rapid printout it can perform (200 to 600 cps or 2.5 to 7.5 ppm); however, the quality is poor because there are few dots per inch. The near-letter-quality print has more dots per inch, is sharper but is slower to produce (60–80 cps or 1 ppm). The ink-jet printer is a type of dot matrix printer that uses a head that sprays tiny droplets of ink onto print material. Ink-jet printers are much quieter than standard dot matrix printers, can make smaller dots to improve print quality, and the liquid ink can be mixed for color printing capability. However, they print more slowly than standard dot matrix printers and since they do not print by impact, they cannot print carbon copies.

**Laser printers** are quieter, nonimpact, and use the electrophotographic technology of copy machines to print a page at a time. They generally cost more, produce sharper images, and print faster than other printers. Laser printers print letter quality images of 300 or greater dpi. Laser printers have enabled a high quality in printing. Postscript is a page description language from Adobe Corporation. An application program uses the postscript language to describe text fonts and graphics images. For a printer to print a postscript document, it must have a CPU and memory to follow the application program's description in designing fonts and graphics. Both application program and printer must have postscript capabilities.

Other types of printers include thermal printers that burn images into a special paper. Thermal printers were quite common on instruments produced in the 1990s.

## Modems

A **modem** is shortened terminology for a **modulator-demodulator,** which is a device that transforms digital data from the computer to analog data for transmission over normal telephone lines and analog data from the telephone line to digital data for use by a computer. Modems allow computers to communicate with other computers over telephone, wireless, and cable systems. Eventually, this modulation and demodulation will be unnecessary when digital transmission systems are more widely used. The digital signal level of a normal telephone line is 0 (zero) and allows for a maximum transmission rate of 64 kilobytes per second (Kbps).[1] To create lines capable of carrying a digital signal, copper wire used for telephone lines can be twisted into two pairs to create a **T-1** line capable of 155 megabytes per second (Mbps) transmission and can carry 24 phone lines.[1] A **T3** line combines 28 T-1 lines and can carry 672 different phone (voice) lines or up to 44.7 Mbps of data. Most **internet service providers** utilize T3 lines to connect to the main backbones of the Internet. Fiberoptic wires are also capable of carrying a digital signal.

## Central Processing Unit

The **central processing unit** (CPU) is the brain of the computer where instructions are read, decoded and executed. Sometimes called the central processor, microprocessor, or processor chip, the CPU controls, coordinates, and performs computer operations including calculations, comparisons, and data transfer. Even though operations may actually be accomplished on other elements (e.g., a video card, a math coprocessor), the CPU directs data to and from those units and tells those units what to do and when to do it.

CPUs are characterized or rated according to the size of data (bits) they can process at one time and the clock speed (MHz) at which they process. Through the years, CPUs have technologically advanced from 8-bit (8088 chip) to 16-bit CPUs (80286 chip), 32-bit CPUs (386 and 486 chips), and

64-bit CPUs (Pentium and x86–64 chips). A 16-bit CPU can process twice as much data in a single step as an 8-bit CPU. It should be noted that for the larger CPU chip capacity to be realized, the software or program that instructs the computer must be written for that chip. CPUs are based on **complex instruction set computer** (CISC) or **reduced instruction set computer** (RISC) architecture. RISC-based computers split big complex operations into simple, tiny operations that can run 15% to 50% faster than CISC computers, and RISC chips are cheaper to produce.

    **Clockspeed** of a computer is the speed of generated and spaced pulses that are sent throughout the computer. The CPU's clock or internal timing device governs the rapidity of machine cycles or speed of the processor. Computers with faster clockspeeds are able to perform more operations per second. Clockspeed is often used as a rating for the CPU. **Megahertz** (MHz, $1 \times 10^6$ cycles per second) is the unit for measuring clockspeed.

    CPUs continue to be designed with faster clockspeeds, larger bit ratings, and smaller physical size. Early microcomputers use the 8-bit CPU (8088 chip) capable of processing 8 bits of data at a time and run at 4.7 to 10 MHz. The 386 machines run at 25 MHz and 33 MHz and 486 microcomputers run at speeds from 25 to 66 MHz. In the summer of 2000, chip manufacturers began to release chips with clockspeeds exceeding 1 gigahertz (GHz) and desktop computers will now far exceed the capabilities of even the largest minicomputers of just a few years ago.

## Power Supply

All computers require a direct current (DC) power supply. Alternating current output from commercial electrical outlets is converted to DC by the power supply. The required wattage (size of power supply) varies with the number of boards and accessory devices that are plugged into or connected to the computer. Memory chips use 5 to 10 watts; each disk drive uses from 10 to 50 watts and each accessory board may use 15 to 25 watts. A typical microcomputer power supply is between 100 and 250 watts.

## Bus

The **bus** is the computer's major circuitry or electrical paths along which data move between the various components. When purchasing any new card or board, one must match it to the bus. An industry standard architecture (ISA) is a 16-bit architecture of the older AT computers. The extended industry standard architecture (EISA) bus was 32-bit and accommodated EISA and ISA cards but no MCA cards. The VL-Bus and PCI (peripheral computer interconnect) have largely replaced the ISA and EISA cards. PCI though is limited in the number of slots that can be placed on a motherboard, and machines requiring a large number of peripheral devices will use the EISA system.

## Types of Computers

Computers are usually classified by size and power into supercomputers, mainframe, mini, workstation, and personal computers. Advances in microelectronics now make distinctions ambiguous and the personal computers of today have far more computing power than the mainframes of even 10 years ago. The following definitions, then, will be generalities rather than absolutes.

### SUPERCOMPUTERS

**Supercomputers are the** fastest type of computer available. These computers are very expensive and used in specialized applications requiring tremendous mathematical calculations. For example, weather forecasting requires a supercomputer. Other uses of supercomputers include animated movies, physics research, and medical modeling. In comparison to mainframe computers described below, the supercomputer uses its power to execute a few programs as fast as possible, whereas the mainframe computer is used to run many programs at the same time.

### MAINFRAME COMPUTERS

The first computers were mainframes, e.g., Univac. Users interact or control mainframes via workstations called terminals, which may be either "dumb" or "smart." **Dumb terminals** are terminals without processing or computing capabilities. They consist of a keyboard by which the user gives commands to the mainframe and a monitor that displays user-entered commands and processing results. All calculations, processing, and storage are executed on the mainframe. In contrast, **smart terminals** are workstations that, in addition to the display and keyboard capabilities of the dumb terminals, provide some processing and memory capabilities independent of the mainframe.

### MINICOMPUTERS

A midsize computer (minicomputer) in terms of size and power lies between the workstation and the mainframe. Technology advances have blurred the distinction between large minicomputers and small mainframes and between small minicomputers and workstations. In general, a minicomputer is a multiprocessor system capable of supporting from 4 to about 200 users simultaneously.

### WORKSTATIONS

Workstations are typically used for applications that require moderate computing power and high-quality graphics. Examples include desktop publishing, computer-assisted design (CAD), computer-assisted manufacturing (CAM), and software development. Workstations generally come with a large, high-resolution graphics screen, large amounts of random access memory (RAM), networking capabilities, and a graphical user interface (GUI). Most workstations also have a mass storage such as a disk drive, but a special type of workstation called a diskless workstation comes without a disk drive. The most common operating systems for workstations are UNIX and Windows NT. In terms of computing power, workstations lie between personal computers and the minicomputer. High-end personal computers are equivalent to low-end workstations and high-end workstations are equivalent to minicomputers.

Like personal computers, most workstations are single-user computers. However, workstations are typically linked together to form a local-area network, although they can also be used as stand-alone systems.

In networking, *workstation* refers to any computer connected to a local-area network. It could be a workstation or a personal computer.

## PERSONAL COMPUTERS

The last category of computers is the personal computer **(microcomputer),** which is the most numerous and well known. Microcomputers are easily moved, are able to stand alone (complete computers capable of processing, storage, calculating); however, they may also be connected to mainframe or minicomputers and they may also support a small number of user terminals. There is no temperature or humidity control requirement and costs range from $500 to $25,000. Examples of microcomputers are the IBM PS/2 series, Compaq, Dell, Gateway, and many more.

## Software

**Software** is a written set of instructions for the computer. **Programs** are software that perform a specific task such as instructing the computer how to interact with a mouse, e.g. the mouse driver. Software is classified according to the task that it performs.

## OPERATING SYSTEMS

An **operating system** is a master control program that organizes all activities of the computer and instructs the computer how to interact with peripheral devices, for example, disk drives, keyboard, and monitor. It is the minimum software required to run a computer. Some parts of the operating system are in ROM. Core parts of the operating system are loaded into the computer RAM from the disk on **booting** (turning the computer on) and are thereafter available from memory for immediate access. Other parts of the operating system are seldom used and may be loaded into memory as needed.

Operating systems set specifications to which application programs must be written in order for them to function. Some examples of earlier operating systems include: DOS, OS/2, and XENIX. Operating systems in common use today include various versions of Windows (95, 98, NT, 2000), UNIX, Linux, and the Mac OS. Application programs, e.g., word processing packages, written for one operating system will not run in any

other operating system. OS/2 is an exception in that it does have a multitasking function that allows a user to run application programs written for DOS. UNIX and variations are largely run on mainframe and minicomputers, even though there is a version, called XENIX, that runs on microcomputers. It is expected that in the future operating systems will allow application programs to run on all types of computers. The tendency to interface all types of computers in networks is driving this trend for standardization of software.

## LANGUAGES

A **language** is a system of symbols that is used for communication. There are different levels of languages for communication with computers. **Machine language** is the only symbolic code that the computer understands. For the computer to understand an instruction, it must be in machine language. Commands in machine language, however, are meaningless to most humans.

**Assembly language** was developed for the convenience of programmers. It resembles English and is more understandable to most humans than machine language. Instructions written in assembly language must first be assembled (translated) into machine language before a computer can understand them. Assembly language is sometimes called a **low-level language** because it is not far removed from machine language, e.g., one word in assembly language is translated into one word in machine language.

Pascal, BASIC, C++, and structured query language (SQL) are **high-level languages** that closely resemble English but are far removed from machine language, e.g., one word in high-level languages may be translated into several words in machine language. Instructions written in these high-level languages must be compiled (translated) to machine language before the computer can understand and execute them. C++ language can be compiled into machine language for almost any computer; therefore, C++ is a **transportable language** because it may be transported or run on almost any computer.

## DRIVERS

A **driver** is a program that instructs the computer on interaction with a peripheral device. In addition to correctly interfacing or connecting a peripheral device with a computer, one must load a driver for each peripheral device before the computer is able to utilize it.

## APPLICATION PROGRAMS

An **application program** is a program that is written for a specific purpose. There are many commercially available programs for general laboratory chores. If a laboratory can locate application software that does exactly what it needs, that software may be used. However, most likely, some tailoring of available software is required to match the individual clinical environments.

**Word processing** programs are programs for managing text documents and their printout. These packages may contain a spell checker, a thesaurus, and even a grammar checker. Most now contain a view-page function, which allows the user to view the layout of a page before printing. Because text is easy to move around, copy, delete, and correct, word processing has greatly decreased the time required to write documents. Some more common examples of word processing programs are Word Perfect™, Lotus WordPro™, and Microsoft Word™.

**Electronic spreadsheet** programs are programs that simulate paper worksheets of columns and rows of numbers for budgets and other financial bookkeeping. The spreadsheet is much larger than a single screen and can be scrolled through for viewing. Mathematical formulas may be added in a row or column of a spreadsheet and thereafter they are automatically calculated and the calculated result, not the formula, is displayed in that column or row. Electronic spreadsheets are useful and save time in planning, forecasting, and predicting because a manual change in a single value is automatically carried throughout the entire spreadsheet. Lotus 1-2-3™, Microsoft Excel™, and Quaatro Pro™ are popular electronic spreadsheets.

**Database management** programs are programs that organize, store, and retrieve data in a database. Common examples are FileMaker™, Microsoft Access™, Lotus Approach™, dBASE™, and Paradox™. Databases are used in numerous applications in the clinical laboratory, e.g., inventory and personnel scheduling.

**Personal information manager** (PIM) programs are programs that are designed to organize or manage one's personal job functions and calendar of events. Sidekick Plus™, Microsoft Outlook™, and Lotus Organizer™ are examples of PIM programs.

**Lecture or seminar presentation** software is a program used to prepare a series of computer illustrations to accompany a presentation. Usually, an overhead projector is used to display the computer output on a large screen for the audience. Microsoft Powerpoint™, Visio™, and Astound™ are examples of presentation software.

**Statistical** programs are written to perform statistical calculations. A common example is Statistical Analysis System or SAS™.

**Netware** programs are programs that organize and control communications over a network. Netware is also the commercial name for a commercial vendor's netware program. Examples of these types of programs are Novell's Netware and 3-Com's Ethernet Share.

**Internet Browsers** are programs that allow users to look at pages from the World Wide Web. Examples of these programs are Microsoft Internet Explorer, Netscape Navigator, Mosaic, and Opera. More specifically, these programs read Hypertext Transfer Protocol (HTTP) pages, usually from the Internet. The pages are written using Hypertext Markup Language (HTML) and allow the communication of text, graphics, and multimedia objects over the Internet. The Web is the channel of the Internet used to distribute these documents. More about the Internet will be discussed later in this chapter.

## NETWORKING AND COMMUNICATION

### Computer Networks

Today, computers almost never operate as stand-alone computers and are usually **networked** to other computers to share data, applications, and peripheral devices. The simplest configuration consists of several computers linked together in what is termed a local area network (LAN). This could be the computers within a "local" area like an office, laboratory, home, or even a small building. LANs are limited to physical distances between computers of less than 2 kilometers and usually use one protocol for communication. When computers are farther apart or multiple LANs are linked to each other, these networks are usually called wide area networks (WANs).

The ability to share expensive peripherals like laser printers, large mass storage, or Internet connections make networks a cost-effective solution to purchasing such devices for every computer. Bridges, routers, and switches are used to connect LANs together (to form WANs) or to connect segments of LAN that are separated by distances greater than those allowed. The bridges, routers, and switches route the data packets traveling through the cables to the proper segment of the LAN or across LANs based on the destination address found within the data packet. When data must travel across networks using different communication protocols (like a LAN to the Internet), then a gateway must be utilized. The gateway is a computer that is connected to both networks and translates the data from one before transmitting to the other. The connection of your laboratory network to the Internet would be handled by a gateway.

Networks are categorized by three characteristics: architecture, protocol, and topology. Peer-to-peer and server/client are two architectures commonly found in networks. The simplest architecture is the peer-to-peer network that connects small numbers of computers. This system allows the hardware (printer, CD-ROM, fax-modem) attached to any computer on the network, to be shared with other computers on the network. Users can also share data stored on their hard drives. The peer-to-peer network is easy to configure and most personal computers come with the necessary software. Additional hardware requirements are a network card and cabling to connect the network cards. Security of information is a concern with peer-to-peer networks. The peer-to-peer system works well only with limited numbers of computers, usually less than 12.

Server/client systems have one central computer (server) that provides various services like e-mail, printers, and Internet access to the other computers on the network (clients). In this system, the data and programs are held on the server and not the individual user computers. While providing a higher level of security, this system is more vulnerable to power failures and hardware failure. If the server is not functional, all data and programs stored there are unavailable. Critical data and programs may be mirrored on other computers within the network to provide backup if the main server crashes. The client/server system is the most common network architecture.

Protocol refers to the common set of signals and rules that the network uses for communication. Your choice of protocol is dependent on what system you are using. **Ethernet** was one of the first protocols developed for connecting computers.[1] Various modifications have been made on the original since its development in 1972 and is still in common use today. **NetBEUI** was developed by IBM for use with small- to medium-sized networks and is very easy to configure.[1] The protocol suffers from network congestion when you have more than 20 machines on the network. The **IPX/SPX** protocol was developed by Novell for use with its Netware systems. This is usually the default protocol when you are using the Microsoft Operating systems on networked computers. IPX/SPX is more difficult to configure and is largely being replaced by **Transmission Control Protocol/Internet Protocol** (TCP/IP). TCP/IP was originally developed as the transfer protocol for the Internet and has now been adapted for controlling transmission in LANs. It allows communication between dissimilar computer systems and can be easily scaled up to handle increasing numbers of machines.

Topology refers to the geometry used in configuring the network. Common topologies are star, ring, and bus. See Figure 9–1

for examples of these topologies. The Internet is actually a network topology and does not physically exist without the connections between the millions of computers using TCP/IP to communicate.

Computers that are attached to the network require a network interface card (NIC) to which the network cable is connected. In a peer-to-peer network, these cards are connected to each other via the cable. In an Ethernet network, the cables are attached to network hubs that manage the receipt and transmission of data from the various computers. Ethernet networks can use three different types of cabling. Unshielded twisted-pair (UTP) is the most common and least expensive. Shielded twisted pair and coaxial cable can also be used. Both of these cables are shielded from electromagnetic interference (EMI). EMI is usually not a problem in offices or homes but within the clinical laboratory, significant EMI can be generated with the number of motors, instruments, and other devices present. Be sure to consider the possibility of EMI when selecting cabling for use in the clinical laboratory environment. Coaxial cabling, also called thin Ethernet, must be configured in the ring topology, making it more difficult to set up. Additionally, the cables and connectors must be protected because any break in the chain will cause the network to fail.

## Communications

Communication or transmission of data between a computer and any other device, whether it is a laboratory analyzer, a laboratory specimen identification label printer, a patient identification plate printer or even another computer, utilizes similar technology and communication parameters. The goal of this section is to provide the laboratorian with sufficient information to understand communications between computers and with laboratory instrumentation.

All input to computers is converted into binary numbers made up of the two digits 0 and 1. Binary code is made up of the two digits 0 and 1. The 1 bit is transmitted as pulses of electricity of high voltage; the 0 bit is transmitted as no pulse or low voltage. In memory, the 1s and 0s are stored as a series of charges (on) and no charges (off). The American Standard Code for Information Interchange (ASCII) is a binary code for data that is used in most minicomputers and in all microcomputers. Another binary code, Extended Binary Coded Decimal Interchange Code (EBCDIC), is used by IBM mainframe and some minicomputers. ASCII has 256 different characters, of which the first 128 are standardized for all computer platforms. The first 32 are control codes used for communications, text formatting, and printing controls, such as making the computer beep. The next 96 characters are used for numbers, letters, and standard punctuation marks. Codes 128 and higher are nonstandard at the present time and are therefore highly vendor dependent. Character data such as letters and punctuation marks are stored in memory or files as the ASCII bit notation, but numbers must be converted to binary bit notation for the computer to utilize them (Table 9–1).

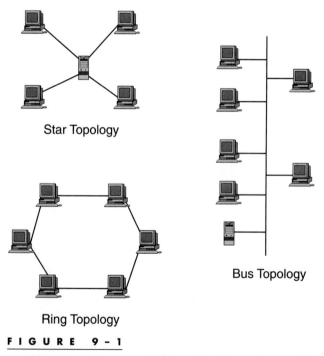

Star Topology

Ring Topology

Bus Topology

**F I G U R E   9 – 1**

Microcomputers connected in various types of network topology.

TABLE 9 - 1

**Binary Bit Notation for Decimal Number 10**

| Bit number | 7 | 6 | 5 | 4 | 3 | 2 | 1 | 0 | |
|---|---|---|---|---|---|---|---|---|---|
| Value of bit | 128 | 64 | 32 | 16 | 8 | 4 | 2 | 1 | |
| Binary value | 0 | 0 | 0 | 0 | 1 | 0 | 1 | 0 | |
| Decimal value | 0 | 0 | 0 | 0 | 8 | 0 | 2 | 0 | |
| Sum in Decimal | 0 | +0 | +0 | +0 | +8 | +0 | +2 | +0 | = 10 |

## Types of Computer Communications

In addition to collecting and processing analytical data, clinical laboratory computers are largely used for communicating those data. The International Standards Organization (ISO) has defined a communications reference model, the **Open System Interconnection (OSI),** which is a 7-layer standard for computer communications protocol (Figure 9–2). This model was developed to encourage standards in communications software and hardware so that multivendor products might be interchangeable and interconnectable. Of the 7 protocol layers, 1 and 2 describe basic communication of a computer with any other device and in the clinical laboratory and are most likely the responsibility of clinical laboratorians.

Layer 1 defines the **physical layer** or the actual set of wires, plugs, and electrical signals for sending and receiving devices. Layer 1 is the cable connection of computers to peripheral devices and is dictated by the protocol used in layer 2.

Layer 2 describes the **data link layer** or the transmission of a block of data from one device to another. Data are packaged in blocks of specific length. Codes for start of data block, for end of data block, and for error checking are appended to each block before transmission.

The types of data link layers are asynchronous transmission and synchronous transmission. **Asynchronous transmission** originated with the mechanical teletype machines and is the transmission of one character at a time over a single wire. The serial port on a microcomputer is the normal asynchronous communication channel. This is the type of communications commonly used between two computers, between two modems, and between most laboratory instruments and computers.

**Synchronous transmission** was developed for higher speeds and higher volumes of transmission and is the transmission of blocks of data over multiple wires with both sending and receiving stations synchronized to each other. Synchronous transmission involves extensive error checking. This is the type of communications used to transfer data internally by the computer and used to send data from computer to printer.

## Transmission Types

Transmission of data may be either parallel or serial. **Parallel transmission** is the concomitant transfer of multiples of 8 data bits or bytes at once over 8 parallel lines. **Synchronous communication** is parallel transmission and requires both sender

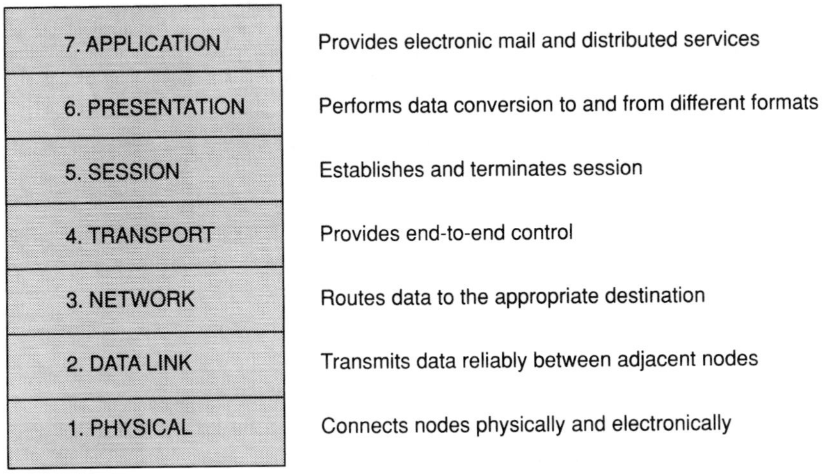

| 7. APPLICATION | Provides electronic mail and distributed services |
| 6. PRESENTATION | Performs data conversion to and from different formats |
| 5. SESSION | Establishes and terminates session |
| 4. TRANSPORT | Provides end-to-end control |
| 3. NETWORK | Routes data to the appropriate destination |
| 2. DATA LINK | Transmits data reliably between adjacent nodes |
| 1. PHYSICAL | Connects nodes physically and electronically |

**FIGURE 9 - 2**

Open System Interconnection (OSI) communications reference model. The 7 layers are shown with short descriptions. Layers 1 and 2 are required for any transmit and receive communications.

and receiver to be synchronized. Parallel transmission is used to transmit data within a computer and to transmit computer output to a printer. All internal computer data transmission is parallel. The CPU determines what size **word** (bit size of transmission) may be transmitted at a time, e.g., 8088 CPU transmits 8 bits at a time, 486 CPU transmits 32 bits at a time. Although parallel communication is more rapid, the cost of its multiwire cabling is more expensive than that for single-wire serial communication. The OSI standard for parallel interface is the **Centronics** 36 pin. Originally, the parallel port on computers was a 36-pin connector and used a ribbon cable to interface with peripheral devices. Today, a 25-pin female D socket, **DB-25S**, serves as the parallel port on most computers. Some printers still have the Centronics 36-pin connector, whereas many have the 25-pin connector. The parallel port is relatively slow for data transmission and is limited to 512 Kbps.

**Serial transmission** is data transfer bit by bit or one bit behind another over a single wire. **Asynchronous communication** is serial transmission and does not require synchronization of sender and receiver. Although parallel communication meets the needs for higher speed data transfer, it is most cumbersome, expensive, and difficult to implement over long distances (300 to 500 feet). Modems, mice, and most laboratory instruments utilize serial communications. A communications card converts data from the parallel format within the computer to serial format that is sent to peripheral devices. That same card receives serial formatted data (from laboratory instruments) and converts it to parallel data for use within the computer. The **RS-232** (Figure 9–3) or RS-232-C is the OSI

interface standard for serial asynchronous communications. Most microcomputers have two serial and one parallel port. The RS-232 port on a computer is a 25-pin male or DB-25 port. Since all of the 25 pins are not used in communications, a 9-pin male DB-9 serial port has been developed and is also used on microcomputers. DB-25 to DB-9 converters are available, if needed, to accommodate or match serial cables, sockets, and ports. The universal serial bus (USB) connector is replacing the serial and parallel cable for data transmission at low and medium bandwidth requirements. USB can achieve transfer rates of 12 Mbps and the cable can also be used to transfer power to the peripheral device. The ability to add and remove peripherals without shutting down the computer is also allowed with USB. This is called "hot swapping." Additionally the USB system takes full advantage of the "plug and play" capabilities most operating systems now employ and no longer requires opening the hardware to add new peripheral boards, setting of switches inside the computer, and other elaborate configuration processes.

## Communication Parameters

Sending and receiving devices must be matched or set to the same communication parameters, which are:

1. Baud rate
2. Parity
3. Data bits
4. Stop bits
5. Duplex (full or half) or echo (on or off)

When running communications software, the parameter information must be entered before transmitting and receiving. A description of the parameters follows.

**Baud rate** is the switching speed of a communications line. Originally baud rate was equivalent to the transmission speed of asynchronous communications in **bits per second** (bps). Newer technology provides more rapid transmission rates and allows one baud or one electrical switching of a communications line to transmit more than one bit. Therefore, at today's higher transmission speeds, baud no longer is equivalent to bps.

A **start bit** is a bit that is added to the beginning of a character before it is transmitted in asynchronous (start/stop) communications. A start bit signals the beginning of a transmission and alerts the receiving device that a character is coming. The start bit is a logical 0 and has a negative voltage.

A **stop bit** is a bit that is added to the end of a character before it is transmitted in asynchronous (start/stop) communications. A stop bit signals the end of a transmission to a receiving device. Communications programs must know how many stop bits are being used. The stop bit is a logical 1 and thus has a positive voltage.

The **number** of data bits is the number of bits used to represent data in communications. For most microcomputer asynchronous communications, 7 data bits are used to repre-

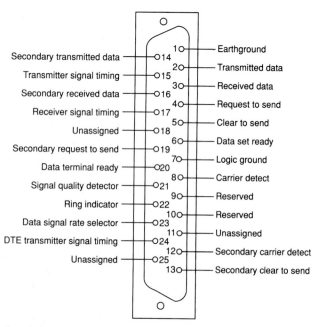

**F I G U R E    9 - 3**

RS232 Standard. The pin numbers and functions assigned in the RS232 standard are shown. Some of the 25 pins are reserved and some are unassigned.

sent a character and one bit is a stop bit. The number of data bits used by laboratory instruments is generally given in the accompanying manual.

**Parity** is the quality of being odd or even. In asynchronous transmission, parity is an error detection method. The sending device checks the number of 1s or 0s and, when necessary, adds an extra parity bit to make the number odd or even. The receiving device then checks for odd or even parity. A **parity bit** is an extra bit attached to the byte, character, or word for error detection in transmission.

A **frame** is the bit length or size of a package of data that is transmitted at one time. Although the length of a frame can vary, nearly all modern clinical laboratory instruments and all microcomputers use a frame of 10 bits. Because the communication is asynchronous and may be sent at any time, there is no clock pulse. For the receiving device to be able to read the communication, it must be given the parameters (baud rate, number data bits, and number stop bits). The start bit signals the beginning of a frame and thereafter the given parameters tell the receiving device what bits to read as data.

**Duplex** is a term describing the direction of communication between two computers. Full duplex is simultaneous two-way communication, e.g., telephone communication. In **full duplex,** characters sent are reflected back from the receiver before being displayed on the sender's screen. In **half duplex,** data travel only one way, and therefore cannot be transmitted and received simultaneously. In half duplex, data are simultaneously sent to the receiver and to the sender's screen. The receiver does not echo back the data for display.

**Echo** is a method whereby the transmitting device may view the outputted communication. When transmitting and not seeing the outputted transmission, turn **echo on.** If everything is displayed in duplicate, turn **echo off.**

**Uploading** is the sending of a file to a central computer from a computer at a remote site. **Downloading** is the copying of a file from a central computer to a computer at a remote site.

## LABORATORY INFORMATION SYSTEMS

The term **Laboratory Information System (LIS)** can be used to describe a system that uses computers to connect laboratory instruments and computers and process the data associated with requesting tests and reporting results. Laboratory information systems can be very simple or highly complex but all have the basic components of a network as discussed in the previous section. The system requires hardware (computers, input/output devices, and peripherals), connections between devices and computers, operating system software, a communication protocol, and a format for data transmitted through the network. In addition, the LIS may be connected to other systems like the Hospital Information System (HIS), other laboratory LISs, or the Internet.

Because many of these systems were originally designed in isolation from the others, there are significant differences between protocols and data formats. Attempts have been made to standardize the format of data within clinical information systems so that LISs and HISs and others can all communicate without error. One example of this is the **Health Level 7 (HL-7)** message protocol. Another example of attempts to standardize the data between laboratory systems is the **Logical Observational Identifiers Names and Codes (LOINC)** database developed at the Regenstrief Institute. This database provides a standard set of names and codes for laboratory results (e.g., bilirubin, amylase, calcium).

## MEDICAL INFORMATICS

Although data and information generated by the clinical laboratory constitute a large part of health care data, it is not the only contributor to these data. Radiology reports, patient history, electrocardiogram reports, and journals all contribute to the massive amounts of data generated in the health care system. Perhaps one of the most important roles for computers has been and will be the management of this information so that health care professionals can effectively acquire, store, retrieve, and utilize the available data and information. Out of this need to access and utilize health care information emerged the field of medical informatics. Although early pioneers in this field began work in the 1950s and 1960s, it was not until the 1980s and 1990s with improvements in computer technology and telecommunications that medical informatics became widely recognized. The term *informatics* originated in 1968 to describe the concept of information science and was later defined to be "the discipline of science which investigates the structure and properties of scientific information."[2] As such, medical informatics would then investigate the structure and properties of medical information.[3]

The term *medical informatics* is often used to describe the use of computers in medicine. However, medical informatics goes beyond the use of computers and the relatively simple collection, storage, and retrieval of data and information. The field is not concerned with the equipment that is used but the information and how it is acquired, utilized, and stored. Medical informatics attempts to bring together information and the necessary tools to the decision-making process in health care.

Informatics (and medical informatics) views the computer as a tool, much like the microscope is a tool in the clinical laboratory.[3] Computer technology is viewed as "enabling us to explore and better understand the informational and cognitive foundations of medicine."[4] The field of medical informatics is rapidly evolving as computer and communication technologies allow access to greater numbers and larger databases of information. The field is actively working to provide health care practitioners the information they need, when they need it, and in a form that is easily interpreted and used for problem solving and decision making.

In the clinical laboratory, informatics can be used to help determine how data should be presented to the user. Some examples of clinical laboratory questions that can utilize informatics:

- Is a bar graph better than simple text to present lab results?
- Should reference ranges be included with lab results?
- How should critical values be displayed to attract attention on a report form?
- What additional laboratory tests should be ordered to complement the current results?
- How can we present large data sets to technologists and technicians to rapidly scan for errors, trends, or other problems?
- How can we acquire data from all laboratory tests performed on a patient over time at different locations so a physician has all results applicable to the decisions without overwhelming them with data?

The clinical laboratory provides a wealth of information, and informatics is the process through which we can assure the most efficient utilization of the information. As genetic information is added to the output of laboratory data, we will be faced with even greater demands for "processing information." The laboratory cannot simply provide numbers but must provide a value-added resource of information to the health care practitioner. By adapting a definition used in nursing informatics,[5] we can define clinical laboratory informatics as a combination of computer technology, information science, and clinical laboratory science used to assist in the management and processing of clinical laboratory data, information, and knowledge to support the practice and delivery of health care.

## SUMMARY

Because the systematic processing of information is critical to the health care delivery system and because computers play a substantial role in this information processing, clinical laboratory personnel must have a basic knowledge of computers and computer communications.

Basic components of a microcomputer include the power supply, the central processing unit (CPU), memory (RAM and ROM), video cards, monitors, storage devices (floppy drives, hard drives, CD ROM drives), input devices (bar code readers, mice), printers, and busses. Most of the computer components are rated according to their throughput speed. For best comparison of computers, one should select a software program that performs a task and run that program on all computers being compared. Because all components of a computer contribute to the total efficiency, timing the performance of a specific software task is the only valid method to compare efficiency of different computers.

Operating systems and languages are used to instruct the computer in its activities as well as in its interaction with peripheral devices such as laboratory instrumentation. Each peripheral device requires a driver (software instructions) be installed to inform the computer of interactive procedures.

Various application programs are commercially available to perform tasks. Major categories are word processing, personal information management, spreadsheet, statistics, and communications. The clinical laboratorian will evaluate the task and then select appropriate software to perform that task. Very seldom is a tailored commercial product available. Most likely, a generic program will have to be altered to meet the individual laboratory's specifications.

Computers are usually networked to other computers to share data, applications, and peripheral devices. Networks can be local (LAN), cover wide areas (WAN), or span the globe (Internet). Networks are classified by their architecture, communication protocol, and topology.

The Laboratory Information System can be used to describe a network of computers connected to each other and laboratory instruments to acquire, validate, interpret, and communicate the information generated by the testing process. Laboratory Information Systems are often connected to other clinical information systems. To assist in the communication of information between these systems, standardized message protocols like HL-7 and LOINC have been developed.

Medical informatics studies the structure and properties of medical information. It works to optimize how data is acquired, stored, and retrieved so the large amounts of data and information generated are available to health care professionals when and where they need it. The use of computer and communication technology is a key aspect of medical informatics practice, but it also is concerned with the human aspects of how information is used in decision making.

### REFERENCES

1. Technical Glossary. Available at: www.Ugeek.com. July 28, 2000.
2. Collen MF. Origins of medical informatics. West J Med 145:778–785, 1986.
3. Hogarth M. (1997) Medical Informatics: An Introduction. Available at: informatics.ucdmc.ucdavis.edu/concepts/intro.htm. July 17, 1997.
4. Blois M. What is medical informatics? West J Med 145: 776–777, 1986.
5. Graves JR, Corcoran S. An overview of nursing informatics. J Nurs Scholarship 21, 227–231, 1989.

# C H A P T E R   1 0
# Carbohydrates

*Margot Hall*

## DEFINITIONS AND BASIC PRINCIPLES

Carbohydrates and their catabolism provide an important source of energy for the human body. The term *carbohydrate*, or hydrates of carbon, and was derived from early observations that the empirical formula of most carbohydrates is $(CH_2O)_n$. Since those early observations, complex carbohydrates containing other chemical moieties and not showing carbon, hydrogen, and oxygen in a ratio of 1:2:1 have been found.

Carbohydrates are more descriptively defined as aldehyde or ketone compounds with multiple hydroxyl groups. Carbohydrates containing an aldehyde group are called aldoses and those with a ketone group are called ketoses. As shown in Figure 10–1, an aldose has the carbonyl (C=O) group at the end of the carbon chain; a ketose has the carbonyl group on an internal carbon atom. Glucose and fructose are examples of an aldose and a ketose, respectively.

Aldoses with three or more carbon atoms and ketoses with four or more carbon atoms contain asymmetric centers that are formed by carbon atoms with four different substituents. Carbohydrate nomenclature is thus based on the configuration about each center of asymmetry. In the straight-chain structural formulas given in Figure 10–2, carbon atom 1 is at the top nearest the aldehyde or ketone group and the other atoms are numbered successively, as shown by the numbers at the left of the formulas. The configurational designation D- or L- refers to the position of the hydroxyl group on the carbon atom next to the bottom $-CH_2OH$ or the asymmetric carbon farthest from the aldehyde or ketone group. By convention, the D-sugars are written with the hydroxyl group on the right and the L-sugars are written with the hydroxyl group on the left. Both D- and L-glucose are shown in Figure 10–2. Note that they are mirror images. Compounds such as these that are identical in composition but differ in spatial configuration are called stereoisomers or enantiomers. The majority of sugars in the body are of the D-configuration.

The predominant forms of sugars in solution are not open chains as shown for D- and L-glucose but rather cyclic or ring structures in which the carbonyl group has formed a covalent bond with one of the hydroxyl groups along the chain. Aldehyde (or ketone) and alcohol groups react to form hemiacetals (or hemiketals). In the case of glucose, the aldehyde group re-acts with the hydroxyl group on carbon 5 to form a hemiacetal, as shown in Figure 10–3. The hydroxyl group on carbon 1 can be written to the right as in Figure 10–3**a.** (referred to as the $\alpha$ form) or to the left as in Figure 10–3**b.** (referred to as the $\beta$ form). This sugar ring can be better represented by the Haworth formula (Figures 10–3**c.** and 3**d.**) in which glucose is referred to as a pyranose because of its similarity to the six-membered ring compound pyran. The designation $\alpha$ means that the hydroxyl group in carbon-1 (the carbonyl carbon, referred to as the anomeric carbon) is below the plane of the ring (Figure 10–3**c.**), $\beta$ means that the hydroxyl group is above the plane of the ring (Figure 10–3**d.**). The $\alpha$ and $\beta$ forms are anomers and differ with respect to optical rotation of polarized light. Common anhydrous crystalline glucose is in the $\alpha$-D-form. An aqueous solution of glucose is an equilibrium mixture containing about one-third $\alpha$-D-glucose, two-thirds $\beta$-D-glucose, and a very small amount of straight-chain compound.

## CLASSIFICATION

There are three main classes of carbohydrates: monosaccharides, oligosaccharides, and polysaccharides.

### Monosaccharides

**Monosaccharides** are simple sugars that contain only one aldehyde or ketone group and two or more hydroxyl groups. They have the empirical formula $(CH_2O)_n$, where n = 3 or more. Sugars with 3, 4, 5, 6, and 7 carbon atoms are trioses, tetroses, pentoses, hexoses, and heptoses, respectively. The hexoses, especially D-glucose, are the most abundant monosaccharides in nature. The three hexoses with the most biological importance are D-glucose and D-fructose (shown in Figure 10–1) and D-galactose. D-galactose is an aldose which differs from D-glucose only in its configuration at carbon atom 4, thus it is an epimer of D-glucose with respect to carbon 4.

Since monosaccharides contain a free aldehyde or ketone group, they can readily reduce oxidizing agents such as cupric ion, ferricyanide, or hydrogen peroxide. In such reactions, the sugar is oxidized in an alkaline solution at the carbonyl group and the oxidizing agent becomes reduced. Sugars capable of reducing oxidizing agents are called reducing sugars. This property provides one basis for the analytical determination of glucose.

```
        H—C=O              CH2OH
          |                  |
        H—C—OH             C=O
          |                  |
      HO—C—H             HO—C—H
          |                  |
        H—C—OH             H—C—OH
          |                  |
        H—C—OH             H—C—OH
          |                  |
        CH2OH              CH2OH
        Aldose             Ketose
       (Glucose)          (Fructose)
```

**F I G U R E    1 0 - 1**

Example of an aldose and a ketose.

## Oligosaccharides

**Oligosaccharides** consist of a few short chains of monosaccharide units joined by covalent bonds. The simplest and most abundant oligosaccharide is a disaccharide.

**Disaccharides** consist of two monosaccharides covalently bound to each other by a glycosidic bond. A glycosidic bond is formed between the aldehyde or ketone group (the carbonyl or anomeric carbon) of one monosaccharide with either the hydroxyl group or the anomeric carbon of the other monosaccharide with loss of a molecule of water.

Figure 10–4 shows the formation of maltose, one of the simplest disaccharides. Maltose is formed from two D-glucose residues by a glycosidic bond between the anomeric carbon of the first glucose residue and carbon atom 4 of the second glucose. Since the configuration of the anomeric carbon is α, the linkage is called an α-1,4 glycosidic bond. Maltose is a reducing sugar since it has one potentially free carbonyl group on the second monosaccharide.

Two other common disaccharides are lactose and sucrose (Figure 10–5). Lactose, which occurs only in milk, is com-

posed of glucose and galactose. Lactose is a reducing sugar because it has a potentially free aldehyde group on the glucose residue. Sucrose, or cane sugar, is composed of glucose and fructose. The linkage of these two monosaccharides involves both anomeric carbon atoms so that there is no free carbonyl group. For this reason sucrose is not a reducing sugar.

## Polysaccharides

**Polysaccharides** are composed of many monosaccharide units linked together. The most important polysaccharides in nature are starch, the main storage carbohydrate of plant cells, and glycogen, the main storage carbohydrate of animal cells. Both contain 25 to 2500 glucose units linked together and are therefore called glucosans.

Starch consists of two kinds of glucosans called amyloses and amylopectins (Figure 10–6). Amylose consists of long, unbranched chains of 25 to 300 glucose units linked together by α-1,4 glycosidic linkages. Amylopectin is a branched polysaccharide composed of 1000 or more glucose units. The successive glucose units in the amylopectin chain are joined by α-1,4 linkages but the branch points are α-1,6 linkages. The different structure of amylose (unbranched) and amylopectin (branched) is important in the selection of starch substrate for amylase determination since α-amylase hydrolyzes only α-1,4, not 1,6 glycosidic bonds.

```
1       H—C=O              H—C=O
          |                  |
2       H—C—OH           HO—C—H
          |                  |
3     HO—C—H             H—C—OH
          |                  |
4       H—C—OH           HO—C—H
          |                  |
5       H—C—OH           HO—C—H
          |                  |
6       CH2OH              CH2OH
        D-Glucose          L-Glucose
```

**F I G U R E    1 0 - 2**

Stereoisomers of glucose.

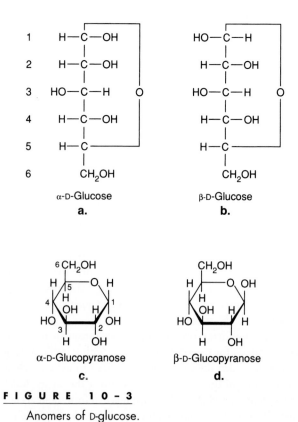

**F I G U R E    1 0 - 3**

Anomers of D-glucose.

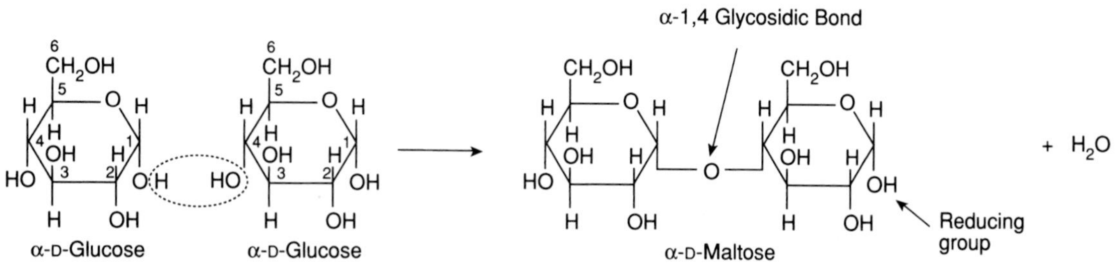

**FIGURE 10-4**

Formation of α-D-maltose.

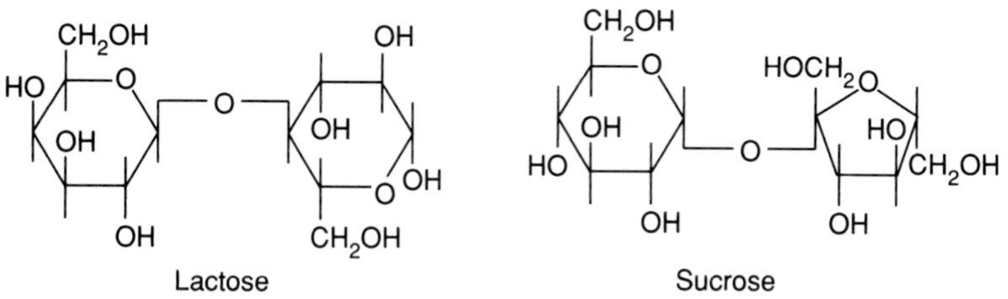

**FIGURE 10-5**

Structures of lactose and sucrose.

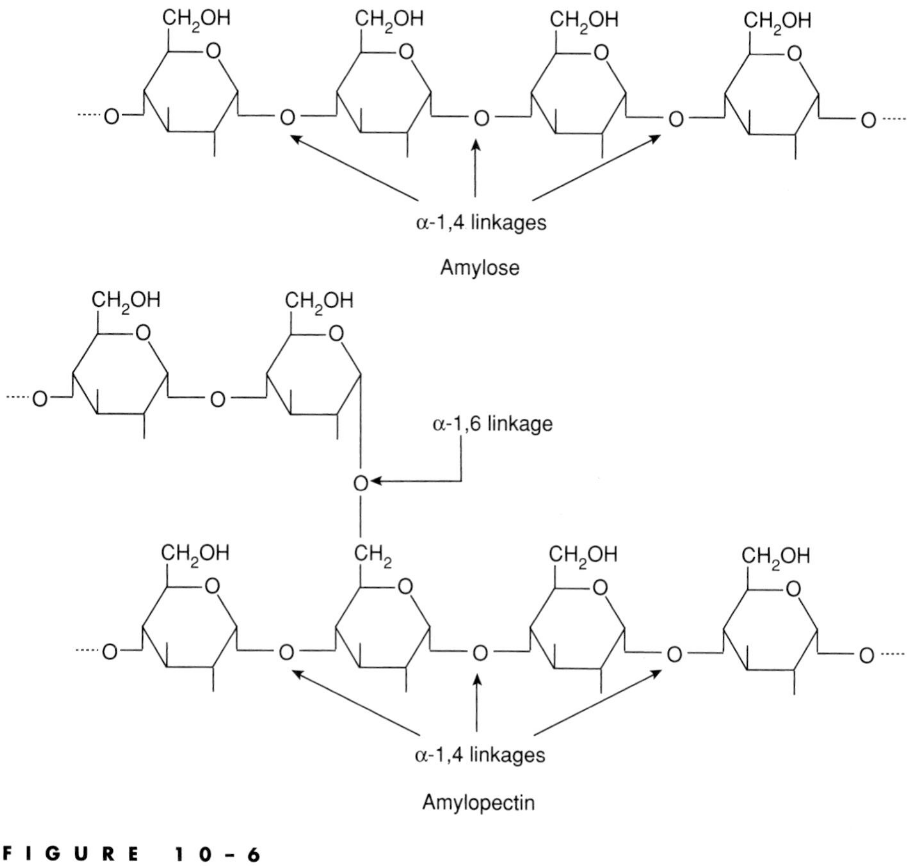

**FIGURE 10-6**

Structures of amylose and amylopectin.

155

Glycogen, like amylopectin, is a branched polysaccharide of D-glucose units but it is more highly branched. Glycogen is present in the liver and skeletal muscle.

## METABOLISM

Carbohydrates are one of the major components of the human diet. Before carbohydrates can be absorbed and used for

energy, they must be broken down to monosaccharides. This breakdown occurs in the process of digestion.

**Digestion** begins in the mouth where salivary amylase hydrolyzes starch to form intermediate dextrins and maltose (Figure 10–7). In the stomach, salivary amylase is inactivated by the acid pH of gastric juice. The pH of the small intestine is more alkaline so digestion of starch and glycogen to maltose is completed there by pancreatic amylase. The maltose, along with any ingested lactose and sucrose, is then hydrolyzed by

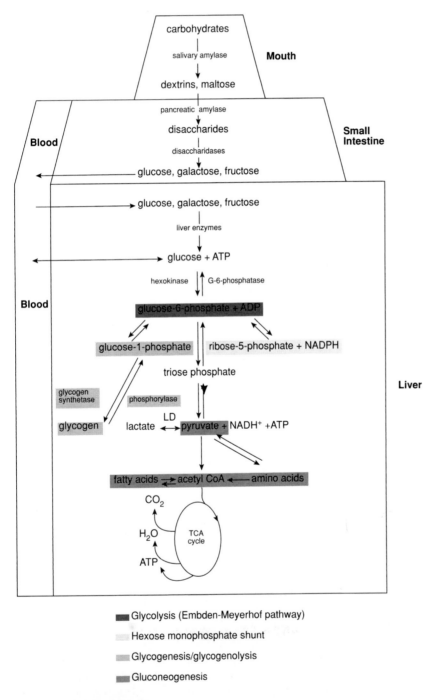

**FIGURE 10-7**

Absorption and metabolism of glucose.

enzymes from the intestinal mucosa (disaccharidases) to form the monosaccharides glucose, galactose, and fructose. These monosaccharides are then absorbed through the intestinal wall into the blood stream and are transported to the liver via portal circulation.

Since glucose is the only monosaccharide that is used by the body for energy, galactose and fructose are converted by liver enzymes to glucose. In the first step of glucose utilization, the glucose in the liver reacts with adenosine triphosphate (ATP) in the presence of hexokinase to form glucose-6-phosphate. The glucose-6-phosphate serves as a pivotal point for three possible metabolic pathways by which glucose is metabolized. It can enter (1) the hexose monophosphate shunt pathway, (2) the glycolytic pathway for energy production, or (3) the glycogenesis pathway for glucose storage.

If the body needs energy, glucose is metabolized completely to carbon dioxide and water with the formation of energy via ATP production. There are two main pathways (Figure 10–7) for this breakdown of glucose: (1) the glycolytic or Embden-Meyerhof pathway, and (2) an alternate hexose monophosphate (HMP) shunt pathway.

In the Embden-Meyerhof pathway, the glucose-6-phosphate is cleaved through a series of steps to a triose phosphate and finally to two molecules of pyruvate. The conversion of glucose into pyruvate or lactate is called **glycolysis.** This process is anaerobic (does not require oxygen), occurs in the cytoplasm of the cell, and provides two molecules of ATP per molecule of glucose. The pyruvate can be converted back to glucose-6-phosphate by a different pathway or it can be converted into lactate by the enzyme lactate dehydrogenase (LD). Under aerobic conditions, pyruvate undergoes oxidative decarboxylation to form acetyl coenzyme A (CoA).

The oxidation of acetyl CoA provides cells with most of the energy potentially available from the oxidation of glucose. As shown in Figure 10–7, acetyl CoA enters the tricarboxylic acid (TCA) cycle, also known as the Krebs cycle or citric acid cycle. The TCA cycle is part of the aerobic phase of glucose metabolism and occurs in the mitochondria of the cell. It consists of a sequence of oxidation-reduction reactions in which acetyl CoA is ultimately oxidized to $CO_2$ and $H_2O$ with the production of 24 molecules of ATP (12 ATPs per molecule of acetyl CoA) primarily due to the coupling of glucose oxidation to the mitochondrial electron-transport system. The complete oxidation of one molecule of glucose in the liver provides 38 molecules of ATP (2 directly from glycolysis, 2 directly from the TCA cycle, and the remainder from oxidation of NADH and $FADH_2$) as a form of energy. Different tissues produce either 36 ATP (muscle and brain) or 38 ATP (liver, heart, kidney) from the complete oxidation of glucose. This is due to their selective use of two different shuttle mechanisms (glycerol phosphate shuttle or malate-aspartate shuttle) for transporting the electrons of NADH produced during glycolysis from the cytosol into the mitochondria.

As stated above, an alternate pathway for the oxidation of glucose is the hexose monophosphate (HMP) pathway, also called the pentose shunt. In this pathway, glucose-6-phosphate

is converted to ribose-5-phosphate (a pentose) with the production of NADPH (Figure 10–7). The NADPH generates reducing power and is important as an energy source for many anabolic reactions such as fatty acid and steroid synthesis. The HMP pathway also plays a key role for glycolysis in the red blood cell since erythrocytes lack mitochondria and thus are not capable of oxidative phosphorylation in the TCA cycle. The ribose-5-phosphate can be further converted to a triose phosphate that can join the glycolytic pathway.

If glucose is not needed by the body for immediate energy, it can be stored in the liver in the form of glycogen. In this process, as illustrated in Figure 10–7, the glucose-6-phosphate is enzymatically polymerized by a series of steps to form glycogen. The process of glycogen formation from glucose is referred to as **glycogenesis.** Glycogenesis occurs when there is an elevated blood glucose such as after a meal. When the blood glucose begins to drop, the glycogen is converted back to glucose by a different set of enzymes. The breakdown of glycogen to form glucose and other intermediate products is called **glycogenolysis.** The glycogenesis–glycogenolysis reactions are important mechanisms for regulating the blood glucose level. Glycogen can also be formed and stored in muscle. Only hepatic glycogen, however, is available to the blood since muscle lacks the glucose-6-phosphatase enzyme necessary for the conversion of glycogen back to glucose.

**Gluconeogenesis** is another pathway that is important in maintaining the blood glucose level, especially during long-term fasting. Gluconeogenesis is the formation of glucose from noncarbohydrate sources such as amino acids, lactate, or the glycerol portion of lipids. Gluconeogenesis is not an exact reversal of anaerobic glycolysis but rather a process sharing certain steps with glycolysis and bypassing others. In this fashion, glucose is formed from lactate, lipids, and proteins. Additionally, as illustrated in Figure 10–7, fatty acids, amino acids, and lactate can be converted to acetyl CoA and then oxidized completely in the TCA cycle.

The concentration of glucose in the blood is maintained remarkably constant under ordinary circumstances. During a brief fast, a drop in the level of blood glucose can be avoided by the formation of glucose via glycogenolysis. During long-term fasting, gluconeogenesis becomes more important as a source of glucose. As blood glucose levels increase, glycogenolysis is replaced by glycogenesis. These pathways have delicate control mechanisms such as feedback inhibition and hormonal control that keep the blood glucose concentration within a narrow range despite changes in feeding and fasting.

## HORMONAL REGULATION

Hormones regulate the blood glucose concentration by affecting one or more of the metabolic pathways illustrated in Figure 10–7. Several hormones work together to maintain the narrow range of blood glucose concentration: insulin lowers the blood glucose; other counterregulatory hormones such as

TABLE 10 – 1

**Effects of Hormones on Blood Glucose Concentration**

| HORMONE | ORIGIN | EFFECT ON GLUCOSE CONCENTRATION | HORMONAL ACTION |
|---|---|---|---|
| Insulin | Beta cells in pancreas | ↓ | Cell membrane, glycogenesis |
| Glucagon | Alpha cells in pancreas | ↑ | Glycogenolysis, gluconeogenesis |
| Epinephrine | Adrenal medulla | ↑ | Glycogenolysis |
| Thyroxine | Thyroid gland | Insignificant | Glycogenolysis |
| Growth hormone | Anterior pituitary | ↑ | Antagonist to insulin |
| ACTH | Anterior pituitary | ↑ | Antagonist to insulin |
| Cortisol | Adrenal cortex | ↑ | Gluconeogenesis, antagonist to insulin |
| Somatostatin | Delta cells in pancreas, other tissues | Minor | Inhibits release of insulin and glucagon |
| Somatomedins | Liver | Minor | Insulinlike activity |

ACTH = adrenocorticotropic hormone; ↓ = decrease; ↑ = increase

glucagon, epinephrine, cortisol, and growth hormone elevate glucose levels. The action of these hormones is summarized in Table 10–1.

**Insulin** is a small peptide secreted by the beta cells of the pancreatic islets of Langerhans in response to an elevated blood glucose level. It is the only hormone that lowers the blood glucose. It does so by increasing membrane permeability to glucose by binding to receptors on cell surfaces, thus enhancing the entry of glucose into liver, muscle, and adipose tissue. It also alters the metabolic pathways of glucose metabolism by enhancing the synthesis of glycogen, lipid, and protein while inhibiting the breakdown of glycogen.

Insulin secretion is controlled by the blood glucose concentration. If the blood glucose is increased, insulin is secreted. A decrease in blood glucose inhibits the release of insulin. The amount of insulin required for a specific decrease of blood glucose varies in individuals. For example, an overweight individual with normal carbohydrate metabolism requires a higher concentration of insulin than does a normal-weight individual.[1]

Insulin is synthesized from a precursor called proinsulin, a single chain polypeptide. Proinsulin is converted into active insulin by action of specific peptidases to form A and B chains of insulin, which are connected by two disulfide bonds and a middle segment called C-peptide (Figure 10–8). The C-peptide is liberated with insulin in essentially equimolar amounts during secretion. Serum insulin levels thus correlate with C-peptide levels.

**Glucagon** is a polypeptide hormone secreted by the alpha cells of the pancreatic islets of Langerhans in response to a low blood glucose level. It is the principal hormone for producing a rapid increase in the concentration of glucose in the blood. It does so by stimulating hepatic glycogenolysis and gluconeogenesis, but it has no effect on muscle glycogen.

**Epinephrine,** also known as adrenaline, is a catecholamine secreted by the adrenal medulla. It increases the blood glucose level by stimulating glycogenolysis and lipolysis while inhibiting the release of pancreatic insulin. It serves as a backup for glucagon and its release is triggered by physical or emotional stress. This causes an immediate increase in the production of glucose for energy along with an increase in heart rate, blood pressure, and other physiologic effects.

**Thyroxine (T₄)** is a tetraiodinated amino acid secreted by the thyroid gland. It promotes glycogenolysis and can lead to a depletion of glycogen stores in the liver. It also accelerates the rate of glucose absorption from the intestine and may lead

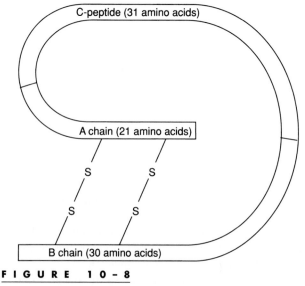

**FIGURE 10 – 8**

Structure of human insulin.

to a mildly abnormal, diabetic type of glucose intolerance in hyperthyroid individuals even though their fasting blood glucose is usually normal. Although the action of thyroxine is hyperglycemic, it has an insignificant role in regulating the blood glucose concentration.

**Growth hormone (GH),** also called somatotropin, is a polypeptide secreted by the anterior pituitary. The action of GH is antagonistic to that of insulin in that it inhibits glucose uptake by the tissues and stimulates liver glycogenolysis, thus raising the blood glucose concentration.

**Adrenocorticotropin (ACTH),** also called corticotropin, is a small polypeptide secreted by the anterior pituitary. Like GH, it increases the concentration of blood glucose because of its antagonistic action to insulin. ACTH stimulates the release of cortisol from the adrenal gland thereby increasing blood glucose.

**Cortisol** and other 11-oxysteroids secreted by the adrenal cortex raise the blood glucose concentration primarily by stimulating gluconeogenesis. They also have some metabolic effects that are antagonistic to insulin and are sometimes referred to as diabetogenic hormones.

**Somatostatin** is a polypeptide hormone formed for the most part in the delta (D) cells of the pancreatic islets of Langerhans. It inhibits secretion of insulin and glucagon, thereby modulating their reciprocating action. Somatostatin thus has only a minor effect on the blood glucose concentration.

**Somatomedins** are peptides produced in the liver in response to stimulation by growth hormone. Somatomedins are a group of hormones, including somatomedin-A, somatomedin-C, and insulinlike growth factors I and II, that directly promote growth. In addition to their growth-promoting effects, somatomedins show insulinlike activity in some tissues such as adipose tissue. It has since been shown that insulinlike growth factor I has a structure similar to that of insulin.[2]

## CLINICAL APPLICATIONS

Various disorders of carbohydrate metabolism may be associated with (1) an increased plasma glucose concentration (**hyperglycemia**), (2) a decreased plasma glucose concentration (**hypoglycemia**), and (3) a normal or decreased plasma glucose concentration, often with the excretion of a nonglucose-reducing sugar in the urine (**inborn errors of carbohydrate metabolism**).

## Hyperglycemia

### CLASSIFICATION

The National Diabetes Data Group proposed, in 1979, a classification for diabetes mellitus and other hyperglycemic disorders.[3] According to this classification, hyperglycemic disorders were divided into five categories: insulin-dependent diabetes mellitus (IDDM), non-insulin–dependent diabetes mellitus (NIDDM), impaired glucose tolerance (IGT), gestational diabetes mellitus (GDM), previous abnormality of glucose tolerance (PrevAGT), and potential abnormality of glucose tolerance (PotAGT). This classification scheme used 140 mg/dL (7.8 mmol/L) fasting plasma glucose as the diagnostic cutoff for diabetes and emphasized the results of the oral glucose tolerance test (OGTT). Since then, in 1997, the American Diabetes Association (ADA) introduced a new classification scheme proposed by the International Expert Committee on the Diagnosis and Classification of Diabetes Mellitus.[4] The adoption of this method of classification and diagnostic criteria has been retained with only minor variations by the ADA in their Clinical Practice Recommendations of 1998[5] and 2000.[6] In contrast with the 1979 classification scheme, the current method of classification is predicated on disease etiology rather than treatment modality. They retained the categories of type 1 and type 2 diabetes mellitus using Arabic numerals in lieu of Roman numerals and eliminating the terms IDDM and NIDDM. Likewise, they retained the category of GDM and developed a new category known as other specific types of diabetes. For the diagnostic criteria, the most notable changes are a shift away from the OGTT with an emphasis on the fasting plasma glucose (FPG) test and a new diagnostic threshold of 126 mg/dL (7.0 mmol/L). This classification is shown in Table 10–2.

**Diabetes mellitus** is the most important disease associated with hyperglycemia. It is not a single, well-defined disease entity but rather a heterogeneous group of disorders. It is characterized by a deficiency of insulin secretion or action resulting in hyperglycemia and the probable development of complications over time. The types of diabetes mellitus listed in Table 10–2 are based in part on whether the deficiency of insulin is absolute, relative, or associated with certain other conditions or syndromes.

**Type 1 diabetes mellitus** (formerly IDDM) is a severe form of diabetes characterized by an absolute deficiency of insulin because of autoimmune destruction or degeneration of the pancreatic islet beta cells. Beta cell injury appears to be precipitated by a heterogeneous group of factors including a permissive genetic background and environmental agents that might be either viral or chemical. Genetic determinants are thought to be important because of the associated increased or decreased frequency of certain human leukocyte antigens (HLA) on chromosome six. The disease is associated with DQA and DQB genes and appears to be influenced by the DRB genes.[7–8] The majority of persons with type 1 diabetes present with one or more of the following: islet cell autoantibodies, insulin autoantibodies, glutamic acid decarboxylase autoantibodies, and tyrosine phosphatase IA-2 and IA-2B autoantibodies.[9–12] Less frequently, one observes other autoantibodies.

Type 1 diabetes mellitus is usually characterized clinically by abrupt onset of symptoms, often following a viral infection, and proneness to ketosis. These patients therefore require insulin treatment to prevent ketosis and sustain life. Patients present with a history of rapid weight loss accompanied by

**TABLE 10-2**

**Classification of Diabetes Mellitus and Other Hyperglycemic Disorders**

| DISORDER | CHARACTERISTIC |
|---|---|
| I. Type 1 diabetes mellitus<br>  A. Immune mediated<br>  B. Idiopathic | Absolute deficiency of insulin |
| II. Type 2 diabetes mellitus<br>  Insulin resistance with insulin secretory defect | Relative deficiency of insulin |
| III. Other specific types of diabetes<br>  A. Genetic defects of beta cell function<br>  B. Genetic defects in insulin action<br>  C. Diseases of the exocrine pancreas<br>  D. Endocrinopathies<br>  E. Drug or chemical induced<br>  F. Infections<br>  G. Uncommon forms of immune-mediated diabetes<br>  H. Other genetic syndromes sometimes associated<br>    with diabetes | Varies with underlying pathologic condition |
| IV. Gestational diabetes mellitus | Glucose intolerance with onset during pregnancy |

From the American Diabetes Association Committee Report[4]

polyphagia, polydipsia, polyuria, and neurological symptoms including confusion, disorientation, and loss of consciousness. Laboratory findings include: hyperglycemia, polyuria, increased serum osmolality, increased urine osmolality and specific gravity, ketonemia, ketonuria, acidosis (acidemia and aciduria), and electrolyte imbalance including an increased anion gap. Over time, these patients will develop renal, cardiac, retinal, neurological, and microvascular complications. Severe complications are more frequently found in the poorly controlled diabetic. Type 1 diabetes mellitus can occur at any age but most frequently occurs in juveniles, thus it was formerly termed *juvenile diabetes*. It accounts for about 10% of all cases of diabetes mellitus.

A small subset of type 1 diabetes mellitus patients have no known cause. They present with insulinopenia and ketoacidosis, are usually of Asian or African descent,[13] but lack evidence of autoimmunity.

**Type 2 diabetes mellitus** (formerly NIDDM) is a milder form of diabetes characterized by a relative deficiency of insulin activity due to insulin resistance (insulin levels may be normal but there is an insufficient peripheral response to the insulin) and an insulin secretory defect.[14] Some may exhibit predominantly insulin resistance with relative insulin deficiency, and others will have predominantly secretory defect with insulin resistance. Patients with type 2 diabetes mellitus exhibit increased amyloid deposition in their islet cells and their glucose intolerance increases in parallel with that deposition.[15] Amyloid is a starchlike protein-carbohydrate complex that can be deposited in tissues, especially during chronic dis-

ease. Type 2 has a stronger genetic basis than type 1, as evidenced by a more frequent familial pattern of occurrence. Environmental factors, such as the intake of excessive calories leading to weight gain and obesity, and lack of physical exercise may also be important in the pathogenesis of type 2 diabetes mellitus. Unlike type 1 diabetes mellitus, no relationship to viruses has been postulated in type 2 diabetes mellitus and no consistent islet cell antibodies or HLA associations have been found.

Patients with type 2 diabetes mellitus are not prone to ketosis and usually do not require insulin, although some may require insulin to control symptomatic hyperglycemia. These patients exhibit increased risk of developing vascular complications and hyperosmolar coma.[16] Patients with type 2 diabetes mellitus are often obese; weight loss may improve their glucose tolerance.[17] Type 2 diabetes mellitus usually first presents in adults after age 40 and progresses slowly. This is the most common form of diabetes mellitus and accounts for 80% to 90% of patients.

**Other specific types of diabetes** are secondary to certain other conditions such as: (1) genetic defects of beta cell function, (2) genetic defects of insulin action, (3) pancreatic exocrine disease, (4) endocrine disease, (5) drug or chemically induced conditions, (6) infections, (7) anti-insulin receptor antibodies, and (8) other genetic syndromes.

Two genetic defects that alter the beta cell function are maturity onset diabetes of youth (MODY) characterized by impaired insulin secretion,[18] and mitochondrial diabetes mellitus (MtDM) characterized by maternal transmission of diabetes with deafness.[19] There are also genetic mutations that prevent the conversion of proinsulin to insulin[20] and those that result in a mutated insulin molecule with poor receptor binding.[21]

In addition to genetic defects of insulin, there are genetic defects of insulin action that include any miscoding for the insulin receptor or post-receptor signal molecules such as enzymes. Examples of the former include type A insulin resistance[22] and the two pediatric syndromes: leprechaunism and Rabson-Mendenhall.[23] An example of a post-receptor signal molecule mutation is insulin-resistant lipotrophic diabetes.[24]

Widespread pancreatic injury can cause diabetes due to decreased or damaged beta cells. Both pancreatitis[25] and pancreatic carcinoma[26] have been associated with hyperglycemia; whereas cystic fibrosis,[27] hemochromatosis,[28] and fibrocalculous pancreatopathy[29] are less frequently found in combination with diabetes.

Endocrinopathies such as Cushing's disease (increased cortisol), glucagonoma (increased glucagon), acromegaly (increased growth hormone), and pheochromocytoma (increased epinephrine) often cause hyperglycemia due to their antagonistic action on insulin.[30-33] Somatostatinoma and aldosteronoma can sometimes inhibit insulin secretion.[33-34]

The administration of anti-insulin hormones or any of a number of drugs (e.g., dilantin, thiazides, pentamidine, beta adrenergic agonists) that impair pancreatic beta cell function will cause hyperglycemia.[35] Poisons such as Vacor[36] can cause irreversible destruction of beta cells with ensuing diabetes.

Two infections that have long been associated with diabetes are cytomegalovirus[37] and congenital rubella.[38] Additionally, coxsackie-B4, adenovirus, and mumps have been implicated.[39]

Antibodies directed at the insulin receptor can block insulin binding and cause hyperglycemia.[23] This has been called type B insulin resistance. Occasionally, one also finds anti-insulin receptor antibodies in patients with systemic lupus erythematosus. It should be noted, however, that some insulin receptor antibodies mimic insulin and cause hypoglycemia. In some cases, patients with the autoimmune disorder known as stiff-man syndrome can develop diabetes.[40]

An increased incidence of diabetes is observed in a variety of genetic defects such as Down's syndrome, Klinefelter's syndrome, Turner's syndrome, and Wolframs syndrome.[41-42] Finally, certain malnourished patients, especially those with high circulating fatty acids, may present with hyperglycemia.

**Gestational diabetes mellitus (GDM)** is characterized by the onset of diabetes or impaired glucose tolerance (IGT) during pregnancy due to hormonal and metabolic changes.[43] GDM is often accompanied by a family history of diabetes mellitus, a clinical history of recurrent monilial infections, or a reproductive history of large babies (>4000 g) or infants with congenital anomalies. Maternal symptoms of GDM are usually mild; however, the effects of hyperglycemia on the fetus can be devastating.[44] These include congenital malformations and perinatal mortality. After delivery, the patient may revert to normal or develop diabetes mellitus later in life. In either case, the woman must be reclassified following delivery depending on her 6-week postpartum plasma glucose levels.

Two terms that have been retained by the ADA guidelines[4] are **impaired glucose tolerance (IGT)** and **impaired fasting glucose (IFG).** IGT is characterized by plasma glucose levels following an oral glucose load (OGTT) that are not normal yet not sufficiently abnormal to be classified in the category of diabetes mellitus. The analogous IFG is characterized by plasma glucose levels following an 8-hour fast that are greater than normal but not sufficiently elevated to be classified as diabetic. These patients may revert to normal or remain borderline but do have a greater risk for the development of diabetes mellitus.

## PATHOPHYSIOLOGY

In diabetes mellitus, the low levels of insulin cause alterations in the normal metabolic pathways (shown in Figure 10–7). Because insulin is deficient, the entry of glucose into cells is impaired, resulting in elevated blood glucose levels. When the elevated blood glucose levels exceed the renal reabsorptive capacity, glucose is excreted in the urine. This condition is called **glycosuria** (or **glucosuria**). Since water is excreted with the glucose, untreated diabetic patients are thirsty and hungry. Characteristic symptoms of diabetes are **polyuria** (frequent urination), **polydipsia** (the intake of large volumes of water), and **polyphagia** (excessive desire for eating). Since excess glucose is excreted in urine rather than being stored as fat, weight loss is common.

In addition to a low insulin level, untreated diabetes is characterized by an increased level of glucagon, resulting in further metabolic changes shown in Figure 10–9. Glycolysis is inhibited and glycogenolysis, lipolysis, and gluconeogenesis are stimulated. The accelerated catabolism of amino acids and fatty acids causes increased amounts of acetyl CoA. This acetyl CoA does not enter the TCA cycle but rather is converted to cholesterol or the ketoacid, acetoacetic acid, and its derivatives, $\beta$-hydroxybutyric acid and acetone. The overproduction of these three ketone bodies, called ketosis, results in their appearance in the blood (**ketonemia**) and in the urine (**ketonuria**). Since acetone is volatile, it may be present in the breath of diabetic patients, giving the breath a characteristic sweet "organic" odor.

In uncontrolled diabetes mellitus, the overproduction of ketoacids causes acidosis or a lowered blood pH. The body compensates for this lowered pH by decreasing the concentration of bicarbonate in the bicarbonate-carbonic acid-buffering system to yield carbon dioxide and water. Depletion of the bicarbonate may lead to metabolic acidosis. The respiratory center is stimulated, producing rapid, deep breathing and increased excretion of carbon dioxide by the lungs. Coma may result and prompt therapy with insulin is necessary to avoid death.

One difference between type 1 and type 2 diabetic patients is their relative glucagon to insulin ratios. In type 1

**Blood**

**Liver**

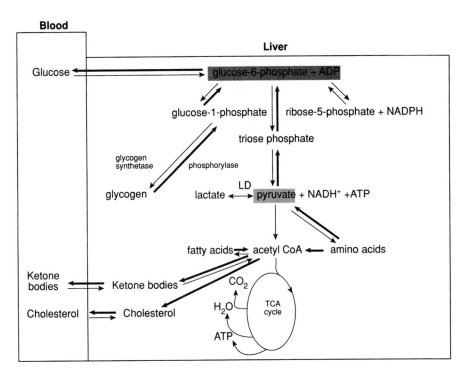

**FIGURE   10-9**

Metabolic changes characteristic of diabetes mellitus.

diabetes mellitus, patients have an absolute deficiency of in-sulin leading to a high glucagon to insulin ratio and the de-velopment of **ketoacidosis** (ketonemia with low pH). In con-trast, type 2 diabetic patients have only a relative decrease in insulin, so the effects of the glucagon are modulated and keto-acidosis is rarely seen. Although fatty acid oxidation with the attendant production of ketones is usually inhibited, the pro-duction of increased triglycerides and very low density lipopro-teins (VLDL) is commonly seen. In contrast to patients with type 1 diabetes, type 2 diabetic patients more frequently pre-sent with **hyperglycemic hyperosmolar nonketotic coma.** This condition is the result of hyperglycemia leading to uri-nary losses of water, glucose, and electrolytes (**osmotic diure-sis**) without sufficient fluid replacement. The resulting dehy-dration can lead to extremely high blood glucose levels and finally coma. It is more frequently seen in elderly patients and may be precipitated by other concomitant medical conditions.

The management of individuals with hyperglycemia con-sists of dietary measures and the administration of insulin or oral hypoglycemic agents when indicated. A complication of treatment with hypoglycemic agents is hypoglycemia, which can also result in coma. Rapid laboratory testing is essential to distinguish between hypoglycemic coma and hyperglycemic coma resulting from the associated ketoacidosis.

Despite treatment with insulin, many individuals with type 1 and some with type 2 diabetes mellitus still develop se-rious complications within 10 to 15 years. Complications may include retinopathy leading to blindness, kidney failure (ne-phropathy), neurologic defects (neuropathy) and microvascu-lar and macrovascular disease. Although life expectancy has in-creased for patients with diabetes, heart attacks and strokes due to vascular complications have resulted in premature mortal-ity. Overall, the risk of death from coronary artery disease is doubled by the presence of diabetes.[45] Diminished blood flow to the legs and feet because of arteriosclerosis is increased four-to sevenfold in diabetic patients. This is a major cause of lower limb amputations along with loss of response to normal pres-sure, minor trauma, susceptibility to infections, and other de-fects in the microcirculation of the leg and foot resulting in gangrene.

The cause of late degenerative complications in diabetes mellitus remains obscure. Many diabetologists believe in the glycemic hypothesis, that is, that elevated glucose itself is the mediator of these complications.[46] This view is supported by the fact that nonenzymatic glycosylation of proteins such as hemoglobin and albumin is common in the body and that the rate of glycosylation increases in direct proportion to plasma glucose concentrations.[47] In 1982, a large multicenter, ran-domized, long-term clinical trial called the Diabetes Control and Complications Trial (DCCT) was initiated to determine whether an intensive treatment regimen directed at maintain-ing blood glucose concentrations as close to normal as possi-ble will affect the development of vascular complications in patients with type 1 diabetes mellitus.[48]

## LABORATORY DIAGNOSIS

The 1997 ADA guidelines[4] for the diagnosis of diabetes mellitus stress the results of the fasting plasma glucose as opposed to those of the OGTT. To obtain a diagnosis of diabetes mellitus, one of the following three criteria must be met and confirmed on a subsequent day by any one of the three criteria:

1.  Symptoms of diabetes plus a random plasma glucose concentration ≥200 mg/dL (11.1 mmol/L)
2.  A fasting plasma glucose ≥126 mg/dL (7.0 mmol/L)
3.  During the OGTT, a 2-hour after oral glucose load plasma glucose ≥200 mg/dL (11.1 mmol/L)

Confirmation is not required if the patient presents with either a hyperosmolar or ketotic crisis. The criteria apply to both adult and pediatric patients. The ADA recommends FPG testing every 3 years for all people over 45 years of age and more frequently if they fall into one of the following high-risk groups: obese people, people with a family history of diabetes mellitus, people in a high-risk racial group (African, Hispanic, Asian, or Native Americans), women with a history of large babies or gestational diabetes, people with hypertension, people with low concentrations of high-density lipoprotein (HDL) cholesterol, people with high concentrations of triglycerides, and people with a history of IFG or IGT.

Diagnosis of type 1 diabetes mellitus is usually straightforward based on history, clinical symptoms and the demonstration of significant hyperglycemia. Diagnosis of type 2 diabetes mellitus may be more difficult and early diagnosis is important to avoid later development of microvascular disease. The clinical laboratory tests described below are important in the diagnosis and treatment of both types of diabetes mellitus.

### Casual (Random) Plasma Glucose

The 1997 ADA guidelines[4] define a casual (random) plasma glucose sample as one which is collected irrespective of when the last meal was ingested or the time of day. Polydipsia, polyuria, and unexplained weight loss are considered to be symptomatic of diabetes mellitus, and a glucose result of 200 mg/dL (11.1 mmol/L) or greater in the presence of these symptoms is presumptive of diabetes mellitus.

### Fasting Plasma Glucose

In normal individuals, a 10- to 16-hour fasting plasma glucose (FPG) concentration is maintained at 80 to 90 mg/dL (4.4 to 5.0 mmol/L),[49] although it tends to increase with age.[50] An elevation of the fasting plasma glucose is indicative of diabetes mellitus. The 1997 ADA guidelines[4] define fasting as 8 hours or more without any caloric intake. According to their criteria, an FPG result that is less than 110 mg/dL (6.1 mmol/L) is normal, values between 110 and 125 mg/dL (6.1–6.9 mmol/L) imply impaired fasting glucose, and values that are greater than or equal to 126 mg/dL (7.0 mmol/L) indicate diabetes mellitus.

### Urine Glucose

In disease states such as diabetes mellitus, glucose appears in the urine when the blood glucose level exceeds the renal threshold for glucose. The renal threshold varies among patients, but usually begins at 160 to 180 mg/dL (8.9 to 10.0 mmol/L), preventing urinary assessment of lower blood glucose values. Urine glucose measurement has been used as a screening test for detection of diabetes mellitus and as a guide to insulin therapy, but its clinical role has become less important with increased use of self-monitoring of blood glucose.[49]

### Two-Hour Postprandial Plasma Glucose

This is a simple loading test in which the plasma glucose is measured 2 hours after the patient consumes a standard load of glucose (75 g of glucose in solution). A plasma glucose level of ≥200 mg/dL (11.1 mmol/L) is indicative of diabetes mellitus when it is confirmed on another day by either an elevated fasting plasma glucose or random plasma glucose value. A value of <140 mg/dL (7.8 mmol/L) is considered normal and values between 140 and 199 mg/dL (7.8 to 11.0 mmol/L) constitute impaired glucose tolerance. Like the fasting plasma glucose, values tend to increase with age.[50] Under the 1979 guidelines,[3] this test was performed following a meal, but the new guidelines[4] require a standard oral load of glucose.

### Oral Glucose Tolerance Test

The 1997 ADA guidelines[4] do not recommend the use of this test. However, they indicate that if it is used, it should be performed according to the original guidelines. It consists of serial measurement of plasma glucose before and after oral administration of glucose.

The following procedure has been recommended by the American Diabetes Association[51] and re-endorsed (with a change in the glucose dose) by the National Diabetes Data Group[3] to standardize the OGTT and updated by the 1997 ADA guidelines:[4]

1.  The patient should have unlimited physical activity and an unrestricted diet containing at least 150 g of carbohydrates for 3 days before the test is performed.
2.  The test should be performed in the morning after the patient has fasted for 10 to 16 hours; only water is permitted.
3.  A fasting plasma glucose is collected.
4.  A glucose dose of 75 g dissolved in flavored water is administered orally to nonpregnant adults. Alternatively, 1.75 g of glucose per kg of ideal body weight is used for pediatric patients and 100 g of glucose for pregnant women. The concentration of the solution should be ≤25 g/dL. The drink should be ingested in approximately 5 minutes and the test is timed from the commencement of drinking.

5.  Plasma glucose is measured every 30 minutes for 2 hours. The patient should remain seated throughout the test. Samples should be collected in sodium fluoride preservative, separated and frozen or assayed within 4 hours.

Typical glucose-tolerance curves for a normal subject and a diabetic patient are shown in Figure 10–10. In a normal patient, the glucose level rises to about 150 mg/dL (8.3 mmol/L) or even higher within 30 to 60 minutes and then decreases as insulin secretion is stimulated by the increase in plasma glucose. The glucose level tends to drop slightly below fasting levels before the effect of the increased insulin level wears off and then returns to normal in approximately 3 hours. In a diabetic subject, glucose levels start high and rise higher than in a normal patient because the diabetic patient has an insufficient supply of insulin and is thus unable to efficiently utilize the administered glucose. Levels remain higher for a longer period before slowly returning to the initial level. According to the 1997 ADA guidelines,[4] a plasma glucose level ≥200 mg/dL (11.1 mmol/L) on the 2-hour sample when confirmed by either the FPG or RPG test is diagnostic of diabetes mellitus. Once again, a value of <140 mg/dL (7.8 mmol/L) on the 2-hour sample would indicate a normal glucose tolerance, whereas values between 140 and 199 mg/dL (7.8–11.0 mmol/L) imply impaired glucose tolerance. The complete tolerance curve is still recommended for pregnant women and samples are collected for 3 hours. If any two of the following conditions are met, the patient is diagnosed as a gestational diabetic: (1) a fasting plasma glucose ≥105 mg/dL (5.8 mmol/L), (2) a 1-hour plasma glucose value ≥190 mg/dL (10.6 mmol/L), (3) a 2-hour value of ≥165 mg/dL (9.2 mmol/L, or (4) a 3-hour value of ≥145 mg/dL (8.1 mmol/L).

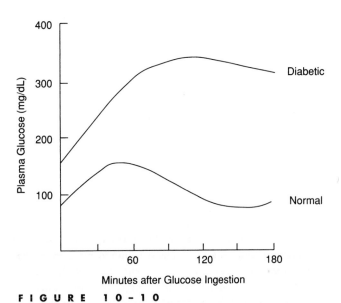

**F I G U R E   1 0 - 1 0**

Glucose tolerance curves for normal subject and a diabetic.

Although a normal OGTT excludes diabetes mellitus, abnormal OGTT values may occur in the absence of diabetes mellitus if the conditions described above are not carefully followed. Other factors, such as illness, trauma, stress, endocrinopathies, and certain drugs that induce hyperglycemia, may also impair glucose tolerance. The test can be useful, however, in the further evaluation of individuals with borderline fasting or postprandial plasma glucose levels and in the diagnosis of gestational diabetes mellitus and impaired glucose tolerance.

### Screening Test for Gestational Diabetes Mellitus

This test is designed to obviate doing a full 3-hour OGTT, which requires a 100-g glucose load and can cause nausea in many pregnant women. It should be performed between 24 and 28 weeks of gestation. The patient need not fast. One uses an oral glucose load of 50 g and collects a 1-hour sample. A plasma glucose of 140 mg/dL (7.8 mmol/L) or greater on the 1-hour sample mandates a complete 3-hour OGTT.[52]

### Intravenous Glucose Tolerance Test

An intravenous glucose tolerance test[53] may be performed on some patients rather than an oral glucose tolerance test because of poor absorption of orally administered glucose or the inability to tolerate the oral carbohydrate load.

A glucose dose of 0.5 g/kg body weight is administered intravenously and glucose levels are determined every 10 minutes for 1 hour. Insulin levels are also often requested with this test.

### Glycated Hemoglobin

Adult hemoglobin is composed mainly of hemoglobin (Hb) A, with a small amount of Hb $A_2$ (2.5%) and Hb F (0.5%). Hb A contains several minor hemoglobin components, identified as Hb $A_{1a}$, Hb $A_{1b}$, and Hb $A_{1c}$. These are modifications of Hb A and are collectively referred to as glycated hemoglobin, glycosylated hemoglobin, Hb $A_1$, "fast hemoglobin," and more recently, glycohemoglobin.[54]

Hb $A_{1c}$ is the major fraction (about 80%) of Hb $A_1$ and is the best defined. As is shown in Figure 10–11, HbA$_{1c}$ is formed by a nonenzymatic reaction, referred to as glycation, between glucose and the N-terminal valine amino acid of each beta chain of Hb A to form a labile Schiff base (pre-A$_{1c}$) with an aldimine structure. As the red cell circulates, some of the aldimine undergoes a slow, irreversible Amadori rearrangement to yield a stable ketoamine (Hb $A_{1c}$).

This reaction is continuous over the 120-day life span of the red blood cell and is proportional to the concentration of glucose in the blood. Diabetic patients thus have a higher proportion of Hb $A_{1c}$ than do normal individuals. Because the measurement of glycated hemoglobin provides an index of the patient's average blood glucose over a 2-month period, the test is useful in determining compliance with therapy and the extent to which satisfactory diabetic control has been achieved.

There are a variety of methods currently available for the measurement of glycated hemoglobin and the validity of this measurement depends in part on the method used. Neverthe-

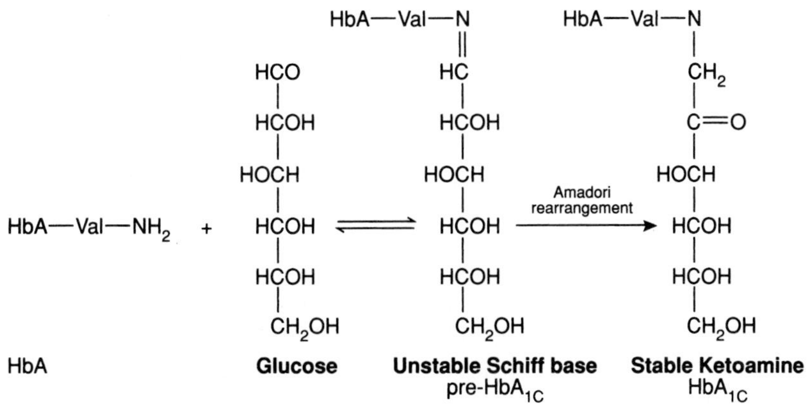

**FIGURE  10-11**

Formation of glycated hemoglobin.

less, measurement of glycated hemoglobin has become an important strategy for assessing glycemia. It is more convenient than the OGTT because it requires only one blood sample and no patient preparation. In addition, it measures glycemic control under real-life conditions.[49] It has been shown that regular measurements of Hb $A_{1c}$ lead to changes in diabetes treatment and improvement of metabolic control as indicated by a lowering of Hb $A_{1c}$ values.[55] It is recommended that the laboratory report the results of their test standardized to the Hb $A_{1c}$ assay results when using assays that measure total glycohemoglobin.[56] This helps the physician interpret the results. The desired therapeutically achieved results are ≤7% Hb $A_{1c}$.[57]

### Fructosamine

Other serum proteins in addition to hemoglobin can bind glucose in the glycation reaction to form ketoamine linkages. The term **fructosamine** refers to the ketoamine linkage between glucose and protein and is used most often as an expression for the sum of all glucose-protein ketoamine linkages in the sample. Fructosamine is unrelated to fructose except that the resulting sugar chain resembles the configuration of fructose.[58]

Since all serum proteins can be glycated and albumin is the most abundant protein in serum, measurement of fructosamine is largely a measurement of glycated albumin. Fructosamine is thus a measure of glycemic control during the 3-week period prior to sampling, since the half-life of albumin is 2 to 3 weeks.

Measurement of fructosamine is easier than that of glycated hemoglobin because it is a simple colorimetric procedure based on the ability of fructosamine linkages to reduce the dye nitroblue tetrazolium. Fructosamine also responds more quickly to changes of glucose control than does glycated hemoglobin and is not affected by abnormal hemoglobins or rapid hemoglobin turnover. There are still controversies, however, concerning whether the fructosamine assay has adequate specificity and how the test should be implemented.[58]

### Self-Monitoring of Blood Glucose

Improvements in diabetic control and insulin therapy have been achieved with self-monitoring of blood glucose by patients at home.[59] Testing glucose concentration in blood is preferred to testing in urine since the renal threshold must be exceeded before glucose appears in the urine. Many patients use insulin pumps rather than daily insulin injections; however, their use necessitates frequent monitoring of blood glucose. Home monitoring of blood glucose has thus become useful. It requires that a patient obtain a drop of his or her own capillary blood and be well trained in the proper use of the glucose monitoring system[60] but most prefer this to urine testing. If urine testing is preferred, self-monitoring should still be used at the time of expected insulin peak or after exercise to help detect and prevent hypoglycemia. Home monitoring blood glucose devices use capillary whole blood, whereas the laboratory instruments typically use either plasma or serum. The serum or plasma glucose values run about 12% higher than the capillary whole blood levels. Thus, when comparing results obtained by home monitoring (whole blood) with those obtained in the laboratory (plasma or serum), one should convert the whole blood results to those of plasma or serum (serum glucose mg/dL = 1.12 × whole blood glucose mg/dL) or vice versa (whole blood glucose mg/dL = 0.89 × serum glucose mg/dL).

### Urine Microalbumin Test

Diabetes mellitus can lead to renal complications with loss of albumin into the urine. In the early reversible stage of diabetic nephropathy, low concentrations of albumin are seen in the urine (**microalbuminuria**). This is treatable by better control of the patient's blood glucose levels and blood pressure. The 1997 ADA guidelines[4] recommend that patients be screened annually for microalbuminuria (30 to 300 mg/day) using one of the following tests: a random urinary albumin to creatinine ratio, a 24-hour urinary albumin concentration, a 4-hour urinary albumin concentration, or a first morning void urinary albumin concentration.

As renal disease progresses, proteinuria (≥550 mg/day) increases, which is detectable by standard urine dipstick tests.[61] Unfortunately, it is usually not reversible at this stage.

### Serum and Urine Ketone Tests

Patients with type 1 diabetes mellitus are frequently tested for serum and urine ketones. The presence and relative concentration of the ketones are indicators of the degree of ketoacidosis. The most frequently used tests employ nitroprusside with and without glycerin to detect acetoacetic acid and acetone or acetoacetic acid alone. In acute cases of ketoacidosis, the equilibrium between acetoacetic acid and beta-hydroxybutyric acid is shifted toward the latter, which is detected using an enzymatic test ($\beta$-hydroxybutyrate dehydrogenase).[62]

### Other Less Common Tests

Autoantibodies are frequently observed in type 1 diabetes mellitus and tests for them exist.[63] They are currently used to screen relatives of patients with type 1 diabetes to detect patients at high risk for developing this disease and to determine the cause of the disease in patients who have recently developed the disease. Insulin testing[64] is occasionally used to help discriminate between type 1 and 2 diabetes mellitus in patients who are progressing from the latter to the former. C-peptide[64] can be used to detect endogenous insulin production in patients being treated with exogenous insulin during the "honeymoon period" of type 1 diabetes. Glucagon, epinephrine, growth hormone, and cortisol can be tested to rule out these alternative sources of hyperglycemia.

## Hypoglycemia

Hypoglycemia is a syndrome characterized by low plasma glucose levels, usually less than 50 mg/dL (2.8 mmol/L), although not all investigators agree on the exact cutoff values. Merimee reported lower reference limits of 35 mg/dL (1.9 mmol/L) in healthy premenopausal women who had fasted for 24 hours.[65] It is possible to have an occasional low plasma glucose without symptoms or disease; knowledge of the clinical setting is necessary for accurate interpretation of a low plasma glucose value.

### CLASSIFICATION

The most common example of hypoglycemia is the diabetic patient who miscalculates insulin dosage. Hypoglycemia that occurs because of some stimulus is referred to as **reactive hypoglycemia.** It is caused by excessive administration of insulin or other hypoglycemic agents (**factitious hypoglycemia**) or by a reduction in gluconeogenesis as a result of ethanol ingestion. Reactive hypoglycemia may occur several hours after a meal (**postprandial hypoglycemia**) in individuals who have had gastrointestinal surgery or in mild diabetics. Relief is obtained by food intake.

Hypoglycemia can also occur as a response to fasting. This is referred to as **fasting** or **spontaneous hypoglycemia.** It is uncommon, but when it does occur, there is usually a serious underlying organic disease. Fasting hypoglycemia can be caused by excessive insulin secreted by insulin-producing pancreatic islet cell tumors (insulinomas), nonpancreatic tumors that produce substances with insulinlike activity, hepatic dysfunction, glucocorticoid deficiency, sepsis, or depleted glycogen stores.

Symptoms of hypoglycemia in adults can be divided into two groups depending on whether the fall in plasma glucose is rapid or gradual. A rapid fall in plasma glucose triggers the release of epinephrine and symptoms caused by epinephrine such as sweating, weakness, shakiness, trembling, nausea, hunger, rapid pulse, lightheadedness, and epigastric discomfort occur. These symptoms are referred to as adrenergic symptoms. They may occur even though the plasma glucose does not drop below the reference range.

A gradual fall in plasma glucose to levels less than 20 or 30 mg/dL (1.1 or 1.7 mmol/L) causes impairment of central nervous system function since the brain depends on an adequate supply of glucose for its energy. Symptoms, known as neuroglycopenia, include headache, confusion, lethargy, seizures, and unconsciousness. Irreversible brain damage or death may occur if the hypoglycemia and coma persist too long.

Infants are less sensitive to a decreased concentration of plasma glucose but values less than 30 mg/dL (1.7 mmol/L) in a term infant and less than 20 mg/dL (1.1 mmol/L) in a premature infant are generally accepted as abnormal. Some conditions causing hypoglycemia in neonates and children include maternal diabetes or eclampsia, prematurity, polycythemia, respiratory distress syndrome, glycogen storage disorders, gluconeogenic enzyme or counterregulatory hormone deficiencies, galactosemia, or hereditary fructose intolerance.

### LABORATORY DIAGNOSIS

### Plasma Glucose

Glucose levels below 50 mg/dL (2.8 mmol/L) are uncommon and should be investigated, especially if the individual is symptomatic. When diagnosing fasting hypoglycemia, samples for plasma glucose should be drawn frequently (every 4 hours) during the fast to anticipate a dangerously low value before it occurs. Most patients with fasting hypoglycemia have an abnormally low value within 12 hours of starting the fast. If no hypoglycemia is demonstrated after a 48-hour fast, fasting or spontaneous hypoglycemia is probably not indicated. If hypoglycemia is triggered by the ingestion of food, it is best to obtain a random plasma glucose at the time the patient has the symptoms. A normal glucose value strongly suggests that the symptoms are not related to hypoglycemia.[64]

### Five-Hour Glucose Tolerance Test

The five-hour glucose tolerance test (5-h GTT) has been the standard test to diagnose postprandial hypoglycemia but it is not an ideal test because it is insensitive and nonspecific.[66] As in the

OGTT, glucose is administered orally. Because symptoms of hypoglycemia are so transient, glucose specimens are obtained every 30 minutes for 5 hours or when the patient develops symptoms of hypoglycemia. Interpretation of the test is difficult because there is no clear-cut distinction between a normal and a hypoglycemic 5-h GTT. The observation of glucose levels of <50 mg/dL (2.8 mmol/L) associated with hypoglycemic symptoms may suggest postprandial hypoglycemia; however, the test is not highly reproducible in any particular individual. The test is prolonged an additional 2 hours beyond the 3-hour OGTT used for the diagnosis of hyperglycemia to detect glucose levels that continue to drop below the fasting glucose level during the last 2 hours. This finding is known as the "hypoglycemia tail" but is not observed in all hypoglycemia patients.

### Insulin Levels

The radioimmunoassay for insulin is useful in the evaluation of excessive insulin production in fasting hypoglycemia. An elevated fasting plasma insulin level in the presence of a low plasma glucose suggests the presence of an insulin-producing pancreatic islet cell tumor. The ratio of insulin to glucose after an overnight or 72-hour fast is referred to as the **insulin/glucose ratio.** This ratio is normally less than 0.30 (insulin expressed as $\mu$U/mL, and glucose in mg/dL) and is important in defining inappropriate insulin secretion.[67]

### C-peptide

Like insulin levels, the C-peptide radioimmunoassay[62] is useful in diagnosis of insulinomas. C-peptide is the connecting peptide in proinsulin and its presence in plasma indicates endogenous insulin secretion such as would occur with an insulinoma. Since commercial insulin preparations have the C-peptide removed during purification, a high insulin level with a decreased or absent C-peptide level indicates that the hypoglycemia may be due to exogenous insulin administration.

The measurement of C-peptide is also useful in insulin-treated diabetic patients. These patients commonly develop anti-insulin antibodies that interfere with immunoassays for insulin. C-peptide measurements can therefore be used as an alternative to insulin assays to evaluate residual beta cell secretory function in these patients.

In addition, C-peptide levels rather than insulin levels are used to indicate the presence of residual pancreatic tissue in post-pancreatectomy patients who require exogenous insulin. When pancreatectomy is performed for removal of an insulinoma, increasing C-peptide levels suggest either recurrence of the tumor or the presence of functioning metastases.

### Insulin Tolerance Test

This test is used to evaluate patients with resistance to administered insulin or with certain other endocrine disorders.[64] A fasting glucose level is determined, insulin is injected intravenously, and glucose levels are determined at several intervals for 2 hours after the insulin is given. It is important to have a physician available to inject glucose intravenously if a hypoglycemic reaction should occur.

The normal response to insulin administered intravenously is a decrease in the plasma glucose level to about half of the fasting level within 30 minutes and then a return to normal by 90 to 120 minutes. If the patient is resistant to insulin, as in the case of adrenal cortical hyperfunction, acromegaly, and some cases of diabetes, there is only a slight or delayed decrease in plasma glucose in response to the insulin. If there is hypofunction of the anterior pituitary or adrenal cortex, as in the case of dwarfism or Addison's disease, the blood glucose level decreases normally in response to the insulin but the subsequent rise is delayed or does not occur at all. This test should be used discriminately in these types of patients because of the risk of severe and prolonged hypoglycemia. Glucose solutions or fruit juices should be given to the patient following completion of the test.

### Tolbutamide Tolerance Test

The tolbutamide tolerance test[64] is used to differentiate insulinomas from other hyperinsulinemic states. After a fasting glucose sample is collected, tolbutamide is injected intravenously and plasma glucose levels are measured at intervals for up to 2 hours. As with the insulin tolerance test, the patient must be observed for signs of severe hypoglycemia and the test terminated if necessary.

Tolbutamide (1-butyl-3-(p-tolylsulfonyl)urea) stimulates the pancreas to produce and secrete insulin. The normal response is therefore similar to that observed with the insulin tolerance test: a rapid fall in plasma glucose to about 50% of the fasting value followed by a return to normal in about 2 hours. In diabetic patients, the plasma glucose will not decrease to levels as low as those seen in normal individuals because the pancreas is unable to secrete adequate insulin. Patients with hypoglycemia caused by insulinomas show an exaggerated response to the tolbutamide and have persistent hypoglycemia for up to 3 hours.

## Inborn Errors of Carbohydrate Metabolism

### GLYCOGEN STORAGE DISEASES

Glycogen storage diseases include a group of inheritable disorders that result from a deficiency of one or more enzymes involved in the metabolism of glycogen. These genetic abnormalities may present themselves as disorders primarily of the liver, heart, or musculoskeletal system. There are 10 distinct types of glycogen storage diseases; however, some are extremely rare. The glycogen storage diseases, referred to by the Roman numerals I to X and in the case of some diseases by eponyms, are listed in Table 10–3. The enzyme deficiency causing each abnormality and the major clinical symptoms of each disease are also given.

Type I (von Gierke's) glycogen storage disease is one of the more common types of glycogen storage disease. Children

TABLE  10-3

**Glycogen Storage Diseases**

| TYPE | ENZYME DEFICIENCY | CLINICAL SYMPTOMS |
|---|---|---|
| I (von Gierke's) | Glucose-6-phosphatase | Severe hepatomegaly and hypoglycemia, lactic acidosis, hyperlipidemia, failure to thrive |
| II (Pompe's) | $\alpha$-1,4-glucosidase | Infant—cardiomegaly, muscle weakness, early death<br>Adult—muscle weakness |
| III (Cori's) | Amylo-1,6-glucosidase (debrancher) | Hepatomegaly, muscle weakness, hypoglycemia |
| IV (Anderson's) | $\alpha$-1,4-Glucan: $\alpha$-1,4-Glucan, 6-glucosyl-transferase (brancher) | Hepatomegaly, cirrhosis, failure to thrive, early death |
| V (McArdle's) | Muscle phosphorylase | Muscle cramps after exercise, myoglobinuria in half the patients |
| VI (Hers') | Hepatic phosphorylase | Hepatomegaly, mild clinical course |
| VII (Tauri's) | Muscle phosphofructokinase | Muscle cramps after exercise, myoglobinuria in some patients |
| VIII | Adenyl kinase | Spasticity, decerebration, high urinary catecholamine, death in infancy |
| IX | Hepatic phosphorylase b kinase | Hepatomegaly, increased liver glycogen concentrations |
| X | Cyclic AMP–dependent kinase | Hepatomegaly only |

with this disease have short stature and a huge abdomen because of massive enlargement of the liver. In addition to hepatomegaly and a general failure to thrive, the disease is characterized by severe hypoglycemia, increased plasma concentrations of lactic acid, and hyperlipidemia. These abnormalities are caused by a deficiency or absence of the enzyme glucose-6-phosphatase in the liver, the enzyme needed for the final step in the formation of glucose from hepatic glycogen. The major product of glycogenolysis in these patients is lactic acid rather than glucose. As would be anticipated with a deficiency of glucose-6-phosphatase activity, these patients have a much diminished rise in plasma glucose and a further increase in lactate concentration after administration of glucagon or epinephrine. This disease can be diagnosed by the intramuscular injection of 0.5 mg glucagon. In a normal individual, there should be a rise in plasma glucose with no change in lactate; a patient with type I glycogen storage disease shows no increase in glucose with an increase in lactate.[62]

The **epinephrine tolerance** test is also used to evaluate this form of glycogen storage disease.[68] Epinephrine is injected intramuscularly and glucose levels are measured at various intervals over a 2-hour period. Since epinephrine stimulates the breakdown of glycogen to glucose, the plasma glucose in a normal individual increases within 1 hour and then returns to the fasting level by 2 hours. A patient with type I glycogen storage disease shows little or no increase in the plasma glucose after administration of epinephrine. Definitive diagnosis of all glycogen storage diseases is based on enzyme assays from the appropriate tissue and by microscopic appearance of the affected tissues.

## GALACTOSEMIA

Galactosemia is a rare genetic disorder characterized by the inability to metabolize galactose because of a deficiency or absence of one of the three enzymes involved in the metabolism of galactose. These enzymes include galactokinase, galactose 1-phosphate uridyl transferase, and uridyl diphosphate glucose-4-epimerase. Classic galactosemia involves the transferase.

Because galactose is contained in milk as a constituent of lactose, classic galactosemia is diagnosed in infants. After ingestion of milk, they develop vomiting, diarrhea, cirrhosis of the liver, cataracts, and mental retardation. The infants fail to thrive and may die unless they receive artificial milk containing no lactose.

Diagnosis of galactosemia is made by identifying galactose in the urine or serum and confirmed by finding a deficiency of 1-phosphate uridyl transferase in the erythrocyte. Screening programs for galactosemia are based on measuring transferase activity in the red blood cells.[62]

## DISORDERS OF FRUCTOSE METABOLISM

Fructose may appear in the urine after eating fruits, honey, and syrups and has no clinical significance. Fructose is also seen in the urine in patients with disorders of fructose metabolism in which a specific enzyme necessary for the metabolism of fructose is lacking. There are three groups of disorders of fructose metabolism; all are transmitted as autosomal recessive traits.

Hereditary fructose intolerance is caused by a deficiency of fructose-1-phosphate aldolase, thus causing the accumulation of fructose-1-phosphate in cells. The ingestion of fruit or sucrose produces vomiting, hypoglycemia, hepatomegaly, and failure to thrive. Laboratory diagnosis is made by finding fructose in the urine and by decreased plasma glucose and phosphate levels after administration of an oral or intravenous fructose tolerance test.

Fructose-1,6-diphosphatase deficiency results from a genetically inherited lack of fructose-1,6-diphosphatase, an enzyme necessary in the formation of glucose from pyruvate. Infants with this rare disease have fasting hypoglycemia, lactic acidosis, hepatomegaly, and a poor prognosis.

Essential fructosuria is a benign condition caused by a deficiency of hepatic fructokinase. It is characterized by high fructose levels in serum and urine after ingestion of sucrose or fructose. It is important not to confuse this defect with diabetes mellitus. Measuring glucose by both a specific and nonspecific method to determine if the urinary sugar is glucose or fructose may be helpful.[62]

## MUCOPOLYSACCHARIDE STORAGE DISEASES

Mucopolysaccharides are structural components of cartilage, bone, skin, and other connective tissues. They consist of repeating disaccharide units that contain a hexosamine (usually acetylated), a uronic acid, and often a sulfate group attached to the hexosamine. They are degraded by lysosomal enzymes.

The mucopolysaccharide storage diseases, referred to as mucopolysaccharidoses, are hereditary disorders caused by a deficiency of one or more of these lysosomal enzymes. The mucopolysaccharides (glycosaminoglycans) accumulate in various tissues and are excreted in the urine. The three classes of mucopolysaccharides involved are dermatan sulfate, heparan sulfate, and keratan sulfate.

Hurler's syndrome is the prototype for all mucopolysaccharide storage diseases. It is a severe, progressive disorder characterized by corneal clouding and death, usually before the age of 10. Individuals with this disorder have coarse facies, skeletal abnormalities, developmental delay, and hepatosplenomegaly. Diagnostic laboratory tests include screening for urinary mucopolysaccharides, quantitative estimation of mucopolysaccharides in urine by measurement of hexuronic acid content, and electrophoretic identification of the mucopolysaccharide excretion pattern. Definitive diagnosis can be made by direct assay of the particular enzyme in leukocytes or cultured skin fibroblasts.[69]

## CEREBROSPINAL FLUID GLUCOSE

The concentration of glucose in cerebrospinal fluid (CSF) is about 60% to 75% of that in plasma, or 40 to 70 mg/dL (2.2 to 3.9 mmol/L). Glucose in CSF is in equilibrium with that in plasma; however, the concentration of CSF glucose is less because of its utilization by the central nervous system and because of facilitative transport across the epithelial membrane by a stereospecific carrier moiety. It takes approximately 2 to 3 hours for a change in plasma glucose concentration to oc-

cur in the CSF; this lag is probably related to the transport of glucose across the blood–CSF barrier.

Increased CSF glucose levels are not very useful and usually only confirm hyperglycemia. The CSF glucose concentration does not increase proportionally with increasing plasma glucose levels. With plasma glucose concentrations as high as 800 mg/dL (44.7 mmol/L) or more, the CSF glucose is only about 30% to 40% of plasma levels.

Decreased CSF glucose levels are useful in the diagnosis of bacterial, tuberculous or fungal meningitis, systemic hypoglycemia, and other diseases involving the central nervous system. In these cases, the CSF glucose is usually decreased to less than 40 mg/dL (2.2 mmol/L). This decrease may be due to (1) impaired transport of glucose from blood to CSF, (2) increased glucose utilization by the brain tissue, or (3) increased glucose utilization by bacteria, leukocytes, or neoplastic cells in the infected CSF. Because of the possible presence of bacteria or cells in CSF, it is important to analyze the specimen immediately or to preserve it with an antiglycolytic agent.[64]

A plasma glucose level should be obtained at the same time as a CSF glucose level to aid in the clinical interpretation of the CSF value. Both plasma and CSF glucose concentrations are determined by the same analytical methods.

## ANALYTICAL PROCEDURES

### Serum and Cerebrospinal Fluid Glucose

#### SPECIMEN

In the past, glucose analysis was usually performed on whole blood. Today, unhemolyzed serum or plasma is the specimen of choice. The use of whole blood measurements is again gaining importance, however, because whole blood specimens are used in home glucose monitoring devices. Glucose values in serum or plasma are about 10% to 15% higher than those in whole blood because of the difference in water content between the two specimen types. Glucose is evenly distributed between the cell and plasma water but whole blood with a normal hematocrit contains only about 80% as much water as does the same volume of plasma.

There are several advantages to using serum or plasma over whole blood. First, serum or plasma is more suitable for automated methods. Also, the hematocrit does not interfere with serum or plasma glucose, but an increased hematocrit will result in lower blood glucose levels because the aqueous content of the blood is decreased. Erythrocytes also contain nonglucose-reducing substances that could interfere with the measurement of glucose when using a reducing method. Finally, the use of serum or plasma eliminates the need for a preservative.

When whole blood is allowed to stand, the glucose is metabolized by erythrocytes, leukocytes, platelets, and any bacterial contaminants so that the concentration of glucose decreases at a mean rate of approximately 7% (5 to 10 mg/dL, 0.3 to 0.6 mmol/L) in 1 hour at room temperature.[70] This glycolysis can be inhibited by adding sodium fluoride to the specimen. Fluoride ions prevent glycolysis by inhibiting enolase and fructose-1,6-diphosphatase. They also inhibit coagulation by binding calcium but clotting may occur after several hours. For this reason, a combined fluoride-oxalate mixture is usually used. Iodoacetate may also be used as an antiglycolytic agent. It inhibits the glycolytic enzyme phosphoglyceraldehyde dehydrogenase. With these preservatives, glucose is stable in whole blood for 24 hours at room temperature. However, the preservatives may inhibit enzymatic reactions making the specimen unsuitable for analysis by some procedures such as a urease method for urea nitrogen.

When no preservative is used, serum or plasma must be separated from the cells within 1 hour after the blood is drawn. Once they are separated, the glucose concentration is stable up to 8 hours at 25°C and 72 hours at 4°C if the specimen is free of cells and bacterial contaminants.

Venous serum or plasma is preferred for glucose analysis. During fasting, the glucose concentration in capillary and arterial specimens is approximately 3 mg/dL (0.2 mmol/L) higher than in venous specimens. When samples were taken 15 to 90 minutes after carbohydrate loading, capillary samples averaged 32 mg/dL (1.8 mmol/L) higher than the corresponding venous sample.[71] For this reason, blood should always be collected from the same source during a glucose tolerance test. A sample should never be collected from a limb while the patient is receiving an intravenous (IV) infusion into that limb since the infusate will markedly change the results.

Since CSF specimens are often contaminated with bacteria or other cellular constituents, they should be analyzed for glucose without delay or preserved with an antiglycolytic agent.

## METHODS

The same analytical methods can be used to determine glucose concentration in serum and CSF. Methods for determination of glucose have been reviewed by Cooper[72] and, more recently, by Burrin and Price.[73] Ten methods have been evaluated and compared with the hexokinase reference method performed on a protein-free filtrate.[74]

Procedures commonly used can be classified as chemical or enzymatic. Enzymatic methods show increased specificity compared to chemical methods. Most chemical measurements are no longer used because of their lack of specificity and their cumbersomeness, but they are briefly discussed because of their historical interest.

Chemical methods are typically less expensive and today are used more frequently with urine specimens because they have a simpler matrix than serum specimens do. The following are the most commonly seen methods.

Older chemical methods were based on oxidation-reduction techniques. In hot, alkaline solution glucose reduces cupric ions ($Cu^{++}$) to cuprous ions ($Cu^+$). The enol form (Figure 10–12) of glucose is favored in alkaline solution and the double bond and negative charge present in the enol anion make glucose an active reducing substance. Since glucose, fructose, and mannose differ only in the second carbon atom, they all form the same enediol and are all measured by any method based on the reducing properties of glucose. Other nonsugar-reducing substances, such as uric acid, ascorbic acid, and creatinine, are also measured. Differences in specificity of the reducing methods depend on how effectively interfering substances are removed during deproteinization and on the nature of the color-producing reaction.

In the **Somogyi-Nelson** method, proteins are precipitated by barium hydroxide and zinc sulfate and the color reagent arsenomolybdate is reduced by the cuprous ion to form a blue molybdenum compound. It is the most specific of the oxidation-reduction methods because uric acid and some creatinine are precipitated with the protein. The **Folin-Wu** procedure employs a tungstic acid filtrate and a phosphomolybdate color reagent but lacks specificity because of the presence of nonglucose-reducing substances in the filtrate. The alkaline ferricyanide method, in which glucose reduces a yellow ferricyanide ion to a colorless ferrocyanide ion, was widely used when glu-

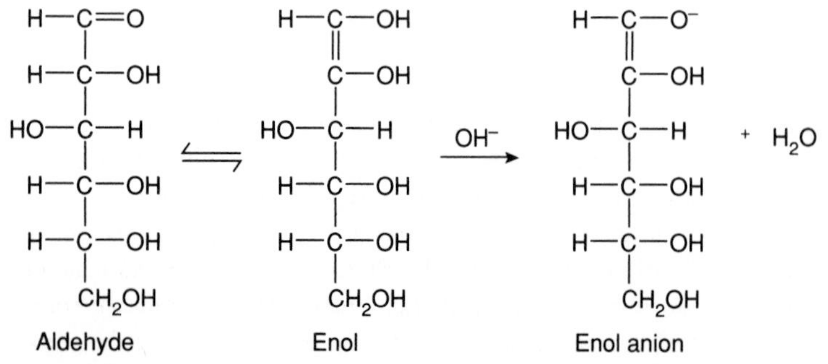

**FIGURE 10-12**

Aldehyde and enol forms of glucose.

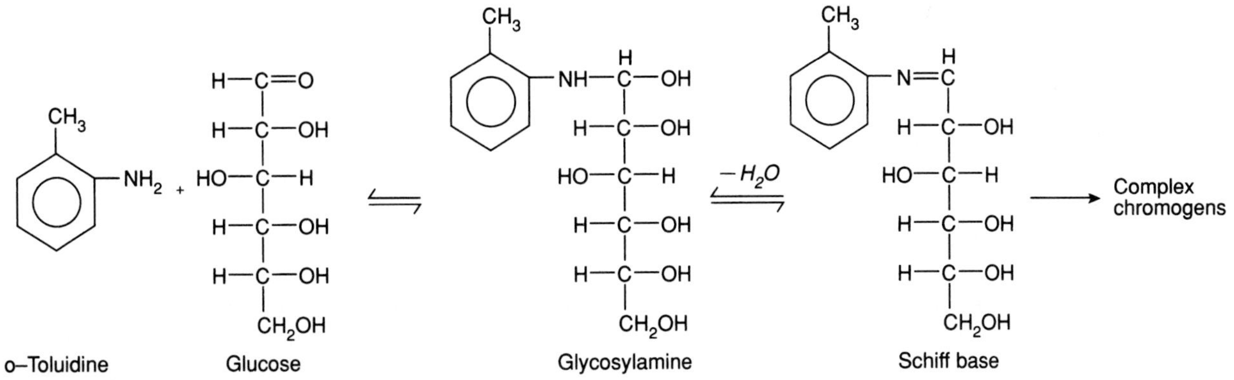

**FIGURE 10-13**

Reaction of glucose with o-toluidine.

cose determinations were performed on the Technicon Auto-Analyzer, but again, other reducing substances interfered.

The o-toluidine method is the most specific of the chemical methods; however, its use presents a health hazard because o-toluidine is now classified as a carcinogen. O-toluidine is an aromatic amine that condenses with the aldehyde group of aldohexoses such as glucose in hot acetic acid solution to form an equilibrium mixture of a glycosylamine and the corresponding Schiff base (Figure 10–13). Further rearrangements take place to produce a green chromogen whose absorbance is measured at 630 nm. O-toluidine reacts with other aldohexoses, such as galactose and mannose, but only galactose can occur naturally in serum (galactosemia). Pentoses, such as xylose, react with o-toluidine to form an orange color that absorbs at 480 nm.

The method may be used with or without protein precipitation. Moderate hemolysis does not interfere significantly with the method. Bilirubin gives falsely elevated values since it may be partially converted to the green pigment biliverdin. Turbidity in the final solution due to the presence of lipemia or the plasma expander Dextran in the specimen likewise causes falsely high results. Sodium fluoride and EDTA also contribute to the final color of the reaction. The major disadvantage of the method is the toxicity of its reagents.

Because the method is relatively specific for glucose, reference values are essentially the same as those listed below for the enzymatic methods. Somewhat higher values are obtained in patients with uremia.

The enzymatic methods use enzymes as reagents to increase the reaction specificity for glucose. They measure true glucose, not reducing compounds. They are the most widely used methods because they are simple and rapid to perform, are easily automated, use a small sample volume, and are highly specific. The two enzymatic systems used are hexokinase and glucose oxidase. The generally accepted reference method for glucose determination is based on the hexokinase system.[74]

The hexokinase system involves two coupled reactions:

$$Glucose + ATP \xrightarrow{HK, Mg^{++}} G\text{-}6\text{-}PO_4 + ADP$$

$$G\text{-}6\text{-}PO_4 + NADP^+ \xrightarrow{G\text{-}6\text{-}PD} 6\text{-}Phosphogluconate + NADPH + H^+$$

Hexokinase (HK) catalyzes the phosphorylation of glucose by adenosine triphosphate (ATP) to form glucose-6-phosphate (G-6-PO$_4$) and adenosine diphosphate (ADP). A second enzyme, glucose-6-phosphate dehydrogenase (G-6-PD), is used to catalyze the oxidation of glucose-6-phosphate by nicotinamide adenine dinucleotide phosphate (NADP$^+$) to form NADPH. The increase in absorbance of NADPH is measured at 340 nm and is directly proportional to the concentration of glucose in the sample. NADP$^+$ is required as the cofactor when the G-6-PD is derived from yeast; NAD$^+$ is used instead of NADP$^+$ when the source of G-6-PD is bacterial (*Leuconostoc mesenteroides*).

The Proposed Product Class Standard (1974) glucose reference method based on this principle uses a protein-free filtrate as the sample[74] but this is too time-consuming for use as a routine method. Serum or plasma can be used directly with a specimen blank to correct for interfering substances that absorb at 340 nm. To save time, many laboratories do not run a blank, thus obtaining slightly higher values than with the proposed reference method. Most methods using commercially prepared lyophilized reagents are adapted to discrete analyzer systems. Hexokinase and glucose-6-phosphate dehydrogenase can be co-immobilized on the inner surface of plastic tubing for use in certain continuous-flow automated systems.

The combined specificities of the enzymes hexokinase and glucose-6-phosphate dehydrogenase limit interference by other carbohydrates. Hexokinase phosphorylates mannose and fructose but these sugars are not present in sufficiently high concentrations in serum to interfere.

Hemolysis interferes with the hexokinase system because

red blood cell glucose-6-phosphate dehydrogenase and 6-phosphogluconate dehydrogenase use $NADP^+$ as a substrate. Most methods today use bacterial enzyme to reduce interference from hemolysis. Either serum or plasma may be used as a specimen. Sodium fluoride and anticoagulants such as heparin, EDTA, and oxalate do not interfere. Blank corrections, which are often omitted in this method, are high for grossly hemolyzed, icteric, or turbid specimens. The main disadvantage of the hexokinase system is the cost of the enzyme.

The hexokinase system can also be coupled to an indicator reaction using phenazine methosulfate (PMS) and an iodonitrotetrazolium salt (INT) so that absorbance may be measured in the visible range. The INT is reduced by NADPH to form a colored product with maximum absorbance at 520 nm.

The enzyme glucose oxidase catalyzes the oxidation of glucose to gluconic acid and hydrogen peroxide ($H_2O_2$):

$$\beta\text{-Glucose} + O_2 \xrightarrow{\text{Glucose oxidase}} \text{D-Glucono-}\delta\text{-lactone} \xrightarrow{H_2O, O_2}$$
$$\text{Gluconic acid} + H_2O_2$$

Glucose oxidase is highly specific for $\beta$-D-glucose. An aqueous solution of glucose contains about one third of $\alpha$-D-glucose and two thirds of $\beta$-D-glucose in equilibrium. For this reason, it is important that glucose standards used in the glucose oxidase method stand for at least 2 hours to reach an equilibrium mixture. As $\beta$-glucose is oxidized by glucose oxidase, $\alpha$-glucose is converted to the $\beta$ form by the law of mass action. Glucose oxidase preparations sometimes contain the enzyme mutarotase, which hastens this process. This precaution is not necessary for the hexokinase method. The glucose concentration is proportional to the $H_2O_2$ produced or to the oxygen consumed, both of which may be measured.

The $H_2O_2$ may be measured by coupling it with a peroxidase indicator reaction:

$$H_2O_2 + \text{Reduced chromogen} \xrightarrow{\text{Peroxidase}} \text{Oxidized chromogen} + H_2O$$

The enzyme peroxidase catalyzes the oxidation of a chromogenic oxygen acceptor, such as orthodianisidine, to form a colored product that can be measured photometrically. This reaction is less specific than the glucose oxidase reaction. Various reducing substances in serum, such as uric acid, ascorbic acid, bilirubin, and glutathione, inhibit the reaction by competing with the chromogen for $H_2O_2$, thus causing falsely low results. Other dyes such as 3-methyl-2-benzolinone hydrazone (MBTH) oxidatively coupled with N,N-dimethylaniline (DMA) (Gochman method) or 4-aminophenazone oxidatively coupled with phenol (Trinder method) are subject to less interference by high concentrations of creatinine, uric acid, or hemoglobin. Low results may be obtained if the glucose oxidase preparation contains catalase as a contaminant since catalase decomposes $H_2O_2$. The main advantage of the glucose oxidase method is its low cost.

The coupled glucose oxidase procedure has been adapted to a wide range of automated instruments including those that use dry chemistry reagents either in a strip or film form. The Vitrios 950 Chemistry System (Ortho-Clinical Diagnostics, a Johnson & Johnson Co., Raritan, NJ), formerly the Kodak Ektochem system, uses glucose oxidase layered on a dry multilayer film with an indicator system similar to that used in the Trinder method. The intensity of a colored end product dye is measured through a lower transparent film by reflectance spectrophotometry.[75]

Many home monitoring devices depend on the glucose oxidase-peroxidase chromogenic reaction. In these methods, a small surface of a test strip is impregnated with combined reagent in dry form. A drop of blood is placed on the reagent pad, washed or wiped off, and the strip is read on a reflectance colorimeter or compared with a colored chart.[76] Results with whole blood are approximately 10% less than results obtained on plasma or serum primarily because of the difference in water content between the two specimen types. Reliable results are obtained only when directions are followed precisely.

Interferences encountered in the peroxidase step of the glucose oxidase method can be eliminated by measuring the rate of **oxygen consumption.** Some instruments use a **polarographic oxygen electrode** that measures the rate of oxygen consumption after addition of sample to a solution containing glucose oxidase. The $H_2O_2$ generated is removed by reaction with ethanol or iodide to prevent the reversal of the reaction:

$$\beta\text{-Glucose} + O_2 \xrightarrow{\text{Glucose oxidase}} \text{D-Glucono-}\delta\text{-lactone}$$
$$\xrightarrow{H_2O, O_2} \text{Gluconic Acid} + H_2O_2$$

$$H_2O_2 + C_2H_5OH \xrightarrow{\text{Catalase}} CH_3CHO + 2\,H_2O$$
$$\text{Ethanol} \qquad\qquad \text{Acetaldehyde}$$

$$H_2O_2 + 2\,H^+ + 2\,I^- \xrightarrow{\text{Molybdate}} I_2 + 2\,H_2O$$

The latter two reactions are necessary to prevent formation of $O_2$ from $H_2O_2$ by catalase, which is present as a contaminant in some preparations of glucose oxidase. Whole blood should not be used since viable cells utilize oxygen. This method is precise, linear, free from interferences, and was found to correlate best with the Proposed Product Class Standard Hexokinase Method.[74]

The polarographic oxygen electrode method was originally available to the laboratory in a manual or semiautomated form as the Beckman Glucose Analyzer. It is now the basis of the automated CX instrument series (CX-3, CX-7, CX-9) from Beckman (Beckman Coulter Inc., Brea, CA).[77] A variation on this is the i-STAT Portable Clinical Analyzer (i-STAT Corporation, Princeton, NJ) which measures the $H_2O_2$ produced amperometrically.[78]

Reference ranges for fasting (10 to 16 hours) glucose, determined by specific enzymatic methods, are listed in Table 10–4.[79] There is no gender difference in the ranges and the normal adult ranges given are applicable to children after the first

TABLE 10 – 4

**Reference Ranges for Fasting Glucose**

| SPECIMEN | mg/dL | mmol/L |
|---|---|---|
| Serum or plasma | 70–105 | 3.9–5.8 |
| Whole blood | 65–95 | 3.6–5.3 |
| Full-term neonate | 30–60 | 1.7–3.3 |
| CSF | 40–70 | 2.2–3.9 |
| Urine–random | <30 | <1.7 |

few weeks of life. Fasting plasma glucose values increase about 2 mg/dL (0.1 mmol/L) per decade in an adult and as much as 8 to 13 mg/dL (0.4 to 0.7 mmol/L) per decade following a glucose challenge.

Cerebrospinal fluid glucose values are usually about 60% to 75% of plasma values and should be compared with plasma values for accurate clinical interpretation.

Methods for measuring glucose in urine are discussed below. The amount of glucose excreted in urine is often determined in a timed rather than a random specimen and is less than 0.5 g/d (27.8 mmol/d).

## Urine Glucose

Glucose appears in the urine in disease states such as diabetes mellitus. Other sugars may also appear in the urine in certain conditions. For example, galactose appears in the urine of infants with galactosemia.

### SPECIMEN

Urine should be analyzed for glucose promptly since urine frequently contains bacteria or other cellular constituents responsible for glycolysis. Glucose may be preserved in a 24-hour urine collection by adding glacial acetic acid or sodium benzoate to the container before starting the collection. Glucose is measured in the urine qualitatively (or semiquantitatively) and/or quantitatively.

### METHODS

Both chemical and enzymatic test formats exist for both the qualitative and quantitative methods.

For qualitative measurement, glucose is measured as a reducing substance in urine. The test is based on the Benedict's copper reduction reaction. Glucose and other reducing substances reduce cupric ions to cuprous ions with formation of yellow cuprous hydroxide or red cuprous oxide. A blue color of $Cu^{++}$ is negative for reducing substances. The Clinitest tablet (Ames Co., Elkhart, IN) is an adaptation of this procedure. This test is not specific for glucose since all reducing sugars (glucose, fructose, galactose, maltose, lactose, xylose, ribose, arabinose) react. Other reducing substances, such as ascorbic acid, uric acid, and creatinine, also contribute significantly to the to-

tal reducing substances present. Because the lower limit of glucose detection is 200 mg/dL (11.1 mmol/L), the qualitative measurement of glucose in a normal individual is negative.

Another qualitative measurement is based on strips impregnated with glucose oxidase, peroxidase, and a chromogen. The strips are dipped into urine and checked for color at the appropriate time. These dipsticks are more sensitive than the copper reduction tablets and are specific for glucose. False-negative results may be caused by ascorbic acid and urates that inhibit the reaction. False-positive results occur when urine is contaminated with hydrogen peroxide or a strong oxidizing agent such as hypochlorite (bleach). Clinistix (Ames Co., Elkhart, IN) is a widely used dipstick.

Quantitative measurement of glucose in urine can be made by the o-toluidine or hexokinase methods or by the glucose oxidase method that measures the rate of oxygen consumption in the same manner described for serum. Glucose oxidase procedures that use the hydrogen peroxide-peroxidase reaction cannot be used because of the high concentration of substances, especially uric acid, that interfere with the peroxidase reaction and produce falsely low results. The urine usually needs to be diluted with water before quantitation.

Identification of urinary reducing sugars can be made by paper chromatography or thin-layer chromatographic techniques. The sugars are separated by ascending or descending chromatography and located after color development with a reagent such as dinitrosalicylic acid, which is specific for reducing sugars.

Reference ranges for fasting (10 to 16 hours) glucose, determined by specific enzymatic methods, are listed in Table 10–4.[79] These vary slightly depending on the method used.

## Glycated Hemoglobin

The measurement of glycated hemoglobin complements more traditional measures of glucose testing in urine and serum by providing an index of the mean concentration of blood glucose over the preceding 2 months.

### SPECIMEN

Blood should be collected with EDTA, heparin, or fluoride as the anticoagulant. A hemolysate of saline-washed red cells is used for determination of glycated hemoglobin. Whole blood may be stored at 4°C for 1 week; hemolysate may be stored for 4 to 7 days at 4°C and up to 30 days at −70°C.

As discussed earlier, the formation of glycated hemoglobin is a two-stage process, with initial formation of a labile Schiff base, called pre-Hb $A_{1c}$, followed by slow formation of the stable ketoamine Hb $A_{1c}$. Since there is a rapid change in the concentration of the labile form of Hb $A_{1c}$ in response to changes in plasma glucose levels, the labile form should be removed for accurate analysis of Hb $A_{1c}$ or total Hb $A_1$. This may be accomplished by incubating erythrocytes in saline or in buffer solutions at pH 5 to 6.

## METHODS

The major assay methods for glycated hemoglobin can be divided into three major categories based on the manner in which glycated and nonglycated hemoglobin components are separated. They can be separated according to (1) differences in charge, (2) differences in chemical reactivity, and (3) differences in structure.[80]

The most commonly encountered clinical glycated hemoglobin methods based on charge differences are described below:

The ion-exchange chromatography method uses short columns filled with weakly acidic cation-exchange resin or negatively charged carboxymethyl cellulose resin. Hemolysate is applied to the column. Because glycated hemoglobin species, primarily Hb $A_{1a}$, $A_{1b}$, and $A_{1c}$, are less positively charged at neutral pH than is Hb A and bind less well to a negatively charged resin, they elute first. A second buffer may be used to elute the main hemoglobin fraction, Hb A. Absorbances of the two eluates are used to calculate percent of total glycated hemoglobin. Many commercial kits with prefilled disposable columns based on this principle are available. Most separate only Hb $A_1$ from Hb A but a few separate Hb $A_{1c}$ from Hb $A_{1a+b}$.

In all ion-exchange methods, it is important to control assay conditions such as temperature, pH, ionic strength, and column size. Labile pre-$A_{1c}$ elutes with the stable form of hemoglobin; therefore, pre-$A_{1c}$ must be removed before assay. Fetal hemoglobin (Hb F) also elutes with Hb $A_1$ and produces falsely elevated results. The presence of other hemoglobinopathies, such as Hb C or Hb S, results in falsely low test values since these hemoglobins and their glycated derivatives do not elute, causing the relative concentration of Hb A to be decreased.

High performance liquid chromatography (HPLC) is a form of ion-exchange chromatography but has additional resolution to separate Hb $A_{1c}$. Hemolysate is injected onto a small glass column filled with cation-exchange resin. A buffer is pumped through the column to elute Hb $A_{1c}$ and the various other minor hemoglobin fractions. After their elution, a second buffer of lower pH and higher sodium concentration is pumped through the column to elute Hb A. The absorbance of the column is monitored continuously.

HPLC is the most generally accepted reference method. HPLC shows excellent assay precision and permits rapid separation of Hb $A_{1c}$ from the other minor hemoglobin components and from Hb A; however, it requires meticulous laboratory technique and expensive equipment. As with other ion-exchange methods, temperature, pH, ionic strength, and column size must be controlled. Labile pre-$A_{1c}$ must be removed before assay and hemoglobin variants may interfere, as in ion-exchange chromatography.

HPLC systems dedicated to the measurement of Hb $A_{1c}$ have been marketed. The Diamat HPLC System (Bio-Rad, Hercules, CA) is a microprocessor-controlled step-gradient HPLC technique that is capable of separating hemoglobins F, S and C, along with other hemoglobin variants, from glycated hemoglobin.[81]

In the electrophoresis method, hemolysate is applied to an agar gel support medium and an electrical potential is applied across the support. The hemoglobin components are separated according to their charge differences: the minor hemoglobin fractions migrate further than Hb A, thus they are referred to as fast hemoglobin. Hb F and labile intermediates migrate to the same region as Hb $A_1$ and cause falsely elevated results. Hemoglobins S and C and their glycated components are resolved and do not interfere. Minor variations in pH, ionic strength, and temperature do not significantly affect the results. Quantitation can be accomplished by scanning the gel with a densitometer.

Isoelectric focusing in polyacrylamide gels is a special type of electrophoresis that separates hemoglobins according to their isoelectric points. Ampholines are used to establish a specific pH gradient on the gel. Hemolysate is applied to the gel and each hemoglobin component separates as a single band at its specific isoelectric point. Hb $A_{1c}$ is resolved from hemoglobins $A_{1a}$, $A_{1b}$, S, C, and F but pre-$A_{1c}$ does interfere.

The most commonly encountered clinical glycated hemoglobin method based on chemical reactivity is described below:

Colorimetric methods are based on the release and quantitation of the bound sugar moieties rather than on the separation and quantitation of the glycated hemoglobins. The most widely used colorimetric method is the hydroxymethylfurfural (HMF)/thiobarbituric acid method. Sugar attached to hemoglobin is converted to 5-HMF during treatment with heat and oxalic acid and is quantitated by its color reaction with thiobarbituric acid at 443 nm. This method is specific for ketoamine-linked glucose; therefore, labile Hb pre-$A_{1c}$, Hb F, and other hemoglobin variants do not interfere. Free glucose, however, interferes and must be removed by dialysis.

The most commonly used clinical glycated hemoglobin method is described below:

The affinity chromatography technique separates large molecules on the basis of their chemical structure. The affinity gel column consists of an insoluble, inert cellulose or agarose matrix covalently bound to a ligand, usually *m*-aminophenylboronic acid. When a blood hemolysate passes through the column, boronic acid reacts with the *cis*-diol groups of glycated hemoglobin to form a reversible 5-membered ring complex that is selectively bound to the column. Nonglycated hemoglobin, as well as pre-Hb $A_{1c}$, is not bound to the column and is eluted first by addition of a buffer. A second buffer, usually sorbitol, dissociates the bound fraction permitting elution of glycated hemoglobin. The absorbance of hemoglobin in both tubes is measured at 415 nm. Glycated hemoglobin is calculated as a percent of the total hemoglobin.

The main advantage of affinity chromatography is the lack of interference from nonglycated hemoglobins, hemoglobin variants, and labile Schiff base intermediates. The method is not as sensitive to temperature or pH fluctuations as ion-

## TABLE 10–5

### Reference Ranges for Glycated Hemoglobins

| SUBFRACTION | RANGE, % |
|---|---|
| HbA$_1$ | 5.0–8.0 |
| HbA$_{1c}$ | 3.0–6.0 |

exchange chromatography. Values tend to be higher by affinity chromatography than by methods based on charge differences because the affinity method can determine glycated hemoglobins that are not charge-modified. Kits containing prepacked columns and the appropriate buffers are available from several manufacturers.

Glycated hemoglobin values are usually expressed as a percentage of total blood hemoglobin. Reference ranges vary with the type of procedure used, the subfractions measured (Hb A$_1$ or Hb A$_{1c}$) and whether the labile fraction is included in the assay. The suggested reference ranges are listed in Table 10–5.[79]

## Ketones

Ketone bodies consist of acetoacetic acid and its derivatives, $\beta$-hydroxybutyric acid and acetone. They are present in blood in the relative proportions of 78% $\beta$-hydroxybutyric acid, 20% acetoacetic acid, and 2% acetone. Excessive formation of ketone bodies results in increased concentrations in the blood (ketonemia) and their excretion in the urine (ketonuria). This happens in persons on starvation diets or in uncontrolled diabetes mellitus.

### SPECIMEN

The specimen can be either fresh serum or urine. Collection vessels should be tightly stoppered and samples should be assayed within 1 hour or refrigerated. If refrigerated, the specimen should come to room temperature before being assayed. No centrifuge or preservative should be used with the sample. Some drugs may cause false positives and therefore should be mentioned on the accompanying slips.

### METHODS

None of the methods used for the determination of ketone bodies in serum or urine reacts with all three ketone bodies. Tests employing **nitroprusside** are the most frequently used semiquantitative measurements of ketone bodies in serum and urine. In this reaction, acetoacetic acid and acetone form a purple color with nitroprusside under alkaline conditions. The test is 15 to 20 times more sensitive for acetoacetic acid than for acetone and does not react with $\beta$-hydroxybutyric acid. Ames (Ames Co., Elkhart, IN) markets this assay in the form of a tablet (Acetest) or a reagent strip (Ketostix). Fresh urine, serum, or plasma, free of visible hemolysis, should be used.

Acetoacetic acid and $\beta$-hydroxybutyric acid can be quantitated in serum by a more specific **enzyme assay** catalyzed by $\beta$-hydroxybutyrate dehydrogenase ($\beta$-HBD):

$$NADH + H^+ + Acetoacetate \xrightleftharpoons{\beta\text{-HBD}} \beta\text{-Hydroxybutyrate} + NAD^+$$

When the reaction is performed at pH 7.0, the reaction proceeds to the right and the concentration of acetoacetic acid present is determined by measuring the decrease in absorbance at 340 nm as NADH is oxidized to $NAD^+$. At pH 8.5 to 9.5, the reaction proceeds to the left and the concentration of $\beta$-hydroxybutyric acid is proportional to the increase in absorbance at 340 nm as $NAD^+$ is reduced to NADH.

Reference ranges for acetoacetic acid and $\beta$-hydroxybutyric acid are less than 3mg/dL (0.3 mmol/L).[79] At these levels, serum and urine will be negative by the nitroprusside semiquantitative screening tests.

## SUMMARY

Carbohydrates are aldehydes or ketones with two or more hydroxyl groups. They are classified as monosaccharides (one aldehyde or ketone group), oligosaccharides (a few monosaccharides bound to each other), or polysaccharides (many monosaccharides linked together). The most abundant and important monosaccharide in nature is the 6-carbon sugar D-glucose.

D-glucose is the principal and almost exclusive carbohydrate circulating in the blood. Blood glucose is derived from the hydrolysis of dietary starch, from the conversion of other dietary hexoses into glucose by the liver, and from the synthesis of glucose from amino acids, fatty acids, or lactate. Glucose serves as the principal fuel for peripheral tissues except during prolonged fasting. The blood glucose concentration is closely maintained by metabolic processes and hormonal control.

Disorders of carbohydrate metabolism may result in blood glucose concentrations that are increased (hyperglycemia) or decreased (hypoglycemia). Diabetes mellitus, the most common and serious cause of hyperglycemia, is produced by an insufficiency of insulin and an excess of glucagon relative to the needs of the patient.

The detection, identification, and quantitation of glucose in serum and urine are vital in the diagnosis of diabetes and in the management of the diabetic patient. Analytical procedures most frequently used for the determination of glucose are the enzymatic glucose oxidase and hexokinase methods because they are specific for glucose. The oral glucose tolerance test is used to confirm the diagnosis of diabetes mellitus or to detect gestational diabetes in pregnant women. Glycated hemoglobin, a conjugate formed by the nonenzymatic addition of glucose to terminal amino groups, is a valuable indicator of the blood glucose level over a period of 2 months and is therefore useful in the management of the diabetic patient.

## REFERENCES

1. Genuth SM: Plasma insulin and glucose profiles in normal, obese and diabetic persons. Ann Intern Med 79: 812, 1973.
2. Rinderknecht E, Humbel RE: The amino acid sequence of human insulin-like growth factor I and its structural homology with proinsulin. J Biol Chem 253:2769, 1978.
3. National Diabetes Data Group: Classification and diagnosis of diabetes mellitus and other categories of glucose intolerance. Diabetes 28:1039, 1979.
4. American Diabetes Association: Report of the expert committee on the diagnosis and classification of diabetes mellitus. Diabetes Care 20:1183, 1997.
5. American Diabetes Association: Clinical Practice Recommendations 1998. Diabetes Care 21(Suppl 1):1, 1998.
6. American Diabetes Association: Clinical Practice Recommendations 2000. Diabetes Care 23(Suppl 1):1, 2000.
7. Cantor AB, Krischer JP, Cuthbertson DD, et al.: Age and family relationship accentuate the risk of IDDM in relatives of patients with insulin dependent diabetes. J Clin Endocrinol Metab 80:3739, 1995.
8. Huang W, Connor E, DelaRosa T, et al.: Although DR3-DQB1 may be associated with multiple component diseases of the autoimmune polyglandular syndromes, the human leukocyte antigen DR4-DQB1I0302 haplotype is implicated only in beta cell autoimmunity. J Clin Endocrinol Metab 81:1, 1996.
9. Schott M, Schatz D, Atkinson M, et al.: Antibodies to GAD and tryptic fragments of islet 64K antigen as distinct markers for development of IDDM: Studies with identical twins. Diabetes 41:782, 1992.
10. Myers MA, Rabin DU, Rowley MJ: Pancreatic islet cell cytoplasmic antibody in diabetes is represented by antibodies to islet cell antigen 512 and glutamic acid decarboxylase. Diabetes 44:1290, 1995.
11. Lan MS, Wasserfall C, Maclaren NK, et al.: IA-2, a transmembrane protein of the protein tyrosine phosphatase family, is a major autoantigen in insulin-dependent diabetes mellitus. Proc Natl Acad Sci USA 93:6367, 1996.
12. Lu J, Li Q, Xie H, et al.: Identification of a second transmembrane protein tyrosine phosphatase, IA-2B, as an autoantigen in insulin-dependent diabetes mellitus: precursor of the 37-kDa tryptic fragment. Proc Natl Acad Sci USA 93:2307, 1996.
13. Banerji M, Lebovitz H: Insulin sensitive and insulin resistant variants in IDDM. Diabetes 38:784, 1989.
14. Olefsky JM, Kolterman OG, Scarlett JA: Insulin action and resistance in obesity and noninsulin-dependent type II diabetes mellitus. Am J Physiol 243:E15, 1982.
15. Yagui K, Yamaguchi T, Kanatsuka A, et al.: Formation of islet amyloid fibrils in beta-secretory granules of transgenic mice expressing human islet amyloid polypeptide/amylin. Eur J Endocrinol 132:487, 1995.
16. Anderson DKG, Svaardsudd K: Long term glycemic control relates to mortality in type II diabetes. Diabetes Care 18:1534, 1995.
17. Wing RR, Blair EH, Bononi P, et al.: Caloric restriction per se is a significant factor in improvements in glycemic control and insulin sensitivity during weight loss in obese NIDDM patients. Diabetes Care 17:30, 1994.
18. Herman WH, Fajans SS, Oritz FJ, et al.: Abnormal insulin secretion, not insulin resistance is the genentic or primary defect of MODY in the RW pedigree. Diabetes 43:40, 1994.
19. Kadowaki T, Kadowaki H, Mori Y, et al.: A subtype of diabetes mellitus associated with a mutation of mitochondrial DNA. N Engl J Med 330:962, 1994.
20. Gruppuso PA, Gorden P, Kahn CR, et al.: Familial hyperproinsulinemia due to a proposed defect in conversion of proinsulin to insulin. N Engl J Med 311:629, 1984.
21. Given BD, Mako ME, Tager HS, et al.: Diabetes due to secretion of an abnormal insulin. N Engl J Med 302:129, 1980.
22. Kahn CR, Flier JS, Bar RS, et al.: The syndromes of insulin resistance and acanthosis nigricans. N Engl J Med 294:739, 1976.
23. Taylor SI: Lilly lecture: Molecular mechanisms of insulin resistance: Lessons from patients with mutations in the insulin-receptor gene. Diabetes 41:1473, 1992.
24. Jones DR, Varela-Nieto I: The role of glycosylphosphatidylinositol in signal transduction. Intl J Biochem Cell Biol 30:313, 1998.
25. Larsen S, Hilsted J, Tronier B, et al.: Metabolic control and B cell function in patients with insulin-dependent diabetes mellitus secondary to chronic pancreatitis. Metabolism 36:964, 1987.
26. Cerosimo E, Pister PWT, Pesola G, et al.: Insulin secretion and action in patients with pancreatic cancer. Cancer 67:486, 1991.
27. Handwerger S, Roth J, Gorden P, et al.: Glucose intolerance in cystic fibrosis. N Engl J Med 281:451, 1969.
28. Phelps G, Chapman I, Hall P, et al.: Prevalence of genetic haemochromatosis among diabetic patients. Lancet 2:233, 1989.
29. Yajnik CS, Shelgikar KM, Naik SS, et al.: The ketoacidosis-resistance in fibro-calculous pancreatic diabetes. Diabetes Res Clin Pract 15:149, 1992.
30. Soffer LJ, Iannaccone A, Gabrilove JL: Cushing's syndrome. Am J Med 30:129, 1961.
31. Jadresic A, Banks LM, Child DF, et al.: The acromegaly syndrome. Q J Med 202:189, 1982.
32. Stenstrom G, Ernest I, Tisell L: Long-term results in 64 patients operated upon for pheochromocytoma. Acta Med Scan 223:345, 1988.
33. Berelowitz M, Eugene HG: Non-insulin dependent diabetes mellitus secondary to other endocrine disorders.

In LeRoith D, Taylor SI, Olefsky JM (eds.): Diabetes Mellitus. New York, Lippincott-Raven, 1996, p. 496.

34. Conn JW: Hypertension, the potassium ion and impaired carbohydrate tolerance. N Engl J Med 273:1135, 1965.

35. O'Byrne S, Feely J: Effects of drugs on glucose tolerance in non-insulin dependent diabetes (parts I and II). Drugs 40:203, 1990.

36. Eposti MD, Ngo A, Myers MA: Inhibition of mitochondrial complex I may account for IDDM induced by intoxication with rodenticide Vacor. Diabetes 45:1531, 1996.

37. Pak CY, Eun H, McArthur RG, et al.: Association of cytomegalovirus infection with autoimmune type 1 diabetes. Lancet 2:1, 1988.

38. Forrest JA, Menser MA, Burgess JA: High frequency of diabetes mellitus in young patients with congenital rubella. Lancet 2:332, 1971.

39. Karjalainen J, Knip M, Hyoty H, et al.: Relationship between serum insulin antibodies, islet cell antibodies, Coxsackie-B4, and mumps virus-specific antibodies and the clinical manifestation of type I (insulin-dependent) diabetes. Diabetologia 31:146, 1988.

40. Solimena M, Folli B, Aparisi R, et al.: Autoantibodies to GABA-nergic neurons and pancreatic beta cells in stiff-man syndrome. N Engl J Med 41:347, 1992.

41. Rimoin DL: Genetic syndromes associated with glucose intolerance. In *The Genetics of Diabetes Mellitus*. Berlin, Springer-Verlag, 1976.

42. Barrett TG, Bundy SE, Macleod AF: Neurodegeneration and diabetes: UK nationwide study of Wolfram (DID-MOAD) syndrome. Lancet 346:1458, 1995.

43. Metzger BE, Organizing Committee: Summary and recommendations of the Third International Workshop-Conference on Gestational Diabetes Mellitus. Diabetes 40:197, 1991.

44. Langer O, Rodriguez DA, Xenakis EMJ, et al.: Intensified versus conventional management of gestational diabetes. Am J Obstet Gynecol 170:1036, 1994.

45. Santiago JV: Overview of the complications of diabetes. In Ninth Annual Arnold O. Beckman Conference in Clinical Chemistry. Diabetes mellitus: from theory to therapy. Clin Chem 32 #10B:B48, 1986.

46. Hollander P: Approaches to the treatment of type I diabetes. Lab Med 21:522, 1990.

47. Vlassara H, Brownlee M, Cerami A: Nonenzymatic glycosylation: Role in the pathogenesis of diabetic complications. In Ninth Annual Arnold O. Beckman Conference in Clinical Chemistry. Diabetes mellitus: from theory to therapy. Clin Chem 32 #10B:B37, 1986.

48. The DCCT Research Group: Diabetes Control and Complications Trial (DCCT): Results of feasibility study. Diabetes Care 10:1, 1987.

49. Singer DE, Coley CM, Samet JH, Natlan DM: Tests of glycemia in diabetes mellitus. Ann Intern Med 110:125, 1989.

50. O'Sullivan JB: Age gradient in blood glucose levels. Diabetes 23:713, 1974.

51. Klimt CR, Prout TE, Bradley RF, et al., Committee on Statistics, American Diabetes Association: Standardization of the oral glucose tolerance test. Diabetes 18:299, 1969.

52. Coustan DR: Screening and diagnosis of gestational diabetes. Semin Perinatol 18:407, 1994.

53. Elahi D, Andersen DK, Tobin JD, et al.: Discrepant performance on oral and intravenous glucose tolerance tests: The role of gastric inhibitory polypeptide. J Clin Endocrinol Metab 52:1199, 1981.

54. IUPAC-IUB Joint Commission on Biochemical Nomenclature (JCBN). Nomenclature of glycoproteins, glycopeptides and peptidoglycans (Recommendations 1985). Eur J Biochem 159:1, 1986.

55. Larsen ML, Horder M, Mogensen EF: Effect of long-term monitoring of glycated hemoglobin levels in insulin-dependent diabetes mellitus. N Engl J Med 323:1021, 1990.

56. Eckfeldt JH, Bruns DE: Another step towards standardization of methods for measuring hemoglobin $A_{1c}$. Clin Chem 43 #10:1811, 1997.

57. Peters AL, Davidson MB, Schriger DL, et al.: A clinical approach for the diagnosis of diabetes mellitus: an analysis using glycosylated hemoglobin levels. JAMA 276:1246, 1996.

58. Koch DD: Fructosamine: How useful is it? Lab Med 21:497, 1990.

59. Consensus statement on self-monitoring of blood glucose. Diabetes Care 10:95, 1987.

60. American Diabetes Association: Tests of glycemia in diabetes. Diabetes Care 21(Suppl 1):S69, 1998.

61. Stehouwer CDA, Donker AJM: Clinical usefulness of measurement of urinary albumin excretion in diabetes mellitus. Neth J Med 42:175, 1993.

62. Threatte GA, Henry JB: Carbohydrates. In Henry JB (ed.): *Clinical Diagnosis and Management by Laboratory Methods.* 19th ed. Philadelphia, W.B. Saunders, 1996, p. 194.

63. Levy-Marrhal C, Dubois F, Noel M, et al.: Immuno-genetic determinants and prediction of IDDM in French school children. Diabetes 44:1029, 1995.

64. Tietz NW: *Clinical Guide to Laboratory Tests.* 3rd ed. Philadelphia, W.B. Saunders, 1995.

65. Merimee TJ, Tyson JE: Stabilization of plasma glucose during fasting. N Engl J Med 291:1275, 1974.

66. Johnson DD, Dorr KE, Swenson SM, et al.: Reactive hypoglycemia. JAMA 243:1151, 1980.

67. Fajans SS, Floyd JC, Jr.: Fasting hypoglycemia in adults. N Engl J Med 294:766, 1976.

68. Caraway WT, Watts NB: Carbohydrates. In Tietz NW (ed.): *Textbook of Clinical Chemistry*. Philadelphia, W.B. Saunders, 1986, p. 814.

69. Hopwood JJ, Muller V, Smithson A, et al.: A fluorometric assay using 4-methylumbelliferyl alpha-L-iduronide

for the estimation of alpha-L-iduronidase activity and the detection of Hurler and Scheie syndromes. Clin Chem Acta 92: 257, 1979.

70. Weissman M, Klein B: Evaluation of glucose determinations in untreated serum samples. Clin Chem 4:420, 1958.

71. Larsson-Conn U: Differences between capillary and venous blood glucose during oral glucose tolerance tests. Scan J Clin Lab Invest 36:805, 1976.

72. Cooper GR: Methods for determining the amount of glucose in blood. Crit Rev Clin Lab Sci 4:101, 1973.

73. Burrin JM, Price CP: Measurement of blood glucose. Ann Clin Biochem 22:327, 1985.

74. Passey RB, Gillum RL, Fuller JB, et al.: Evaluation and comparison of 10 glucose methods and the reference method recommended in the proposed product class standard (1974). Clin Chem 23:131, 1977.

75. Curme HG, Columbus RL, Dappen GM, et al.: Multi-layer film elements for clinical analysis: General concepts. Clin Chem 24:1335, 1978.

76. Symposium on home glucose self-monitoring. Diabetes Care 4:392, 1981.

77. Kadish AH, Little RA, Sternberg JC: A new and rapid method for the determination of glucose by measurement of rate of oxygen consumption. Clin Chem 14:116, 1968.

78. Spencer WW, Sylvester D, Nelson GH: Evaluation of a glucose method in which a hydrogen peroxide electrode is used. Clin Chem 24:386, 1978.

79. Caraway WT, Watts NB: Carbohydrates and Appendix 20, Table 25. In Tietz NW, (ed.): *Textbook of Clinical Chemistry.* Philadelphia, W.B. Saunders, 1986, pp. 796, 807, 1810–1850.

80. Goldstein DE, Little RR, Wiedmeyer H, et al.: Glycated hemoglobin: Methodologies and clinical applications. Clin Chem 32:B64, 1986.

81. Delahunty T: Convenient screening for hemoglobin variants by using the Diamat HPLC system. Clin Chem 36: 903, 1990.

# C H A P T E R  1 1
# Lipids

*Richard C. Mroz, Jr.*

The lipids are essential biologic molecules whose role in cell structure and metabolism are still under intensive investigation. The lipids display a great range of chemical variation and function but may be summarized in a few general statements.

Lipids are composed almost exclusively of carbon, hydrogen, and oxygen in a manner that precludes them from interacting with molecules of water to form solutions. Water-insoluble lipids are usually soluble in other organic solvents such as alcohols, acetone, benzene, chloroform, and similar solvents. The hydrophobic (water repelling) nature of the lipids is essential to function of cellular membranes.

Lipids are important in energy storage, providing more than twice the caloric energy in equivalent amounts of protein or carbohydrate. At the same time, lipids tend to be more compact since water of hydration is excluded from the storage form of these molecules.

In recent years the public awareness of the importance of dietary lipids and cholesterol has increased to such a point that numerous popular periodicals and books include quite detailed descriptions of the chemistry, physiology, and clinical significance of lipids, which are often confusing and disquieting to nonscientific readers.

The nature of lipids suggest a useful definition for them: **Lipids** are organic compounds that are actually or potentially esters of fatty acids, utilized by living organisms, and soluble in organic solvents but insoluble in water. In terms of human health and physiology there are four major functions of lipids:

- Critical structural components of biological membranes
- Provide readily available energy reserves
- Serve as essential vitamins and hormones
- Aid in solubilization of dietary lipids

Since good health depends not only on the avoidance of harmful substances but also on the proper functioning of our body cells, the harmful effects of hyperlipidemias seem to be at odds with the need for lipids to preserve function. The nature and function of lipids as a metabolic fuel, material for membrane construction, and as critical biochemicals for use in numerous pathways make them indispensable.

The exclusion of water due to differences in polarity mean that lipids tend to associate with each other. We find small groups of them congregating in micelle formation to facilitate their movement through the polar aqueous medium of our bodies. On a slightly larger scale, mixtures of lipids associate with proteins forming the various lipoproteins. Finally, large masses of lipids gather in specialized cells to comprise the adipose tissues that serve both for insulation from the highly variable external environment and as visceral and subcutaneous cushioning to protect our internal organs.

## CLASSIFICATION OF LIPIDS

Lipids may be classified by various characteristics, but there is no common system such as that seen in classifications of enzymes.

### Fatty Acids

There are two major functions of the fatty acids:

1. They are the components of more complex lipids found in membranes, hormones, and vitamins.
2. They store large amounts of energy, especially in the form of triglycerides.

**Fatty acids** have the general formula R—COOH, where R is a long chain (12 to 26 carbon atoms in length) hydrocarbon. The terminal carboxyl group is easily ionizable and is usually found in the form of $COO^-$ in body fluids, conferring a weak negative charge to fatty acids. Fatty acids are described by the number of carbon atoms in the "backbone" of the molecule. For example, a C18 fatty acid contains 18 carbon atoms. The numbering of the carbons begins with the carbon of the terminal carboxyl group.

The bonds between the carbon atoms are also used to characterize the fatty acid. If all the bonds between the carbons are single bonds, then the molecule is a **saturated fatty acid** (Figure 11–1). Fatty acids with a single double bond between any two carbons are called **monounsaturated fatty acids,** and those with two or more double bonds are known as **polyunsaturated fatty acids.**[1]

The positions and numbers of double bonds in fatty acids can be further designated by the number of sites of unsaturation. For example, stearic acid is an 18 carbon fatty acid with no unsaturation and is designated as C18:0. The presence of double bonds in a fatty acid is indicated by the symbol D and the number of the first carbon of the double bond, such as in oleic acid, which has a single double bond between carbons 9 and 10, is designated as C18:1D9. Multiple double bonds in

**Saturated Stearic Acid C18:0**
$CH_3(CH_2)_{16}COOH$
**Monounsaturated Oleic Acid C18:1D9**
$CH_3(CH_2)_7CH{=}CH(CH_2)_7COOH$
**Polyunsaturated Linoleic Acid C18:2D10,13**
$CH_3(CH_2)_4CH{=}CHCH_2CH{=}CHCH_2(CH_2)_7COOH$
**Polyunsaturated Linolenic Acid C18:3D9,12,15**
$CH_3CH_2CH{=}CHCH_2CH{=}CHCH_2CH{=}CH(CH_2)_7COOH$

FIGURE 11-1

Saturated and unsaturated fatty acids. All 4 fatty acids have 18 carbons, but the number and location of double bonds differentiate them.

polysaturated fatty acids would be indicated as shown in Figure 11–1.

## Glycerol Esters

**Triglycerides**, also known as triacylglycerols, are lipids that combine fatty acids to 3 carbon atoms of the glycerol backbone (Figure 11–2). A simple triglyceride contains three identical fatty acids whereas a mixed triglyceride contains different fatty acids. These compounds are the prevalent glycerol ester in plasma and tissue storage fat (95% triglycerides).

Triglycerides from animal sources tend to have fatty acid chains, which are shorter and saturated and tend to solidify at room temperatures. Those from plants tend to have longer chains, which are polyunsaturated and remain liquid (oils) even at refrigerator temperatures.

Mono and diglycerides are similar compounds generated during the emulsification and digestion of fatty acids from food. Monoglycerides contain a single fatty acid, whereas diglycerides contain two.

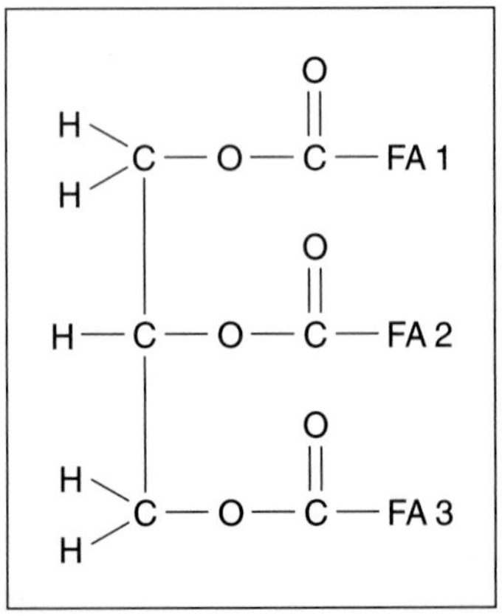


FIGURE 11-2

Triglyceride molecule. Three fatty acids are esterified to the 3 carbon glycerol backbone. This is the major form of fat absorbed in the intestinal tract.

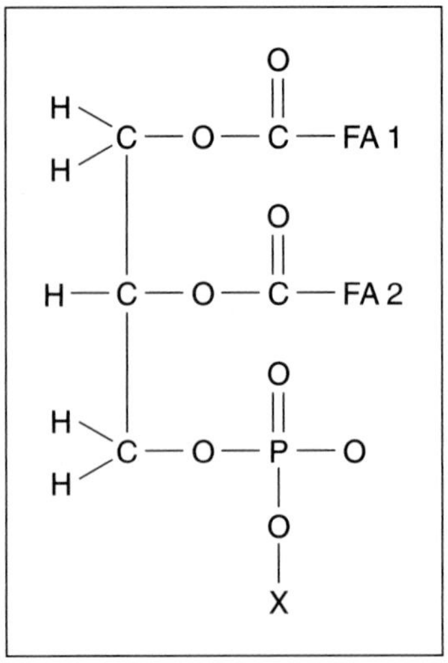


FIGURE 11-3

Basic Phosphoglycerides. FA1 and FA2 are fatty acids. When X is a hydrogen, the compound becomes phosphatidic acid. Phospholipids in which X is ethanolamine are called phosphatidylethanolamine; when substituted with serine they become phosphatidylserine; when substituted with inositol they become phosphatidylinositol. These 3 compounds are known collectively as the cephalins. When X is choline $[(CH_2)_2N(CH_3)_3]$ then the compound becomes a lecithin. Lecithins are important components of lipoproteins, cell membranes, as well as liver and brain. They are also essential for the production of lung surfactants.

**Phosphoglycerides** are glycerol esters that contain a phosphoric acid group on one of the end carbons of the glycerol backbone (Figure 11–3). Other groups may be attached to the phosphate portion to form various phosphoglycerides. Hence, a choline molecule attached to the phosphate group forms phosphatidylcholine **(lecithin).** Similarly, ethanolamine, serine, and inositol side groups comprise the **cephalins,** which are found primarily in the brain.[2] **Cardiolipins** tend to be even more complex. These have two phosphoglycerate portions attached to the glycerol backbone.

## Sphingolipids and Derivatives

Another alteration in the structure of the basic triglyceride results in **sphingosine** (Figure 11–4), an amino dialcohol, which serves as a precursor to other sphingolipids.[2] When sphingosine is combined with a C18 or a longer fatty acid at the amino group, a **ceramide** is formed. Ceramides are the basis of three important sphingolipids: sphingomyelin, galactosylceramide and glucosylceramide. These three lipids are of primary importance in the structure of the cell membranes and the central nervous system.

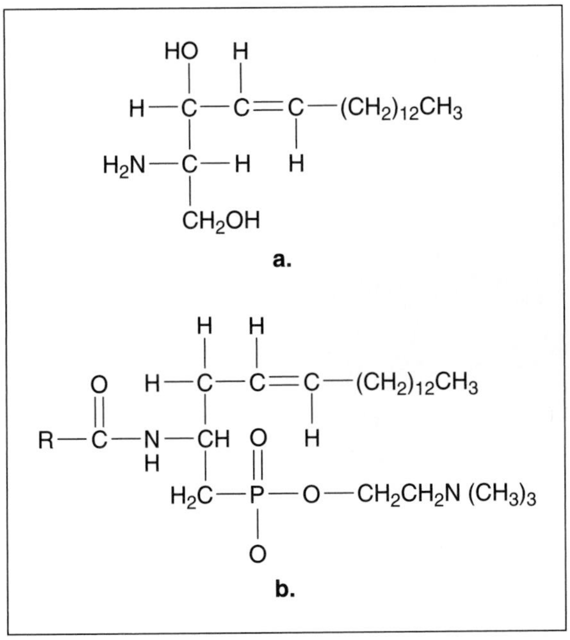

FIGURE  11-4

Sphingolipids **a.** Sphingosine, an amino alcohol, is
a precursor to the ceramides. **b.** Sphingomyelin is an
important ceramide in cell membranes and as a sheath
for nerves in both central and peripheral nervous
systems.

## Plasmalogens

**Plasmalogens** are glycerol ether phospholipids that resemble
the phospholipids with the major difference being that the fatty
acid at C1 of glycerol contains either an O-alkyl or O-alkenyl
ether species. There are three known types of plasmalogens:
choline, ethanolamine, and serine plasmalogens.[3] **Platelet activating factor (PAF)** is a choline plasmalogen, 1-alkyl, 2-acetyl

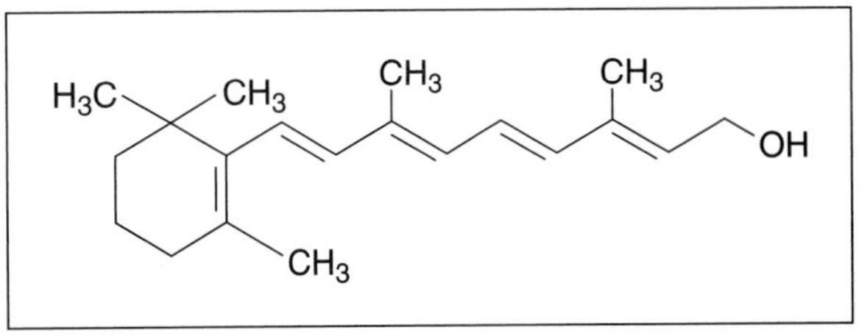

FIGURE  11-5

Retinol is one form of vitamin A and an example of
a terpene.

phosphatidylcholine, and is found in granulocytes, especially
basophils, as well as in mast cells and monocytes. PAF is a potent mediator of hypersensitivity and anaphylaxis and stimulates platelet aggregation.

## Terpenes

**Terpenes** are 5 carbon branched chain units (isoprenoids).
They are seen as intermediates in the metabolic production of
cholesterol. The fat-soluble vitamins A (Figure 11–5), E, and
K are classified as terpenes.[3]

## Sterol Compounds and Derivatives

Sterols are complex lipids derived from the tetracyclic solid alcohol known as **cholesterol** and closely related cholesterol esters. The cholesterol molecule is based on the sterane nucleus
known as perhydrocyclopentanophenanthrene (Figure 11–6a.).
Cholesterol (Figure 11–6b.) and its esters are the basis of the
bile acids, steroid hormones (Chapters 29 and 31), and vitamin D.

About 70% of total cholesterol in humans is found in the
form of esterified cholesterol.[4] Cholesterol esters are formed
when long chain fatty acids, transferred from triglycerides, bind

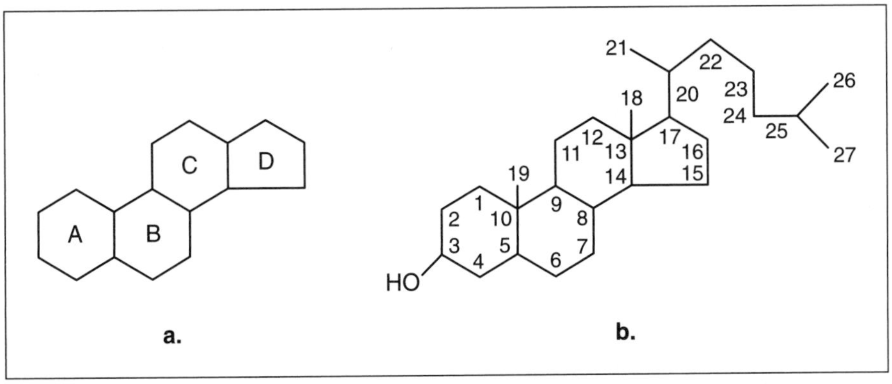

FIGURE  11-6

Sterol derivatives. **a.** Ring structure of perhydrocyclopentanophenanthrene.
**b**. Cholesterol molecule with common site of esterification, hydroxyl (—OH)
group at C3.

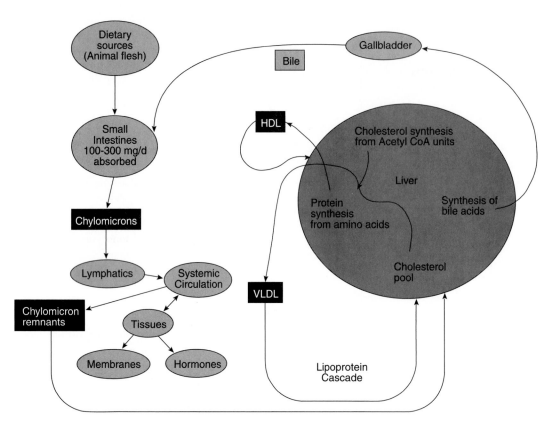

Metabolic pathways of cholesterol.

to the hydroxyl group located at C3. Esterification of the cholesterol molecule can occur both in cytoplasm and in plasma. The plasma reaction requires the enzyme **lecithin-cholesterol acyltransferase (LCAT),** and the intracellular reaction utilizes **acyl-cholesterol acyltransferase (ACAT).**[4] Other modifications of cholesterol, such as hydroxylation necessary for bile acid production or isomerization for steroid hormone metabolism, occur either at the double bond between C5 and C6 or at C7. Figure 11–7 presents a summary of the general metabolic pathways in which cholesterol takes part.

## METABOLISM OF LIPIDS

### Exogenous Lipids

Approximately 40% of the caloric intake of a typical American diet consists of lipids, about 35% from saturated animal lipids, and 5% polyunsaturated vegetable lipids. Triglycerides (fats) comprise a major portion (98% to 99%) of the animal lipids with the remainder being cholesterol and other lipids. Cholesterol from plant sources is called phytosterol. The phytosterols are poorly absorbed in the intestinal mucosa but the presence of phytosterols will compete with the uptake of the

animal cholesterols. This means that the more phytosterols consumed, the less dietary cholesterol from animal sources may be absorbed.[4]

In general, the incorporation of exogenous lipids occurs in 3 phases: (1) digestive, (2) absorption, and (3) transport. The **digestive phase** occurs inside the lumen of the intestines and involves altering the chemical nature of the lipids in a process known as **emulsification.** The gall bladder is critical to the digestive phase. Bile, composed of conjugated bile acids, lecithin and cholesterol, is released from the gall bladder into the small intestine through the bile duct. The highly **amphipathic** properties (strongly hydrophilic and hydrophobic at the same time) of the bile acids break up lipid globules into smaller units, called **micelles,** rendering them more vulnerable to the action of three digestive enzymes produced by the pancreas and secreted into the duodenum. **Lipase** acts on triglycerides to release free fatty acids forming monoglycerides, diglycerides, and glycerol; **cholesterol esterase** cleaves the ester linkages to release free fatty acids and free cholesterol and **phospholipase A** hydrolyzes the exogenous phospholipids.

During the **absorption phase,** the digested lipids diffuse into the intestinal mucosal cells, primarily in the form of mono- and diglycerides, free fatty acids (FFAs), and glycerol. Cholesterol and other lipids are also absorbed. Within the mucosal cells, the FFAs will bind to coenzyme A (acyl or acetyl

CoA) by the action of an enzyme known as **fatty acid CoA ligase.** This enzyme preferentially binds long chain FFAs to the CoA molecule, which then donates the fatty acids to reesterify glycerols and mono- and diglycerides. The resulting triglyceride molecules are packaged into micelles called **chylomicrons,** which also contain lipoproteins, cholesterol, and various phospholipids.[4]

In the **transport phase** the chylomicrons are moved to the mucosal cell membrane and released by a reverse pinocytosis mechanism. Short- and medium-chain FFAs are also released bound to albumin and transported in the portal circulation while chylomicrons are released into the thoracic duct of the lymphatic system eventually to enter the circulatory system.[4,5]

Figure 11–8 summarizes the metabolic fates for dietary lipids in the body. Please note that fatty acids are also used to produce essential phospholipids, to help maintain cell membranes, and to produce milk in the mammary glands of the female. Mixed into the complex picture are the essential fatty acids derived from vegetable sources, e.g., linoleic, linolenic, and arachidonic acids, which the body is unable to produce but requires for the synthesis of prostaglandins and leukotrienes.

## Endogenous Lipids

It is interesting to note that the human body produces most of its cholesterol endogenously. Dietary sources contribute a mere 150 to 300 mg daily, whereas the liver synthesizes 1.5 g per day. In fact, excess carbohydrates and proteins from the diet are used to produce CoA (coenzyme A) molecules, which then may be used to produce endogenous cholesterol and fatty acids.[2,3]

## Lipid Utilization and Storage

Chylomicrons are removed quickly from circulation by tissues cells, usually within 30 minutes of release. Cellular enzymes, most notably **lipoprotein lipase,** will hydrolyze the fatty acids from the triglycerides within the chylomicrons and release the chylomicron remnants, consisting mainly of cholesterol, phospholipids, and lipoproteins, back into circulation where hepatocytes will remove the remnants. Lipoprotein lipase is activated by the presence of **apolipoprotein CII,** which is present in the chylomicron.[5] The FFAs will be used by the cells for energy or end up stored for later use in adipose (fat) cells.

Regardless of the source of the lipids, the principal site of storage of these compounds is in the adipose tissues. Despite the vast amounts of energy stored in adipose tissues, the human body preferentially uses sugars and glycogen for energy needs. Only as these carbohydrates approach depletion does the body begin to utilize fats. Thus, with an average daily intake of 140 g of fat and constant amounts being excreted, fat accumulation occurs quite easily.

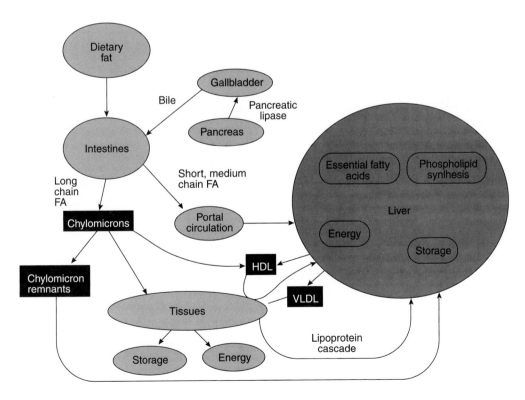

### FIGURE 11-8

The various fates of dietary fats and their utilization in metabolic pathways.

## LIPOPROTEINS

Lipids are, by their chemical nature, insoluble in water, which renders them unable to be transported in aqueous solutions such as plasma. The addition of a variety of proteins, called lipoproteins, enables the lipids to remain partially soluble in plasma and facilitates their transport and utilization. The lipoproteins, when separated from lipids, are known as **apolipoproteins** or **apoproteins**.

The basic properties of the five basic **lipoproteins**[4–7] are summarized in Table 11–1.

### Electrophoretic Mobility of the Lipoproteins

Lipoprotein electrophoresis (LPE) can be used to separate the various lipoproteins by differences in their net charges.[4] The method is very similar to protein electrophoresis but the fractions must be stained with a lipid stain such as Oil Red 7B rather than a protein stain such as Ponceau S. The lipoprotein bands are produced by differences in the migration rate of each lipoprotein. The bands are identified by comparison to the serum protein bands (Figure 11–9). **High-density lipoprotein** (HDL) is an alpha lipoprotein, **low-density lipoprotein** (LDL) is a beta lipoprotein, **very low-density lipoprotein** (VLDL) is a pre-beta lipoprotein, and **intermediate-density lipoprotein** (IDL) is found in the "floating beta" band located between beta and pre-beta, which in some instances blend together to form one broad beta band. Chylomicrons are found at or near the point of application.[4]

In current laboratory practice, LPE is used primarily in reference laboratories due to its relatively high cost in terms of technologist time. There are a variety of methods specific for individual lipoproteins, which can be run on automated instruments at considerable cost savings.

Lipoproteins are metabolized through a series of steps, beginning with the chylomicrons, into the five specific types of lipids described in Table 11–1.

### Chylomicrons

**Chylomicrons** represent the largest of the lipoprotein fractions. Because of a high triglyceride and low protein content, they also have the lowest density. This low density permits high concentrations of chylomicrons to "float" on top of the serum or plasma. This layer is observable in some lipemic serum specimens when allowed to stand at 4 to 6°C for 12 hours. Assembled in the intestinal epithelial cells, chylomicrons are released into the lymphatic system and eventually enter the systemic circulation via the thoracic duct and jugular vein.[4,5] Along the way, the chylomicrons, which are relatively poor in apolipoproteins, pick up molecules of apolipoprotein C-II and apo E through interactions with HDL particles. Apo C-II activates lipoprotein lipase which in turn catalyzes the hydrolysis of triglycerides in the chylomicrons. The chylomicrons then interact with tissues to provide them with monoglycerides, glycerol and free fatty acids.

After losing most of its triglyceride content, the chylomicron again interacts with HDL, this time yielding its apo AI, apo AII, apo C and some of its lipid content to become a

---

TABLE 11–1

### Summary of Lipoprotein Properties

| COMMON NAME | CHYLOMICRONS | VLDL | IDL | LDL | HDL |
|---|---|---|---|---|---|
| Electrophoretic mobility | None | Pre-beta | Beta | Beta | Alpha |
| Density (g/mL) | <.95 | 0.95–1.006 | 1.006–1.019 | 1.019–1.063 | 1.063–1.21 |
| Size (nm) | 80–500 | 40–80 | 24.5 | 20 | 7.5–12 |
| Protein content (%) See Table 11–3 | 2 | 8 | 15 | 21 | 50 |
| Phospholipid content (%) | 7 | 18 | 20 | 23 | 28 |
| Triglyceride content (%) | 82 | 52 | 20 | 9 | 3 |
| Cholesterol content (%) | 9 | 22 | 35 | 47 | 19 |
| Comments | Forms creamy top layer when serum left standing | Converted to LDL in the plasma | Transitional form between VLDL and LDL | Major transporter of cholesterol in the plasma | Major transporter of cholesterol from the cells to the liver Two different forms. |

VLDL = very low-density lipoprotein; IDL = intermediate-density lipoprotein; LDL = low-density lipoprotein; HDL = high-density lipoprotein.

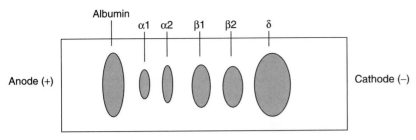

a. Stained with Ponceau S protein stain

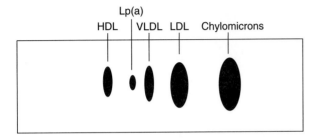

b. Stained with Amido Black lipid stain

**FIGURE  11–9**

Serum protein and lipoprotein electrophoresis. **a.** Migration of serum protein fractions. **b.** Same specimens using lipid stain to indicate relative locations of lipoprotein fractions.

**chylomicron remnant.**[4] The remnant contains primarily cholesterol esters, apo B-48 and apo E. Apo E receptors in the liver recognize the remnant and facilitate endocytosis and eventual hepatic degradation of the chylomicron remnant to produce VLDL.

### Very Low-Density Lipoproteins

Synthesized in the liver from chylomicron remnants, triglyceride-laden VLDL contains apoproteins B-100, C-I, C-II, C-III, and E. As in the chylomicrons, C-II serves as a required cofactor for lipoprotein lipase to hydrolyze triglycerides, which are passed on to the tissues.[6] This results in the catabolism of VLDL to produce IDL. As it is consumed, the VLDL particle also transfers apo C and free cholesterol to HDL.

### Intermediate-Density Lipoproteins

As VLDL loses its lipid content, it is transformed into IDL particles. IDLs persist for short periods of time and contain approximately equal amounts of cholesterol and triglycerides and apoproteins B100 and E. As with the chylomicron remnants, apo E is required for the liver uptake and further degradation of IDL to LDL by the action of hepatic lipase.[4] A deficiency of apo E results in elevation of both chylomicron remnants and IDL.

### Low-Density Lipoproteins (LDL)

The LDLs are formed as the IDLs are degraded. The size of the LDL particle is also smaller and denser than the VLDL and IDL predecessors. Utilization of the LDLs occurs in most cells by way of surface LDL receptors (LDLr) found on membranes of hepatocytes and peripheral tissue cells that possess a high affinity for apolipoprotein B-100. Increased numbers of the LDLr are found on cells that require cholesterol for synthesis of other compounds such as the adrenal and gonadal hormones.

LDL plus its apoprotein, B100, will bind to LDLr on the surface of cells (step 1, Figure 11–10). Receptor bound LDL particles are phagocytized (step 2) into the cells to be further metabolized within the cell. Inside the lysosomes (step 3), various enzymes convert the cholesterol esters into free (nonesterified) cholesterol and degrade apolipoprotein B-100 into its component amino acids (step 4). Free cholesterol is deposited into the cytoplasm of tissue cells (step 5), especially in vascular endothelial cells. The appearance of free cholesterol in the cells has several effects on the cell's lipid metabolism by:

- activating ACAT, which reesterifies the cholesterol for storage within the cell (step 6).
- inhibiting the activity of 3-hydroxy-3-methylglutaryl-CoA (HMG-CoA) reductase, which limits synthesis of endogenous cholesterol (step 7).

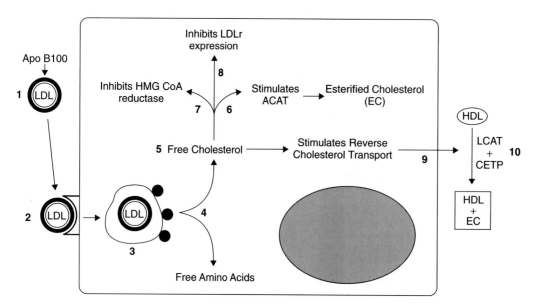

**FIGURE 11–10**

Uptake and processing of HDL (steps 1 to 4) results in formation of free cholesterols (step 5), which then stimulates formation of cholesterol esters (step 6) that are stored and used in the cell. The free cholesterols also inhibit the cell from producing its own cholesterol (step 7) and expressing additional LDL receptors (step 8). Finally, the free cholesterol stimulates reverse cholesterol transport (step 9), resulting in its removal to nascent HDL (step 10) and eventual disposal in the liver.

• reducing expression of the LDLr on the cell surface to prevent intake of further LDL (step 8).

## High-Density Lipoproteins (HDL)

HDLs are produced in both the liver and intestinal walls and contain proportionally more protein and less cholesterol than any of the lipid fractions. The apolipoproteins associated with HDL are apo A-I, apo A-II and apo C (C-I, C-II, and C-III).

There are actually two somewhat different forms of HDL. HDL$_2$ is a larger but less dense (1.063 to 1.11 g/mL) molecule than is HDL$_3$ (1.11 to 1.21 g/mL). HDL$_2$ also contains more apo A-I. Another form of HDL, known as HDLc, is associated with a deficiency of cholesteryl ester transfer protein (CETP), an important intermediate in lipid metabolism.[4,5] The HDLc is also associated with apolipoprotein E, which enables it to bind to LDL receptors.

Nascent, disc-shaped HDL particles containing apo A-I, apo A-II, lecithin, and free cholesterol are initially released into the plasma from liver and intestinal sources. Lecithin-cholesterol acyltransferase (LCAT), activated by the presence of apo A-I, catalyzes the esterification of cholesterol, forming the functional spherical form that actively participates in reactions with the lipoproteins. The half-life of HDL in plasma is about 3 to 6 days.

HDL plays an important role in the reverse cholesterol transport (RCT) mechanism[8,9,10] (step 9, Figure 11–10) in which HDL, in association with CETP and LCAT, esterifies

and then removes cholesterol from cells (step 10). The HDL particles are transported to the liver where the action of hepatic lipase (HL) degrades the HDL. HL appears to directly regulate HDL by both stimulating uptake of HDLs by liver cells and hydrolyzing the lipids.[9] The HDL cholesterol is converted into bile salts for emulsification of dietary fats.

HDL, along with LCAT, CETP, apo A-I and HL, provides protection against coronary artery disease (CAD) by reducing the formation of atherogenic plaques of cholesterol. As mentioned earlier, HDL interactions with triglyceride-rich chylomicrons and VLDL are also important in their eventual degradation.[8,9]

## Lipoprotein (a)

Lipoprotein (a) **[Lp(a)]** is a similar lipid to LDL.[4] Elevations of both LDL and Lp (a) often occur concurrently because both compete for the same LDL receptor sites on cells. This lipid has been identified as another risk factor for CAD because elevated levels of Lp(a) and its associated apolipoprotein, apo (a) are linked to initiation of myocardial infarctions.[11–16] Apo (a) migrates in the "fast" pre-beta region of the lipoprotein electrophoresis.[4]

## Oxidized Lipids

Reactive oxygen species (ROS) such as superoxides ($O_2{}^-$), peroxides ($H_2O_2$), and others ($OH^-$, $ROO^•$) are formed during normal aerobic metabolism. Their levels may be increased due to underlying disease (e.g,. diabetes mellitus) or smoking. The free oxygen radicals rapidly bind to proteins and lipids, especially those containing polyunsaturated fatty acids. The initial oxidation sets off a chain reaction, catalyzed by metallic ions such as Fe and Cu, resulting in continuous release of the oxygen radical.[17-19] Heme compounds and lipooxygenases in platelets and granulocytes also contribute to the ROS in blood. Neutrophils generate superoxides to kill phagocytized material and then die from the effects of those same ROS. LDL is most commonly oxidized but HDL may become oxidized as well.[15] The oxidized lipids are far more likely to initiate and promote cardiovascular diseases such as myocardial infarction. This will be discussed in more detail in the Pathophysiology section.

## Antioxidants

Antioxidant enzymes and vitamins in plasma and cells are essential in controlling the ROS.[18,19] Superoxide dismutase (SOD) and glutathione peroxidase (GPX) will break chain reactions of lipid oxidation. GPX requires selenium as a cofactor and acts in concert with glutathione reductase (GR) and thioredoxin reductase.[20] Antioxidant vitamins such as $\beta$ carotene (provitamin A) traps ROS in tissues where $PO_2$ levels are lowest. Vitamin C (ascorbic acid) is a natural reducing agent and easily binds molecular $O_2$ and nitrates/nitrites.[21,22] This is especially important at cell membranes. Vitamin E ($\alpha$ tocopherol) is concentrated in mitochondria, endoplasmic reticulum, and membranes where $PO_2$ levels are highest, e.g., lung, red blood cells, and retina. Vitamin E tends to break the free radical chain reactions.

## Apolipoproteins

As indicated in Table 11–1, all lipoproteins contain varying amounts of protein. These apolipoproteins vary in structure and function. Five major groups and many subgroups of apolipoproteins have been described. Table 11–2 summarizes the apolipoproteins.[7]

### APOLIPOPROTEIN A

**Apo AI** is the major protein constituent of HDL. It activates the plasma enzyme lecithin-cholesterol acyltransferase (LCAT), which catalyzes the formation of cholesterol esters. Apo AI in combination with **apo AII** and **apo CI** is responsible for the removal of free cholesterol from extrahepatic tissues.[5,23,24]

### APOLIPOPROTEIN B

Two forms of apo B have been described: A large 100 amino-acid long structure called **apo B-100** and smaller 48-amino-acid form known as **apo B-48.** The latter form is the result of alteration of B100 mRNA in the intestinal mucosa. Apo B-48 tends to be associated with chylomicrons found in the lymph. As these chylomicrons are cleared, B-48 is also removed and is not detected in appreciable amounts in fasting plasma except in patients with defects in clearing chylomicron remnants.

TABLE 11-2

### Apolipoproteins

| APOLIPOPROTEIN | ASSOCIATED LIPIDS | MOLECULAR WEIGHT (kDa) | FUNCTION/COMMENTS |
|---|---|---|---|
| Apo A-I | Chylomicrons, HDL | 29 | The major protein of HDL<br>Activates LCAT |
| Apo A-II | Chylomicrons, HDL | 17.4 | Enhances hepatic lipase activity |
| Apo A-IV | Chylomicrons, HDL | 46 | Found in triglyceride-rich lipoproteins |
| Apo B-100 | VLDL, IDL and LDL | 513 | The major protein of LDL<br>Binds to LDL receptors |
| Apo B-48 | Chylomicrons | 241 | Found only in chylomicrons<br>Derived from B-100 gene, it lacks the ability to bind LDL receptors |
| Apo C-I | Chylomicrons, VLDL, HDL | 7.6 | Activates LCAT |
| Apo C-II | Chylomicrons, VLDL, HDL | 9 | Activates lipoprotein lipase |
| Apo C-III | Chylomicrons, VLDL, IDL, HDL | 8.7 | Inhibits lipoprotein lipase |
| Apo D | HDL | 20 | Only found with HDL |
| Apo E | Chylomicron remnants<br>VLDL, IDL and HDL | 34 | At least 4 alleles exist.<br>Binds to LDL receptor, |
| Apo(a) | LDL | 300–800 | Associated with Lp(a) |

HDL = high-density lipoprotein; LCAT = lecithin-cholesterol acyltransferase; IDL = intermediate-density lipoprotein; LDL = low-density lipoprotein; Lp(a) = lipoprotein(a).

**Apo B-100,** the more common plasma form, is synthesized in the liver and found primarily in LDL but may be found in VLDL and IDL as well.[4] It functions as the recognition site for LDL to bind to LDL receptors on cell membranes.[25]

## APOLIPOPROTEIN C

The primary activity of **apo C** is to activate lipoprotein lipase (LPL) leading to the breakdown of triglycerides at the cellular level with subsequent release of fatty acids to the cells for metabolism and storage. Three major forms have been identified: apo CI, apo C-II, and apo CIII, which have 57, 78, and 79 amino acids, respectively.[5] Synthesized in the liver, apo C tends to associate mostly with VLDL and HDL.

Of particular importance, apo C-II is a required cofactor for extrahepatic lipoprotein lipase activity. To ensure extrahepatic clearance of VLDL and chylomicrons, apo C-II apparently prevents these particles from binding to hepatic receptors, the first step in hepatic clearance.[26,27] Apo C-III apparently inhibits the action of LPL, in spite of the presence of apo C-II.[28] Apo C is not detected in IDL or LDL suggesting that HDL transfers its apo C molecules to chylomicrons and VLDL and later picks them up again.

## APOLIPOPROTEIN D

**Apo D** is a glycoprotein and apparently involved in the movement of cholesterol esters and triglycerides among the various lipoproteins. These transfer proteins are different from the earlier described CETP and phospholipid transfer protein (PLTP). Apo D appears to be largely responsible for the binding and transport of unconjugated bilirubin by HDL in plasma.[29,30]

## APOLIPOPROTEIN E

**Apo E** is crucial to regulation of lipids in plasma through regulation of receptor-mediated uptake and clearance and stimulation of lipolysis. Three major forms of Apo E are expressed by at least 3 alleles, called E2, E3, and E4.[31-34] E3 appears to be predominant among most human populations surveyed.[31]

Synthesized in the liver, apo E is incorporated into HDL, which then transfers apo E molecules to VLDL and chylomicrons. As these particles are subsequently degraded to IDL and chylomicron remnants, apo E3 and apo E4 are recognized by hepatic receptors to initiate binding and catabolism of lipids in the cells but apo E2 does not bind to these hepatic receptors.[31]

Polymorphic gene expression among the E alleles is a growing area of research, especially in the areas of atherosclerosis and neurologic disease. Some examples of these disease interactions are:

1. Homozygous apo E2 individuals are unable to clear the chylomicron remnants and IDLs, resulting in a type III hyperlipoproteinemia disorder and increased risk of coronary heart disease.[32]
2. Heterozygous E2 individuals have lower lipoprotein (a) levels. Elevation of Lp (a) is associated with increased risk of coronary heart disease.[33-38]

3. Apo E2 and E3 are associated with improved neurologic function, especially neuronal repair, but E4 is far less effective in this role. Homozygous E4 is considered a major risk factor in development of early-onset Alzheimer disease, whereas homozygous expression of E3 is associated with a reduced risk of Alzheimer disease.[39]

## APOLIPOPROTEIN (a)

**Apo (a)** regulates the expression of **Lp (a)** in the liver. Apo (a) has at least 19 known alleles and produces apoproteins in the range of 300 to 800 kDa.[40] Apo (a) has a structure similar to the plasminogens but apparently does not share the amino acid sequences that activate coagulation and fibrinolysis.[41] Lp (a) is attached to apo B but appears to have no specific function.[4] It is strongly implicated as a risk factor in coronary artery disease.[12-16,42] Increased Lp (a) levels correlate with smaller apo (a) proteins and may be modulated by apo E.[36]

## PLASMA LIPID TRANSFER PROTEINS

There are two proteins that transfer lipids among various lipoproteins, cholesteryl ester transfer protein (CETP) and phospholipid transfer protein (PLTP). CETP plays a crucial role in the reverse cholesterol transport.[43-46] Increased levels of CETP correlate to reduction of HDL levels due to the action of hepatic lipase.[47]

Humans with a genetic deficiency of CETP have both elevated HDL and apolipoprotein A-I levels as well as decreased LDL and apolipoprotein B levels. The CETP-deficient individuals have substantially increased rates of LDL breakdown due to increased LDL receptor efficiency in binding and clearing of these lipids. Despite the elevation of HDL and reduction of LDL, humans who are CETP deficient display a greater rate of coronary artery disease.[48,49]

# ANALYTICAL PROCEDURES FOR LIPIDS

Lipid profiles are an important diagnostic tool to categorize the various disorders of lipids, commonly known as the **hyperlipidemias.** In 1975, a lipid profile consisted of a total cholesterol, triglycerides, and the serum appearance after standing in the refrigerator for several hours. It was generally observed that high levels of cholesterol were associated with increased risk of CAD and atherosclerosis. Improved technology and continuing research have added much to the understanding of the lipids and cardiovascular disease. Today, lipid profiles, consisting of specific tests for cholesterol, HDL, LDL, apo A, apo B, and triglycerides, along with family history and patient's nutrition and lifestyle habits all contribute to paint a more realistic and reliable risk assessment than was possible in 1975.

## Samples

Serum is the sample of choice for all lipid determinations. Usually the serum is collected after a 12- to 14-hour fast in order to minimize dietary impact on the triglyceride levels.[4,50] Cholesterol levels do not change to any significant degree in response to daily dietary intake. Plasma samples collected in dry EDTA may be used as well.

## Serum or Plasma Appearance

The appearance of a serum or plasma sample after it has remained undisturbed for 4 to 6 hours at 4 to 8°C may prove to be helpful in classifying and ultimately treating hyperlipidemic patients.[5] However, the appearance reveals little about the HDL and LDL cholesterol levels. This test is inexpensive and simple to perform but requires that specimens be stored in clear tubes with very little of the label obstructing the cross-sectional view through the tube, especially at the meniscus of the specimen. A creamy layer forming at the surface of the serum contains chylomicrons, which is an indication of either a nonfasting specimen or a serious defect in lipoprotein lipase production or function. Varying degrees of cloudiness, called lipemia, are usually associated with elevated triglyceride levels. In such cases, a dilution of the specimen may be required to bring the triglyceride levels within the linear range of the analytical method. Consequently, the appearance provides observable data that aid in the correlation and validation of laboratory results.

## Total Cholesterol

Early methods for cholesterol analysis were subject to a high degree of analytical variance, primarily due to the poor reac-

tivity of many of the cholesterol esters. Newer methods now utilize cholesterol esterase as a pretreatment, which breaks all of the ester linkages to generate free cholesterol and eliminate much of the previous problems in testing. Oxidation of lipids does not affect cholesterol measurements; only fatty acids are oxidized and these are removed by the cholesterol esterase reaction. However, there are certain factors that affect the accuracy of cholesterol results. These factors, referred to as preanalytical factors, are outlined in Table 11–3.

An understanding of these preanalytical factors is important in terms of the laboratory service concept. Quite often a total cholesterol may be utilized as a screening test for further lipid studies. As a result of an abnormally high value, the patient may be redrawn for a full lipid profile. Factors may affect the accuracy of these tests, resulting in varying degrees of discrepancy, which may cast doubt on the credibility of the laboratory results. Ultimately, it may fall on the clinical laboratory scientist to decide whether the discrepancy is statistically significant, and if it is, sort out the information to propose a plausible explanation for the discrepancy.

## CHEMICAL METHODS

Some of the earlier methods for cholesterol testing called for the production of colored products (chromagen) by reacting cholesterol with strongly acidic reagents. The color produced depended on the type and concentration of acid used along with whatever other reagents were present. The classic **Liebermann-Burchard method** measured the cholesterol extracted into cold chloroform and then treated with

TABLE 11–3

**Preanalytical Factors That Influence Cholesterol Results**

| FACTOR | EFFECT | COMMENT |
|---|---|---|
| Age | Increases with age | Low levels (<100 mg/dL) at birth double during the first few days of life, then remain fairly stable until age 20. After age 20, levels steadily increase. |
| Sex | Different trends for males and females | Levels no different up to ages 30 to 35 years, at which point male levels begin to increase faster than female levels. After age 55, male levels decline, and female levels continuously increase until at the age of 60, when female levels are usually higher than males. |
| Menstruation | Peaking effect (10%–25% variation) | Increase prior to menstruation, peak at ovulation, then decline. |
| Fasting | Negligible | Less than 3% increase after a meal. |
| Stress | Increases | May remain elevated for several hours after a highly stressful episode. |
| Time of specimen | Variable | Diurnal fluctuations about 10%. Day-to-day variation anywhere from 5–200 mg/dL. Average of 35 mg/dL higher in the months of December and January. |
| Hemolysis | Negligible or decreases | Since erythrocytes have a lower (10%–30%) cholesterol concentration than serum, some dilutional effects may occur with gross hemolysis. |

acetic anhydride, acetic acid, and concentrated sulfuric acid to form a green complex.

**Liebermann-Burchard Reaction**

Dehydration step

$$\text{Cholesterol} \xrightarrow{\text{strong acids}} 3,5 \text{ Cholestadiene}$$

Two oxidation steps

$$3,5 \text{ Cholestadiene} \longrightarrow \text{Cholestahexaene sulfonic acid}$$

(Absorbs @ 410 nm)

The other classic color reaction of cholesterol incorporated the use of iron salts and sulfuric acid to produce a reddish purple complex. This has been referred to as the **Salkowski reaction.**

These earlier methods were time-consuming and hazardous, requiring manual organic phase extractions and manipulations using strong acids, considerable skill, and technologist time. The strong acid reagents necessitated working in fume hoods, careful manipulation to prevent spills, and logistical problems in storage and transport of reagents. It was later discovered that cholesterol esters and free cholesterol did not produce equivalent amounts of color, so saponification was added to convert cholesterol esters into free cholesterol.

## ENZYMATIC METHODS

The disadvantages of the earlier chemical methods necessitated the development of faster and safer methods that led to the use of enzymes as reagents for cholesterol testing.[51] The earliest method carried out the analysis in three enzymatic steps:

1. Hydrolysis of the cholesterol esters by cholesterol esterase (CE)

$$\text{Cholesterol-esters} \xrightarrow{\text{CE}} \text{Cholesterol} + \text{Fatty acids}$$

2. Oxidation of cholesterol by cholesterol oxidase (CO) to form hydrogen peroxide and cholestone

$$\text{Cholesterol} + O_2 \xrightarrow{\text{CO}} \text{Cholest-4-3-one} + 2 H_2O_2$$

3. Catalysis of $H_2O_2$ by horseradish peroxidase (HRP) to produce free oxygen radical that oxidizes a reduced dye to the colored end product:

$$H_2O_2 + \text{4-Aminophenazone} + \text{Phenol} \xrightarrow{\text{HRP}}$$

$$\text{Quinoneimine} + 2H_2O \text{ (Absorbs @ 500 nm)}$$

This coupled enzyme reaction is fast, easily automated, and has relatively few interferences. Endogenous reducing substances such as uric acid, ascorbic acid, bilirubin, and glutathione may react with hydrogen peroxide and produce falsely decreased cholesterol levels. Bilirubin also absorbs at 500 nm so a sample with excessive levels of that pigment may be falsely interpreted as having an elevated cholesterol level. This coupled enzyme method, or variations of it, is now the major method used for analysis for total cholesterol.

An alternative enzymatic method for cholesterol is the polarographic oxygen electrode method that measures the decrease in oxygen tension during the reaction as cholesterol is oxidized in step 2. Since oxygen consumption is actually being measured, hydrogen peroxide interactions with other reducing substances will not interfere. However, this requires the use of a different type of instrument (nonspectrophotometric) and the additional burden of maintaining the electrode and its membrane.

The expected reference range for total cholesterol is based on recommended values of the **National Cholesterol Education Program Expert Panel (NCEP).**[52] Although there are well-documented variations in total cholesterol values based on age and sex (Table 11–3), these reference values are most widely applied in monitoring:

| <200 mg/dL | (<5.18 mmol/L) | Desirable |
|---|---|---|
| 200–239 mg/dL | (5.18–6.19 mmol/L) | Borderline high |
| ≥240 mg/dL | (>6.22 mmol/L) | High |

## Cholesterol Fractions

The various forms of cholesterol (HDL, LDL, VLDL) may be separated by a variety of techniques. Chemical precipitation using salts and organic solutions is relatively simple but may result in interferences to the determination of the cholesterol fraction. Ultracentrifugation is a cumbersome method requiring expensive, high-speed centrifuges, long spin times and considerable technologist time. It is used now primarily for research and as the gold standard reference method but is rarely used in clinical laboratories.[5]

Lipoprotein electrophoresis (LPE) is another method of separating and measuring all of the lipoproteins but has largely been replaced by specific assays for HDL and LDL. Newer high resolution gel electrophoresis methods are now becoming available that provide greater reliability in determining all lipoprotein fractions.[53,54]

### HDL CHOLESTEROL

HDL may be separated by a variety of selective precipitation methods that use divalent cations such as $Ca^{+2}$, $Mg^{+2}$, or $Mn^{+2}$ in solutions of buffer, heparin, dextran sulfates or polyethylene glycol. The lower density lipoproteins, e.g., LDL, IDL, and VLDL, will tend to float on top of the serum where they may be aspirated away.[4] The remaining sample, known as the infranatant, will contain only HDLs. Determination of the HDL would then be accomplished using the same method as used for total cholesterol above. Excessive levels of cations used in HDL separation, especially $Mn^{2+}$ may interfere with the enzymes used in the cholesterol assay method. Manipulating the concentrations of these cations and salts in the precipitation reagents will minimize interferences with the cholesterol assay. Excessive levels of triglycerides may not be fully precipitated and remain in the infranatant.[4]

Newer HDL methods have been described over the last 5 years. One type of immunoprecipitation assay involves use of antibodies to apo B, which does not occur in HDLs. These antibodies will remove all those fractions (e.g., LDL, VLDL, and chylomicrons) that contain apo B. Homogeneous enzymatic assays make use of cholesterol oxidase and cholesterol esterase that are modified by polyethylene glycol (PEG). These enzymes, under specific conditions of cation and dextran concentration, will react with HDLs only, eliminating the need for pretreatments to separate the HDL. Comparative studies demonstrate excellent agreement with the older precipitation method[55] but there is some greater susceptibility to interfering substances.[56,57]

HDL levels do vary due to age and gender. Females tend to have slightly lower HDL levels than do similarly aged males. The NCEP reference range for HDL cholesterol has been established at a minimal value of 40 mg/dL (1.02 mmol/L).[52] Persons with values below this minimum are considered to be at greater risk of developing coronary artery disease.

## LDL CHOLESTEROL

LDL cholesterol may also be separated using such methods as ultracentrifugation or electrophoresis[4,5] but the problems involved with these methods has led NCEP to recommend the use of the Friedewald calculation method.[58] This method to calculate LDL requires prior determination of the total cholesterol, triglyceride and HDL cholesterol. LDL is estimated using the formula:

$$LDL = Total\ cholesterol - (HDL + [triglyceride/5])$$

This calculation assumes that TG (triglycerides)/5 is a relatively accurate estimate of VLDL. The Friedewald method works well under most circumstances but it does have limitations. Even moderately elevated levels of triglycerides (>200 mg/dL) or the appearance of abnormal types of lipoproteins (e.g., increased IDL in type III hyperlipidemia) will invalidate the results of this calculation, resulting in falsely decreased LDL.[59-60]

The problems of LDL calculation led to the development of newer methods to fractionate and directly measure the LDL. An immunoprecipitation method using antibodies to apo A and apo E will remove HDL and VLDL fractions, leaving the remaining LDL to be directly assayed using the cholesterol oxidase method explained earlier.[61] Chemical precipitation of only LDL can be accomplished using a buffered heparin solution. In this assay, the remaining HDL and VLDL are measured and then subtracted from the total cholesterol. This calculation method is less susceptible to hypertriglyceridemia than is the Friedewald method. Homogeneous LDL cholesterol methods are also available in which LDL selectively reacts with the reagents. As with the selective HDL method, the elimination of the pretreatment step reduces analytical time and reduces costs while maintaining the reliability of the assay, even when faced with high triglycerides.[61-63]

The NCEP recommended value for LDL is ≤100 mg/dL (2.60 mmol/L).[52] Lower levels of LDL are associated with reduced risk of coronary artery disease.

## TRIGLYCERIDES

Triglyceride determination is essential in evaluating hyperlipidemias and the risk of cardiovascular disease. Early methods were long and tedious procedures and involved extractions with organic solvents that were not easily adaptable to automation. As with cholesterol testing, the advent of enzymatic methods represented tremendous savings in terms of technologist time and safety.

Most current methods for triglycerides commonly employ coupled enzymes[64] in four basic analytical steps:

1. The breakdown of triglyceride by lipase (LPS):

$$Triglyceride \xleftrightarrow{LPS} Glycerol + Free\ fatty\ acids$$

2. The phosphorylation of glycerol catalyzed by glycerol kinase (GK):

$$Glycerol + ATP \xleftrightarrow{GK} Glycerol\text{-}3\text{-}phosphate + ADP$$

3. The oxidation of glycerol-3-phosphate by glycerol phosphate oxidase (GPO) to dihydroxyacetone phosphate (DHAP):

$$Glycerol\text{-}3\text{-}phosphate + O_2 \xleftrightarrow{GPO} DHAP + H_2O_2$$

4. The catalysis of $H_2O_2$ by horseradish peroxidase (HRP) to produce free oxygen radical that oxidizes a reduced dye to the colored end product:

$$H_2O_2 + Reduced\ dye \xleftrightarrow{P} oxidized\ dye^* + H_2O$$

An alternative method varies step 3 by using glycerol-3-phosphate dehydrogenase (GPD) plus $NAD^+$, which is reduced to $NADH + H^+$.

3a. $$Glycerol\text{-}3\text{-}phosphate + NAD^+ \xleftrightarrow{GPD} DHAP + NADH + H^+$$

NADH is then measured at 340 nm (near UV). The major problem with this type of assay is the ability of the spectrophotometer to distinguish absorbance differences at that wavelength. Sample blanks are necessary to reduce interferences from other UV-absorbing pigments in the sample. This type of interference is less likely to occur when using chromagens that absorb light in the visible range.

NCEP reference ranges for adults in general (slight variations are seen with age):

| | | |
|---|---|---|
| <200 mg/dL | (<2.83 mmol/L) | Acceptable |
| 200–400 mg/dL | (2.83–5.65 mmol/L) | Borderline high |
| >400 mg/dL | (>5.65 mmol/L) | High |

## APOLIPOPROTEINS

Apolipoproteins, also called apoproteins, play a critical role in the metabolism of lipids and are now recognized as important indicators of disease. The measurement of specific apoproteins,

---

*Absorbance measured at visible wavelength of light depending on the indicator (chromagen) used.

as part of a lipid profile, provides useful data in evaluating a patient's risk for cardiovascular disease. The most common methods used today are immunoprecipitation.[5] Reaction of a specific antibody and the apolipoprotein in the sample results in the formation of partially insoluble immune complexes that are composed of antigen bound to antibody. Radial immunodiffusion methods were among the first methods applying this principle, but this technique had been replaced by rate nephelometry that measures light scattering by large immune complexes. As in other nephelometric methods, the scattering of light by the complexes is directly proportional to their concentration and permits quantitation of a wide variety of apoproteins with test specificity conferred by the use of a specific antibody to a given protein.

Apo A-I has often been proposed as an alternative to HDL testing because of its association with HDL but not with LDL. Since Apo A-I is also associated with VLDL and chylomicrons, exclusive use of A-I may provide misleading results in the presence of substantial amounts of these lipids. Normal fasting specimens have only trace amounts of VLDL and chylomicrons, however, and for these samples, apo A-I testing may provide a reasonable approximation of HDL levels. Apo B is found primarily in VLDL and LDL. Owing to its LDL association, determination of apo B is an alternative to calculated LDL.[65] When used in such a manner, apo A-I and apo B may indicate the relative relationship between HDL and LDL levels, respectively.

The reference values for apolipoprotein are:

Apo A-I    1.20–1.52 g/L (females)    1.12–1.38 g/L (males)
Apo B      0.92–1.38 g/L (females)    0.99–1.36 g/L (males)

The level of both A-I and B tend to increase between the ages of 20 and 59 years in both sexes. After age 60, apo B levels increase markedly until about age 70 when they begin to decline. Apo A-I levels remain steady until age 70 when they also begin to decline.

Until recently, it was difficult to properly quantitate apo (a), which is a fast pre-beta lipoprotein. Newer and more sensitive, high-definition electrophoretic methods are now able to reliably measure apo (a).[54,66] Of nearly 30 studies already published, there is little agreement as to optimal plasma levels of Lp(a), however all of these studies do assert that lower levels (under 50 mg/dL) of this lipoprotein are associated with reduced risk of CAD and correlate high levels to increased risk or recent evidence of acute myocardial infarction (AMI).[11–16,67,68] Some studies seem to indicate that elevated Lp (a) may be associated primarily with coronary artery disease but has little predictive value for other forms of cardiovascular diseases such as cerebrovascular accidents (stroke).[67] Apo(a) will be elevated after surgery or AMI and remains elevated for as long as 10 days after the AMI.[5]

## PATHOPHYSIOLOGY

There are 6 to 8 million Americans who suffer from the symptoms of coronary artery disease (CAD), one form of cardiovascular disease (CVD), resulting in about 500,000 deaths each year. CAD is a result of a life-long process of **atherosclerosis,** the deposition of lipids in various tissues within the body. Lipid deposits will form plaques that occlude blood vessels throughout the body but are most dangerous in blood vessels of the heart, liver, and kidney. Other deposits may also occur in the skin where they are known as xanthomas. This process may take decades to develop. Atherosclerosis can be seen in postmortem examinations of blood vessels in children as young as 9 years of age.

The major pathophysiology of atherosclerosis is associated with plaque formation that reduces blood flow and initiates formation of a clot (thrombus). The complete obstruction of blood circulation may be manifested in different types of symptoms. Occlusion of arteries in the heart will result in a myocardial infarction (MI). If such an obstruction occurs in a vessel supplying blood to the brain, then a stroke or cerebrovascular accident occurs. Renal or liver infarctions occur by similar mechanisms. The loss of blood flow, unless reversed quickly, will culminate in tissue ischemia and eventual death, often damaging the affected organ beyond the ability to repair itself.

## Pathophysiology of Atherosclerosis

There are two mechanisms to explain the pathophysiology of atherosclerosis: (1) chronic endothelial injury,[69] and (2) elevated lipids.[5,11,23,24,37] The endothelium (epithelial lining of blood vessels) may become damaged by various mechanisms such as smoking, hypertension, microbial infection, drug use, and underlying disease. Infections by herpesvirus and *Chlamydia pneumoniae*, both of which were previously considered to cause innocuous infections, have been implicated in creating the initial endothelial damage that then develops into atherosclerotic lesions over a period of 20 to 40 years.

The loss of vascular endothelium along with increased adhesion of platelets to subendothelium will result in aggregation of platelets and the chemotaxis of monocytes and T lymphocytes to the site of endothelial injury. Once in place, there is a release of platelet-derived and monocyte-derived growth factors that induce migration of smooth muscle cells into the injury site. The resulting plaque, also called the "fatty" plaque, features cells loaded with lipids. Oxidative stress has been established as a significant causative mechanism of chronic endothelial injury that then triggers a variety of responses, especially oxidation of lipids, which manifests as atherosclerosis.

### ATHEROGENESIS

Elevation of plasma LDL levels results in penetration of LDL into the arterial wall, leading to lipid accumulation in smooth muscle cells and local macrophages (fatty streak). The macrophages are called "foam cells" due to the appearance of lipids, mainly LDL, within them. LDL augments smooth muscle cell hyperplasia in response to growth factors from aggregated platelets and forms an enclosed lesion that begins to occlude the blood vessel. As the lesion grows and more smooth muscle cells appear, the plaque becomes a "fibrous" plaque as contrasted to the early fatty plaque.

Both LDL and oxidized LDL (LDLox) accumulate in the plaque but LDLox[70-72] is chemotactic to certain monocytes and promotes their migration into the wall of the blood vessel and eventual differentiation into macrophages, essentially producing an inflammatory lesion. Autoantibodies to oxidized LDL may be used to indicate an active coronary artery disease process.[73,74]

A group of unusual receptors, known as CD 36, are found on the surface of the macrophages in the atherosclerotic lesion. Generically called "scavenger" receptors, these CD 36 receptors actively bind oxidized lipoproteins.[75-77] The scavenger macrophages are not inhibited by increasing intracellular concentrations of cholesterol and accumulate huge amounts of lipids, transforming the macrophages into so-called foam cells. LDLox is also cytotoxic to endothelial cells and may be responsible for their dysfunction or loss from the more advanced atherosclerotic lesions.[78] Oxidized HDL loses its ability to remove cholesterol from atherosclerotic plaques.[79]

## RISK FACTORS FOR CAD

Providing data that can help predict the potential risk of CAD is a crucial function of the clinical chemistry laboratory. A lipid profile should include determinations of total cholesterol, HDL, LDL, apo A and apo B plus triglycerides. However, lipid profiles are only one aspect of assessing risk factors associated with cardiovascular disease. Some risk factors may be due to genetics or lifestyle choices.

Risk factors are classified as nonmodifiable and modifiable. Nonmodifiable factors are those that cannot be changed by the clinician or patient and include: gender, age, and family history of cardiovascular disease. A number of other well-known risk factors that can be altered include hypertension, cigarette smoking, obesity, physical inactivity, and diet.[80,81]

### Lipids Levels

Abnormally elevated levels of LDL, Lp(a), and reduced levels of HDL predispose a person to atherosclerosis. The correlation of increased total serum cholesterol, LDL cholesterol, and Lp(a) levels with the risk of CAD is direct and indisputable, whereas HDL levels are inversely correlated with CAD risk. If the source of the lipids is dietary, this becomes a modifiable factor; if the hyperlipidemia is inherited, it is not.

### Hypertension

Elevated diastolic or systolic blood pressure is associated with endothelial damage. This, in turn, provides initial lesions into which inflammatory cells infiltrate. If LDL levels are elevated, the fatty streak begins to form.

### Smoking

Cigarette smoking increases the risk of both CAD and peripheral artery disease. There is a dose relationship between the risk of CAD and the number of cigarettes smoked daily. Passive smoking may also increase the risk of CAD. Men and women are both susceptible but the risk for women may be greater. Nicotine and other tobacco-derived chemicals are toxic to vascular endothelium. Cigarette smoking increases LDL and decreases HDL levels, raises blood carbon monoxide (which produces endothelial hypoxia), promotes vasoconstriction of arteries already narrowed by atherosclerosis, increases platelet thrombus formation, and increases plasma fibrinogen concentration. It also promotes formation of peroxides, one of the major reactive oxygen species.

### Diabetes Mellitus

Diabetes mellitus is associated with earlier and more extensive development of atherosclerosis as part of a widespread metabolic disorder. Diabetes is a particularly strong risk factor in women and effectively negates the protective effect of female hormones. The myocardium is especially sensitive to oxidative stress in hyperglycemia while hyperinsulinemia damages vascular endothelium.[82,83]

### Obesity

Obesity is an independent risk factor for CAD. Hypertriglyceridemia is commonly associated with obesity and may presage diabetes mellitus by increasing specific lipids. Not all triglyceride elevations are likely to be atherogenic; LDL is associated with greater risk. Diet plays a crucial role in obesity. A diet that is high in saturated fatty acids or calories will contribute to hypertriglyceridemia.

### Exercise

Physical inactivity and a sedentary lifestyle are linked with increased risk of CAD and studies have shown that regular exercise is protective and reduces such risk.

### Oxidative Stress

Oxidative stress can arise through the increased production of reactive oxygen species or a deficiency of antioxidant defenses. Oxidative stress appears to amplify the other risk factors identified with development of coronary artery diseases.

### Inflammation

Atherogenesis is, after all, an inflammatory process involving the migration of phagocytes into the atherosclerotic plaque and replacement of normal tissue cells with other cell types. This inflammation can be detected by using the **high sensitivity CRP (hs-CRP) test.** This assay is a modification of the older C-reactive protein (CRP) test. CRP is an acute phase reactant that increases during inflammatory disease, and the hs-CRP been shown to be a good predictor of impending myocardial infarction, especially in diabetic subjects.

### Homocysteine

Over the last 25 years, there has been an increasing body of evidence indicating that elevated plasma levels of the amino acid homocysteine, also called hyperhomocysteinemia, is an independent risk factor in coronary artery disease (CAD).[84-88] Accumulation of homocysteine promotes vascular endothelial injury that predisposes blood vessels to atherosclerosis.

There are four potential causes of elevated plasma homocysteine:

1. Deficiencies of three critical enzymes; cystathionine $\beta$-synthase, methylenetetrahydrofolate reductase, and methionine synthase result in a childhood onset of disease that includes early atherosclerosis, retardation, and skeletal abnormalities. This rare disease is often indicated by the presence of homocystine crystals in urine (homocystinuria).
2. Mutations in the gene that codes for the enzyme methylenetetrahydrofolate reductase (MTHFR), the crucial enzyme that converts folic acid into methylenetetrahydrofolate. This disorder appears to produce a form of hyperhomocysteinemia that manifests in adulthood.
3. Low levels of vitamins B$_6$, B$_{12}$, and especially folic acid owing to poor diet or malabsorption is associated with small to moderate elevations of homocysteine.
4. Reduced renal function, especially glomerular filtration rate, will result in elevated homocysteine levels. Homocysteine may play a role in the development of albuminuria.

Homocysteine is derived from the essential amino acid methionine and is a sulfur-bearing (thiol), nonessential amino acid. It is enzymatically converted into the amino acid cysteine, which is then degraded (transsulfuration) into sulfates that are excreted in urine. Although the mechanism is not well understood, homocysteine may play a role in formation of reactive oxygen species, which are then able to oxidize lipids, multiplying their atherogenic potential.[84,85] It may also alter vascular endothelium and promote thrombosis formation. Even small increases in homocysteine levels are associated with increased risk; reduction of normal plasma levels of homocysteine will reduce the risk of CAD due to this compound.

Tetrahydrofolate (folic acid) is converted into methylenetetrahydrofolate, an important intermediate in the metabolism of homocysteine from methionine. Use of folate as a dietary supplement has been repeatedly demonstrated as an effective therapy. Vitamins B$_6$ (pyridoxone) and B$_{12}$ (cyanocobalamin) are enzymatic cofactors that assist in the reduction of homocysteine levels, but their therapeutic role is less uncertain than that of folate.[87,88]

Homocysteine is transported in blood in two major forms: protein bound (~80–90% of total) and free forms complexed with cysteine. These two forms may be in either reduced form (~99% of total) or oxidized form. The oxidized form is known as homocystine; many citations use the spelling homocyst(e)ine to imply both forms.[87]

Laboratory analysis for homocyst(e)ine is far from standardized. Immunoassay, fluorometric, and chromatographic methods have all been utilized. Newer immunoassays for homocyst(e)ine, primarily fluorescence polarization methods, require conversion of protein-bound homocyst(e)ine into the free form, which is then measured.[89,90] Reference values for homocyst(e)ine in plasma are 5 to 15 $\mu$mol/L, but there is continuing controversy over the upper limit. Patients with homocyst(e)ine levels between 10 and 15 $\mu$mol/L do have a somewhat greater risk of CAD.[87,89] Homocyst(e)ine levels do increase with age. Patients with the enzyme deficiency form of hyperhomocysteinemia may have levels as high as 500 $\mu$mol/L.[88]

## LIPIDS AND CAD

Results of the decades-long Framingham study, as well as many other similar studies, have been used to set guidelines for use in assessment of risk of CAD. In terms of laboratory-measured factors, increased risk of CAD has been associated with low levels of HDL cholesterol and elevated levels of LDL cholesterol.[91] Table 11–4 summarizes the most widely applied guidelines.

## OTHER DIAGNOSTIC TESTING

Other measures of cardiovascular risk include the use of the ratio of total cholesterol to HDL cholesterol. Clinicians consider a ratio of 5 or less to be optimal, but this measure suffers from the inherent inaccuracy of a calculated LDL value when triglyceride values are even moderately elevated. The use of directly measured LDL values restores the reliability of the TC/HDL ratio as another risk factor to be evaluated.

## Disorders of Lipid Metabolism

### HYPERLIPOPROTEINEMIAS

The terms **hyperlipidemia** or **hyperlipoproteinemia** (HLP) are used interchangeably to describe disorders that are the result of elevated lipids. For nearly 30 years, the Fredrickson and

TABLE 11–4

### Guidelines for Laboratory Assessment of Coronary Artery Disease

| TEST | DESIRABLE | BORDERLINE | UNDESIRABLE |
|---|---|---|---|
| Total Cholesterol | <200 mg/dL | 200–239 mg/dL | ≥240 mg/dL |
| HDL Cholesterol | ≥60 mg/dL | 35–59 mg/dL | <35 mg/dL |
| LDL Cholesterol | <130 mg/dL | 130–159 mg/dL | ≥160 mg/dL |
| Triglycerides | <200 mg/dL | 200–400 mg/dL | >400 mg/dL |

Levy classification of HLPs has been used to group these disorders on the basis of laboratory findings.[5] This classification system is predicated on the patient's phenotype as determined by lipids in serum. It is important to note that the lipoprotein patterns of Fredrickson and Levy for an individual may change over time, or as a result of disease onset, weight gain or weight loss, and certain drug interventions.

HLPs can be further classified as primary or secondary. In **primary** or familial HLP, there is no apparent underlying disease present, and it may be related to an inherited disorder. In **secondary** HLP, the abnormal pattern is caused by an underlying disorder. The classification of lipid disorders has varied in past years but the most useful approach for interpretation of laboratory data would be the categorization of inherited disorders of cholesterol metabolism. The following discussion presents the Fredrickson-Levy classification as well as the terminology used to indicate the type of inherited disorder of cholesterol metabolism.

## Elevated Chylomicrons (Familial Chylomicronemia or Fredrickson Type I)

Chylomicrons formed at the intestinal wall following a meal are normally cleared from the plasma fairly rapidly by the activity of lipoprotein lipase (LPL). Patients with ineffective or insufficient LPL will accumulate abnormal amounts of chylomicrons.[92] The primary disorder is inherited as an autosomal recessive trait and generally detectable early in a patient's life. Secondary disorders that affect the function or production of LPL may be discovered in older patients.

Accumulation of chylomicrons results in extremely elevated triglyceride levels. As triglyceride levels exceed 2000 mg/dL, deposits may result in xanthoma formation in various regions of the body, or in the retina. Some patients may experience mild to severe (sometimes fatal) pancreatitis as well as hepatomegaly, splenomegaly, or both. The symptoms subside only when triglyceride values are brought under control.

Apoprotein CII is a required cofactor of LPL and ineffective or deficient apo CII would have similar but somewhat different clinical manifestations. Although CII deficiencies are rare, such patients tend to be 10 years of age or older and do not present with the eruptive xanthomas or hepatosplenomegaly. However, apo CII–deficient individuals do have recurrent episodes of acute abdominal pain and pancreatitis following ingestion of a fatty meal.

The sera of patients with chylomicronemia show initially a characteristic creamy layer forming at the surface of a fasting specimen. Triglyceride levels are markedly elevated, often requiring dilution before results are obtained. Despite the pancreatitis, the serum amylase level may initially be falsely normal. Repeating the amylase test with serum diluted with normal saline may restore the expectedly elevated activity.

Lipoprotein electrophoresis will often be helpful in demonstrating the presence of chylomicrons with a normal to slightly increased VLDL and decreased HDL. Serum cholesterol levels may be slightly elevated.

## Increased LDL or Primary Hypercholesterolemia (Fredrickson Type II)

Type II disease, also called familial hypercholesterolemia (FH), is the result of literally hundreds of different mutations of the LDL receptors.[93-95] This reduces the cellular intake of LDL with resulting serum cholesterol values exceeding 800 mg/dL (>21 mmol/L). There are two major forms of FH. Homozygous hypercholesterolemia (type IIa) manifests as early or premature atherosclerosis with a striking increase in occurrence of myocardial infarction in both men and women before the age of 30. In the Helsinki Heart Study, low HDL was identified as a better predictor of early onset CAD in female type IIa patients than an increased LDL.[94] Dietary restrictions of fat intake are usually ineffective and drug therapy is necessary to reduce the LDL cholesterol. The heterozygous form of FH (type IIb) also presents with elevated LDL and risk of CAD but this occurs later in life. Type IIb disorders are, however, treatable with dietary changes. A third type of FH has also been described that is not related to mutations of LDL receptors or apo B.[96] Laboratory data will demonstrate elevations in total cholesterol and LDL (β lipoprotein). VLDL (pre-β lipoprotein) will also be elevated in type IIb disease.

## Increased IDL (Familial Dysbetalipoproteinemia or Fredrickson Type III)

Familial dysbetalipoproteinemia is associated with individuals who are homozygous for apo E2.[5] This rare inherited disorder is characterized by the inability to degrade chylomicron remnants and IDLs; apo E2 cannot bind to the hepatic receptors that signal uptake and eventual catalysis of these lipids.[97,98] Patients accumulate chylomicron remnants and IDL since normal chylomicron and VLDL synthesis still occurs and exhibit xanthoma formation along with CAD and other atherosclerotic vascular diseases.

LPE is necessary for differential diagnosis of this disorder since the presence of the normally absent IDL causes a broad beta band to appear. Laboratory lipid determinations would include elevated total cholesterol and triglycerides owing to increased IDL, VLDL and chylomicrons, and low LDL levels. Determination of the VLDL level by ultracentrifugation will be helpful to elucidate this problem. A VLDL/total plasma triglyceride ratio exceeding 0.25 is a strong indication of type III disease.

## Increased VLDL (Familial Hypertriglyceridemia or Fredrickson Type IV)

This disorder is relatively common and appears as both primary and secondary disease. The primary type IV disease is autosomal recessive, whereas the secondary disorder may be the result of drug therapy, estrogen therapy, alcoholism/alcohol abuse, glycogen storage disorders, obesity, diabetes mellitus, or hypothyroidism. Both primary and secondary hypertriglyceridemias display increased triglycerides and cholesterol due to either increased VLDL production in liver, decreased VLDL clearance, or a combination of both. HDL and LDL may both be reduced in type IV disease but reductions of HDL and apo E seem to be linked to the disease.[99]

Characteristic clinical symptoms are not usually manifested in childhood but may appear at a later age. Premature CAD as a disorder has been debated but generally evidence indicates that an elevated VLDL is not an independent risk factor. Laboratory results show elevated triglyceride and VLDL levels with a normal or only slightly increased cholesterol. In LPE, increased VLDL levels cause a heavy pre-beta band along with the absence of a chylomicron band.

### Increased VLDL with Increased Chylomicrons (Fredrickson Type V)

This disorder results in markedly elevated triglyceride levels either due to an impaired ability to remove the triglyceride-rich lipoproteins, excess production of these particles, or a combination of both. Although occurring less frequently than type IV, similar disease states are associated with the secondary form of both disorders. The type V disorder also has a familial form, the genetics of which are yet unknown, but it is associated with increased apo C-III, which inhibits lipoprotein lipase. Patients usually present with symptoms over the age of 20, including eruptive xanthomas and episodic bouts of abdominal pain with or without pancreatitis. Premature CAD has not been a clearcut problem in these patients.

Elevations of both chylomicrons and VLDL give the standing serum a creamy top layer with a turbid infranate. On LPE, heavy chylomicron and pre-beta bands are the prominent features. LDL and HDL cholesterol may be normal to low while total cholesterol and triglyceride levels are increased.

### Familial Combined Hyperlipidemia (FCH)

This disorder is the result of the inheritance of an autosomal dominant gene that usually appears in adult years. Although similar to type IIb or type IV hyperlipidemias, this disorder is far more common than either. The major laboratory findings include elevated total cholesterol, LDL, apo B, and markedly increased triglycerides and are associated with excessive production of LDL by the liver. As expected, patients with FCH have an increased risk of CAD.

### Increased HDL or Familial Hyperalphalipoproteinemia

Familial hyperalphalipoproteinemia patients display a reduced risk for CAD due to elevated HDL cholesterol and apo AI levels. The elevation of HDL also results in a slightly elevated total cholesterol. These patients show enhanced LPL activity and hence clearance of VLDL and chylomicrons due to an autosomal dominant trait.

### HYPOLIPOPROTEINEMIAS

With all the attention on hyperlipoproteinemias, one might get the impression that the less lipids in the serum the better. This seems to be true to a certain degree but once the levels get too low, another type of lipid problem could be occurring. Very low lipid levels probably indicate an abnormality in lipid metabolism that has similar or even worse implications than hyperlipidemias.

### Reduced LDL (Hypobetalipoproteinemia)

The familial form of this disorder is inherited as an autosomal dominant trait and appears to be an inability to synthesize apo B-100 and apo B-48. With low total and LDL cholesterol levels and normal to low triglyceride levels, patients usually have a significant increase in life expectancy.

### Absent LDL (Abetalipoproteinemia)

This rare autosomal recessive trait results in no LDLs due to a lack of apolipoprotein B. Homozygous expression results in virtually no detectable triglycerides, phospholipids, and apo B with very low total cholesterol, nearly all in HDL form. Heterozygotes appear normal but have low (but not absent) LDL levels with normal levels of chylomicrons, VLDL, or LDL.

Patients with abetalipoproteinemia (homozygotes) cannot absorb fats and accumulate large lipid-filled vacuoles in the intestinal mucosal cells that block the absorption of the essential fat soluble vitamins (A, K, E, and D). These malabsorption problems could result in failure to thrive in infancy, progressive degeneration of the nervous system and loss of night vision. Vitamin K deficiency is especially troublesome; most infants are born with an 8-hour supply. A lack of K could then manifest as prolonged prothrombin time. The unabsorbed fats remaining in the intestine will be metabolized by microbial organisms and produce steatorrhea, foul-smelling, soft stools. Peripheral blood smears may demonstrate as many as 50% to 70% of erythrocytes with spiny projections (acanthocytosis).

### Decreased HDL (Hypoalphalipoproteinemia)

This disorder results in low levels of HDL usually associated with very high triglycerides or hypertriglyceridemia. Obesity, diet, excessive alcohol consumption, and lack of exercise have all been linked to reduced HDL levels. These factors are all modifiable and lifestyle changes may correct the condition that would lead to increased risk of CAD.

The familial form of the disorder is the result of autosomal dominant inheritance, with reduced HDL and apo AI, but there is some evidence that atherosclerosis is not present. Therefore, it is necessary to properly determine the cause of the reduced HDL.

### Absent HDL (Tangier Disease)

Tangier disease is the complete absence of HDL with very low levels of apo AI and apo AII due to inheritance of homozygous recessive alleles. As a result, cholesterol esters tend to accumulate in various tissues including liver, spleen, lymph nodes, cornea, skin, and intestinal endothelium with apparently little effect on normal function. Some patients report peripheral nerve damage. Heterozygotes have reduced HDL levels but do not accumulate the cholesterol esters in tissues. The major problem with Tangier patients seems to be an increased risk of atherosclerosis.

Laboratory results usually indicate low LDL, low total cholesterol levels with undetectable amounts of HDL, low or absent apoprotein AI or AII, and lack of an alpha band on lipoprotein electrophoresis. The patient will also display normal to slight hypertriglyceridemia.

## LIPID LYSOSOMAL ABNORMALITIES

Inborn errors of metabolism are inherited disorders that affect biochemical pathways, usually through missing or nonfunctioning enzymes, and result in the accumulation of intermediate compounds (substrates) from those pathways in tissues or cells. Many of these intermediates may be toxic to the cells. Lysosomes contain the enzymes that catalyze many of the biochemical pathways within cells. Lipid metabolism may be disturbed by lysosomal disorders in which catabolic enzymes necessary for lipid utilization may be lacking or are ineffective. The term *lipid lysosomal disorders* may be used to describe the general category of lipid abnormalities, but it is important to remember the primary defect in these disorders results in abnormal accumulation of the intermediate substrates of the lipid pathways.

In lipid lysosomal disorders that manifest in early childhood, there is generally psychomotor deterioration and developmental retardation leading to early death. Lipid substrate accumulates in reticuloendothelial cells in the liver and spleen, which results in hepatosplenomegaly and lipid-laden cells in the bone marrow. Lipids may also accumulate in the central nervous system, resulting in the neurologic problems associated with each disorder. The majority of these disorders are inherited as autosomal recessive traits and, as such, are rarely found. Table 11–5 describes several disorders plus the known defect and metabolite.

Early detection of the lipid storage disorders has been a focus on ongoing research since most of these syndromes produce irreversible damage by the time they are diagnosed. There are some newer screening assays now in use. Lysosome-associated membrane protein (LAMP-1) has been demonstrated to be increased in the plasma in 70% of individuals with lysosomal storage disorders. A second lysosome-associated membrane protein (LAMP-2)[100] has also been described as a marker for this group of disorders.

### Gaucher's Disease

The most common lipid storage disease is Gaucher's disease, caused by a deficiency of $\beta$-glucocerebrosidase resulting in an accumulation of glucocerebroside. Three types are known; chronic, nonneuropathic (type I), infantile neuropathic (type II), and juvenile neuropathic (type III). Type I is more common and occurs primarily in adults, resulting in normocytic or hypochromic anemia with thrombocytopenia, leukopenia, bone pain (with erosion of the cortices of the long bones), hepatosplenomegaly, and pigmentation of the skin.

Laboratory diagnosis includes the presence of Gaucher's cells, which are lipid-laden macrophages, in the bone marrow and elevated serum acid phosphatase. Lack of cerebral involvement (nonneuropathic) in type I indicates a better prognosis than neuropathic cases with rapid deterioration of the central nervous system. Patients with type II Gaucher's usually survive no more than 2 years; those with type III disease may survive into adolescence.

### Niemann-Pick Disease (Sphingomyelin Lipidosis)

In Niemann-Pick disease a deficiency of sphingomyelinase results in an accumulation of sphingomyelin. Four types have been differentiated (A, B, C, and D) with types A, C, and D being more acute neuropathic disorders resulting in fatal psychomotor and intellectual deterioration. Splenomegaly and hepatomegaly are associated with the disorder, but the presence of Niemann-Pick cells, which are macrophages loaded with sphingomyelin, are diagnostic.

The different Niemann-Pick disorders vary mainly in their time of onset. Type A tends to affect newborn infants, whereas type C has a later onset. Type D is a Nova Scotia variant similar to type C. Type B tends to be chronic with no neurologic

TABLE 11–5

**Lipid Lysosomal Disorders**

| DISORDER | ENZYME DEFICIENCY | ACCUMULATING SUBSTRATES |
|---|---|---|
| Gaucher's | $\beta$-Glucocerebrosidase | Glucocerebroside |
| Niemann-Pick | Sphingomyelinase | Sphingomyelin |
| Krabbe's | Galactocerebroside-$\beta$-galactosidase | Galactocerebroside |
| Metachromatic leukodystrophy | Arylsulfatase A | 3-Sulfato-galactosyl-cerebroside |
| Fabry's disease | $\alpha$-Galactosidase A | Ceramide trihexoside |
| Tay-Sachs disease | Hexosaminidase A | $G_{M2}$ ganglioside |
| $G_{M1}$ gangliosidosis | $G_{M1}$ $\beta$-galactosidase | $G_{M1}$ gangliosides, galactose-containing oligosaccharides |
| Fucosidosis | $\alpha$-Fucosidase | Fucose-containing sphingolipids |

involvement. In contrast to Gaucher's disease, anemia and thrombocytopenia are uncommon and the serum acid phosphatase level is normal.

### Krabbe's Disease (Galactocerebroside Lipidosis or Globoid Cell Leukodystrophy)

Krabbe's disease is the result of galactocerebroside accumulation due to a deficiency of the enzyme galactocerebroside-beta-galactosidase. This disorder primarily affects the central nervous system and results in severe mental and motor deterioration. Blindness and deafness are common. Laboratory findings may show elevated protein and the presence of globoid cells (large multinucleated macrophages) in the cerebrospinal fluid. A number of types have been described varying in age of onset and severity of the symptoms. The disease is usually fatal within 6 to 12 months of onset.

### Metachromatic Leukodystrophy

This disorder is due to a deficiency of arylsulfatase A, which results in an accumulation of 3-sulfato-galactosylcerebroside (sulfuric acid esters of cerebrosides). Clinically, the disease is characterized by progressive paralysis and mental deterioration.

### Fabry's Disease (Angiokeratoma Corporis Diffusum Universale)

In Fabry's disease, a deficient alpha-galactosidase A results in the accumulation of ceramide trihexoside in the central nervous system cells. This results in severe pain in the extremities and characteristic angiokeratoma (reddish lesions) on buttocks and around the navel. Hypertension and heart problems are also common due to accumulation of ceramide trihexoside, which promotes narrowing of the arteries. Unlike many of the other lipid lysosomal disorders, Fabry's is inherited as an X-linked trait.

### Tay-Sachs Disease ($G_{M2}$ Gangliosidosis)

Primarily found in families with Ashkenazi Jewish ancestry, Tay-Sachs (TSD) patients accumulate $G_{M2}$ ganglioside in the neurons of the central nervous system due to a deficiency in hexosaminidase A. TSD culminates in psychomotor deterioration and often dementia. The most severe form occurs in infants and usually results in death within 5 years. Adult and juvenile-onset forms of TSD have also been described. A common finding is blindness associated with a cherry red spot in the retina.

A number of different mutations in the genes which code for hexosaminidase subunits have been identified. Hexosaminidase has two isoenzymes, A and B; the A isoenzyme is heat labile and the B form is heat stable. Related disorders have also been identified:

1. Bernheimer-Seitelberger disease, which has a juvenile onset
2. Adult-chronic gangliosidosis, which has a juvenile to adult onset without dementia
3. Sandhoff's variant is similar to TSD and results from a deficiency in both hexosaminidase A and B.

### $G_{M1}$ Gangliosidosis

With this disorder, $G_{M1}$ gangliosides and galactose-containing oligosaccharides accumulate due to a deficiency of $G_{M1}$ beta-galactosidase. Two types have been studied primarily varying in the severity of the disorder with type I being the more severe and type II being more progressive.

### Fucosidosis

A deficiency in alpha-fucosidase results in the accumulation of fucose-containing sphingolipids and glycoprotein fragments. Two types have been differentiated: type I associated with frequent respiratory infections, progressive psychomotor retardation, thick skin that secretes abnormal amounts of sweat with elevated salinity and cardiomegaly, and a milder type II where the unusual sweating is absent but angiokeratomas are present.

## SUMMARY

Lipids are critical molecules to human metabolism and structure. The unique nature of the lipids requires highly specialized biochemical pathways for in vivo absorption, transport and processing, and poses special problems for in vitro analytical processes.

The many and varied forms of lipids, from the simplest fatty acids to the highly complex terpenes and sphingosines, are still the subject of investigation and discovery as more new forms are found and described. Even more exciting is the discovery of new functions of known lipids. The Fredrickson classification scheme serves as a basis to understanding the relationship of lipids and disease, but this is only the starting point in an expanding body of information.

The importance of lipids in clinical laboratory diagnosis is increasing as more lipid moieties are found to be clinically significant. As methodologies improve, lipid assays are more easily and reliably incorporated into routine laboratory testing. The diagnostic applications of lipid testing have greatly expanded our understanding of diseases. A lipid profile in 1975 was used primarily for diagnosis of cardiovascular disease and consisted of a few relatively simple tests, including simple observations. Today that lipid profile may include 5 different lipid fractions plus 2 or 3 apolipoproteins and antibodies to oxidized LDL. This wealth of information permits a greater degree of reliability in predicting cardiovascular diseases as well as various other types of lipid disorders. It is safe to say that we are only now realizing the potential for lipid testing. The clinical laboratory of the near future may offer a lipid profile as different as the modern lipid profile of today differs from its 1975 ancestor.

### REFERENCES

1. Mayes PA: Lipids of physiological significance. In Murray RK, Granner DK, et al.( eds.): *Harper's Biochem-*

*istry*, 24th ed. Stamford, CT, Appleton & Lange, 1996, pp 146–157.

2. Naito HK. Lipids. In Kaplan LA, Pesce AJ (eds.): *Clinical Chemistry: Theory, Analysis and Correlation*, 3rd ed. St. Louis, CV Mosby, 1996, pp 1041–1052.

3. Voet D, Voet JG: Lipid metabolism. In Voet D, Voet JG (eds.): *Biochemistry*. New York, John Wiley and Sons, 1990, pp 619–677.

4. Naito HK: Coronary artery disease and disorders of lipid metabolism. In Kaplan LA, Pesce AJ (eds.): *Clinical Chemistry: Theory, Analysis and Correlation*, 3rd ed. St. Louis, CV Mosby, 1996, pp 642–682.

5. Stein EA, Myers GL: Lipids, apolipoproteins and lipoproteins. In Burtis CA, Ashwood ER (eds.): *Tietz Fundamentals of Clinical Chemistry*, 4th ed. Philadelphia, WB Saunders, 1996, pp 375–401.

6. Mann WA, Meyer N, Weber W, et al.: Apolipoprotein E and lipoprotein lipase co-ordinately enhance binding and uptake of chylomicrons by human hepatocytes. Eur J Clin Invest 25:880–882, 1995.

7. Marshall WJ: Lipids and lipoproteins. In Marshall WJ (ed.): *Clinical Chemistry*, 3rd ed. London, CV Mosby, 1995, pp 213–228.

8. Murdoch SJ, Breckenridge WC: Influence of lipoprotein lipase and hepatic lipase on the transformation of VLDL and HDL during lipolysis of VLDL. Atherosclerosis 18:193–212, 1995.

9. Thuren T: Hepatic lipase and HDL metabolism. Curr Opin Lipidol 11:277–283, 2000.

10. Bruce C, Chouinard RA Jr, Tall AR: Plasma lipid transfer proteins, high-density lipoproteins, and reverse cholesterol transport. Annu Rev Nutr 18:297–330, 1998.

11. Austin MA, Hokanson JE: Epidemiology of triglycerides, small dense low-density lipoprotein, and lipoprotein (a) as risk factors for coronary heart disease. Med Clin North Am 78:99–115, 1994.

12. Duriez P, Dallongeville J, Fruchart JC: Lipoprotein (a) as a marker for coronary heart disease. Br J Clin Pract Suppl 77A:54–61, 1996.

13. Danesh J, Collins R, Peto R: Lipoprotein (a) and coronary heart disease. Circulation 102:1082–1085, 2000.

14. Rhoads GG, Dahlen G, Berg K, et al.: Lp (a) lipoprotein as a risk factor for myocardial infarction. JAMA 256:2540–2544, 1986.

15. Marcovina SM, Hegele RA, Koschinsky ML: Lipoprotein (a) and coronary heart disease risk. Curr Cardiol Rep 1(2):105–111, 1999.

16. Marcovina SM, Koschinsky ML: Lipoprotein (a) as a risk factor for coronary artery disease. Am J Cardiol 82:57U–66U, 1998.

17. Singh RB, Niaz MA, Bishnoi I, et al.: Diet, antioxidant vitamins, oxidative stress and risk of coronary artery disease: The Peerzada Prospective Study. Acta Cardiol 49:453–467, 1999.

18. Siow RC, Sato H, Leake DS, et al.: Vitamin C protects human arterial smooth muscle cells against atherogenic lipoproteins: Effects of antioxidant vitamins C and E on oxidized LDL-induced adaptive increases in cystine transport and glutathione. Arterioscler Thromb Vasc Biol 18:1662–1670, 1998.

19. Diaz MN, Frei B, Vita JA, Keaney JF Jr.: Antioxidants and atherosclerotic heart disease. N Engl J Med 337:408–416, 1997.

20. Mustacich D, Powis G: Thioredoxin reductase. Biochem J 15:346(Pt 1):1–8, 2000.

21. Jarvinen R, Knekt P, Seppanen R, et al.: Antioxidant vitamins in the diet: Relationships with other personal characteristics in Finland. J Epidemiol Community Health 48:549–554, 1994.

22. Kelly FJ: Use of antioxidants in the prevention and treatment of disease. J Int Fed Clin Chem 10(1):21–23, 1998.

23. Sniderman AD: Apolipoprotein B and apolipoprotein AI as predictors of coronary artery disease. Can J Cardiol Jul(4)(Suppl A):24A–30A, 1988.

24. Srivastava RA, Srivastava N: High density lipoprotein, apolipoprotein A-I, and coronary artery disease. Mol Cell Biochem 209(1–2):131–144, 2000.

25. Yla-Herttuala S: Expression of lipoprotein receptors and related molecules in atherosclerotic lesions. Curr Opin Lipidol 7:292–297, 1996.

26. Jong MC, Hofker MH, Havekes LM: Role of Apo Cs in lipoprotein metabolism: Functional differences between ApoC1, ApoC2, and ApoC3. Arterioscler Thromb Vasc Biol 19:472–484, 1999.

27. Ginsberg HN, Le NA, Goldberg IJ, et al.: Apolipoprotein B metabolism in subjects with deficiency of apolipoproteins CIII and AI. Evidence that apolipoprotein CIII inhibits catabolism of triglyceride-rich lipoproteins by lipoprotein lipase in vivo. J Clin Invest 78:1287–1295, 1986.

28. Sacks FM, Alaupovic P, Moye LA, et al.: VLDL, Apolipoproteins B, CIII, and E, and risk of recurrent coronary events in the cholesterol and recurrent events (CARE) trial. Circulation 102:1886–1892, 2000.

29. Goessling W, Zucker SD: Role of apolipoprotein D in the transport of bilirubin in plasma. Am J Physiol Gastrointest Liver Physiol 279:G356–G365, 2000.

30. Morton RE, Zilversmit DB: The separation of apolipoprotein D from cholesteryl ester transfer protein. Biochim Biophys Acta 663:350–355, 1981.

31. Wiebe C, Holzem G, Wielckens K, et al.: Apolipoprotein E polymorphism: Automated determination of apolipoprotein E2, E3, and E4 isoforms. Lipids 35:99–104, 2000.

32. Horita K, Eto M, Saito M, et al.: Effects of apolipoprotein E polymorphism on plasma lipoprotein (a) levels. Artery 20(6):324–336, 1993.

33. Wang T, Nakajima K, Leary ET, et al.: Ratio of remnant-like particle-cholesterol to serum total triglycerides

is an effective alternative to ultracentrifugal and electrophoretic methods in the diagnosis of familial type III hyperlipoproteinemia. Clin Chem 45:1981–1987, 1999.

34. Horejsi B, Ceska R: Apolipoproteins and atherosclerosis. Apolipoprotein E and apolipoprotein (a) as candidate genes of premature development of atherosclerosis. Physiol Res 49(Suppl 1):S63–S69, 2000.

35. de Knijff P, Kaptein A, Boomsma D, et al.: Apolipoprotein E polymorphism affects plasma levels of lipoprotein (a). Atherosclerosis 90:169–174, 1991.

36. Pati U, Pati N: Lipoprotein (a), atherosclerosis, and apolipoprotein (a) gene polymorphism. Mol Genet Metab 71:87–92, 2000.

37. Ozturk IC, Killeen AA: An overview of genetic factors influencing plasma lipid levels and coronary artery disease risk. Arch Pathol Lab Med 123:1219–1222, 1999.

38. Davignon J, Gregg RE, Sing CF: Apolipoprotein E polymorphism and atherosclerosis. Arteriosclerosis 8: 1–21, 1988.

39. Mahley RW, Huang Y: Apolipoprotein E: From atherosclerosis to Alzheimer's disease and beyond. Curr Opin Lipidol 10:207–217, 1999.

40. Sandholzer C, Saha N, Kark JD, et al.: Apo (a) isoforms predict risk for coronary heart disease. A study in six populations. Arterioscler Thromb 12:1214–1226, 1992.

41. Sangrar W, Koschinsky ML: Characterization of the interaction of recombinant apolipoprotein (a) with modified fibrinogen surfaces and fibrin clots. Biochem Cell Biol 78:519–525, 2000.

42. Seman LJ, DeLuca C, Jenner JL, et al.: Lipoprotein (a)-cholesterol and coronary heart disease in the Framingham Heart Study. Clin Chem 45:1039–1046, 1999.

43. Kinoshita M, Arai H, Fukasawa M, et al.: Apolipoprotein E enhances lipid exchange between lipoproteins mediated by cholesteryl ester transfer protein. J Lipid Res 34:261–268, 1993.

44. Moulin P: Cholesteryl ester transfer protein: An enigmatic protein. Horm Res 45(3–5):238–244, 1996.

45. Quintao EC, Medina WL, Passarelli M: Reverse cholesterol transport in diabetes mellitus. Diabetes Metab Res Rev 16:237–250, 2000.

46. Quintao EC: Is reverse cholesterol transport a misnomer for suggesting its role in the prevention of atheroma formation? Atherosclerosis 116:1–14, 1995.

47. Marcel YL, McPherson R, Hogue M, et al.: Distribution and concentration of cholesteryl ester transfer protein in plasma of normolipemic subjects. J Clin Invest 85:10–17, 1990.

48. Yamashita S, Sprecher DL, Sakai N, et al.: Accumulation of apolipoprotein E-rich high density lipoproteins in alphalipoproteinemic human subjects with plasma cholesteryl ester transfer protein deficiency. J Clin Invest 86:688–695, 1990.

49. Ikewaki K, Nishiwaki M, Sakamoto T, et al.: Increased catabolic rate of low density lipoproteins in humans with cholesteryl ester transfer protein deficiency. J Clin Invest 96:1573–1581, 1995.

50. Lehman CA: Lipids and lipoproteins. In Lehman CA (ed.): Saunders Manual of Clinical Laboratory Science. Philadelphia, WB Saunders, 1998, pp 59–76.

51. Flegg HM: An investigation of the determination of serum cholesterol by an enzymatic method. Ann Clin Biochem 10:79–83, 1973.

52. Executive Summary of the Third Report of the National Cholesterol Education Program (NCEP) Expert Panel on Detection, Evaluation, and Treatment of High Blood Cholesterol in Adults (Adult Treatment Panel III). JAMA 285:19, 2486–2497, 2001.

53. Benlian P, Cansier C, Hennache C, et al.: Comparison of a new method for the direct and simultaneous assessment of LDL- and HDL-cholesterol with ultracentrifugation and established methods Clin Chem 46: 493–505, 2000.

54. Nauck M, Winkelr K, März W, et al.: Quantitative determination of high-, low- and very-low-density lipoproteins and lipoprotein (a) by agarose gel electrophoresis and enzymatic cholesterol staining. Clin Chem 41:1761–1767, 1995.

55. Cobbaert C, Zwang L, Ceriotti F, et al.: Reference standardization and triglyceride interference of a new homogeneous HDL-cholesterol assay compared with a former chemical precipitation assay. Clin Chem 44: 779–789, 1998.

56. Nauck M, März W, Wieland H: New immunoseparation-based homogeneous assay for HDL-cholesterol compared with three homogeneous and two heterogeneous methods for HDL-cholesterol. Clin Chem 44: 1443–1451, 1998.

57. a Simó JM, Castellano I, Ferré N, et al.: Evaluation of a homogeneous assay for high-density lipoprotein cholesterol: limitations in patients with cardiovascular, renal, and hepatic disorders. Clin Chem 44:1233–1241, 1998.

58. Friedewald WT, Levy RI, Fredrickson DS: Estimation of the concentration of low density lipoprotein cholesterol in plasma without use of the preparative ultracentrifuge. Clin Chem 18:499–502, 1972.

59. Warnick RG, Knopp RH, Fitzpatrick V, et al.: Estimating low density lipoprotein cholesterol by Friedewald equation is adequate for classifying patients on the basis of nationally recommended cutpoints. Clin Chem 36:15–19, 1990.

60. Vrga L, Contacos C, Li SCH et al.: Comparison of methods for measurement of apolipoprotein B and cholesterol in low-density lipoproteins. Clin Chem 43: 390–393, 1997.

61. Esteban-Salán M, Guimón-Bardesi A, de la Viuda-Unzueta JM,et al.: Analytical and clinical evaluation of two

homogeneous assays for LDL-cholesterol in hyperlipidemic patients. Clin Chem 46:1121–1131, 2000.

62. Jialal I, Hirany SV, Devaraj S, et al.: Comparison of an immunoprecipitation method for direct measurement of LDL-cholesterol with beta-quantification (ultracentrifugation). Am J Clin Pathol 41:232–240, 1995.

63. Rifai N, Iannotti E, DeAngelis K, et al.: Analytical and clinical performance of a homogeneous enzymatic LDL-cholesterol assay compared with the ultracentrifugation-dextran sulfate-Mg$^{2+}$ method. Clin Chem 44:1242–1250, 1998.

64. Stavropoulous WS, Crouch RD: A new colorimetric procedure for the determination of serum triglycerides. Clin Chem 20:857, 1974.

65. Graziani MS, Zanolla L, Righetti G, et al.: Plasma apolipoproteins A-I and B in survivors of myocardial infarction and in a control group. Clin Chem 44:134–140, 1998.

66. Tate JR, Rifai N, Berg K, et al.: International federation of clinical chemistry standardization project for the measurement of lipoprotein(a). Phase I. Evaluation of the analytical performance of lipoprotein (a) assay systems and commercial calibrators. Clin Chem 44:1629–1640, 1998.

67. Nguyen TT, Ellefson RD, Hodge DO, et al.: Predictive value of electrophoretically detected lipoprotein (a) for coronary heart disease and cerebrovascular disease in a community-based cohort of 9936 men and women. Circulation 96:1390–1397, 1997.

68. Kronenberg F, Kronenberg MF, Kiechl S, et al.: Role of lipoprotein (a) and apolipoprotein (a) phenotype in atherogenesis: Prospective results from the Bruneck study. Circulation 100:1154–1160, 1999.

69. Liao JK: Endothelium and acute coronary syndromes. Clin Chem 44: 1799–1808, 1998.

70. Grundy SM: Role of low-density lipoproteins in atherogenesis and development of coronary heart disease. Clin Chem 41:139–146, 1995.

71. Kita T, Yokode M, Ishii K, et al.: The role of oxidized lipoproteins in the pathogenesis of atherosclerosis. Clin Exp Pharmacol Physiol Suppl 20:37–42, 1992.

72. Jialal I: Evolving lipoprotein risk factors: Lipoprotein (a) and oxidized low-density lipoprotein. Clin Chem 44:1827–1832, 1998.

73. Liang KW, Huang JL, et al.: Significantly higher levels of oxidized LDL autoantibody in coronary artery disease patients. Chung Hua I Hsueh Tsa Chih (Taipei) 63(2):101–106, 2000.

74. Vaarala O: Autoantibodies to modified LDLs and other phospholipid-protein complexes as markers of cardiovascular diseases. J Intern Med 247:381–384, 2000.

75. Endemann G, Stanton LW, Madden KS, et al.: CD 36 is a receptor for oxidized low density lipoprotein. J Biol Chem 268:11811–11816, 1993.

76. Nakata A, Nakagawa Y, Nishida M, et al.: CD36, a novel receptor for oxidized low-density lipoproteins, is highly expressed on lipid-laden macrophages in human atherosclerotic aorta. Arterioscler Thromb Vasc Biol 19:1333–1339, 1999.

77. Podrez EA, Febbraio M, Sheibani N, et al.: Macrophage scavenger receptor CD36 is the major receptor for LDL modified by monocyte-generated reactive nitrogen species. J Clin Invest 105:1483, 2000.

78. Gillotte KL, Horkko S, Witztum JL, et al.: Oxidized phospholipids, linked to apolipoprotein B of oxidized LDL, are ligands for macrophage scavenger receptors. J Lipid Res 41:824–833, 2000.

79. Santamarina-Fojo S, Lambert G, Hoeg JM, Brewer HB Jr: Lecithin-cholesterol acyltransferase: Role in lipoprotein metabolism, reverse cholesterol transport and atherosclerosis. Curr Opin Lipidol 11:267–275, 2000.

80. Gordon T, Kannel WB, Castelli WP, Dawber TR: Lipoproteins, cardiovascular disease and death. The Framingham Study. Arch Intern Med 141:1128–1130, 1981.

81. Folsom AR: 'New' risk factors for atherosclerotic diseases. Exp Gerontol 34:483–490, 1999.

82. Guerci B, Antebi H, Meyer L, et al.: Increased ability of LDL from normolipidemic type 2 diabetic women to generate peroxides. Clin Chem 45:1439–1448, 1999.

83. Polidori MC, Mecocci P, Stahl W, et al.: Plasma levels of lipophilic antioxidants in very old patients with type 2 diabetes. Diabetes Metab Res Rev 6:15–19, 2000.

84. Fallon UB, Ben-Shlomo Y, Elwood P, et al.: Homocysteine and coronary heart disease in the Caerphilly cohort: A 10 year follow up. Heart 85:153–158, 2001.

85. Fallon UB, Elwood P, Ben-Shlomo Y, et al.: Homocysteine and ischaemic stroke in men: the Caerphilly study. J Epidemiol Community Health 55(2):91–96, 2001.

86. Gale CR, Ashurst H, Phillips NJ, et al.: Renal function, plasma homocysteine and carotid atherosclerosis in elderly people. Atherosclerosis 154(1):141–146, 2001.

87. Jacobsen DW: Homocysteine and vitamins in cardiovascular disease. Clin Chem 44: 1833–1843, 1998.

88. Taylor BV, Oudit GY, Evans M: Homocysteine, vitamins, and coronary artery disease. Comprehensive review of the literature. Can Fam Physician 46:2236–2245, 2000.

89. Ueland PM, Refsum H, Stabler SP, et al.: Total homocysteine in plasma or serum: Methods and clinical applications. Clin Chem 39:1764–1779, 1993.

90. Powers HJ, Moat SJ: Developments in the measurement of plasma total homocysteine. Curr Opin Clin Nutr Metab Care 3:391–397, 2000.

91. Caudill SP, Cooper GR, Smith SJ, Myers GL: Assessment of current National Cholesterol Education Program guidelines for total cholesterol, triglyceride, HDL-cholesterol, and LDL-cholesterol measurements. Clin Chem 1998 44:1650–1658, 1998.

92. Medh JD, Bowen SL, Fry GL, et al.: Lipoprotein lipase

binds to low density lipoprotein receptors and induces receptor-mediated catabolism of very low density lipoproteins in vitro. J Biol Chem 271:17073–17080, 1996.

93. Frikke-Schmidt R, Arlien-Soborg P, Thorsen S, et al.: LDL receptor mutations and ApoB mutations are not risk factors for ischemic cerebrovascular disease of the young, but lipids and lipoproteins are. Eur J Neurol 6(6):691–696, 1999.
94. Goldstein JL, Brown MS: The LDL receptor defect in familial hypercholesterolemia. Med Clin North Am 66:335–362, 1982.
95. Day IN, Whittall RA, O'Dell SD, et al.: Spectrum of LDL receptor gene mutations in heterozygous familial hypercholesterolemia. Hum Mutat 10(2):116–127, 1997.
96. Haddad L, Day IN, Hunt S, et al.: Evidence for a third genetic locus causing familial hypercholesterolemia. A non-LDLR, non-APOB kindred. J Lipid Res 40:1113–1122, 1999.
97. Pedersen JC, Berg K. Interaction between low density lipoprotein receptor (LDLR) and apolipoprotein E (apoE) alleles contributes to normal variation in lipid level. Clin Genet 35(5):331–337, 1989.
98. Tacken PJ, Beer FD, Vark LC, et al.: Very-low-density lipoprotein binding to the apolipoprotein E receptor 2 is enhanced by lipoprotein lipase, and does not require apolipoprotein E. Biochem J 347(Pt 2):357–361, 2000.
99. Dergunov AD, Smirnova EA, Merched A, et al.: Structural peculiarities of the binding of very low density lipoproteins and low density lipoproteins to the LDL receptor in hypertriglyceridemia: Role of apolipoprotein E. Biochim Biophys Acta 1484(1):29–40, 2000.
100. Hua CT, Hopwood JJ, Carlsson SR, et al.: Evaluation of the lysosome-associated membrane protein LAMP-2 as a marker for lysosomal storage disorders. Clin Chem 44:2094–2102, 1998.

## BIBLIOGRAPHY

Burtis CA., Ashwood ER: *Tietz Fundamentals of Clinical Chemistry*, 4th ed. Philadelphia, WB Saunders, 1996.

Marshall WJ: *Clinical Chemistry*, 3rd ed. London, CV Mosby, 1995.

Kaplan, LA, Pesce AJ: *Clinical Chemistry: Theory, Analysis and Correlation*, 3rd ed. St. Louis, CV Mosby, 1996.

Murray RK, Granner DK, et al.: *Harper's Biochemistry 24th ed.* Stamford, CT, Appleton & Lange, 1996.

# CHAPTER 12
# Proteins

*Joan Radtke*

**Proteins** are polymers of amino acids produced by living cells in all forms of life. Each form of life is defined in large measure by the protein it produces. An amazing variety of proteins exist with diverse functions, sizes, shapes, and structures but each is composed of only 20 different amino acids in varying numbers and sequences.[1,2] The sequence of amino acids, which ultimately determines the characteristics of the protein, is determined by genetic information contained in the nucleus of the cell. All proteins contain carbon, hydrogen, oxygen, sulfur, and nitrogen. The presence of nitrogen differentiates proteins from carbohydrates and lipids and contributes approximately 16% of protein mass.

Protein is composed of L-alpha–amino acids. The nucleus of the amino acid is the alpha carbon to which the carboxylic acid ($-COOH$) and amine ($-NH_3$) groups are attached. Also attached to the alpha carbon is a hydrogen molecule and one other group frequently referred to as an R group. This means that except for glycine, where the other group is another hydrogen, the amino acid is asymmetric and two isomers are possible. The isomer found in nature has the L configuration. The D- and L-alpha–amino acid structures (stereoisomers) can be seen in Figure 12–1. Complete hydrolysis of all protein yields only 20 amino acids, although many others are found in nature. In higher forms of life, like humans, some amino acids are not synthesized and must be ingested. Amino acids that must be present in the diet are called essential amino acids and in humans they include: valine, leucine, isoleucine, phenylalanine, tryptophan, threonine, methionine, and lysine.

All 20 amino acids have the structure indicated in Figure 12–1. Amino acids are **amphoteric,** meaning that they contain 2 ionizable sites and, depending on the pH of their environment, the sites can be negative, positive, or neutral. At physiologic pH, approximately 7.4, both sites are ionized, the COOH easily loses a hydrogen ion and becomes $COO^-$, and the $NH_2$ easily gains the hydrogen ion and becomes $NH_3^+$. When both sites are ionized, the amino acid is called an **ampholyte** or **zwitterion.** The R group on each amino acid is different and may also have ionizable groups. In highly acidic solutions (low pH), amino acids have a net positive charge and in highly alkaline solutions (high pH), amino acids have a net negative charge.

Each amino acid has a pH at which it is neutral, having no net surface charge. This is called the **isoelectric point** (pI) and is a function of the R group. The isoelectric points for amino acids range from approximately pH 3 to 10, so there is no pH at which all 20 amino acids will be neutral at the same time. Individual protein molecules, like amino acids, also have unique isoelectric points.

Amino acids are linked to each other through **peptide bonds,** which are illustrated by the following reaction:

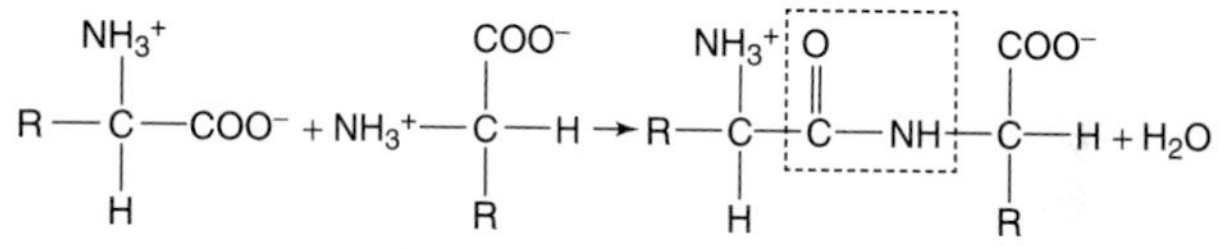

$$NH_3^+ \quad\quad COO^- \quad\quad NH_3^+\ O \quad\quad COO^-$$
$$R-\underset{H}{\overset{|}{C}}-COO^- + NH_3^+-\underset{R}{\overset{|}{C}}-H \rightarrow R-\underset{H}{\overset{|}{C}}-\overset{\|}{C}-NH-\underset{R}{\overset{|}{C}}-H + H_2O$$

The covalent peptide bond is formed when the carboxyl group of one amino acid joins the amino group of another. A molecule of water is formed as a byproduct. Equilibrium favors hydrolysis so energy is expended in activating the carboxyl group and causing the reaction to go forward.

## CLASSIFICATION

Proteins are structurally diverse molecules having many unique functions. Although there is no universally satisfactory classification system, a number of systems have been developed and are useful to clinical laboratory scientists.

### Structure

The **primary structure** of a protein is determined by the type and number of amino acids and the amino acid sequence linked by covalent peptide bonds. The amino acid sequence for all proteins is determined by DNA coding. Even in a very large protein, one amino acid substitution can alter biologic activity. The **secondary structure** is the one dimensional shape the strand of amino acids takes as amino acids interact with adjacent amino acids through hydrogen bonds, disulfide linkages between the cysteine amino acids, and other polar and nonpolar R group interactions. The peptide bond is not free to rotate. Many of the bonds associated with the R groups, however, can rotate and this rotation allows conformational changes that cause the secondary shape to form. The secondary shapes are described as pleated sheet, alpha helix, or random coil. The **tertiary structure** is the three-dimensional structure that forms as the amino acids interact with more

L Alpha Amino Acid                          D Alpha Amino Acid

$$H_2N-\underset{\underset{R}{|}}{\overset{\overset{COOH}{|}}{C}}-H \qquad\qquad H-\underset{\underset{R}{|}}{\overset{\overset{COOH}{|}}{C}}-NH_2$$

**FIGURE 12-1**

D and L structures of amino acids.

distant members of the chain, causing it to fold and take its characteristic shape. The tertiary shape of the protein is mainly the result of hydrophobic interactions, but electrovalent linkages, hydrogen bonds, disulfide bridges, and van der Waals forces also play a role. The **quaternary structure** is formed when two or more chains attract to form aggregates. These chains are called monomers or subunits and the final proteins formed are called dimers, tetramers, or oligomers. Disruption of the bonds holding the secondary, tertiary, or quaternary structures together is called **denaturation** and can cause **inactivation** or loss of function of the protein. Denaturation is accomplished by heat, pH changes, chemicals such as detergents, metals and solvents, and by mechanical forces. The bonds that hold the protein's tertiary and quaternary structure together are very weak. It is important in the clinical laboratory setting to note that excessive heat, a freeze–thaw cycle, or vigorous mixing can break these bonds and thus denature the protein. An enzyme can lose its activity, a receptor can lose its ability to bind, and an antigen can lose its antigenicity and fail to be recognized by the antibody if these proteins are denatured before being assayed.[2]

## Shape

Proteins are classified by shape as globular and fibrous. Globular proteins are compact, tightly folded, and coiled chains. The majority of serum proteins are globular. Fibrous proteins such as hair, collagen, and fibrin are mostly structural proteins.[1]

## Solubility

Fibrous proteins are insoluble in aqueous solution. Globular proteins are generally soluble in water or weak salt solutions. Insoluble proteins form precipitates that can easily be separated from soluble proteins by centrifugation or filtration. Loss of solubility occurs when the solute, in this case protein, loses its attraction to the solvent. Properties of the solute that influence solubility include: pH, ionic strength, temperature, and dielectric constant. Differences in solubility can be used to separate the major plasma fractions, **albumin** and **globulins,** from each other. This separation or salting out of proteins involves precipitating them in saturated ammonium sulfate. When the concentration of the ammonium sulfate is reduced to about 50% saturated, the albumin dissolves and the globulins remain precipitated. The varying solubilities of proteins are helpful in some clinical applications, such as preparation of protein free filtrates or isolation of proteins from a solution, but are of limited use in classification.[2]

## Composition

**Simple proteins** are proteins composed only of amino acids. Some proteins, however, that contain permanently associated non–amino acid groups are termed **conjugated proteins.** The amino acid portion of the conjugated protein molecule is called the **apoprotein** and the non–amino acid portion is called the **prosthetic group.** The name of the conjugated protein is derived from the prosthetic group as shown in Table 12–1. Most plasma proteins are glycoproteins. Albumin, however, which represents about half of the total serum protein concentration, is a simple protein.[2]

## Electrophoretic Mobility

A protein molecule retains some of the electrical charge characteristics of the amino acids. Most of the charges are from the R groups since the amino and carboxylic acid terminals are involved in the peptide bonds that form the protein. The

**TABLE 12-1**

**Classification of Complex Proteins**

| CLASSIFICATION | PROSTHETIC GROUP | EXAMPLE |
|---|---|---|
| Lipoprotein | Lipid | High-density lipoprotein (HDL) |
| Glycoprotein | Carbohydrate (<4% of molecule) | Immunoglobulin G |
| Mucoprotein | Carbohydrate (>4% of molecule) | Hemopexin |
| Metalloprotein | Metal | Hemoglobin: iron |
| | | Ferritin: iron |
| | | Ceruloplasmin: copper |
| | | Alcohol dehydrogenase: zinc |
| Phosphoprotein | Phosphate | Casein of milk |

TABLE 12-2

**Electrophoretic Fractions: Major Constituent Proteins and Approximate Reference Values for Relative Percentage and Concentration\*,3**

| FRACTION | RELATIVE PERCENT (%) | CONCENTRATION (G/DL) |
|---|---|---|
| Prealbumin (Transthyretin) | Usually not detected by routine SPE | 0.01–0.04 |
| Albumin | 50 | 3.2–5.5 |
| Alpha-1 | 5 | 0.1–0.3 |
|   Alpha-1-acid glycoprotein | | |
|   Alpha-1antitrypsin | | |
|   Alpha-1-fetoprotein | | |
|   Alpha-1-lipoprotein (HDL) | | |
| Alpha-2 | 10 | 0.6–1.0 |
|   Haptoglobin | | |
|   Alpha-2-macroglobulin | | |
|   Ceruloplasmin | | |
| Beta | 15 | 0.7–1.1 |
|   Transferrin | | |
|   Hemopexin | | |
|   Beta-lipoprotein (LDL and VLDL) | | |
|   Beta-2-microglobulin | | |
|   Complement (C3 and C4) | | |
|   Fibrinogen (plasma only) | | |
| Gamma | 20 | 0.8–1.6 |
|   IgG | | |
|   IgM | | |
|   IgA | | |
|   IgD | | |
|   IgE | | |
|   C-Reactive protein | | |

\*Assuming a usual total protein reference interval of 6.0 to 8.3 g/dL.

SPE = serum protein electrophoresis; HDL = high-density lipoprotein; LDL = low-density lipoprotein; VLDL = very low-density lipoprotein.

**electrophoretic mobility** of the protein is determined by the **charge** and **size** of the molecule and by other factors that will be discussed later in this chapter. The traditional electrophoretic mobility classification of serum, urine, and cerebrospinal fluid proteins is based on electrophoresis on cellulose acetate media at pH 8.6. At pH 8.6, most body fluid proteins carry a net negative charge and migrate toward the anode (positive pole). The proteins separate into 5 fractions or bands based on their movement in an electrical field. The albumin fraction migrates the farthest because it has the lowest pI and is therefore the most negatively charged. Each fraction contains proteins that are different functionally but similar electrophoretically. Table 12–2 is a list of the proteins found in each major body fluid fraction.

## Function

Proteins are commonly classified, or grouped, according to their function in the body. Table 12–3 lists the most important

protein functions that testify to the tremendous role of proteins in biochemical processes.[1]

TABLE 12-3

**The Classification of Proteins According to Function**

1. Catalysts (enzymes)
2. Regulatory proteins: receptors, hormones, repressors, and inhibitors
3. Transport proteins: albumin, transferrin, and haptoglobin
4. Structural proteins: contractile, fibrous, and keratinous proteins
5. Protective proteins: immunoglobulins and complement
6. Oncofetal and placental proteins: alpha$_1$-fetoprotein
7. Proteins that have unknown functions

## Size, Density, and Mass

Proteins are sometimes categorized by their size, density, and mass. Techniques that sort proteins using these characteristics include ultracentrifugation, gel filtration, and sodium dodecyl sulfate polyacrylamide gel electrophoresis (SDS PAGE). These techniques will be discussed later in this chapter.

---

## METABOLISM: SYNTHESIS AND DEGRADATION

Digestion of protein begins in the stomach. Gastric secretions include **hydrochloric acid** (with a pH of 1) and **pepsin.** The strong acid unfolds or denatures the protein and exposes the peptide bonds to the gastric proteolytic enzyme, pepsin. Pepsin acts specifically on the peptide bonds between those amino acids containing an aromatic ring or carboxylic acid in their R group, breaking the proteins into shorter polypeptides. As the polypeptides move into the small intestine, the pH changes from acidic to basic, and pepsin is inactivated. The digestive enzymes of the small intestine such as trypsin, chymotrypsin, and carboxypeptidase function at an alkaline pH and continue the process of breaking down dietary protein into its amino acid building blocks. Digestion is completed as free amino acids are absorbed across the intestinal wall, a process that requires active transport and is energy dependent. The amino acids absorbed into circulation are available to all types of body tissues undergoing protein synthesis.[3]

In a process similar to digestion, proteins of living cells are constantly being degraded and resynthesized. This process is called **protein turnover.** The daily turnover rate involves 1% to 2% of the total protein in the body. Infants and children have higher turnover rates since they experience rapid growth.

Many proteins are turned over in the cells where they exist by the action of peptidases and proteases. Plasma proteins, however, are bound by specific receptors on the cells of the liver, internalized and degraded there. Protein turnover, or degradation rate, is described as the **half-life** and defined as the time required to reduce the concentration by half if no new protein is produced. Individual proteins have different rates of turnover. Enzymes have very short half-lives, whereas muscle tissue and other structural proteins have long half-lives.[3]

Protein metabolism is partially regulated by many **hormones.** Triiodothyronine, cortisol, aldosterone, somatotropin, and growth hormone play a significant role in protein production in tissues that they target by regulating the induction or repression of protein synthesis. For example, bone-forming cells (osteoblasts) have receptors for parathyroid hormone (PTH), activated vitamin D, and estrogen. These hormones stimulate the structural genes that specify the amino acid sequence for synthesis of insulinlike growth factor I (IGF-I), a protein that regulates bone formation and modeling.[3]

Synthesis of most plasma proteins such as albumin, fib-

rinogen, lipoproteins, haptoglobin, and many more occurs in the liver. The immunoglobulins and hemoglobin in the adult, produced by plasma cells and red blood cells, respectively, are the only exception.[2,3]

Urea, a major nitrogenous waste product, is the end product of protein catabolism. Excess amino acids, those not needed to build new proteins, have the amine group removed by transaminases specific for one amino acid–alpha keto acid pair as illustrated in this general reaction:

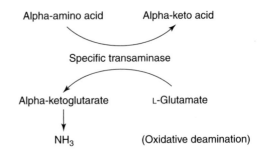

The **ammonia** produced by oxidative deamination is converted to **urea** in the liver. Urea is filtered by the kidney and becomes a major constituent of urine, accounting for about half of the dissolved solids.[4] After deamination of the amino acid, the remaining remnant, a carbon chain, is converted to fat or is used to produce energy by processes similar to those utilized in carbohydrate metabolism.

---

## GENERAL ANALYTICAL PROCESSES

The proteins that are most frequently analyzed in a clinical laboratory setting are those present in serum or plasma. Proteins in other body fluids such as urine and cerebrospinal fluid (CSF) may also be tested. Protein analyses, depending on the method used, can be qualitative, semiquantitative, or quantitative. Some methods measure all proteins, whereas others measure groups of proteins or specific individual proteins. Summarized below are the analytical processes routinely used for protein analysis in the clinical laboratory. Also mentioned are methods used in research settings that provide fundamental information on proteins that are useful for the development, evaluation, and understanding of routine methods.

### Spectrophotometry, Turbidimetry, Nephelometry, and Refractometry

Serum total protein and serum albumin tests are frequently ordered and commonly measured using automated quantitative procedures based on **spectrophotometry.** These methods will be detailed later in the chapter. Although rarely used, refractometry can roughly quantitate serum proteins and is based on the refractive index varying with protein concentration.

In research settings, spectrophotometers, capable of accurate measurements in the ultraviolet range, are used to measure the protein concentration of solutions with low protein levels such as CSF and specific protein standards. Since tryptophan and tyrosine absorb light at 280 nm, absorbance measurements taken at this wavelength are used to estimate the protein concentration of a sample.

**Turbidimetry** and **nephelometry,** as described in Chapter 6 on spectrophotometry, are related techniques that involve passing a beam of light through a suspension of insoluble particles and measuring the amount of light blocked or scattered. Nephelometry is generally more sensitive than turbidimetry. **Laser nephelometry,** which uses a laser beam as a light source, improves the sensitivity even more. Quantitative and semiquantitative procedures for urine protein and CSF are based on the measurement of insoluble complexes (turbidity) that forms when acids such as sulfosalicylic acid (SSA) or trichloroacetic acid (TCA) are used to denature the proteins present in these dilute protein solutions. A spectrophotometer can be used to measure the turbidity or, alternatively, a simple nephelometer can be used to measure the scatter of light. These measurements are then used to estimate or quantitate the solution's protein concentration.[2]

Some immunochemical reactions can be detected using nephelometry. Proteins, such as IgG and IgA, are so large that when they react with specific antisera, large complexes or particles form that are detected using laser nephelometry. A laser beam is directed at the suspensions and the amount of light scattered or the rate of increased scatter (rate nephelometry) is compared to that of known protein standards.

## Immunochemical

Immunochemical assays utilize antibodies to bind and thus identify the protein being measured. Laboratory testing based on this simple immunologic process has extremely wide application in the clinical laboratory and is used to measure hundreds of different types of proteins in biologic fluids. The exquisite specificity and sensitivity of immunologic methods, such as nephelometric and turbidimetric imunoassays, enzyme-linked immunoassays, and chemiluminescent immunoassays to name but a few, allow us to measure small concentrations of unique proteins such as ferritin, C-reactive protein, parathyroid hormone, and lipoproteins. A full discussion of immunochemical techniques is presented in the Chapter 7.

## Electrophoresis

**Electrophoresis** is the migration of charged molecules through a buffered medium in response to an electrical field. In the clinical laboratory, the purpose of performing electrophoresis on body fluids such as serum, red blood cell hemolysates, urine, and CSF is to separate the constituent protein into major fractions. Once the proteins are separated, selective staining can be used to visualize all protein or groups of serum proteins such as lipoproteins and enzymes. Laboratory professionals are trained to interpret electrophoretic patterns and correlate abnormal findings with disease states.[5,6]

Proteins, like the amino acids they are composed of, are amphoteric. Since each protein molecule is composed of many amino acids with ionizable groups, the net amount or surface charge on the molecule is variable. The pI of the protein and the pH of the buffer solution together determine the overall charge on the amphoteric protein molecule. Protein molecules can be positively charged (cations), negatively charged (anions), or they can be neutral, depending on the pH of the solution and their unique pI. Recall that the pI, or **isoelectric point,** is the pH at which the protein is neutral. Neutral proteins will not migrate in an electrical field. If the pH of the solution is higher or more basic than the pI (pH > pI), the protein carries a net negative charge and migrates toward the anode (+pole). If the pH is lower or more acidic than the pI (pH < pI), the protein carries a net positive charge and will migrate toward the cathode (−pole). For example, using routine electrophoresis (buffer pH = 8.6), albumin migrates the farthest because it has the lowest pI (around 4.7) and is therefore the most negatively charged. The slowest migrating gamma globulin fraction contains proteins with isoelectric points as high as 7.3.

The **rate of migration** during electrophoresis depends not only on the net charge of the molecule but also on the size and shape of the molecule, the strength of the electrical field, the porosity, viscosity, and temperature of the support media and electroendosmosis. Heat production and velocity of migration must be carefully balanced. Diffusion of the protein into the gel increases with time, causing poor **resolution** of bands; thus better resolution is possible with faster migration rates. Production of excess amounts of heat may denature the protein and cause changes in the consistency of the support media. Denatured proteins do not migrate in an electrical field and can cause a background artifact known as **trailing.** Heat removal, facilitated by an effective cooling system, allows for better resolution without protein denaturation or destruction of the separation media.

**Electroendosmosis** (EEO) is a buffer flow effect that results in the displacement of the separated proteins toward the cathode (−pole). The effect is due to a negatively charged support media that attracts positively charged buffer ions. The positive buffer ions migrate toward the cathode when exposed to an electrical field. The proteins at pH 8.6 are negative (anions) and migrate toward the anode against the buffer flow. The rate of buffer flow or EEO varies among different support media. Some EEO is helpful as it tends to separate the gamma region from the proteins of other regions. Electroendosmosis is what causes the gamma region to be cathodic to the point of application in cellulose acetate protein electrophoresis. The gamma globulins are negatively charged but

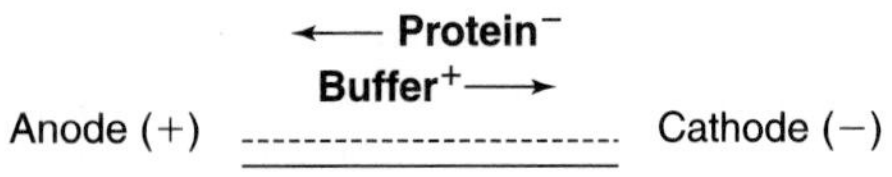

←—— **Protein⁻**

**Buffer⁺**——→

Anode (+) -------------------------- Cathode (−)

**FIGURE 12-2**

Diagram illustrating electroendosmosis. ----------- represents the negatively charged support media. Since the negative charges are attached, they do not migrate. The positively charged buffer ions migrate when the current is applied, causing a flow of buffer ions toward the cathode. The negative proteins move against the buffer flow toward the anode.

they are also large and the charge is not sufficient to overcome the effect of the buffer flow (Figure 12–2).

The basic steps involved in electrophoresis are:

1. Apparatus and support media preparation. The electrophoretic cell and voltage meter are prepared following manufacturer specifications. The buffer most commonly used for electrophoresis of proteins is barbital buffer having a pH near 8.6. Some support media, cellulose acetate for example, must be soaked in buffer before applying the sample (Figure 12–3).
2. Sample application. Sample is applied to the media in a narrow band or spot using the method appropriate for the type of media used. Diffusion of the applied sample must be avoided by starting the electrophoresis immediately after applying the sample.
3. Electrophoresis. The support media is placed in the electrophoretic cell and voltage is applied. For protein migration to occur, conductivity between the support media

and the cell buffer chambers must be continuous, so it is important to check the positioning of the support media within the cell.

4. Protein fixation and visualization. After completion of the electrophoresis, the media is treated to allow visualization of the proteins. This step involves protein fixation and staining. Fixation may be accomplished by precipitating the proteins with acids, salts, or antibody, or by blotting the proteins onto a nitrocellulose membrane. This is done so that the proteins will not diffuse into the gel and the bands will remain sharp. Staining may be done using stains or labeled antibody. If the protein is an enzyme, a substrate that will form a colored product may be used. Protein stains commonly used include Coomassie brilliant blue, amido black, ponceau S, silver stain, and immunostains labeled with horseradish peroxidase. In the case of capillary electrophoresis, the proteins, as they are eluted, pass through a detector that directly measures the UV absorbance of the peptide bonds. The fixation and staining steps in capillary electrophoresis are therefore eliminated.
5. Densitometry. A densitometer is an instrument that scans a separated and stained electrophoretogram to measure the absorbance or fluorescence of the bands. The instrument directly determines the percentage that each band contributes to the entire pattern. When provided with the total concentration in terms of weight/volume or U/L of the proteins being separated, the instrument can calculate the concentration of the protein within each band. As shown in Figure 12–4 with serum protein electrophoresis, the instrument prepares a tracing showing the intensity of each band relative to others and the percentage and concentration of protein under each major fraction.[5]

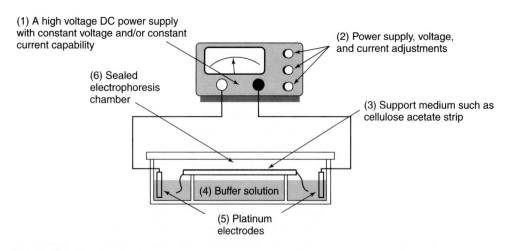

(1) A high voltage DC power supply with constant voltage and/or constant current capability

(2) Power supply, voltage, and current adjustments

(6) Sealed electrophoresis chamber

(3) Support medium such as cellulose acetate strip

(4) Buffer solution

(5) Platinum electrodes

**FIGURE 12-3**

A simple diagram of an electrophoresis chamber. (Redrawm from Karselis TC: *The Pocket Guide to Clinical Laboratory Instrumentation*, Philadelphia, FA Davis, 1994. Reprinted with permission.)

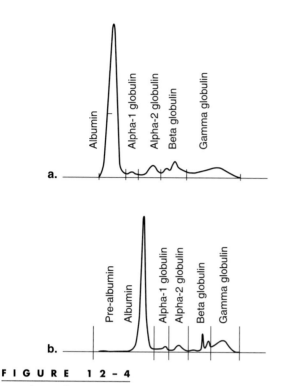

F I G U R E   1 2 - 4

Electrophoretic pattern of a normal serum. **a.** Electrophoretic pattern obtained by densitometric scanning of
a stained agarose gel. **b.** Electrophoretic pattern of
the same serum obtained in the Paragon CZE 2000.
(Redrawn from Thormann W, Wey AB, Lurie IS, et al.:
Capillary electrophoresis in clinical and forensic
analysis: Recent advances and breakthrough to routine
applications. Electrophoresis 20:3203, 1999. Reprinted
with permission.)

## Zone Electrophoresis

Zone electrophoresis uses a porous medium to support the
buffer and allow migration of the charged protein molecules
through it. Cellulose acetate, agarose gel, and polyacrylamide
gel are the types of zone electrophoresis media used in a clinical laboratory setting. The type of equipment needed, the resolution (sharpness of the bands and the degree of separation
of bands from each other), and the buffers and visualization
techniques utilized vary with the type selected.

**Cellulose acetate** is commonly used for electrophoresis
of serum proteins and red blood cell hemoglobins. It has the
advantages of being inexpensive, easily automated, and does
not require a cooling apparatus or an expensive power supply.
It has a high amount of EEO, which may work well for some
applications but leads to diffuse bands. High-resolution separation using cellulose acetate is therefore not possible. The
medium has the disadvantage of being opaque and requires
chemical treatment to partially clarify it before densitometry.

It also has the disadvantage of having a small pore size, which
limits its usefulness for separation of large molecules.

**Agarose gel** has several advantages over cellulose acetate.
The medium comes in various purities, which makes it possible to adjust for the amount of EEO needed. The pore size is
also variable, depending on the concentration of agarose used.
A larger pore size makes possible the separation of large molecules such as lipoproteins and nucleic acids. Agarose gel can
be used for immunochemical applications because antibody
may easily be added to the agarose before the media is poured
or antibody may be allowed to diffuse into the gels after electrophoresis is complete. The resolution possible with agarose,
which varies with voltage, is also much better than the resolution obtained with cellulose acetate. During high-voltage
electrophoresis, it is necessary to keep the gel cool. The equipment is therefore more expensive than that used for cellulose
acetate electrophoresis. More sensitive densitometry is possible with agarose gel because the media is clear. Agarose gel
medium is fragile, so the gels must be handled carefully.

**Polyacrylamide gel** is less fragile than agarose gel and it
allows even better resolution of the protein fractions. Pore size
is variable but is not as large as that of agarose, so electrophoresis of large molecules like nucleic acids is not possible.
The separated molecules, since they are restricted by the pore
size as well as electrophoretic properties, achieve better resolution. Gradient gels, with large pore size on the cathodic end
(application area) and small pore size on the anodic end, are
available to further aid in the separation of molecules based
on size as well as electrophoretic mobility. The optical clarity
of the gel is similar to that of agarose. Polyacrylamide gel has
no EEO.

### CAPILLARY ELECTROPHORESIS

Capillary electrophoresis (CE) is the newest method of separation based on movement of a molecule in an electrical field
(Figure 12–5). This technique is changing the way many proteins and polypeptides are studied in diagnostic and forensic
laboratories because it is rapid, sensitive, and adaptable to automation. Clinical laboratories performing electrophoresis in
high volume are replacing cellulose acetate and agarose-gel
manual systems with automated CE systems. Capillary electrophoresis also promises to be useful for the evaluation of
hemoglobin variants and the quantitation of hemoglobin $A_2$,
hemoglobin F, and glycated hemoglobins.[7]

Proteins are separated in a capillary of fused silica. Capillaries containing gel or ampholyte solutions are also used. The
internal diameter of the columns range from 20 to 200 $\mu$m
and are 10 to 100 cm in length. The empty capillaries have a
negatively charged surface, contributing to a high EEO. The
buffer flows in the direction of the cathode. The anions in the
solution migrate toward the anode, which is in opposition to
the flow of the buffer. The sample is loaded at the cathode and
then both ends of the capillaries are immersed in the buffer
containing electrode chambers. The technique has very small

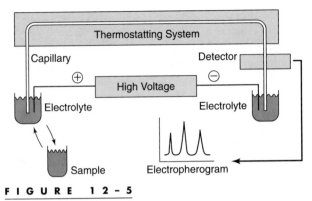

A schematic diagram of a typical capillary electrophoresis instrument. (Redrawn from Karcher RE, Nuttall K: Electrophoresis. In Burtis CA, Ashwood ER (eds.): *Tietz Textbook of Clinical Chemistry*, 3rd ed. Philadelphia, WB Saunders, 1999. Reprinted with permission.)

sample volume requirements and proteins are not denatured during the process.

Capillary electrophoresis has very efficient heat transfer, allowing the use of high voltage and resulting in rapid separation and high resolution. The Paragon CZE 2000 (Beckman Instruments, Palo Alto, CA) was designed for separation and analysis of serum proteins. The system features 7 parallel capillaries (20 $\mu$m ID-fused silica, 20 cm length), operates with primary tubes, has a throughput of 42 samples per hour, and has a computerized data management system. During CE, proteins migrate past a detection window in the capillary, where UV absorbance measurements are taken. The amount of light absorbed at 214 nm by peptide bonds is directly related to protein concentration. Serum protein electrophoresis patterns produced using CE are very similar to those produced using cellulose acetate and agarose gel. The high resolution of CE, however, demonstrates distinct transferrin and complement peaks in the beta region.[6]

## IMMUNOFIXATION ELECTROPHORESIS

Immunofixation electrophoresis is a two-step process involving agarose gel electrophoresis followed by the use of specific antibody that is layered over the separated proteins. The antibody serves to fix the antigen in the gel and to identify it. After staining, the resulting patterns confirm the identity of monoclonal proteins that were initially found on routine serum protein electrophoresis.

To identify the most common monoclonal proteins, the specimen (serum, urine, or CSF) is placed in the wells of an agarose-gel membrane that can accommodate 6 electrophoretic separations. Each individual separation is then covered with a porous material containing antiserum to one of the following: a mixture of human proteins, IgG, IgA, IgM, lambda chain, and kappa chain. If the antigen is present in the specimen, the

antibody reacts with it, forming an insoluble complex that adheres to the gel and is easily stained.[2]

## ISOELECTRIC FOCUSING

Isoelectric focusing, used primarily in a research setting, is a high-resolution technique that separates proteins on the basis of their isoelectric point (pI). This is accomplished by adding ampholytes to a support media such as agarose or polyacrylamide gels. Ampholytes are small amphoteric molecules of varying pIs that, when exposed to an electrical field, migrate to form a pH gradient. The protein sample, when applied to the isogel, migrates in an electrical field until the proteins reach the area of the gel where the pH is equal to the pI of the protein. At this point, migration stops and the proteins are "focused" or distributed in very narrow bands based on their pI (Figure 12–6).[1]

## SDS PAGE

SDS PAGE is another electrophoretic technique commonly used to estimate the size of a protein or determine the **purity** of protein solution. A detergent, sodium dodecyl sulfate (SDS), is added to the polyacrylamide gel and electrophoresis is performed after application of the proteins. SDS coats the protein, making it more soluble and increasing the negative charge until the charge is directly proportional to the size of the protein. SDS PAGE is used primarily in research to characterize proteins during purification.[1]

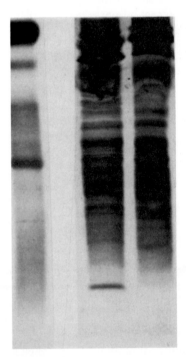

Agarose isogel pH 4 to 5 used for A1A phenotyping, and pH 3 to 10 used for CSF oligoclonal banding (stained with silver stain).

## TWO-DIMENSIONAL ELECTROPHORESIS

Two-dimensional electrophoresis allows the resolution of complex mixtures of proteins by combining the processes of isoelectric focusing (pI) with SDS page (size). Proteins are first separated by isoelectric focusing. A gel that is cylindrical in shape is used. After the proteins are focused, the gel is placed on the sample application area of a rectangular-shaped SDS PAGE system and electrophoresed a second time. The resulting electrophoretogram would have proteins separated by their **pI** in one dimension and by their **size** in the other. Since two-dimensional patterns are so complicated, typically over a thousand proteins for a normal serum specimen, computers are commonly used to analyze the pattern. Two-dimensional electrophoresis is performed in research settings.[5]

## Column Chromatography

Gel, affinity, and ion exchange column chromatography are used for protein separation in the research setting and have some application in the clinical laboratory. Gel filtration chromatography is based on the **size** of the protein and is most often used to **purify** proteins for purposes other than clinical analysis. The gel is selected based on the size of its pores. When the protein is applied to the column, small molecules are freer to interact with the gel and flow slowly through the column. Larger molecules are unable to enter the pores and therefore pass through the column rapidly. **Affinity chromatography** is based on reversible adsorption to the column. There are many types of adsorbents to choose from, including enzyme substrate, inhibitor or cofactor, antigen, lectin, nucleic acid, hormone, or cellular surface material. The technique, therefore, can be adjusted to isolate or purify many specific types of proteins. Elution from the column is accomplished by changing the ionic strength, pH, or polarity of the buffer. **Ion exchange chromatography** separates proteins based on the net surface charge of the proteins and is used in the clinical setting for separation and analysis of hemoglobin variants and glycated hemoglobins.[8]

## CLINICAL APPLICATIONS

The proteins that are most frequently analyzed in the clinical laboratory are the plasma proteins. However, proteins in other body fluids such as urine and CSF may also be analyzed. Most plasma proteins are synthesized in the liver with the immunoglobulins being the major exception. Immunoglobulins are produced by plasma cells. Serum contains the same proteins as plasma with the exception of fibrinogen, which is consumed in the clotting process.

## Total Protein

### PATHOPHYSIOLOGY

Total protein is measured in serum as a part of routine chemistry profiles. The total serum protein reference interval for an ambulatory adult is between 6.4 and 8.3 g/dL (64 to 83 g/L).[8] This interval may vary since each laboratory must establish its own ranges for analytes based on methodology and patient population. A major collective function of the serum proteins is to maintain the **colloidal osmotic pressure** of plasma. Plasma osmotic pressure prevents the loss of fluid into the tissues. The total protein content of serum is influenced by an individual's nutritional status, hepatic function, renal function, and presence of metabolic errors or diseases such as multiple myeloma. Even though total serum protein can be easily quantitated by the biuret method, it is the variations in the specific protein fractions that are most useful for diagnosing a disease.

**Dehydration** causes all fractions of protein to be increased by the same percentage. A dehydrated patient commonly has hyperproteinemia. Dehydration may be caused by decreased fluid intake or by increased water loss in diseases such as Addison's disease, diabetic acidosis, or severe diarrhea. Multiple myeloma is a malignancy causing an overproduction of one protein fraction. An increase in the serum total protein is a common finding.[2]

**Hypoproteinemia** may be due to increased protein loss or to low protein intake as found in starvation or malabsorption disorders. Accelerated protein loss may be due to a disease such as nephrotic syndrome where albumin is lost through damaged tubules. Hypoproteinemia may also be due to blood loss that occurs as the result of a traumatic injury. In this case, water is replaced more rapidly than the proteins. Serum protein levels also decrease in patients with extensive burns.

### METHODOLOGY

Total protein is measured in serum, plasma, CSF, cytosol preparations, and other body fluids. Historically, the **Kjeldahl method** for total protein determination, based on the measurement of **nitrogen,** is of interest but this reaction is not used clinically since it is labor intensive and time consuming. Sixteen percent of the mass of protein is assumed to be nitrogen. Individual protein fractions vary in nitrogen content, making total protein measurements, in reality, estimated values. In practice, the Kjeldahl method is used to determine the protein level of commercially prepared standards required for the routinely performed biuret method.[2]

The **biuret reaction** is the serum total protein assay commonly used in today's highly automated clinical laboratory environment. The simple reagent contains copper sulfate as the major reactant, sodium hydroxide to establish an alkaline environment, and stabilizers to keep copper in the $Cu^{+2}$ state.

Biuret is an organic compound with the structure:

$$NH_2 - C - NH - C - NH_2$$
$$\parallel \qquad\qquad \parallel$$
$$O \qquad\qquad\quad O$$

The molecule reacts with $Cu^{+2}$ in an alkaine solution to form a colored chelate that absorbs light at 540 nm. The **peptide bonds** of proteins are structurally similar to biuret and react in the same way. Therefore, when the reaction is applied to the measurement of serum total protein, the amount of light absorbed by the complex is directly proportional to the number of **peptide bonds,** which is directly related to protein concentration. Since at least two peptide bonds are required for this reaction, amino acids and dipeptides do not react.[2]

Total protein is measured in other body fluids such as urine and in CSF. The usual concentration of protein in urine (1 to 14 mg/dL) and CSF (15 to 45 mg/dL)[8] is much lower than that found in serum. Total protein procedures, more sensitive than those used for serum total protein, are therefore required. **Dye-binding methods** utilize the ability of protein to bind dyes such as Coomassie brilliant blue and pyrogallol red. A colored complex is formed that is measured spectrophotometrically. **Precipitation methods** use acids such as benzethonium chloride, sulfosalicylic acid, or trichloroacetic acid to denature the proteins in dilute body fluids. The finely precipitated proteins, when suspended, block or reflect light in a manner directly related to the protein concentration in the specimen. Quantitation of the acid precipitation methods therefore involves nephelometry or turbidimetry.[3]

## Albumin

### PATHOPHYSIOLOGY

Albumin has a molecular weight of approximately 66000. Albumin normally comprises more than one half of all serum proteins. Plasma osmotic pressure is therefore dependent on the concentration of plasma albumin. Albumin also serves as a **transport molecule** for less soluble substances such as fatty acids, bilirubin, hormones, calcium, metals, drugs, and vitamins. The serum albumin concentration is normally between 3.4 to 5.0 g/dL (34 to 50 g/L)[8]. Dye-binding methods are most commonly used.

Decreased serum albumin is seen in liver disease (decreased production), glomerulonephritis or nephrosis (increased loss), gastrointestinal disease (malabsorption), starvation, and in burn patients (increased loss). There is also a rare condition called hereditary **analbuminemia** in which albumin is not produced. Increased serum albumin usually denotes dehydration, although it may result from albumin therapy. Many plasma proteins are polymorphic owing to genetic variability in their expression. One example of this occurrence is **bisalbuminemia,** a congenital condition characterized by a split or double albumin band observed following protein electrophoresis. The two albumin peaks are generally antigenically identical and cannot be differentiated by immunoassay. There are no clinical symptoms associated with bisalbuminemia.[2]

Albumin is considered a negative acute phase reactant protein. During inflammatory processes and chronic inflammatory disorders, albumin levels decrease as a result of decreased synthesis and increased catabolism. The body directs its anabolic functions toward the synthesis of other proteins that have a more direct role in fighting and repairing the inflammatory process.

### METHODOLOGY

Serum albumin is most often assayed using **dye-binding** techniques. Albumin preferentially binds to anionic dyes that do not attract globulins. Bromcresol purple (BCP) and bromcresol green (BCG) are most commonly used. The amount of light absorbed by the albumin-dye complex is proportional to the amount of albumin present. Dye-binding methods for serum albumin are inexpensive and easy to automate. Serum albumin can also be calculated using serum protein electrophoresis and total protein analysis data. Immunochemical methods have also been developed.[3]

## Prealbumin (Transthyretin)

Prealbumin, also called transthyretin, has a molecular weight of approximately 54000. The major function of this protein is to **transport thyroxine** and **triiodothyronine.** Prealbumin is a sensitive indicator of nutritional status because it has a very short half-life. The level falls rapidly if caloric and protein intake levels decrease. Prealbumin is also classified as a **negative acute phase reactant.** Therefore, prealbumin levels decrease in inflammation and malignancy and also during liver disease as a result of decreased synthesis. Prealbumin levels may rise during renal disease if the glomerular filtration rate is diminished. When performing serum protein electrophoresis, prealbumin migrates faster than albumin but since the concentration of prealbumin is so low, it is not detectable with routine techniques. Prealbumin can be measured using immunochemical methods.[2]

## Retinol-Binding Protein

Retinol-binding protein (RBP) is another **transport** protein. It combines with prealbumin to transport vitamin A (retinol) to a target cell.[9] Retinol-binding protein also migrates more rapidly than albumin and is quantitated using immunochemical methods.

## Alpha$_1$-Antitrypsin

Alpha$_1$-antitrypsin (AAT) is a group of serine protease inhibitors synthesized in the liver. Several phenotypic expressions are possible owing to the presence of multiple alleles. The function of AAT is to inactivate proteases, such as elastase. As an anti-elastase, AAT prevents breakdown of connective tissue after elastase has been released from neutrophils in an area of inflammation. AAT deficiencies are inherited in either a homozygous or heterozygous state. Depending on the phenotype, deficiency of AAT can result in severe hepatic disease in infants, leading to fatal cirrhosis or in emphysema of early onset (in patients ranging in age from late 20s to 40 years). The damage is due in part to the uninhibited proteases causing structural damage in these tissues. Alpha-1-antitrypsin is an **acute phase reactant.**[2]

**Acute phase reactants** are those plasma proteins that elevate in response to acute inflammation. This elevation frequently happens as a result of infection, myocardial infarction, tumor growth, surgery, or trauma. It is assumed that all acute phase reactants play a part in host defense. Since the acute phase reaction is associated with many diseases, measurements of acute phase reactants have little diagnostic value. They may, however, be used to monitor progression or the treatment of a specific disease. As the acute phase reactants rise, levels of the so-called negative acute phase reactants, albumin, prealbumin, and transferrin fall. The total serum protein concentration, as a result, changes very little.

Screening for AAT deficiency may be done using protein electrophoresis because approximately 90% of the alpha-1 band is composed of this protein. It should be noted that a normal alpha-1 band may be seen in AAT deficiency during an acute phase reaction. AAT is quantitated using immunochemical methods such as immunonephelometry and phenotyping is done using isoelectric focusing.[2]

## Alpha₁-Acid Glycoprotein

Alpha₁-acid glycoprotein (AAG) has a molecular weight of approximately 44000 and is produced in the liver. There is evidence that its primary function is to inactivate progesterone but it may also bind basic drugs and affect pharmacokinetics. Alpha₁-acid glycoprotein is an **acute phase reactant** and is therefore elevated in inflammation, especially during autoimmune reactions such as rheumatoid arthritis and systemic lupus erythematosus. Elevations of AAG may be a reliable indicator of patients with ulcerative colitis.[2] Decreased levels are seen in nephrotic syndrome due to its relatively small size. Alpha₁-acid glycoprotein is measured using immunochemical techniques such as nephelometry.

## Alpha₁-Fetoprotein

Alpha₁-fetoprotein (AFP) is synthesized by the fetal liver and is a major plasma protein in the fetus during the second trimester of pregnancy. Alpha₁-fetoprotein is one of the triple marker tests performed on maternal serum, along with unconjugated estriol and human chorionic gonadotropin (HCG), to **screen fetuses** that have a high risk for open neural tube defects (ONTD) and/or Down's syndrome. High concentrations of AFP in the maternal serum during the second trimester are associated with ONTD, whereas low concentrations, together with increased levels of HCG and low levels of unconjugated estriol, are associated with Down's syndrome.[10] AFP is also used as a **tumor marker** and is elevated in serum if cancers of the liver and germ cell tumors are present. The protein is assayed using immunochemical techniques.

## Alpha₂-Macroglobulin

Alpha₂-macroglobulin (AMG) is noted for its large size (around 725 kD) and is a protease inhibitor. It is not an acute

phase reactant. AMG, along with haptoglobin, is a major component of the alpha₂ fraction on routine serum protein electrophoresis. The protein functions in the kinin, complement, coagulation, and fibrinolytic pathways. AMG is mildly depressed in acute inflammation and prostate cancer before treatment and is significantly depressed in severe attacks of acute pancreatitis.

AMG is elevated in **nephrotic syndrome.** These patients typically demonstrate a prominent increase in the alpha₂ fraction when routine serum protein electrophoresis is performed. In nephrotic syndrome, there is a large loss of protein into the urine since the diseased kidneys are unable to retain proteins, such as albumin, that have a relatively small molecular weight. The large size of AMG prevents its loss and elevates the alpha₂ fraction on serum protein electrophoresis. Synthesis of AMG is increased by estrogens, so it may be elevated during pregnancy and in patients on estrogen therapy. Immunochemical methods are used to quantitate AMG.[2]

## Haptoglobin

Haptoglobin (HAP) is a glycoprotein that can manifest as three different phenotypes. The function of haptoglobin is to **transport free hemoglobin** in the plasma to the reticuloendothelial system where hemoglobin is degraded. Hemoglobin not bound to HAP is filtered through the glomerulus and precipitates in the tubules, causing severe kidney damage. However, hemoglobin bound to haptoglobin is too large to be filtered and thus adequate levels of haptoglobin prevent kidney damage and retain the hemoglobin iron stores that would otherwise be lost. The entire haptoglobin-hemoglobin complex is degraded by the liver or reticuloendothelial system, which explains why the level of HAP is generally diminished following a **hemolytic crisis.** The level of haptoglobin is therefore decreased in patients with hemolytic anemias and congenital hemoglobin defects such as megaloblastic anemia, sickle cell anemia, glucose-6-phosphate dehydrogenase deficiency, hereditary spherocytosis, thalassemia, and during hemolytic transfusion reactions. Haptoglobin also behaves as an acute phase protein and is elevated during infection, neoplasia, trauma, myocardial infarction, and other inflammatory processes. Haptoglobin migrates electrophoretically in the alpha₂ band on serum protein electrophoresis. The protein can be quantitated using immunochemical methods and is used clinically to screen for or to monitor the progression of hemolytic disorders.[2]

## Hemopexin

Hemopexin is a beta-1 globulin. It functions as a **transport** protein that binds **free heme** after hemoglobin has been catabolized to its component parts. The heme-hemopexin complex travels to the liver where the heme portion is converted to bilirubin. Hemopexin synthesis is less affected than haptoglobin by factors such as estrogen therapy and inflammation.[2] In cases where intravascular hemolysis is being considered and inflammation or estrogen use is known to exist, it may be advisable to monitor hemopexin.

## Ceruloplasmin

Ceruloplasmin (Cp) is a **copper** containing alpha-2 globulin synthesized in the liver. Six copper molecules are bound tightly to each ceruloplasmin molecule, producing a faint blue-colored complex. About 95% of the plasma copper is attached to ceruloplasmin. The remaining copper is bound to albumin. Ceruloplasmin functions in critical plasma **redox reactions** and plays an important role in regulating the ionic state of iron necessary for the incorporation of iron into the transferrin molecule.

Serum Cp levels are most commonly used to diagnose **Wilson's disease.** Wilson's disease, along with dietary copper deficiency and Menke's disease, is classified as a secondary hypoceruloplasminemia. Wilson's disease is due to the absence of a hepatocellular P-type ATPase needed to incorporate copper into apoCp. Without the functional holoprotein, the body is unable to excrete copper in the bile and a toxic accumulation of copper in the liver, brain, kidneys, eyes and red blood cells results. The level of Cp is decreased in Wilson's disease while dialyzable or free serum copper levels and urinary copper are increased. Copper that deposits in the cornea produces the characteristic Kayser-Fleischer rings. A definitive diagnosis of Wilson's disease requires DNA analysis or confirmation of increased tissue copper. Lifelong drug therapy is used to control the disease.[2]

Ceruloplasmin is an **acute phase reactant** with modest elevations occurring during inflammation. It is also elevated during pregnancy and with oral contraceptive usage since estrogen stimulates Cp synthesis. Along with other proteins, ceruloplasmin levels may be decreased in patients suffering from malnutrition and chronic hepatitis. Ceruloplasmin is quantitated using immunochemical methods or a spectrophotometric measurement of oxidase activity. The former method measures the functional or copper containing protein, whereas the immunochemical methods do not differentiate the apoprotein from the copper containing protein. The oxidase activity method is more difficult to perform and less specific but it may provide better clinical information.[2]

## Transferrin

Transferrin (TRF) is a beta glycoprotein that functions as an **iron transport** protein. Ferric ions from heme degradation in the liver and those absorbed from the diet are transported by transferrin to the sites of erythrocyte production in the bone marrow. Transferrin levels are used to diagnose different types of anemia and to monitor treatment (see Chapter 21). Elevated levels of transferrin, with low iron saturation, are found in iron deficiency anemia because the body synthesizes more transferrin in an attempt to transport more iron into those cells actively making hemoglobin. Normal or low levels of TRF, with increased iron saturation, are found in anemias due to

the failure of red cells to incorporate iron. Transferrin is a **negative acute phase** protein. Levels are decreased in infections, following severe burns, neoplasia, liver disease, kidney disease, and hereditary atransferrinemia. TRF levels are elevated during pregnancy when a greater demand on the iron stores is made and during estrogen usage.[2]

## Beta₂-Microglobulin

Beta₂-microglobulin (BMG) has a molecular weight of approximately 11800. Its small size allows the protein to pass through the glomerulus into the glomerular filtrate. If kidney function is normal, very little BMG appears in the urine. The protein is almost entirely reabsorbed and broken down in the proximal tubules. BMG is used to assess **renal tubule function,** especially in kidney transplant patients when rejection is suspected. Elevated plasma levels are seen in renal failure, inflammation, and malignancies.

Beta₂-microglobulin is a component of the cell membrane of all nucleated cells, particularly lymphocytes and tumor cells. In HIV, when lymphocytes are being destroyed by the virus, BMG elevates in the plasma. Elevated CSF levels of BMG are found in acute leukemia and lymphoma when there is central nervous system involvement.[2,9]

## C-Reactive Protein

C-reactive protein (CRP), so named because it reacts with the C polysaccharide of the cell wall of pneumococci, is an **acute phase protein** synthesized in the liver. The protein is involved with the immune system and plays a role in complement activation. C-reactive protein recognizes substances released from damaged tissue as potentially toxic, binds to them, and facilitates clearing them from the blood. C-reactive protein is considered to be the most sensitive APR, but it is not very specific.

C-reactive protein is elevated in infections and with tissue damage and cellular necrosis. It is used clinically to detect infections in susceptible conditions such as leukemia, systemic lupus erythematosus (SLE) and post-surgery. Repetitive measurements are often helpful in monitoring therapy during an inflammatory disease such as rheumatoid arthritis. C-reactive protein is also used to detect kidney transplant rejection in allograft recipients. Various immunochemical methods are used to measure CRP when monitoring an acute phase response. C-reactive protein shows potential as an early marker for acute myocardial infarction. When used for this purpose, a sensitive immunochemical method, one that detects very low level increases of the protein, is required.[2,11]

## Complement Proteins

The complement system is composed of at least 20 proteins that participate in the body's **immunologic defense.** C3 and C4 are the more frequently analyzed serum complement proteins. Both proteins migrate in the beta fraction of serum protein electrophoresis but are present in concentrations too low to make estimation possible with routine electrophoresis procedures. Increased and decreased levels of C3 and C4 have clinical significance and are used for the diagnosis of disorders such as SLE, rheumatoid vasculitis, subacute bacterial endocarditis (SBE), glomerulonephritis and bacteremias. Immunochemical methods, especially immunoturbidimetry or nephelometry, are commonly used to measure the complement proteins.[2]

## Fibrinogen

Fibrinogen is a soluble glycoprotein made by the liver. Fibrinogen serves as the substrate for the coagulation enzyme thrombin. Fibrinogen is also an acute phase protein. It is decreased during disseminated intravascular coagulation (DIC), in patients with liver disease or hereditary afibrinogenemias. Fibrinogen is most commonly assessed in the coagulation laboratory using clot-detection techniques. If plasma instead of serum is used for routine serum protein electrophoresis, fibrinogen produces a very sharp peak in the beta region that may lead to a confusing interpretation of the pattern.

## Immunoglobulins

The immunoglobulins (antibodies) are the major group of serum proteins distinguished by the fact that they are not produced by the liver. They are produced by **plasma cells** from B lymphocyte lineage in the bone marrow. All immunoglobulins have two identical heavy chains and two identical light chains. This tetramer is held together by disulfide bonds. The immunoglobulins are classified as IgG, IgA, IgM, IgD, and IgE. Light chains are classified as either kappa or lambda. The immunoglobulins are directly involved in the immune response. This response involves the interaction of several systems, which include humoral immunity (antibody production), cell-mediated immunity (T lymphocytes), phagocytosis, and complement proteins.

Serum immunoglobulins are roughly identified by electrophoresis and confirmed using immunofixation electrophoresis. They are quantitated by immunochemical techniques such as turbidimetry, nephelometry, enzyme immunoassay (EIA) or radial immunodiffusion (RID).

### IMMUNOGLOBULIN DISORDERS

Decreased levels of immunoglobulins, immunodeficiency, can be genetic or acquired. Disorders of this type are discussed in the chapter entitled Immunologic Disorders. Increased levels of the immunoglobulins may be classified as **monoclonal,** coming from one cell line, or **polyclonal,** coming from multiple cell lines. All cells from the same clone produce identical antibody. If a clone multiplies, antibody production can become so elevated that an increased gamma fraction is visible following electrophoresis. The abnormal protein produced is called a paraprotein and is a characteristic finding in malignancies such as multiple myeloma and Waldenström's macro-

globulinemia. It is possible to differentiate polyclonal increases from monoclonal increases by electrophoretic separation. A monoclonal paraprotein is visible as a discrete band somewhere in the gamma region, whereas a polyclonal increase appears as a heavy homogeneous gamma fraction or as multiple bands, depending on the resolving capability of the media used and the abnormality leading to the protein production. Polyclonal hypergammaglobulinemias can result from many disorders, some of which include infectious diseases, liver disease, hypersensitivities such as asthma, and autoimmune connective tissue disorders such as SLE.[2]

### IgG

IgG is the immunoglobulin found in the highest concentration in adults. It diffuses into extravascular spaces because of its small size and is capable of crossing the placenta. Its functions are to **neutralize toxins, bind antigens** (including microorganisms), and **activate complement.** IgG has a molecular weight of approximately 160000 and in adults, is found at concentrations between 650 and 1600 mg/dL (6.5 to 16.0 g/L).[8] Because infants do not immediately begin to produce IgG, the infant depends on the maternal IgG that crossed the placenta before birth. The levels fall off gradually and then begin to rise as the infant begins to produce IgG. At 3 months of age, the infant level is 200 to 700 mg/dL (2.0 to 7.0 g/L);[8] at 1 year, it is 340 to 1200 mg/dL (3.4 to 12.0 g/L),[8] and the level gradually rises until adult levels are reached. Polyclonal IgG increases are associated with liver disease, autoimmune collagen diseases (such as SLE and rheumatoid arthritis), and bacterial and viral infections.[2]

### IgA

IgA has a molecular weight of about 160000. It is a **secretory** antibody and is present primarily in saliva, tears, sweat, colostrum, and nasal secretions. It provides external surface protection against microorganisms. It is present as a dimer in these fluids and is stabilized against proteolysis by a component called secretory protein. In the plasma, it is present as a monomer. Infants usually have roughly 20% of the adult level, by age 3, 50%, and by age 12, 100% of the adult level. IgA does not cross the placenta and in cord blood the normal level of IgA is less than 1 mg/dL. Polyclonal IgA levels are increased in patients with cirrhosis and various infectious diseases. On serum protein electrophoresis, IgA migrates between the beta and gamma fractions. High elevations of IgA, as seen in liver cirrhosis, are demonstrated by the spectrophotometric pattern described as beta-gamma bridging.[2]

### IgM

IgM is a pentamer with a molecular weight of 900000. It is the first immunoglobulin to be produced during the immune response, the so-called **primary response** to an antigen. It is also the first immunoglobulin produced by the fetus during development. Because of its large size, it does not pass into extravascular spaces nor is it transported across the placenta. It is, therefore, not involved in hemolytic disease of the newborn. The adult reference range is 50 to 300 mg/dL (0.5 to 3.0 g/L).[8] By age 4 months, the infant will have about 50% of adult levels, and by age 9, the child will have close to 100%. Cord blood has <25 mg/dL (<0.25 g/L).[8] Polyclonal increases are seen in cirrhosis and various infectious diseases.[2]

### IgD AND IgE

IgD and IgE account for less than 1% of the serum immunoglobulins. IgD is similar in structure to IgG. The function of IgD has not been clearly defined. IgE is usually firmly bound to mast cells and may be increased in **allergic reactions.**[2]

### Monoclonal Gammopathies

Monoclonal increases of the immunoglobulins are known as monoclonal gammopathies. They can be classified as either malignant or benign types. Disorders classified as malignant monoclonal gammopathies include multiple myeloma, Waldenström's macroglobulinemia, and heavy-chain diseases.

Multiple myeloma is a malignant neoplastic disease involving a clone of plasma cells in the bone marrow. It typically affects individuals older than 60 years of age. It was named multiple myeloma in reference to the multiple bone tumors that are a feature of the disease. Multiple myeloma is associated with a variety of immunoglobulin classes. IgG myeloma is the most commonly involved immunoglobulin class and represents approximately 50% of cases, whereas IgA represents about 25%. IgD and IgE involvement is quite rare, representing 2% and 0.1%, respectively, of cases. A monoclonal production of light chains represents approximately 20% of multiple myeloma cases. If the monoclonal peak is identified as an IgM immunoglobulin, the disorder is probably Waldenström's macroglobulinemia.[2]

Multiple myeloma is characterized by a wide spectrum of clinical manifestations. As the malignancy develops, bone lesions occur causing pain and decreasing bone strength. **Skeletal pains** are the presenting and predominant symptoms. X rays of the bone demonstrating lytic or **punched out** lesions is a characteristic finding in 76% of the patients at the time of diagnosis.[12] Plasma cells produce abnormal amounts of immunoglobulins and/or light chain fragments known as Bence-Jones protein. The abnormal paraprotein appears as a sharp band, or **M spike,** in the normally homogeneous gamma region during protein electrophoresis. Other bone marrow products such as red and white blood cells, platelets, and normal immunoglobulins are diminished, causing **anemia** and the inability of the body to fight infection.[12]

There are a number of routine laboratory analyses that are abnormal in this disease. The **total protein** level is usually increased and may reach as high as 10 to 12 g/dL (100 to 120 g/L). The increase is due to the elevated gamma fraction, whereas the albumin level is often decreased. Proteinuria is a frequent finding because of the presence of **Bence Jones** pro-

tein. These excess free light chains, being of small molecular weight, are excreted by the kidney in the urine. They can cause renal damage by precipitating in the renal tubules. Bence Jones proteins are usually not present in the serum unless renal damage has occurred because they are filtered by the glomerulus.

Laboratory diagnosis of multiple myeloma should include both **serum** and **urine electrophoresis** since 15% of myelomas secrete light chains only. The diagnosis can be missed if only serum electrophoresis is performed because the light chains are commonly found only in the urine. Protein electrophoresis cannot differentiate the type of immunoglobulin class involved. An additional test, such as **immunofixation electrophoresis,** is ordered that uses antisera specific for the immunoglobulin classes or light chains. The light chains may also be measured as a ratio (K/L) and used as a tumor marker. Serum levels of the polyclonal IgG, IgA, and IgM are also measured. They are used to confirm the identity of the spike and to determine if the patient is susceptible to an infection.[2]

The proliferation of abnormal plasma cells in the marrow produces excessive bone destruction and **calcium** is released. The hypercalcemia, which occurs in some cases, may contribute to the renal damage. **Uric acid** levels are frequently elevated due to increased cell proliferation and destruction. Cryoglobulins may also be elevated. **Cryoglobulins** are gamma globulins that precipitate in the cold and redissolve when warmed to body temperature. These may be associated with any of the heavy chain classes and may be secondary to multiple myeloma as well as other disorders such as macroglobulinemia, leukemia, SLE, rheumatoid arthritis, polycythemia, or a number of other inflammatory diseases. When patients with cryoglobulins are exposed to extreme cold, precipitation of these proteins causes hyperviscosity of the plasma, spasms in the capillaries, pallor and cyanosis, pain, and in severe cases, leads to skin ulcers and gangrene. This is called **Raynaud's** phenomenon. Serum is tested for the presence of cryoglobulins by placing a sample in the cold (4°C for up to 72 hours), checking for precipitate at the end of the cold incubation, and redissolving the precipitate, if any, at 37°C.

Patients may also experience symptoms related to the **hyperviscosity** syndrome. Owing to the high concentration of immunoglobulins, the serum becomes very thick and viscous, resulting in decreased rate of blood flow through the small blood vessels of the brain and heart. The increased workload placed on the heart may lead to congestive heart failure. All the immunoglobulin classes can cause a hyperviscosity syndrome if the serum level rises sufficiently. However, the **IgM** class, because of its large size and number of immunoglobulin units, causes a much higher increase in viscosity than the other immunoglobulins. The hyperviscosity syndrome is therefore most commonly found with elevations of IgM.[12]

A number of hematologic abnormalities are also characteristic findings in multiple myeloma. Anemia is present due to bleeding, marrow replacement by malignant cells, and shortened red blood cell life span. Some degree of leukopenia and thrombocytopenia may also be apparent. The most striking hematologic finding is **rouleaux,** in which the red blood cells appear to adhere to each other microscopically due to the increased paraprotein concentration.[12]

**Multiple myeloma** is a progressive and ultimately fatal disease, although remissions have been achieved in some cases. The median survival in only 36 months. Conventional treatment consists of the use of marrow suppressive agents such as melphalan and prednisone.[13] Alternative treatments include high-dose chemotherapy regimens, autologous and allogenic transplantation, and immunotherapy.[14]

**Waldenström's macroglobulinemia,** also known as primary macroglobulinemia, is a gammopathy involving the production of **IgM** globulins. It is almost entirely a disease of the elderly, with a peak incidence in the sixth and seventh decades. In contrast to multiple myeloma, bone pain is not a prominent symptom and bone lesions are rarely seen. Patients do experience vague symptoms of ill health such as weakness and weight loss that may precede more serious manifestations for many years. The most common and predominant features are related to the increased serum viscosity, which is more pronounced in Waldenström's macroglobulinemia because of the large size of the IgM molecules. Anemia, cryoglobulinemia, and bleeding are common manifestations. Accelerated blood cell destruction and decreased erythropoiesis account in part for the anemia, while the bleeding problems are due to the circulatory impairment of the viscous blood and IgM interference with coagulation factors. Exchange transfusions may be used to treat the symptoms. Renal disease is much less common in Waldenström's macroglobulinemia than in multiple myeloma even in the presence of Bence Jones proteinuria, which occurs in approximately 80% of cases.[2]

Benign monoclonal gammopathies are common conditions in which unexplained abnormal serum proteins occur. M components can be commonly found in individuals of 70 years or older. In many of these patients, there is a history of some type of chronic disease. **Monoclonal gammopathy of undetermined significance** (MGUS) and **smoldering multiple myeloma** (SMM) need to be differentiated from overt diseases such as multiple myeloma and Waldenström's disease. The most useful approach to the evaluation of an unexplained monoclonal gammopathy is careful follow-up study of the patient by monitoring immunoglobulin levels, the presence of Bence Jones protein and patient symptoms.[2]

## AMYLOIDOSIS

Amyloidosis is a group of diseases characterized by the deposition of a fibrillar protein substance, called amyloid, between the cells of various organs. The deposits, which can be localized or systemic, put pressure on the organs where deposits are found and may eventually cause death. Amyloid deposits can be secondary to another disease or they can be an inherited (primary) disorder. Amyloid means starchlike. The protein's name is related to the fact that the protein stains with iodine, which also stains starch. However, a definitive identification of amyloid in tissue is made with Congo red stain. Amyloid,

all molecular types, binds Congo red and emits an apple-green fluorescence under polarized light.[2]

The AL type of amyloid protein is the most common type and is often composed of light chains associated with immunoglobulins (Bence Jones protein). This type of amyloidosis occurs in both multiple myeloma and a primary type of amyloidosis. Both disorders are associated with excessive production of plasma cells that produce monoclonal light chains. With AL amyloidosis, deposits may occur in the tongue, heart, lymph nodes, spleen, joints, peripheral nerves, and skin.

The AA type of amyloidosis demonstrates deposits mainly of AA proteins and a small amount of light chains. AA protein deposits, found in the kidney, liver, and spleen, commonly cause a nephritic syndrome and/or hepatosplenomegaly. AA amyloidosis is associated with chronic inflammatory diseases such as rheumatoid arthritis, inflammatory joint diseases, and in some granulomatous infectious diseases like tuberculosis.

Senile amyloidosis protein deposits are found most often in the heart but have also been found in the pancreas and brain tissue. A few genetically transmitted forms of amyloidosis have also been described.[2]

The reference ranges for serum proteins in adults are listed in Table 12–4 and Figure 12–7 illustrates electrophoretograms in various disease states.

## Cardiac-Related Proteins

Myoglobin and the troponins are proteins measured in serum to detect and evaluate acute myocardial infarction. For more information, please refer to the chapter discussing enzymes.

TABLE 12-4

**Interim Consensus Reference Ranges for Plasma Proteins in Adults between the Ages of 20 and 60 Years[2]**

| CONSTITUENT | RANGE (mg/dL) |
| --- | --- |
| Prealbumin (transthyretin) | 20–40 |
| Albumin | 3500–5200 |
| Alpha-1-antitrypsin | 90–200 |
| Alpha-1-acid glycoprotein | 50–120 |
| Alpha-2-macroglobulin | 130–300 |
| Haptoglobin | 30–200 |
| Transferrin | 200–360 |
| Ceruloplasmin | 20–60 |
| C3 | 90–180 |
| C4 | 10–40 |
| C-reactive protein | <0.5 |
| IgG | 700–1600 |
| IgA | 70–400 |
| IgM | 40–230 |

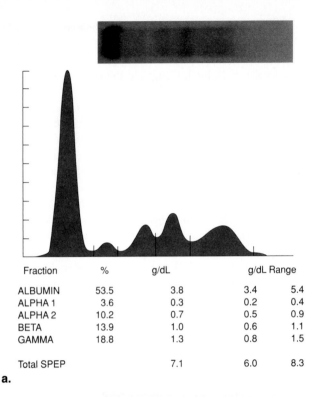

| Fraction | % | g/dL | g/dL Range | |
|---|---|---|---|---|
| ALBUMIN | 53.5 | 3.8 | 3.4 | 5.4 |
| ALPHA 1 | 3.6 | 0.3 | 0.2 | 0.4 |
| ALPHA 2 | 10.2 | 0.7 | 0.5 | 0.9 |
| BETA | 13.9 | 1.0 | 0.6 | 1.1 |
| GAMMA | 18.8 | 1.3 | 0.8 | 1.5 |
| Total SPEP | | 7.1 | 6.0 | 8.3 |

**a.**

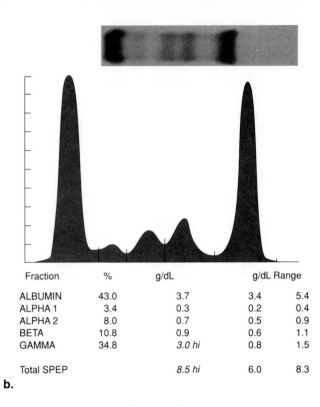

| Fraction | % | g/dL | g/dL Range | |
|---|---|---|---|---|
| ALBUMIN | 43.0 | 3.7 | 3.4 | 5.4 |
| ALPHA 1 | 3.4 | 0.3 | 0.2 | 0.4 |
| ALPHA 2 | 8.0 | 0.7 | 0.5 | 0.9 |
| BETA | 10.8 | 0.9 | 0.6 | 1.1 |
| GAMMA | 34.8 | *3.0 hi* | 0.8 | 1.5 |
| Total SPEP | | *8.5 hi* | 6.0 | 8.3 |

**b.**

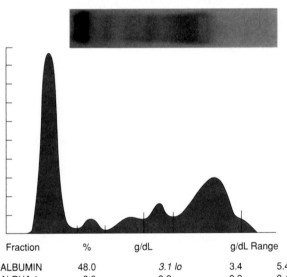

| Fraction | % | g/dL | g/dL Range | |
|---|---|---|---|---|
| ALBUMIN | 48.0 | *3.1 lo* | 3.4 | 5.4 |
| ALPHA 1 | 3.9 | 0.3 | 0.2 | 0.4 |
| ALPHA 2 | 6.4 | *0.4 lo* | 0.5 | 0.9 |
| BETA | 9.0 | 0.6 | 0.6 | 1.1 |
| GAMMA | 32.6 | *2.1 hi* | 0.8 | 1.5 |
| Total SPEP | | 6.5 | 6.0 | 8.3 |

**c.**

| Fraction | % | g/dL | g/dL Range | |
|---|---|---|---|---|
| ALBUMIN | 44.6 | *2.5 lo* | 3.4 | 5.4 |
| ALPHA 1 | 8.1 | *0.5 hi* | 0.2 | 0.4 |
| ALPHA 2 | 17.2 | *1.0 hi* | 0.5 | 0.9 |
| BETA | 15.7 | 0.9 | 0.6 | 1.1 |
| GAMMA | 14.5 | 0.8 | 0.8 | 1.5 |
| Total SPEP | | *5.6 lo* | 6.0 | 8.3 |

**d.**

**FIGURE 12-7**

Electrophoretograms of various disease states. **a.** Normal serum electrophoresis. **b.** Monoclonal gammopathy. The intensely stained spike in gamma region is indicative of an increase in one immunoglobulin class typically seen in monoclonal gammopathies such as multiple myeloma. **c.** Polyclonal gammopathy (seen in several conditions that enlist antibody production): A diffuse, broad gamma band suggests a polyclonal increase in immunoglobulin fractions as seen in chronic inflammatory disorders, liver disease, and infectious disorders. **d.** Acute-phase pattern: The typical acute inflammatory pattern is characterized by a decrease in the albumin fraction with an increase in both the $\alpha_1$ and $\alpha_2$ fractions. *(Continued.)*

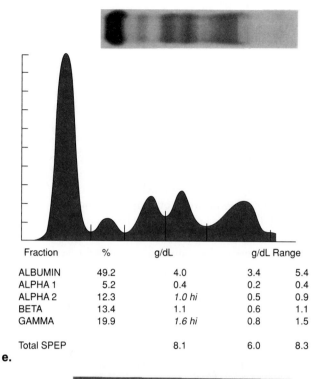

| Fraction | % | g/dL | g/dL Range | |
|---|---|---|---|---|
| ALBUMIN | 49.2 | 4.0 | 3.4 | 5.4 |
| ALPHA 1 | 5.2 | 0.4 | 0.2 | 0.4 |
| ALPHA 2 | 12.3 | *1.0 hi* | 0.5 | 0.9 |
| BETA | 13.4 | 1.1 | 0.6 | 1.1 |
| GAMMA | 19.9 | *1.6 hi* | 0.8 | 1.5 |
| Total SPEP | | 8.1 | 6.0 | 8.3 |

e.

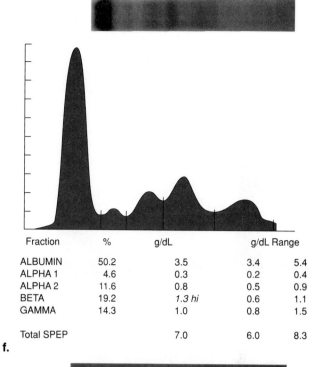

| Fraction | % | g/dL | g/dL Range | |
|---|---|---|---|---|
| ALBUMIN | 50.2 | 3.5 | 3.4 | 5.4 |
| ALPHA 1 | 4.6 | 0.3 | 0.2 | 0.4 |
| ALPHA 2 | 11.6 | 0.8 | 0.5 | 0.9 |
| BETA | 19.2 | *1.3 hi* | 0.6 | 1.1 |
| GAMMA | 14.3 | 1.0 | 0.8 | 1.5 |
| Total SPEP | | 7.0 | 6.0 | 8.3 |

f.

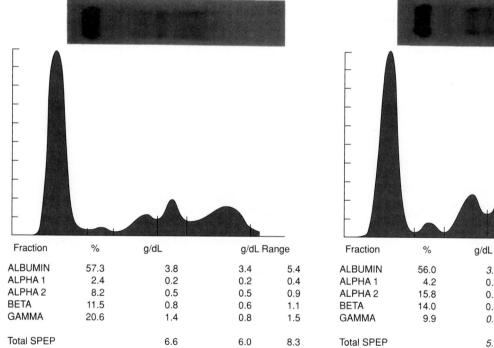

| Fraction | % | g/dL | g/dL Range | |
|---|---|---|---|---|
| ALBUMIN | 57.3 | 3.8 | 3.4 | 5.4 |
| ALPHA 1 | 2.4 | 0.2 | 0.2 | 0.4 |
| ALPHA 2 | 8.2 | 0.5 | 0.5 | 0.9 |
| BETA | 11.5 | 0.8 | 0.6 | 1.1 |
| GAMMA | 20.6 | 1.4 | 0.8 | 1.5 |
| Total SPEP | | 6.6 | 6.0 | 8.3 |

g.

| Fraction | % | g/dL | g/dL Range | |
|---|---|---|---|---|
| ALBUMIN | 56.0 | *3.2 lo* | 3.4 | 5.4 |
| ALPHA 1 | 4.2 | 0.2 | 0.2 | 0.4 |
| ALPHA 2 | 15.8 | 0.9 | 0.5 | 0.9 |
| BETA | 14.0 | 0.8 | 0.6 | 1.1 |
| GAMMA | 9.9 | *0.6 lo* | 0.8 | 1.5 |
| Total SPEP | | *5.7 lo* | 6.0 | 8.3 |

h.

**FIGURE 12–7 (CONT.)**

**e.** Chronic inflammation pattern: Chronic inflammation is characterized by a decreased albumin and increased $\alpha_1$ and $\alpha_2$ fractions as seen in acute inflammatory reactions as well as by an increase in the gamma fractions. **f.** Pattern seen in microcytic anemia: An increased $\beta$ fraction in microcytic anemia is due to an increased synthesis of transferrin, the iron transport protein. **g.** $\alpha_1$-Antitrypsin deficiency: $\alpha_1$-antitrypsin deficiency appears as either a decrease or complete absence of the $\alpha_1$ band depending on whether the condition is heterozygous or homozygous. **h.** Nephrotic syndrome: the nephrotic syndrome pattern is characterized by decreases in all protein fractions except $\alpha_2$. $\alpha_2$-macroglobulin is retained by the kidney due to its large molecular size. *(Continued.)*

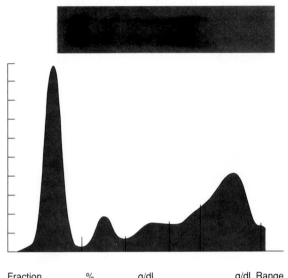

| Fraction | % | g/dL | g/dL Range | |
|---|---|---|---|---|
| ALBUMIN | 38.6 | *2.4 lo* | 3.4 | 5.4 |
| ALPHA 1 | 8.5 | *0.5 hi* | 0.2 | 0.4 |
| ALPHA 2 | 9.8 | 0.6 | 0.5 | 0.9 |
| BETA | 9.1 | 0.6 | 0.6 | 1.1 |
| GAMMA | 34.0 | *2.1 hi* | 0.8 | 1.5 |
| | | | | |
| Total SPEP | | 6.3 | 6.0 | 8.3 |

i.

**FIGURE 12-7 (CONT.)**

**i.** Cirrhosis: The typical electrophoretic pattern of cirrhosis shows a merging of the β and γ fractions known as the β-γ bridge.

---

## PROTEIN IN OTHER BODY FLUIDS

### Urine

Protein in urine is normally present in negligible amounts (20 to 150 mg/d).[2] Most of the protein is albumin because of its small size and high plasma concentration. The rest of it is Tamm-Horsfall protein, which is secreted by the tubules and is a constituent of urinary casts.[4] The renal glomeruli serve as molecular sieves for the plasma. With normal kidney function, the majority of plasma proteins are held back and do not enter the protein-free filtrate. Those proteins that enter the filtrate have relatively low molecular weights and most will be actively reabsorbed and conserved by the body for synthesis of new proteins.

Elevated urinary protein is an early indicator of **renal impairment.** As the disease progresses, the amount of urinary proteins and their relative sizes increase. Dipstick tests are used to economically screen for renal disease. The most common procedure uses a buffered indicator (bromphenol blue, pH 3.0) on the reaction pad that changes color intensity as the level of

protein increases. A more sensitive method is needed to detect diabetic nephropathy early in the course of the disease. For this reason, an immunologically based dipstick method is used that qualitatively detects very low level increases in urinary albumin. The name of the test is **microalbumin.** The "micro" refers to smaller amounts of albumin in the fluid, not to any changes in the size of the molecule.[9] The presence of microalbuminuria is an indicator of the development of renal disease in patients with diabetes mellitus.

Quantitation of urine total protein using acid precipitation and dye-binding methods have been discussed. Immunologic procedures such as immunonephelometry and RID are used to quantitate individual urinary proteins such as albumin, IgG, or BMG. This information can be used to estimate glomerular selectivity and to evaluate tubular proteinuria.

The presence of light chains in the urine, as found in multiple myeloma and Waldenström's macroglobulinemia, can be detected by electrophoresis and classified using immunofixation electrophoresis. To improve sensitivity, the urine may need to be concentrated prior to applying the sample onto the electrophoresis support media.

### Cerebrospinal Fluid

Cerebrospinal fluid (CSF) protein levels are normally very low. The range in a CSF specimen collected from around the lumbar spine is approximately 15 to 45 mg/dL (150 to 450 mg/L).[2] Elevated levels of total protein may be caused by damage to the **blood–brain barrier** during disease or following trauma. Elevations may also be caused by increased production of protein in the central nervous system secondary to diseases such as neoplasia, infection, and multiple sclerosis. The quantitation of individual protein fractions is useful when evaluations of CSF total protein are found or when the clinical picture suggests a central nervous system abnormality. This is done using the same sensitive procedures for quantitating serum proteins such as nephelometry, RID, RIA, and EIA.

**Myelin Basic Protein** (MBP) is a structural component of the myelin sheath. The myelin sheath functions as an electrical insulator for the nerve axon. Nerve impulses are conducted more readily when it is intact. Myelin basic protein is normally not present in the CSF, but in demyelinating disease states, like multiple sclerosis, resulting in necrosis or breakdown of myelin, it may be present. Myelin basic protein is measured by immunochemical methods or immunostaining techniques. The rise and fall of MBP in the CSF is helpful in assessing the amount of active demyelination.[2,15]

Abnormal paraproteins may be present in the CSF and may be evaluated using the same techniques used for evaluation of serum proteins after the CSF is concentrated or may be examined directly using unconcentrated CSF and silver stain. CSF is commonly evaluated for the presence of **oligoclonal bands** in the immunoglobulin region. These are defined as one or more bands in the CSF that are not present in the serum. At least one oligoclonal band is present in over 90% of patients with multiple sclerosis.[15]

**Multiple sclerosis** (MS) is a disease of many and varied symptoms including vision problems, muscle weakness or numbness, and urinary urgency. The occurrence of the symptoms is quite variable. They may last for weeks to months, with months to years of remission interspersed between. The progression of the disease is also equally unpredictable, although it usually involves increasing neurologic abnormalities. Multiple sclerosis commonly begins in young adults but can be found in children and in patients over 40 years of age.

At the cellular level, the disease is characterized by lesions, inflammation, and demyelination of the nerves of the spinal cord, brain stem, or eyes. The cause of the MS is still unknown but viral agents and autoimmune processes have been suggested. Patients with MS have an increased CSF IgG that is produced in the central nervous system. The abnormal IgG tends to separate into oligoclonal bands after high-resolution electrophoresis, isoelectric focusing, or capillary electrophoresis. The protein is first concentrated to ensure adequate visualization or the electrophoretogram is stained using special, very sensitive staining techniques (silver or immunostains).

**CSF IgG** may be produced within the central nervous system or it may be plasma in origin, showing up in the CSF after the blood–brain barrier is damaged. There are two calculations that are helpful in evaluating the source of elevated CSF IgG. The first is the **IgG/albumin ratio,** which is normally less than 25%. Elevations of the IgG/albumin ratio indicate increased CSF IgG. The second is the **IgG index,** which is (CSF IgG/serum IgG)/(CSF albumin/serum albumin) and is normally less than 0.66. Elevations of the IgG index indicate blood–brain barrier damage rather than increased production of IgG in the CSF.[15]

## Other Fluids

As previously discussed, alpha-fetoprotein (AFP) is a protein present in the fetus and infant in very large amounts but in the normal adult it is found in very small amounts. AFP is commonly used as a tumor marker but is also used to screen maternal serum and **amniotic fluid** for fetal defects (mainly open neural tube defects). This can be done because fetal levels of AFP are very high. Some of the fetal AFP is normally passed into the amniotic fluid and a small amount of this makes its way into the maternal circulation. Calculation of normal maternal serum levels is very complex because gestational age of the fetus, maternal weight, age, and race are all factors that must be taken into consideration. If the fetus has an open neural tube defect, an abdominal wall defect, or anencephaly, the amniotic fluid AFP levels will be much higher than normal, as will the maternal serum AFP levels, because more fetal AFP is lost through the open defect. AFP levels vary with gestational age so it is extremely important that this be considered when interpreting AFP results.

Unique proteins that are released by tumors and are measurable in body fluids are known as **tumor markers.** Some tumor markers are measured in cytosol preparations as well as in serum, urine, CSF, and other body fluids. For more details on tumor markers, consult the chapter discussing this topic.

## SUMMARY

Protein assays have been used to diagnose and monitor disease for many years. Technological developments, especially monoclonal antibody technologies, have greatly improved the sensitivity and specificity of protein measurements. As the technologies associated with monoclonal antibodies, protein separation, and protein sequencing are more fully developed, new protein analyses will be added to the clinical laboratory's test menu. Indeed, there are many things yet to be learned about the genetic causes of protein abnormalities and what can be done to solve these problems.

## REFERENCES

1. Nelson DL, Cox MM: *Leninger Principles of Biochemistry*, 3rd ed. New York, Worth Publishers, 2000.

2. Johnson AM, Rohlfs EM, Silverman LM: Proteins. In Burtis CA, Ashwood ER (eds.): *Tietz Textbook of Clinical Chemistry*, 3rd ed. Philadelphia, W. B. Saunders Co., 1999; pp 477–540.

3. Kaplan LA, Pesce AJ: *Clinical Chemistry: Theory, Analysis and Correlation*, 3rd ed. St. Louis, Mosby, 1996.

4. McBride LJ: *Textbook of Urinalysis and Body Fluids.* Philadelphia, Lippincott-Raven, 1998.

5. Love JE, Ward KM: Electrophoretic instrumentation systems. In Ward KM, Lehmann CA, Leiken AM (eds.): *Clinical Laboratory Instrumentation and Automation: Principles, Applications and Selection.* Philadelphia, W. B. Saunders, 1994, pp 155–183.

6. Karcher RE, Nuttall K: Electrophoresis. In Burtis CA, Ashwood ER (eds.): *Tietz Textbook of Clinical Chemistry*, 3rd ed. Philadelphia, W. B. Saunders, 1999, pp 150–163.

7. Thormann W, Wey AB, Lurie IS, et al.: Capillary electrophoresis in clinical and forensic analysis: Recent advances and breakthrough to routine applications. Electrophoresis 20:3203, 1999.

8. Burtis CA, Ashwood ER (eds.): *Tietz Textbook of Clinical Chemistry*, 3rd ed. Philadelphia, W. B. Saunders, 1999.

9. Bishop ML, Duben-Engelkirk JL, Fody EP: *Clinical Chemistry: Principles, Procedures and Correlations*, 4th ed., Philadelphia, Lippincott Williams & Wilkins, 2000.

10. Benn PA, Clive JM, Collins R: Median for second-trimester maternal serum alpha fetoprotein, and uncon-

jugated estriol; differences between races or ethnic groups, Clin Chem 43:333–337, 1997.

11. Williams LR, Sedrick R, Moulton L, et al.: Evaluation of four automated high-sensitivity C-reactive protein methods: implications for clinical and epidemiological applications, Clin Chem 46:461–468, 2000.

12. Long JM: Multiple myeloma and related plasma cell disorders. In Harmening, DM (ed.): *Clinical Hematology and Fundamentals of Hemostasis*, 3rd ed. Philadelphia, FA Davis, 1997, pp 404–423.

13. Morgan GJ: Advances in the biology and treatment of myeloma, Br J Haematol 105(Suppl):4–6, 1999.

14. Kyle RA: The role of high-dose chemotherapy in the treatment of multiple myeloma: A controversy. Ann Oncol 11(Suppl):S55–S58, 2000.

15. Corsaut K: Degenerative processes. In Davis BG, Mass D, Bishop ML (eds.): *Principles of Clinical Laboratory Utilization and Consultation*. Philadelphia, W. B. Saunders, 1999, pp 404–423.

# CHAPTER 13

# Inherited Metabolic Disorders

*Jane Adrian*

The opportunity to cope with and potentially cure abnormalities rooted in the genetic material requires a framework for discussing this topic in the present and for the future. To appreciate where these disorders fit into a much larger scope, this chapter begins with an overview of genetic disorders. Second, the chapter focuses specifically on the inherited metabolic disorders. These are often referred to as the **inborn errors of metabolism.** A number of these are of particular interest because of ongoing debates regarding their inclusion in newborn screening programs. The technologies past, present, and developing to aid in the diagnosis and monitoring of these disorders are considered. The summary includes a number of ethical issues embedded, debated, and surrounding genetic testing and newborn screening.

It may be that any one clinical laboratorian may not encounter all or even any of the relatively rare disorders discussed in this chapter unless one would work in a specialty laboratory or with individuals with special needs. Nonetheless, the professional laboratorian remains ever vigilant of the possibility that one may observe by sight or odor or other indicator a clue that may lead to an early diagnosis and treatment and thus save an individual from life-altering disability or death. The content of this chapter changes daily. A part of ongoing professional responsibility is to remain abreast of breakthroughs where prevention or gene therapies will surely replace the tragic reality of these conditions.

## OVERVIEW OF GENETIC DISORDERS

**Genetics** is defined as the study of the patterns of inheritance. A **genetic disease** can be defined as a disorder that is caused by a variation in genetic material. A disease results when a mutation in one or more genes arises spontaneously or is inherited. When expressed, the mutant gene either causes the synthesis of an abnormal protein or alters the level of production of a normal protein.

In 1997, the National Institutes of Health and the Department of Energy published Promoting Safe and Effective Genetic Testing in the United States: Final Report of the Task Force on Genetic Testing. This document is designed to provide guidelines for performing and safeguarding laboratory test results that reveal genetic information. In that regard, clinical

laboratorians are in a unique position to appreciate the intent and scope of the definition. A **genetic test** is

> the analysis of human DNA, RNA, chromosomes, proteins, and certain metabolites in order to detect heritable disease-related genotypes, mutation, phenotypes or karyotypes for clinical purposes. Such purposes include predicting risk of disease, identifying carriers, and establishing prenatal and clinical diagnosis or prognosis. Prenatal, newborn and carrier screening, as well as testing in high risk families, are included. Tests for metabolites are covered only when they are undertaken with high probability that an excess or deficiency of the metabolite indicates the presence of heritable mutations in single genes. Tests conducted purely for research are excluded from the definition, as are tests for somatic mutations and testing for forensic purposes.[1]

This definition clarifies for the laboratory scientist that all testing relating to metabolic disorders is, by definition, genetic testing. Therefore, the dissemination of the results of this testing requires the utmost prudence and confidentiality on the part of the professional. The information revealed through genetic related tests can be life altering to the individual as well as family members.

One way of thinking about genetic diseases is to divide them into three generalized groups based on the time of onset of their phenotypic expression:

- Group I defects are the congenital defects that are manifested in utero.
- Group II defects are hereditary and degenerative diseases that often develop later in life and may be influenced by environmental factors.
- Group III defects are inherited biochemical disorders that are expressed through the endocrine, metabolic, nutritional, or immunologic systems.

This delineation mirrors the *International Classification of Diseases, Ninth Revision* (ICD-9).[2]

### Group I: Congenital Defects Manifest in Utero

Congenital abnormalities refer here to a wide variety of structural anomalies in which the number and/or form of the chromosome is in some way altered.

T A B L E  1 3 – 1

**Tests Included in Various State Newborn Screening Programs**

| INHERITED DISORDER | INCIDENCE | SYMPTOMS | CAUSE | ANALYTE MEASURED | INTERVENTION |
|---|---|---|---|---|---|
| Phenylketonuria | 1:10,000 | Developmental delay, mental retardation, seizures, autisticlike behavior, peculiar mousy odor | Deficient enzyme phenylalanine hydroxylase, or impaired synthesis, or recycling of the biopterin (BN4) cofactor | Phenylalanine | Dietary restriction of protein |
| Congenital hypothyroidism | 1:3600 to 1:5000 | Neonatal jaundice; otherwise asymptomatic. Damage irreversible. Poor growth, goiter, low metabolic rate, constipation. Poor peripheral circulation, bradycardia, and myxedema | Inadequate production of thyroid hormone | Thyroxine (T4) Thyroid-stimulating hormone (TSH) | Oral hormone replacement |
| Galactosemia Galactose-1-uridyltransferase deficiency (GALT) | 1:60,000 to 1:80,000 | Failure to thrive, vomiting, liver disease, cataracts, mental retardation, death | Deficiency of one of the enzymes that catalyze galactose to glucose: galactokinase, galactose-1-phosphate uridyl transferase, or uridine diphosphate-galactose-4-epimerase | Galactose-1-phosphate uridyl transferase; Uridyl-1-transferase; Free galactose | Lactose/galactose-free diet |
| Maple syrup urine disease; Branched-chain ketoaciduria | 1:200,000 to 1:250,000 | Lethargy, irritability, and vomiting, progressing to coma and death if untreated | Deficient decarboxylases and other enzymes prevent the conversion of keto amino acids to fatty acids | Leucine, isoleucine, valine, and corresponding ketoacids also accumulate | Dietary restriction and monitoring of branched chain amino acids |
| Homocystinuria | 1:50,000 to 1:150,000 | Increased concentrations of homocystine in body tissues; thromboembolism, dislocation of the ocular lens, scoliosis, osteoporosis, developmental and mental retardation, seizures, psychiatric disturbances, myopathy, marfanoid habitus. | Absent or deficient cystathionine $\beta$-synthetase prevents the conversion of homocystine to cystathionine, resulting in increased concentrations of homocystine in body tissues | Methionine | Depends on which of the more than 9 genetic disorders is implicated; may indicate a methionine-restricted, cystine-supplemented diet; or folic acid and betaine therapy; or $B_6$; $B_{12}$ |

| Disorder | Incidence | Clinical Features | Pathophysiology | Screening Test | Treatment |
|---|---|---|---|---|---|
| Biotinidase deficiency | 1:70,000 to 1:100,000 | Seizures, hypotonia, dermatitis, alopecia, ataxia, hearing loss, optic nerve atrophy, metabolic acidosis, mental retardation, coma, death within 3 months of birth | Deficiency in the enzyme prevents the recycling of biotin, specifically, biocytin and biotinyl peptides cannot be cleaved, resulting in multiple carboxylase deficiency | Biotinidase | Oral biotin supplements |
| Congenital adrenal hyperplasia | 1:10,000 to 1:15,000 | "Salt wasting" type: severe dehydration; vascular shock. "Virilizing form": masculine features in the female | Deficiency in the enzyme 21-hydroxylase | 17-hydroxyprogesterone | Cortisol or analogs; surgery to correct ambiguous genitalia |
| Hemoglobinopathies | Hb SS: 1:375 Trait: 1:10 in blacks. Other Hb variants: F,A,G,D,J,N, Barts: 1:1000 | Initially, asymptomatic and nonemergent. With time, the following symptoms may appear: aseptic necrosis of bones, leg ulcers, neoproliferative retinopathy, infections, cerebral thrombosis, renal concentrating defects, and delayed growth and sexual maturation | Abnormal hemoglobins are synthesized or decreased synthesis of a beta globulin chain | Hemoglobin electrophoresis | Antibiotic prophylaxis, immunizations, pain management, screening for anemia, selected oxygen therapy |
| Glucose-6-phosphate dehydrogenase deficiency | 1:10 to 1:50 | Neonatal hyperbilirubinemia, chronic congenital nonspherocytic hemolytic anemia, drug- or viral-induced hemolytic anemia | Defect in the pentose phosphate pathway that protects hemoglobin from oxidant hemolysis | Glucose dehydrogenase activity | Avoid oxidant drugs; fava beans; aspirin |
| Tyrosinemia, types I and II | 1:250 in neonates weighing <2500 g; 1:500 in neonates weighing >2500 g | Failure to thrive, vomiting, diarrhea, hepatomegaly, renal tubular dysfunction, hypophosphatemic rickets, corneal lesions, linguistic delay, mental retardation; In addition, type II: hyperkeratosis with blisters | Type I: Reduced fumarylacetoacetase hydroxylase leading to inhibited multiple transport functions and enzymatic activity; Type II: Reduced hepatic tyrosine aminotransferase | Immunoassay for enzyme | Diets restricted in tyrosine and phenylalanine |

(continued)

**Tests Included in Various State Newborn Screening Programs (Continued)**

| INHERITED DISORDER | INCIDENCE | SYMPTOMS | CAUSE | ANALYTE MEASURED | INTERVENTION |
|---|---|---|---|---|---|
| Cystic fibrosis | 1:2000 in Europeans, 1:17,000 in blacks, 1:9000 in Hispanics | Poor growth with chronic respiratory infections, malabsorption, and gastrointestinal abnormalities; high level of sweat sodium and chloride; cirrhosis of liver | Generalized disturbance in exocrine function related to an abnormal transmembrane regulator protein that has properties of a chloride channel | Immunoreactive trypsin; sweat test for sodium and chloride | Oral nutrition, fat-soluble vitamins, predigested formula, pancreatic enzyme replacement. Pulmonary care with anti-*Pseudomonas* antibiotics. Gene therapy using recombinant DNA placed with a viral vector |
| Fatty acid oxidation disorders (FOD) | | Lethargy, hypotonia, vomiting, hypoglycemia leading to coma, encephalopathy, hepatic failure or death | Enzyme defect interrupts the fatty acid metabolic pathway so that the infant cannot use this store for an energy source. Condition is triggered by fasting, vomiting, and infection | Specific acylcarnitine(s) | Low fat diets, carnitine supplements, frequent meals, and no fasting. |
| Medium chain acyl-CoA dehydrogenase deficiency (MCAD) | 1:10,000 | | | | |
| Long chain 3-hydroxyacyl CoA dehydrogenase (LCHAD) | 1:50,000 | | | | |
| Very long chain acyl-CoA dehydrogenase deficiency (VLCAD) | Unknown | | | | |
| Short chain acyl CoA dehydrogenase deficiency (SCAD) | Unknown | | | | |
| Carnitine palmitoyl-transferase deficiency type II (CPT-II) | Unknown | | | | |

226

| Disorder | Incidence | Clinical Features | Pathophysiology | Laboratory Findings | Treatment |
|---|---|---|---|---|---|
| Glutaric acidemia type II (GA-II) 2,4 dienoyl-CoA reductase deficiency | Unknown | | | | |
| Organic aciduria disorders (OA) | | Vomiting, metabolic acidosis, ketosis, dehydration, coma, hyperammonemia, lactic acidosis, hypoglycemia, failure to thrive, hypotonia, sepsis, developmental delay, and hematologic disorders | Enzymatic deficiencies that lead to accumulation of organic acids in biologic fluids. This accumulation causes acid-base imbalances and altered pathways. | Abnormal acylcarnitine(s) | Low-protein diets, carnitine and/or vitamin supplements; avoid fasting. |
| Glutaryl CoA dehydrogenase deficiency type I (GA-I) | 1:30,000 | | | | |
| Propionyl CoA carboxylase deficiency (PA) | 1:50,000 | | | | |
| Methylmalonic acidemia (MMA) | 1:50,000 | | | | |
| Isovaleryl CoA dehydrogenase deficiency (IVA) | 1:50,000 | | | | |
| 3-Methylcrontonyl CoA carboxylase deficiency (3-MMC) | Unknown | | | | |
| Mitochondrial acetoacetyl CoA thiolase deficiency (b-KT) | Unknown | | | | |
| 3-Hydoxy-3-methylglutaryl-CoA lyase deficiency (HMG) | Unknown | | | | |

The diagnosis of these disorders is often made initially through prenatal counseling[3] that may include a thorough family history, ultrasound, or chromosome analysis of amniotic fluid. For example, the risk of an individual with spina bifida or other neural tube defects continues to be screened through nonspecific biochemical markers such as increases in alpha-fetoprotein. The higher the concentration of the marker, the greater the risk of the phenotypic expression of the condition in the infant. Ultrasound followed by amniocentesis allows for the confirmation of the most obvious of these defects. Fortunately, in some of these cases, the focus clinically is beginning to shift from diagnosis to prevention.

For example, evidence exists that neural tube defects such as spina bifida and anencephaly can to be prevented by supplementation of folic acid prior to conception.[4,5] In 1998, the Institute of Medicine recommended 0.4 mg (400 $\mu$g) of B vitamin folic acid from synthetic supplements and fortified foods in addition to a balanced diet of folate rich foods such as beans, orange juice, and leafy green vegetables for all women of childbearing age. The infants of women who have a family or personal history of neural tube defects have been shown to benefit from 4.0 mg of folic acid daily, beginning at least 3 months before conception and continuing through the first trimester.[6]

## Group II: Hereditary and Degenerative Diseases Manifest Later in Life

The symptoms of this group of inherited diseases appear in adolescence or adult life. For the degenerative diseases of the central nervous system, no curative treatments currently exist.

There are, however, a number of hereditary and degenerative diseases for which there are growing regimens of prevention and treatment.

Individuals with family histories of these disorders may request testing prior to the onset of the associated symptoms. In these cases, such as with Huntington's chorea, the individual may be tested for the gene mutation specific to the particular disease. The same opportunity exists for some types of cancer. For example, a woman who has lost her mother and a sibling to ovarian or breast cancer may wish to know if she carries the BRCA gene. If tests are positive, she could, among a number of other preventive measures, be assessed more frequently by medical personnel, increase the number of breast self-examinations in a month, or choose a semiannual mammogram or prophylactic mastectomy.

## Group III: Defects Expressed through the Endocrine, Metabolic, Nutritional, or Immunologic Systems

Historically, the **inborn errors of metabolism** represent the first understood subgroup of inherited and biochemical disorders that interrupt physiologic pathways. These disorders typically show no readily observable defects at birth. Within

days, however, the effects of the block in the physiologic pathway express themselves in one of three ways:

- excess toxic precursors
- excess toxic metabolites
- deficient metabolites

Infants with these defects become lethargic, fail to thrive, may experience vomiting, diarrhea, various neurologic symptoms, or overwhelming illness due to infection. If left undiagnosed and untreated, a number of these disorders result in poor growth, mental retardation among other developmental disabilities, and death. However, if the biochemical abnormality can be detected early before the excess or deficiency affects the child's brain, nervous system, or physical development, excess morbidity, mental retardation, or premature death may be avoided. For this reason, a number of these disorders are included in newborn screening programs, some of which are government mandated. Currently, newborns are screened for different diseases in different states.[7,8] The American Academy of Pediatrics advocates for the adoption of uniform testing standards. Table 13–1 lists the test menu included in various state newborn screening programs.[9,10]

Note that in addition to the inherited metabolic disorders, some state screening programs require universal hearing screening, whereas several state programs currently screen for 2 infections: toxoplasmosis and human immunodeficiency virus. These have been noted here only to complete the current listing.

## CLINICAL APPLICATIONS IN DETECTING METABOLIC RELATED DISORDERS

The inherited disorders selected for specific discussion in this chapter are based on either the potential significance for prevention or intervention through recommended newborn screening programs, or by startling laboratory observations that may aid in the diagnosis of relatively rare conditions. These disorders are grouped into the following categories by the ICD-9.

### Disorders of the Endocrine System

The disorders of interest include congenital hypothyroidism and congenital adrenal hyperplasia. Other disorders of the endocrine system such as diabetes mellitus, diabetes insipidus, acromegaly, gigantism, and dwarfism are discussed elsewhere in this text.

#### CONGENITAL HYPOTHYROIDISM

Congenital hypothyroidism, with an incidence of 1:3600 to 1:5000 births, represents the most common and preventable cause of mental retardation. The affected infants (formally referred to as cretins) are unable to produce adequate amounts of thyroid hormone due to thyroid aplasia or hypoplasia or its development in an abnormal location (ectopic). All newborn screening programs in the United States currently require a test for $T_4$ or thyroxine followed with a thyroid-stimulating hormone (TSH). In affected infants, the TSH is elevated and the $T_4$ values are decreased. If detected early and treated through life-long thyroid replacement hormone, between 70% and 80% of these infants may achieve an IQ of 85 or greater.[10,11]

## CONGENITAL ADRENAL HYPERPLASIA

Congenital adrenal hyperplasia, with an incidence of 1:10,000 to 1:15,000 births, is an autosomal recessive disorder. Several states include screening for this disorder by measuring 17-hydroxyprogesterone in a Guthrie blood spot (described later) by immunoassay or radioimmunoassay. Congenital adrenal hyperplasia is an inborn error of steroid biosynthesis that causes a lack of cortisol production and may also cause a lack of aldosterone production. A deficiency in 21-hydroxylase production is the cause of 90% to 95% of these cases. The blocked enzymatic step causes an overproduction and accumulation of precursors that are then shunted into the androgen biosynthetic pathway. The consequences of this deficiency are expressed most often in a "salt wasting type" or a virilizing form. Infants severely affected with the salt wasting type may present to the emergency room with severe dehydration and vascular shock characteristic of adrenal crisis. In the case of the virilizing form, the increased fetal adrenal androgens in the female infant may be expressed in masculine features, resulting potentially in the wrong sex assignment at birth. Infants with this deficiency presenting with the salt-losing diagnosis are treated with aldosterone, cortisol, or analogs. Infants presenting with the virilizing form are treated with cortisol; surgical correction of ambiguous genitalia may be indicated.

## Disorders of the Metabolic Systems

The disorders associated with metabolic pathways, or the inborn errors of metabolism, that are relevant to this discussion may be grouped as follows:

- disorders of amino-acid transport and metabolism
- disorders of carbohydrate and lipid transport and metabolism

## DISTURBANCES OF AMINO-ACID TRANSPORT

More than 150 amino acids have been described. Of those 21 are necessary for human life. Of the 21, 10 of the amino acids depend on diet as a source; these are often referred to as the essential amino acids. The remaining 11 amino acids can be synthesized.

A disorder may arise when a disturbance occurs in any of the amino acid structures or pathways. These disturbances regularly result in aminoaciduria. Traditionally, the aminoacidurias have been termed either renal aminoacidurias or overflow aminoacidurias. The **renal aminoacidurias** are characterized by normal levels of the amino acid in the plasma but increased levels in the urine; these are often triggered by decreased renal tubular reabsorption. The malfunction in reabsorption may result due to a congenital abnormality of renal tubular function or it may occur as a result of, or in association with, some acquired disease.

The **overflow aminoacidurias** are characterized by increased concentration of one or more of the amino acids or their metabolites in the plasma and in the urine as a result of normal renal clearance.

Another way to characterize the aminoacidurias is to consider if the finding is primary or secondary. **Primary aminoaciduria** results from an enzyme defect in the pathway by which a specific amino acid is metabolized. **Secondary aminoaciduria** results when the defect is located in the renal tubular transport mechanism. Secondary aminoaciduria may also arise when the diseased organ, such as the kidney, has developed a generalized renal tubular dysfunction. Liver disease or starvation may additionally result in secondary aminoaciduria.

Cystinuria, cystinosis, and Hartnup syndrome are examples of **disturbances of amino acid transport.** Laboratory findings leading to a diagnosis of cystinuria and Hartnup syndrome are seldom life threatening. However, these same findings leading to a diagnosis of cystinosis result in death.

### Cystinuria

Although it is now understood that cystinuria is the result of an error in amino acid transport and not metabolism per se, it stands as one of the original "inborn errors of metabolism" described by Sir A.E. Garrod in 1908. The disorder occurs with an incidence of 1:10,000 births and is inherited as an autosomal recessive disorder. In cystinuria, the carrier protein responsible for transporting the amino acids cystine, lysine, ornithine, and arginine across the epithelial cell membrane into the renal tubules and into the intestinal wall is defective. All of these amino acids are alpha amino acids and have in common a second amino group in the molecule. This feature is illustrated in Figure 13–1.

The defect in the renal tubular reabsorption mechanism results in a renal aminoaciduria because the amino acids cannot be reabsorbed from the glomerular filtrate. Excessive amounts of these amino acids are excreted, and renal calculi occur.[11]

The remarkable laboratory finding in these cases is the colorless, hexagonal cystine crystals that precipitate in acid urine. The characterization of these crystals as cystine has in the past been identified by the cyanide/nitroprusside test. In this analysis, the cystine is reduced to cysteine by sodium cyanide; the resulting free sulfhydryl groups react with nitroprusside to produce a red purple color. Today, the presence of cystine can further be confirmed by high-pressure liquid chromatography. The cystine concentration can be quantified if a 24-hour specimen is submitted. Quantitative ion exchange amino acid analysis can detect not only the increased amount

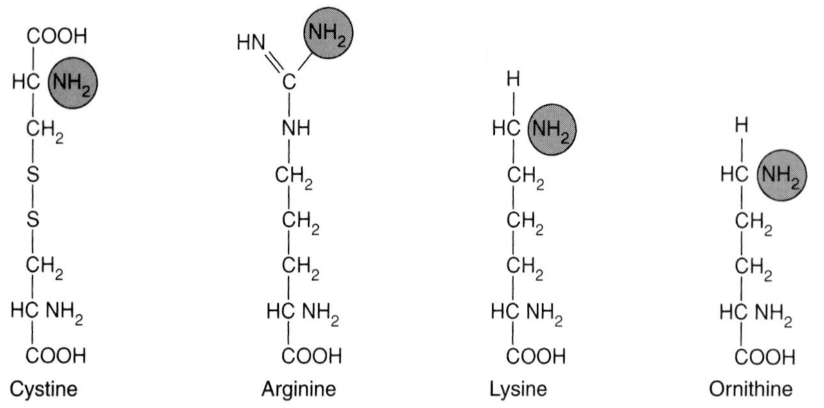

**FIGURE 1 3 - 1**

Structural similarity between cystine and the basic amino acids arginine, lysine, and ornithine.

of cystine but also the amount of lysine, arginine, and ornithine present.

Finding the cystine crystals may indicate the individual's potential to form cystine calculi or nephrolithiasis. The calculi are yellow-white in color and have a characteristic waxy luster. These stones are often soft but at the same time, densely granular. Cystine stones account for 1% to 3% of renal calculi. These renal calculi may occur throughout childhood and peak in the third decade of life. They tend to recur following removal. Cystinuria may be a marker for an individual with renal tubular disease.

Therapy for cystinuria currently includes restricted diet, hydration, maintaining the urine pH above 7.5, chelation, chemolysis, and surgery. For those individuals in whom the cystine stones are resistant to dissolution, shock-wave destruction (percutaneous ultrasonic lithotripsy) has proven a possible alternative.

## Cystinosis

While in cystinuria, the amino acid crystallizes in the urine, in cystinosis, the cystine crystals are deposited in the kidneys, eyes, bone marrow, liver, spleen, and macrophages. As such, cystinosis is considered a lysosomal storage disorder that is thought to result from a defect in the transport process for the passage of cystine across lysosomal membranes. This condition occurs in about 1:40,000 births. The systemic manifestations of this condition are life threatening.

Three forms of cystinosis have been described based on the time of onset of symptoms: nephropathic infant onset, intermediate or adolescent onset, and benign adult onset. Individuals with infantile nephropathic cystinosis display neurologic deficits, failure to thrive, photophobia, rickets, acidosis, and generalized renal dysfunction as evidenced by increased renal excretion of potassium, glucose, and phosphate as well as amino acids. When proximal tubular defects result in glycosuria, aminoaciduria, phosphaturia, proteinuria, and acidosis, the condition is referred to as **Fanconi syndrome**. Cysti-

nosis is only one potential cause of Fanconi syndrome. Individuals experiencing late onset, intermediate, or adolescent cystinosis manifest symptoms anywhere between 18 months and 17 years of age. The kidney damage is less severe and Fanconi syndrome does not surface.

Benign or adult-onset cystinosis results in cystine crystals deposited in the cornea, leukocytes, and bone marrow. The condition is often diagnosed through an incidental finding during an eye examination and tends not to result in renal dysfunction or retinopathy.

## Hartnup Syndrome

With an incidence of 1:18,000 births, Hartnup syndrome is characterized by general aminoaciduria. Most of the amino acids excreted are the neutral monocarboxylic structures and include alanine, threonine, glutamine, serine, asparagine, valine, leucine, isoleucine, phenylalanine, tyrosine, tryptophan, histidine, and citrulline.

Individuals with Hartnup syndrome often present with gait difficulty, emotional lability, delusions, tremor, and a red, scaly pellagralike rash that appears within the first decade of life. This rash is the result of a nicotinamide deficiency that results when tryptophan, which is normally converted to nicotinic acid and nicotinamide, is malabsorbed. Tryptophan serves as a precursor for nicotinamide. With more than 400 mg of nicotinamide daily, the tryptophan malabsorption becomes less of a problem.

## DISTURBANCES OF AMINO ACID METABOLISM

### Phenylketonuria

The incidence of phenylketonuria, leading to an increase in plasma and urinary phenylalanine, is 1:10,000 to 1:25,000 births. Phenylketonuria (PKU) is an autosomal recessive disorder resulting in a deficiency of the liver enzyme phenylalanine hydroxylase or of impaired synthesis or impaired recycling of the biopterin (BN4) cofactor. Normally the amino acid phenylalanine is converted to tyrosine through a complex pathway requiring phenylalanine hydroxylase (Figure 13–2).

The dysfunction within this pathway results in an accumulation of phenylalanine in the blood and urine (phenylketonuria). Other abnormal metabolites of phenylalanine, namely phenyllactic, phenylpyruvic, and phenylacetic acids also appear in the urine. Infants appear entirely normal after birth. However, undiagnosed and untreated PKU results in progressive developmental delay in the first year of life, followed by severe mental retardation, seizures, a peculiar mousy odor, hypopigmentation, eczema, and autisticlike behavior including self-injury. The hypopigmentation develops because phenylalanine is a competitive inhibitor of tyrosinase, the enzyme that initiates the pathway for the production of melanin. The impairment of the central nervous system is due to the excess phenylalanine and the consequential reduction of norepinephrine, myelin, and serotonin levels, leading to convulsions and extreme hyperactivity. The peculiar mousy odor is due to the increased phenylacetic acid excreted in the sweat and urine.

In 1962, Robert Guthrie developed the Guthrie test to detect this inborn error of metabolism.[12] The test relied on a blood-soaked filter paper sample taken from the infant after feeding between the first and the seventh days of life. A disk of the dried blood sample is placed on culture media containing β-2-thienylanaine, which has been inoculated with *Bacillus subtilis* spores. Normally, the β-2-thienylanaine inhibits this particular strain. Increased concentrations of phenylalanine allow the organism to overcome the inhibition and grow. After an overnight incubation, the zones of bacterial growth are compared with control disks containing known amounts of phenylalanine. In 1963, Massachusetts was the first state to implement newborn screening. Today all 50 states include newborn screening for PKU.[13]

The qualitative bioinhibition assay developed by Guthrie is being replaced by quantitative automated fluorometric assays. These and other assays in the newborn screening menu still rely on the Guthrie blood-soaked filter-paper technique. Clinical laboratorians have a shared responsibility to ensure that the preanalytical conditions of timing and technique of the specimen collection are correct.[14] Screening must occur in newborns older than 24 hours and younger than 7 days of age. Infants who are screened prior to the first 24 hours of life, those who have received blood transfusions, and those who are born prematurely are candidates for retesting. It is important for laboratorians to know which screening test method is being used in individual state laboratories. For example, antibiotic therapy can affect results by inhibiting bacterial growth in the traditional Guthrie bioinhibition assay. Moreover, the screening cutoff values for diagnosis varies from state to state. Clinical laboratorians will want to watch for changes in technology and to monitor cutoff limits as result reporting for the diagnosis of PKU becomes standardized. They will also want to play a role in assuring that test results are reported to responsible parties in an immediate turnaround time so that therapies may commence at once.

Initial results suggestive of PKU require confirmation through quantitative analysis of serum phenylalanine, tyrosine, urinary pteridines, and blood dihydropteridine reductase. The results of these tests assist the clinician in prescribing therapy. The American Academy of Pediatrics recommends that all infants with phenylalanine levels above 6 mg/dL should be considered for dietary restriction.[10] Infants who begin early reduction of phenylalanine levels through a protein-restricted diet and special formulas and who avoid aspartame, often found in diet drinks and nonglucose sweeteners, may achieve normal intelligence. Follow-up requires periodic serum assays for phenylalanine and tyrosine. The National Institutes of Health most recent consensus panel recommends a comprehensive approach to lifelong care for individuals with PKU. The target phenylalanine level for infants and children through 12 years is 2–6 mg/dL and for individuals over age 12 is 2–15 mg/dL.

Newborn screening for the presence of PKU and a restricted diet to avoid the most morbid of outcomes represents a breakthrough in genetic medicine. For the first time, a form of mental retardation that had been considered therapeutically hopeless is now in fact treatable. Affected individuals born since the mid-1960s have benefitted. Now that these individuals have reached childbearing age, a secondary phenomenon has surfaced—maternal PKU. Women who have ceased dietary restriction of phenylalanine will give birth to infants already compromised and mentally retarded. Today it is understood that women affected by this genetic disorder must return to the protein-restricted diets prior to conception and throughout the pregnancy to avoid a morbid outcome for the infant.

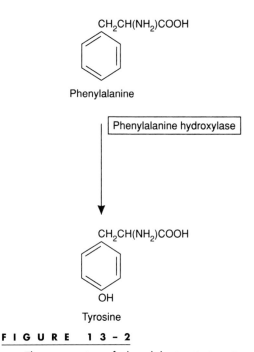

$CH_2CH(NH_2)COOH$

Phenylalanine

Phenylalanine hydroxylase

$CH_2CH(NH_2)COOH$

OH

Tyrosine

**FIGURE 13-2**

The conversion of phenylalanine to tyrosine.

Prenatal diagnosis and carrier testing are available by DNA analysis.

**Alkaptonuria** and **tyrosinemia** (formally tyrosinosis [type I] and tyrosinuria [type II]) are other examples of disorders of aromatic amino-acid metabolism that result from a deficiency or absence of an enzyme that leads to the accumulation of a compound in the metabolic pathway. The accumulation of the compound is toxic and results in symptoms that are characteristic of the disease (Figure 13–3). **Albinism** is an example of an absent enzyme; the characteristic symptoms result from the absence of a compound that should have been produced.

## Albinism

There are two types of albinism. Although both are inherited as autosomal recessive traits, each type is caused by separate recessive gene defects. The incidence of oculocutaneous albinism type I is about 1:10,000 births. The condition arises due to the absence of tyrosinase, the enzyme that converts tyrosine to melanin (Figure 13–4).

Because no melanin is produced, eyesight is extremely poor and color of the hair, skin, and eyes is lacking. The in-

cidence of oculocutaneous albinism type II is about 1:60,000 births. The condition results due to a quantitative deficiency of tyrosinase. Associated symptoms are less acute.

## Alkaptonuria

The incidence of this rare condition is about 1:250,000 births. Historically, alkaptonuria was one of the original inborn errors of metabolism described by Garrod. Normally, phenylalanine and tyrosine are metabolized to homogentisic acid, which is further oxidized to maleylacetoacetic acid. If the liver enzyme homogentisic acid oxidase is missing or deficient, homogentisic acid accumulates (Figure 13–5).

Infants with this condition may present with darkened urine after it is exposed to air, sunlight, or the addition of alkali. Later in life, adults may present with characteristic arthritis. These individuals may develop dark blue or black pigments in their cartilage and connective tissue due to the accumulation of homogentisic acid polymers.

## Tyrosinemia: Types I and II

Tyrosinemia is currently the single term used to describe two types of autosomal recessive conditions, both of which are

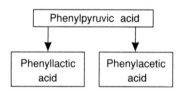

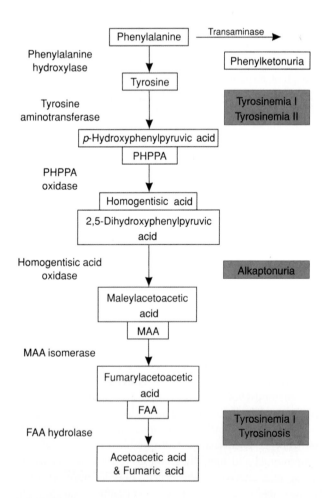

## FIGURE   13 - 3

Metabolic pathway of phenylalanine.

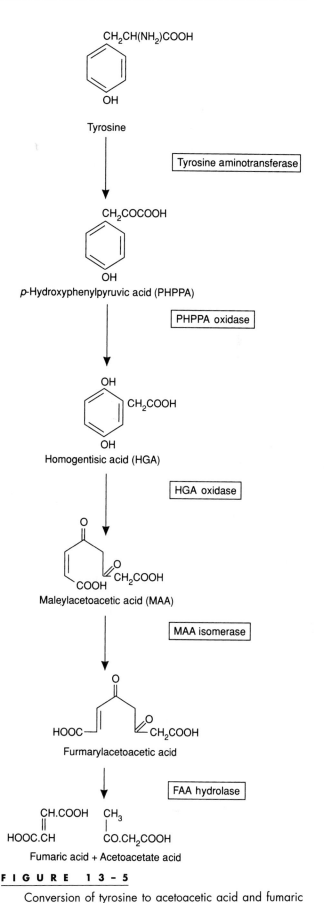

**FIGURE 13-4**

Conversion of tyrosine to melanin.

characterized by elevated tyrosine levels detectable in the blood and urine. Elevated tyrosine levels are not uncommon in premature infants. Tyrosinemia can be diagnosed using the Guthrie blood spot and an immunoassay. The sample should be taken 48 to 72 hours after milk feeding. States vary regarding whether this test is a part of the mandatory newborn screening program. Affected infants may present with vomiting, diarrhea, failure to thrive, hepatomegaly, renal tubular dysfunction that may lead to Fanconi syndrome, hypophosphatemic rickets, corneal lesions, mild retardation, and linguistic delay. Tyrosinemia with increased levels of tyrosine and phenylalanine appears as a result of enzyme deficiencies that lead to a relative deficiency of *p*-hydroxyphenylpyruvate (PHPPA) when the individual is stressed via a high-protein diet. In the case of tyrosinemia type I, commonly referred to as tyrosinosis, the enzyme activity of furmarylacetoacetate acid hydrolase (FAH) is deficient. Tyrosinemia type I may occur in an acute or chronic form. In addition to the symptoms listed earlier, infants with the acute form have a cabbagelike odor. Moreover, increased levels of tyrosine in the blood and urine, and increased blood levels of methionine can be detected. The incidence is 1:250 among premature infants weighing <2500 g. The highest incidence of 1:16 can be observed in Canadian Inuits who do not breastfeed their infants. Infants of Scandinavian decent and French Canadians are also at increased risk.

**FIGURE 13-5**

Conversion of tyrosine to acetoacetic acid and fumaric acid.

Tyrosinemia type II is sometimes called Richner-Hanhart syndrome and is characterized by hyperkeratosis with painful, nonpurulent blisters and an oculocutaneous syndrome, resulting in lacrimation, photophobia, and redness. The deficient enzyme in type II is the hepatic enzyme tyrosine aminotransferase (TAT), the rate-limiting enzyme of tyrosine catabolism. This deficiency results in lifetime tyrosinemia, tyrosinuria, and increases in urinary phenolic acids, N-acetyltyrosine and tyramine. The incidence of this particular disorder has not been established. Both types I and II tyrosinemia appear to respond to diets low in tyrosine, phenylalanine and methionine. Transient tyrosinemia in neonates may be controlled by reducing the protein.[10] Laboratory findings associated with tyrosinemia may include generalized aminoaciduria, with a marked loss of glucose, ketones, proteins, and phosphate. In the most severe of cases of liver involvement, tyrosine crystals may be observed in the urinary sediment.

## Maple Syrup Urine Disease

**Maple syrup urine disease (MSUD) is an example of a disturbance of branched-chain amino-acid metabolism.** Of this class of disorders, maple syrup urine disease, with an incidence of 1:200,00 to 1:250,000 births, is the one sometimes included in newborn screening programs. This genetic autosomal recessive disorder includes the disruption of the metabolism of the branched-chain amino acids leucine, isoleucine, and valine.

The defect is rooted in the second step of decarboxylation wherein the keto acid decarboxylase enzyme fails to function. This disorder leads to a build up of leucine, isoleucine, valine, and their corresponding keto acids in the serum, spinal fluid, and urine of the infant. In classic cases of MSUD, the body fluids of the infant, including the urine, the sweat, and the ear cerumen, cast a characteristic burnt maple sugar odor. Symptoms, including lethargy, irritability, and coma resulting in mental retardation and death, appear usually between 3 and 7 days after birth. In addition to the sweet odor in the urine, other laboratory findings may include hypoglycemia and acidosis. Increased levels of keto acids in the urine can be detected by the presence of a yellow-white precipitate with the dinitrophenylhydrazine test and a gray-blue color with the ferric chloride test. Screening methods employ the bacterial inhibition assay, 4-azaleucine, to detect increased levels of leucine in the Guthrie dried blood spot. Preanalytical concerns include the need for a collection of the specimen between 14 and 24 hours of age. Specimens obtained earlier may not detect an increase in leucine. Positive results must be reported immediately because mental retardation can occur within the first week of life unless dietary restriction of the branched-chain amino acids is implemented without delay. Dietary management can aid in reducing mental retardation and death.

## Homocystinurias

**Homocystinurias** are examples of **disturbances of sulfur-bearing amino-acid metabolism.** The **homocystinurias** are a group of autosomal recessive disorders that are characterized by increased concentrations of homocystine in body tissues due to a defect in the catabolism of sulfur-containing amino acids. The incidence of homocystinuria is approximately 1 in 50,000 to 1 in 150,000.[10] The classic homocystinuria is due to an absence or deficiency in cystathionine β-synthetase, the enzyme which converts homocysteine to cystathionine (Figure 13–6). Specifically, the enzyme deficiency affects the transsulfuration pathway that converts the sulfur atom of methionine into the sulfur atom of cysteine. This is the primary pathway through which methionine is disposed. The defect results in a buildup of homocysteine, homocystine metabolites and methionine, which can be detected through a Guthrie blood spot test. In the past, the increased methionine was detected by a bacterial inhibition assay using methionine sulfoximine. As with many of these inborn errors of metabolism, timing of the collection of the specimen may be critical. Diagnostic levels of methionine may not be present until after 3 days of life, when there is adequate protein intake.[10] Newer diagnostic methods include direct methionine assays by tandem mass spectrometry. Of potential interest in the clinical laboratory is that urine with increased methionine and homocysteine will produce a reddish color with the cyanide-nitroprusside spot test.

At birth, the infant with homocystinuria appears normal. With age, the following symptoms emerge: thromboembolism, dislocation of the ocular lens, scoliosis, osteoporosis, developmental disabilities including mental retardation, seizures, psychiatric disturbances, myopathy, and a marfanoid habitus (a tall and lean body type with long extremities). After identification of homocystinuria, treatment depends on which of the at least 9 specific genetic disorders constitutes the underlying cause. If the underlying deficiency is the cystathionine β-synthase, treatment includes a methionine-restricted, cystine-supplemented diet. Folic acid and betaine therapy have been

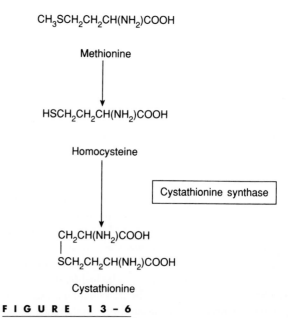

**F I G U R E    1 3 - 6**

Conversion of methionine to cystathionine.

reported to help in these cases. If pyridoxine is the underlying metabolic defect, then treatment includes large doses of vitamin $B_6$. If cobalamin metabolism and transport in which methylmalonic acid and homocystine appear in the urine, then these individuals may be treated with hydroxycobalmin or vitamin $B_{12}$.

## DISTURBANCES OF CARBOHYDRATE AND LIPID TRANSPORT AND METABOLISM

This chapter has focused on disorders of amino-acid transport and metabolism that are of interest due to special findings in the clinical laboratory and those for which newborn screening is recommended by the American Academy of Pediatrics. The discussion of which metabolites to include in newborn screening programs is currently at the forefront of scientific and political debate at national and state levels. Because clinical laboratorians have a role to play in these important public health issues, and in the interest of being complete, the following discussion briefly mentions the other metabolites that if detected and treated early in the newborns life may prevent developmental disabilities, mental retardation, and death.

### Galactosemia

This inherited disorder is an example of a **disorder of carbohydrate transport and metabolism** that is expressed as a cellular deficiency of galactose-1-phosphate uridyl transferase, galactokinase, or uridine diphosphate-galactose-4-epimerase. All of these enzymes catalyze the reaction in the unique pathway by which galactose is converted to glucose. Infants may present with failure to thrive, vomiting, liver disease, cataracts, and mental retardation in untreated survivors. Newborn screening programs screen for increased galactose using either *Escherichia coli* (or *E. coli*) in combination with a bacteriophage (Paigen test), or a fluorescent spot screening test (Beutler test) and a fluorometric assay (Hill test). The early and rapid onset of symptoms require a rapid turnaround time so that follow-up care in specialized metabolic and genetic clinics can be initiated.

### Fatty Acid Oxidation Disorders

The **fatty acid oxidation disorders** are 7 of the newest tests to be included in public health laboratory menus. The acquisition of the tandem mass spectrometer has made the expanded screening tests possible. These **disorders of lipid metabolism** represent a class of inborn errors characterized by an enzyme defect in the fatty acid metabolic pathway, which inhibits the body's ability to utilize stored fat. These disorders are listed in Table 13–1. Clinical symptoms include hypotonia, lethargy, and vomiting. Resulting hypoglycemia can result in coma, encephalopathy, hepatic failure, or death. Once diagnosed, treatment includes a low-fat diet and supplementing the diet with therapeutic levels of carnitine. Acute episodes are managed by administering intravenous glucose.

For example, medium chain acyl-CoA dehydrogenase is an 8-carbon fatty acid known as octanocylcarnitine or C8, one of the acylcarnitines. A deficiency of this enzyme, known as MCAD, is an autosomal recessive inherited disorder that occurs with a frequency of 1 in 10,000 births. Newborns with this deficiency often die because of the resulting defect of fatty acid oxidation. In other words, these infants lack the enzyme to metabolize fat to provide energy between feedings or during acute episodes of infection or vomiting. It is now suspected that perhaps 2% to 3% of all deaths attributed to sudden infant death syndrome may be caused by MCAD. Once diagnosed, infants may survive and live a healthy normal life. Typically meals are spaced no more than 10 hours apart. Additionally, the diet may be supplemented with carnitine.

## OTHER AND UNSPECIFIED DISORDERS OF METABOLISM

### Cystic Fibrosis

**Cystic fibrosis** is an example of an **unspecified disorder of metabolism.** It is an autosomal recessive disorder of exocrine function that results because of an abnormal transmembrane regulator protein that has properties of a chloride channel. Incidence in offspring of Northern Europeans may be as common as 1 in 2000; in African Americans, 1 in 17,000; and in Hispanics, 1 in 9000.[10] The defective cystic fibrosis transmembrane regulator protein results in thick mucus secretions, chronic obstructive lung disease, recurrent pulmonary infection, cor pulmonale, and death. In addition to a general failure to thrive, the clinical laboratory may see evidence of high levels of sweat sodium and chloride, cirrhosis of the liver, and an abnormal glucose tolerance.

Newborns can be screened for this disorder using the Guthrie blood spot. The immunoreactive trypsin (IRT) test uses an immunoassay method. Elevations of immunoreactive trypsin decline in the first few months of birth; therefore timing of the collection of the specimen is not as critical for diagnosis and treatment as in some other metabolic disorders. Genetic counseling and prenatal diagnosis for cystic fibrosis are available. Carrier screening is available through DNA mutation analysis. Gene therapy for this condition is under investigation.

### Biotinidase Deficiency

**Biotinidase deficiency** is classified as a **deficiency of other circulating enzymes.** Biotinidase deficiency is an autosomal recessive disorder of biotin recycling with an incidence of approximately 1 in 10,000 to 1 in 15,000 births. The enzyme biotinidase liberates biotin, an essential cofactor, from biocytin and biotinyl peptides so that it can be used by the body. When a deficiency of biotinidase exists, then the body cannot use biotin efficiently and several enzyme systems are slowed or halted. A multiple carboxylase deficiency results. The individual may present with ketoacidosis and acidemia. Left untreated, the child may exhibit seizures, dermatitis, alopecia, ataxia, hearing loss, optic nerve atrophy, developmental delay, and metabolic acidosis. Coma and death may result. The infant's serum is assayed for a deficiency of biotinidase by a colorimetric method on a dried blood spot. The effects of this deficiency disappear when the child is given therapeutic levels of biotin.

## Organic Acidurias

**Organic acidurias** are a group of inherited metabolic disorders that lead to an accumulation of organic acids in biologic fluids such as blood and urine. Table 13–1 lists 7 now screened for disorders using the tandem mass spectrometer. The buildup of organic acids in the blood and urine produces disturbances in the acid-base balance and causes alterations in pathways of intermediary metabolism.[15] These disorders can cause intoxication-like symptoms such as episodes of vomiting, metabolic acidosis, ketosis, dehydration, or coma. Infants may present with hypoglycemia, lactic acidosis, or hyperammonemia. Chronic symptoms include recurrent vomiting, failure to thrive, hypotonia, and global developmental delay. Individuals found to suffer from these inborn errors of metabolism may be treated by restricting protein in the diet and with vitamin supplements and/or carnitine to relieve symptoms.

In addition to these disorders, newborn screening programs may include tests for the infection toxoplasmosis and the hemoglobinopathies, specifically sickle cell diseases: SS, SC, and S/$\beta$-thalassemia.

---

## ANALYTICAL PROCEDURES: PAST, PRESENT, AND ANTICIPATED

The clinical laboratorian continues to play a critical role in the identification of an individual with inherited metabolic disorders. Until the standard test menu for newborn screening is accepted in every state, laboratory personnel should be vigilant for indicators of conditions not included in the screen. Even for those tests included in the screening menu, the turnaround time from specimen collection to result reporting may not be optimum for alerting the clinician and initiating corrective therapies in the most timely manner. Consequently, the laboratory reporting of classic urine observations could still play a role in identifying the underlying cause of an individuals failure to thrive, jaundice, poor appetites, abnormal body odors, vomiting, and delayed development.

The classic observations include the color, odor, and identification of crystals present in the urine. Table 13–2 summarizes these classic laboratory findings in some of these disorders. The principles of these tests are reviewed briefly.

The **ferric chloride test** is classic for its detecting aromatic hydroxyl groups. The urine is acidified with dilute hydrochloric acid; 10% ferric chloride solution is added. In the presence of phenylpyruvic acid, the toxic byproduct of unmetabolized phenylalanine, a dark green color fades to yellow. The presence of tyrosine and $p$-hydroxyphenylpyruvic acid (PHPPA) yields a green color. The alpha-ketoisocaproic acid resulting from the maple sugar urine disease yields a blue-gray color. Homogentisic acid associated with alkaptonuria yields a blue color. The ferric chloride test is nonspecific; therefore certain drugs such as phenothiazines and salicylates can result in a false positive.

The Phenistix, developed originally by Ames Company in Elkhart, IN, was an adaptation of the ferric chloride test, directed more specifically to detect phenylpyruvic acid. The reagent pad contained ferric ammonium sulfate, magnesium sulfate, and cyclohexylsulfamic acid. The Guthrie bacterial

TABLE  13 – 2

**Classic Laboratory Observations of Inherited Metabolic Disorders**

| DISORDER | COLOR | ODOR | CRYSTAL | CHEMICAL/COLORIMETRIC |
|---|---|---|---|---|
| Cystinuria |  | Sulfurous | Cystine | Cyanide/nitroprusside (red) |
| Cystinosis |  |  | Cystine | Cyanide/nitroprusside (red) |
| Phenylkenoturia |  | Mousy/Musty |  | Ferric chloride (dark blue-green) |
|  |  |  |  | 2,4-Dinitrophenylhydrazine (yellow-white precipitate) |
| Tyrosinemia I & II | Dark brown |  | Tyrosine | Ferric chloride (green) |
|  |  |  |  | Nitrosonaphthol (orange) |
|  |  |  |  | 2,4-Dinitrophenylhydrazine (yellow-white precipitate) |
| Alkaptonuria | Dark brown |  |  | Ferric chloride (blue) |
| Maple syrup urine disease |  | Maple syrup |  | Ferric chloride (blue-gray) |
|  |  |  |  | 2,4-Dinitrophenylhydrazine (yellow-white precipitate) |
| Homocystinuria |  | Sulfurous |  | Cyanide/nitroprusside (red) |
| Galactosemia and related pentoses, fructoses, lactoses |  |  |  | Glucose oxidase negative/copper reduction test positive |

inhibition assay, as described earlier in the chapter, typically replaced the generalized use of the Phenistix product. Currently, phenylalanine levels characteristic of PKU are detected through a fluorometric reaction. In this procedure, phenylalanine, copper, and ninhydrin are enhanced by any number of method specific dipeptides. The product of this reaction is measured fluorometrically. Phenylalanine and tyrosine as well as leucine and isoleucine (characteristic of MSUD) among other amino acids are detectable by tandem mass spectrometry as well.

Carbonyl groups of $\alpha$-keto amino acids in urine react with **dinitrophenylhydrazine** to produce insoluble hydrazones. A positive result is displayed in a yellow or yellow-white precipitate and is characteristic of phenylketonuria and MSUD. Tyrosine forms a soluble red complex with **nitrosonaphthol**. Positive results may suggest tyrosinemia or phenylketonuria.

**Cyanide (sodium or ferro) nitroprusside** reacts in the presence of dilute alkali with free sulfhydryl groups to produce a reddish-purple color. Cysteine, cystine, and homocystine yield a positive result.

The results of the nonspecific chemical tests have long required confirmation of a specific amino acid or metabolite by paper or thin layer chromatography, or high-pressure liquid chromatography. These technologies are further enhanced today with polymerase chain reaction,[16] DNA microarray,[17] and tandem mass spectrometry.[18,19] The tandem mass spectrometer represents the technology that has allowed the organic acidemias and the fatty acid oxidation disorders to be added to newborn screening menus. Periodically checking with the newborn screening programs in each state and territory is the only way to remain current regarding this topic.

What remains the same, however, is that most of this testing is accomplished with the same Guthrie blot spot cards devised in the 1960s. Collection of these specimens remains critical. The National Committee on Clinical Laboratory Standards has prepared a guideline. **Time and Technique of Collection** remain critical preanalytical features of these screenings. Each analyte has a somewhat different optimum time of collection. Transfusions, premature births, and time of feeding are all critical to ensuring that the metabolite has had an opportunity to raise to measurable levels in the infant's blood. These samples must be collected, sent to the public health laboratory, and results obtained. Getting specimens to the public health laboratories in a timely fashion remains a problem. Typically, there is a minimum of 48 to 72 hours of time lapse between collection and resulting. This system suffers also from incomplete collections, lost specimens, and other technical error. Consequently, the traditional role that laboratorians have played in first-line observation remains important to the overall scheme of early diagnosis and prevention.

## SUMMARY

The unraveling of the human genome has opened vistas of possibility as well as reason for caution. To date, more than

300 inherited errors of metabolism have been described. These are usually inherited as an autosomal recessive trait. A missing or deficient enzyme can cause a block in the metabolic pathway and result in toxic metabolites. Many of these disorders produce nonspecific symptoms in the newborn that, if undetected and untreated, may lead to developmental delay and mental retardation. The clinical laboratory can provide valuable information ranging from simple screening tests on urine samples to more sophisticated amino acid and metabolic identification and quantification. As the technologies continue to evolve, the challenge will be to balance the benefit of screening and needed therapies with the costs and risks. In the meantime, the clinical laboratorian will be required to maintain the highest standards of confidentiality. Laboratories will no doubt be required to ensure that consent forms for genetic testing have been explained and signed. Technical issues include discussions of sensitivity and specificity of screening tests and the determination of reportable ranges. Moreover, the laboratorian must also be concerned that funding and appropriate programs are available for supportive therapies. Clinical laboratorians have an opportunity to support public health departments by remaining aware of issues surrounding newborn screening and efforts to standardize screening menus.

## REFERENCES

1. Holtzman NA, Watson MS: *Promoting Safe and Effective Genetic Testing in the United States: Final Report of the Task Force on Genetic Testing.* Washington, D.C., National Institutes of Health, Department of Energy, September, 1997.
2. *International Classification of Diseases, Ninth Revision—Clinical Modification, Sixth Edition.* Los Angeles, CA, Practice Management Information Corporation. October, 2000.
3. Simonoff E: Mental retardation: Genetic findings, clinical implications and research agenda. J Child Psychiatry 37:359, 1996.
4. Knowledge and use of folic acid by women of childbearing age–United States 1995 and 1998. Morb Mortal Wkly Rep 48:April 30, 1999.
5. Neural tube defect surveillance and folic acid intervention—Texas-Mexico border, 1993–1998. Morb Mortal Wkly Rep 49: January 14, 2000.
6. Isabel JM, Miller SM: Detection, prevention of birth defects. Adv Lab 73–76, March, 2000.
7. *Newborn Screening–1996: An Overview of Newborn Screening Programs in the United States, Canada, Puerto Rico and the Virgin Islands.* Maternal and Child Health Program (Title V, Social Security Act). Washington, D.C., Maternal and Child Health Bureau, Health Resources and Services Administration, U.S. Department of Health and Human Services.
8. Serving the family from birth to the medical home—newborn screening: A blueprint for the future. Executive

summary: Newborn screening task force report. Pediatrics 106:386–388, 2000.

9.  A call for a national agenda on state newborn screening programs. Pediatrics 106:393, 2000.

10. Newborn screening fact sheets: American Academy of Pediatrics Committee on newborn screening. Pediatrics 98:473–501, 1996.

11. Lashley FR: *Clinical Concepts in Nursing Practice.* New York, Springer Publishing Co., 1998.

12. Paul DB: The history of newborn phenylketonuria acreening in the U.S. Appendix 5: In Holtzman NA, Watson MS (eds.): *Promoting Safe and Effective Genetic Testing in the United States: Final Report of the Task Force on Genetic Testing.* Washington, D.C., National Institutes of Health, Department of Energy, September, 1997.

13. Joseph F, Russo TM: Origins of spurious organic acidurias. Lab Med 31:622–624, 2000.

14. National Committee on Clinical Laboratory Standards: *Making a Difference Through Newborn Screening: Blood Collection on Filter Paper [video].* Wayne, PA, NCCLS, 1997.

15. Korf BR. *Human Genetics: A Problem-Based Approach.* Malden, MA, Blackwell Science, 2000.

16. Heath EM, O'Brien DP, Banas R, et al.: Optimization of an automated DNA purification protocol for neonatal screening. Arch Pathol Lab Med 123:1154–1160, 1999.

17. Dobrowolski SF, Banas RA, Naylor EW, et al.: DNA microarray technology for neonatal screening. Acta Pedriatr Suppl 432:61–64, 1999.

18. American College of Medical Genetics and American Society of Human Genetics Test and Technology Transfer Committee Working Group: Tandem mass spectrometry in newborn screening. Genet Med 2:267–269, 2000.

19. Levy HL: Newborn screening by tandem mass spectrometry: A new era. Clin Chem 44:2401–2402, 1998.

# CHAPTER 14

# Immunologic Disorders

*Audrey E. Hentzen*

The generalized purpose of the immune system is to maintain the integrity of "self" by distinguishing it from nonself and to defend the body against foreign material. Many different mechanisms work in harmony to defend the host. These are divided into natural and acquired immunity. Natural immunity is innate, nonspecific, and the first line of defense in the host. Acquired immunity is a host response specifically directed against foreign antigens. Both responses involve cellular and soluble components. Natural immunity utilizes phagocytic cells (macrophages, neutrophils, and mast cells), complement, and the acute inflammatory response to fight off invading organisms or substances. Lysozyme and interferon are also naturally occurring cellular substances that act in nonspecific ways to digest intracellular phagosomes and block viral replication in infected cells, respectively. Acquired immunity requires the recognition of nonself substances as foreign antigens, which leads to cellular and humoral responses. T lymphocytes, B lymphocytes and plasma cell responses generate specific antibodies, immune memory, and a permanent adaptation or change in the immune system. An important difference between the natural and acquired response is that the innate response is not altered by repeated exposure to a given infectious agent, whereas the acquired immune system remembers the infectious agent and can mount a defensive response that prevents repeated infection.

## AUTOIMMUNITY

### Theories of Origin

The science of immunology has proliferated at an astounding rate. This new era was ushered in by the discovery of monoclonal antibodies, which can identify markers on the surface of cells. This discovery revolutionized the study of lymphocytes and made it possible to recognize subpopulations within this cell line. T and B lymphocytes were described with T cells being further classified into T helper (T4) and T suppressor (T8) cells. T helper cells assist in antibody production by B cells, whereas T suppressor cells inhibit antibody production. Monocytes or macrophages also play a critical role in antigen processing (antigen presenting cell, APC) and presentation to

T helper cells for more efficient antibody production. These effector cells are regulated by numerous control mechanisms and, by working in concert, these control mechanisms establish an immunoregulatory balance for maintaining self-tolerance.[1–3]

Normal individuals are tolerant of their own self-antigens, which are inherited like all genes. Tolerance is an unresponsiveness to self-antigens expressed on circulating and tissue cells. Self-tolerance requires a harmonious group of players and events to maintain a safe environment for normal tissue function. Mechanisms are in place to provide this safe environment within the body.[4] The first is a centralized tolerance within the lymphoid tissue (thymus and bone marrow), where negative selection of T and B lymphocytes occurs. Negative selection is a deletion of immature lymphocytes that carry receptors that recognize self-antigens or produce antibody against self-antigens. These cells are killed and eliminated to remove these populations of lymphocytes that are potentially dangerous. The second is peripheral tolerance that targets mature lymphocytes for apoptotic cell death (programmed cell death) or anergy (functional inactivation). To inhibit immune responses directed toward self, mature T lymphocytes, which act through APC activation, are rendered inactive, or T suppressor cells that are activated are inhibited through cytokine production. B cells, which recognize self-antigen, may be rendered anergic or excluded from lymphoid follicles, which prevents them from being activated to produce antibody.

An immune reaction against "self-antigens" (autoimmunity) was at one time considered not to occur in normal healthy individuals. However, it is now evident that the production of autoantibodies is a relatively common occurrence in response to aging, certain drugs, and some infections. This failure of the self-tolerance mechanisms or sensitivity to self-antigens is a type of hypersensitivity. Hypersensitivity may also result from uncontrolled responses to foreign antigens.[5] Effector mechanisms for autoimmune disease are the same as host defense humoral and cell-mediated responses to microbes and other foreign antigens. Circulating autoantibodies, immunocomplexes, and reactive T lymphocytes may play a significant role in tissue injury.

Mechanisms associated with the loss of self-tolerance and the development of autoimmune disease may be related to lymphocyte abnormality and loss of self-tolerance, genetic factors that predispose individuals for autoimmunity, infectious agents

TABLE 14-1

**HLA-Linked Immunologic Diseases**

| HLA ALLELE | DISEASE |
|---|---|
| DR4 | Rheumatoid arthritis |
| DR3, DR4, DR3/4 heterozygote | Insulin-dependent diabetes mellitus |
| DR2 | Multiple sclerosis |
| B8/DR3 | Polymyositis/dermatomyositis |
| DR2/DR3 | Systemic lupus erythematosus |
| B8/DR2/DR3 | Sjögren's syndrome |
| DR4 | Pemphigus vulgaris |
| B27 | Ankylosing spondylitis |

that stimulate an autoantibody production, and other changes in normal tissue such as inflammation, ischemia, and trauma that may expose otherwise concealed antigens.[5] Autoimmunity is a failure or breakdown of the self-tolerance mechanisms in which a combination of factors may be operating in different

disorders to generate the pathophysiology. Autoimmune disorders may be organ-specific or systemic depending on the types of autoantibody formed.[6]

Failure of central tolerance may result in the release of T and B cells that recognize self-antigens. This leads to auto-antibody production either directly through antigen exposure or indirectly through antigen presentation by APC and the assault on normal healthy tissue. Additionally, the loss of regulation of the antibody-producing cells by a decrease in T suppressor cells can lead to autoimmunity.[7,8] Furthermore, mutations that interfere with apoptotic signaling may block cell death and allow clonal expansion of harmful cell lines.[9]

Genetic factors seem to play a significant role in familial clustering in several of the autoimmune disorders.[1] Studies of these family units have shown association with the HLA-DR and HLA B27 alleles (Table 14–1).[10] The strongest association is between ankylosing spondylitis, an inflammatory disease of the vertebral joints. Individuals who have ankylosing spondylitis are HLA B27 positive in 90% of the cases.[11] However, presence of disease-associated HLA types are found in healthy individuals. Expression of a particular HLA gene alone may not be the causative agent for autoimmunity, and may be

TABLE 14-2

**Classification of Autoimmune Disorders**

| DISEASE | TARGET ANTIGEN |
|---|---|
| Organ-specific autoimmune disease | |
| Addison's disease | Adrenal cell cytoplasm |
| Allergic asthma | $\beta_2$-adrenergic receptors |
| Autoimmune thyroiditis | Thyroglobulin |
| Graves' disease | TSI and TSH receptor |
| Insulin-resistant diabetes | Insulin receptor |
| IDDM | Islet cells (cytoplasmic), GAD, and IA-2 |
| Primary myxedema | Cytoplasmic microsome |
| Premature ovarian failure | Interstitial cells and corpus luteum |
| Thyrotoxicosis | Thyroperoxidase enzyme |
| | |
| Systemic autoimmune disease | |
| Dermatomyositis/polymyositis | Nuclear antigens including DNA, PM-1, and Jo-1 |
| Drug-induced lupus | Histone |
| Lupus erythematosus | Nuclear antigens including DNA, histone, Sm, RNP, SS-A, SS-B, and nucleolar |
| Mixed connective tissue | RNP |
| Rheumatoid arthritis | γ-globulin, RA-associated nuclear antigen RA-33 filaggrin and citrulline |
| Scleroderma/CREST syndrome | Nuclear antigens including nucleolar DNA, and RNP, Scl-70 and centromere |
| Sjögren's syndrome | Nuclear antigens including nucleolar, SS-A, and SS-B |

TSI = thyroid-stimulating immunoglobulin; TSH = thyroid-stimulating hormone; IDDM = insulin-dependent diabetes mellitus; GAD = glutamic acid decarboxylase; IA = islet cell antigen; Sm = Smith; SS = Sjögren's syndrome; RNP = ribonucleoprotein; Scl = DNA topoisomerase I; PM = polymyositis-associated nucleolar antigen; Jo = histidal t RNA synthetase; RA = rheumatoid arthritis.

in association with other factors or other abnormalities present in unknown major histocompatibility DNA sequences.

Viral and bacterial infections may be associated with autoimmune disease through host response to infectious agent, tissue injury, or immune deregulation by the microbe.[7,12] Effector mechanisms may become dysfunctional or self-antigens may be altered, causing a host response directed toward self-antigens. Additionally, molecular mimicry may occur, that is, infectious organisms may contain antigens that induce host responses and antibodies that cross-react with self-antigens. Many of these mechanisms for autoimmunity are still being researched and evidence supporting specific alterations in cellular activities or molecular changes is being gathered.

## Classification of Autoimmune Disease

Traditionally, autoimmune disorders were classified by whether they were organ-specific or acted in a systemic manner (Table 14–2). More recent advancement and understanding of molecular mechanisms for autoimmunity have led to more detailed classifications based on final effector mechanisms such as antibody and aberrant APC or T cell function (Table 14–3). Diseases caused by autoantibodies are produced either by

antigen-antibody complexes that form in the circulation and are deposited in vessel walls or by antibodies that bind antigens in particular cells or tissues. Disease caused by T lymphocyte mediation cause tissue injury either by secretion of cytokines and triggering inflammation (type 1 diabetes mellitus, multiple sclerosis, rheumatoid arthritis, and inflammatory bowel disease) or by killing target cells directly (myocarditis and type 1 diabetes mellitus).[13]

During the past several years, our knowledge of immunology and molecular biology has heightened our understanding of mechanisms involved in the various autoimmune disorders. Although much is left to be learned, efforts from intense research have provided new clinical practice and significant information for the diagnosis and management of autoimmune diseases. Clinical testing for specific antigens and antibodies was made significantly more sensitive and specific with the discovery and production of monoclonal antibodies and automation.

## Antinuclear Antibodies

Antinuclear antibodies (ANA) have been described in a variety of autoimmune diseases. Specific ANAs, although not

TABLE 14-3

### Classification of Autoimmune Disorders by Effector Mechanisms

| DISEASE | TARGET ANTIGEN | MECHANISM OF PATHOPHYSIOLOGY |
|---|---|---|
| Diseases caused by cell or tissue specific antibodies | | |
| Hemolytic anemia | RBC membrane proteins | Opsonization and phagocytosis |
| Thrombocytopenic purpura | Platelet membrane proteins | Opsonization and phagocytosis |
| Pemphigus vulgaris | Epidermal cadherin | Activation of proteases |
| Vasculitis | Neutrophil granule proteins | Neutrophil degranulation and inflammation |
| Goodpasture's syndrome | Noncollagenous protein | Complement and Fc receptor inflammation |
| Acute rheumatic fever | Streptococcal cell wall antigen | Macrophage activation |
| Myasthenia gravis | Acetylcholine receptor | Antibody inhibition |
| Graves' disease | TSH receptor | Thyroid stimulation |
| Insulin resistant diabetes | Insulin receptor | Antibody inhibition |
| Pernicious anemia | Intrinsic factor | Neutralization of intrinsic factor |
| Disease caused by immune complex | | |
| Systemic lupus erythematosus | DNA, nucleoproteins, others | Complement and Fc receptor inflammation |
| Polyarteritis nodosa | Hepatitis B surface antigen | Complement and Fc receptor inflammation |
| Poststreptococcal glomerulonephritis | Streptococcal cell wall antigens | Complement and Fc receptor inflammation |
| Disease caused by T cell mediation | | |
| IDDM | Islet cell antigens | In mice, T helper cytokines |
| Rheumatoid arthritis | Unknown antigen in joint | T lymphocyte cytokines |
| Experimental allergic Encephalomyelitis | Myelin/proteolipid protein | T helper cytokines and interleukins |
| Chronic hepatitis | Contractile proteins | T helper cytokines and interleukins |

IDDM = insulin-dependent diabetes mellitus.

pathognomonic for a given disease, occur in high frequency, becoming marker antibodies that contribute greatly to the diagnostic process. ANAs are a group of circulating autoantibodies targeted at antigens within a cell's nucleus. Many of the ANAs fix complement and thereby damage target tissue, whereas others play a pathologic role through T lymphocytes. The clinical significance of the ANAs is not only associated with their pathogenic role in immune complex formation of systemic rheumatic diseases but also in assisting with the diagnostic process.[8,14] Antinuclear antibodies have been identified in the following:

1. Systemic lupus erythematosus (SLE)
2. Sjögren's syndrome
3. Polymyositis and dermatomyositis
4. Systemic sclerosis
5. Mixed connective tissue disease
6. Rheumatoid arthritis

Each of these autoimmune disorders is characterized by circulating autoantibodies to either nuclear antigens, extractable nuclear antigens (ENA), histones, nonhistones, or the centromere. All of the antigens are associated with the nucleus. Several are in the nucleolus, others are intranuclear and, perhaps a few, may be on the nuclear membrane.[15]

Many theories or mechanisms have been proposed as to the origin of ANAs. Fundamental derangements of the immune system demonstrating a variety of immunologic abnormalities have been described: (1) decreased suppressor T cell function, (2) alteration of the self-antigens that escape tolerance at the T cell level, (3) enhanced helper T cell function, (4) polyclonal B cell activation, and (5) impaired macrophage Fc-receptor-mediated uptake of circulating immune complexes, allowing tissue deposition and inflammatory response.[15,16]

Various methods of ANA analysis are available but the indirect immunofluorescent antinuclear antibody test is the standard screening test used in most laboratories. This assay is based on the use of a fluorescein-conjugated antiglobulin to detect the formation of immune complexes. A serum specimen or control is layered into a well on a microscope slide containing mouse kidney or liver cells with intact nuclei. Newer cell substrates using human epithelial cell lines (HEp-2) have been developed to employ cells of human origin with larger nuclei for pattern identification and to obtain cells in various phases of mitotic division. This provides for greater detection of a variety of antibodies that react with specific nuclear antigens. The serum is allowed to react with the various nuclear components of the cell nuclei and then patient or control serum is washed away. The slide is then overlaid with fluorescein-conjugated antiglobulin to detect any immune complexes that have formed. Unbound antiglobulin is washed away and then slides are read by fluorescent microscopy to detect and distinguish patterns of fluorescence. The indirect immunofluorescent ANA test uses screening dilutions that are diluted further if

the test is positive to determine antibody titers. These titers are important for diagnosis and monitoring patient therapy.

Four fluorescent patterns are recognized and described with this indirect immunofluorescent technique: (1) homogeneous or diffuse, (2) peripheral, shaggy, rim, ring, or membranous, (3) speckled, and (4) nucleolar (Figure 14–1).[16] Attempts have been made to correlate certain patterns with distinct disorders. None of the ANAs are 100% specific for a disease but their presence and titer have great diagnostic value.

The homogeneous pattern is the most common and the least specific. The pattern in the nucleus is diffuse and uniform, staining the nucleus in a solid manner. It is associated with antibodies to the DNA protein histone, and this antibody can be found in many of the connective tissue disorders. The peripheral pattern outlines or forms a shaggy ring about the nucleus and is best seen when human leukocytes are used as a substrate. It is affiliated with antibodies directed against double-stranded (ds) DNA and is characteristic of active systemic lupus erythematosus. The speckled pattern represents antibodies most commonly directed against the centromere DNA component and other non–DNA nuclear constituents. These are often grouped together and called anti-extractable nuclear antigen (anti-ENA). The saline ENA include the Smith antigen (Sm), ribonucleoprotein (RNP), rheumatoid-associated nuclear antigen (RANA), nuclear antigen induced by Epstein-Barr virus, and other nuclear proteins such as histidal tRNA synthetase (Jo-1) and DNA topoisomerase I (Scl). Anti-ENAs are also directed against acid-extractable nuclear antigens that can be found in Sjögren's syndrome. These include Sjögren's syndrome nuclear antigen A and B (SS-A, SS-B, respectively). The nucleolar pattern is reflected by a homogeneous staining of the nucleolus within the nucleus. It has been suggested that the antigen may be the ribosomal precursor of ribonucleoprotein.[17]

The nuclear staining patterns must be interpreted with caution for several reasons: (1) collagen vascular diseases may have multiple autoantibodies so one pattern may obscure another, (2) the titer of the various autoantibodies will differ, and (3) each antigen has different responses to fixation and denaturation, which influences the pattern produced.[17]

Anti-DNA antibodies are of two types:

1. Antibodies to single-stranded (denatured) DNA (sDNA)
2. Antibodies to double-stranded (native) DNA (dsDNA)

Anti-ENA antibodies are divided into six subclassifications. All of these antigens are extractable from the nuclear extract but contain no DNA.

1. Anti-RNP is an antiribonucleoprotein. Ribonucleoprotein consists of RNA and a nonhistone.[18]
2. Anti-Sm is a nonhistone antibody that reacts with a soluble glycoprotein. This antibody was first observed in a patient named Smith and is thus designated Sm.[18]

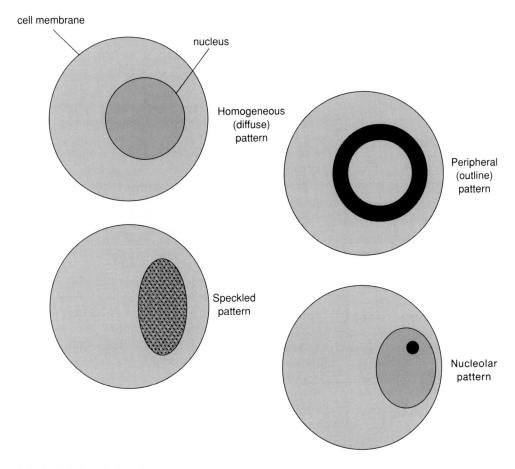

cell membrane

nucleus

Homogeneous
(diffuse)
pattern

Peripheral
(outline)
pattern

Speckled
pattern

Nucleolar
pattern

**FIGURE  14-1**

Antinuclear antibody staining patterns.

3.  Anti-SS-A/Ro is an antibody directed against acidic gly-coprotein. The SS comes from Sjögren's syndrome.
4.  Anti-Ha is an antibody to nuclear antigen and has been documented as being identical to SS-B/La.[19]
5.  Anti-PM-1 (prototype serum Mi) is an antibody that re-acts with an antigen found in calf thymus nuclear extract.[16]
6.  Anti-MA-1 is a recent antibody found to react with dis-tinct nuclear acidic protein antigen.[16]

Antihistones are a group of basic proteins complexed with DNA.

Anti-RNA antibodies can react with cytoplasmic antigens or nuclear RNA protein (Mo).[2] Anti-double-stranded RNA (ds-RNA) and DNA-RNA hybrid molecules exist in this group. The ds-RNA is commonly associated with certain viruses.[17]

Anticytoplasmic antibodies are antibodies directed against mitochondrial, ribosomal, and lysosomal antigens.[10]

Anticentromere antibodies are directed against kineto-chore bound to centromeric DNA.[20] Rheumatoid-associated

nuclear antigen (RANA) is a newer nuclear antigen produced when B cells are infected with the EB virus.

Anti-Jo-1 is an antibody directed against histidal tRNA synthetase enzyme.[8]

Anti-Scl-70 is an antibody directed against the enzyme DNA topoisomerase 1, which assists in arranging DNA con-figurations.[20]

Anti-RNA polymerase 1 is an antibody to the enzyme RNA polymerase 1 located within the nucleolus.[20]

The numerous antinuclear antibodies are important mark-ers in the various autoimmune disorders (Table 14-4). It is quite common for a variety of antibodies to be present, mak-ing it necessary for further investigation to help clarify the clin-ical significance of the ANA and diagnosis.

Immunologic testing has become more sensitive and spe-cific as our knowledge of immunology, molecular biology, and bioengineering advances. Autoantibody-detection meth-ods have been developed utilizing patient tissue sections, cell lines, pooled natural and recombinant nuclear antigens, and cell extracts as antigen sources, making way for monoclonal

## TABLE 14-4

**Disease-Associated Antinuclear Antibody (ANA) Markers**

| ANA PATTERN | ANTIGEN | DISEASE |
|---|---|---|
| Homogeneous | Histone-DNA complex | Systemic lupus erythematosus (SLE) Connective tissue disease |
| Peripheral | ds-DNA | SLE |
| Speckled | Sm | SLE |
| | MA, MA-1 | SLE |
| | RNP | Mixed connective tissue disease SLE Sjögren's syndrome Scleroderma Polymyositis |
| | SS-A | Sjögren's syndrome SLE |
| | SS-B | Sjögren's syndrome SLE |
| | Jo-1 | Polydermatomyositis |
| | Scl-70 | Scleroderma/CREST |
| | Centromere | Scleroderma/CREST |
| | RANA | Rheumatoid arthritis |
| | RA-33 | Rheumatoid arthritis |
| Nucleolar | RNA | Scleroderma/CREST |
| | PM-Scl | Polymyositis |

antibody production.[9,12,13] With the development and utilization of monoclonal antibodies, immunofluorescence, enzyme immunoassay, and microparticle agglutination, assays have been linked with nephelometry, turbidometry, and spectrophotometry in automated immunoassay instruments, leading to more specific and sensitive testing for autoimmune disorders (see Chapter 7).

## CLINICAL APPLICATIONS

### Autoimmune Disorders

#### SYSTEMIC LUPUS ERYTHEMATOSUS

Systemic lupus erythematosus (SLE) is a multisystem disease characterized by the formation of various autoantibodies that react with nuclear, cytoplasmic, and cell surface antigens. The onset is acute or chronic, remitting or relapsing with periods of febrile illness. The skin, joints, kidney, and serosal membranes are the most commonly affected areas in SLE but, during periods of active aggressive disease, injury can occur to any organ of the body. The incidence of SLE is 1 in 2000, predominantly in females (4:1 over males) and is more prevalent

in nonwhites. The peak age of onset is the second or third decade of life, although clinical manifestations may begin in childhood.[21,22]

The multisystem organ and tissue involvement in SLE is due to the autoantibodies and a disseminated vasculitis. The vasculitis develops when complement-activated immune complexes lodge in and around vascular structures, initiating local inflammation through complement-mediated chemotaxis of neutrophils. These immune complexes are composed of nuclear antigens and antinuclear antibodies.

It appears that SLE is a disease with defects in the regulatory mechanisms of the immune system. Antibody production by B lymphocytes, ordinarily regulated by T suppressor cells, seems to be defective in SLE. Additionally, there are deficiencies in complement C2 and C4 in about 10% of patients with SLE. This may contribute to ineffective clearance of immunocomplexes that form.[13,21] Genetic factors are implicated in the incidence, onset, and nature of SLE. The HLA antigens of DR2, DR3, A1, and B8 have all been described as being associated with SLE. Some nongenetic factors have also been described as causes of SLE. Drugs such as hydralazine and procainamide and sometimes quinidine, chlorpromazine, methyldopa, isoniazid, and phenytoin are also known to produce an SLE-like response in humans.[22] Viruses have been implicated due to their ability to disrupt T suppressor cell function and population, but no direct viral cause has been demonstrated. Estrogen enhances anti-DNA antibody formation and increases the severity of renal disease in animal models.[21,22]

Presentation of the disease is extremely variable, making it a diagnostic dilemma. SLE may begin with fever and malaise and approximately 90% of patients present with articular symptoms such as intermittent arthralgias and acute polyarthritis. When these symptoms occur, the disorder is often confused with rheumatoid arthritis. Another common finding is the malar erythema (butterfly rash) associated with regions most commonly exposed to ultraviolet light such as the face, neck, upper chest, and back.[23]

The poorest prognosis is associated with central nervous system (CNS) involvement and the nephrotic syndrome. However, bacterial and viral pneumonia along with pericarditis and endocarditis are life-threatening complications. Remission is common with eventual reoccurrence of the disease in a variety of forms. The course at this time is unpredictable from patient to patient. Physical and emotional stresses such as surgery, infections, pregnancy, exposure to sunlight, and the use of oral contraceptives can adversely affect the course of the disease.

Anemia is found in approximately 75% of SLE patients due to bone marrow suppression. In 10% of the SLE cases, warm autoimmune hemolytic anemia (AIHA) occurs. The antibody is predominately IgG.[24] Leukopenia can be found in one half of patients with SLE. The total number and function of granulocytes or lymphocytes or both may be depressed. Antigranulocyte antibody, peripheral destruction, and central bone marrow suppression of granulopoiesis are proposed mechanisms for the granulocytic leukopenia. The absolute or relative lymphopenia occurs due to circulating cytotoxic anti-lymphocyte antibodies.

Thrombocytopenia occurs in 14% to 26% of patients with 75% to 80% of SLE patients exhibiting an antiplatelet antibody.[8,22] Additionally, an antiphospholipid antibody, termed the lupus anticoagulant, inhibits the procoagulant functions of phospholipids used in many of the activated partial thromboplastin time (APTT) reagent systems. Antiphospholipid antibody possesses activity against cardiolipin and is often associated with false-positive VDRL testing. Partial thromoboplastin and prothrombin time are prolonged but hemorrhagic episodes are rare. Paradoxically, it appears that patients with the antiphospholipid antibody are at a higher risk for thrombotic episodes, vasculitis, lysis of erythrocytes, and spontaneous abortions.[22] The precise mechanism for the thrombotic event is unknown but some of the possible explanations proposed are: (1) inhibited release of prostacyclin from blood vessels, (2) increased activity of related von Willebrand–factor VIII complex activity, (3) decreased release of plasminogen activator, (4) inhibited protein C activation, (5) inhibited antithrombin III activity, (6) inhibited prekallikrein activation, (7) increased production of antibodies directed against cardiolipin membranes, and (8) inhibited endothelial cell function.[25]

Diagnosis of SLE is usually made by ANA screening, where approximately 99% of patients demonstrate circulating

antibodies to at least one nuclear antigen. Antibodies are directed against double- and single-stranded DNA, RNA, RNA-associated proteins, histone, nucleoli, ENA, and Sm. Testing for ANAs is usually done by immunofluorescence.[21] Since some of these antibodies are also found in other connective tissue disorders, a differential diagnosis must be made. The presence of antibody against native dsDNA, producing peripheral immunofluorescent pattern or Sm antigen, displayed by the speckled pattern, provides good evidence for a diagnosis of SLE. Table 14–5 lists the incidence of various antibodies found in patients with SLE.

ANA testing may be diagnostic for SLE but it does not provide information concerning the progress or severity of the disease. It appears that no single test can serve as a universal indicator for the extent of the disease process. Tests for anti-DNA antibodies, cryoglobulins, C-3 levels, and immune complexes along with renal biopsy have been used to monitor the course of the disease.[26]

Treatment of SLE remains controversial. Each patient must be evaluated and treated independently, since the management of the disease depends upon the severity of the disease and specific organ lesions involved. Therapy is aimed at optimizing the patient's quality of life. Skin lesions and musculoskeletal involvement can often be controlled with nonsteroidal anti-inflammatory agents such as salicylates and antimalarial drugs. When renal involvement is present, corticosteroid therapy is often required. In end-stage renal disease (ESRD) it is necessary to use hemodialysis and perhaps transplantation. When the CNS is involved, corticosteroids and specific psychotropic drugs are used. When there is occurrence of severe hemolytic anemia, thrombocytopenia, or lupus crisis, an acute fulminant event, high-dosage corticosteroid treatment and pulse therapy of immunosuppressive cytotoxic drugs such as cyclophosphamide, chlorambucil, or azathioprine are effective.[22,27]

Prognosis is extremely variable from patient to patient. The most common cause of death is renal failure and central nervous system lupus, followed by secondary infections. With

TABLE 14–5

**Antinuclear Antibodies Profile for Systemic Lupus Erythematosus (SLE)**

| ANTIGEN-ANTIBODY SYSTEM | INCIDENCE (%) |
|---|---|
| DNA | 50–60 |
| DNP | 70 |
| Sm antigen | 30 |
| Histones | 60 (95% drug induced SLE) |
| Other antigens | |
| SS-A | 30–40 |
| SS-B | 15 |
| RNP | 30–40 |

the use of corticosteroids and cytotoxic agents, the 5-year survival rate now approaches 80% to 90%.[22]

## SJÖGREN'S SYNDROME

Sjögren's syndrome is a systemic connective tissue disease with atrophy of the lacrimal and salivary glands. It is characterized by dry eyes (keratoconjunctivitis sicca) and dry mouth (xerostomia), also known as sicca syndrome.[28,29] Additional symptoms may include dryness of the nose, trachea, bronchi, vagina, and skin. This chronic inflammatory disorder is often associated with another connective tissue disease (secondary form).[2] Approximately 50% of the patients with a diagnosis of Sjögren's syndrome have rheumatoid arthritis, but associations with lupus erythematosus occur 15% of the time, and Sjögren's syndrome also occurs with systemic sclerosis and polymyositis.[22] When Sjögren's syndrome is associated with other connective tissue diseases, it is referred to as the sicca complex.

Patients with Sjögren's syndrome appear to have a higher incidence of developing a generalized lymphadenopathy, pseudolymphoma, or a lymphoid malignancy.[30,31] Ninety percent of the patients are female between the fourth and sixth decades of life.[32] The disorder has rarely been documented in children.

The exact cause of this disorder is unknown, although many factors are implicated. Genetic, viral antigens, or viral-altered autoantigens, hormonal and immunologic-based causes are all possibilities. Factors such as sex hormones, latent viruses, infectious agents, and drugs may all play a part in altering the immune response. Genetic studies indicate that sicca syndrome is frequently associated with HLA-B8, DR3, whereas the secondary form when associated with rheumatoid arthritis has a positive correlation with DR4.[33]

The fibrosis of the lacrimal and salivary glands is a result of lymphocyte infiltration. Although the infiltrate is predominantly T cells of the CD4 (helper) subset, there is good evidence to support a B cell infiltration as well. B cell and plasma cell hyperactivity manifests as polyclonal hypergammaglobulinemia (increases in IgG, IgA, and IgM) and production of rheumatoid factors, antinuclear antibodies, cryoglobulins, and antisalivary duct antibodies.[22,34]

Symptoms of keratoconjunctivitis sicca include chronic burning of the eyes in conjunction with feelings of irritation, grittiness, and blurring. The eyelids may have a tendency to stick together. Xerostomia (dry mouth and lips) may inhibit chewing and phonation. Often there is difficulty in swallowing dry foods and the voice may even become hoarse or weak. Vaginal dryness may also be present. Lack of salivary function promotes tooth decay and the ability to taste and smell may subside.[31,35] Impaired mucus secretion in the lung may lead to bouts with pneumonia. Enlargement of the parotid glands and submaxillary glands may occur but is usually painless.[32]

There is a normochromic, normocytic anemia in approximately 25% of patients and leukopenia and eosinophilia in 25% to 30%. The ESR is elevated above 30 mm/h in over 90% of the cases. Hypergammaglobulinemia is present and

cryoglobulinemia may also be present. Antibodies to tissue antigens that are organ-specific such as gastric, parietal, thyroglobulin, thyroid, microsomal, mitochondrial, smooth muscle, and salivary duct antigens have been described.[33]

Rheumatoid factor is found in 75% to 95% of the patients regardless of the presence of rheumatoid arthritis or other connective tissue disorders. Homogeneous or speckled ANA patterns occur in 60% to 70% of the patients.[36] Antibodies are directed toward 2 acid extractable nuclear antigens, SS-B (also termed La) is found in 60% to 70% of the patients with the primary form of the disease, and in the secondary form associated with lupus erythematosus, 70% to 80% of patients have anti-SS-A (also termed Ro). However, SS-A is only considered specific for Sjögren's syndrome when SS-B is also present (Table 14–6).[34]

Treatment is dependent on the symptoms and severity of the disorder. The restoration of glandular secretions has not been demonstrated. Artificial tears (methylcellulose eye drops) help with eye lubrication. Artificial salivas, sipping of water, or chewing sugarless gum may give temporary relief to dry mouth. Fluoride gel trays and remineralizing solutions may equilibrate the chemical balance of the mouth. Radiation was used to decrease enlarged salivary glands but an increase in the incidence of lymphoma ended its use.[33,35] The disease is usually confined to salivary and lacrimal glands, resulting in chronic xerostomia and xerophthalmia. Development of extraglandular lymphoid infiltration or neoplasia is rare.

## POLYMYOSITIS AND DERMATOMYOSITIS

Polymyositis and dermatomyositis are characterized by inflammatory and degenerative changes in muscles (polymyositis) and a skin rash (dermatomyositis).[37] Weakness of neck, pelvic girdle, and proximal muscles is the dominant feature of the disease.[36,38] Because various clinical expressions of polymyositis exist, subclassifications have been developed to categorize the disorder, depending on whether the myopathy occurs alone, in association with a malignancy, in childhood, or in association with a collagen vascular disease.[39]

This disorder has a female to male ratio of 2:1 with the peak age of onset occurring between the fourth and sixth decade of life. It is more common in the black population.[40] The childhood form occurs between 5 and 15 years of age. It is classified as an autoimmune disorder owing to the presence of autoantibodies in the majority of the patients.

TABLE 14 – 6

**Antinuclear Antibodies Profile for Sjögren's Syndrome**

| ANTIGEN-ANTIBODY SYSTEM | INCIDENCE (%) |
| --- | --- |
| SS-A | 70 |
| SS-B | 60 |

Etiology is unknown, although cell-mediated immunity has been strongly implicated. Cytotoxic T lymphocytes as well as macrophages are present in the inflammatory infiltrate. The damage to the muscle fibers may occur by T lymphocyte infiltration and cytotoxicity or when muscle antigens are exposed to soluble lymphotoxins.[41] The cause of autosensitization is obscure but microbial agents are prime suspects. Primary idiopathic polymyositis and dermatomyositis have an increased prevalence for the histocompatibility antigens of HLA-B8 and DR3.[38] Many autoimmune autoantibodies are present, although none appear to be responsible for the tissue damage.[42]

Symmetric muscle weakness is present and is associated with variable degrees of pain, swelling, or atrophy of muscles. Muscular atrophy may be totally disabling. A dusky lilac suffusion around the eyes, and erythematous telangiectatic rash around the face and exterior surfaces of the limbs is associated with the term dermatomyositis. In addition, a similar eruption is present on the V of the neck, forehead, shoulders, upper chest, and back.[40,43] The skin rash may develop into a dermal fibrosis, producing stiffness of the fingers.[43] A smooth or scaly erythematous lesion may also be present over the knuckles, knees, or elbows and is referred to as Gottron's sign.[39,42] Raynaud's syndrome (intermittent attacks of pallor followed by cyanosis and then redness of the digits) and arthritis are common findings in these patients.[39]

Patients note difficulty in rising from a sitting or reclining position or climbing the stairs. They also complain of extreme difficulty in raising and maintaining the arms over the head. Weakness can also occur in the neck flexors and pharyngeal area. When the pharyngeal muscles are involved, dysphagia and regurgitation result.[40] Other systems may be involved. Cardiac involvement with congestive heart failure, arrhythmias, and conduction disturbances is not uncommon and contributes to the mortality rate.

Associated malignancies increase with age. A diligent search for a neoplasm by the physician should take place when the patient is over 40 years of age because of a 25% to 50% incidence of an occult neoplasm. Tumors most commonly found are lung, breast, prostate, and colon.[39,42]

Most of the routine clinical laboratory tests are normal. The ESR is increased. Elevated values are found in the muscle-associated enzymes such as the transaminases, creatine kinase, lactate dehydrogenase, and/or aldolase activities. Serum enzyme elevation reflects the muscle mass involved and the severity of damage. However, normal enzyme results may be found in patients with widespread muscle atrophy or during periods of remission.

Myoglobinemia and myoglobinuria are found, especially with active muscle damage. To separate polymyositis from other muscle disorders, electromyography and nerve conduction velocity studies are of some value. These studies help to eliminate disorders due to denervation.[43]

The autoantibodies present are anti-Jo-1 (directed against the enzyme histidyl-t RNA synthetase), anti-RNP, anti-PM, Anti-Scl, anti-SS-A, and anti-SS-B.[42] Preliminary evidence

### TABLE 14-7

**Antinuclear Antibodies Profile for Polymyositis and Dermatomyositis**

| ANTIGEN-ANTIBODY SYSTEM | INCIDENCE (%) |
| --- | --- |
| PM-Scl | Polymyositis (50%) |
| | Dermatomyositis (10%) |
| Jo-1 | May be present |

implies that anti-Jo-1 may be fairly specific for polymyositis (Table 14–7).[44]

Recent studies report survival rates of 70% to 80% at 6 to 7 years following diagnosis. Intermittent periods of remissions and exacerbations can spontaneously occur. Patients with cardiac and pulmonary involvement have a higher incidence of mortality.[40,42]

Corticosteroid therapy significantly improves the course of the myopathy in approximately 75% of the patients with dermatomyositis and polymyositis. Creatinuria is the most sensitive index for therapy, followed by serum enzyme levels. The nonresponding 25% are put on cytotoxic immunosuppressive drugs. Plasmapheresis has been of some value in those patients refractory to steroid and immunosuppressive agents. Exercise helps restore strength, but no known therapy improves interstitial pulmonary fibrosis or cardiac involvement.[42]

## PROGRESSIVE SYSTEMIC SCLEROSIS

Progressive systemic sclerosis, also known as systemic sclerosis and scleroderma, is a disorder of the connective tissue associated with degenerative and inflammatory changes capable of developing into a diffuse fibrosis. Scleroderma (skin thickening) is a basic hallmark of the disease owing to collagenous sclerosis (collagen deposition).[45] Numerous tissues and organs can be involved (skin, blood vessels, synovium, skeletal muscle, GI tract, lungs, heart, and kidneys.[46,47]

The variants of systemic sclerosis are defined according to the degree and extent of skin thickening. Diffuse cutaneous scleroderma has widespread skin involvement that includes the distal and proximal extremities and trunk. Because of its aggressiveness, early development of serious visceral involvement occurs.[48,49]

The CREST syndrome (calcinosis, Raynaud's phenomenon, esophageal dysmotility, sclerodactyly and telangiectasia) is confined to the face and fingers demonstrating only limited skin involvement. This limited cutaneous scleroderma can remain localized in the skin for one or more decades.[48] Scleroderma overlaps many of the other connective tissue disorders.

Systemic sclerosis occurs 2 to 4 times more frequently in women from the third to the sixth decade of life.[48,49] It has also been documented in infants and children, but is extremely rare. The disease appears to be more severe in the black population, especially in black women.[50]

The cause of systemic sclerosis is unknown. An immunologic basis for this disorder is indicated by the various autoantibodies found in a patient's serum (ANA, rheumatoid factor, polyclonal hypergammaglobulinemia) but evidence to support this is indirect. A mechanism being considered is an activation through humoral factors that may stimulate fibroblasts to produce collagen.[22,51] A positive feedback cycle then occurs. T cell–directed autoimmune events against microvasculature endothelial cells may lead to fibroblast activation and fibrosis.[22,45] Other investigators have suggested the presence of immune complexes as a possible cause of the vascular lesion.[52]

The first symptoms are usually associated with the "swelling or puffiness" of the hands referred to as Raynaud's phenomenon or polyarthritis in the joints of the hands. Skin thickening usually follows the initial symptoms by several months, but Raynaud's phenomenon may antedate systemic sclerosis by years or even decades.[48] With continual collagenization, complete immobilization of the joints will occur. Muscle atrophy sets in next with proximal muscle weakness and even muscle wasting.[45] A consistent finding in systemic sclerosis is esophageal hypomotility with difficulty in swallowing food and pills. Gastrointestinal disturbances in the form of heartburn and dysphagia will eventually occur. Respiratory complaints of dyspnea and chronic cough referred to as "stiff lung syndrome" develop and can even progress to pulmonary hypertension.[53] Myocardial fibrosis leads to congestive heart failure and left-sided heart failure. Cardiac arrhythmias and conduction dysfunction lead to pericardial effusion and tamponade.[54] Two thirds of the patients have renal abnormalities. Should hyperplasia of interlobular arteries develop, it can provide a renal crisis of malignant arterial hypertension requiring immediate attention or irreversible renal insufficiency will result in death.[55] Physical examination is the most reliable method of diagnosing scleroderma. Skin biopsy reveals compact collagen fibers and approximately 50% of biopsies demonstrate focal collections of T lymphocytes.

The normochromic, normocytic anemia of chronic disease is usually present, although it is possible to find a microangiopathic or autoimmune hemolytic anemia component. The ESR is usually elevated associated with a mild polyclonal hypergammaglobulinemia.[56]

Rheumatoid factor is found in 30% of the patients with systemic sclerosis. Antinuclear and/or antinucleolar antibodies are present in 90% or more of the cases.[55] Anti-RNA polymerase 1 is relatively specific for the diffuse form of the disease and presents as a nucleolar pattern on immunofluorescence.[57] Anticentromere antibody is a fairly sensitive and specific indicator of the limited cutaneous form of scleroderma with a centromere immunofluorescent pattern.[57] Anti-Scl-70 assists in identifying diffuse cutaneous disease in 30% to 40% of patients and has a diffuse fine-speckled immunofluorescent pattern.[53,57] Table 14–8 and Table 14–9 describe the ANA profiles for scleroderma and CREST.

The course in systemic sclerosis is extremely variable in each patient, but the overall 10-year survival rate is approximately 65%.

## TABLE 14-8
### Antinuclear Antibodies Profiles for Scleroderma

| ANTIGEN-ANTIBODY SYSTEM | INCIDENCE (%) |
| --- | --- |
| Scl-70 | 10–20 |
| Nucleolar antigens | 40–50 |

The disease remains limited in the (CREST) syndrome but causes of mortality can be associated with pulmonary hypertension and intestinal malabsorption. In the course of diffuse scleroderma, mortality is often a consequence of early involvement of the kidney, heart, or lungs.[48]

Several considerations must be evaluated by both the patient's family and physician. The natural history of the disease must be stressed especially in the CREST syndrome because of its relatively benign course.

Treatment should be carefully evaluated owing to the lack of a drug or combination of drugs with proven effective results. Patients need to be educated about their disorder so preventive measures may be taken to avoid exacerbation of symptoms. These preventive measures include (1) a lanolin-based cream and reduced bathing to prevent dry skin, (2) altered eating habits to include less food at more frequent intervals to assist digestion, (3) avoidance of cold exposure and tobacco, (4) physical therapy to maintain musculoskeletal function, and (5) judicious use of antibiotics and nonsteroidal anti-inflammatory drugs.[45,58]

D-penicillamine has been used to reduce skin thickening but is poorly tolerated by many patients.[55] Corticosteroids have been used during inflammatory manifestations.[48] Severe renal involvement with malignant hypertension responds well to antihypertensive drugs if used immediately.[59]

## MIXED CONNECTIVE TISSUE DISEASE

Mixed connective tissue disease (MCTD) is a disease process characterized by coexisting features of scleroderma, rheumatoid arthritis, SLE, polymyositis, and polymyositis-dermatomyositis. Very high titers of circulating anti-RNP with immunofluorescent speckled pattern are present.[60] Some feel MCTD is not a distinct clinical entity, yet many continue to support it as a primary disorder. Although the controversy continues, it is difficult to dispute the high titer of anti-RNP without the presence of native DNA or Sm antigen normally found in SLE. The abnormal T cell regulatory function of MCTD

## TABLE 14-9
### Antinuclear Antibodies Profile for CREST Syndrome

| ANTIGEN-ANTIBODY SYSTEM | INCIDENCE (%) |
| --- | --- |
| Centromere antigens | 80–90 (high titers) |

differs from other rheumatic diseases.[61] Patients with MCTD also have minimal renal involvement and an exceedingly good response to corticosteroids. This contributes to a good prognosis that contrasts significantly with SLE. MCTD has a female-to-male ratio of 12:1 with disease presentation occurring between the third and the sixth decade of life.[62]

As in so many immune disorders the etiology is unknown. A strong suspicion toward an immune mechanism is supported by several findings: (1) high titers of anti-RNP that persist, (2) mild or moderate degree of hypocomplementemia, (3) immune complex formation during active disease, (4) deposition of IgG, IgM, or complement in affected tissues, (5) abnormal T suppressor activity during active disease, (6) infiltration of lymphocytes and plasma cells in involved tissues, and (7) hypergammaglobulinemia.[61]

Often the patient's initial complaints are arthritis, swollen hands, Raynaud's phenomenon, and abnormal esophageal motility myositis. Lymphadenopathy and hepatosplenomegaly may also be pronounced.[61] Other symptoms are those normally characterized by each of the overlapping features most commonly observed in SLE: systemic sclerosis, polymyositis, and RA.

High titers of ANA (often >1:1000) producing a speckled pattern are characteristic of MCTD. High titers of anti-RNP (Table 14–10) exceeding 1:100,000 are also characteristic findings. Complement is decreased in 25% of cases. Polyclonal hypergammaglobulinemia is found in 75% of cases, resulting in an elevated ESR. If active myositis is present, the serum levels of aldolase and creatine kinase will be elevated. Anemia and leukopenia are present in less than half the cases treated.

The overall mortality rate is 13% with a mean survival of 6 to 12 years. Death is usually associated with vascular complications. Remissions of several years have been documented with little or no therapy.

Response to corticosteroid treatment is usually good. Additionally, salicylates, anti-inflammatory drugs, and antimalarial drugs are often effective in treating less severe cases. If the disease is progressive, cytotoxic drugs may enhance clinical improvement.[61]

## RHEUMATOID ARTHRITIS

Rheumatoid arthritis is a chronic immune-mediated systemic inflammatory disorder of the synovial membranes in the peripheral joints. Characteristic joint deformities and radiologic

changes begin to occur and eventually destroy the joint cartilage and supporting structures such as ligaments and tendons. In some cases, a lesion in the subcutaneous tissue adjacent to the joint develops and is referred to as a rheumatoid nodule.[63]

The disorder occurs in approximately 2.5% of the population with a female-to-male ratio of 3:1. The peak onset of the disorder occurs between the fourth and sixth decades of life.[63]

Rheumatoid arthritis is caused by an inflammatory process resulting from an immunologic response taking place in the joints.[64] The trigger for some patients may be an immune reaction generated by an Epstein-Barr viral infection.[65] Both humoral and cell-mediated immunity appear to be involved in the pathogenesis. T helper cells and activated B lymphocytes and plasma cells are found in the inflamed synovium. In some severe cases, well-formed lymphoid follicles with germinal centers may be present.[22] Additionally, many cytokines, interleukins and tumor necrosis factor have been identified in synovial fluid. Susceptibility and high risk to this disease appear to be related to genetic predisposition and the presence of the HLA-DR4 haplotype.[65,66] Inheritance patterns have not been completely defined nor have protein sequences been fully characterized.[67]

An unknown primary stimulus causes synovial lymphocytes to produce an IgG immunoglobulin that is recognized as foreign. This elicits an immune response that is heterogeneous, with the production of rheumatoid factor (RF), autoantibodies of the IgG, IgM, or IgA immunoglobulin classes.[22] IgM is the major immunoglobulin class in the circulation. RF is found in the circulation and the joints of 75% to 80% of all patients with rheumatoid arthritis.[64,68] The exact role played by rheumatoid factors in the pathogenesis of the disease is unknown but the presence of IgG aggregate or rheumatoid factor complexes results in the activation of the complement system via the classic pathway.[22,68] Complement breakdown components activate the alternative complement systems, resulting in many inflammatory processes including histamine release, chemotaxis, membrane damage, and cell lysis. The inflammatory response is well underway as neutrophils accumulate and phagocytize the immune complexes.[69] Prostaglandins and leukotrienes produced by the inflammation mediate the inflammatory process to continue the production of RF, therefore perpetuating and amplifying the inflammation.

Clinical symptoms include low-grade fever, malaise, and fatigue may precede the joint pain. The most common complaints on initial presentation are manifestations of bilateral and symmetrical peripheral arthritis. The arthritis involves areas such as wrists, metacarpophalangeal, knee, and ankle. Morning stiffness lasting longer than 30 minutes after rising or after exercise is often present. Onset may be insidious or abrupt. Duration of the clinical symptoms helps to differentiate it from other arthritides.[70] Joint tenderness and swelling may develop into subcutaneous nodules in 30% to 40% of the cases.[71] The course of the disease is not predictable but lung involvement and small vessel obliterative vasculitis may lead to neuropathy or ischemic ulceration of the skin.

TABLE 14–10

**Antinuclear Antibodies Profile for Mixed Connective Tissue Disease**

| ANTIGEN-ANTIBODY SYSTEM | INCIDENCE (%) |
| --- | --- |
| RNP | 95–100 (high titers) |

A normochromic or hypochromic, normocytic anemia and thrombocytosis are associated with a chronic disorder. Elevated serum immunoglobulins may be present and an elevated ESR can be demonstrated in 90% of the cases.[71] C-reactive protein is also increased.

Latex-agglutination tests for detection of RF include hemagglutination tests, such as Rose-Waaler, which have a high sensitivity but are fairly nonspecific for rheumatoid arthritis.[67] Serial dilutions of patient sera may be prepared and used when performing the latex-agglutination tests to obtain RF titers. However, the titer for RF does not correlate well with the prognosis. Newer techniques using radioimmunoassay (RIA), indirect immunofluorescence, enzyme-linked immunosorbent assay (ELISA), and laser nephelometry allow for characterizing specific RF subclasses.

Synovial fluid analysis shows a poor mucin clot and an inflammatory infiltrate of neutrophils phagocytizing immune complexes.[68] Synovial fluid complement levels are decreased.

Patients with rheumatoid arthritis may have positive speckled pattern ANA tests. Anti-RANA is present in 85% to 95% of patients, with anti-RA-33 filaggrin showing less incidence and in even fewer cases, anti-histone is present.[6,22] In patients with classic articular changes in small joints with a positive RF test, the diagnosis is clear. However, when other extraarticular manifestations are present, they disguise the clinical picture, and ANA patterns and specific antibody identification are useful for differentiating the rheumatoid diseases.

Because of the variable course of the disease from patient to patient, or even within the same patient, a prognosis is difficult to predict. The majority of patients have a chronic indolent course with increasing pain and disability. However, a small group of patients may remit after one acute attack with no reoccurrence.[69,72]

Four treatment objectives must be addressed with each patient: (1) relieve the pain, (2) minimize inflammation to maintain as much muscle and joint function as possible, (3) prevent as many undesirable side effects as possible, and (4) reinstate a productive and desirable life style.[65]

Conservative therapy is utilized early in the disease process. Careful balance between physical therapy followed by heat or cold therapy is used to maintain active range of motion, strength, and mobility. Salicylates are commonly employed anti-inflammatory drugs. A group of nonsteroidal anti-inflammatory drugs (NSAIDs) may be substituted for salicylates when aspirin fails to be effective or is poorly tolerated. These drugs include fenprofen, ibuprofen, naproxen, sulindac, tolmetin, mefenamic acid, ketoprofen, diclofenac, carprofen, indomethacin, piroxicam, etodolac, and nabumatone. If these fail to provide necessary relief for the patient, antimalarial drugs, gold therapy (chrysotherapy), and D-penicillamine are administered. Corticosteroids are used to suppress the inflammatory aspects, but long-term administration is limited by the undesirable side effects. Immunosuppressive drugs may be required when severe active RA is in progress.[71] Surgery (arthro-plasty) may be employed to correct joint deformity and maintain movement.

## POLYARTERITIS NODOSA

Polyarteritis nodosa (PN) is a necrotizing vasculitis of the small- to medium-sized blood vessels in muscle tissue. It can result in ischemia of the tissue being supplied by the affected vessel with resultant multi-organ involvement. The involved organs include the skin, joints, peripheral nerves, kidney, liver, heart, and intestines.[73,74] The disorder is fairly rare with 0.9/100,000 incidence found in one study.[75] No hereditary or racial predisposition is evident and frequency of disease is 2 to 3 times higher in men than in women.[76]

The disease is of unknown etiology, although associating infections with hepatitis B, tuberculosis, and streptococcal infections, and otitis media have been linked with supplying an exogenous antigen to initiate the immunologic mechanism.[77] Also, the finding of hepatitis B surface antigen (HBsAg) circulating in the blood and deposited in the immune complex supports hepatitis B virus as the initiating agent in one third of the cases.[78] Immune complexes activate the complement system generating chemotactic factor C5a, which promotes the migration of neutrophils to the vascular site for phagocytosis. Other complement components of C3a, C4a, along with C5a cause degranulation of the mast cells and basophils. These cells release histamine and arachidonic acid metabolites that are capable of promoting vascular permeability. The resultant swelling exposes the basement membrane. Upon engulfing the complexes, the neutrophil releases lysosomal enzymes such as collagenase, elastase, and oxygen metabolites that are capable of injuring the exposed vessel wall.[78,79] Hypersensitivity reactions to some drugs such as sulfonamides or penicillin are also potential initiating factors.[76,80]

Fever, malaise, and weight loss are common presenting features. Often a recent illness or a drug reaction is documented prior to the onset of symptoms. Skin rash, peripheral neuropathy, joint pain, and renal involvement are some of the clinical manifestations of organ involvement.[73] Abdominal pain, nausea, diarrhea, and bleeding ulcer indicate gastrointestinal involvement.[78] Cardiac involvement is apparent on autopsy, but is rarely recognized clinically in conjunction with polyarteritis. Coronary insufficiency may develop into congestive heart failure.[73]

A moderate leukocytosis of 20,000 to 40,000 cells/$\mu$L is found in approximately 80% of the patients. Renal involvement manifested by proteinuria and hematuria is present in 50% of the cases. An elevated ESR, normochromic and normocytic anemia, and mild thrombocytosis are commonly present. Elevated levels of serum gamma globulins may be present, although the demonstration of autoantibodies is rare.[74,76]

Other laboratory findings include rheumatoid factors, reduced level of complement, presence of cryoglobulins and anti-neutrophil cytoplasmic antibodies with a perinuclear ANA pattern. Diagnosis is based on biopsy of the vessel involved to establish necrotizing arteritis. Visceral angiographic displays can demonstrate vascular involvement and assist in the diagnostic process especially when clinically accessible tissue is not available for biopsy.[73]

The disease course is directly related to involved organs and the extent of involvement. The course of the disease ranges from an acute process to a more chronic course with recurrent episodes over a period of months to years or until major organ involvement occurs. Without treatment, 33% of the patients die within 1 year and 88% do not survive beyond 5 years. Hypertension control is essential with renal failure being the major cause of death.[74]

Often a multifaceted treatment approach is followed that correlates with the disease process. Corticosteroids provide some success for less fulminant cases, whereas immunosuppressive drugs, especially cyclophosphamide and azathioprine in conjunction with corticosteroids, have been used to treat the more aggressive form of polyarteritis showing significant benefit.[78,79] With corticosteroid and immunosuppressive therapy, approximately one half of the patients can achieve a 5-year survival rate.

## OTHER AUTOIMMUNE DISORDERS

Other chronic progressive inflammatory disorders have been identified:

- Behçet's disease manifests as apthous stomatitis, iritis, and genital ulcers
- Ankylosing spondylitis is a chronic inflammatory disorder of the sacroiliac joints, spine, and large peripheral joints
- Reiter's syndrome is characterized by a triad of arthritis, urethritis, and conjunctivitis
- Psoriatic arthritis is an asymmetric, erosive polyarthritis
- Relapsing polychondritis is characterized by recurrent episodes of inflammatory necrosis of the cartilaginous tissues
- Relapsing panniculitis or Weber-Christian disease is a rare syndrome of recurrent episodes of discrete nodular inflammation and necrosis of subcutaneous fat
- Complement deficiencies and collagen vascular disease leading to increased susceptibility to infection.[22]

These disorders have specific clinical characteristics that are related to their autoimmunity to specific self-antigens. Etiology may be related to genetic predisposition (characterized by HLA alleles), hereditary complement deficiencies, or exposure to viral or infectious agents. These disorders do not exhibit ANA patterns but instead are diagnosed by clinical symptoms and disease-specific immunoassays.

## IMMUNODEFICIENCY

An intact immune system is critical for survival and defense against the onslaught of infectious agents. Defects in any components of the immune system can lead to inability to mount a host response and fight off infection. Defects in immune function can be classified as primary or congenital, and secondary or acquired immunodeficiencies.[81] Primary immuno-

deficiency occurs as a result of genetic defects or gene mutations that lead to development of a defect in the host's immune system and increased susceptibility to infection. Secondary or acquired immunodeficiency results from a detrimental effect on the host's immune system due to malnutrition, disease, disseminated cancer, cancer therapy or infection, especially infection by the human immunodeficiency virus (HIV). Primary immunodeficient disorders generally affect the infant and childhood age groups with a strong male preponderance owing to X-linkage. The secondary immunodeficiency disorders occur at any age with no significant sex prevalence.[82] In either classification, the finding of increased frequency, severity, and duration of infection are strong clinical clues to direct the physician toward investigating an immunodeficient disorder. Complications or unusual manifestations in the infection's course may be the most helpful indication of immunodeficiency, especially if the infection is caused by organisms not typically pathogenic.[82]

Whether the immunodeficiency is congenital or acquired, similar manifestations occur. There is increased susceptibility to infection and incidence of certain types of cancer with immunodeficiency being the result of defects in lymphocyte maturation or activation of effector mechanisms of the innate and adaptive immune system.[81] The following are classified as immunodeficient disorders:

### Defects in Lymphocyte Maturation
1. Severe combined immunodeficiency (SCID)
   A. Mutation in the cytokine receptor
   B. Adenosine deaminase deficiency
   C. Reticular dysgenesis
   D. X-linked agammaglobulinemia
2. DiGeorge syndrome
3. Nezelof's syndrome

### Defects in Lymphocyte Activation
1. Selective IgA deficiency
2. Selective IgG deficiency
3. X-linked hyper IgM syndrome
4. X-linked lymphoproliferative disease

### Wide-Spectrum Defects
1. Wiskott-Aldrich syndrome
2. Ataxia telangiectasia

### Defects in Innate Immunity
1. Chronic granulomatous disease
2. Leukocyte adhesion deficiency
3. Chédiak-Higashi syndrome

### Acquired Immunodeficiency Syndrome
1. Human immunodeficiency virus (AIDS)
2. Malnutrition, iatrogenic, and other infections

## CONGENITAL IMMUNODEFICIENCY

Immunodeficiency, a defect of humoral or cell-mediated immunity, was not recognized as a clinical entity before 1952 when

Dr. Ogden Bruton first described the inability of a child to produce antibodies.[81] This sex-linked agammaglobulinemia was caused by a defect in B lymphocyte maturation and consequential loss of humoral response. Congenital immunodeficiencies have been described and the genetic bases of many of these disorders are now characterized, making gene replacement therapy a viable option. Congenital abnormality may be a defect in a specific stage of lymphocyte maturation, differentiation, or in their activation. Abnormalities that exist in B lymphocyte lineage lead to deficient antibody production and increased susceptibility to infection. Abnormal T cell maturation and function may lead to deficient cell-mediated immunity as well as the ability to induce B cells to produce antibody.[81]

## SEVERE COMBINED IMMUNODEFICIENCY

Disorders affecting both B and T lymphocytes resulting in defective humoral or cell-mediated immunity are called severe combine immunodeficiencies (SCID). Approximately 50% of SCID are X-linked, recessive, and due to mutation in the gene encoding the shared gamma protein found in receptors for IL 2, 4, 7, 9, and 15.[81] Phenotypically, these T cells have impaired maturation and the absolute number is reduced in the peripheral circulation. These T cells lack the ability to induce B cell antibody production. The other 50% of SCID patients have a deficiency of adenosine deaminase (ADA) due to an autosomal recessive pattern of inheritance.[81] ADA deficiency leads to toxic buildup of deoxyadenosine and S-adenosylhomocysteine, which inhibits lymphocyte maturation and overall reduction of B and T cells. An even rarer, severe form of SCID, named reticular dysgenesis, is characterized by a defect of the hematopoietic stem cells leading to the absence of myeloid cells (granulocytes) and T and B lymphocytes.[81]

X-linked agammaglobulinemia, also named Bruton's agammaglobulinemia (for Dr. Bruton's discovery in 1952), is due to a defect in B cell maturation that blocks B cell development beyond the pre-B stage.[81] These patients have reduced or absent serum IgG and absence of B cells in the peripheral circulation and lymphoid tissue. The defect has been traced to a mutation or deletion in the gene encoding the B cell tyrosine kinase, which is involved in the signaling for pre-B cells to mature.[81] Patients are susceptible to infection and 20% develop autoimmune disorders.

Administration of human serum immunoglobulin is a lifelong form of treatment. Antibiotics are required to assist with each infectious episode. Replacement therapy of serum globulin has greatly prolonged the life of these patients to the second or third decade, although many develop chronic lung disease. There is also a higher incidence of leukemia and lymphoma documented for this disorder.[83]

## DIGEORGE SYNDROME

DiGeorge syndrome is due to developmental failure of the third and fourth pharyngeal pouch, giving rise to a hypoplastic or absent thymus and parathyroid glands with midline cardiac defects and facial abnormalities. A total absence of T cells with no ability to mount a cell-mediated response is evident.[84] Immunoglobulin levels are normal and T-cell-independent humoral immunity is intact.

An interruption of the development of normal pharyngeal pouch structures from which the thymus and parathyroid tissues are derived occurs near the 8th to the 12th week of gestation. Inheritance is uncertain and a nonhereditary mutation occurring during embryogenesis may be caused by physical or chemical trauma such as maternal use of alcohol.[85,86] Owing to the absence of the thymus gland, precursor T cells are not able to differentiate and mature normally.[87]

The physical characteristic features of abnormal facies are depicted by low set prominent ears, fish-shaped mouth, and an antimongoloid slant of the eyes.[84] Patients develop tetany within the first 24 to 48 hours owing to lack of the parathyroid glands and consequent hypocalcemia.[86] Congenital heart disease is also common. Recurrent infections begin soon after birth because of viral, bacterial, fungal, or protozoan agents.

Laboratory findings include a lymphocytopenia with no circulating mature T cells. Cell-mediated immune responses are depressed, although there are normal levels of immunoglobulins.[88]

Thymic hormone treatment has helped to improve the condition. Early transplantation of fetal thymus or thymic epithelium has initiated normal mature T cell numbers and function. When the transplanted fetal thymus is less than 12 weeks' gestation, no graft-versus-host disease develops.[87] Bone marrow transplants have also been used.[88]

Absent parathyroid function leads to a hypocalcemia that does not respond well to conventional calcium supplementation. Calcium administered in conjunction with vitamin D and parathyroid hormone provide the most improvement.[89] A congenital heart condition requires immediate surgical correction, but caution must be given when blood is transfused to avoid graft-versus-host disease.[89]

## NEZELOF'S SYNDROME

Nezelof's syndrome is normally categorized under the combined immunodeficiency diseases with marked T cell deficiency and variable B cell deficiency with poor antibody response to vaccination.[90] The cause is unknown and no defined genetic pattern is apparent and most cases occur sporadically. A defect appears to be associated with thymic hypoplasia and poor B cell to T cell interaction. Because of the lack of uniformity of this disorder, it is basically a catch-all category after other combined immunodeficiency disorders have been excluded.[90]

Patients develop chronic or recurrent infections to bacterial, fungal, viral, and protozoan agents. On some occasions, a marked hepatosplenomegaly or lymphadenopathy becomes clinically evident.[91] A lymphopenia exists with abnormal cellular and humoral immune responses. T cells are decreased, although the B cell numbers are usually normal. Levels of immunoglobulin may be decreased, normal, or elevated with normal or abnormal immunoglobulin class distribution.

Nezelof's syndrome is less severe and patients have survived to their late adolescence. Long-term complications include chronic lung disease, chronic fungal infection, and the development of some malignancies.[91] Infection requires aggressive antibiotic therapy. Bone marrow transplants are the only possible cure, although thymus transplants have shown some success.[90,92]

## SELECTIVE HYPOGAMMAGLOBULINEMIA

Selective hypogammaglobulinemia, also known as selective IgA deficiency, is characterized by a marked decrease or even lack of IgA immunoglobulin in the serum with other immunoglobulin levels being normal.[81] There may also be a deficiency of secretory IgA. Cellular immunity is generally normal.[93]

It is the most common of the immunodeficiencies with an incidence of 1 in 700 people. IgA levels are less than 5 mg/dL. Most cases occur sporadically when a block occurs in the B cell's maturation at the terminal differentiation phase to IgA antibody-secreting plasma cells. A possible increase in T cell suppressor activity selective for IgA may cause the block.[94,95]

Patients are usually asymptomatic, but some may have an increased incidence of sinopulmonary disease, celiac disease, and autoimmune diseases. A few patients have severe allergies when IgE is elevated and are significantly more difficult to control than a patient without IgA deficiency. If anti-IgA antibodies develop, severe hypertensive reactions or even fatal anaphylaxis may occur following a blood transfusion. IgA-deficient donors or washed red blood cells must be used in this situation.[95,96] Serum and secretory IgA levels are absent or severely depressed. Serum immunoelectrophoresis is a definitive diagnostic indicator.

Treatment is not normally required. However, antibiotic therapy is initiated when respiratory infections persist. Selective replacement of IgA is not available and pooled human immunoglobulin is usually contraindicated owing to the patient's ability to form normal amounts of antibody of other immunoglobulin classes. This could allow them to develop anti-IgA antibodies.[96,97]

Selective IgG subclass deficiencies have been found in patients with normal total serum IgG levels. Deficiency of IgG3 is the most common subclass deficiency in adults, whereas subclass IgG2 deficiencies are more common in children.[81] These subclass deficiencies usually result from abnormal B cell differentiation rather than mutations of the gene encoding the constant region of IgG molecules.

Hyper IgM syndrome is a rare disorder associated with defective B cell switching of IgM to IgG and IgA isotypes.[81] The defect is caused by mutation in the gene encoding the T cell effector molecule responsible for stimulating B cells to undergo heavy chain isotype switching. Clinical symptoms are similar to those for patients with hypogammaglobulinemias, except these patients show increased susceptibility to infection by intracellular microbes such as *Pneumocystis carinii*.

X-linked lymphoproliferative disease is a disorder caused by mutations in the gene encoding an adapter molecule re-

quired for T cell activation and function reducing cell-mediated immunity.[81] The disease is characterized by an inability to eliminate Epstein-Barr virus leading to fulminant infectious mononucleosis and the development of B cell tumors and hypogammaglobulinemia.

## WISKOTT-ALDRICH SYNDROME

Wiskott-Aldrich syndrome is an X-linked recessive disorder of male infants characterized by thrombocytopenia, eczema, and immunodeficiency with recurrent infections usually resulting in death.[98] Both cellular and humoral abnormalities exist.[99] Infectious agents commonly involved are pyogenic bacteria, viruses, fungi, and *P. carinii*.

A gene that encodes a cytosolic protein expressed predominantly in the bone marrow is defective.[81] Phenotypically, this is characterized by reduced expression of cell surface glycoproteins and altered trafficking of leukocytes to sites of inflammation. Reduced T cell surface glycoprotein reduce B cell responses and ability to produce antibodies. Patients are especially susceptible to infection with encapsulated pyogenic bacteria.

Patients usually present with bloody diarrhea, middle ear infection, or other recurrent infections. A higher incidence of malignancy including lymphoma and lymphocytic leukemia occurs after the first decade if they survive this long.[100]

Antibiotics on a continuous basis assist in the recurrent infections. Bone marrow transplantation, especially from a matched sibling, has been very encouraging.[100] The only cure is replacement of the lymphoid tissue and hematopoietic stem cells.[98] Corticosteroids are contraindicated for thrombocytopenia because they enhance susceptibility for infections, and splenectomy has a high fatality rate.[101]

## ATAXIA TELANGIECTASIA

Ataxia telangiectasia is an autosomal recessive disorder characterized by cerebellar lesions leading to ataxia (irregularity of muscle action), telangiectasias (dilated blood vessels) of the skin and eyes, persistence of upper respiratory tract infections, and variable immune and endocrine abnormalities.[102,103]

The defect may be in the repair mechanism for DNA.[104] It is also postulated that an alteration in the endodermal maturation or its interaction with the mesoderm may explain the systemic abnormalities. The immune abnormalities are associated with decreased IgG4, IgG2, IgA, and IgE immunoglobulin levels plus decreased numbers of T cells yielding depressed T cell immunity.[105]

The patient typically presents with problems by the age of 2, although ataxia may occur as early as 9 months.[106] Recurrent sinopulmonary infections are followed by ataxia. Neurologic symptoms develop as the patient becomes older. The telangiectasias may appear as early as 2 years of age or as late as 9 years of age. The area most commonly affected are the face, ears, arms, and the sclera of the eyes. The endocrine abnormalities include gonadal dysgenesis, testicular atrophy, and an unusual form of diabetes mellitus that is insulin resistant.

Progeric signs such as premature aging and graying of the hair may develop.[105] Progressive mental retardation may occur associated with the neurologic involvement. A high incidence of malignancy is found in these patients, with the most common forms being leukemia, brain tumors, and gastric cancers.[103] A decrease in immunoglobulins occurs with serum IgA being absent in approximately 40% of the patients. A reduced number of T cells in association with an increased alpha-fetoprotein and carcinoembryonic antigen (CEA) assist in the diagnosis. The confirmation of the diagnosis may be delayed for long periods in an effort to differentiate it from selective IgA deficiency or other immune disorders.

The patient normally follows a course of progressive neurologic deterioration manifested by choreoathetosis and muscle weakness and eventually succumbs to one of the many manifestations of the disease.[103] Infections in early childhood and malignancies are the chief cause of death.[106] Antibiotics are used to treat the recurrent infections, but for the numerous other problems no effective therapy is available.[103]

## CHRONIC GRANULOMATOUS DISEASE

Defects in the innate immune system remove the first line of defense against infectious organisms. Congenital disorders of the cellular (mast cells, neutrophils, macrophages) and humoral immunity (complement, lysozyme, interferon) result in recurrent infection with varying severity. Chronic granulomatous disease (CGD) is a rare X-linked recessive disorder characterized by recurrent intracellular bacterial and fungal infections.[81] There is a mutation in the gene encoding the phagocyte oxidase enzyme, leading to defective production of superoxide anion production that is required for microbiocidal killing activity. Because of poor microbiocidal activity on intracellular organisms, chronic cell-mediated immune responses are triggered that result in the formation of granulomas composed of activated macrophages.

## LEUKOCYTE ADHESION DEFICIENCY

This is a rare autosomal recessive disorder characterized by poor leukocyte adhesion ability.[81] Leukocyte adhesion function includes adherence to endothelium, neutrophil aggregation, chemotaxis, phagocytosis, and interaction with T lymphocytes, especially natural killer cells. Leukocyte adhesion deficiency (LAD-1) has deficient expression of the $\beta_2$-integrins that participate in the adhesion of leukocytes to other cells. Leukocyte adhesion deficiency (LAD-2) defects are phenotypically similar, but the defective leukocyte adhesion results from absent sialyl groups located on the leukocyte cell surface. These sialyl groups interact specifically with cytokine-activated endothelium. Both abnormal adhesion-dependent functions lead to recurrent bacterial and fungal infections and impaired wound healing.

## CHÉDIAK-HIGASHI SYNDROME

The Chédiak-Higashi syndrome is characterized by giant cytoplasmic granules in neutrophils, monocytes, lymphocytes, melanocytes, platelets, and cells of the nervous system. The disease is due to a cellular abnormality leading to fusion of cytoplasmic granules and reduced lysosomal action and natural killer function.[81] Patients experience recurrent infections by pyogenic bacteria, partial oculocutaneous albinism nerve defects, bleeding disorders, and infiltration of organs by non-neoplastic lymphocytes. Cytolytic T lymphocyte function remains intact.

Therapeutic approaches for congenital immunodeficiencies are directed toward infection control and defective component replacement. Passive immunization with pooled gamma globulin provides short-term, life-saving therapy for acute episodes. Bone marrow transplantation for SCID, ADA, Wiskott-Aldrich syndrome, and LAD is most successful with HLA matching to prevent graft-versus-host disease. Enzyme replacement therapy has produced temporary relief but gene therapy may provide long-lasting relief from disease states.

## ACQUIRED IMMUNODEFICIENCY SYNDROME

Acquired immunodeficiency syndrome (AIDS) is characterized by severe cell-mediated immune deficiency resulting in opportunistic infections, malignancies, and neurologic symptoms in previously healthy individuals. CD4 cells of the immune system, macrophages, follicular dendritic cells, and Langerhans' cells are infected by HIV virus.[81] It is characterized by progressive defects in the humoral and cell-mediated immunity, a marked lymphopenia with a deficiency of the CD4+ subset of T cells referred to as T helper cells, and polyclonal activation of B lymphocytes and increased immunoglobulin production.

The causative agent in AIDS has been identified as a **retrovirus** referred to as human immunodeficiency virus (HIV). HIV-1 and HIV-2 are the causative agents, both of which cause similar clinical syndromes, but HIV-1 is the most common cause of AIDS. HIV-1 and HIV-2 are closely related but do differ in genomic structure and antigenicity.[81] *Retroviridae* are a family of RNA viruses characterized by the possession of reverse transcriptase and the ability to make DNA copies of itself.[107] The virus invades the CD4 (T helper subset) lymphocyte and through reverse transcriptase produces DNA that integrates into the cell genome. Cytokine stimulation of the CD4 lymphocyte stimulates normal cellular activities and an associated transcription of the HIV genome sequence.[81] HIV RNA is transported to the cytoplasm for viral protein synthesis and viron assembly. Some viral proteins (HIV gp120/gp41) are directed to the lymphocyte membrane surface. HIV core particles push through the cell membrane, producing a membrane envelope that contains viral proteins. Viral production leads to lysis of the host cell and an in vivo depletion of these cells, thus destroying the host immune response machinery.[81,107,108] HIV begins with an acute infection of the CD4 T cell that is only partially controlled by the adaptive immune response. HIV then becomes a chronic progressive disease of the peripheral lymphoid system with concomitant recurrent episodes of secondary infections, neoplasms, and declining CD4 T cell lymphocytes. Advanced stages of HIV infection show viral replication in lymph nodes and the spleen. When destruction of the peripheral lymphoid tissue is complete and blood CD4 T cell counts drop below 200 cells/mm3, patients suffer from opportunistic infections, neoplasms, wasting syndrome, kidney failure, central nervous system degeneration, and death.[81]

AIDS is transmitted by sexual contact, intravenous drug administration by contaminated needles, transfusion of blood and blood products, and the passage of the virus from infected mothers to their newborn children.[109]

Six high-risk groups for the development of AIDS have been identified in the United States.

1. Homosexual and bisexual males
2. Intravenous drug abusers
3. Hemophiliacs requiring factor VIII concentrates
4. Recipients of blood products
5. Offspring of the first 3 high-risk groups
6. Heterosexual partners of high-risk individuals
7. Unknown

Fevers, rash, flulike symptoms, neurologic manifestations, weight loss, and persistent generalized lymphadenopathy are initial presenting features. A latent period between seroconversion and clinical expression of AIDS is common and this period varies from months to years. During the initial asymptomatic period, the CD4:CD8 T cell ratio (T4:T8) is usually decreased and lymphadenopathy is evident and viral antibody is produced. Full-blown AIDS patients have bouts with opportunistic infections, the most common of which are: *Pneumocystis, Candida, Cryptococcus, Nocardia, Strongyloides, Toxoplasma, Zygomycetes,* and *Mycobacterium avium.* Viral infections that are particularly troublesome are cytomegalovirus, herpes simplex, herpes zoster, and hepatitis.[107,108,110]

Secondary cancers such as Kaposi's sarcoma, non-Hodgkin's lymphoma, and Burkitt's lymphoma may occur.[110] Because the AIDS virus can infect the nervous system, the appearance of neurologic symptoms such as encephalitis, meningitis, focal deficits, hallucinations, and progressive dementia may be additional concerns for the patient.[81,109] Thrombocytopenia and purpura have been associated with increased platelet-bound IgG in AIDS patients.

A variety of immunologic abnormalities are present on testing. Most of the abnormalities can be traced to the pronounced cell-mediated immune deficiency directly associated with the decreased number of CD4 T helper cells. A delayed hypersensitivity response to common antigens, a poor T cell proliferative response to mitogens and antigens, polyclonal hypergammaglobulinemia, circulating immune complexes, inability to produce antibody after immunization, decreased natural killer function, and depressed virus-specific cytotoxic T cell function are all characteristic findings.[109] CD8 T suppressor cells are normal or increased. Therefore, a decreased T4:T8 ratio of <1 is present in patients with AIDS. With the destruction of the CD4 T helper population, some other immune alterations directly related to the absence of this T subset occur. Interleukin 2, gamma interferon, macrophage

chemotactic growth factor, and B cell growth factor are all depressed.[109]

A specific diagnosis can be made on the isolation of HIV from serum, cells, or lymph nodes, but these viral cell cultures are not commonly performed. The presence of HIV antibodies is diagnostically useful. The techniques utilized in antibody testing are ELISA and the Western blot. Molecular-based testing utilizing amplification systems has increased sensitivity and specificity (Chapter 7). The ability to test for HIV nucleic acid reduces the window of time between initial infection and the ability to detect the presence of the replicating virus. This is essential for a safe blood supply for transfusion services.

Mortality approaches 100% with 92% of the deaths being directly associated with opportunistic infections. No complete recoveries from AIDS have been documented, although several long-term survivals are on record.[110]

Even with the discovery and extensive scientific study directed at the causative virus, no vaccine is yet available. The degree of polymorphism in the viral isolates from patient to patient helps to account for its diverse behavior and the difficulty in vaccine preparation.[81]

The major thrust in trying to control the epidemic is focused at educating the public, counseling high-risk groups, and using preventive measures. Additionally, careful screening of blood products is now available. Biosynthetic clotting factors can be substituted in some situations for those requiring treatment for bleeding problems.

Administration of two classes of drugs, used in combination, target molecules for which there are no human homologs. Drugs such as 3'-azido-3'-deoxythymidine (AZT) or 2'3'-dideoxyiosine and 2'3'-dideoxycytidine are nucleotide analogs that inhibit reverse transcriptase and block the replication of HIV.[81] Use of two of these drugs in combination with an additional protease inhibitor, which blocks the processing of viral precursor proteins, is commonly called triple drug therapy or highly active antiretroviral therapy (HAART). Drugs that block viral entry are being investigated with extensive work being focused on providing an effective, safe vaccine.

Acquired immunodeficiencies are also caused by malnutrition, neoplasm, infections, and secondary effects from other disease processes (autoimmune disease).[81] Iatrogenic immunodeficiencies may develop following splenectomy or immunosuppressive therapy for transplant rejection, inflammatory disease, or cancer therapy.[81] Other viral infections have similar clinical manifestations. Human T cell lymphotropic virus 1 and measles have immunosuppressive effects. Additionally, chronic parasitic infections may also lead to immunosuppression.

## SUMMARY

Intense research has provided significant information about the immune system and mechanisms of the host innate and acquired immunity. This information is critical for the management and diagnosis of autoimmune diseases. Antinuclear antibodies have been described in a variety of autoimmune diseases with specific ANAs present in given disease states.

This chapter has reviewed many of the autoimmune disorders, their clinical presentations, diagnoses, and treatment. The pathogenesis of autoimmune diseases is still being characterized but viral involvement, genetic predisposition, and chemical and drug exposure are strongly implicated in the loss of self-tolerance and development of autoimmunity. Immunodeficiency may be congenital or acquired, with loss of immunity being traced to the loss of B or T cell function, developmental maturation, or individual cell lines.

In general, the various autoantibodies found in these disorders give only supporting evidence for diagnosis. Within themselves, they are not confirmatory nor does the absence exclude them from the associated disease. As we gain a greater understanding for the molecular basis of immunity, immune self-tolerance and autoimmunity, we will be able to address clinical diagnostic and treatment issues more effectively.

## REFERENCES

1. Tizard IR: *Immunology: An Introduction.* 2nd ed. Philadelphia, Sanders College Publishing, 1988, pp 514–520.
2. Theofilopoulos AN: Autoimmunity. In Stites DP, Abba IT, Parslow TG (eds.): *Basic and Clinical Immunology,* 5th ed. Los Altos, CA, Lange Medical Publications, 1984, p 1952.
3. Turgeon ML: *Immunology and Serology.* 2nd ed. St. Louis, Mosby, 1996, p 4–5.
4. Abbas AK, Lichtman AH, Pober JS: *Cellular and Molecular Immunology.* 4th ed., Philadelphia, WB Saunders, 2000, pp 208–230.
5. Abbas AK, Lichtman AH, Pober JS: *Cellular and Molecular Immunology.* 4th ed., Philadelphia, WB Saunders, 2000, p 404.
6. Nakamura RM: Human autoimmune diseases: Progress in clinical laboratory tests. Med Lab Observer 32:32, 2000.
7. Robbins SL, Cotran RS, Kumar V: *Pathologic Basis of Disease.* 3rd ed. Philadelphia, WB Saunders, 1984, p 177.
8. Tan EM: Antinuclear antibodies in diagnosis and management. Hosp Pract 18(1):79, 1983.
9. Abbas AK, Lichtman AH, Pober JS: Disease caused by immune responses: Hypersensitivity and autoimmunity. In Abbas AK, Lichtman AH, Pober JS (eds.): *Cellular and Molecular Immunology.* 4th ed. Philadelphia, WB Saunders, 2000, pp 418–420.
10. Sinha AA, Lopex MT, McDevitt HO: Autoimmune disease: The failure of self tolerance. Science 248:1380–1388, 1990.
11. Hang LM, Nakamura RM: Current concepts and advances in clinical laboratory testing for autoimmune disease. Crit Rev Clin Lab Sci 34:275–311, 1994.
12. Abbas AK, Lichtman AH, Pober JS: *Cellular and Molecular Immunology.* 4th ed., Philadelphia, WB Saunders, 2000, pp 422–423.
13. Abbas AK, Lichtman AH, Pober JS: *Cellular and Molecular Immunology.* 4th ed. Philadelphia, WB Saunders, 2000, pp 410–417.
14. Alspaugh M, Maddison P: Resolution of the identity of certain antigen-antibody systems in systemic lupus erythematosus and Sjögren's syndrome: An inter-laboratory collaboration. Arthritis Rheum 22:796, 1979.
15. Maddison PJ, Reichlin M: Deposition of antibodies to a soluble cytoplasmic antigen in the kidneys of patients with systemic lupus erythematosus. Arthritis Rheum 22:858, 1979.
16. Greenwald CA, Peebles CL and Nakamura RM: Laboratory tests for antinuclear antibody ANA in rheumatic diseases. Lab Med 9(4):19–28, 1978.
17. Beck JS: Variations in the morphological patterns of "autoimmune" nuclear fluorescence. Lancet 1:1203, 1961.
18. Tan EM: Antinuclear antibodies in diagnosis and management. Hosp Pract 17:84, 1983.
19. Smith HR, Stinberg, AD: Autoimmunity—A perspective. Ann Rev Immunol 1:175, 1983.
20. Reimer G, Rose KM, Scheer U, et al.: Autoantibody to RNA polymerase 1 in scleroderma sera. J Clin Invest 79:65–72, 1987.
21. Robbins SL, Cotran RS, Kumar V: *Pathologic Basis of Disease.* 3rd ed. Philadelphia, WB Saunders, 1984, pp 180–189.
22. Stites DP, Terr AI, Parslow RG: *Basic and Clinical Immunology.* 8th ed., Stamford, CT, Appleton & Lange, 1994, pp 387–411.
23. Lambert PH, Perrin L, Izui S: *Recent Advances in Systemic Lupus Erythematosus.* New York, Academic Press, 1984, pp 225–229, 279.
24. Shoenfeld Y, Isenberg D: Anti-DNA antibody idiotypes: Their pathogenic role and prognostic significance in systemic lupus erythematosus (SLE). Res Diagn Clin Test 427:52–55, 1989.
25. Rapaport SI: *Introduction to Hematology.* 2nd ed. Philadelphia, JB Lippincott, 1987, pp 553–556.
26. Budman DR, Steinberg AD: Hematologic aspects of systemic lupus erythematosus. Ann Intern Med 86:220–229, 1977.
27. Blatt PN, Martin SE: The lupus anticoagulant. Arch Pathol Lab Med 111:113, 1987.
28. Talal N: Sjögren's syndrome. In Rose N, Mackay I (eds.): *The Autoimmune Diseases.* New York, Academic Press, 1985, pp 145–159.
29. Talal N, Moutsopoulos H, Kassan S (eds.): *Sjögren's Syndrome: Clinical and Immunological Aspects.* West Germany, Springer-Verlag, 1987.
30. Talal N: Sjögren syndrome and pseudolymphoma. Hosp Pract 23(9):71–80, 1988.

31. Talal N: Sjögren's syndrome. In Schumacher, RH (ed.): *Primer on the Rheumatic Diseases.* 9th ed. Atlanta, Arthritis Foundation, 1988, p 136.

32. Townes AS, Stevens MB: Sjögren's syndrome. In Harvey AM, Johns RJ, McKusick VA, et al. (eds.): *The Principles and Practice of Medicine.* 20th ed. New York, Appleton-Century-Crofts, 1980, pp 1133–1135.

33. Talal N: Sjögren's syndrome. In Schumacher, RH (ed.): *Primer on the Rheumatic Diseases.* 9th ed. Atlanta, Arthritis Foundation, 1988, pp 137–138.

34. Robbins SL, Cotran RS, Kumar V: *Pathologic Basis of Disease.* 3rd ed. Philadelphia, WB Saunders, 1984, p 189.

35. Berkow R: Sjögren's syndrome. In *The Merck Manual of Diagnosis and Therapy.* 15th ed. Rahway, NJ, Merck and Co., 1987, pp 1249–1250.

36. Barwick DD, Walton JN: Polymyositis. Am South J Med 35:646, 1963.

37. Peter JB: Polymyositis and dermatomyositis. In Stein, J (ed.): *Internal Medicine.* Vol 1. Boston, Little Brown, and Co., 1983, p 1063.

38. Pachman LM, Maryjowski MC: Juvenile dermatomyositis and polymyositis. Clin Rheum Dis 10:95–115, 1984.

39. Townes AS, Stevens MB: Polymyositis. In Harvey AM, Johns RJ, McKusick VA, et al. (eds.): *The Principles and Practice of Medicine.* 20th ed. New York, Appleton-Century-Crofts, 1980, pp 1125–1127.

40. Berkow R: Polymyositis/dermatomyositis. In *The Merck Manual of Diagnosis and Therapy.* 15th ed. Rahway, NJ, Merck and Co., 1987, pp 1280–1282.

41. Dawkins RL, Silko PJ: Polymyositis and myasthenia gravis: Immunodeficiency disorders involving skeletal muscle. Lancet 1:200, 1975.

42. Cronin ME, Miller FW, Plotz PH: Polymyositis and dermatomyositis. In Schumacher, RH (ed.): *Primer on the Rheumatic Diseases.* 9th ed. Atlanta, Arthritis Foundation, 1988, pp 121–123.

43. Robbins SL, Cotran RS, Kumar V: *Pathologic Basis of Disease.* 3rd ed. Philadelphia, WB Saunders, 1984, p 194.

44. McCarty GA: Autoantibodies and their relation to rheumatic diseases. Med Clin North Am 70:237, 1986.

45. Peter JB: Polymyositis and dermatomyositis. In Stein, J (ed.): *Internal Medicine.* Vol 1. Boston, Little Brown and Co, 1983, pp 1053–1056.

46. Medsger TA, Jr: Systemic sclerosis (scleroderma), eosinophilic fasciitis, and calcinosis, in McCarty, DJ: *Arthritis and Allied Conditions.* 10th ed. Philadelphia, Lea & Febiger, 1985, pp 994–1036.

47. LeRoy EC: Scleroderma (systemic sclerosis). In Kelley WN, Harris ED, Ruddy, S, et al.: *Textbook of Rheumatology.* Philadelphia, WB Saunders, 1981, pp 1183–1205.

48. Medsger TA: Systemic sclerosis and localized scleroderma. In Schumacher, RH (ed.): *Primer on the Rheu-*

*matic Diseases.* 9th ed. Atlanta, Arthritis Foundation, 1988, pp 111–116.

49. Medsger TA, Masi AT: Epidemiology of systemic sclerosis. Ann Intern Med 74:714, 1971.

50. Robbins SL, Cotran RS, Kumar V: *Pathologic Basis of Disease.* 3rd ed. Philadelphia, WB Saunders, 1984, pp 192–193.

51. Haynes DC, Gershwin ME: The immunopathology of progressive systemic sclerosis (PSS). Semin Arthritis Rheum 11:331, 1982.

52. McCoy R, et al: The kidney in progressive systemic sclerosis: Antibody elution studies. Lab Invest 35:124, 1976.

53. Tan EM: Antinuclear antibodies. In Stein, J (ed.): *Internal Medicine.* Vol 1. Boston, Little Brown, pp 947–948.

54. Robbins SL, Cotran RS, Kumar V: *Pathologic Basis of Disease.* 3rd ed. Philadelphia, W.B. Saunders Co., 1984; p 194.

55. Berkow R: Progressive systemic sclerosis. In *The Merck Manual of Diagnosis and Therapy,* 15th ed. Rahway, NJ, Merck and Co., 1987, pp 1277–1279.

56. Fudenberg HH, Stites DP, Caldwell JL, Wells JV: *Basic and Clinical Immunology.* 3rd ed. Los Angeles, CA, Lange Medical Publications, 1980, p 458.

57. Penning CA, Steen VD, Reimer G, et al.: An analysis of systemic sclerosis patients with autoantibodies to the nucleolar proteins PM-Scl, RNA polymerase 1 and fibrillarin. Arthritis Rheum 30:S96, 1987.

58. Townes AS, Stevens MB: Polmyositis. In Harvey AM, Johns RJ, McKusick VA, et al. (eds.): *The Principles and Practice of Medicine.* 20th ed. New York, Appleton-Century-Crofts, 1980, p 1125.

59. Traub YM, Shapiro AP, Rodnan GP, et al.: Hypertension and renal failure (scleroderma renal crisis) in progressive systemic sclerosis: Report of a 25 year experience with 68 cases. Medicine 62:335–352, 1984.

60. Sharp JC, et al.: Mixed connective tissue disease—an apparently distinct rheumatic disease syndrome associated with specific antibody to a ribonucleoprotein antigen. Am J Med 52:148, 1972.

61. Berkow R: Mixed connective tissue disease. In *The Merck Manual of Diagnosis and Therapy,* 15th ed. Rahway, NJ, Merck and Co., 1987, pp 1288–1289.

62. Robbins SL, Cotran RS, Kumar V: *Pathologic Basis of Disease.* 3rd ed. Philadelphia, WB Saunders Co., 1984, p 195.

63. Townes AS, Stevens MB: Rheumatoid arthritis. In Harvey AM, Johns RJ, McKusick VA, et al. (eds.): *The Principles and Practice of Medicine.* 20th ed. New York, Appleton-Century-Crofts, 1980, pp 1135–1138.

64. Stites DP, Terr AI: *Basic and Clinical Immunology,* 3rd ed. Norwalk, CT, Appleton & Lange, 1991, pp 444–446.

65. Schumacher HR: Rheumatoid arthritis. In Schu-

macher, HR (ed.): *Primer on the Rheumatic Diseases.* 9th ed. Atlanta, Arthritis Foundation, 1988, pp 84–96.

66. Hazelton RA, et al: Immunogenetic insights into rheumatoid arthritis: A family study. Q J Med 51 (New Series):336, 1982.

67. Robbins SL, Cotran RS, Kumar V: *Pathologic Basis of Disease.* 3rd ed. Philadelphia, WB Saunders, 1984, p 1351.

68. Stites DP, Terr AI: *Basic and Clinical Immunology,* 3rd ed. Norwalk, CT, Appleton & Lange, 1991, p 447.

69. Robbins SL, Cotran RS, Kumar V: *Pathologic Basis of Disease.* 3rd ed. Philadelphia, WB Saunders, 1984, p 1354.

70. Horwitz CA: Laboratory diagnosis of rheumatoid diseases. Postgrad Med 67(5):193–203, 1980.

71. Berkow R: Rheumatoid arthritis. In *The Merck Manual of Diagnosis and Therapy.* 15th ed. Rahway, NJ, Merck and Co. 1987, pp 1239–1245.

72. Townes AS, Stevens MB: Rheumatoid arthritis. In Harvey AM, Johns RJ, McKusick VA, et al. (eds.): *The Principles and Practice of Medicine.* 20th ed. New York, Appleton-Century-Crofts, 1980, pp 1139–1140.

73. Conn DL: Polyarteritis. In Schumacher HR (ed.): *Primer on the Rheumatic Diseases.* 9th ed. Atlanta, Arthritis Foundation, 1988, p 125.

74. Berkow R: Polyarteritis nodosa. In *The Merck Manual of Diagnosis and Therapy.* 15th ed. Rahway, NJ, Merck and Co., 1987, p 1285.

75. Kurland LT, Chuang TKY, Hunder GG: The epidemiology of systemic arteritis. In Lawrence RC, Shulman LE (eds.): *Epidemiology of the Rheumatic Diseases.* New York, Gower Medical Publishing, Ltd., 1984, pp 196–206.

76. Townes AS, Stevens MB: Polyarteritis. In Harvey AM, Johns RJ, McKusick VA, et al. (eds.): *The Principles and Practice of Medicine.* 20th ed. New York, Appleton-Century-Crofts, 1980, pp 1128–1130.

77. Stites DP, Terr AI, Parslow RG: *Basic and Clinical Immunology.* 8th ed., Stamford, CT, Appleton & Lange, 1994, pp 447–449.

78. Peter JB: Polyarteritis nodosa. In Stein, J (ed.): *Internal Medicine.* Vol 1. Boston, Little Brown and Co., 1983, pp 1048–1049.

79. Kaufman LD, Kaplan AP: Microscopic polyarteritis. Hosp Pract 24(6):85–97, 1989.

80. Bennington JL: *Dictionary and Encyclopedia of Laboratory Medicine and Technology.* Philadelphia, WB Saunders, 1984, p 1164.

81. Abbas AK, Lichtman AH, Pober JS: *Cellular and Molecular Immunology.* 4th ed. WB Saunders Co., 2000, pp 445–467.

82. Stites DP, Terr AI: *Basic and Clinical Immunology.* 3rd ed. Norwalk, CT, Appleton & Lange, 1991, pp 341–354.

83. Tizard IR: *Immunology: An Introduction.* 2nd ed. Philadelphia, Saunders College Publishing, 1988, p 388.

84. Humphrey AL, The immunodeficiency diseases. In Harvey AM, Johns RJ, McKusick VA, et al. (eds.): *The Principles and Practice of Medicine.* 20th ed. New York, Appleton-Century-Crofts, 1980, p 1100.

85. Stites DP, Terr AI: *Basic and Clinical Immunology.* 3rd ed. Norwalk, CT, Appleton & Lange, 1991; pp 335–339.

86. Berkow R: DiGeorge syndrome. In *The Merck Manual of Diagnosis and Therapy.* 15th ed. Rahway, NJ, Merck and Co., 1987, p 284.

87. DiGeorge AM: Congenital absence of thymus and its immunologic consequences: Concurrence with congenital hypoparathyroidism. In Bergsma D (ed.): *Immunologic Diseases in Man.* Birth Defects 4:116, 1968.

88. Robbins SL, Cotran RS, Kumar V: *Pathologic Basis of Disease.* 3rd ed. Philadelphia, WB Saunders, 1984, p 284.

89. Williams WJ: *Hematology,* 4th ed. New York, McGraw-Hill, 1990, p 972.

90. Bennington JL: *Dictionary and Encyclopedia of Laboratory Medicine and Technology.* Philadelphia, WB Saunders, 1984, p. 1071.

91. Stites DP, Terr AI: *Basic and Clinical Immunology.* 3rd ed. Norwalk, CT, Appleton & Lange, 1991, pp 343–345.

92. Steihm ER, Fulginiti VA: *Immunologic Disorders in Infants and Children.* Philadelphia, WB Saunders, 1980.

93. Tizard IR: *Immunology: An Introduction.* 2nd ed. Philadelphia, Saunders College Publishing, 1988, pp 329–330.

94. Tizard IR: *Immunology: An Introduction.* 2nd ed. Philadelphia, Saunders College Publishing, 1988, p 398.

95. Wintrobe MM: *Clinical Hematology.* 8th ed. Philadelphia, Lea & Febiger, 1981, p 1398.

96. Berkow R: Selective IgA deficiency. In *The Merck Manual of Diagnosis and Therapy.* 15th ed. Rahway, Merck and Co, 1987, p 284.

97. Robbins SL, Cotran RS, Kumar V: *Pathologic Basis of Disease.* 3rd ed. Philadelphia, WB Saunders, 1984, p 206.

98. Williams WJ: *Hematology.* 4th ed. New York, McGraw-Hill, 1990, p 970.

99. Peter JB: Wiskott-Aldrich syndrome. In Stein, J (ed.): *Internal Medicine.* Vol 1. Boston, Little Brown, 1983, p 971.

100. Berkow R: Wiskott-Aldrich syndrome. In *The Merck Manual of Diagnosis and Therapy.* 15th ed. Rahway, NJ, Merck and Co, 1987, p 285.

101. Fudenberg HH, Stites DP, Caldwell JL, Wells JV: *Basic and Clinical Immunology.* 3rd ed. Los Angeles, Lange Medical Publications, 1980, p 429.

102. Tizard IR: *Immunology: An Introduction.* 2nd ed. Philadelphia, Sanders College Publishing, 1988, p 389.

103. Berkow R: Ataxia Telangiectasia. In *The Merck Manual of Diagnosis and Therapy.* 15th ed. Rahway, Merck and Co, 1987, p 286.

104. Stites DP, Terr AI: *Basic and Clinical Immunology.* 3rd ed, Norwalk, CT, Appleton & Lange, 1991, p 345–340.

105. Bluestein HG: Ataxia telangiectasia. In Stein, J (ed.): *Internal Medicine.* Vol 1. Boston, Little Brown, 1983, p 971–972.

106. Stites DP, Terr AI: *Basic and Clinical Immunology.* 3rd ed. Norwalk, CT, Appleton & Lange, 1991, pp 341–346.

107. Haseltine WA, Wong-Staal F: The molecular biology of the AIDS virus. Sci Am 259:52–62, 1988.

108. Tizard IR: *Immunology: An Introduction.* 2nd ed. Philadelphia, Sanders College Publishing, 1988; p 394.

109. Stites DP, Terr AI: *Basic and Clinical Immunology.* 3rd ed. Norwalk, CT, Appleton & Lange, 1991, pp 699–700.

110. Berkow R: Sjögren's Syndrome. In *The Merck Manual of Diagnosis and Therapy.* 15th ed. Rahway, NJ, Merck and Co, 1987, p 291.

# C H A P T E R   1 5

# Clinical Enzymology

*Joan E. Aldrich*

Enzymes are organic molecules that accelerate biochemical reactions so that the reactions proceed fast enough to sustain life. Essentially, all the steps in cellular metabolic pathways proceed because enzymes catalyze them. In typical enzyme-catalyzed reactions, each molecule of enzyme reacts with $10^2$ to $10^7$ molecules of substrate each second.[1] The distinguishing feature of an enzyme is that it emerges from a reaction in the same form and concentration as it was when it entered the reaction.

## MEASURING ENZYMES

### Significance of Enzyme Measurement

Inborn errors of metabolism are a group of diseases in which a genetic mutation results in an abnormal enzyme in a metabolic pathway. The mutation alters the amino acid sequence of the enzyme protein. If this change in primary structure causes a change in the secondary or tertiary shape of the enzyme, its activity level or reaction specificity is likely to be altered. The clinical consequences of such mutations range from innocuous to incompatible with life. Altered enzyme activity in a metabolic pathway is usually detected by measuring abnormal concentrations of the enzyme's metabolites.

Instead of measuring metabolic pathways, the clinical laboratory usually measures enzymes that have leaked into plasma from damaged cells. Detecting and quantitating the amount of enzyme in plasma can monitor the presence and amount of damaged tissue and, in several cases, the pattern of elevated plasma enzymes can identify the specific tissue that is damaged. The clinical laboratory also measures enzymes whose major functions are carried out in plasma but, historically, the study of these coagulation factors lies in the realm of the hematology laboratory.

### Properties of Enzymes

Enzymatic activity is always associated with a protein. In most cases, the activity is a consequence of reaction by a part of the protein itself, although there are examples in which an associated group actually performs the reaction while the protein holds the reacting groups in proximity to each other. These associated groups include small RNA molecules and derivatives

of vitamins. Study of the protein itself and the conditions that affect it are common ways to examine an enzyme reaction.

An enzyme, like any protein, has a specific shape that is determined by its primary, secondary, and tertiary structures; a few clinically important enzymes require quaternary structure for their activity. The location on the protein where the enzyme reacts with its substrate is called the **active site.** The specificity of an enzyme for a particular substrate and the nature of the reaction catalyzed both rely on the exact spatial relationship of the side chains of the amino acids that are present in the protein's active site. A well-studied example is the hydrolysis of a peptide bond by chymotrypsin[1] (Figure 15–1). The active site of chymotrypsin is a groove on the surface of the enzyme in which specific residues of serine and histidine are exposed. When the aromatic amino acid side chain of the substrate is held in the groove, the adjacent peptide bond is attacked and hydrolyzed by the serine and histidine side chains of the active site. Only aromatic amino acids have the correct size and polarity to fit the active site tightly enough to be acted on. This requirement for a certain size, shape, and polarity confers specificity on an enzyme-catalyzed reaction because any condition that alters the size or shape of the groove or the ionization state of the serine and histidine will obliterate the activity of the enzyme.

Most enzymes act on only one or a small group of closely related compounds and they only conduct one narrowly prescribed reaction. In fact, modern protein-modeling experiments have demonstrated that, in some cases, the enzyme changes shape when the correct substrate binds to its active site.[1] This "induced fit" brings the reactive centers into close proximity and allows the reaction to proceed.

An alternate mechanism for changing the proximity between substrate and active site is called **allosterism.** In this case, a separate compound reacts with a distant site on the enzyme molecule and alters the shape of the active site, thus altering its fit with the substrate. The distant site is called an allosteric site. The altered active site may be either more or less reactive. Allosterism is a common mechanism for regulating the activity of a key enzyme in a metabolic pathway. It is also a source of activation or inhibition in an enzyme assay.

Some enzymes require the presence of nonprotein activators or cofactors to be active. These cofactors may participate in the reaction or may stabilize a particular conformation of the enzyme molecule. A cofactor that is tightly bound to the enzyme is referred to as a **prosthetic group.** In the absence of

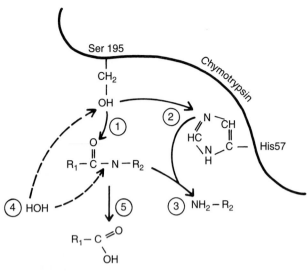

**FIGURE 15-1**

The mechanism of hydrolysis by chymotrypsin. ① Oxygen from the alcohol group of serine residue 195 attacks the peptide bond and forms a serine-peptide intermediate. ② Hydrogen from the alcohol group of serine 195 is passed through histidine 57 to the amino group of the freed peptide ③. ④ Hydrogen from water restores H to the alcohol of serine, and donates OH for the carboxyl of the freed peptide ⑤. A nearby aspartic acid residue (not shown) participates by stabilizing histidine residue 57.

the prosthetic group, the enzyme is referred to as an **apoenzyme,** and the active combination of the two is called a **holoenzyme.** The prosthetic group may be a vitamin derivative (e.g., nicotinamide-adenine dinucleotide, $NAD^+$, or pyridoxal-5-phosphate, P5P), or a metal ion (e.g., $Zn^{++}$ or $Mg^{++}$), or a complex moiety (e.g., heme).

Many enzymes are present in the body as **isoenzymes.** These are different physical forms of an enzyme that all conduct the same reaction. In some cases, isoenzymes result from tissue-specific post-translational differences in the enzymes. An example of this kind of variation is amylase where the carbohydrates that are attached to the amylase protein in pancreatic tissue are different from the carbohydrates attached in salivary tissue; thus the isoenzymes can be differentiated by reagents such as lectins or antibodies that recognize carbohydrate motifs.

In other isoenzymes, the physical difference is caused by variable quaternary structure. For example, the association of two peptide components comprises the active form of creatine kinase (CK). The three isoenzymes of CK are composed of two B peptides (BB), one B peptide and one M peptide (MB), or two M peptides (MM). A separate gene codes each type of peptide and different tissues express each gene to a different extent. This property is used to distinguish between CK released from skeletal muscle (MM) and CK released from car-

diac muscle (both MM and MB). The three isoenzymes of CK can be differentiated from each other by their different electrophoretic mobilities or by different antigenic epitopes.

## Mechanism of Enzyme Reactions

For a chemical reaction to proceed, the total energy of the reaction must proceed downhill. In most cases, this means that the energy in the chemical bonds of the product is less than the energy in the bonds of the substrate. Substrate molecules are kept from spontaneously becoming product molecules by the energy contained in the chemical bond that must be altered by the reaction. This energy barrier is referred to as **energy of activation** (Figure 15–2). In the absence of enzyme, very few molecules of substrate have sufficient kinetic energy to surpass the energy of activation and thus the reaction proceeds slowly or not at all.

The mechanism by which an enzyme enhances the rate of a reaction is through forming a covalent bond with the substrate (Equation 15–1). The chemical bond formed in this intermediate enzyme-substrate (ES) complex contains less energy, which allows molecules with less kinetic energy to surpass the energy of activation and become product. Thus, even at body temperature (37°C), enzyme-catalyzed metabolic reactions can proceed rapidly.

$$E + S \leftrightarrow ES \rightarrow E + P \qquad (15-1)$$

The reaction between enzyme and substrate is reversible. The enzyme-substrate complex can either revert to the original molecules or complete the reaction and form product and regenerated enzyme (Equation 15–1). Since the energy in the bonds of the product is lower than those of the complex, the

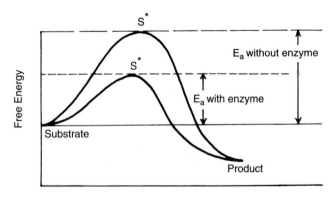

**FIGURE 15-2**

Enzymes increase the speed of a reaction by lowering the energy of activation ($E_a$). $S^*$ represents substrate molecules with sufficient kinetic energy to alter their chemical bonds and become molecules of product. In the presence of enzyme, $S^*$ is in the form of ES complex.

final reaction is usually treated as if it were irreversible. It is recognized, however, that when equilibrium concentrations are achieved, the net forward reaction equals the net backward reaction. This state occurs frequently in intracellular metabolic pathways where several of the enzymatic steps are near equilibrium. However, the point is moot in laboratory measurement of enzyme reactions because substrate is always added in great excess and the reaction is assessed long before equilibrium is attained.

## Enzyme Kinetics

The amount of enzyme present in a patient's sample is assayed by measuring its effect on the rate of a chemical reaction: the more enzyme that is present, the faster the reaction proceeds. For this to be true, all other conditions that affect the rate of the reaction must be controlled. Those conditions include providing constant pH and constant temperature as well as excess amount of substrate (and any other chemicals that are used up in the reaction). In addition, physiologic ionic strength and sufficient activators or cofactors must be provided.

In general, conditions are used that produce the maximum rate of reaction, i.e., optimal conditions. A rapid reaction rate is desirable for several reasons: (1) it produces a measurable reaction with only a small aliquot of sample, (2) it is very sensitive to small amounts of (or small variations in) enzyme concentration, and (3) patients' results are available quickly. Frequently, optimal conditions simulate conditions in the body, i.e., pH 7.4 and 37°C but sometimes a different pH or temperature provides better reaction conditions.

The **effect of pH** on the rate of an enzyme-catalyzed reaction varies with the ionization state of the enzyme protein (including its active site), ionization of substrates or cofactors, and (on occasion) production or utilization of $H^+$ in the reaction. For example, the reaction catalyzed by lactate dehydrogenase (LD) is reversible:

$$lactate^- + NAD^+ \leftrightarrow pyruvate^- + NADH + H^+$$

The forward reaction mixes LD with $lactate^-$ and $NAD^+$ and measures the rate of formation of NADH. The optimum pH for this reaction is 8.3 to 8.9. The alternate reverse reaction mixes LD with $pyruvate^-$ and NADH and measures the rate of disappearance of NADH. The optimum pH for this reaction is 7.1 to 7.4. The difference in pH optimum reflects the participation of $H^+$ in the reaction.

The choice of buffer and the regulation of pH reflect knowledge of the optimal pH and the shape of the pH activity curve. The pH-activity curve for an enzyme assay is determined by performing the assay with all parameters held constant except the pH of the reaction. The pH where the reaction rate is fastest is the optimum. The shape of the curve determines how tightly the pH of the assay must be controlled.

**Ionic strength** of the medium has an effect on the 3-dimensional shape of an enzyme. The effect is seen mostly at extremes of very strong or very weak solutions that denature some proteins. In practice, this effect is most often relevant when analyzing a patient's sample that contains such a high concentration of enzyme that it must be diluted to obtain an accurate result. For very stable enzymes, diluting with water is allowed because the shape and activity of the enzyme is retained at low ionic strength but other enzymes require diluting with isotonic saline, 7% albumin, or inactivated serum to maintain the active shape of the enzyme. The sensitivity of an enzyme molecule to changes in ionic strength can be determined by comparing the results of assays in which diluents with various ionic strengths are used. If enzyme activity decreases with decrease in ionic strength, then care must be taken to maintain isotonicity in the reaction.

At a **temperature** lower than optimal, substrate and enzyme molecules have less kinetic energy; thus fewer enzyme-substrate complexes are able to overcome the energy barrier and the rate of reaction is slowed. At a temperature higher than optimal, the enzyme begins to denature, which reduces its effective concentration and thus reduces the rate of the reaction. This is a crucial point for some enzymes that are particularly unstable at elevated temperatures. For example, the method for analyzing creatine kinase at 37°C must be rapid because, at that temperature, denaturation of the enzyme is fast enough to affect the result after just a few minutes of incubation. Except when otherwise specified, reports of enzyme activity are assumed to reflect a reaction performed at 37°C.

The **length of time** that an enzyme is reacting with its substrate must be closely monitored. The purpose of an enzyme assay is to measure the amount of enzyme; therefore the amount of enzyme must be the only variable in the measurement. Theoretically, the initial rate (velocity) of the reaction is the best measure of the amount of enzyme but, in practice, the rate is measured over a span of seconds to a few minutes. To ensure that enzyme concentration is the only variable during this incubation period, most assays measure the reaction continuously. This is called a **kinetic assay.** Figure 15–3a. demonstrates the multiple measurements from a kinetic assay that are used to calculate the amount of product formed per minute. The consistent increase in absorbance at each time interval confirms that the amount of product formed per minute is constant. This is experimental evidence that all conditions that affect the reaction are also constant and the assay is measuring enzyme concentration only.

If the enzyme assay is incubated too long, substrate concentration becomes limiting and there is a decrease in the rate at which product is being formed. This is referred to as **substrate exhaustion** (Figure 15–4). Correcting the situation so that only enzyme concentration limits the reaction will require using a higher concentration of substrate, a lower concentration of enzyme, or a shorter incubation period so that the substrate is not used up.

In some enzyme assays, there is a delay between mixing the enzyme with substrate and the initial formation of product. This is called the **lag phase** (Figure 15–4). This source of

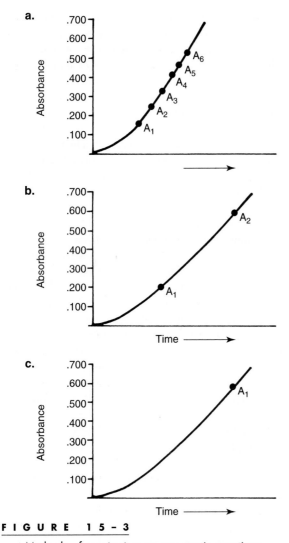

**a.**

**FIGURE  15-3**

Methods of monitoring an enzymatic reaction:
**a.** kinetic assay, **b.** two-point assay, **c.** end-point
assay.

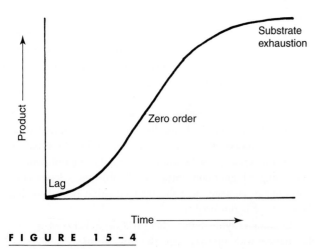

**FIGURE  15-4**

Reaction phases seen in enzymatic reactions.

error can be avoided by using either a kinetic assay or a **two-point assay,** i.e., taking two measurements during the incubation and calculating the reaction rate between them (Figure 15–3**b.**). A kinetic assay is always preferable because even in a two-point assay there is an assumption of constant reaction rate between the two readings. Some enzyme assays rely on a single measurement after a fixed length of incubation. These **end-point assays** (Figure 15–3**c.**) are least reliable since there are no data to measure the initial concentration of product or to ensure constant reaction conditions.

Most modern, high-volume clinical instruments use kinetic measurements of enzyme assays. Using computer-driven cuvette arrays or several reading stations, multiple measurements of many samples can be taken efficiently. Alternatively, the advantage of two-point assays is that one operator working manually can analyze a large number of samples concurrently.

The effect of increasing the **concentration of substrate** (and other consumables) on the rate of an enzyme reaction is typically a hyperbolic curve (Figure 15–5). At low substrate concentrations, only a fraction of the active sites of the enzyme are participating in the reaction and the rate of reaction is mostly dependent on the concentration of substrate. At greater substrate concentrations, all of the active sites are participating in the reaction for the duration of the assay and the rate of the reaction is dependent on the concentration of the enzyme. Nomenclature for this situation follows the convention that proportionality between concentration and reaction rate is called **first-order,** whereas a reaction rate that is independent of concentration is called **zero-order.** The nomenclature is derived from this equation:

$$\text{reaction rate} \propto \text{concentration}^n$$

For an enzyme assay, the reaction rate should depend only on the concentration of enzyme ($n = 1$) and be independent of the concentration of the substrate ($n = 0$). In other words, the reaction should be first order with respect to enzyme concentration and zero order with respect to substrate concentration.

The substrate activity curve (Figure 15–5) is determined by assaying an enzyme sample at several concentrations of substrate while holding all other conditions constant. The maximum reaction rate ($V_{max}$) is proportional to enzyme concentration and is independent of substrate concentration. This is the desired situation for measuring the amount of enzyme. The **Michaelis-Menten equation** (Equation 15–2) describes the effect that substrate concentration has on the rate of an enzyme reaction. This equation demonstrates that when $S$ and ($K_m + S$) are essentially equal, $\nu \cong V_{max}$. In other words, at large substrate concentration (where S is at least 50 times greater than $K_m$), the reaction rate ($\nu$) is measuring the concentration of enzyme ($V_{max}$).

$$\nu = \frac{V_{max}\, S}{K_m + S} \qquad (15\text{--}2)$$

where $\nu$ is the rate of the reaction (measured), $V_{max}$ is the maximum reaction rate that reflects the amount of enzyme, S is the concentration of substrate, and $K_m$ is a constant.

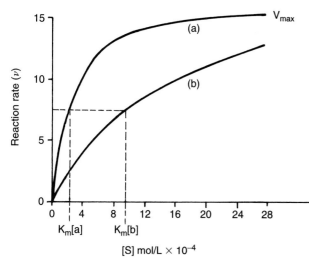

**FIGURE 15-5**

Michaelis-Menten plot of reaction rate (velocity) versus substrate concentration for two different substrates (a and b). The $K_m$ for substrate a is $2 \times 10^{-4}$ mol/L, and the $K_m$ for substrate b is $9.5 \times 10^{-4}$ mmol/L.

The Michaelis-Menten constant, $K_m$, represents the affinity of an enzyme for a particular substrate. In practical terms, it can be defined as the substrate concentration where $v = \frac{1}{2} V_{max}$ (Figure 15-5). Therefore, knowledge of $K_m$ allows prediction that the zero-order substrate concentration will be 50 times $K_m$. $K_m$ can also be used to compare the efficacy of two alternative substrates for an enzyme assay (Example 15-1). The substrate that is used most efficiently by the enzyme is the one with the lower $K_m$ since less of it is required to allow maximum reaction rate.

*Example 15-1*

In Figure 15-5, the reaction rate ($v$) appears to be approaching the value 15 ($V_{max}$) when a high concentration of either substrate a or substrate b is used. However, the concentration needed to achieve $\frac{1}{2} V_{max}$ differs markedly between the two substrates. For substrate a, $K_m = 2 \times 10^{-4}$ mol/L; therefore $100 \times 10^{-4}$ mol/L (i.e., $50 \times K_m$) will insure that $v$ equals $V_{max}$ in the assay. On the other hand, $K_m$ for substrate b = $9.5 \times 10^{-4}$ mol/L. Its higher $K_m$ reflects a lesser affinity with the enzyme and the requirement for much higher concentration to achieve $V_{max}$.

It is technically difficult to obtain sufficient data over a wide range of concentrations so that the substrate activity curve can be drawn accurately. The inverse of the Michael-Menten equation, called the **Lineweaver-Burk transformation,** provides a convenient tool to remedy this problem (Equation

15-3). The Lineweaver-Burk equation is the familiar equation of a straight line, y = ax + b, and a straight-line graph can be easily drawn from experimental data (Figure 15-6). From this graph, both $K_m$ and $V_{max}$ can be determined with accuracy since the x-intercept (a) = $-1/K_m$, and the y-intercept (b) = $1/V_{max}$. This method of graphing data is the most common way to determine $K_m$.

$$\frac{1}{v} = \frac{K_m + S}{V_{max} S} = \frac{K_m}{V_{max} S} + \frac{S}{V_{max} S} = \frac{K_m}{V_{max}} \times \frac{1}{S} + \frac{1}{V_{max}}$$

$$(15-3)$$

There is an additional use of the Lineweaver-Burk plot when studying the effect or mechanism of **inhibitors** (Figure 15-7, Table 15-1). An inhibitor that temporarily occupies the active site of an enzyme will compete with the substrate for binding and will interfere with the desired reaction. In the presence of this inhibitor, the affinity between enzyme and substrate will appear to be decreased ($\uparrow K_m$). However, by increasing the concentration of substrate, competition for the active site can be overcome and at high substrate concentrations, the expected $V_{max}$ can be achieved. This phenomenon is referred to as **competitive inhibition.** Competitive inhibitors are rarely a problem in the clinical laboratory because enzyme assays are routinely performed using a large excess of substrate.

Of greater concern are **noncompetitive** and **uncompetitive inhibitors** that may be present in a patient's sample or may form in an unstable reagent. A noncompetitive inhibitor effectively destroys the active site by causing the enzyme to change its shape or by irreversibly binding to the active site. Although the remaining active sites have the usual affinity for substrate ($K_m$ is unchanged), some of the enzyme is destroyed ($\downarrow V_{max}$) and an accurate result of enzyme activity in the sample cannot be obtained. An uncompetitive inhibitor combines with the enzyme-substrate complex and prevents formation of product. Thus, the reaction acts as if there was less enzyme-substrate complex ($\downarrow V_{max}$) and there is less apparent affinity for the substrate ($\uparrow K_m$).

When trouble-shooting a low result for an enzyme assay in the clinical laboratory, increasing the concentration of sub-

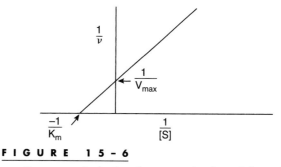

**FIGURE 15-6**

Lineweaver-Burk plot of reciprocal values: $1/v$ and $1/[S]$ derived from a Michaelis-Menten plot. This plot is used for the experimental evaluation of $K_m$ and $V_{max}$.

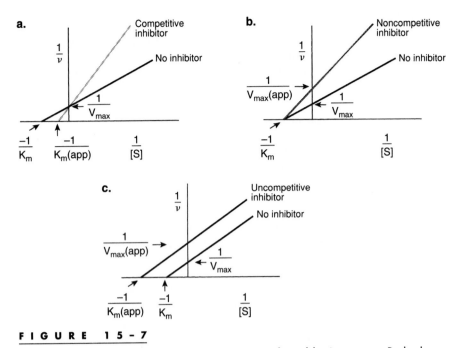

**FIGURE 15-7**

Effect of inhibitors on an enzyme reaction evaluated by Lineweaver-Burk plots:
**a.** competitive inhibitor increases $K_m$ but does not change $V_{max}$. **b.** Noncompetitive inhibitor decreases $V_{max}$ but does not change $K_m$. **c.** Uncompetitive inhibitor changes both $K_m$ and $V_{max}$.

strate will help differentiate between a competitive inhibitor and the other two kinds. If increased substrate concentration does not restore $V_{max}$, then a new sample or fresh reagent sometimes can avoid a noncompetitive or uncompetitive inhibitor.

## Calculating Enzyme Activity

The amount of enzyme in a patient's sample is measured by its effect on the rate of a reaction. Although there may be some denatured inactive enzyme in a sample, enzyme that is freshly released from damaged tissue is assumed to retain its activity and therefore to be an accurate measure of the presence and amount of tissue damage.

The amount of enzyme is reported in **International Units** per liter of patient's sample. An International Unit (U) is defined as the amount of enzyme that will catalyze the reaction of 1 $\mu$mol of substrate per minute in an assay with defined parameters such as pH, temperature, excess substrate, etc. The SI unit of enzyme activity is the **katal,** which is defined as the amount of enzyme that will catalyze the reaction of one mole of substrate per second. The two units are easily interconverted by using the number of micromoles per mole and the number of seconds per minute.

**Calibrators** that contain a known amount of enzyme are generally not available owing to instability and cost. Instead of using calibrators, the parameter that is measured in most enzyme assays is the rate of change in absorbance in a defined period (e.g., 1 minute). Then the molar absorptivity ($\varepsilon$) of the

measured product is used to convert change in absorbance to change in micromoles. Many current methods of enzyme analysis utilize the absorbance characteristics of the coenzyme $NAD^+$. $NAD^+$ has the optical property of absorbing light at 340 nm when in its reduced form, NADH. The oxidized form, $NAD^+$, however, has no absorbance peak at this wavelength (Figure 15–8). Thus, the progress of an enzymatic reaction can be followed by measuring either an increase or decrease in absorbance at 340 nm as NAD is reduced or NADH is oxidized. Since 340 nm is in the ultraviolet portion of the spectrum, these methods are often referred to as UV methods.

Many enzymes, especially the dehydrogenase enzymes whose activity involves $H^+$ transfer, require $NAD^+$ or $NADP^+$ as a coenzyme. Many enzymes that do not require $NAD^+$ can be linked or coupled to additional enzymatic reactions that do require these coenzymes and thus can also be measured by this technique.

One common example of an enzymatic reaction requiring $NAD^+$ as a coenzyme is:

$$lactate \xrightarrow{\text{LD}} pyruvate$$

$$NADH \quad NAD^+$$

The oxidation of lactate to pyruvate is catalyzed by the enzyme lactate dehydrogenase (LD). $NAD^+$ is reduced to NADH as it accepts the $H^+$ from lactate. An increase in absorbance at 340 nm can be observed. The amount of NADH produced is directly related to the extent of LD enzymatic ac-

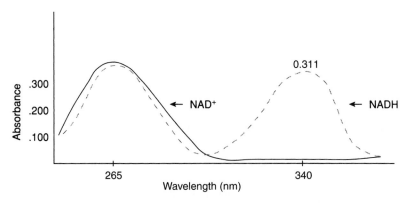

Absorption spectra of 50 $\mu$mol/L solutions of NAD$^+$ and NADH (1-cm cuvette).
Note: NADP$^+$ and NADPH give spectra identical to NAD$^+$ and NADH.

tivity. The higher the enzymatic activity, the greater will be the absorbance value. The enzymatic activity can be calculated from the absorbance characteristic of NAD$^+$ by use of the following formula:

$$\frac{\Delta A}{\varepsilon \times l} \times 10^6 \times \frac{1}{T} \times \frac{TV}{SV} = U/L$$

where $\Delta A$ = change in absorbance of sample over specified time period; $\varepsilon$ = molar absorptivity coefficient of NADH (moles/liter $\cdot$ cm$^{-1}$); $l$ = length of light path (cm); $T$ = time of reaction (minutes); $TV$ = total volume of reaction mixture; $SV$ = sample volume; $10^6$ = conversion factor to convert from moles to micromoles.

This calculation is based on the molar absorptivity coefficient ($\varepsilon$) of the reaction product, which is NADH in this example. Recall from Chapter 6 that $\varepsilon$ can be calculated from Beer's law $A = \varepsilon l c$. By rearranging the equation using the data listed in Figure 15–8, the molar absorptivity of NADH can be calculated as:

$$\varepsilon = \frac{0.311}{0.05 \times 10^{-3} \text{ moles/liter} \times 1 \text{ cm}}$$

$$\varepsilon = 6.22 \times 10^3 \text{ mol/L} \cdot \text{cm}^{-1}$$

The value of $6.22 \times 10^3$ moles/L $\cdot$ cm$^{-1}$ is the molar absorptivity coefficient of NADH obtained at a wavelength of 340 nm. This is a constant value for NADH and will always remain the same as long as the same reaction conditions are employed. Most notably a change in the wavelength and reaction temperature will affect the value.

The following values for a hypothetical reaction can be used to demonstrate the use of the formula to calculate enzymatic activity.

$$\Delta A/2 \text{ min} = 0.120, \qquad T = 2 \text{ minutes}$$

$$TV = 3.1 \text{ mL}, \qquad SV = 0.100 \text{ mL}$$

$$l = 1 \text{ cm}, \qquad \varepsilon = 6.22 \times 10^3$$

$$\frac{0.120}{6.22 \times 10^3 \times 1} \times 10^6 \times \frac{1}{2} \times \frac{3.1}{0.100} = 299 \text{ U/L}$$

By making use of the optical properties of NAD$^+$ and measuring a change in absorbance over a specified time period, the enzymatic activity can be determined. Example 15–2 illustrates the use of the molar absorptivity of $p$-nitrophenol to calculate enzyme activity.

## Coupled Reactions

Frequently, neither the substrate nor the product of an enzyme reaction has a distinctive absorption spectrum to use for measuring the rate of the reaction. Modern commercial kits for enzyme assays solve this problem by adding additional substrates and enzymes to link the measured reaction to other reactions that culminate in a colored product. As long as the patient's enzyme concentration is the only limiting factor in the sequence of reactions and all the auxiliary substrates and enzymes are present in excess, then the rate of production of the final colored product will reflect the amount of enzyme (Example 15–3).

## Enzymes as Reagents

While the topic of this chapter is measurement of enzymes, modern methods in clinical laboratories also utilize enzymes as reagents to **measure the concentration of a substrate.** The sensitivity and specificity of enzyme reactions make them ideal for rapid, precise measurement of substrate concentrations. Examples include using glucose oxidase to measure serum glucose concentration, using urease to measure serum urea concentration, and using lipase to measure serum triglyceride concentration.

*Example 15–2*

The molar absorptivity of an alkaline solution of *p*-nitrophenol at 405 nm is 18,450 (1 cm cuvette). When assaying a serum sample for alkaline phosphatase activity, 1.5 mL of a solution containing the substrate *p*-nitrophenylphosphate is incubated with 50 $\mu$L of serum, producing *p*-nitrophenol. The following absorbance readings for the assay were taken from continuous (kinetic) monitoring.

| Incubation Time (sec) | Abs$_{405}$ | $\Delta$Abs/15 sec |
|---|---|---|
| 15 | 0.025 | |
| | | 0.027 |
| 30 | 0.052 | |
| | | 0.043 |
| 45 | 0.095 | |
| | | 0.045 |
| 60 | 0.140 | |
| | | 0.045 |
| 75 | 0.185 | |
| | | 0.045 |
| 90 | 0.230 | |

First, calculate the change in absorbance per 15-sec incubation to ensure that the reaction rate is constant. In these data there is a lag during the initial 45 seconds of incubation, after which the absorbance changes at the constant rate of 0.045 per 15 seconds. This zero order reaction rate is equal to 0.180 $\Delta$Abs per minute. Using the zero-order reaction rate, calculate the amount of enzyme in international units per liter.

$$U/L = \frac{0.180\ \Delta A/min}{18,450\ \Delta A/mol/L} \times \frac{10^6\ \mu mol}{mol} \times \frac{1.55\ mL}{0.05\ mL} = 302$$

Whether using an enzyme to measure substrate concentration or using a substrate to measure enzyme concentration, all the same considerations for optimizing enzymatic activity pertain. Thus pH, ionic strength, temperature, activators, and inhibitors must all be controlled in the reaction; the only difference is that the rate of reaction is limited by the concentration of substrate (first order) while the concentration of enzyme is not limiting (zero order). This requirement for excess amount of enzyme is not difficult since it is not used up by the reaction. Therefore, minimal amount of enzyme is sufficient as long as the length of incubation allows all of the substrate to be used up and the reaction goes to completion (equilibrium).

Unlike reactions that measure the amount of enzyme, reactions that use enzymes to measure the amount of substrate can usually be calibrated by parallel analysis of known concentrations of substrate. Like enzyme assays, several reactions can be linked together to produce a colored product. In this

*Example 15–3*

Creatine kinase catalyzes the reversible phosphorylation of creatine by ATP. The reaction is measured by linked reactions that produce NADPH, which increases the absorbance at 340 nm:

$$\text{creatine-phosphate} + \text{ADP} \xleftrightarrow{\text{CK}} \text{creatine} + \text{ATP}$$

$$\text{ATP} + \text{glucose} \xrightarrow{\text{hexokinase}} \text{glucose-6-phosphate} + \text{ADP}$$

$$\text{glucose-6-phosphate} + \text{NADP}^+ \xrightarrow{\text{G-6-PD}}$$

$$\text{6-phosphogluconate} + \text{NADPH} + \text{H}^+$$

The reagent contains excess amounts (zero-order concentrations) of creatine phosphate, ADP, glucose, hexokinase, NADP$^+$, and G-6-PD. Therefore the rate of production of NADPH is only limited by the rate of the creatine kinase reaction. NADPH absorbs 340 nm light but NADP$^+$ does not (Figure 15–8). The number of international units of creatine kinase can be calculated from the rate of change in absorbance at 340 nm by using the molar absorptivity of NADPH.

case, the concentration of the final colored product reflects the concentration of the initial substrate.

Another application of enzymes as reagents involves their use as **labels for immunoassay reactions.** For example, an enzyme may be covalently attached to an antibody that is used as a reagent. Here, advantage is taken of the fact that enzymes are not used up in a reaction and thus a small amount of the enzyme-labeled antibody can be detected by letting the enzyme incubate with its substrate for a longer time. For example, in immunosorbent assays, the antibody is frequently labeled with horseradish peroxidase (HRP) or calf intestinal alkaline phosphatase. When there is only a small amount of patient's antigen in these "sandwich assays," there will be only a small amount of conjugated enzyme-antibody bound in the immunoassay. But even this small amount of enzyme can be quantitated by a longer, although timed, incubation with excess substrate. In this case, the amount of bound enzyme is proportional to the amount of patient's antigen.

A recent addition to the enzymatic measurements in clinical laboratories is the use of **restriction endonucleases.** These enzymes, derived from bacteria, hydrolyze specific sites on double-stranded DNA molecules. These specific restriction sites are palindromic sequences of nucleic acid bases, i.e., 4 to 10 A, T, G, C bases in a sequence that is symmetrical around a center point (Figure 15–9). Several inherited disorders and malignancies can be detected and identified by using specific restriction endonucleases to search for base sequences that are expected in the DNA of abnormal cells. The

| Enzyme | Recognition Sequence and Hydrolysis Site |
|--------|-------------------------------------------|
| BamH1 | 5'-GG↓ATCC-3'<br>3'-CCTAG↑G-5' |
| HaeIII | 5'-GG↓CC-3'<br>3'-CC↑GG-5' |
| NotI | 5'-GC↓GGCCGC-3'<br>3'-CGCCGG↑CG-5' |

**FIGURE 15-9**

The base sequences in double-stranded DNA that are recognized as substrate sites by three common restriction endonucleases and their sites of hydrolysis (↓). Restriction endonucleases are named sequentially for the bacterial species where they occur; e.g., HaeIII is the third endonuclease isolated from *Haemophilus influenzae*.

DNA fragments produced by the enzymes are then separated electrophoretically and the length of each fragment found is used diagnostically.

## CLINICALLY SIGNIFICANT ENZYMES

During the explosive growth of clinical laboratories in the 1950s and 1960s, the number of published assays for different enzymes became unmanageable. To meet this challenge, the Enzyme Commission of the International Union of Biochemists wrote a set of nomenclature rules.[2] This work established a nomenclature system that assigns a unique EC number and name for each enzyme (Table 15-1) and also consolidated different reporting methods by defining the International Unit of enzyme activity. The name of an enzyme, according to the Enzyme Commission rule, is composed of a first name that lists its substrate(s) and a last name that describes the type of reaction catalyzed. Since all enzyme reactions are theoretically reversible at equilibrium, the compound selected as substrate is based on the equilibrium constant. For example, in the reaction A ↔ B, if the equilibrium constant favored turning B into A then the enzyme would be named "B-ase." In the clinical laboratory, common abbreviations and nicknames for enzymes are often used but publications always specify official names and numbers. Thus, all readers of a publication know that an enzyme whose first number is "1" conducts an oxidation-reduction reaction or an enzyme whose last name is "kinase" uses ATP to phosphorylate a substrate.

## Aspartate Aminotransferase and Alanine Aminotransferase

The aminotransferases (also known as transaminases) are cytoplasmic enzymes that play an important metabolic role in exchanging the carbon-skeleton between amino acids and ketoacids. There is a wide variety of aminotransferase enzymes but only two of them, aspartate aminotransferase (AST, EC 2.6.1.1) and alanine aminotransferase (ALT, 2.6.1.2), are measured in clinical laboratories. These two enzymes are present in all tissues and their concentrations are especially high in hepatocytes, cardiac and skeletal muscle cells, and renal parenchymal cells. ALT is predominantly a liver-specific enzyme (Figure 15-10). Damage to one of these tissues can be detected by measuring the amount and type of aminotransferase in serum. Mitochondria have a distinct isoenzyme of AST, which may be found in serum when tissue damage is severe. Assays used in clinical laboratories do not distinguish the mitochondrial form from the cytoplasmic form.

Each aminotransferase enzyme catalyzes the reversible transfer of an amino group from a specific amino acid to α-oxoglutarate producing a new amino acid (glutamate) and the keto acid analogue of the original amino acid. Thus, aspartate aminotransferase produces oxalacetate from aspartate and alanine aminotransferase produces pyruvate from alanine. Pyridoxal-5-phosphate (P5P) is required as prosthetic group for both enzymes. It temporarily carries the amino group of the substrate until the α-oxoglutarate acceptor becomes available.[3]

Neither AST nor ALT has substrates or products with distinctive absorption spectra. Therefore, both assays use coupled reactions for spectrophotometric monitoring.[4] The rate of pyruvate production by ALT is linked to a reaction catalyzed by lactate dehydrogenase (Equation 15-4). This coupled reaction converts the cofactor NADH to NAD$^+$; therefore absorbance at 340 nm decreases as pyruvate is produced by ALT. The rate of oxalacetate production by AST is measured by linking to a reaction catalyzed by malate dehydrogenase (Equation 15-5). This coupled reaction converts NADH to NAD$^+$; therefore absorbance at 340 nm decreases as oxalacetate is produced by AST.

$$\text{L-alanine} + \alpha\text{-oxoglutarate} \xrightarrow{\text{ALT}} \text{L-glutamate} + \text{pyruvate}$$

$$\text{pyruvate} + \text{NADH} + \text{H}^+ \xrightarrow{\text{LD}} \text{lactate} + \text{NAD}^+ \quad (15\text{-}4)$$

$$\text{L-aspartate} + \alpha\text{-oxoglutarate} \xrightarrow{\text{AST}} \text{L-glutamate} + \text{oxalacetate}$$

$$\text{oxalacetate} + \text{NADH} + \text{H}^+ \xrightarrow{\text{MDH}} \text{malate} + \text{NAD}^+ \quad (15\text{-}5)$$

Some automated clinical instruments use an alternate set of coupled reactions to measure the oxalacetate product of AST[5] (Equation 15-6). The first reaction uses a decarboxylase to convert oxalacetate to pyruvate. In the next reaction, the pyruvate is oxidized with hydrogen peroxide as a product. In the third reaction, peroxidase uses the hydrogen peroxide to

TABLE 15-1

TABLE 15-1

**Enzyme Classification**

| CLASS | REACTION | NAME | ABBREVIATION | EC CODE |
|---|---|---|---|---|
| 1. Oxidoreductases | Catalyze oxidation-reduction reactions between two substrates | Lactate dehydrogenase | LD | 1.1.1.27 |
| | | 3-Hydroxybutyrate dehydrogenase | HBD | 1.1.1.30 |
| | | Glucose-6-phosphate dehydrogenase | G-6-PD | 1.1.1.49 |
| 2. Transferases | Catalyze the transfer of a group other than hydrogen between two subunits | Gamma glutamyltransferase | GGT | 2.3.22 |
| | | Aspartate aminotransferase (transaminase) | AST | 2.6.1.1 |
| | | Alanine aminotransferase (transaminase) | ALT | 2.6.1.2 |
| | | Creatine kinase | CK | 2.7.3.2 |
| 3. Hydrolases | Catalyze the hydrolytic cleavage of compounds | Triacylglycerol acylhydrolase (lipase) | LPS | 3.1.1.3 |
| | | Cholinesterase | CHS | 3.1.1.8 |
| | | Alkaline phosphatase | ALP | 3.1.3.1 |
| | | Acid phosphatase | ACP | 3.1.3.2 |
| | | 5'-Nucleotidase | 5'-NT | 3.1.3.5 |
| | | $\alpha$-Amylase | AMS | 3.2.1.1 |
| | | Leucine aminopeptidase | LAP | 3.4.11.1 |
| 4. Lyases | Catalyze the removal of groups from substrates without hydrolysis, leaving double bonds in the product | Fructose bisphosphate aldolase | ALS | 4.1.2.13 |
| 5. Isomerases | Catalyze the interconversion of isomers | Phosphohexose isomerase | PHI | 5.3.1.1 |
| 6. Ligases | Catalyze the joining of two molecules coupled with the hydrolysis of a pyrophosphate bond in ATP or similar component | Carbamoyl-phosphate synthase | | 6.3.5.16 |
| | | Acetyl-CoA carboxylase | | 6.4.1.2 |

catalyze the oxidation of a dye-precursor producing a colored product.

$$\text{oxalacetate} \xrightarrow{\text{oxalacetate decarboxylase}} \text{pyruvate} + CO_2$$

$$\text{pyruvate} + \text{phosphate} + O_2 \xrightarrow{\text{pyruvate oxidase}} \text{acetyl-phosphate} + H_2O_2$$

$$H_2O_2 + \text{colorless leuco-dye} \xrightarrow{\text{peroxidase}} H_2O + \text{colored dye}$$

$$(15-6)$$

The preferred sample for both AST and ALT assays is nonhemolyzed serum. Since erythrocytes contain 5 times (ALT) to 15 times (AST) as much enzyme as normal serum, even a small amount of hemolysis can cause a falsely elevated result. Serum samples are stable for several hours at room temperature and for at least 1 week at refrigerator temperature.

The reference range for serum level of AST in adults[6] is approximately 15 to 40 U/L. Values for healthy infants are up to twice as high. The reference range for serum level of ALT in both adults and infants is approximately 10 to 40 U/L.

## Alkaline Phosphatase

The enzyme activity in serum that is referred to as alkaline phosphatase (ALP, EC 3.1.3.1) is actually the aggregate of a group of enzymes. In contrast to the classic definition of isoenzymes, these enzymes are not produced from allelic genes. Instead, they are enzymes from various organs that all happen to hydrolyze organic phosphate esters, have an optimum pH near 10 (although they are partially active at pH 7.4), and require $Mg^{++}$ for optimal activity (Equation 15–7). The physiologic

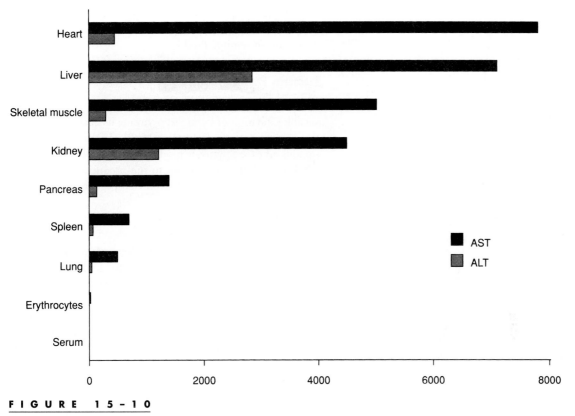

**FIGURE 15-10**

Tissue sources of AST and ALT.

substrates of alkaline phosphatase enzymes are not known. They are present in high concentrations in bone and biliary tract; the major clinical application for measuring ALP is to detect disease in these two tissues.

$$\text{organic-phosphate} \xrightarrow[\text{Mg}^{++}, \text{ pH } 10]{\text{ALP}} \text{organic-alcohol} + \text{HPO}_4^{=}$$

$$(15\text{--}7)$$

The study of ALP isoenzymes has been complicated by their nonallelic origin. Electrophoretic separation of the isoenzymes of ALP using cellulose acetate shows that most of them migrate in a broad band with $\alpha_2$-globulins. This area of migration appears to include both the bone and biliary forms found in normal serum. Neither cellulose acetate nor polyacrylamide gel electrophoresis separates the isoenzymes of alkaline phosphatase sufficiently for reliable diagnostic use. Inhibition assays and immunochemical assays for differentiating the tissue origin of an elevated level of serum ALP have not gained wide acceptance. The most commonly used method for differentiating ALP isoenzymes tests for heat stability. When a serum sample that has an elevated level of ALP is heated to 56°C for 10 minutes, activity from the bone isoenzyme is virtually destroyed (<20% activity remains), whereas activity from the biliary isoenzyme is moderately resistant (≥50% activity remains). Other isoenzymes that are not normally pre-

sent in significant amounts in serum include intestinal ALP, placental ALP, and tumor markers (Regan and Nagao ALP). These forms of the enzyme generally are quite resistant to heat inactivation (>90% activity remains).

Most commercially available assays for ALP measure the rate of production of colored *p*-nitrophenol by hydrolysis of its colorless phosphate ester at pH 10.4 and 37°C (Equation 15–8).[7] *p*-Nitrophenol has a fairly wide absorption peak around 380 to 410 nm (Figure 15–11) and a high molar absorptivity ($\varepsilon$), which make it suitable for rapid, sensitive assay.

$$\textit{p}\text{-nitrophenyl-phosphate} \xrightarrow[\text{Mg}^{++}]{\text{ALP}} \textit{p}\text{-nitrophenol} + \text{HPO}_4^{=}$$

$$(15\text{--}8)$$

Although ALP is classified as a hydrolase (EC class 3), it has much higher activity when the buffer used to control pH is a phosphate acceptor; therefore the buffer aminomethyl-propanol, which can accept the phosphate moiety, is commonly used. The combination of requirement for $\text{Mg}^{++}$ and enhanced activity in the presence of a phosphate acceptor suggest that the mechanism of action of ALP may resemble the mechanism of kinase enzymes.

Serum and heparinized plasma are acceptable samples for ALP assay. Calcium-binding anticoagulants are not acceptable;

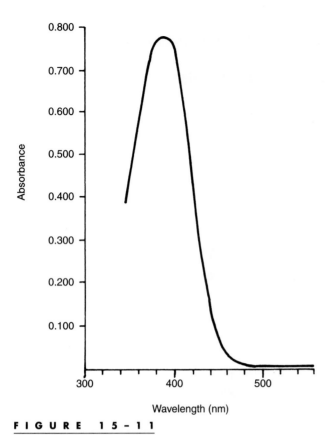

**FIGURE   15-11**

Absorption spectrum of *p*-nitrophenol in alkaline solution.

they result in plasma that has a lower ALP result presumably due to binding the $Mg^{++}$ activator. Hemolysis must be avoided since erythrocyte membranes contain ALP. Fasting serum is preferred because of reports that people with blood group B or O show a rise in intestinal ALP during food absorption.[6] A serum sample for ALP can be stored for a few days at refrigerator temperature. Freezing and lyophilizing should be avoided because they cause variation in ALP activity. Although clinical samples are not generally lyophilized, sera used for quality control frequently are. Those samples must "age" for at least 30 minutes after reconstitution so they will contain a predictable amount of ALP activity.

Serum from healthy adults contains approximately 40 to 125 U/L when using the method outlined above.[6] Infants and children (including adolescents) have significantly higher values that are related to rapid bone growth. During pregnancy, ALP value is increased owing to the contribution of the placental isoenzyme.

## Acid Phosphatase

Historically, clinical laboratories have measured a different set of phosphatase isoenzymes that have a pH optimum of approximately 5. These **acid phosphatases** were used as a marker of prostatic hypertrophy and prostatic carcinoma but have been superseded by the assay for prostate-specific antigen (PSA).

The remaining application of acid phosphatase assay is in the forensic investigation of alleged rape because of its high concentration in seminal fluid.

## Lactate Dehydrogenase

Lactate dehydrogenase (LD, EC 1.1.1.27) catalyzes the reversible oxidation of lactate to pyruvate; its cofactor $NAD^+$ is the oxidizing agent (Equation 15–9). LD activity in cells siphons off excess pyruvate produced by anaerobic glucose metabolism and also contributes to the production of NADH, which the cell uses in the electron transport chain.

$$\text{L-lactate}^- + NAD^+ \xrightarrow{\text{LD}} \text{pyruvate}^- + NADH + H^+ \qquad (15\text{–}9)$$

The enzyme is present in all cells, and is found in high concentration in muscle cells (both cardiac and skeletal), liver, kidney, erythrocytes and leukocytes, lungs, lymph nodes, spleen, and brain. Increased LD activity in serum is not specific for disease of any tissue, although it may support a diagnosis that is based on other findings, e.g., myocardial infarction, renal infarction, hepatitis, megaloblastic anemia, muscular dystrophy, or metastatic cancer.

LD requires the association of four peptides for activity. The two genes that code for the peptides, H and M, have different rates of activity in different tissues. Cardiac myocytes, renal parenchymal cells, and erythrocytes all contain relatively large amounts of LD composed of the tetramers HHHH and HHHM, whereas skeletal myocytes and hepatocytes contain relatively large amounts of the tetramers MMMM and MMMH (Figure 15–12). Most other visceral tissues synthesize both peptides and thus have mixtures of HHHM, HHMM, and HMMM.

The LD tetramers differ in their net charge and can be separated by electrophoresis. The convention for numbering electrophoretically separated isoenzymes is: isoenzyme number 1 travels farthest toward the anode, and the rest are numbered in order (2, 3, 4, . . . ) back toward the cathode. Thus HHHH is also known as LD-1, HHHM as LD-2, . . . MMMM as LD-5. The relative amounts of LD isoenzymes in normal serum are LD-2 > LD-1 > LD-3, with only minor amounts of LD-4 and LD-5. In the clinical laboratory, electrophoretic separation of LD isoenzymes has been supplanted by other diagnostic tests that are more organ-specific and more efficient.

Even though the equilibrium constant favors the pyruvate to lactate direction at neutral pH, clinical assays for lactate dehydrogenase use the forward reaction (Equation 15–9) at pH 8.3 to 8.9.[8] Using this reaction, the amount of enzyme is measured by the rate of increase in absorbance at 340 nm as NADH is produced. Note that the alkaline pH pulls the reaction forward by removing the $H^+$ product.

Nonhemolyzed serum or heparinized plasma is appropriate for LD analysis. Red blood cells should be removed promptly to prevent artifactual leakage of LD into the serum. Serum is stable for a few days at room temperature; refrigera-

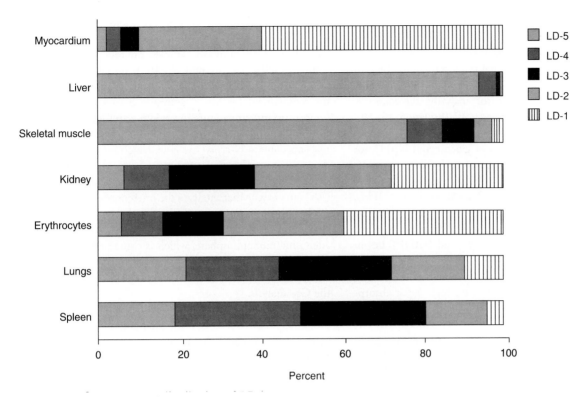

**FIGURE  15-12**

Distribution of lactate dehydrogenase (LD) isoenzymes in different tissues.

tion and (especially) freezing should be avoided because they cause instability of the M peptide and its isoenzymes. This instability will alter both total LD activity and the relative amount of the isoenzymes present if the sample is frozen.

Healthy adult serum has approximately 100 to 200 U/L LD when assayed by the reaction outlined above. Infants and children have values up to 4 times higher.[6]

## Creatine Kinase

In cells, creatine kinase (CK, EC 2.7.3.2) catalyzes the reversible phosphorylation of creatine using ATP as cofactor (Equation 15–10). As with most kinases, the active form of the cofactor is actually $Mg\text{-}ATP^{-4}$, which explains the requirement for $Mg^{++}$ as activator. CK appears to have sulfhydryl groups that are required for its active shape because samples that are not analyzed promptly lose their activity, but activity can be restored by the addition of N-acetyl-cysteine.

$$\text{creatine-phosphate} + \text{ADP} \xLeftrightarrow[\text{Mg}^{++}]{\text{CK}} \text{creatine} + \text{ATP}$$

$$\text{ATP} + \text{glucose} \xrightarrow[\text{Mg}^{++}]{\text{hexokinase}} \text{glucose-6-phosphate} + \text{ADP}$$

$$\text{glucose-6-phosphate} + \text{NAD}^+ \xrightarrow{\text{G-6-PD}} \text{NADH} + \text{H}^+$$
$$+ \text{6-phosphogluconate} \qquad (15\text{–}10)$$

CK is present in highest concentration in skeletal muscle but is also present in significant amount in cardiac muscle, brain, intestinal tract, kidney, uterus, and prostate. Notably, it is absent from liver, erythrocytes, placenta, and thyroid, a fact that is sometimes useful in differential diagnosis. In muscle cells, creatine phosphate acts as a temporary form of stored energy so that, when the cell is using energy rapidly, it can react with ADP to produce ATP for continued contractions. Resting muscle cells have up to 5 times as much creatine phosphate as ATP.

Two genes code for peptides that combine to form active CK dimer. The activity of the two genes differs in different tissues, resulting in three isoenzymes: MM, MB, and BB. The MM form is present in high concentration in both skeletal muscle cells and cardiac muscle cells, whereas the MB form is characteristic of cardiac muscle cells. The BB form is found in brain and intestinal cells and also has been found as a tumor marker. CK isoenzymes can be separated electrophoretically, resulting in alternate nomenclature: CK-1 (BB), CK-2 (MB), and CK-3 (MM) that describes their relative migration from anode toward cathode. Electrophoretic separation has also demonstrated CK enzymes with altered mobility including a mitochondrial isoenzyme (CK-mito) and two immunoglobulin-bound forms (CK-macro I and CK-macro II, which are bound to IgG or IgA, respectively). The mitochondrial isoenzyme appears to reflect severe tissue damage and predicts a poor prognosis. The immunoglobulin-bound form has no known relationship to disease but migrates close to CK-MB, and therefore may be a source of interference in interpretation of an electrophoretic pattern. CK-BB from brain is rarely seen in serum electrophoretic patterns of CK due to its inability to cross the blood–brain barrier. Its presence in serum is most often due to disease of the intestinal tract, prostate, kidney, or bladder or breast.

The most common method for analyzing the total CK activity of serum is the reverse reaction[9] (Equation 15–10). In addition to creatine-phosphate, ADP, and $Mg^{++}$, this coupled reaction adds excess amounts of glucose and $NAD^+$ (or $NADP^+$), as well as hexokinase and glucose-6-phosphate dehydrogenase (G-6-PD), in order to follow the rate of the CK reaction by the rate of production of NADH (or NADPH). The reaction is conducted at pH levels of 6.8 to 6.9. The coupled reaction sequence demonstrates a lag phase of up to 2 minutes. The choice between $NAD^+$ and $NADP^+$ lies in the biologic source of the G-6-PD used; the animal enzyme uses $NADP^+$ as cofactor, whereas bacterial G-6-PD uses $NAD^+$. Both NADH and NADPH have high molar absorptivity at 340 nm.

An alternate coupled reaction[10] uses ATP produced by CK to oxidize glycerol, producing glycerol phosphate (Equation 15–11). The glycerol phosphate is then oxidized by glycerol phosphate oxidase, producing hydrogen peroxide. The hydrogen peroxide is then used by peroxidase to oxidize a colorless leuco dye, producing a colored product.

$$ATP + glycerol \xrightarrow{glycerol\ kinase} glycerol\text{-}1\text{-}phosphate + ADP$$

$$glycerol\text{-}1\text{-}phosphate + O_2 \xrightarrow{GP\ oxidase} H_2O_2$$
$$+ \ dihydroxy\text{-}acetone\text{-}phosphate$$

$$H_2O_2 + leuco\text{-}dye \xrightarrow{peroxidase} H_2O + colored\ dye \quad (15\text{--}11)$$

The isoenzymes of CK separate clearly by electrophoresis on agarose at the pH 8.6. They can be detected by incubating the agarose with the same reaction mixture that is used for quantitative assay: the separated bands of CK isoenzymes produce fluorescent NADH (or NADPH) at the sites of their migration. A fluorometric densitometer can be used to scan the fluorescent bands and calculate their relative amounts. This method for measuring the isoenzymes of CK has fallen into disuse because it has a large standard deviation, is relatively insensitive, and takes much longer than alternate immunoassay methods and alternate tests (see discussion on troponin in the section on myocardial infarction).

Immunoassay methods for measuring CK isoenzymes focus completely on measuring the amount of MB isoenzyme (CK-2) in a serum sample. A popular immunosorbent assay uses an antibody with specificity for B peptide as the sorbent and an enzyme-labeled secondary antibody with specificity for M peptide.[11] Only MB isoenzyme will bind to both antibodies and be measured when the label is activated. An alternate immunoassay for the MB isoenzyme uses an anti-M

antibody to inhibit the MM isoenzyme and then measures residual CK activity.[12] Since even normal serum contains MB, and BB is only seen in rare samples, the residual activity is assumed to reflect the amount of MB in the sample.

Calcium-binding anticoagulants are prohibited because of the requirement for $Mg^{++}$ activator. Serum is stable several hours at room temperature, overnight at refrigerator temperature, and for at least 1 month at $-20°C$. Most commercial reagents contain N-acetyl-cysteine, which restores activity lost during storage. Grossly hemolyzed samples should be avoided because erythrocytes contain large amounts of adenylate kinase (AK), an enzyme that catalyzes the interconversion of ATP and ADP and thus interferes with the coupled reactions. This enzyme can be inhibited by the presence of large amounts of adenosine monophosphate, which is contained in most commercial reagents; however, gross hemolysis may contribute sufficient AK to overcome the inhibition and cause an error in the CK analysis.

The amount of CK in serum of healthy adults is approximately 40 to 170 U/L for men and 25 to 150 U/L for women.[6] The higher value in men reflects their greater muscle mass. Healthy infants may have values 2 to 3 times those of adults.

The amount of CK-MB that is measured in serum is extremely dependent on the method used, and methodology is currently in a state of flux. Local reference ranges should be determined using the reagent manufacturer's suggestions appropriately. Many clinical laboratories also report the ratio of CK-MB to total CK, called a CK-MB index. This ratio is intended to clarify diagnostic interpretation between increased absolute amount of CK-MB caused by damage to massive amount of skeletal muscle or increased absolute amount caused by damage to cardiac muscle. Here, too, the reference range is method-dependent and must be determined locally.

## Gamma-Glutamyl Transferase

Gamma-glutamyl transferase (GGT, EC 2.3.2.2) has an important role in cellular metabolism by reacting with the membrane transport molecule that brings amino acids into the cell.[3] It is present in high concentration in cells that line the biliary tract (including intrahepatic canaliculi) and is also found in kidney, pancreas, and intestine. Notably, it is not found in cardiac or skeletal muscle, and therefore can help distinguish liver damage from muscle damage, a feat not shared by AST, ALT, or LD.

In the body, GGT transfers the γ-glutamyl group of glutathione to almost any amino acid. This lack of specificity is advantageous in devising a clinical assay for the enzyme by synthesizing a derivative of glutamic acid with a dye bound to the γ carboxyl group. A γ-glutamyl-p-nitroanilide substrate donates its γ-glutamyl moiety to glycylglycine and releases colored p-nitroaniline[13] (Equation 15–12). Both substrates are soluble and colorless; thus, the rate of the GGT reaction is measured by the rate of production of *p*-nitroanilide, which causes an increase in absorbance at 410 nm.

$$\gamma\text{-glutamyl-}p\text{-nitroaniline} + \text{glycylglycine} \xrightarrow{\text{GGT}}$$

$$p\text{-nitroaniline} + \gamma\text{-glutamyl-glycylglycine} \quad (15\text{--}12)$$

The preferred sample is serum, which can be stored up to a month in the refrigerator. Hemolysis does not interfere with the reaction because erythrocytes do not contain GGT.

The serum of healthy adults contains up to approximately 40 U/L GGT.[6] Infants often have values several-fold higher.

## Amylase

Amylase (AMS, EC 3.2.1.1) is secreted into pancreatic juice and hydrolyzes complex dietary carbohydrates in the intestinal lumen. It is also present in high concentration in saliva, and is secreted in minor amounts by several other tissues (fallopian tubes, lactating breast, cervical mucosa, and endometrium). However, its clinical use is almost exclusively for the diagnosis of pancreatitis.

In the intestinal lumen, dietary starch and glycogen, which are branched polymers of glucose molecules, are attacked by amylase, which hydrolyzes alternating $\alpha$-1,4-glycosidic bonds. Amylase is an endohydrolase, which means that it attacks its substrate anywhere in the molecule, i.e., not only at the end of a branch as an exohydrolase would. Thus, the action of amylase rapidly breaks the large, complex, insoluble substrate molecules into small, soluble pieces. The ultimate products are maltose (two glucose moieties connected by an $\alpha$-1,4-glycosidic bond) and limit dextrins (several glucose moieties that surround an $\alpha$-1,6-glycosidic bond). Note that amylase is unable to hydrolyze $\beta$-glycosidic bonds, which accounts for the inability to digest cellulose as well as the custom of calling the enzyme $\alpha$-amylase.

Amylase requires both $Ca^{++}$ and $Cl^-$ for activity, a consideration that becomes important when using a single method to analyze serum, urine, and dilutions of both fluids. Care must be taken to ensure that the reagent or diluent provides sufficient activating ions. The pH optimum is 6.9. Although it is a protein, amylase is small enough that it is efficiently filtered by kidneys and is cleared from plasma rapidly. Thus, normal urine contains a measurable amount of amylase.

Starch is a difficult reagent because it has variable composition (molecular weight, number and length of branches) and is not water soluble. Thus, reagent manufacturers have devised artificial substrates for the measurement of amylase. Coupling a colored dye to the alcohol groups of a starch molecule can be used to measure amylase activity by the rate of production of soluble dye. The unit of activity that is measured is micromoles of dye formed per minute, which assumes that each $\alpha$-1,4-glycosidic bond that is hydrolyzed produces a soluble product.

One of the most popular methods for measuring amylase[14] measures the hydrolysis of maltotetraose, an oligosaccharide of four glucose moieties coupled by $\alpha$-1,4-glycosidic bonds (Equation 15–13). The maltose molecules produced by amylase action are linked to a series of reactions that culminate in the production of NADH and increased absorbance at 340 nm.

$$\text{maltotetraose} + H_2O \xrightarrow[Ca^{++},\,Cl^-]{\text{amylase}} 2\text{ maltose}$$

$$\text{maltose} + \text{phosphate} \xrightarrow{\text{maltose phosphorylase}} \text{glucose}$$
$$+ \text{glucose-1-phosphate}$$

$$\text{glucose-1-phosphate} \xrightarrow{\text{phosphoglucomutase}} \text{glucose-6-phosphate}$$

$$\text{glucose-6-phosphate} + NAD^+ \xrightarrow{\text{G-6-PD}} NADH + H^+$$
$$+ \text{6-phosphogluconate} \quad (15\text{--}13)$$

A popular alternate method uses maltotrioside, an artificial oligomer of glucose to which chloro-nitrophenol (CNP) has been conjugated[15] (Equation 15–14). The rate of production of CNP products is measured.

$$\text{CNP-maltotrioside} \xrightarrow[Ca^{++},\,Cl^-]{\text{amylase}} \text{CNP} + \text{CNP-maltose}$$
$$+ \text{glucose} + \text{maltotriose} \quad (15\text{--}14)$$

Amylase methods must be applicable to either serum or urine samples since both are used for the diagnosis of acute pancreatitis. Serum or heparinized plasma is stable for several days at room temperature and for extended period when refrigerated or frozen. A urine sample for amylase assay can be a random sample for emergency cases or a timed sample (1 h or 24-h) if serial samples are to be compared. If urine is stored before analysis, it should be adjusted to neutral pH for stability and then care be taken to prevent degradation from bacterial growth. If amylase clearance is to be measured, the urine sample must be a timed collection and the serum sample must be obtained during the urine collection. Clearance is calculated using the usual formula UV/P, where U is the urine AMS concentration, V is the urine volume, and P is the plasma AMS concentration.

Owing to the extreme variability of methods in use in clinical laboratories, local reference ranges should be determined using the reagent manufacturer's suggestions appropriately. Typical ranges using the maltotetraose method are approximately 35 to 125 U/L for serum and up to 17 U/h for urine. The ratio of amylase clearance to creatinine clearance is sometimes used as an aid to interpreting amylase results in a patient with renal disease. Reference range for the ratio is approximately 1% to 4%.

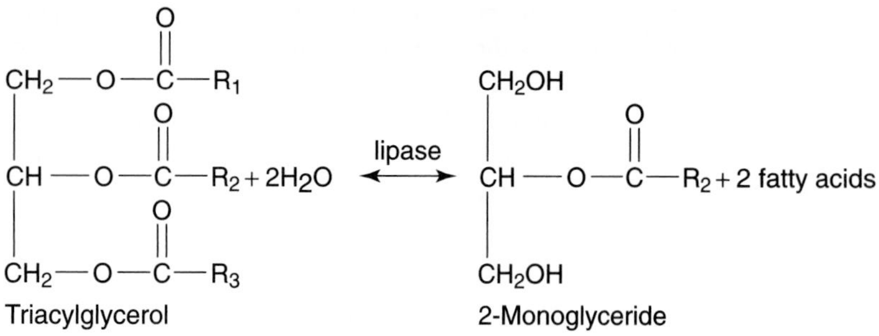

**FIGURE 15-13**

Hydrolysis of triglyceride (triacylglycerol) substrate by pancreatic lipase.

## Lipase

Lipase (LIP, EC 3.1.1.3), like amylase, is used in the diagnosis of acute pancreatitis, although it is present in small quantities in several other tissues including stomach, leukocytes, and adipose tissue. In the body, lipase is secreted into pancreatic juice where it acts on dietary triglycerides (triacylglycerols) in the intestinal lumen. Lipase hydrolyzes the two terminal fatty acids from a triglyceride molecule, producing free fatty acids and monoglyceride that can be absorbed by the intestinal mucosa (Figure 15–13).

Lipase is a water-soluble enzyme and its substrate is not water soluble. Therefore, cofactors that act like detergents are required to bring the enzyme and substrate together for reaction; bile salts (e.g., cholic acid, deoxycholic acid) perform this function in the intestine. Along with lipase, pancreatic acinar cells also secrete colipase, its protein cofactor.

The insolubility of triglycerides and the variability of the fatty acids they contain have led to the development of artificial substrates for the analysis of lipase. The products of the lipase-catalyzed reaction are then linked to a series of coupled reactions to produce a product that absorbs light. Several methods are available; two popular examples will suffice.

A colored dye, methylresorufin, is conjugated to the artificial substrate 1,2-O-dilauryl-RAC-glycero-3-glutaric acid.[16] The action of lipase separates glutaric acid–dye conjugate from the diglyceride moiety and then alkaline pH hydrolyzes the conjugate producing free dye. The rate of production of colored dye is used to monitor the lipase reaction. An alternate popular method[17] hydrolyzes 1,2-diglyceride and uses a series of coupled reactions to produce a colored product (Equation 15–15). Here, too, the rate of production of colored dye is used to monitor the lipase reaction. Turbidimetric assays have fallen into disuse because of the difficulty in preparing a reproducible, homogeneous substrate and because they cannot be reported in International Units of enzyme activity.

$$1,2\text{-diglycerol} \xrightarrow[\text{cholic \& deoxycholic acids}]{\text{lipase}} \text{fatty acid} + 2\text{-monoglycerol}$$

$$2\text{-monoglycerol} \xrightarrow{\text{monoglycerol lipase}} \text{fatty acid} + \text{glycerol}$$

$$\text{glycerol} + \text{ATP} \xrightarrow{\text{glycerol kinase}} \text{glycerol-3-phosphate} + \text{ADP}$$

$$\text{glycerol-3-phosphate} + O_2 \xrightarrow{\text{glycerol phosphate oxidase}} H_2O_2 + \text{dihydroxy-acetone-phosphate}$$

$$H_2O_2 + 4\text{-amino-antipyrine} + \text{dye precursor} \xrightarrow{\text{peroxidase}} H_2O + \text{quinonimine dye} \quad (15\text{-}15)$$

Serum is the preferred sample. It is stable for several days at room temperature. Although lipase that reaches the plasma is rapidly filtered by the kidneys, it is almost completely restored to the plasma by tubular reabsorption. Therefore, urine samples are not used for diagnostic assays.

Like amylase, there is considerable variability in reported reference ranges due to the variety of methods in use. Typical ranges for serum are approximately 10 to 200 U/L using the methylresorufin method and 7 to 60 U/L using the 1,2 diglyceride method.

## Plasma Cholinesterase

In contrast to virtually all other enzymes measured in the clinical laboratory, cholinesterase is measured to indicate poisoning instead of tissue damage. The enzyme found in plasma arises from liver, heart, and white matter of the brain. It has no known function. Its clinical importance is that it acts as a surrogate for acetyl-cholinesterase (AChE), which is active at neural synapses. Both plasma cholinesterase (PChE, EC 3.1.1.8) and AChE hydrolyze esters of choline; thus persons exposed to organophosphate insecticides, as well as patients anesthetized with succinyl-choline, rely on their cholinesterase enzymes to destroy the poisons or drug and restore synaptic function. The poisons and drug act as competitive inhibitors of the natural substrate, and therefore their effects should wear off as they are gradually hydrolyzed by the enzymes.

Patients with normal alleles of PChE are able to hydrolyze the poisons or drugs within a few minutes to hours and only require supportive therapy for that period. However, some patients have alleles that act extremely slowly. These alleles can be detected using the inhibitors dibucaine or fluoride. While the usual ($E^u$) allele is inhibited by either of these reagents, the allele $E^a$ resists inhibition by dibucaine, $E^f$ resists inhibition by fluoride and $E^s$ is an inactive enzyme. Other allelic isoenzymes have been reported.

The substrate used to assay plasma cholinesterase is butyryl-thiocholine, which is hydrolyzed to butyric acid and thiocholine (Equation 15–16). The thiocholine is measured by producing a colored derivative with dithiobis-nitrobenzoate.[18]

$$\text{S-butyryl-thiocholine} \xrightarrow{\text{cholinesterase}} \text{butyric acid + thiocholine}$$

$$\text{thiocholine + 5,5-dithiobis-2-nitrobenzoate} \longrightarrow$$
$$\text{mercapto-nitrobenzoate + mercaptothiocholine-nitrobenzoate}$$
$$(15–16)$$

Serum is the preferred sample. Hemolysis is not acceptable because erythrocytes contain acetylcholinesterase which acts on the same substrates as PChE. Serum is stable for several hours at room temperature and up to 1 week in the refrigerator.

Using the nitrobenzoate-coupled reaction, serum from healthy adults has approximately 5 to 12 U/L.[6] Specific inhibition ranges for distinguishing mutant alleles should be obtained from primary references.[19]

## Glucose-6-Phosphate Dehydrogenase

Measurement of glucose-6-phosphate dehydrogenase (G-6-PD, EC 1.1.1.49) by clinical laboratories differs from the normal routine in two ways: (1) the enzyme activity is being measured in order to detect abnormal alleles to aid the investigation of hemolytic anemia instead of detecting tissue damage, and (2) the sample used is erythrocytes rather than serum or plasma.

The physiologic function of G-6-PD is production of NADPH in the pentose-phosphate pathway of glucose metabolism (Equation 15–17). The body uses the NADPH for several purposes including maintaining the reducing nature of erythrocyte cytoplasm so that metabolically produced peroxides do not oxidize hemoglobin (and other proteins). The most common dietary source of metabolically produced oxidative stress is fava beans, a common staple is some parts of the world. Numerous drugs, including common antimalarials, also cause oxidative stress in erythrocytes. In the presence of an inactive or weakly active form of G-6-PD, an oxidative challenge (drug or diet) can oxidize hemoglobin forming precipitated Heinz bodies that induce splenic removal of the damaged cells.

$$\text{glucose-6-phosphate + NADP}^+ \xrightarrow{\text{G-6-PD}}$$
$$\text{NADPH + H}^+ + \text{6-phosphogluconate} \qquad (15–17)$$

Immature erythrocytes have the most G-6-PD activity and the activity normally declines to a normal average value as the cells age in the circulation. Thus, any condition that alters the average life span of circulating erythrocytes will in-

fluence the result of a G-6-PD assay. The assay is intended to detect the presence of one of the numerous mutants of G-6-PD that have decreased or absent enzymatic activity. Generally, the mutant enzymes can be classified into those that are synthesized with normal activity but with a short half-life, and those that are synthesized as an inactive protein. In the United States, the most common example of the first type is called $A^-$, which denotes its fast electrophoretic mobility (A) and its low activity in circulating erythrocytes (minus). This mutation is common in Americans of African ancestry. When an oxidative stress occurs, there is a transient hemolytic anemia that is usually self-limiting because the hemolytic crisis causes reticulocytosis and the young erythrocytes (reticulocytes) contain a normal amount of enzyme activity.

The most common examples of the second type are $B^-$, which is prevalent in Americans of Mediterranean ancestry and a form prevalent in Americans of Southeast Asian ancestry. When people with these mutations are exposed to an oxidant, their hemolytic anemia can reach severe proportions because both their circulating erythrocytes and their reticulocytes are deficient in G-6-PD activity and thus are subject to oxidative damage and removal from the circulation.

The gene for G-6-PD is located on the X chromosome. Thus, men who inherit a mutant form are G-6-PD deficient because they have only one X chromosome per cell, whereas women who inherit a mutant form are most often silent carriers. Only rarely does a woman inherit two mutant alleles and thus become homozygous for G-6-PD deficiency. Interestingly, normal men and normal women have the same amount of G-6-PD activity in each cell due to the inactivation of all but one X chromosome in female cells. This is also the reason why a woman who is heterozygous for a mutant allele most often has approximately 50% of normal activity when a sample of her erythrocytes is measured.

Both the qualitative spot-test for G-6-PD and the quantitative assay use the same reaction (Equation 15–17), which produces NADPH. For both assays, erythrocytes collected with any convenient anticoagulant are washed with saline to remove plasma proteins. The erythrocytes are then lysed and the hemolysate is centrifuged to remove ghosts (erythrocyte membranes) and produce a sparkling clear red solution. G-6-PD in erythrocytes is stable for a few days at room temperature and can be reliably measured in blood stored for over a month in the blood bank. Hemolysate is stable for several months at $-20°C$.

For the qualitative assay,[20] an aliquot of hemolysate is incubated with the mixture of substrate and cofactor and at timed intervals a drop of the reaction mixture is transferred to a filter paper and dried rapidly. The dried aliquots are examined under long wavelength UV light (Wood's lamp) in a dark room. Normal G-6-PD produces enough NADH for visible fluorescence within a few minutes of incubation, but mutants with deficient activity take much longer. Heterozygotes for G-6-PD mutations and artifactually elevated levels due to reticulocytosis cannot be distinguished by this assay.

The quantitative assay for G-6-PD activity[21] is identical except that the rate of formation of NADH is continuously monitored in a fluorometer or by increasing absorbance at 340 nm in a spectrophotometer. By measuring both the activity (U/L) and the number of erythrocytes in the aliquot, the activity per cell can be calculated and compared to the reference range. Using the quantitative assay, artifactual levels due to reticulocytosis cannot be distinguished. Values for heterozygotes can usually be distinguished from homozygous normals, but this only contributes to diagnosis indirectly since heterozygotes are not subject to oxidative hemolytic anemia.

Normal alleles in erythrocytes of normal average age have approximately 300 to 400 U per $10^{12}$ erythrocytes.[6] Infants have higher values due to the young age of their circulating erythrocytes as they replace their hemoglobin F-laden cells with cells containing hemoglobin A.

## CLINICAL APPLICATIONS

### Myocardial Infarction

Damage to cardiac myocytes allows leakage of a variety of intracellular constituents into the plasma. Since early detection of myocardial infarction correlates with improved prognosis, several laboratory tests are applied to this diagnostic problem.

Cardiac muscle cells have high concentrations of CK-MM, CK-MB, LD-1, AST, and ALT. Historically, all of these have been used to detect and monitor myocardial infarction but current practice only measures CK-MB and total CK from this list. Creatine kinase isoenzymes leak from ischemic cardiac cells and the serum levels usually rise above the reference range within 8 hours (Figure 15–14). The levels of both the MM and MB isoenzymes usually peak 12 to 24 hours later at a level 5 to 20 times the upper limit of normal, which is commensurate with the amount of damaged tissue. Their levels return to reference ranges in 2 to 4 days.

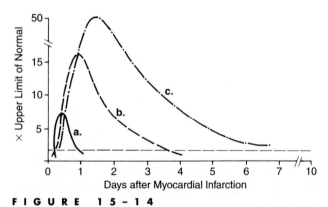

**FIGURE 15-14**

Typical serum levels following an acute myocardial infarction. **a.** Myoglobin. **b.** Total CK and CK-MB. **c.** Troponin I and troponin T.

Since cardiac myocytes are virtually the only cells with a large proportion of MB isoenzyme, measurement of either the absolute amount of CK-MB or calculating the MB index is usually a reliable indicator of myocardial infarction. The MB index compares the absolute amount of CK-MB to the total CK activity in serum (% CK-MB = CK-MB activity/total CK × 100%). This comparison allows distinction between increased total CK activity due to myocardial damage and that due to skeletal muscle or neural damage. The reference range for the CK-MB index is <1.5%. Modern methods are based on CK-2 mass measurement rather than enzyme activity. The availability of monoclonal anti-CK-2 antibody has facilitated automated and rapid test results. The ratio of CK-2 mass to total CK activity can also be calculated as the percent relative index (%RI = CK-2 mass/total CK activity × 100%). Increases in either % CK-2 or % RI are an indication that the heart is the source of the elevated CK activity. Since the amount of both total CK and CK-MB return to reference ranges rapidly, they are also useful in detecting onset of a second myocardial infarction where new peaks in serum levels will occur. Other causes of myocardial damage such as heart surgery, myocarditis or late stages of muscular dystrophy also cause increases in serum levels of CK-MB (Table 15–2). In the latter two cases, the time course of rising and falling levels that is seen in myocardial infarction is absent because the tissue damage is ongoing.

Recently, the serum levels of two nonenzymatic proteins have become the recommended laboratory tests for diagnosis of myocardial infarction. The cardiac isoforms of **troponin I** (cTnI) and **troponin T** (cTnT) show greater sensitivity and specificity than CK isoenzymes for detecting myocardial infarct. Both types of troponin are involved in transmitting the calcium signal to the actin-myosin complex to initiate muscle contraction. Troponin isoforms are measured by immunoassays using monoclonal antibodies that are specific for the cardiac types. Their serum levels rise above the reference range within 8 hours after myocardial infarction (like CK) and rise to levels 20 to 50 times the upper limit of normal (Figure 15–14). Like CK-MB, the serum level of troponin reflects the amount of damaged cardiac tissue. Five to 10 days pass before the level of troponin returns to the reference range. There does not seem to be any clinical advantage between measuring cTnI or cTnT.

The improved sensitivity of troponin measurements when compared to CK lies in the higher serum levels achieved and the duration of elevated levels. The improved specificity is due to the fact that cardiac forms of troponins differ from their skeletal muscle counterparts so that antibodies can distinguish between the two tissue sources. On the other hand, since a small proportion (approximately 2%) of skeletal muscle creatine kinase is the CK-MB isoenzyme, damage to a large quantity of skeletal muscle can cause significant elevation in the absolute amount of CK-MB in serum. While the calculated CK-MB index is designed to eliminate this confusion, interpretation of its value can be complicated when both skeletal

TABLE 15-2

**Changes in Serum Creatine Kinase (CK) and CK Isoenzymes in Certain Disease States and Traumas**

| CONDITION | TOTAL CK | CK ISOENZYMES |
|---|---|---|
| **INCREASED ACTIVITY** | | |
| Myocardial infarction | CK first appears 6–15 hours after the MI; peaks in 24 hours; returns to normal in 1–4 days. Activity is 7–12 × normal | Mostly due to rises in CK-MM with a simultaneous rise in CK-MB. CK-MB rises 3–15 hours after MI; peaks at 12 hours; returns to normal within 2–3 days |
| Myocarditis | May be markedly increased | Associated with a relative increase in CK-MB |
| Therapeutic electric countershock | Up to 6 × normal in roughly 50% of all patients | CK-MB is normal |
| Cardiac catheterization and coronary arteriography | Moderate increases can be seen | CK-MB is usually unchanged |
| Exercise stress testing in patients with suspected coronary artery disease | Negligible | CK-MB is unchanged |
| Muscular dystrophy (Duchenne and Becker) | Symptomatic Duchenne patients have values 50+ × the upper limit; female Duchenne carriers have values 3–6 × the upper limit | Due to CK-MM and CK-MB |
| Neurologic muscle disorders | CK is normal | No increase in isoenzymes |
| Malignant hypothermia | Marked increase | Due to CK-MM |
| Muscle trauma (crushing injury; physical exertion; seizures, surgery; injections; viral infections, alcohol, and toxin induced) | Rise is dependent on extent of injury May rise to >200 × normal in severe cases | Due to CK-MM |
| Reye's syndrome | Up to 70 × normal | Due to CK-MM |
| Cerebrovascular accident or disease | Rise correlates with extent of injury | CK-BB increases |
| Cerebral ischemia | Rise correlates with extent of injury | CK-BB increases |
| Hypothyroidism | Up to 50 × normal | CK-MM is the major isoenzyme involved |
| **DECREASED ACTIVITY** | | |
| Decreased muscle mass | Variable | Due to CK-MM |
| Bedridden individuals | Variable | Due to CK-MM |
| Metastasis | Variable (some individuals) | Due to CK-MM |
| Steroid therapy | Variable (some individuals) | Due to CK-MM |
| Hyperthyroidism | Low to borderline normal | Due to CK-MM primarily |

MI = myocardial infarction.

muscle and cardiac muscle are damaged. Measuring serum troponin levels aids in distinguishing between the various causes of elevated CK-MB levels. Many laboratories currently measure both troponin and CK-MB levels on serum from patients with myocardial infarctions.

Unfortunately, several hours elapse between onset of a myocardial infarction and the initial rise in serum levels of either the CK isoenzymes or troponins. Also, both proteins are reported to have transient elevations in some cases of angina. Recently, measurement of serum **myoglobin** has been recommended as a screening test for earlier detection of myocardial infarction. Myoglobin is the major heme-containing protein found in all muscle cells where it functions as an oxygen carrier. Owing to its ubiquitous occurrence, elevated serum levels of myoglobin do not distinguish between skeletal muscle and cardiac muscle damage. However, its serum level rises within approximately 2 hours of a myocardial infarction. Therefore, a negative result for serum myoglobin in the first few hours after the onset of chest pain is useful to rule out myocardial infarction and leads to the search for another cause of the pain. On the other hand, a positive result only indicates muscle cell damage and does not specify cardiac muscle.

Elevated levels of **C-reactive protein** (CRP) and the amino acid **homocysteine** are touted as indicators of the arterial inflammation that is associated with plaques that precede myocardial infarctions. Although CRP has long been known as an acute phase protein, recent evidence shows a correlation between levels near the upper limit of normal and propensity for myocardial infarction or stroke.[22] Homocysteine is an intermediate in the metabolic pathway between methionine and cysteine. In elevated concentrations, it causes damage to arterial walls, which presages the formation of cholesterol-laden plaques.[23] Vitamins, especially pyridoxal and folic acid, decrease the serum level of homocysteine, which may account for their positive effect on reducing the incidence of heart disease and myocardial infarction. Neither CRP nor homocysteine is recommended for diagnosis or prognosis of an acute myocardial infarction.

## Muscle Disease

Damage or disease of muscle, other than cardiac muscle, is associated with increased levels of AST, LD isoenzyme 5, and CK-MM. Depending on the amount of muscle tissue involved, the enzyme values can reach extraordinary levels in serum. Examples of this situation include extreme physical exertion, trauma due to accident or surgery, **polymyositis** and **dermatomyositis** (connective tissue diseases), and **muscular dystrophy.** CK-MM is present in such high concentrations in patients with X-linked Duchenne's muscular dystrophy that it has been suggested as a method to screen for female carriers. Although the level in the serum of known carriers is statistically indicative of their status, it is not a reliable predictor of carrier status. Conversely, these enzymes show normal or only slightly elevated activity when there is a muscle disorder of neurologic origin. Examples of neurogenic muscle disorders include myasthenia gravis, multiple sclerosis, and poliomyelitis.

## Liver Disease

Liver diseases can be divided into two classes: diseases that affect hepatocytes, and diseases that affect the biliary tree including the bile duct. Each of these two classes is associated with a particular pattern of serum enzyme elevations. Note, however, that inflammation of hepatocytes usually causes swelling that can irritate and occlude bile canaliculi, and inflammation of the biliary tree usually causes stagnation of bile solutes in the liver that can irritate the hepatocytes. Therefore, the enzyme patterns in the two classes of liver disease differ in degree rather than absolute amounts of serum enzymes.

In general, serum enzyme levels are more sensitive to hepatic disease than tests that reflect liver function such as albumin, bilirubin, or coagulation factor measurements. By combining the elevations of various liver-associated enzymes into a pattern, the nature and degree of liver disease can often be discerned. The pattern that is usually assessed is AST and ALT for hepatocyte disease and ALP and GGT for biliary disease.

Hepatocytes are rich in both AST and ALT (Figure 15–10) and inflammation of the liver leads to elevations in the serum level of both enzymes with the level of AST usually exceeding that of ALT (AST > ALT). This is the pattern seen in hepatic hypoxia (such as is caused by **congestive heart failure**), **toxic hepatitis** (such as chemical poisoning, or **Reye's Syndrome**), **infectious mononucleosis,** and active **cirrhosis** (such as is caused by alcohol abuse) (Table 15–3). In these diseases, the serum level of AST rises to 5 to 20 times normal and the ALT level is not elevated as high. While transaminase levels are not necessarily an indicator of the number of damaged liver cells, the levels return to normal as the disease resolves.

Note that AST content exceeds ALT content in all tissues that are rich in the transaminases (Figure 15–10) but only in liver and kidney cells does the ALT content exceed 25% of the AST content. Therefore, the presence of elevated serum levels of ALT is much more specific for hepatocyte damage than AST levels and a rise in the serum level of ALT sometimes precedes discernible rise in AST. Furthermore, in patients with **acute viral hepatitis,** the serum level of ALT characteristically exceeds that of AST (AST < ALT) with ALT levels sometimes reaching 100 times normal. The magnitude of elevation in serum level and the inverted ratio of transaminase levels is a useful diagnostic tool for diagnosing acute viral hepatitis, although it does not distinguish between the different viral causes of hepatitis.

Liver disease also causes increased levels of other enzymes in plasma. Lactate dehydrogenase and isoenzymes four (MMMH) and five (MMMM) can become significantly elevated in plasma, whereas the levels of biliary enzymes ALP and GGT show only slight to moderately increased levels. After detecting hepatocyte damage by the pattern of enzyme levels, the degree of impaired liver function can then be assessed by measuring bilirubin, albumin, coagulation factors, and performing serum protein electrophoresis.

The cells of the vessels in the biliary tree are rich in ALP and GGT. Inflammation, stagnation, or occlusion of these vessels has been lumped into a class called cholestasis or obstructive jaundice (because of the accumulation of bilirubin in plasma and tissues). Inflammation of the bile canaliculi or bile ducts causes both release of ALP into plasma and enhanced synthesis of ALP in the inflamed cells. Values 3 to 10 times

TABLE　15–3
## Clinical Causes of Decreased or Increased Serum AST and ALT Activity

| CONDITION | AST | ALT |
|---|---|---|
| **DECREASED ACTIVITY** | | |
| Uremia | Suppression of activity in some patients | Not applicable |
| Vitamin B$_6$ deficiency | Low normal to below normal; corrected by some methods | Low normal to below normal; corrected by some methods |
| **INCREASED ACTIVITY** | | |
| Myocardial infarction | 4–5 × normal; >10–15 × normal is associated with fatal infarcts | Normal to slight increase in uncomplicated infarcts |
| Congestive heart failure | 4–5 × normal | Normal to slight increase |
| Pericarditis | 4–5 × normal | Normal to slight increase |
| Myocarditis | 4–5 × normal | Normal to slight increase |
| Heart failure with liver congestion | >10 × normal | 5–10 × normal |
| Viral hepatitis | 10–100 × normal | 10–100 × normal |
| Toxic hepatitis | Up to 20 × normal | Up to 20 × normal |
| Reye's syndrome | 3–5 × normal | 3–5 × normal |
| Infectious mononucleosis | Up to 20 × normal | Up to 20 × normal |
| Obstructive jaundice, cholangitis | Up to 5 × normal | Up to 5 × normal |
| Cirrhosis | Variable increases, usually up to 2 × normal | Variable increases, usually up to 2 × normal |
| Muscular dystrophies | Up to 8 × normal | Up to 8 × normal |
| Gangrene | 2–5 × normal | Normal to slight increase |
| Skeletal muscle injury | 2–5 × normal | Normal to slight increase |
| Pulmonary emboli | Up to 3 × normal | Normally not affected |
| Acute pancreatitis | 2–5 × normal | Normally not affected |
| Malignancies of brain or spinal cord | Variable amount | Normally not affected |

normal are seen in biliary diseases. The pattern of clinical findings and other laboratory tests distinguishes between increased ALP due to cholestatic disease and that due to bone disease (see section entitled bone disease).

GGT is a microsomal enzyme present in high concentration in the cells that line the biliary tract. Its synthesis is enhanced by the presence of several drugs including alcohol. The degree of elevation of serum GGT is greater in obstructive biliary disease than in hepatic disease, but it is also increased significantly by recent alcohol intake or hepatotoxic drugs. GGT is a useful adjunct to ALP because of its different tissue distribution. While ALP can be increased by biliary or bone disease as well as pregnancy and normal bone growth, GGT is found in biliary vessels, kidney, pancreas, and intestine but not in bones or placenta.

Because of the proximity of the pancreatic duct to the bile duct, obstruction of the bile duct can also result in elevated levels of amylase and lipase in plasma from inflammation of the pancreas (see following section on pancreatic disease).

## Bone Disease

Elevated levels of ALP in plasma are found when there is a high rate of turnover of bone tissue because osteoblasts are rich in alkaline phosphatase. Examples of normal causes for increased amounts of bone ALP are normal growth (infants and children have higher reference ranges than adults) and normal healing of fractured bone. Abnormal causes include bone cancer (primary or metastatic), rickets and osteomalacia, primary hyperparathyroidism, acromegaly, and Paget's disease (Table 15–4). In all of these diseases, osteoblasts are more active than normal as they attempt to rebuild bone that is being destroyed and thus their ALP isoenzyme is present in serum at higher level. In bone cancers, the tumor is destroying bone tissue by encroachment; in rickets and osteomalacia, there is increased bone remodeling due to lack of vitamin D; in primary hyperparathyroidism, excessive parathyroid hormone is actively causing bone resorption; in acromegaly, there is abnormal enhanced growth of bone tissue; and in Paget's disease, there is increased

TABLE 15-4

**Increases in Serum ALP by Isoenzyme in Certain Clinical States**

| BONE ORIGIN | PLACENTAL ORIGIN | INTESTINAL ORIGIN | LIVER ORIGIN | UNIDENTIFIED ISOENZYMES (REGAN OR NAGAO) |
|---|---|---|---|---|
| Paget's disease<br>Osteomalacia<br>Bone tumors<br>Bone fractures<br>Hyperparathyroidism<br>Pulmonary infarct<br>Chronic renal failure<br>Hyperphosphatemia | During the 3rd trimester of pregnancy | Lesions of the small intestine<br>Individuals with blood types B or O | Acute and chronic pancreatitis<br>Cardiac failure with hepatic congestion<br>Cirrhosis | Malignancies: carcinoma of lung, breast, ovary, and colon |

turnover and abnormal remodeling of bone tissue. If clinical signs and other laboratory tests do not distinguish the source of elevated ALP, the heat instability test is probably the most convenient method for identifying the bone isoenzyme.

Decreased levels of ALP have been reported in cases in which bone metabolism is suppressed, e.g., hypothyroidism, hypophosphatemia, vitamin C deficiency (scurvy), kwashiorkor (protein malnutrition), and severe anemia. Normal bone metabolism requires adequate calcium and phosphate metabolism as well as vitamin C for collagen synthesis and sufficient nutrition and metabolic rate.

## Pancreatic Disease

Pancreatic acinar cells produce the enzymes required for the intestinal digestion of carbohydrates, lipids, proteins, and nucleic acids. These include amylase, lipase, trypsin, chymotrypsin, elastase, and several nucleases. Of these, only amylase and lipase are measured for the diagnosis of **acute pancreatitis.**

Inflammation of the pancreas, whether obstructive, viral, or idiopathic, is a severe disease with a significant rate of mortality. Acute pancreatitis releases digestive enzymes into the interstitial fluid and plasma, where even a small amount of these enzymes causes significant tissue damage. As an example of this damage, the small, normal escape of trypsin into plasma is the probable cause of hepatic cirrhosis seen in persons who have congenital deficiency of the neutralizing protein, alpha$_1$-antitrypsin. The amount of digestive enzymes released in acute pancreatitis is much greater and causes much more tissue damage.

The serum levels of amylase and lipase often rise above the reference range within an hour of the onset of acute pancreatitis. Both enzymes are filtered through the renal glomeruli, but amylase remains in the urine and lipase is reabsorbed back into the plasma. This accounts for the occurrence of elevated urinary amylase that precedes and succeeds the elevated level in serum and the transient nature of the elevated serum level. The serum level of amylase rises between 5 and 50 times nor-

mal in acute pancreatitis and returns to normal within 3 days if the acute inflammation is resolved (Figure 15–15). The magnitude of increase and its duration do not correlate with the degree of tissue damage. The increase in serum levels of lipase parallels amylase, but lipase remains elevated up to a week following the inflammatory event. Measurement of the ratio of amylase clearance to creatinine clearance has not gained wide

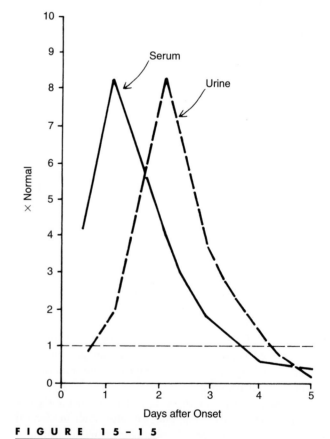

FIGURE 15-15

Serum and urine amylase levels in a case of acute pancreatitis.

use as a diagnostic tool. Some patients with acute pancreatitis experience a precipitous decrease in serum calcium, presumably due to it being sequestered by lipids forming insoluble soaps.

**Chronic pancreatitis** and pancreatic **tumors** are not associated with elevated levels of amylase or lipase in serum. Inflammation of other tissues that are rich in amylase, such as salivary glands and fallopian tubes, may cause increased serum amylase. It is important to note that true increase in serum amylase should always be accompanied by increase in urine amylase. This fact will distinguish between true hyperamylasemia and **macroamylasemia.** Macroamylasemia is a benign, transient condition in which the amylase normally found in serum becomes attached to an immunoglobulin. Conjugation to this large molecule prevents the amylase from being removed by glomerular filtration, resulting in serum levels 2 to 3 times normal but normal or low urine amylase.

## SUMMARY

Enzymes are protein molecules that catalyze biologic reactions. Most clinical laboratory assays for enzymes measure their leakage from damaged cells into plasma.

The active site of a protein is the site where substrate is bound. An enzyme-substrate complex is formed that enhances the rate of production of product by lowering the energy of activation.

The primary, secondary, tertiary, and (in some cases) quaternary structures of the protein contribute to the overall shape of the enzyme and define the conditions necessary for its activity and specificity. These conditions include pH, temperature, ionic strength, and allosteric activators or inhibitors.

Most enzyme assays simulate body conditions except for adding zero-order concentration of substrates. A kinetic assay is preferred because it provides evidence that only enzyme activity is controlling the rate of reaction. The Michaelis-Menten equation and its derivative Lineweaver-Burk transformation describe the velocity substrate curve, facilitate experimental determination of $K_m$ and $V_{max}$, and provide a method for distinguishing between different kinds of enzyme inhibitors.

Enzyme assays are reported in International Units per liter of sample. In many commercial assays, when the substrates, cofactors, or products of an enzyme reaction are not colored, auxiliary enzymes and substrates are added to provide coupled reactions that culminate in a colored product.

Clinically significant enzymes that are measured in virtually all modern laboratories include AST, ALT, ALP, LD, CK, GGT, AMS, LIP, PChE, and G-6-PD. Each of them has a characteristic set of tissues where they are found in high concentration, and some also have tissue-specific distribution of their isoenzymes. By measuring the pattern and time course of serum enzyme levels, damage to specific tissues can often be deduced. Examples include muscle diseases (including both skeletal and cardiac myocytes), liver disease (including both hepatic and biliary cells), bone disease, and pancreatic disease.

## REFERENCES

1. Campbell MK: The behavior of proteins: Enzymes. In *Biochemistry.* 3rd ed. Philadephia, Harcourt Brace, 1999, pp 144–195.
2. Moss DW, Henderson AR: Enzymes. In Burtis CA, Ashwood ER: *Tietz Textbook of Clinical Chemistry.* 3rd ed. Philadelphia, WB Saunders, 1998, pp 617–721.
3. Roskoski R: Membrane transport. In *Biochemistry.* Philadelphia, WB Saunders, 1996, pp 457–467.
4. Wroblewski F, LaDue JS: Serum glutamic pyruvic transaminase in cardiac and hepatic disease. Proc Soc Exp Biol Med 91:569, 1956.
5. Bergmeyer HU, Hørder M, Rej RJ: Approved recommendation (1985) on IFCC methods for the measurement of catalytic concentration of enzymes. Part 2. IFCC Methods for aspartate aminotransferase (L-aspartate: 2-oxoglutarate aminotransferase, EC 2.6.1.1). Clin Chem Clin Biochem 24:497, 1986.
6. Tietz NW: *Clinical Guide to Laboratory Tests.* 3rd ed. Philadelphia, WB Saunders, 1995.
7. Bowers GN, McComb RB: Measurement of total alkaline phosphatase activity in human serum. Clin Chem 21:1988, 1975.
8. Amador E, Dorfman LE, Wacker WEC: Serum lactic dehydrogenase activity: An analytical assessment of current assays. Clin Chem 9:391, 1963.
9. Szasz G, Gerhardt W, Gruber W: Creatine kinase in serum: 3. Further study of adenylate kinase inhibitors. Clin Chem 23:1888, 1997.
10. The Committee on Enzymes of the Scandinavian Society for Clinical Chemistry and Clinical Physiology: Recommended method for the determination of creatine kinase in blood. Scan J Clin Lab Invest 36:711, 1976.
11. Chan DW, Taylor E, Fryl R, et al.: Immunoenzymetric assay for creatine kinase MB with subunit-specific monoclonal antibodies compared with an immunochemical method and electrophoresis. Clin Chem 31:465, 1985.
12. Gerhardt W, Ljungdahl J, Borjesson S, et al.: Creatine kinase B-subunit activity in human serum I. Development of an immunoinhibition method for routine determination of S-creatine kinase B-subunit activity. Clin Chim Acta 78:29, 1979.
13. Szasz G: A kinetic photometric method for serum γ-glutamyl transpeptidase. Clin Chem 15:124, 1969.
14. Pierre KJ, Tung KK, Nadj H: A new enzymatic kinetic method for determination of α-amylase. Clin Chem 22:1219, 1976.
15. Mauck LA: A kinetic colorimetric method for the determination of total amylase activity in serum. Clin Chem 31:1007, 1985.
16. Panteghini M, Pagani F: Characterization of a rapid immunochromatographic assay for simultaneous detection of high concentrations of myoglobin and CK-MB in whole blood. Clin Chem 42:1292, 1996.

17. Imamura S, Hirayama T, Arai T, et al.: An enzymatic method using 1,2-diglyceride for pancreatic lipase test in serum. Clin Chem 35:1126, 1989.

18. Silk E, King J, Whittaker M: Assay of cholinesterase in clinical chemistry. Ann Clin Biochem 16:57–75, 1979.

19. Evans RT: Cholinesterase phenotyping: Clinical aspects and laboratory applications. Crit Rev Clin Lab Sci 23:35, 1986.

20. Beutler E, Mitchell M: UDP glu consumption methods, in Hsia, DYY (ed.): *Galactosemia.* Springfield, Thomas, 1969, pp 72–82.

21. Motulsky AB, Yoshida A: Methods for the study of red cell glucose-6-phosphate dehydrogenase, in J.J. Yunis (ed.): *Biochemical Methods in Red Cell Genetics.* New York, Academic Press, 1969, pp 52–94.

22. Ridker PM, Hennekens CH, Buring JE, et al.: C-reactive protein and other markers of inflammation in the prediction of cardiovascular disease in women. New Engl J Med 342:836, 2000.

23. Nygard O, Nordrehaug JE, Refsum H, et al.: Plasma homocysteine levels and mortality in patients with coronary artery disease. New Engl J Med 337:230, 1997.

# Liver Function

*Lynn R. Ingram*

## LIVER ANATOMY

The liver is a large and complex organ found in the upper right quadrant of the body. It is beneath and attached to the diaphragm and protected by the lower rib cage. The liver accounts for approximately 2.5% of an adult's body weight. Weighing between 1200 and 1600 g, it is unequally divided into two lobes by the falciform ligament, the right lobe being about 6 times larger than the left lobe (Figure 16–1). The lobes have no functional significance, and there is free communication between all portions of the liver.

The liver is a vascular organ with approximately 1500 mL of blood per minute passing through it. The liver is unusual in that it receives a dual blood supply. Blood rich in nutrients and other absorbed substances from the gastrointestinal tract is carried to the liver by the portal vein. Even though the portal vein contributes 80% of the total blood volume of the liver, it supplies only 40% of the oxygen. The hepatic artery, branching from the abdominal aorta, is the primary supplier of well-oxygenated blood to the liver. To complete the hepatic circulation, blood is drained from the liver by a collecting system of veins that empties into the hepatic veins and ultimately into the inferior vena cava.

The excretory system of the liver begins with a collection system of bile canaliculi. These are tiny spaces between the hepatocytes that drain the excretory products of the cells into larger and larger ductules, finally converging into the right and left hepatic ducts. These two ducts then join to form the hepatic duct, which drains the secretions from the liver. The hepatic duct and the cystic duct from the gallbladder unite to form the common bile duct, and the combined digestive secretions are then expelled into the duodenum.

### Liver Lobule

The liver lobule is the basic microscopic unit of the liver and is responsible for all metabolic and excretory functions performed by the liver. Each lobule is roughly hexagonal in shape with 4 to 6 peripherally located portal triads, numerous columns of hepatic parenchymal cells, a continuous system of blood-carrying sinusoids, and a central vein at the center of the unit (Figure 16–2). Each portal triad contains a branch of the portal vein and hepatic artery and a bile duct. Blood is

supplied to the lobule by the branches of the portal vein and hepatic artery and flows through the sinusoids toward the central vein. The sinusoids are the capillary channels lying between the cords of hepatic parenchymal cells. They are lined with two types of cells: modified epithelial cells and macrophages called Kupffer cells.

The hepatic parenchymal cells, or hepatocytes, perform the functions of the liver and are found in radiating columns of cells from the central vein toward the periphery of the lobule. Hepatocytes are large cells that make up approximately 80% of the volume of liver tissue. These cells perform the metabolic, detoxification, excretory, and synthesis functions associated with the liver and are responsible for the regenerative properties of the liver. There is a free exchange of substances between the blood in the sinusoids and the hepatocytes. Blood is drained from the lobule by the central vein, which eventually connects to the hepatic veins and the inferior vena cava. The bile collection system of the lobule flows in the opposite direction from the flow of blood. The excretory products formed by the hepatic parenchymal cells are removed from the cells and collected in the smallest ducts called bile canaliculi. The bile canaliculi are found in the spaces between the hepatocytes and interconnect to form a system of larger and larger bile ductules. These bile ductules converge into interlobular bile ducts and intrahepatic ducts and finally form the hepatic duct, which removes the bile from the liver.

Endothelial cells are flattened cells that line the sinusoids and function as filters to prevent the passage of large molecules into the hepatocytes. Another cell type lining the sinusoids is a fixed macrophage, the Kupffer cell. These cells are active phagocytes that engulf bacteria, aging erythrocytes, toxins, cellular debris, and other substances from the blood flowing through the sinusoids. Other cells that lie beneath the sinusoidal lining in the liver lobule are the lipocytes, which store fat; fibroblasts, which give a supporting structure to the liver; and neurons, which compose unmyelinated nerves and are a part of the autonomic nervous system.

### Subcellular Components of the Hepatocyte

Organelles within the hepatic parenchymal cells are responsible for the individual functions associated with the liver. The Golgi apparatus acts as a packaging plant by assembling and transporting lipoproteins and glycoproteins and is instrumental in the secretion of albumin and bilirubin. Lysosomes within

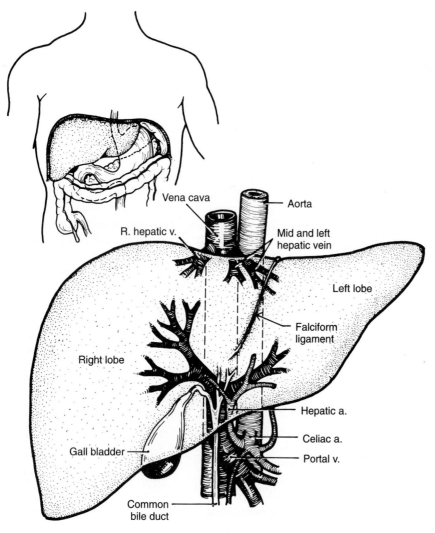

FIGURE  16-1

Gross anatomy of the liver with major blood vessels and bile drainage system and placement of the liver within the body. (From Tietz NW (ed): *Fundamentals of Clinical Chemistry*. 2nd ed. Philadelphia, WB Saunders, 1976, p 1026. Reprinted with permission.)

the cells contain hydrolytic enzymes that digest and catabolize substances such as lipoproteins and ferritin and metabolize iron, copper and bile pigments. Microbodies (peroxisomes) are involved with many functions of the hepatocyte including respiration, lipid and purine metabolism, gluconeogenesis, and the detoxification of alcohol. The mitochondria are the energy sources for the cells and are especially active in oxidative phosphorylation and the oxidation of fatty acids in a variety of metabolic pathways. Endoplasmic reticulum is a system of passageways within the cytoplasm and is probably involved, either directly or indirectly, in every function of the hepatocyte. Both rough and smooth endoplasmic reticulum is present and well defined in the hepatic parenchymal cell. The rough endoplasmic reticulum has many ribosomes scattered along its surface and is involved in the synthesis of albumin, certain coagula-

tion factors, cholesterol, and bile acids and in the metabolism of drugs and steroids. Smooth endoplasmic reticulum does not contain ribosomes but is associated with the deposition of glycogen and with other metabolic processes.

## LIVER FUNCTION

The liver performs many diverse and complex tasks that can be categorized as metabolism, detoxification, excretion or secretion, and storage functions. It is estimated that the liver performs hundreds of separate activities, and if the liver becomes completely nonfunctional, death will occur from hypoglycemia within 24 hours.[1] Every substance that is absorbed from the

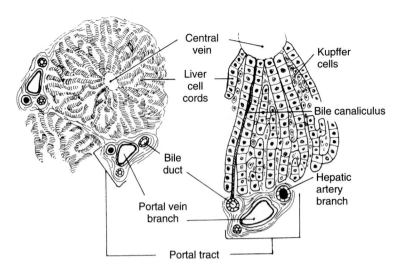

**FIGURE 16-2**

Diagram of a liver lobule **(left)** and a sector of a lobule enlarged **(right).** (From
Raphael SS (ed): *Lynch's Medical Laboratory Technology.* 4th ed. Philadelphia,
WB Saunders, 1983, p 243. Reprinted with permission.)

gastrointestinal tract must first pass through the liver before it
is distributed by the general circulation. During this first pass,
most substances are altered in some way. The liver creates and
distributes life-sustaining compounds from the raw materials
provided by absorption and serves as a protective barrier between many harmful substances and the general circulation. It
acts as a storage compartment for many compounds and has
the ability to release stored materials as the body needs them.
Even when the liver cannot store or use a compound, it can
prepare that compound for use by another part of the body.
The liver can excrete or secrete certain substances and provides
the only route of elimination from the body for many substances. The liver is an organ with full regenerative properties
and it has a tremendous reserve capacity that allows it to function within normal limits until 80% of the hepatocytes have
been destroyed.[2] The integration of each of these functions to
maintain a constant environment within the body is not the
least of the contributions that the liver makes to an individual's health.

## Metabolic Functions

### CARBOHYDRATE METABOLISM

The liver has an important role in the metabolism of many
substances such as carbohydrates, lipids, proteins and amino
acids, and bilirubin. The liver is responsible for the production, catabolism, and storage of glucose and other sugars. Upon
ingestion and absorption of carbohydrate, glucose-rich blood
is received from the portal circulation. The liver can use the
glucose for its own cellular energy requirements, or the glucose can be circulated to peripheral tissues for their immediate use. The liver can also store glucose as glycogen within the

liver or other tissues, or it can be prepared for more permanent storage as adipose tissue by synthesis of free fatty acids
and triglycerides. A steady supply of glucose is necessary to
provide energy for metabolic needs, even though ingestion of
dietary carbohydrates is sporadic. During a fasting period, the
liver becomes the major force in preventing a fall in blood glucose levels. Upon fasting, the liver breaks down stored glycogen through the process of glycogenolysis. When that supply
is exhausted, it creates glucose through **gluconeogenesis.** The
process of gluconeogenesis uses amino acids from muscle tissue, glycerol from the breakdown of triglycerides in adipose
tissue, or lactate or pyruvate provided by **glycolysis** in peripheral tissues to create glucose when needed. The liver exhibits its central role in maintaining stable plasma glucose concentrations by its ability to store glucose while it is available
and then to release it when needed for energy.

### AMINO ACID AND PROTEIN METABOLISM

The liver is instrumental in the metabolism of amino acids.
Amino acids delivered to the liver from the portal vein may
be made into proteins used in the synthesis of small nitrogen-
containing compounds such as creatine, or degraded into constituent moieties if the supply of amino acids exceeds the current requirements. Amino acids are used and often reused to
make essential substances for the body. The liver also regulates
the amount and type of amino acids that are delivered to the
circulation for use by other tissues. The liver is a primary site
of synthesis of most plasma proteins. It generates albumin, the
alpha and beta globulins, and coagulation factors II, V, VII,
IX, and X. The liver also produces specialized proteins such as
transferrin, haptoglobin, ceruloplasmin, fibrinogen, and some
of the acute phase reactants. Most of the proteins are made

from constituent amino acids in various sites within the liver for transport to the circulation. Proteins that are to be exported from the liver cell are thought to be attached to a secretory protein. The combined protein is channeled through the transport mechanism of the smooth endoplasmic reticulum to the Golgi apparatus, where the secretory protein is removed before excretion from the cell. Albumin is made in large quantities (between 120 and 200 mg/kg of body weight per day) by the ribosomes on the rough endoplasmic reticulum and accounts for a major percentage of the synthetic capacity of the liver.

## LIPID METABOLISM

The liver metabolizes both the lipids and the lipoproteins responsible for the transport of lipids. The liver gathers free fatty acids from the diet, those released from fat deposits, and those manufactured within the liver itself and then breaks them down to produce acetyl-CoA. This moiety can enter one of several metabolic pathways to form triglycerides, phospholipids, or cholesterol. By converting free fatty acids into fat, a more stable storage form, energy that is in excess of that needed is conserved and stored for future use. The liver produces cholesterol for cell membranes and other synthetic functions as well as cholesterol metabolic products including adrenal cortical hormones, estrogen, and bile acids. Endogenous cholesterol production accounts for between 1.5 and 2.0 g per day with the average diet providing less than 0.7 g per day.[3] The liver is also responsible for the disposal of cholesterol and is capable of eliminating cholesterol from the body in large quantities through bile excretion into the feces. Lipoproteins are necessary to make the water-insoluble lipids into more soluble compounds, allowing them to be transported to other cells. The liver also provides the apoprotein portion of the lipoprotein molecules, making lipoprotein synthesis dependent on the liver's ability to make apoproteins. Apoproteins are made on the ribosomes of the rough endoplasmic reticulum and are attached to the lipid in smooth endoplasmic reticulum as it is prepared for secretion.

## BILIRUBIN METABOLISM

Bilirubin metabolism is the activity that is most often associated with the liver. It is the only organ that has the capacity to rid the body of heme waste products (Figure 16–3). Approximately 80% of the 250 to 400 mg of bilirubin formed each day comes from the release of hemoglobin from erythrocytes reaching the end of their 120-day life span and the ultimate degradation of that hemoglobin. The remaining 20% of the bilirubin metabolized daily originates in enzymes and other proteins that contain heme, such as cytochromes, and from erythrocytes that are prematurely destroyed or abnormally produced.[4]

Degradation of hemoglobin takes place in the cells of the reticuloendothelial system. This process produces a protein portion, which is returned to the amino acid pool for subsequent use, the iron molecule, which is attached to transferrin or ferritin for transport and recycling into hemoglobin and other iron-containing molecules, and the waste product, porphyrin. The porphyrin is converted into biliverdin by the action of an enzyme, heme oxygenase, and the biliverdin is almost immediately acted on by another enzyme, bilirubin reductase, which converts the biliverdin into bilirubin. Ninety-five percent of the resulting bilirubin becomes reversibly, but firmly, attached to albumin and it is in this form that bilirubin circulates through the blood, eventually arriving at the liver. This form of bilirubin is called **unconjugated** or **indirect bilirubin** and is insoluble in water. The remaining 5% of bilirubin formed at this point does not combine with albumin, and it is significant because it can easily cross cell membranes. This unbound bilirubin has a special affinity for the brain and nervous tissues, is toxic, and in large quantities, can cause brain damage.

The liver is extremely efficient in clearing unconjugated bilirubin from the plasma. When the bilirubin arrives at the liver cell, it flows into the sinusoidal spaces of the liver lobule. At some point, the albumin portion is stripped from the bilirubin molecule and replaced with a carrier protein called ligandin. Ligandin transports the bilirubin into the hepatic parenchymal cells to the microsomes where it is conjugated. An enzyme, glucuronyl transferase, transfers 2 glucuronic acid molecules from uridine diphosphate (UPD)–glucuronic acid to the bilirubin molecule. This conjugation process changes the nonpolar bilirubin molecule to a mixed polar–nonpolar molecule that can cross lipid cell membranes. The bilirubin has become water-soluble and is called **conjugated** or **direct bilirubin.** Water-soluble bilirubin can now be excreted into the bile canaliculi for removal from the body. Conjugated bilirubin can also be reabsorbed by the hepatocytes and released into the systemic circulation, which accounts for the small quantity of conjugated bilirubin that can normally be found in plasma. Since it is water soluble, any conjugated bilirubin in the circulation can also be excreted into the urine as urine bile. After conjugated bilirubin reaches the collecting bile ducts, it cannot cross the mucosal barrier and will no longer be absorbed. The conjugated bilirubin is excreted into the hepatic duct, combined with secretions from the gallbladder through the cystic duct, and expelled through the common bile duct into the duodenum. There bacterial action reduces the bilirubin to one of a group of colorless chromagens called urobilinogen. Most of the urobilinogen formed is excreted in the feces, but approximately 20% will be absorbed by the enterohepatic circulation to be recycled through the liver and reexcreted. An even smaller portion of this absorbed urobilinogen will enter the systemic circulation and be excreted into the urine. Excretion of urobilinogen through the urinary tract accounts for less than 4 mg per day.[5]

A distinct bilirubin fraction, seen only when there is significant hepatic obstruction, is called **delta bilirubin.** Delta bilirubin is conjugated bilirubin that is covalently bound to

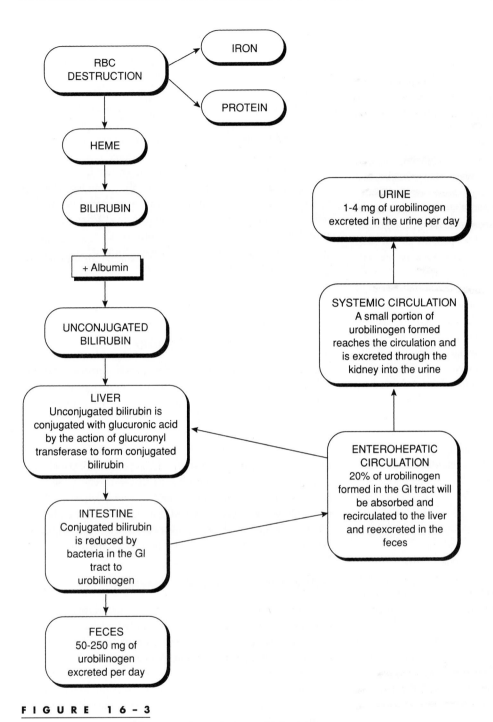

**FIGURE  16-3**

Representation of the normal metabolism of bilirubin.

albumin. It reacts in most laboratory methods exactly as conjugated bilirubin does. The attachment of albumin renders the delta bilirubin insoluble, and the molecule is too large to be filtered by the glomerulus and it is not excreted into the urine. The presence of the delta bilirubin fraction may account for the finding in obstructive jaundice that urine bilirubin will disappear before serum concentrations of conjugated bilirubin return to normal.

## Detoxification Functions

The liver serves as a barrier between potentially harmful substances absorbed from the gastrointestinal tract and the systemic circulation. Its detoxification functions include the processes of hydrolysis, hydroxylation, oxidation, reduction, carboxylation, and demethylation. These mechanisms convert substances into forms that are either less toxic or more water soluble and therefore more easily excreted. The detoxification of drugs is a function of the drug metabolizing enzyme system of cytochrome P450. The cytochrome P450 system is found in the microsomes of the hepatocyte and facilitates the transformation of drugs to more excretable end products by conjugation with such moieties as glycine, glutathione, sulfuric acid, acetate, or glucuronic acid.

The liver also is important in the disposal of potentially toxic exogenous and endogenous compounds. Conjugation of bilirubin with glucuronic acid is a prerequisite to the disposal of bilirubin. This process not only makes the bilirubin water soluble and excretable through the bile and urine but unabsorbable from the gastrointestinal tract and biliary system and thus harmless. Ammonia is a normal by-product of bacterial action on substances found in the gut but is toxic to the central nervous system in excess quantities. The liver is the only organ with the necessary enzymes to convert ammonia to the nontoxic substance, urea. Ingested ethanol, the alcoholic constituents found in many foods, and the endogenous alcohols formed by metabolism of other compounds, must be metabolized by the liver to prevent toxic damage. Most (over 90%) of the alcohol absorbed from the intestines is carried directly to the liver and the remainder is eliminated from the kidney and lungs.[6] The liver will use alcohol for energy because alcohol is the preferred substrate for three enzyme systems used to metabolize alcohol. These enzyme systems are the alcohol dehydrogenase system, the ethanol oxidizing system, and the catalase system. Alcohol is converted to acetaldehyde and then to acetate, which is rapidly metabolized to carbon dioxide and water by the peripheral tissues.

## Excretion Functions

The detoxification and excretion functions of the liver are closely related in that after detoxification the resulting substances must be excreted from the body to prevent further harm. Through the formation of bile, the biliary tract is a frequent route of elimination of solutes from the body. More than 3 L of bile per day are produced, but because bile is reabsorbed through the enterohepatic circulation 2 to 5 times per day, less than 1 L is actually excreted.[1] Bile is primarily composed of conjugated bile acids, phospholipids, cholesterol, bile pigments, hormones, and small amounts of protein as well as absorbed water and electrolytes. The formation of bile is similar to that of urine formation by the kidney in that the fluid is changed as it passes through the collection system of the organ. Conjugated bilirubin is excreted exclusively through the bile and large amounts of cholesterol can be excreted by being converted to the bile acids, cholic acid and chenodeoxycholic acid. Bile acids are then conjugated with glycine or taurine to form bile salts that are excreted into the biliary system through an active transport mechanism using a carrier substance. The bile formed also facilitates digestion through the process of intestinal absorption of lipids and fat-soluble vitamins.

## Storage Functions

Even though the liver performs many diverse functions, there is still space within the liver for the storage of essential compounds. To provide a source of energy during fasting periods, the liver can deposit up to 7% of its weight as glycogen. Almost 10% of the total body content of iron is present in hepatic stores as ferritin, and the liver is a storage site for the fat-soluble vitamins A, E, D, and K and other vitamins such as $B_{12}$. Copper and other metals can be stored in the liver in certain disease states, deposited primarily in the lysosomes. A significant amount of bilirubin normally is stored in the liver cell bound to the cytosolic-binding proteins. When there is an abundance of fatty acids, the liver converts these substances to adipose tissue, the most stable storage form of triglycerides. Therefore, although the liver does not store fatty acids, it is instrumental in their storage elsewhere.

## ANALYTICAL PROCEDURES

The ideal laboratory test is one that is both sensitive and specific and has the capacity to reflect the severity of the abnormality. When assessing the function of the liver, there is no one best analyte to determine the overall function. Therefore, liver profiles have been designed to evaluate several of the major functions of the liver to allow a broad understanding of how well the organ is performing. Liver profiles, or panels, will usually have 4 to 8 laboratory tests that will reflect the liver's ability to metabolize, detoxify, and excrete substances. These tests will aid in the diagnosis of existing liver disease, help to differentiate among the many liver diseases, and determine the extent and severity of the disease process (Table 16–1).

### Indicators of Metabolic Function

Most liver profiles contain one or more laboratory tests that evaluate the liver's ability to metabolize materials. Protein synthesis is a major metabolic function of the liver. Although the liver produces almost all of the plasma proteins, the determination of only albumin and prothrombin time will yield useful information for evaluation of liver function. Albumin and prothrombin time are commonly used tests that reflect hepatic synthesis and release.

#### SERUM ALBUMIN

Albumin is quantitatively the most significant protein synthesized by the liver and is an indicator of overall function but there are factors other than liver function that can alter albumin concentrations. The patient's nutritional status is extremely important since albumin synthesis is dependent on the availability of amino acids from the diet, especially tryptophan. Hormone balance, osmotic pressure, and renal function may also alter albumin concentrations. The liver can synthesize

**TABLE 16-1**

**Laboratory Tests Used in the Evaluation of Liver Functions**

| | |
|---|---|
| **Routine chemistry tests** | Alanine aminotransferase |
| | Total Protein/Albumin |
| | Alkaline phosphatase |
| | Aspartate aminotransferase |
| | Bilirubin—conjugated and unconjugated |
| | Gamma-glutamyltransferase |
| **Special chemistry tests** | Alpha-fetoprotein |
| | Ammonia |
| | Ceruloplasmin |
| | Serum iron and ferritin |
| | Serum bile acids |
| **Urine chemistry tests** | Urine urobilinogen |
| | Urine bilirubin |
| **Immunologic tests** | IgM and IgG antibodies to hepatitis A |
| | Hepatitis B surface antigen |
| | Antibody to hepatitis B surface antigen |
| | IgM and IgG antibodies to hepatitis D |
| | Antimitochondrial antibodies |
| | Antibodies to hepatitis C virus |
| **Hematology tests** | Complete blood count |
| | Reticulocyte count |
| | Red cell enzyme studies |
| | Determination of abnormal hemoglobin types |
| | Prothrombin time |
| | Coagulation factor studies |

albumin at twice the healthy basal rate in certain situations and thus partially compensate for decreased synthetic capacity or increased albumin losses.[7] However, when the liver is diseased, albumin concentrations decrease. This decrease is not seen immediately, because the half-life of albumin is approximately 20 days. The usefulness of this determination is in the evaluation of chronic liver diseases rather than in acute situations. If the plasma albumin concentration is decreased, the liver has had diminished function for a relatively long time. Conversely, a normal albumin concentration does not rule out liver disease. Plasma albumin values of less than 3.0 g/dL may signify considerable hepatic functional impairment and concentrations of less than 2.5 g/dL may be associated with ascites and reflect a poor prognosis.[8]

## PROTHROMBIN TIME

The prothrombin time is often considered in the evaluation of liver function but it is not routinely used for an initial di-

agnosis of liver disease. Serial determinations of prothrombin times are a means of following the progress of the patient's disease and assessing the risk of bleeding. A prothrombin time assesses the extrinsic coagulation pathway so that if any one of the factors produced by the liver (factors II, V, VII, X) is deficient, the prothrombin time will be prolonged. The half-life of the coagulation factors made by the liver ranges from 6 hours to 5 days so that in acute liver problems the prothrombin time will be abnormal early in the progress of the disease and is sensitive to rapid changes in the liver's synthetic function.[7] Prothrombin times that remain prolonged and become increasingly abnormal are prognostic of fulminant liver failure. Although a prolonged prothrombin time is not exclusively associated with liver disease, it is particularly suited to assessing acute liver failure.

## SERUM LIPIDS AND LIPOPROTEINS

There are many abnormalities of lipid and lipoprotein metabolism in liver disease. The typical profile seen is an increased level of triglycerides and fatty acids, decreased levels of cholesterol esters, and the accompanying alterations in lipoprotein concentrations. Many of these abnormalities can be attributed to the deficiencies of two enzymes of liver origin, lecithin-cholesterol acyltransferase (LCAT) and hepatic triglyceride lipase. LCAT catalyzes the esterification of cholesterol and triglyceride lipase clears triglycerides from the plasma. With abnormalities in the concentration of these enzymes, it is clear that the concentration of the end products of these enzymatic reactions will be abnormal also. The liver produces both very low-density lipoproteins and high-density lipoproteins and the concentrations of each of these will be decreased with liver disease. Although these findings are not specific to liver dysfunction, the appearance of an abnormal lipoprotein, called lipoprotein X, is both a sensitive and specific indicator of cholestasis. Lipoprotein X contains free cholesterol and phospholipids and has albumin as its primary apoprotein. In one study, lipoprotein X was found to be present in 98% of patients with mechanical obstruction of the bile duct.[9]

## CARBOHYDRATES

Although the regulation of carbohydrate metabolism by the liver is of utmost importance, rarely are laboratory tests evaluating carbohydrate metabolism used in a liver profile. Carbohydrate concentrations in the plasma are so dependent on factors such as nutritional status, time of the last meal, hormone balance, and pancreatic function that evaluation of plasma glucose concentrations will not give much insight into the quality of the function of the liver. The carbohydrate metabolism abnormalities seen in liver diseases are usually nonspecific and uninformative.

## SERUM BILIRUBIN

An initial determination of the concentration of unconjugated and conjugated bilirubin is a useful approach to the diagno-

TABLE 16-2

### Reference Ranges for Bilirubin Concentrations

| AGE | TOTAL BILIRUBIN | CONJUGATED BILIRUBIN |
|---|---|---|
| Infants <1 month of age | 4.0–8.0 mg/dL<br>68–137 $\mu$mol/L | 0–2.0 mg/dL<br>0–34 $\mu$mol/L |
| Adults | 0.2–1.0 mg/dL<br>3.4–17 $\mu$mol/L | 0–0.2 mg/dL<br>0–3.4 $\mu$mol/L |

sis of jaundice and liver disease. Plasma bilirubin concentrations reflect the balance between production of bilirubin from the breakdown of hemoglobin and the capacity of the liver to clear the bilirubin from the plasma. The average plasma concentration of total bilirubin in apparently healthy adults is less than 1 mg/dL with less than 0.8 mg/dL being of the unconjugated type and less than 0.2 mg/dL being the conjugated type (Table 16–2).

When total bilirubin concentrations rise above the expected level, it is important to specify the concentrations of both conjugated and unconjugated bilirubin to be helpful in

the broad classification of hyperbilirubinemias. Conjugated hyperbilirubinemia occurs when over 50% of the total bilirubin is conjugated, and unconjugated hyperbilirubinemia occurs when more than 80% of total bilirubin is unconjugated (Table 16–3). Once the predominant form of bilirubin is determined, the patient's history, physical findings, and other laboratory tests will further identify the specific cause of the problem.

### Jendrassik-Grof Bilirubin Method

Many current methods for the determination of plasma bilirubin concentration are based on the diazo coupling of bilirubin pigments first described by van den Bergh and Snapper in 1913. Many revisions of the original procedure have been made, and modification of Jendrassik and Grof is now recommended by the National Committee for Clinical Laboratory Standards. This method gives reliable results as judged by the reference method, the high-performance liquid chromatography (HPLC) method of Lauff and colleagues.[10] The Jendrassik-Grof method has advantages over earlier diazo methods in that it is less sensitive to variations in pH, protein, and hemoglobin concentrations in the patient's sample, forms minimal turbidity during the reaction, and is sensitive enough to produce sufficient, reliable color even with very low concentrations of bilirubin.

TABLE 16-3

### Conditions Causing Unconjugated and Conjugated Hyperbilirubinemias

| DISORDER | DEFECT IN BILIRUBIN METABOLISM |
|---|---|
| **UNCONJUGATED HYPERBILIRUBINEMIA** | |
| Hemolysis | Increased production |
| Ineffective erythropoiesis | Increased production |
| Neonatal physiologic jaundice | Increased production<br>Decreased UDP-glucuronyl transferase activity<br>Increased intestinal absorption of bilirubin |
| Crigler-Najjar syndrome, type I | No UDP-glucuronyl transferase activity |
| Crigler-Najjar syndrome, type II | Decreased UDP-glucuronyl transferase activity |
| Gilbert's syndrome | Decreased UDP-glucuronyl transferase activity<br>Decreased hepatic uptake |
| Congestive heart failure | Impaired delivery of bilirubin to the liver |
| **CONJUGATED HYPERBILIRUBINEMIA** | |
| Dubin-Johnson syndrome | Impaired biliary excretion |
| Rotor's syndrome | Decreased hepatic uptake and storage<br>Decreased biliary excretion |
| Hepatic storage syndrome | Decreased hepatic uptake and storage<br>Decreased biliary excretion |
| Intrahepatic cholestasis | Decreased biliary excretion |
| Extrahepatic cholestasis | Decreased biliary excretion |
| Hepatocellular injury | Decreased biliary excretion |

In the Jendrassik-Grof method, bilirubin pigments react with a diazo reagent composed of sulfanilic acid in hydrochloric acid and sodium nitrite. The resulting azobilirubin is measured spectrophotometrically. Individual concentrations of conjugated and unconjugated bilirubin can be determined by treating one aliquot of the patient's sample with the diazo reagent only and treating a second aliquot with diazo reagent after a pretreatment step using an accelerator, such as a caffeine-benzoate reagent. When treating with diazo reagent, only the water-soluble form of bilirubin reacts, resulting in conjugated bilirubin measurements. The addition of the caffeine-benzoate reagent allows both the conjugated and unconjugated bilirubin to become water soluble and react with the diazo reagent to give total bilirubin concentrations. Ten minutes after the reaction of the bilirubins with diazo reagent, solutions of ascorbic acid, alkaline tartrate, and dilute hydrochloric acid are added to both reaction mixtures. These reagents destroy the excess diazo reagent and shift the pH from an acid to an alkaline pH, making the resulting color less subject to interfering chromagens in the sample. The final blue-green azobilirubin formed is then read at 600 nm on a spectrophotometer. To determine the amount of unconjugated bilirubin, the conjugated bilirubin concentration is simply subtracted from the total bilirubin concentration.

The Jendrassik-Grof method uses a serum or plasma sample that should be free of hemolysis and lipemia. Hemolysis decreases the reaction of bilirubin with diazo reagent, producing falsely low concentrations, and lipemia causes error in the spectrophotometric measurements. Bilirubin is both light and temperature sensitive. Allowing serum or plasma to be exposed to fluorescent or natural light reduces bilirubin concentrations by 10% within 30 minutes. Therefore, the samples should be protected from light before and during analysis. Urine and spinal fluid may also be used for this method. Samples may be stored in a dark refrigerator for up to 1 week or in a freezer for 3 months without significant alterations in bilirubin concentrations. Precautions in the collection and storage of the samples for analysis will greatly reduce errors in this method.

The careful preparation of bilirubin standards is critical since bilirubin standards are not stable and may be a source of error in this method. Standards should be protected from light and high temperatures in the same way as samples. It is imperative that instruments be frequently restandardized to maintain reliable results. In obstructive and hemolytic jaundices when larger that normal amounts of biliverdin are produced, other errors may result since biliverdin will not react with diazo reagent and less than expected bilirubin values result. Large serum concentrations of zinc have also been shown to interfere with the diazo reaction.

## Thin-Film Determination of Bilirubin Concentrations

A second type of laboratory test for bilirubin determinations based on the Jendrassik-Grof diazo method uses a thin-film technique developed by Eastman Kodak Company and used

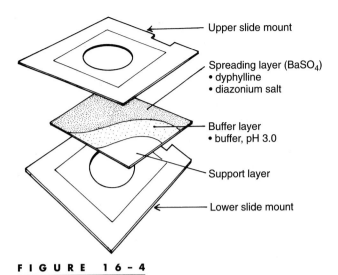

- Upper slide mount
- Spreading layer (BaSO$_4$)
  - dyphylline
  - diazonium salt
- Buffer layer
  - buffer, pH 3.0
- Support layer
- Lower slide mount

**FIGURE  16-4**

Vitros clinical chemistry slide for total bilirubin determination. (From total bilirubin test methodology, Publication MP2-39, Rochester, NY, Johnson and Johnson Clinical Diagnostics, Inc., 1996. Reprinted with permission.)

on the Johnson and Johnson Vitros™ analyzers. The slides used in this method contain 3 separate layers (Figure 16–4). The top layer is a spreading and reaction layer and contains barium sulfate, a diazonium salt, and an accelerator, dyphylline. This layer separates the unconjugated bilirubin from albumin and contains all the necessary components for the quantification of bilirubin. A middle layer is a buffered mordant layer that stabilizes the azo derivatives produced in the reaction layer and increases the sensitivity of the assay. The third layer is a nonreactive transparent support. When the bilirubins in the sample come into contact with the reagents on the slide, a spectral change occurs. The reflectance densities of the azo derivatives of all bilirubin fractions (unconjugated, conjugated, and delta bilirubin) are then measured at 2 wavelengths. The reflectance measurements at 540 nm reflect bilirubin concentrations and the measurement of 460 nm are used to correct for spectral interferences.[11] These results indicate total bilirubin concentrations.

To differentiate the conjugated bilirubin from the unconjugated bilirubin, another type of dry chemistry slide with 4 layers is used (Figure 16–5). This method takes advantage of the fact that conjugated and unconjugated bilirubin have different light absorption spectra when bound to a cationic polymeric mordant. The top layer is a spreading layer that not only allows uniform dispersal of the sample but also contains caffeine, surfactants, and sodium benzoate to disassociate the conjugated bilirubin from albumin. Both the conjugated bilirubin and the bilirubin removed from the albumin migrate through the next layer (the masking layer) on the slide to the third layer, the reagent layer, where the measurements are made. The second masking layer uses selective filtration to trap

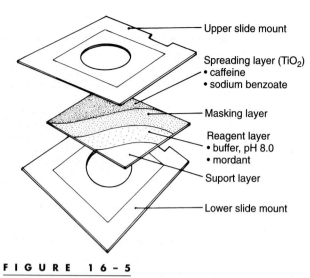

**F I G U R E   1 6 – 5**

Vitros clinical chemistry slide for bililrubin, unconjugated and conjugated determination. (From Total bilirubin test methodology, Publication MP2-40. Rochester, NY, Johnson and Johnson Clinical Diagnostics, Inc., 1996. Reprinted with permission.)

many large molecules. This is especially important because this layer removes hemoglobin, the albumin-bound delta bilirubin, lipids, and lipochromes. These molecules comprise a large group of interfering substances in bilirubin methods and are essentially removed from the final measurement. In the reagent layer, the conjugated and unconjugated bilirubin binds to the buffered mordant. Two separate reflection density measurements are made, one at 400 nm for unconjugated bilirubin and another at 450 nm for conjugated bilirubin.[12]

The dry chemistry slide methods use nonhemolyzed fresh serum or plasma samples for analysis. No special patient preparation is necessary and heparin is the anticoagulant of choice for plasma specimens. Care must be taken with the samples to protect the photosensitive bilirubin from light, and variations in temperature are to be avoided.

Dry chemistry slide bilirubin methods correlate well with the Jendrassik-Grof spectrophotometric method and the HPLC method of Lauff.[13] The methods are stable, precise, easy to perform, and have few common interferences. The use of dual-wavelength measurements eliminates the interferences from hemoglobin and other chromagens that absorb light in the 555-nm region. Patient samples with a carbon dioxide content of less than 15 mmol/L may show a falsely increased total bilirubin.[14]

### Direct Spectrophotometric Measurements of Plasma Bilirubin

Determination of serum bilirubin concentrations is a routine and important evaluation in newborn infants. Since the plasma of newborns does not contain pigments such as carotene that would interfere with this assay, direct measurement of the absorbance of bilirubin at 455 nm is proportional to the con-

centration of total bilirubin. Interferences as a result of hemoglobin in the baby's plasma can be corrected by a second spectrophotometric measurement at 575 nm, which is then subtracted from the absorbance at 455 nm. This direct determination of serum bilirubin can only be used on infants less than 1 month of age and samples must be collected and stored with the same precautions as for other bilirubin assays.

## Indicators of Hepatic Detoxification and Excretion Ability

### PLASMA AMMONIA

In addition to the tests of metabolic function, a liver profile usually evaluates the detoxification and excretion ability of the liver. A plasma ammonia concentration is a reflection of the liver's ability to convert toxic ammonia byproducts into urea and then excrete it. Ammonia is a normal product of bacterial action on the contents of the gastrointestinal tract. The portal vein delivers ammonia to the liver, which is the only organ with the necessary enzymes to synthesize urea. The kidney can then easily excrete urea. Elevated plasma levels of ammonia are associated with advanced liver disease, coma, and other neurologic symptoms. Arterial blood ammonia concentrations are elevated in approximately 90% of patients with hepatic encephalopathy but, obviously, some patients will have normal or borderline ammonia levels. There is poor correlation between the clinical severity of hepatic encephalopathy and the degree of elevation of blood ammonia levels.[15]

The most common laboratory determination of ammonia concentrations in plasma is based on the following enzymatic reaction using glutamate dehydrogenase:

$$\text{2-oxoglutarate} + \text{NH}^+_4 + \text{NADPH} \underset{\text{pH 7.4}}{\overset{\text{glutamate dehydrogenase}}{\rightleftharpoons}} \text{glutamate} + \text{NADP}^+ + \text{H}_2\text{O}$$

The NADP+ formed from the conversion of NADPH is measured at 340 nm. These methods have been shown to be both accurate and precise, easily automated, and to use small sample volumes.

The accuracy of all plasma ammonia concentrations is dependent on a reliable sample. Ammonia contamination of samples can be caused by the patient, the phlebotomist or laboratorian smoking while in contact with the sample, atmospheric ammonia being absorbed into the sample, poor venipuncture technique, and poor handling and storage of the sample. Plasma collected in EDTA, heparin, or potassium oxalate is the preferred sample because serum samples have higher and more variable ammonia concentrations. Samples should be immediately placed on ice to prevent the metabolism of other nitrogenous compounds to ammonia in the sample. Blood ammonia concentrations have been shown to increase at a rate of 0.017 $\mu$g/mL of blood per minute at 25°C. Hemolysis in the sample is unacceptable since red cells have a concentration of ammonia 2 to 3 times higher than that of plasma.[16] If the analysis cannot be done immediately, the plasma should be removed from the cells and placed on ice. A frozen sample will be stable for several days.

## EXOGENOUS DYE TESTS

Exogenous dye tests have traditionally been used to test the liver's detoxification and excretion ability. Dye tests first evaluate the liver's ability to transport exogenous substances into the hepatocyte, then its ability to metabolize the substance, usually by conjugating it to make it more soluble, and finally its excretion into bile. These tests may provide a sensitive picture of the functioning of the liver as a whole. However, they are not routinely performed currently because of the problems associated with the administration of exogenous substances to presumably ill patients. At present, the most frequent tests of detoxification and excretion are based on the determinations of endogenously produced substances such as bilirubin and bile acids.

## BILE ACIDS ASSAYS

Bile acids have two major roles in the body and both are formed exclusively by the liver. They are the final products of the metabolism of cholesterol and play a role in the overall digestion of lipids, allowing for more effective elimination of excess cholesterol and other lipids through the bile. Bile acids help to control the composition of bile by increasing the excretion of substances such as bilirubin, cholesterol, lecithin, and water. Bile acids have an extensive enterohepatic recirculation and almost 90% of bile acids are reexcreted through the liver. Bile acids compose the major group of organic anions excreted by the liver and appreciable amounts are found in the plasma if the liver's uptake or excretory function is impaired. Determination of serum bile acid concentrations adds little diagnostic value to other more routinely used analytes.

The current laboratory methods for the determination of bile acids are based on complex methods such as gas chromatography, enzymatic methods, or immunoassays. These methods are accurate and sensitive enough to measure the very small concentrations normally found in plasma. The plasma concentrations found in a fasting specimen give more relevant information than random or postprandial specimens in the detection of mild liver disease.

## FECAL AND URINE UROBILINOGEN

The formation of a group of colorless compounds known as urobilinogen is the result of the reduction of conjugated bilirubin by the normal bacteria found in the gut. These compounds are readily dehydrogenated to urobilins, resulting in an orange color, and the combination of urobilinogens and urobilins are found in the feces. Urobilinogen undergoes enterohepatic circulation with approximately 10% to 20% of the amount found in the intestines being reabsorbed. Most of the reabsorbed urobilinogen is recirculated to the liver, where it is reexcreted into the bile and eventually into the feces. A fraction of the ab-

sorbed urobilinogen is not accepted by the liver and circulates to the kidney, where it is excreted, resulting in a reference range of 0 to 4 mg/24 h for urinary urobilinogen. Increased fecal and urine urobilinogen concentrations are seen in conditions in which there is an overproduction of heme by-products, causing increased formation and excretion of bilirubin. Decreased concentrations are found in hepatic diseases and intrahepatic and extrahepatic obstructions. When the reference range for urinary urobilinogen is considered, it is obvious that decreased concentrations will be impossible to detect. Visual examination of a fecal specimen with decreased urobilinogen reveals the characteristic gray or clay-colored feces. Tests for fecal urobilinogen concentrations are rarely performed but the same assay for urine urobilinogen can be applied using an aqueous extract of fresh feces.[1]

The laboratory determination of fecal and urine urobilinogen is based on Ehrlich's reaction using acidic paradimethylaminobenzaldehyde to give a red color. Alkaline ferrous hydroxide is added to reduce any urobilin in the sample to urobilinogen and sodium acetate reduces interferences from other chromagens that may react with Ehrlich's reagent. Because bilirubin interferes with this reaction, any significant amounts in the sample must be removed by filtration after the addition of barium chloride. Fresh samples are required since oxidation converts the urobilinogen to urobilin on standing.

## Enzyme Determinations

Enzyme determinations prove to be useful in the diagnosis, prognosis, and evaluation of liver diseases. The most clinically significant enzymes for liver disease are the aminotransferases (both alanine and aspartate aminotransferase), gammaglutamyltransferase, and alkaline phosphatase. Each of these enzymes provides a different perspective on the functioning of the liver but all are used to detect active parenchymal liver cell damage (Table 16–4).

### AMINOTRANSFERASES

Alanine aminotransferase (ALT) is found predominantly in the liver, and aspartate aminotransferase (AST) is found in nearly equal amounts in the heart, skeletal muscle, and liver. Elevations of both of these enzymes result from leakage from damaged or necrotic cells. AST is present in the mitochondria and cytosol of the liver cell and ALT is found only in the cytosol. These enzymes show an early rise in almost all diseases of the liver and remain elevated for a period of 2 to 6 weeks. The highest concentrations (greater than 1,000 IU/mL) are seen in acute conditions such as viral hepatitis, drug and toxin-induced hepatic necrosis, and hepatic ischemia but the elevations do not correlate well with the extent of damage to the liver. Generally the ALT concentrations will be higher than the AST concentrations in acute liver diseases, although it is difficult to differentiate liver diseases based on AST and ALT alone. If the level of AST exceeds that of ALT in a known liver problem, the prognosis is poor and indicates massive cell necrosis.

TABLE  16-4

**Expected Enzyme Activities in Various Liver Diseases**

| ENZYME | ACUTE HEPATITIS | CIRRHOSIS | CHRONIC LIVER DISEASE | ALCOHOLIC LIVER DISEASE | OBSTRUCTIVE DISEASE | HEPATIC TUMORS |
|---|---|---|---|---|---|---|
| Aspartate aminotransferase | ↑↑ | N, ↑ | ↑ | ↑ | ↑ | ↑ |
| Alanine aminotransferase | ↑↑↑ | N, ↑ | ↑ | ↑ | ↑ | ↑ |
| Alkaline phosphatase | ↑ | N, ↑ | N, ↑ | N, ↑ | ↑↑↑ | ↑↑ |
| Gamma-glutamyltransferase | ↑ | N, ↑ | N, ↑ | ↑↑↑ | ↑↑ | ↑↑↑↑ |
| Lactic dehydrogenase | ↑↑ | ↑↑ | N, ↑ | N, ↑ | N | ↑↑↑ |

N = Normal; ↑ = elevated.

Decreasing levels of these enzymes usually correspond with recovery of the liver function but rapid decreases may indicate severe necrosis of the hepatocytes with an inability to produce enzymes and irreversible liver damage. Because both ALT and AST increase with other disease states, it is important to correlate these results with other laboratory tests such as other enzyme levels, serum bilirubin levels, and other tests related to the specific disease states suspected for a definitive diagnosis.

## GAMMA-GLUTAMYLTRANSFERASE

Gamma-glutamyltransferase (GGT) is a microsomal enzyme that is increased in many conditions involving the pancreas, hepatobiliary system, and the kidney. Even though the enzyme is found in the greatest concentrations in the kidney, its usefulness is in the diagnosis of liver diseases. Serum GGT has a high specificity for liver disorders such that abnormal plasma activity is found in about 90% of patients with liver disease.[8] GGT is often used in conjunction with an alkaline phosphatase test to differentiate between liver and bone diseases, especially in children because alkaline phosphatase levels are naturally increased due to rapid bone growth. Hepatic enzyme-inducing drugs such as phenytoin, the tricyclic antidepressants, benzodiazepine tranquilizers, and warfarin cause plasma GGT increases when there is no indication of hepatic malfunction.[8] GGT is particularly useful in the identification of alcoholic damage to the liver with the reported sensitivity of an elevated GGT for detecting alcohol consumption ranging from 52% to 94%.[17] This allows GGT to be used as an early sign of alcoholic damage when there are no other clinical or laboratory signs of cirrhosis.

## ALKALINE PHOSPHATASE

The alkaline phosphatase (ALP) enzyme is actually a group of enzymes made in the liver, bone, placenta, kidney, and intestine. The increases seen are due to the increased synthesis of the enzyme rather than its release from damaged or necrotic cells. ALP found in serum is primarily of liver or bone

origin, and it is important to distinguish the source of the enzyme. ALP is increased in most hepatic diseases and in both intrahepatic and extrahepatic obstructive diseases, but the highest elevations (more than 3 times the upper limit of normal) are more likely to represent obstructive disease. Liver disease resulting in the necrosis of hepatocytes does not usually increase ALP, unless there also is necrosis of the bile canaliculi or ductules. A normal ALP found in a jaundiced patient will essentially rule out an obstruction. Any bone disease associated with increased osteoblastic activity will have correspondingly increased ALP activity, so it is important to remember that growing children and women in the third trimester of pregnancy will have increased concentrations of ALP due to increased bone growth and the presence of ALP placental isoenzyme.

## LACTIC DEHYDROGENASE, LEUCINE AMINOPEPTIDASE, 5'-NUCLEOTIDASE

Lactic dehydrogenase (LD), leucine aminopeptidase (LAP), and 5'nucleotidase (5'NT) are also elevated in patients with liver diseases but give little additional diagnostic information than the enzymes discussed previously. LD-5 is the liver-specific isoenzyme of total LD and usually indicates hepatocellular necrosis or metastatic liver carcinoma. LAP and 5'-NT are enzymes used to increase the specificity of the ALP enzyme. LAP is an enzyme usually associated with pancreatic carcinoma when there is also biliary tract involvement, and 5'-NT can distinguish between the elevated ALP of bone growth from that of liver origin. Both enzyme levels usually correspond to ALP concentrations and give essentially the same information concerning obstructive diseases but do not increase with bone involvement. Interpretation of increased ALP concentrations is easier if paired with either LAP or 5'-NT. If concentrations of both enzymes are increased, hepatic involvement is probable, and if the LAP or 5'-NT is normal while the ALP is increased, other processes are probably responsible for the increase.

## CLINICAL APPLICATIONS

### Jaundice

Jaundice is a condition characterized by a yellow discoloration of the skin, sclera, and mucous membranes. It is most frequently caused by an increase in the concentration of bilirubin in the circulation, although it can be caused by other substances such as carotene or certain drugs. Conjugated bilirubin causes more jaundice than unconjugated bilirubin because of its higher water solubility and easier absorption into tissues. Conjugated bilirubin is easily bound to elastin tissue and other tissues that have a high protein content. Overt jaundice is noticeable in the patient when the bilirubin content rises above 2 to 3 mg/dL of serum (Figure 16–6).

Jaundice is classified into three general categories: prehepatic, hepatic, and posthepatic jaundice. In both prehepatic and posthepatic jaundice types, the function of the liver itself is not impaired. In many of these situations, the liver is, in fact, functioning at its maximum capacity in a compensatory effort to alleviate the problems caused by other factors. This is not the case with hepatic jaundice where the abnormalities are caused by an intrinsic liver defect or disease.

### PREHEPATIC

Prehepatic jaundice is caused by an increased production and release of bilirubin most commonly due to hemolytic processes or ineffective erythropoiesis. Increased hemolysis may be due to a variety of hemolytic anemias, exposure to chemicals, hemolytic antigen-antibody reactions, disease states such as some cancers, and by drugs coating red blood cells (Table 16–5). Ineffective erythropoiesis is a pathologic process where a very low proportion of red cells formed in the bone marrow enter the circulation and those remaining in the bone marrow are prematurely destroyed. An increase in the amount of bilirubin released from the bone marrow results and is called early-labeled bilirubin since it has not been circulating within the red blood cells for 120 days.

The rate of hemolysis and the ability of the liver to transport, conjugate, and excrete bilirubin will determine the degree of jaundice in a patient. In most cases of prehepatic jaundice, the production of bilirubin is well below the capacity of

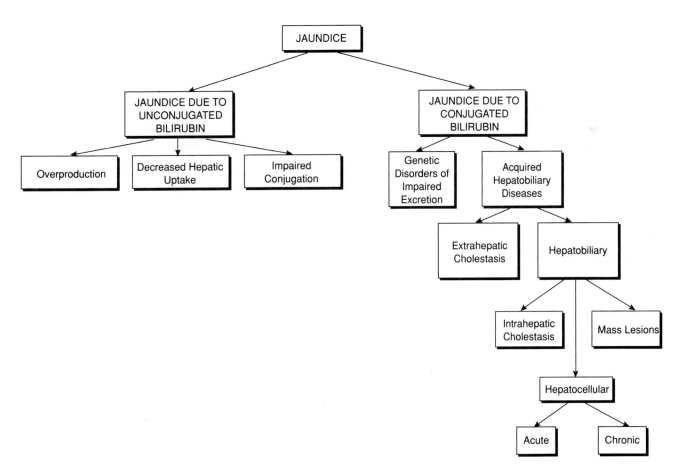

**FIGURE 16-6**

Schematic of the differential diagnosis of jaundiced conditions.

## TABLE 16 - 5

### Causes of Prehepatic Jaundice

| | |
|---|---|
| **Hereditary hemolytic processes** | Hereditary spherocytosis<br>G-6-PD Deficiency<br>Sickle cell disease<br>Thalassemia<br>Hemoglobin C disease |
| **Acquired hemolytic processes** | Hemolytic disease of the newborn<br>Hemolytic transfusion reactions<br>Drug-induced hemolytic anemia<br>Autoimmune hemolytic anemia<br>Paroxysmal nocturnal hemoglobinuria |
| **Ineffective erythropoiesis** | Megaloblastic anemias<br>Sideroblastic anemia<br>Erythroleukemia<br>Lead poisoning |
| **Physiologic jaundice of the newborn** | Prematurity |
| **Impaired delivery of bilirubin to the liver** | Congestive heart failure |

the liver to conjugate and excrete it. Serum bilirubin levels may still be essentially normal when there is a 50% reduction in red cell survival as long as liver function is normal.[18]

Liver function tests are helpful in the diagnosis of prehepatic jaundice (Table 16–6). The increase in bilirubin is the most obvious abnormality, being primarily of the unconjugated type. Depending on the degree of hemolysis, varying amounts of bilirubin enter the liver and corresponding amounts of conjugated bilirubin are found in the intestine. This causes an increased formation of urobilinogen in the gut that is excreted in the feces or absorbed into the enterohepatic circulation and ultimately excreted in the urine. There should be no bilirubin found in the urine because the increase is of the unconjugated type, which is not filtered by the glomerulus of the kidney. Liver enzyme assays should be normal in this condition except in conditions where there is hemolysis. In these situations, LD will be increased due to the high concentration of LD found within red cells that is now released into the plasma.

## HEPATIC

Jaundice of the hepatic type can be subdivided into two types: retention and regurgitation jaundice. **Retention jaundice** results from a defect in the transport of bilirubin into the hepatocyte. **Regurgitation jaundice** occurs when the hepatic cell is damaged or defective or the excretion of products from

## TABLE 16 - 6

### Expected Laboratory Results in Prehepatic, Hepatic, and Posthepatic Jaundice Conditions

| LIVER FUNCTION TEST | PREHEPATIC JAUNDICE | ACUTE HEPATOCELLULAR JAUNDICE | CHRONIC HEPATOCELLULAR JAUNDICE | POSTHEPATIC JAUNDICE |
|---|---|---|---|---|
| Total bilirubin | Normal to Increased | Increased | Increased | Increased |
| Conjugated bilirubin | Normal to Increased | Increased | Increased | Increased |
| Unconjugated bilirubin | Increased | Increased | Increased | Increased |
| Urine urobilinogen | Increased | Increased | Increased | Decreased |
| Urine bilirubin | Normal | Increased | Increased | Increased |
| Albumin | Normal | Normal | Decreased | Normal |
| Globulin | Normal | Normal | Increased | Normal |
| Aminotransferases | Normal | Increased AST<br>Increased ALT | Increased AST<br>Increased ALT | Normal to slight increase in AST and ALT |
| Alkaline phosphatase | Normal | Normal to 3× ULN | Normal to 3× ULN | Increased to 10× ULN |
| Lactic dehydrogenase | Increased when hemolysis is present | Increased | Increased | Normal |
| Prothrombin time | Normal | Normal | Prolonged | Normal |

ULN = upper limits of normal.

the hepatocyte is impaired. In the retention type of jaundice, the conjugated bilirubin level is less than 0.2 mg/dL, the urine bilirubin negative, and the urine urobilinogen is decreased or normal. If there is a regurgitation type of jaundice present, uptake, conjugation, and excretion impairment are present because of damaged liver cells. This condition produces increased total bilirubin, conjugated bilirubin, and urine bilirubin levels. In addition, the urine urobilinogen level is increased because uptake is blocked, even though the fecal urobilinogen may be decreased and stool color is lighter than usual. Conjugation enzyme deficiencies, Gilbert's disease, and Crigler-Najjar syndrome are examples of causes of retention jaundice, and Dubin-Johnson syndrome, Rotor syndrome, viral hepatitis, and neoplastic conditions are examples of regurgitation jaundice (Table 16–7). These disease processes will be discussed in detail later in this chapter.

Laboratory values will vary within the category of hepatic jaundice (Table 16–6). Although the total bilirubin concentration will invariably be increased, the relative amounts of unconjugated and conjugated bilirubin vary according to the defect in the disease process. In general, a decreased amount of bilirubin reaches the intestines because of the malfunctioning liver and results in a decreased amount of urobilinogen being formed and excreted into the feces. This is reflected in less urobilinogen being absorbed into the enterohepatic circulation and a decreased amount of urobilinogen being excreted into the urine. A very small amount of urobilinogen is normally excreted in the urine so a lower than normal value is difficult to determine. If the conjugated bilirubin concentration is increased, an increased urine bilirubin can also be expected.

### TABLE 16–7
#### Causes of Hepatic Jaundice

| Retention jaundice | Physiologic jaundice of the newborn |
|---|---|
| | Gilbert's syndrome |
| | Crigler-Najjar syndrome, types I and II |
| Regurgitation jaundice | Dubin-Johnson syndrome |
| | Rotor's syndrome |
| | Recurrent benign intrahepatic cholestasis |
| | Cholestatic jaundice of pregnancy |
| | Cirrhosis |
| | Viral hepatitis |
| | Alcoholic liver disease |
| | Drug-induced liver disease |
| | Primary biliary cirrhosis |
| | Postoperative jaundice |
| | Hepatocellular carcinoma |
| | Toxic liver injury |
| | Autoimmune liver disease |
| | Inborn errors of metabolism |

### TABLE 16–8
#### Causes of Posthepatic Jaundice

Common bile duct stone
Cancer of the bile ducts, pancreas, ampulla of Vater
Bile duct stricture or stenosis
Sclerosing cholangitis
Choledochal cysts
Biliary atresia in infants

### POSTHEPATIC

Posthepatic jaundice, or obstructive jaundice, is caused by a blockage of the flow of bile from the liver (Table 16–8). Although the liver itself is not the cause of the problem, bile produced by the liver cannot be released into the intestines and overflows back into the blood. Although a complete blockage of the flow of bile is uncommon, partial and intermittent obstructions are likely, and the jaundice found in conjunction with this condition varies. The most common obstructions are stones within the common bile duct, an obstructing neoplasm of the pancreas or other organs in close proximity to the ducts, or strictures severe enough to cause a blockage. Stones are usually formed in the gallbladder and rarely cause symptoms until they travel through the small ducts and lodge there. Strictures can be caused by congenital defects in the ducts or trauma to the ducts during abdominal surgery.

In posthepatic jaundice, the increase in bilirubin is almost entirely of the conjugated type (Table 16–6). Because of the requisite obstruction, the quantity of bilirubin reaching the intestines is decreased, resulting in clay-colored feces. This color is due to the decreased formation of urobilinogen from bilirubin in the intestines and its decreased excretion. There should be little or no urobilinogen but large quantities of bilirubin in the urine. The kidney provides the only route of excretion for the increased levels of conjugated bilirubin in the plasma, and the yellow-orange urine color reflects this excretion of bilirubin. Often there is no correlation between the plasma concentration of conjugated bilirubin and the concentration of bilirubin excreted in the urine. Much of the conjugated bilirubin in obstructive conditions circulates covalently bound to albumin and is called delta bilirubin. Since delta bilirubin is protein-bound, it cannot pass the glomerulus of the kidney, and therefore urinary bilirubin concentrations are less than expected when the serum concentrations of conjugated bilirubin are significantly elevated. When there is prolonged cholestasis, the liver may be damaged, resulting in decreased conjugation ability. Under these circumstances, the unconjugated bilirubin may be increased in a posthepatic jaundice, although rarely to the degree that conjugated bilirubin is elevated.

### NEONATAL

A fourth category of jaundice is a special type of jaundice applicable only to the newborn. Neonatal jaundice is a condition defined as having total serum bilirubin concentrations above 15 mg/dL in the few days following birth or bilirubin levels persisting above 10 mg/dL for more than 2 weeks. The newborn is expected to have a much higher bilirubin concentration than an adult because of the significant amount of hemolysis occurring during birth and the infant's immature liver. Before birth, the fetus is entirely dependent on the mother's liver to perform the necessary functions. The enzymes necessary for metabolism and conjugation are not present in the neonate in sufficient concentrations and do not function efficiently for a few days after birth. These two conditions, as well as an increased rate of absorption of unconjugated bilirubin from the infant's intestinal tract, often cause bilirubin levels to rise to 10 mg/dL before the liver can begin to clear the excess bilirubin from the plasma. In premature and some full-term infants, bilirubin concentrations rise above the expected levels and medical treatment should be considered to assist the removal of excess bilirubin to prevent the development of kernicterus. **Kernicterus** is the deposition of unconjugated bilirubin in the central nervous system that may cause severe neurologic damage. Treatment of this hyperbilirubinemia is usually phototherapy with monochromatic blue light to cause the oxidation of bilirubin to more soluble end products and enhance the renal excretion of the bilirubin.[19] In severe situations, the use of enzyme-inducing drugs such as phenobarbital or exchange transfusions may be used to reduce bilirubin concentrations. Bilirubin levels usually peak at 2 to 3 days postpartum followed by a rapid fall to normal infant concentrations. When the elevated bilirubin levels persist beyond 2 weeks or continue to increase above 15 mg/dL, an aggressive effort should be made to establish the cause of the liver dysfunction. Several pathologic conditions such as biliary atresia, ABO or Rh incompatibility, septicemia, neonatal hepatitis, or inherited metabolic liver diseases cause these symptoms to continue and worsen and the infant should be evaluated immediately.

Although the concentration of unconjugated and conjugated bilirubin in the plasma and urobilinogen and bile in the urine are important in the differential diagnosis of jaundice, the value of information obtained from other departments of the laboratory and hospital should not be underestimated. The hematology department can greatly assist in the diagnosis of prehepatic disorders, the radiology department in the assessment of posthepatic jaundice, and the immunology section for the diagnosis of infectious hepatic problems.

## Congenital Extrahepatic Biliary Atresia

During the first few days after birth, a significant rise in a newborn's serum bilirubin concentration is not unexpected. This is due to hemolysis occurring during birth as well as the natural immaturity of the infant's liver. Total bilirubin concentrations up to 10 mg/dL are common, especially in premature or postmature infants. Such physiologic neonatal jaundice generally resolves itself within the first 2 weeks of life. When the increase in bilirubin is prolonged or exceeds 15 mg/dL, the

possibility of other causes of hyperbilirubinemia should be considered. A very serious and aggressive condition where the extrahepatic bile ducts become inflamed and increasingly nonfunctional is called **extrahepatic biliary atresia.** In most such cases there are no patent biliary ducts from the porta hepatis, where the portal vein and hepatic artery enter the liver, to the duodenum, where the bile empties into the gastrointestinal tract. There are varying degrees of severity of this obstructive situation but if the flow of bile is not corrected within a short period, more damage to the liver will occur owing to the toxic effects of the stagnant bile products. For the most successful results, correction should occur before the infant is 12 weeks old, so it is important that the condition be diagnosed early.

Extrahepatic biliary atresia is an acquired defect not a hereditary one. Several pathogeneses have been proposed for the development of biliary atresia and are currently under study. These mechanisms include occult viral infections with reovirus type 3, cytomegalovirus or group C rotavirus, exposure of pregnant women to toxic substances, a defect in the morphogenesis of the extrahepatic biliary system, inflammatory and/or autoimmune conditions, and circulatory defects in the fetus and newborn that deprives the liver of blood.[20] Females are affected more often than males, and this condition occurs in 1 of 10,000 to 13,000 live births.[21] Increasing jaundice and hepatomegaly are seen within the first 2 to 3 weeks of life and affected infants have diarrhea and steatorrhea from the lack of bile acids to aid in digestion. The disorder results in cirrhotic liver failure and death within 2 years if not treated successfully.

The clinical and laboratory picture is similar to any obstructive liver disease. The key to prompt diagnosis and treatment is the differentiation of extrahepatic biliary atresia from prolonged neonatal jaundice, a true hepatic jaundice or correctable obstructive diseases. One distinguishing feature is that the hyperbilirubinemia is primarily of the conjugated type in biliary atresia (more than 75%), whereas physiologic jaundice results in an unconjugated hyperbilirubinemia. Serum enzymes do not provide specific information because ALP and GGT are elevated in any obstructive biliary disease. The presence of lipoprotein X also indicates cholestasis but will not specifically identify biliary atresia. In patients with physiologic jaundice, the administration of phenobarbital induces liver enzyme activity and a rapid return to reference values for laboratory results is seen. Phenobarbital does not correct biliary atresia. A liver biopsy is a helpful tool in prompt diagnosis and should not be delayed in those infants with a conjugated hyperbilirubinemia persisting beyond 6 weeks after birth.

The Kasai surgical procedure to alter the path of removal of bile from the liver is the primary treatment available for patients with minimal atresia of biliary ducts. For many children affected, this surgery is not indicated because it does not correct the inherent defect and orthotopic liver transplantation is the only effective treatment for these patients. With advances in surgical techniques and immunosuppression therapies, biliary atresia is the most frequent indication for liver transplantation in infants and children.[20]

## Hemolytic Anemias

**Hemolysis** refers to premature erythrocyte destruction and includes both ineffective erythropoiesis and increased lysis. Liver function studies are helpful in the assessment of the severity of the hemolytic process but should not be used for an initial diagnosis. Specific laboratory testing to identify the source of the hemolysis is required. The liver is functioning properly in these situations and only when the liver's ability to dispose of the excess bilirubin is exceeded will liver function studies be abnormal.

There are two categories of processes that will cause increased hemolysis of erythrocytes, **intrinsic** (or **congenital**) **hemolysis** and **extrinsic** (or **acquired**) **hemolysis.** Intrinsic hemolysis is caused by a defect or condition within the cell itself, usually an acute or chronic hemolytic anemia. Abnormalities of the red cell membrane as in hereditary spherocytosis or hereditary elliptocytosis, errors in metabolic pathways in conditions such as glucose-6-phosphate dehydrogenase deficiency and other enzyme deficiencies, and hemoglobinopathies such as sickle cell anemia are characterized by these hemolytic processes. Foreign effects on normal erythrocytes causing hemolysis is called extrinsic hemolysis. Drug-induced, immune, or autoimmune hemolytic anemias are the most common causes of extrinsic hemolysis. Hemolytic transfusion reactions and hemolytic disease of the newborn are also causes of extrinsic hemolysis. Treatment of the cause of the hemolysis corrects related abnormal liver function.

The most prominent abnormal liver function result in a patient with a hemolytic anemia is an increase in total bilirubin concentration, being predominantly of the unconjugated type. The urine does not contain bilirubin because the increase in serum concentration is of the insoluble, albumin-bound fraction. Increases in urine urobilinogen, hemosiderin, and hemoglobin reflects the extent of the hemolysis. Fecal urobilinogen should also be increased because this is the major route of elimination of hemoglobin byproducts. LD is increased because of the high concentration of this enzyme within the red cell that is released during hemolysis, and not because of damage to the liver. Liver enzymes such as AST, ALT, GGT, and ALP are found in normal activities.

## Cirrhosis

Cirrhosis literally means a yellow-orange condition of the liver. The architecture of the liver is permanently destroyed and this condition is the end stage of a number of different disease processes.

### WILSON'S DISEASE

Wilson's disease is an inherited disorder characterized by defective metabolism and excretion of copper. The disease was first described in 1912 but not until the mid-1940s was copper proven to be the causative agent. This inborn error of copper metabolism is caused by a defective gene on chromosome 13 and affects many systems in the body, especially the liver, cornea, kidney, and brain. The prevalence of the disease is from 1 to 3 per 100,000 persons, affecting males and females equally.[22] Copper excretion from the liver is the primary defect in Wilson's disease and is caused by a mutation of the gene for a copper-transporting adenosine triphosphatase, *ATP7B*.[22] Identification of the gene for Wilson's disease has enabled genetic diagnosis of this disorder. However, there are more than 60 disease-specific mutations now described.[23]

Wilson's disease is rarely detected in young children, and is only diagnosed when the accumulated copper begins to show toxic effects. The typical age of presentation for Wilson's disease is 10 to 13 years.[22] Only a small quantity of copper is required for normal metabolic functions, and it is particularly active as a cofactor in certain enzymatic reactions. In Wilson's disease normal amounts of copper are ingested but since the liver is unable to excrete the copper into bile, it accumulates in the liver and other tissues. After many years of ingesting more copper than can be metabolized, normally functioning liver tissue is destroyed by the metal's toxic effect. This results in decreased liver function that resembles chronic viral hepatitis. Copper is released from the damaged hepatocytes into the circulation, resulting in elevated serum copper concentrations. Complicating this situation is the fact that the liver is the primary site of production for the copper-transporting protein, ceruloplasmin. When excess copper damages the liver, it synthesizes minimal amounts of ceruloplasmin, which would help to distribute the excess copper.

Because the physical signs and symptoms are identical in the two conditions, Wilson's disease is often misdiagnosed as viral hepatitis. The most significant problem with this incorrect diagnosis is that specific treatment for Wilson's disease will be withheld. Wilson's disease can be treated effectively with the chelating agents, penicillamine or trientine, or with zinc acetate, which reduces intestinal absorption of dietary copper. These treatments will improve existing symptoms and prevent much of the permanent neurologic damage caused by the toxic effects of copper on nervous tissue if instituted early in the disease process.

Wilson's disease should be investigated in any young patient suspected of having viral hepatitis and presenting hemolysis. Hemolysis is a common finding in Wilson's disease because the excess free copper alters red cell membrane stability by oxidative injury.[22] Younger patients often present with hepatic symptoms and older patients with neurologic symptoms. Common neurologic problems in Wilson's disease include tremors, excessive salivation, loss of fine motor coordination, and psychiatric disorders such as bizarre behavior, schizophrenia, depression, and psychosis.[22] Most patients exhibiting the neurologic and psychiatric manifestations of the disease will also demonstrate Kaiser-Fleischer rings in the eyes. These rings are deposits of copper found in the Descemet's membrane of the cornea and are highly suggestive for Wilson's disease.

Laboratory results expected in Wilson's disease include increased 24-hour urinary copper excretion ($>100$ $\mu$g/24 hours) and decreased ceruloplasmin concentrations ($<20$ mg/dL).[22] A liver biopsy allows for the determination of hepatic copper concentrations that are elevated to more than 250 $\mu$g/g dry weight. Laboratory results indicating liver damage are increased ALT and AST concentrations, hyperbilirubinemia, low serum albumin concentrations, or deficiencies of coagulation factors that may result in bleeding and bruising.

Wilson's disease is progressive and fatal if not treated. Some advanced cases have been treated with liver transplantation with subsequent complete reversal of the disease. Lifelong treatment with penicillamine, trientine, or zinc acetate reverses the hepatic symptoms of the disease, often lessens the current neurologic and psychiatric disturbances, and prevents further complications.

## ALPHA₁-ANTITRYPSIN DEFICIENCY

Alpha₁-antitrypsin deficiency is the most common genetic cause of liver disease in children and the most frequent genetic diagnosis for which children undergo liver transplantation. It is also the most common genetic cause of pulmonary emphysema in adults.[24] The most common genetic mutation resulting in a severe deficiency, PiZZ, is a single amino acid substitution caused by the gene located on the long arm of chromosome 14. The lung damage in this condition is caused by proteolytic attack on lung elastin but damage to the liver involves a different process, one of destruction of liver cells due to accumulation of abnormal alpha₁-antitrypsin in the endoplasmic reticulum of hepatocytes.

Alpha₁-antitrypsin is a glycoprotein formed in the liver that inhibits the action of trypsin and other proteases. It is the major component of alpha₁-globulins, and if this protein is not present in sufficient quantities to prevent the action of these hydrolytic enzymes, tissue damage occurs. This inherited defect causes decreased synthesis of alpha₁-antitrypsin and emphysema or cirrhosis. Many patients with a deficiency of alpha₁-antitrypsin present at a very early age with jaundice and hepatomegaly. These symptoms may disappear within a few months, however, leaving only mildly abnormal liver function test results. Persons with decreased concentrations of alpha₁-antitrypsin will develop chronic obstructive pulmonary disease much earlier in life than those who do not have a deficiency. Studies show that the average age of development of airflow obstruction in patients with alpha₁-antiglobulin deficiency ranges between 45 and 50 years of age, in contrast to normal individuals of 60 to 70 years of age.[25] Invariably the hepatic form of alpha₁-antitrypsin deficiency demonstrates increased bilirubin concentrations as well as AST and ALP increases. Since this protein makes up 80% to 90% of the alpha₁-globulin fraction of serum, routine serum protein electrophoresis demonstrates a significant decrease in the alpha₁-globulin peak. Isoelectric focusing techniques used to identify the specific protein and a liver biopsy are necessary for a definitive diagnosis.

The severity of symptoms and the patient's prognosis are variable, depending on the degree of deficiency of the alpha₁-antitrypsin. Treatment with purified and recombinant plasma alpha₁-antitrypsin by either intravenous or intratracheal aerosol administration has proven effective in treating those patients with emphysema. This therapy is associated with increased serum concentrations of alpha₁-antitrypsin without significant side effects.[24] Replacement of alpha₁-antitrypsin by somatic gene therapy has also been discussed in the literature.[25] There is no specific therapy for patients with alpha₁-antitrypsin–associated liver disease except for supportive care, but this inherited disorder has been essentially corrected in those patients receiving a liver transplant.

## HEMOCHROMATOSIS

Hemochromatosis is a condition characterized by an increase in iron stores and the development of toxic damage due to high concentrations of iron in tissues. This may be inherited as a defect in iron metabolism or acquired from any condition that would increase the availability of iron for metabolism. Acquired hemochromatosis may be found in patients with thalassemia, hereditary spherocytosis, sideroblastic anemia, excessive administration of oral iron supplements, or through multiple blood transfusions.[26] Persons receiving more than 50 transfusions are at high risk for acquired hemochromatosis. Hereditary hemochromatosis is inherited by an autosomal recessive trait and results in increased storage of iron in cells of the liver, heart, pancreas, and other organs. The apparent defect is an increase in the absorption of iron from the gastrointestinal tract in which dietary intake of iron is normal but over many years of increased absorption, the iron accumulates in the cells. Most cases of hereditary hemochromatosis are not identified until the patient is middle-aged, with a mean age at presentation of 50 years.[27] The characteristic features of this condition are not apparent until 20 to 40 g of iron have been stored in the body.[28]

The majority of patients with hereditary hemochromatosis are descended from a common Celtic ancestor who lived 60 to 70 generations ago. They carry a mutation (C282Y) that alters a major histocompatibility complex class I-like protein designated HFE.[29] Homozygous and heterozygous conditions exist and blood donor studies demonstrate that as many as 1 in 10 white Americans carries at least one allele with this mutation.[29] Males with this condition outnumber females by more than 10:1, even though the inheritance pattern is not sex-linked. Females are protected by years of menstruation, which prevents the accumulation of iron that is necessary for the development of symptoms.

The usual clinical symptoms of hemochromatosis include skin pigmentation caused by hemosiderin deposits, hepatomegaly, hypogonadism, and carbohydrate intolerance. The hepatic dysfunction is usually classified as fibrosis or cirrhosis. Serum bilirubin and AST and ALT concentrations are usually only slightly increased. The diabetic state that many patients with hemochromatosis experience is caused by the destruction of the beta islet cells of the pancreas and hepatocytes by the deposition of iron. This may be the same mechanism for the hypogonadism seen in some males with hemochromatosis.

The laboratory diagnosis of hemochromatosis should include serum iron concentrations, total iron-binding capacity, ferritin concentrations, and percent transferrin saturation. The determination of serum iron is neither a sensitive nor specific indication of the hepatic stores of iron, but these values in conjunction with other laboratory values may be of some diagnostic significance. Serum ferritin levels show the greatest correlation with iron stores and may be a guide to the degree of liver damage. A definitive diagnosis requires a liver biopsy and histologic evaluation of storage iron using iron-staining techniques. It is important to identify all affected but asymptomatic family members of known hemochromatosis patients so that treatment can be instituted before there is irreversible damage to tissues. The use of genetic testing is appropriate in all first-degree relatives of known hemochromatosis patients or in cases where the diagnosis is suspected but not certain.[27] Genetic screening of the general population for this condition is not practical.

The preferred therapy for hemochromatosis is regular phlebotomy to remove iron from the body. This forces the body to use stored iron for the synthesis of erythrocytes and depletes the iron stores. Approximately 250 mg of iron can be removed in 500 mL of blood in a weekly phlebotomy. Phlebotomy should be continued until the patient's transferrin saturation is less than 50% and the serum ferritin levels fall to less than 50 ng/mL.[23] Therapy may require 2 to 3 years of weekly phlebotomies before the storage iron can be depleted. Many of the clinical symptoms of hemochromatosis will improve dramatically once the iron concentrations fall into a more normal range, but hepatic fibrosis or endocrine abnormalities usually do not resolve.

## PRIMARY BILIARY CIRRHOSIS

Primary biliary cirrhosis (PBC) is a chronic, progressive, obstructive liver disease characterized by destruction of the intrahepatic bile ducts, the presence of inflammation and scarring, and the eventual development of fibrosis and cirrhosis. There is no known etiology for this condition. Although there seems to be some familial tendency to develop PBC, there is no indication that it is a simple inherited disorder. PBC is primarily a condition of middle-aged women who present with nonspecific complaints of fatigue and itching. At early stages of the disease, jaundice is absent but hepatomegaly and some elevations of ALP are usually present. Other symptoms may be a darkening of the skin due to deposition of melanin, hirsuitism, anorexia, and weight loss. Increased fat excretion in stools with a corresponding decrease in fat-soluble vitamins (vitamins A, E, D, and K) indicates a decrease in the excretion of bile acids from the liver.

The most striking abnormality in PBC is associated with specific humoral and cellular immune responses, which suggests an autoimmune basis. Up to 95% of patients with PBC demonstrate the presence of antimitochondrial antibodies (AMA) in their sera.[30] These antibodies are heterogeneous and react with mitochondria of different organs and different species. The most commonly occurring antibody is anti-M2, which reacts with the inner membrane of mitochondria and is found in more than 95% of patients with PBC. Other antibodies frequently found are anti-M2 with anti-M4 and anti-M8, which indicates a severe form of PBC, and anti-M9, which when found in conjunction with anti-M2 may indicate a mild benign form of the disease.[31] Often abnormalities of the complement system are seen, and complement activation may be responsible for the inflammatory damage to the liver. In one study, 84% of patients with PBC had one disorder of autoimmune origin and 40% had two or more conditions such as autoimmune thyroiditis, scleroderma, or rheumatoid arthritis.[32]

Laboratory findings in patients with PBC include results suggestive of obstructive jaundice such as increased conjugated bilirubin concentrations, increased ALP and GGT, and the appearance of lipoprotein X. Decreased liver function is also indicated by increased serum bile acids levels, increased serum lipid concentrations, especially total cholesterol and phospholipids, and decreased quantities of serum albumin. Confirmation of the presence of antimitochondrial antibodies is a specific diagnostic finding.

Treatment of PBC using ursodeoxycholic acid and low doses of methotrexate is promising in the normalization of laboratory results and slowed progression of the disease.[30] Even so, this treatment has not been shown to improve survival of this condition. Patients who have progressed to complete liver failure have liver transplantation as the only option for treatment. PBC patients are good candidates for transplantation and the procedure offers complete reversal of the disease process.

## Abnormalities of Bilirubin Excretion

### DUBIN-JOHNSON SYNDROME

Dubin-Johnson syndrome produces an obstructive liver disease that reduces biliary excretion of conjugated bilirubin. It is a disorder that is both chronic and benign and is thought to be inherited as an autosomal recessive trait. The liver's uptake, processing, and storage of bilirubin are normal and only the action of removal of bilirubin from the hepatocyte and its excretion into bile are defective. The patient experiences few, if any, symptoms, and often this condition is discovered in the evaluation of other illnesses or in the screening of family members of an already affected individual. Mild hepatomegaly and jaundice may be present. Usually the total bilirubin concentration remains between 2 and 5 mg/dL, with over 50% being the conjugated type, but it may rise to 20 to 25 mg/dL on occasion.[33] Because of the obstructive nature of this condition, much of the conjugated bilirubin circulates bound to albumin as delta bilirubin. This makes laboratory evaluation of the precise concentration of conjugated bilirubin difficult since delta bilirubin reacts as conjugated bilirubin in aqueous solutions of diazo reagent in spite of its combination with albumin. Liver enzymes such as ALP, AST, and ALT are usually normal as well as the concentration of serum bile acids.

The lack of specific laboratory and clinical markers make diagnosis difficult but the use of histologic findings and radiologic examinations of the gallbladder may be helpful. A distinguishing feature of Dubin-Johnson syndrome is the dark pigmented granules found within the liver on biopsy. These are thought to be pigmented lysosomes, and although not specific to this condition, they are a common finding. An unusual finding is that the usual dyes injected for radiologic studies are not excreted by the liver in patients with Dubin-Johnson syndrome so that the biliary system, and especially the gallbladder, are not visible on X-ray film with the use of these dyes. Dubin-Johnson syndrome also demonstrates an abnormal metabolism of the porphyrin waste products, coproporphyrin isomers. A normal individual excretes coproporphyrin through the urine and bile. Seventy-five percent of the total coproporphyrin formed is released in the bile and a majority is coproporphyrin isomer type I. The remaining 25% is excreted in the urine and is predominantly coproporphyrin isomer type III. In Dubin-Johnson syndrome, the total excretion of coproporphyrin is normal, but nearly 80% of the urinary coproporphyrin is isomer type I instead of the usual isomer type III.[4]

More distinctly abnormal laboratory results occur in patients using anabolic steroids and women using oral contraceptives and during pregnancy because these conditions normally increase the excretory load on the liver. But even in these situations, Dubin-Johnson syndrome is a mild disorder with an excellent prognosis and a normal life expectancy. No treatment is necessary.

## ROTOR'S SYNDROME

Rotor's syndrome closely resembles Dubin-Johnson syndrome in that both are characterized by a benign conjugated hyperbilirubinemia that is inherited by an autosomal recessive trait. A reduction in the concentration or activity of the intracellular binding proteins such as ligandin may be the specific defect in this condition. Rotor's syndrome is not progressive, and the only consistent laboratory abnormality is an elevated conjugated bilirubin concentration in both serum and urine. The total bilirubin concentration usually remains between 2 and 5 mg/dL, with over 50% being of the conjugated type. All other liver function tests are normal and patients rarely have complaints other than general fatigue or malaise. In contrast to the Dubin-Johnson syndrome, a liver biopsy does not show the dark pigmentation in Rotor's syndrome. Another distinction between the two conditions is the urinary excretion of coproporphyrin. In Rotor's syndrome there is a 2.5 to 5-fold increase in total coproporphyrin excretion, with up to 65% of the total being of isomer type I.[33] In comparison, Dubin-Johnson syndrome patients excrete normal concentrations of urinary coproporphyrin, 80% being of isomer type I.

Rotor's syndrome is less common than Dubin-Johnson syndrome, has an excellent prognosis, and no treatment is necessary. As with all benign, inherited hyperbilirubinemias, an accurate diagnosis is important to distinguish it from more serious liver diseases that require treatment.

## CRIGLER-NAJJAR SYNDROME

Crigler-Najjar syndrome is a rare, inherited condition caused by a decrease of uridine diphosphate (UDP)–glucuronyl transferase, the primary enzyme responsible for the conjugation of bilirubin. It results from a mutation in one of the 5 exons of the gene coding for this enzyme known as *ugt1*.[34] There are two degrees of severity of this syndrome. Crigler-Najjar syndrome type I is the most severe form, with virtually no detectable level of UDP–glucuronyl transferase in the circulation. Crigler-Najjar syndrome type II is less severe, with activity of UDP-glucuronyl transferase reduced by 90% or more.

Crigler-Najjar syndrome type I is the rarest of the unconjugated hyperbilirubinemias. It is inherited as an autosomal recessive trait and patients will die within the first year of life due to kernicterus, the accumulation of unconjugated bilirubin in the brain and nervous tissue, unless treated. Noticeable jaundice and hepatomegaly are seen early in the life of the infant and become progressively worse. There is no detectable level of UDP–glucuronyl transferase activity in the serum and unconjugated bilirubin concentrations rise to between 20 and 50 mg/dL. The rate of production of bilirubin and its transport into the hepatocyte seem normal but when the liver is unable to conjugate and excrete the bilirubin, it is regurgitated into the blood stream. Since unconjugated bilirubin is not water soluble, it cannot be excreted through the urine. It circulates in higher and higher concentrations and is absorbed into the tissues, with a special affinity for nervous and brain tissues. There is no excretion of conjugated bilirubin in the bile and the concentration of urine and fecal urobilinogen is decreased. Most of the usual laboratory tests for liver function are normal, other than the serum concentrations of unconjugated bilirubin and urobilinogen. The usual therapy for Crigler-Najjar syndrome is to reduce the serum concentrations of bilirubin with exchange transfusions within the first days of life, plasmapheresis, and phototherapy. Ten to 12 hours of phototherapy per 24 hours is required to control bilirubin concentrations even minimally. Treatment with tin-protoporphyrin or zinc-mesoporphyrin decrease the bilirubin temporarily and may reduce the daily requirement for phototherapy.[34] Administration of enzyme-inducing agents such as phenobarbital does not increase enzyme activity and is not an effective treatment for Crigler-Najjar type I. Orthotopic liver transplantation has proven to be successful if performed before the central nervous system complications arise. Liver cell transplantation with normal donor hepatocytes is being investigated with promising results. Normal hepatocytes are administered via percutaneous, transhepatic intraportal route and results show a decrease in the phototherapy required to maintain a total serum bilirubin concentration of approximately

15 mg/dL.[34] Gene replacement and gene repair therapy using recombinant retroviruses and adenoviruses is also an approach to a true cure of Crigler-Najjar syndrome that is currently being investigated.

Crigler-Najjar syndrome type II is also very rare and exhibits a lower than normal activity of UDP–glucuronyl transferase. Most patients have less than 10% of normal activity of this enzyme.[35] Because the liver has minimal conjugating ability, the serum concentration of unconjugated bilirubin usually remains less than 20 mg/dL. Laboratory findings are uniformly normal except for the increased unconjugated bilirubin concentration. Patients have no symptoms other than jaundice and it is rare that treatment is necessary. There have been few deaths due to kernicterus reported in this condition. Phenobarbital administration results in lowered concentrations of unconjugated bilirubin and may be used if clinical jaundice is obvious. Phenobarbital reduces serum bilirubin concentrations in Crigler-Najjar type II by approximately 25%.[34] Treatment must be continued to suppress the return of higher bilirubin concentrations and the attending jaundice.

## GILBERT'S DISEASE

Gilbert's disease is the least serious of the inherited unconjugated hyperbilirubinemias and the most common, affecting 2% to 12.4% of the population.[35] Males are affected more than females, and the inheritance pattern is thought to be one of autosomal dominance with incomplete expressivity. There is some evidence that Crigler-Najjar syndrome type II and Gilbert's disease have a common genetic basis because both conditions have been found within the same families. The activity of UDP–glucuronyl transferase is reduced by 20% to 50% in this condition and the unconjugated bilirubin concentration is only slightly increased, usually between 1 to 3 mg/dL. An unusual finding in this condition is that fasting will increase the bilirubin concentrations significantly. Persons with Gilbert's disease have few symptoms other than mild jaundice and vague complaints such as fatigue, malaise, or abdominal pain. Other laboratory findings such as urobilinogen concentrations and hepatic enzyme activities are normal. The diagnosis is generally made by the persistence of mild unconjugated hyperbilirubinemia, an increase in bilirubin concentrations after a fast, and the lack of any other abnormal liver function tests. No treatment is necessary for this benign condition (Table 16–9).

## Fatty Liver Conditions

### ALCOHOLISM

Ethyl alcohol is a systemic toxin that injures all tissues and, when consumed over a period of time, invariably causes fatty deposits in the liver. Chronic alcohol consumption has been linked with liver disease, especially cirrhosis, since the late 1700s. Since that time, alcohol has been found to have toxic effects on the brain, heart, peripheral nerves, and gastroin-

**TABLE 16-9**

**Heritable, Congenital Disorders of Bilirubin Metabolism**

I. Impaired hepatic uptake
? Gilbert's disease
II. Impaired bilirubin conjugation (decreased glucuronyl transferase deficiency)
1. Gilbert's disease
2. Crigler-Najjar syndrome, types I and II
3. Physiologic jaundice of newborn (normal delayed development of glucuronide conjugating enzyme)
4. Transient familial neonatal hyperbilirubinemia (inhibitory effect of maternal serum on bilirubin conjugation)
III. Impaired hepatic excretion
1. Dubin-Johnson syndrome
2. Rotor's syndrome
3. Cholestasis of pregnancy
4. Recurrent intrahepatic cholestasis

Chen TS, Chen PS: *Essential Hepatology*. Boston, Butterworth Co., 1977. Reprinted with permission

testinal tract as well as the liver. Malnutrition is an additional consideration because alcoholic beverages are deficient in nutrients even though they are high in calories. The body cannot store alcohol, so it must be metabolized, often at the expense of other more vital metabolic functions. The liver has the major role in the metabolism of alcohol, which makes it especially vulnerable to alcohol's toxic effects. Alcoholism is a serious and widespread social and health problem worldwide, and alcohol accounts for about 100,000 deaths per year in the United States.[36]

Alcohol is absorbed from the stomach as well as the large and small intestines. Ninety percent is transported to the liver for oxidation, while the remaining 10% is metabolized and excreted from the kidneys and lungs. Within each hepatocyte, elimination of alcohol requires the cytosolic enzyme system, alcohol dehydrogenase (ADH), to oxidize alcohol to acetaldehyde. This end product is lipid soluble and very reactive and may be more damaging to cells than the original toxin, alcohol. A coenzyme, acetaldehyde dehydrogenase, breaks down the acetaldehyde to acetyl CoA, which is then converted to acetate. The acetate formed can then be oxidized to carbon dioxide and water or enter the citric acid cycle to form other compounds such as fatty acids. $NAD^+$ is an important cofactor and hydrogen ion acceptor in this reaction. A second route of metabolism for alcohol in the liver uses a microsomal ethanol oxidizing system (MEOS). This system becomes most significant in chronic alcohol abusers as a supplement to the alcohol dehydrogenase metabolic pathway. MEOS oxidizes ethanol, oxygen, and NADPH to acetaldehyde, water, and $NADP^+$.

Regular daily consumption of alcohol stresses the liver and the ability of these oxidizing systems to handle the metabolic load is reduced.

Alcoholic injury to the liver can be classified into three groups: alcoholic fatty liver, alcoholic hepatitis, or alcoholic cirrhosis. The earliest stage of liver damage is designated as alcoholic fatty liver, or alcoholic steatosis, and is the most common abnormality following chronic ethanol ingestion. In this condition, the patient rarely has overt symptoms of liver disease, though they may present with hepatomegaly or abdominal pain or tenderness. Patients with more advanced cases may also exhibit nausea, vomiting, anorexia, jaundice, or edema. The typical patient is young to middle-aged with a history of moderate alcohol consumption for 6 months to a year. Alcoholic fatty liver produces very few laboratory abnormalities. A slightly increased AST and ALT activity and an increased GGT activity may be the only laboratory findings of significance. Liver biopsy will show fatty infiltration where fat is collected in vacuoles in the cells' cytoplasm.[37] At this stage of development, a complete recovery within a month is seen with abstinence.

The intermediate stage of liver injury is alcoholic hepatitis. At this point, there is evidence of acute liver inflammation and necrosis, but the clinical picture may vary from a mild syndrome similar to alcoholic fatty liver to the fatal process of liver failure. The typical patient is a middle-aged female with complaints of nausea, vomiting, weight loss, abdominal pain, weakness, and peripheral neuritis. Physical findings often include hepatomegaly, jaundice, ascites, fever, and encephalopathy.[6] Many patients also show signs of malnutrition. Laboratory results reflect more severe liver damage and include increased AST, ALT, GGT, ALP, and total bilirubin concentration of up to 30 mg/dL. Serum proteins, especially albumin, are decreased and the prothrombin time prolonged. This condition may be easily confused with viral hepatitis and it is important to recognize that a history of heavy drinking does not necessarily rule out viral causes of the liver problem. Treatment for this type of liver damage is not specific but avoidance of alcohol ingestion and supportive therapy for any specific complication is indicated. Prognosis is dependent on the type and severity of liver damage.

The most severe damage imposed on the liver by alcohol is alcoholic cirrhosis. It is more common in men than women and most often is discovered when the patient is over 40 years of age. The early symptoms are not specific but classic findings are weight loss, weakness, hepatomegaly, splenomegaly, jaundice, ascites, fever, malnutrition, and edema. Laboratory abnormalities include increased total bilirubin concentrations, decreased albumin levels with increased globulin concentrations, and prolonged prothrombin time. A liver biopsy is the only method by which a definite diagnosis of alcoholic cirrhosis can be made. The prognosis of this condition is affected by complicating factors such as gastrointestinal bleeding or ascites. The 5-year survival of patients with alcoholic cirrhosis and jaundice and/or ascites is approximately 60% in those patients who remain abstinent, but drops to approximately 30%

in persons who continue to drink alcohol.[38] Most frequent causes of death from alcoholic cirrhosis are hepatic failure (27% to 51%), gastrointestinal bleeding (9% to 47%), hepatocellular carcinoma (5% to 16%), infections (3% to 17%), and renal failure (1% to 8%).[6]

## REYE'S SYNDROME

Reye's syndrome is a condition that usually follows an infection with varicella or influenza in children between the ages of 5 and 15.[39] Most frequently, the primary illness runs a natural course for 2 to 4 days and the patient seems to improve when a sudden onset of fever and vomiting and, less commonly, diarrhea develops. Within 24 hours, central nervous system symptoms appear, including lethargy, convulsions, and delirium, and may then progress into coma, respiratory arrest, and death. Reye's syndrome causes a generalized mitochondrial malfunction and results in an acute metabolic disorder of both the central nervous system and liver. There is a strong association between the use of salicylates during viral illnesses and the development of Reye's syndrome. The association has resulted in requiring the use of a warning label on all aspirin and aspirin-containing medications in 1986, and since that time, the incidence of Reye's syndrome has decreased dramatically. Other viruses such as herpesvirus, coxsackievirus, echovirus, and adenoviruses have been implicated, and toxins such as aflatoxin, insecticides, and pesticides are also linked to the syndrome.

Common laboratory findings include a normal total bilirubin concentration, increased AST and ALT activities, a striking increase in serum ammonia concentrations, and a prolonged prothrombin time indicating hepatic necrosis. Other results seen in this condition are decreased serum and spinal fluid glucose concentrations and increased sodium and blood urea nitrogen levels.

Treatment of Reye's syndrome consists of management of the hepatic failure and central nervous system abnormalities that are frequently the cause of death. There is often significant cerebral edema in Reye's syndrome, and reduction in the resultant intracranial pressure with the use of diuretics such as mannitol or glycerol is necessary. The course of this disease is rapid, and even with aggressive medical care, the mortality rate is 42% in recognized cases.[40] The process is reversible in all but the final stages of coma and respiratory arrest, but residual neurologic disorders are seen in many of those who recover from Reye's syndrome.

## THE LIVER IN PREGNANCY

There are normal physiologic changes that make the evaluation of liver function difficult in a pregnant woman. Protein, lipid, and bile acid concentrations are altered, and certain serum enzyme activities reflect both maternal and fetal production. Albumin concentrations are considerably decreased in pregnant women owing to decreased production by the liver and the dilution effect of an increased plasma volume. Peripheral lipolysis accounts for the higher than usual triglyceride, cholesterol, and phospholipids concentrations seen. Significant increases in ALP and LAP activities reflect enzymes of placental origin, not liver origin. GGT activities are generally lower, whereas AST and ALT activities should remain normal during pregnancy. These laboratory values, except for the AST and ALT, can be seen in most mild liver disorders and may not provide much useful information in the evaluation of suspected liver problems during pregnancy. The difficulty lies in making a distinction between the expected variations seen in a normal pregnancy and those variations caused by a true liver disorder.

Acute and chronic hepatitis and alcohol-related liver conditions are common liver disorders in the pregnant woman. The clinical manifestations and outcomes of viral hepatitis, except for hepatitis E, are no different during pregnancy than for the general population, although the viruses may be transmitted to the baby in utero or during delivery. Hepatitis E and hepatitis due to herpes simplex virus is much more dangerous during pregnancy. Hepatitis E has a maternal mortality rate of 15% to 20% and herpes infections, although rare in pregnant women, have a maternal mortality of up to 43%.[41] Alcohol use during pregnancy has more severe consequences for the fetus than the mother. Chronic use may result in fetal alcohol syndrome, which includes facial abnormalities, congenital malformations, growth retardation, central nervous system dysfunctions, and may include abnormal liver function in affected infants.[42] Pregnancy in women with cirrhosis is rare, but when it occurs, morbidity and mortality for mother and infant is high. Cholestasis and common bile duct stones are common causes of jaundice and may require surgery.

There are three unique syndromes that impair liver function during pregnancy. Intrahepatic cholestasis of pregnancy (IHCP) is a rare, benign disorder of late pregnancy and presents with jaundice and pruritus (itching). It resolves rapidly after delivery but is likely to return with future pregnancies. Laboratory test results reflect obstructive liver disease with increased ALP, conjugated bilirubin concentrations, and serum bile acid concentrations. IHCP is associated with an increased risk of prematurity and stillbirth in the baby and an increased risk of postpartum bleeding in the mother.[41]

Acute fatty liver of pregnancy (AFLP) is a rare, but often fatal, disorder of late pregnancy characterized by accumulation of fat within hepatocytes. It occurs in 1 in 13,000 deliveries and is similar to Reye's syndrome in children. The syndrome begins with vomiting and abdominal pain with jaundice and neurologic symptoms appearing within 2 weeks. If untreated, AFLP will progress to fulminent liver failure, uncontrolled bleeding, disseminated intravascular bleeding, coma, and death. Fetal and/or maternal death has been reduced to less than 20% of cases in recent years.[41] AFLP usually does not occur in subsequent pregnancies.

A third complication of pregnancy is called the HELLP syndrome and is seen most frequently in women exhibiting the clinical features of eclampsia or preeclampsia. It occurs in approximately 0.1% to 0.6% of all pregnancies and 4% to 12% of women with severe eclampsia. The mortality rate for women with HELLP is from 1% to 3%.[41] These women have hepatic necrosis and three characteristic laboratory abnormalities, Hemolysis, Elevated Liver enzymes, and Low Platelet counts (HELLP). Hemolysis is due to a microangiopathic hemolytic anemia and both AST and ALT concentrations are increased. Renal dysfunction is another characteristic finding with the HELLP syndrome. A few women develop preeclampsia in more than one pregnancy and therefore are at risk of recurrence of the HELLP syndrome.[42]

## Hepatitis

Hepatitis is characterized by necrosis and inflammation of hepatocytes that results in a decrease in functional ability and abnormal liver function test results. These changes in the liver can be caused by infectious and/or toxic agents. There are now 6 specifically identified hepatitis viruses, known as hepatitis A virus (HAV), hepatitis B virus (HBV), hepatitis delta virus (HDV), hepatitis C virus (HCV), hepatitis E virus (HEV), and hepatitis G virus (HGV) (Table 16–10). A type of hepatitis assumed to be caused by a group of unidentified viruses is designated as non-A, non-E hepatitis (NANE). While there are other viruses that will affect liver tissue, such as cytomegalovirus (CMV) or Epstein-Barr virus (EBV), the liver is the primary, and sometimes exclusive, target of infection for these six viruses. CMV, EBV, and other viruses infect the liver along with other body tissues and hepatic involvement is usually not a predominant feature of the illness.

## Hepatitis A

Hepatitis A is caused by a picornavirus that is a small (27 nm), spherical particle containing single-stranded RNA. The virus replicates in the hepatocyte and is excreted through the bile into the gastrointestinal tract. Hepatitis A virus (HAV) particles are therefore often found in the feces of acutely ill patients, providing the usual fecal-oral route of transmission. HAV is resistant to inactivation by ether, acid, and temperatures up to 60°C for 1 hour but can be inactivated by temperatures of 185°F or higher for 1 minute, ultraviolet irradiation, and formaldehyde solutions. Surfaces can be disinfected with a 1:100 dilution of household bleach in tap water. The virus is quite stable at both refrigerator and freezer storage temperatures.

HAV infection is often associated with poor personal hygiene, a contaminated water supply, or poor public sanitation conditions. HAV can be transmitted parenterally but this is very unusual, and HAV is generally considered to be infectious and spread only by direct, person-to-person contact. Although there is worldwide incidence of HAV, it is found with greater prevalence in underdeveloped countries of the world. In advantaged countries, HAV is frequently seen in epidemic proportions when large numbers of people are confined to common living conditions such as in military facilities, prisons, and psychiatric institutions. Outbreaks are also associated with

**Comparison of Hepatitis Types A, B, C, D, and E**

| ITEM | TYPE OF HEPATITIS | | | | |
|------|------|------|------|------|------|
| | **A** | **B** | **C** | **D** | **E** |
| **TAXONOMY** | | | | | |
| Family | Picornaviridae | Hepadnaviridae | Flaviviridae | Delta viridae | Caliciviridae |
| Genus | Hepatovirus | Ortho hepadnavirus | Unnamed | Deltavirus | Unnamed |
| Genotypes | 7 | 5 | 9 | 3 | 3 |
| **CLINICAL PRESENTATION** | | | | | |
| Age group | Primarily young | All ages | ? All ages | ? All ages | Mostly adults |
| Onset | Abrupt | Insidious | Insidious | Abrupt insidious | Abrupt |
| Inoculation period | | | | | |
| Range (days) | 15–50 | 28–160 | 14–160 | Varies | 15–45 |
| Mean (days) | ±30 | ±80 | ±50 | Varies | ±40 |
| **SYMPTOMS** | | | | | |
| Arthralgias, rash | Uncommon | Common | Uncommon | Uncommon | Common |
| Fever | Common | Uncommon | Uncommon | Common | Common |
| Nausea, vomiting | Common | Common | Common | Common | Common |
| Jaundice | Uncommon in children | Less common than in hepatitis A | Uncommon | Common | Common |
| **LABORATORY DATA** | | | | | |
| Duration of enzymes | Short | Prolonged | Prolonged | Variable | Short |
| **LOCATION OF VIRUS** | | | | | |
| Blood | Transient | Prolonged | Prolonged | Prolonged | Transient |
| Stool | Yes | No | No | No | Yes |
| **OUTCOMES** | | | | | |
| Acute disease | Mild | Moderate | Mild | Can be severe | Severe in pregnant women |
| Mortality | Low | Low | Low | High | As above |
| Chronic hepatitis | No | Yes | Yes | Yes | No |
| Primary hepatocellular carcinoma | No | Yes | Yes | ? No | No |
| **TRANSMISSION** | | | | | |
| Oral | Yes | ? | No | No | Yes |
| Percutaneous | Rare | Yes | Yes | Yes | No |
| Sexual | Yes | Yes | ? | Yes | No |
| Perinatal | No | Yes | ? | No | No |
| *Homologous immunity* | Yes | Yes | Can have second bouts | Yes | ? |
| *Nucleic acid* | RNA | DNA | RNA | RNA | RNA |
| *Size of genome* | 7.5 | 3.2 | 9.4 | 1.7 | 7.5 |
| *Virion size* | 28 | 42 | 38–50 | 43 | 32 |

From Zakem D, Boyer TD: *Hepatology: A Textbook of Liver Disease.* Philadelphia, W.B. Saunders, 1996. p. 1078. Reprinted with permission.

the ingestion of uncooked shellfish harvested from contaminated waters. Persons at special risk in the United States are homosexual men, children, and staff in day care centers and families of children in day care centers. HAV is often underreported since the initial symptoms of the infection are mild and many times go unnoticed. There is serologic evidence that 30% to 50% of the U.S. population has been exposed to HAV but only 3% to 5% can document an illness with symptoms of hepatitis A.[43]

Hepatitis A has an incubation period of 2 to 6 weeks after the initial infection. Fecal shedding of virus particles and the resulting infectivity begins around the last week of the incubation period and usually remains for 2 to 4 weeks. The disappearance of HAV particles in the feces corresponds to the appearance of HAV-antibody in the serum and feces and the increase in aminotransferase activity in the serum. The IgM class of antibody to HAV is the first response to infection and lasts for only a few weeks before the IgG class of HAV antibodies appears. IgG anti-HAV will persist in measurable quantities for many years. It is the basis for proof of infection with HAV and confers absolute immunity to this infection (Figure 16–7).

The physical symptoms of HAV infection are mild and nonspecific. Most are classified as the flulike symptoms of low-grade fever, nausea, vomiting, and muscle aches. Jaundice is seen infrequently but even when noticed is very mild. Generally, children have fewer and milder symptoms than adults. Most infections are acute, self-limited illnesses followed by complete recoveries within 3 to 4 months. Complications are rare and there are no instances of chronic hepatitis or carrier states associated with HAV infections. Fulminant hepatitis A is rare. Abnormal laboratory results may include an increased total bilirubin with approximately equal concentrations of conjugated and unconjugated bilirubin. Increased levels of AST and ALT enzymes may also be seen.

Serologic diagnosis of hepatitis A is based on the identification of the IgM class of HAV antibody in serum of suspected infected individuals. By the time the symptoms of hepatitis are evident, virtually all patients will have detectable levels of this antibody, permitting an accurate diagnosis in 90% to 100% of cases of HAV infections.[43] Total HAV antibody determinations (both IgM and IgG class anti-HAV) are most useful in the determination of the immune status of persons and their resistance to reinfection.

Prevention of hepatitis A consists of maintaining good sanitary conditions and using hepatitis A immune globulin and/or hepatitis A vaccines. Immune globulin affords a passive immunity and is primarily indicated for household contacts of persons with active hepatitis A, for postexposures in known outbreaks of hepatitis A, and for nonimmunized

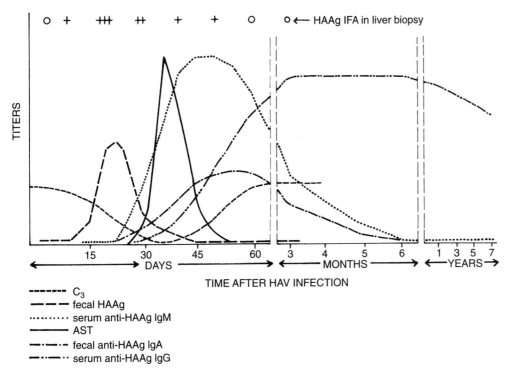

**FIGURE 16–7**

Schematic representation of viral markers in the blood, liver, and feces throughout the course of primary HAV infection. (From Zakim D, Boyer TD: *Hepatology: A Textbook of Liver Disease.* Philadelphia, WB Saunders, 1990. Reprinted with permission.)

international travelers. Two inactivated hepatitis A vaccines have been approved for use in the United States. Both require two doses of vaccine and have a protective efficacy rate of 94% to 100%.[44] Vaccines are recommended for children living in areas where rates of hepatitis are at least twice the national average, for persons traveling to or working in countries that have high endemicity, men who have sex with men, illegal drug users, persons who work with HAV-infected primates or with HAV in a research setting, and persons who have clotting-factor disorders.[44] Treatment of active disease generally consists only of amelioration of symptoms.

## HEPATITIS B

Hepatitis B is a more serious primary illness than hepatitis A and is more likely to result in long-term complications. The hepatitis B virus (HBV) replicates in the hepatocyte and is released from the liver into the peripheral circulation. The primary route of transmission between individuals is through percutaneous and mucous membrane transfer of HBV contaminated blood or blood products. The complete HBV particle, called the Dane particle, is approximately 42 nm in diameter with a surrounding envelope layer and a dense internal core (Figure 16–8). The envelope material is produced in the cytoplasm of the hepatocyte and is composed of lipid and protein. It may be found in the circulation as the coating on the Dane particle, or as incomplete viral strands, or as spheres of envelope material. Its primary antigenic determinant is the hepatitis B surface antigen (HBsAg) and its component subtypes, a, d, y, w, and r. The group-specific determinant (a) is shared by all HBsAg preparations and two pairs of subtype determinants (d,y and w,r) have been demonstrated and act as alleles.[43] The core substance, which is produced in the nucleus of the hepatocyte and has not been demonstrated in plasma, is composed of DNA and DNA polymerase. It is responsible for the hepatitis B core antigen (HBcAg) and the hepatitis B "e" antigen (HBeAg). The presence of the HBeAg correlates with the degree of infectivity and is only present when HBsAg is present. The virus is very stable and has been shown

to retain infectivity for 15 years in serum samples stored at 30 to 32°C.[43] HBV requires heat of 98°C for 20 minutes for inactivation.

Transmission of HBV requires direct contact with blood or body fluids. Common modes of transmission are through transfusions of blood or blood products, punctures with contaminated needles, direct contact of blood with open wounds, intimate contact with sexual partners, or transmission from an infected mother to her newborn infant. Persons with special risks for contracting HBV are percutaneous drug users, health care workers who have frequent contact with blood and/or blood products, patients requiring hemodialysis, hemophiliacs, homosexuals, and persons with multiple sexual partners. Oral transmission has been documented but the inoculum must be large. The Centers for Disease Control and Prevention estimates that there are between 140,000 and 320,000 HBV infections per year in the United States, with approximately 50% of those infections being symptomatic.[45]

Characteristically there is a 1- to 6-month incubation period from the initial exposure to HBV and an average incubation of 6 to 8 weeks. Several weeks before the onset of clinical symptoms, the presence of HBsAg can be demonstrated in serum. Once the clinical symptoms and jaundice appear, the rise in aminotransferases and the appearance of anti-HBc follows. IgM anti-HBc is the first antibody to be detected and persists in high titer for several months. It is then replaced by IgG anti-HBc. The Dane particle markers, HBcAg and DNA polymerase, are present in serum at approximately the same time as HBsAg but do not persist as long as HBsAg. HBsAg can be seen in serum for up to 3 months after the symptoms begin and a rise in anti-HBs is seen only after the disappearance of HBsAg. Anti-HBs is the serologic marker necessary to prove prior infection and resulting immunity to HBV. It is found in 80% to 90% of infected persons and indicates successful resolution of HBV infection. HBeAg rises during the icteric phase of the illness and is followed by the development of anti-HBe, which persists at relatively low titers for several years after infection (Figure 16–9).

Up to 95% of primary infections with HBV are self-limited illnesses and completely resolve within 6 months.[46] Approximately 5% of persons infected with HBV will remain HBsAg positive for more than 20 weeks. A significant number of these patients will clear the antigen over the next year, but many will remain HBsAg positive indefinitely and are designated as chronic HBsAg carriers. These persons retain very high titers of anti-HBc, but there is a wide range of anti-HBs titers detected in the serum. Less than 1% of all persons with HBV infections develop fatal massive hepatic necrosis, but this figure is significantly higher than with HAV infections. There also appears to be a causal relationship between hepatitis B infections and chronic liver disease and hepatocellular carcinoma. In studies of patients with diagnosed liver carcinomas, more than 80% have evidence of previous or current HBV infections. It appears that in geographic areas where there is a high incidence of HBV, the incidence of hepatocellular carcinoma

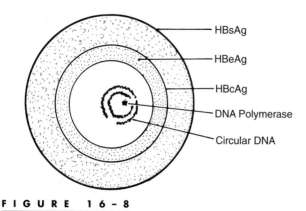

**FIGURE 16-8**

Hepatitis B virus, the Dane particle, with serologic markers identified.

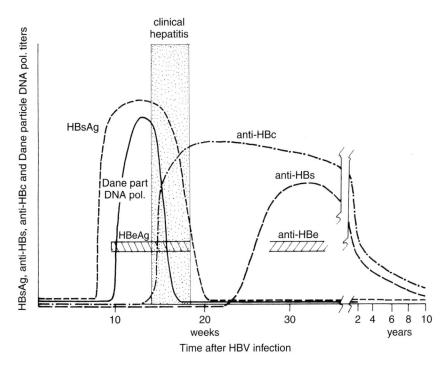

Self-Limited HBsAg Positive HBV Infection

Schematic representation of viral markers in the blood throughout the course of self-limited HBsAg-positive primary HBV infection. (From Zakim D, Boyer TD: Hepatology: *A Textbook of Liver Disease.* Philadelphia, WB Saunders, 1990. Reprinted with permission.)

is also high but the exact mechanism for this relationship is not known.

The clinical course of HBV is variable but uniformly more prolonged and usually more severe than hepatitis A. Symptoms may not be evident in all persons but the most commonly seen include jaundice, fatigue, anorexia, weight loss, malaise, nausea, dark urine and pale stools, and itching. Rashes and muscle and joint pain are seen in some individuals. Abnormal laboratory results reflect the necrotic damage to the liver and include varying degrees of increased serum unconjugated and conjugated bilirubin, increased urine bilirubin, and increased AST, ALT, and ALP enzyme activities. A drop in the serum albumin concentrations indicates a worsening disease.

A specific diagnosis is made through serologic determinations in patients with a clinical and personal history suggestive of hepatitis B infection. A profile of serologic tests, including HBsAg, IgG and IgM anti-HBc, and anti-HBs, provides useful diagnostic information for active infections or to identify past HBV infections. Analysis of a second blood sample drawn 4 to 6 weeks after the initial sample may be necessary to fully establish a diagnosis in patients who do not exhibit an expected serologic pattern on the initial sample. HBV DNA in liver or serum or DNA polymerase in serum is available in a limited number of laboratories. Both of these markers are sensitive in-

dicators of HBV replication. The presence of HBV DNA is the most sensitive marker for ongoing infection; quantification of the amount of DNA may have prognostic significance and has been used as an indicator of response to interferon-alpha-2b therapy.[47]

Until the development of a recombinant technology hepatitis B vaccine, prevention of hepatitis B was based on the prophylactic treatment of exposed individuals with hepatitis B immune globulin (HBIG) and supportive therapy. The Advisory Committee on Immunization Practices (ACIP) recommends the use of hepatitis B vaccine for everyone under 18 years of age and for adults over 18 who are at risk for hepatitis B. These high-risk individuals include sexually active adults with more than one sex partner of the same or opposite sex, illicit intravenous drug users, persons at occupational risk, hemodialysis patients, household and sexual contacts of chronic HBV-infected persons, and clients and staff of institutions for the developmentally disabled. Currently available vaccines show excellent immunogenicity and protective efficacy. Treatment of hepatitis B depends on supportive care and the avoidance of liver damaging substances. Lamivudine is now approved for treatment of hepatitis B, and although the acute response has been good, recurrence of HBV after cessation of therapy has been high.[46] Extended corticosteroid therapy and interferon-alpha-2b has also been used to treat hepatitis B, with little evidence of long-term success.

## Hepatitis D

Hepatitis D is an incomplete RNA virus that requires the presence of HBV in order to replicate. HDV is a 35- to 37-nm particle consisting of an RNA genome and a delta protein antigen, both of which are coated with HBsAg. HDV is transmissible independently; however, because its replication requires the production of HBsAg by HBV, clinical infection with HDV can occur only in the presence of HBV.[48] It is a pathogenic virus causing significant liver damage and producing a more severe illness than is caused by HBV infection alone. The virus is not related to any of the other known hepatitis viruses and was only identified in 1977 as an internal component of certain types of HBsAg particles. Clinical, serologic, and laboratory features are similar to those seen in HBV infections. Although HDV and HBV may occur as simultaneous infections (called coinfection), more frequently HDV infection occurs as a superinfection of persons with established HBV disease. Those with the superinfection are more likely to develop severe liver damage. In North America, HDV is most commonly found in intravenous drug users and in individuals who have received multiple transfusions such as hemophiliacs.[37] The prevalence of HDV varies by geographic region and is therefore more common in areas that are endemic for HBV. HDV is estimated to occur in 1% to 10% of HBsAg carriers in the United States.[43]

The diagnosis of HDV can be made with several serologic assays, including IgM anti-HDV, IgA anti-HDV, HDV Ag, and HDV RNA. In addition to these assays, IgM anti-HBc titers are useful as a means of identifying HDV coinfection because they indicate a recent HBV infection (Figures 16–10 and 16–11).[48] HDV testing should be performed on individuals with an identified HBV infection that is prolonged or more severe than expected.

Since HBV infection is requisite for HDV infection, prevention of HBV through the use of HBV vaccines will also prevent cases of HDV. There is no specific treatment for HDV infections.

## HEPATITIS C

In the late 1980s, a breakthrough in the identification of a specific cause of non-A, non-B (NANB) hepatitis was made. An enveloped, single-stranded RNA virus of the Flaviviridae family was found to be the causal agent of up to 90% of cases of parenterally transmitted NANB. Currently in the United States, 1% to 2% of the general population is believed to have HCV antibodies and approximately 170,000 new cases of hepatitis C are diagnosed annually.[49] Up to 70% of acute infections have no signs or symptoms, which accounts for the fact that the acute phase of HCV infections is not well characterized. The incubation period varies between 2 weeks and 6 months with an average of 45 to 55 days. Fifteen percent of these infections are self-limited and the virus is completely cleared from the body but the remaining 85% become chronic carriers. Exposure to the virus does not confer immunity in

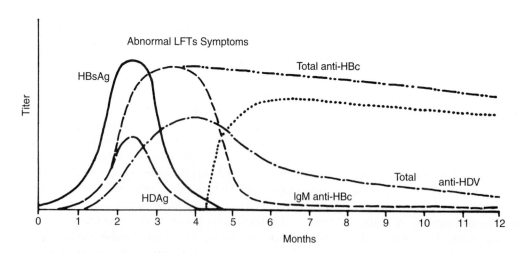

**FIGURE 16-10**

Hepatitis D coinfection serologies (acute HBV and acute HDV). The hepatitis D viral antigen and the HBsAg are both detectable in the blood at approximately the same time. The HDAg and the HBsAg decline in titer in parallel and disappear as their respective antibodies appear. The IgG component of anti-HDV falls much more rapidly than total anti-HBc and becomes negative usually within 1 to 2 years postresolution of acute hepatitis D. (LFT = liver function tests.) (From Krawitt EL, ed.: *Medical Management of Liver Disease.* New York, Marcel Dekker, 1999, p. 49. Reprinted with permission.)

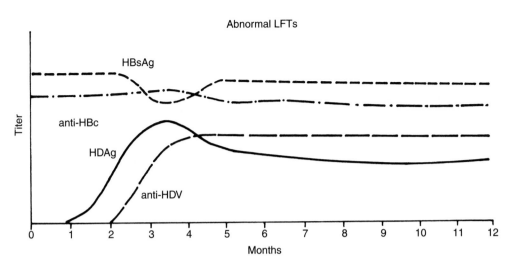

Abnormal LFTs

**FIGURE 16-11**

Hepatitis D superinfection serologies (chronic HBV and acute HDV). The hepatitis D superinfection of a chronic HBV carrier results in transient suppression of the HBV viral replication. This suppression of HBV viral replication causes a decrease in the HBV DNA level in the blood. Since the patient's immune system was unable to clear the original HBV infection, the HDV also invariably becomes chronic as well. Persistent HDV infection is characterized by continuous high levels of both the IgM anti-HDV and IgG anti-HDV. (From Krawitt EL, ed.: *Medical Management of Liver Disease.* New York, Marcel Dekker, 1999, p. 50. Reprinted with permission.)

those few who do not become chronically infected, and persons already infected may become superinfected with different strains of the virus.[50] Most studies report that cirrhosis develops in 10% to 20% of persons with chronic hepatitis C over a period of 20 to 30 years and hepatocellular carcinoma in 1% to 5%.[44] Between 8,000 and 10,000 deaths occur annually in the United States from hepatitis C.[49]

Hepatitis C is transmitted by direct contact through needle inoculation, blood transfusions, organ transplantation, chronic hemodialysis, and nosocomial or occupational exposure. The most common mode of transmission is through intravenous drug use. Transmission by contaminated blood or blood products is rare, calculated to be one in 103,000 units transfused.[50]

HCV infection is most often diagnosed through serologic testing of serum for anti-HCV antibodies by enzyme immunoassay (EIA) or recombinant immunoblot assay (RIBA). These tests detect anti-HCV in more than 97% of infected patients but do not distinguish between acute, chronic, or resolved infection (Figure 16–12).[44] Reverse transcriptase PCR testing for HCV RNA can be performed, although this assay is not currently FDA approved.

Treatment options for HCV are limited. The use of alpha-interferon for 1 year is the recommended treatment for chronic HCV infection but has limited efficacy. Combination therapy of alpha-interferon preparations and ribavirin have had more positive results in preventing the return of viremia but still has less than 50% success.[50] Passive immunization with

intravenous immunoglobulin has not proven effective at all and because HCV has a high rate of mutation, a vaccine has not been developed at this time.

## HEPATITIS E

Hepatitis E is a hepatitis virus identified in 1990 and described as a 27- to 34-nm RNA virus similar to viruses of the Calicivirus family. It is transmitted by the fecal-oral route, and although the acute illness may be severe, it is rarely fatal. Water supplies contaminated with human feces are the most common source of the infection, and person-to-person transmission appears to be very rare. Outbreaks and high seroprevalence of HEV have been reported in India, Pakistan, Afghanistan, Bangladesh, Nepal, Myanmar, Borneo, Algeria, Somalia, Sudan, Ivory Coast, Mexico, China, Vietnam, Thailand, Egypt, and some former Soviet republics.[51] At this time, HEV is not a major threat to developed countries because neither epidemics or sporadic cases of hepatitis E have been documented in the United States or western Europe, although a few cases of HEV acquired in endemic areas have been seen after travelers have returned from these areas.[43]

HEV is similar to HAV in that it is transmitted by the fecal-oral route and does not cause chronic liver disease. Clinical symptoms of HEV infection cannot be distinguished from other forms of viral hepatitis. It affects young adults more frequently than children and has a longer incubation period than HAV. Mortality in the general population is low, at approximately 0.5% to 4%, and fulminant hepatic failure is also rare.

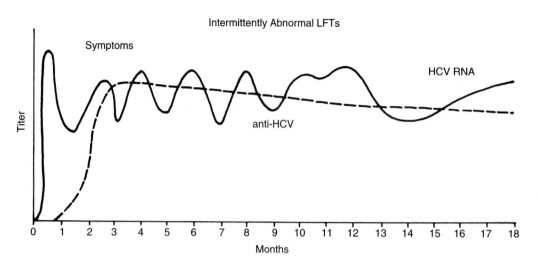

**F I G U R E   1 6 - 1 2**

(Chronic) hepatitis C: Time course of serologies. The HCV RNA rises very rapidly and becomes detectable at high titer within 1 to 2 weeks of the initial exposure. This titer then declines and tends to stabilize at a characteristic level for an individual patient. The HCV antibody (anti-HCV) usually takes 4 to 8 weeks to become positive. This antibody remains positive whether the patient resolves the infection or develops chronic hepatitis. (From Krawitt EL, ed.: *Medical Management of Liver Disease.* New York, Marcel Dekker, 1999, p. 45. Reprinted with permission.)

The most severe disease has been seen in pregnant women, in whom mortality rates range from 20% to 39%.[43] High rates of both infant and maternal mortality are documented in many studies with these deaths, primarily owing to hepatic encephalopathy and disseminated intravascular coagulation.[51]

The diagnosis of acute HEV infection is made by serologic

assays for IgM anti-HEV. EIAs are available using multiple recombinant proteins with high sensitivity for these antibodies. IgM anti-HEV is usually detectable at the time patients present with symptoms and remains positive for several months (Figure 16–13).[37]

There are no passive or active immunizations approved

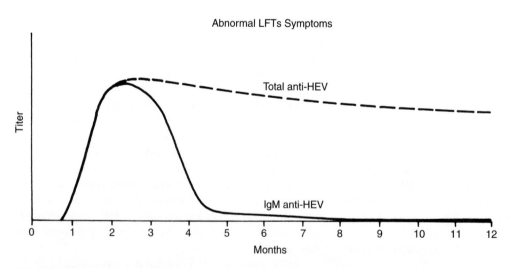

**F I G U R E   1 6 - 1 3**

Generalized time course of clinical events and antiviral serologic response to a hepatitis E infection. The total anti-HEV consists of both the IgM anti-HEV and the IgG anti-HEV. The IgM component declines over time and only the IgG fraction remains detectable after 6 months. (From Krawitt EL, ed.: *Medical Management of Liver Disease.* New York, Marcel Dekker, 1999, p. 50. Reprinted with permission.)

for HEV, and prevention is directed at improving sanitary conditions in underdeveloped countries. Treatment consists of supportive care and most patients recover completely without complications or sequelae.

## HEPATITIS F

One report has identified hepatitis F as a distinct hepatic virus, but confirmation studies have not been able to replicate these findings.

## HEPATITIS G

In 1995–1996, a new virus was recognized as a cause of hepatitis that could not be identified as HAV, HBV, HCV, HDV, or HEV. Designated as HGV or GBV (based on the initials of the surgeon from whom the virus was first isolated), this flavivirus' genome of 9,392 nucleotides has been fully characterized but knowledge of the clinical aspects of this virus is not as complete.[48] HGV has not conclusively been shown to cause clinical disease, and 75% of recipients of HGV-infected transfusions have no biochemical evidence of liver disease.[48] It is distributed worldwide and transmitted parenterally. Those persons at high risk for this infection include intravenous drug users, dialysis patients, multiple-transfusion recipients, and transplant patients. HGV is present in the volunteer blood donor population and active infection has been shown to persist for up to 9 years.[46] The natural history and potential risks of the infection have yet to be fully defined. There is no antibody test for HGV currently and only reverse transcriptase PCR assays can identify infections.

## NON-A, NON-E HEPATITIS

Non-A, non-E hepatitis (NANE) is diagnosed when a patient exhibits all clinical and laboratory signs of a hepatitis infection but the presence of any of the known hepatitis viruses is excluded by serologic testing. Nonviral or toxic damage to the liver must also be ruled out for this diagnosis. NANE was identified as a diagnosis of hepatitis in the 1970s after serologic testing became available for HAV and HBV that allowed for more effective screening of blood donors. The number of cases of post-transfusion hepatitis was predicted to drop dramatically once a screening program was instituted, but this did not occur to the degree expected. It became obvious that another type of virus was causing these illnesses that was not being identified by the available serologic tests. Ninety percent of these cases have since been shown to be caused by HCV. Studies have since shown that there are many antigenically distinct agents causing what is being called NANE hepatitis. Two distinct modes of transmission have been identified for NANE hepatitis: enterically or epidemically transmitted NANE (ET-NANE) hepatitis, and post-transfusion or parenterally transmitted NANE (PT-NANE) hepatitis.

ET-NANE causes a sporadic illness similar in nature to that of HAV and HEV infections. It is a mild disease with few complications. No chronic liver disease develops and most cases can be traced to a single source of infection such as a contaminated water supply. All aspects of this illness are consistent with HAV and HEV epidemics, except that there is no serologic evidence of exposure to either virus.

PT-NANE hepatitis is similar to HBV and HCV infections in mode of transmission and clinical and laboratory aspects. The incubation period is usually 6 to 8 weeks from exposure, and most cases are mild with no significant jaundice. ALT levels increase markedly, an important finding in the absence of serologic markers. The risk of developing chronic hepatitis and serious long-term liver disease is related to the severity of the illness and is a common complication in NANE hepatitis. PT-NANE hepatitis is most often associated with transmission by blood transfusions, although the risk is extremely low (approximately 0.03% per unit transfused) after the addition of anti-HCV screening of blood for transfusion. Less than 10% of post-transfusion hepatitis is now designated as PT-NANE hepatitis.[43] A significant number of persons with NANE hepatitis, however, have no known exposure to a source of infection. It is therefore obvious that there is still much to discover about this disease.

## DRUG-INDUCED AND TOXIC HEPATITIS

Detoxification is one of the major functions of the liver, and for this process to take place, it requires that the entire drug or toxin dose be transported and deposited in the liver. This action makes the liver extremely susceptible to toxic injury. There are a number of toxic substances and therapeutic drugs that will cause direct injury to the liver and result in the inflammatory and necrotic process of hepatitis or cholestasis. Some agents are invariably toxic and will always result in some measure of hepatic injury. Others are harmless in the majority of situations and only a small percentage of persons subjected to the substance will incur liver damage. Known therapeutic agents that are hepatotoxic should be used with caution, and only when the benefits of the drug are judged to be greater than the risk for hepatocellular damage.

Patients with toxic and drug-related hepatitis show symptoms similar to other types of hepatitis. The clinical picture is variable and can range from asymptomatic cases to those with a sudden onset of symptoms that may be severe and life threatening. Onset of symptoms is closely related to the exposure to the toxic agent. Diagnosis is generally made by a history of exposure, consistent clinical, laboratory, and biopsy findings and improvement after removal of the presumed toxin. Treatment is based on removal of the toxin and supportive care while the liver recovers.

The therapeutic use of drugs should be considered when evaluating clinically apparent hepatitis. Many times, recovery with regeneration of the liver will occur when the hepatotoxic drug is discontinued but the liver damage may be irreversible. The case fatality rate of drug-induced liver disease is approximately 5% overall.[52] Of primary importance is the distinction between hepatitis of drug or toxin origin and NANE hepatitis, since the treatment approaches differ greatly.

## CHRONIC HEPATITIS

Chronic hepatitis is diagnosed when an acute case of hepatitis of any origin does not resolve within 6 months to a year. Most persons will completely recover from even the most severe hepatitis within 3 to 4 months, but persistence of elevated enzyme activities, increased bilirubin concentrations, and any applicable serologic markers indicate a progression to the chronic form of hepatitis. The most frequent cases of chronic hepatitis result from HBV and HCV infections, but drug-induced or toxic hepatitis and metabolic diseases such as Wilson's disease or alpha-1-antitrypsin deficiency may also be causes. There is evidence that many cases are an idiopathic autoimmune form of chronic hepatitis. HAV and HEV will not develop into chronic illness, but the presence of HCV or HDV significantly increases the risk for chronicity.

As with acute hepatitis, the symptoms of chronic hepatitis vary with the type of primary infection. Many times the only abnormality is the persistence of elevated ALT activity, but other patients may demonstrate liver dysfunction and jaundice, fatigue, bleeding, arthritis, and renal complications and may progress into cirrhosis. Cirrhosis is a common complication of chronic hepatitis. This condition is a consequence of liver cell death that causes permanent structural damage to the liver. Normally functioning liver tissue is then replaced with fibrous tissue. A liver biopsy is necessary for a definitive diagnosis of cirrhosis, and no treatment has been identified that will alter the progressive course of the condition. A diagnosis of chronic hepatitis can be made by abnormal liver function and serologic findings more than 6 months after diagnosis of an acute case of hepatitis.

Women are more likely than men to develop idiopathic autoimmune chronic hepatitis. These patients usually have several circulating autoimmune antibodies in their sera at the time of diagnosis. The most common autoantibodies seen in this condition are antinuclear antibodies, liver membrane antibodies, autoantibodies against a soluble liver antigen, anti-liver/kidney microsomal antibodies, and smooth muscle antibodies.[53] These atypical antibodies are the only guideline for distinguishing idiopathic autoimmune chronic hepatitis from chronic NANE hepatitis.

There is no specific treatment for chronic hepatitis. Corticosteroid therapy is used with some success in those with severe symptoms.

## Fulminant Hepatic Failure

Fulminant hepatic failure is diagnosed when an apparently healthy patient with no recent history of liver disease suddenly develops serious hepatic dysfunction and neurologic complications. Often, it is a rapidly fatal condition, with death ensuing within 8 weeks of the onset of symptoms. Two categories of this condition have been established, fulminant and subfulminant. Fulminant liver failure reflects the classic definition with encephalopathy developing within 8 weeks of the onset

of illness. The term subfulminant liver failure is applied when the encephalopathy does not develop for 9 to 26 weeks. The frequency of fulminant liver failure is approximately 2000 cases per year in the United States and mortality rates reach more than 80% in those cases who do not receive a liver transplant.[54] Acute necrosis of hepatocytes accounts for the liver failure and the encephalopathy is generally thought to be due to the accumulation of toxic substances in the body that the diseased liver is unable to clear. Other organ systems are often involved in this process and renal complications are common. Cardiac dysfunction, pancreatic lesions, hypoglycemia, and portal hypertension also may be seen in individuals with fulminant hepatic failure.

Although in 15% to 20% of cases of fulminant hepatic failure no known cause can be identified, there are three general categories of causes of this condition.[54]

1. Infections—The most common infectious cause is viral hepatitis, particularly of HAV or HBV origin, with herpes simplex virus and Epstein-Barr virus also being frequently seen.
2. Poisons, chemicals or drugs—Although there are many toxic substances that may produce fulminant hepatic failure, the three most common are ingestion of mushrooms of the *Amanita* species, individual toxic responses to common antibiotics such as tetracycline, and intentional or accidental overdose of acetaminophen.
3. Hepatic ischemia—Heat stroke and prolonged impaired blood flow during surgery may be followed by fulminant hepatic failure. Budd-Chiari syndrome, thrombosis of the hepatic veins, also results in this condition.

Symptoms of fulminant hepatic failure include sudden jaundice, abdominal discomfort, hypotension, and altered personality and behavior. All functions of the liver are equally affected and liver function tests are usually extremely abnormal, especially the activities of AST and ALT enzymes. As the condition worsens, the enzyme concentrations will return to normal as the liver cells exhaust the supply of enzyme. The bilirubin concentration is increased but may not be as elevated as would be expected considering the enzyme levels. Bleeding may also be present due to the liver's inability to synthesize coagulation factors, and some individuals, especially young patients, develop life-threatening hypoglycemia. Neurologic symptoms must be present for a diagnosis of fulminant hepatic failure. These include personality changes, impaired mental function, memory loss, and some motor abnormalities that may progress to decreased consciousness and coma.

Although mortality in this condition is high, those who survive fulminant hepatic failure have a complete return to normal liver function within a very short time considering the extent of the liver damage seen in most cases. It is impossible to predict which patients will recover, although patients who progress to the worst stages of coma have a much lower chance of recovery than those who do not. Management and treatment of the condition consists of treating the symptoms and the prevention of a deepening coma. Exchange transfusions and hemofiltration through activated charcoal filters to cleanse the blood have been studied as treatments to reduce toxicity until the liver has the opportunity to regenerate; however, only minor improvements in the patient's status usually occur. Hemodialysis is recommended for those patients with accompanying renal failure.

If a patient can be supported through the acute phase of fulminant liver failure, the liver can regenerate itself with a complete return to normal liver function. In cases where the assault on the liver is so great that the patient cannot survive through this acute period, liver replacement is the only therapeutic choice. Orthotopic liver transplantation is the preferred treatment for severely affected patients but the availability of donor organs limits that choice in many instances. Other options in these extreme situations include auxillary liver transplantation, xenotransplantation, and the recent development of extracorporeal liver perfusion. Auxillary liver transplantation surgically places a donor liver in the recipient without removing the recipient's native liver. This additional liver mass adequately performs the liver functions and allows the damaged liver to heal and regenerate itself. When the patient's liver has recuperated, the donor liver is either removed or allowed to atrophy by stopping the immunosuppression therapy. This surgical procedure is technically much more difficult than orthotopic liver transplantation, but this option has an advantage of avoiding the need for life-long immunosuppression, requiring it only during that time that the donor liver is expected to function.[55] Xenotransplantation uses porcine livers as donor organs. Extracorporeal liver perfusion mechanisms use human or porcine hepatocytes on various support matrices and involve flowing blood or plasma over 50 to 200 g of hepatocytes.[56] This type of technique would be used to support a patient until orthotopic liver transplantation could be performed or until the patient's own liver could regenerate and support itself.

## Neoplasms

Tumors of the liver can be classified as either benign or malignant and as primary or metastatic in origin. The most common benign tumors are hepatocellular adenomas, seen almost exclusively in women, and hemangiomas, which rarely cause symptoms and are found incidentally during surgery or at autopsy. These tumors must be differentiated from malignant tumors so that the appropriate therapy can be instituted.

Hepatocellular carcinoma (HCC) is by far the most common primary, malignant tumor of the liver and is uniformly fatal within a short time. It affects men more frequently than women. The incidence of HCC varies widely with geographic location but correlates well with the prevalence of HBV infections. HCC is one of the most frequently occurring malignancies in southern Africa, Southeast Asia, Japan, and Greece

but is relatively uncommon in the United States, Great Britain, and Western Europe. The association of HCC and HBV infections is indisputable. Evidence for this strong association comes from epidemiology studies, including geographic distribution, case control studies, prospective studies, and family studies. Studies have also shown that HBV DNA is often integrated into the liver tumor cell itself.[43] More than 80% of patients with HCC also have serologic evidence of HBV infection and cirrhosis is found in the majority of cases of HCC.[57] Other conditions linked with the development of HCC are aflatoxins, anabolic steroid use, ethanol abuse, infections with the Chinese liver fluke (*Clonorchis sinensus*), and alpha$_1$-antitrypsin deficiencies.

HCC often develops in persons with a long history of chronic liver disease, and worsening symptoms may not be noticed early in the disease process. The great reserve capacity of the liver permits normal biochemical function until most of the liver is affected by the malignancy. HCC is an insidious, but progressive, deteriorating condition with the development of abdominal pain, malaise, weight loss, anorexia, and fever. Patients may not be extremely jaundiced and laboratory findings are not at all diagnostic. In fact, laboratory findings are very similar to those found in most other liver diseases, especially chronic viral hepatitis. Serum enzymes are increased and the alkaline phosphatase activity is usually increased more than expected. A sudden change in routine liver function tests in a cirrhotic patient may indicate the development of this malignant process. The presence of alpha-fetoprotein will be found in up to 80% of persons with HCC. This alpha$_1$-globulin is seen in high concentrations in fetal serum and for a short time after birth, but is not normally found in the sera of adults. The demonstration of alpha-fetoprotein is highly suggestive of a primary hepatic tumor. Liver biopsy is usually required for a diagnosis.

Because of the silent nature and lack of early symptoms, it is rare that HCC is diagnosed at a stage that can be treated effectively. The malignancy is usually widespread throughout the liver early in its development so that resection is rarely possible. Even with aggressive treatment, death usually occurs within 1 year of diagnosis. Prevention of HCC through the extensive use of vaccinations for the prevention of HBV is the best defense. Liver transplantation treats both the tumor and the cirrhosis that is most likely present, but there is a high recurrence rate in those patients with large tumors. Since most HCC cases are due to infection with HBV or HCV, reinfection of the transplanted liver is common. A promising treatment for HCC is percutaneous ethanol injection, where absolute alcohol is injected into the tumor causing complete necrosis of the tumor. This treatment is well tolerated and highly effective in small tumors in which more than 90% undergo complete necrosis.[58] Other innovative treatments include intratumoral placement of a microwave electrode to induce tumor necrosis, tumor embolization with gelfoam, or chemotherapeutic agents to cut off the blood supply to the tu-

TABLE 16–11

**Indications for Liver Transplantation in Adults**

| INDICATION | RESULT | RECURRENCE |
|---|---|---|
| Postnecrotic cirrhosis (PNC) (viral) | | |
| A | Excellent | Low |
| B | Poor | High[a] |
| C | Fair to good | Medium[b] |
| Delta | Fair to good | Low |
| Primary biliary cirrhosis (PBC) | Excellent[c] | Low |
| Primary sclerosing cholangitis (PSC) | Very good | Low |
| Ethanol | Good | Variable[d] |
| Fulminant hepatic failure (FHF) | Fair[e] | Low[f] |
| (Viral hepatitis [A, B, C, delta], herpes, adenovirus, Wilson's disease, drugs, Reye's syndrome) | | |
| Metabolic disorders | Excellent | None |
| ($\propto$-1-antitrypsin deficiency, tyrosinemia, Wilson's disease, glycogenosis type IV, familial hypercholesterolemia, Gaucher's disease, hemochromatosis[g]) | | |
| Neoplasms | Fair to poor | High[h] |
| (Hepatoma, APUDomas, hemangioendothelial sarcoma [HES], cholangiocarcinoma) | | |
| Autoimmune hepatitis | Good | Low |
| Budd-Chiari syndrome | Very good | Low[i] |
| Congenital | Very good | None |
| (Caroli's disease, choledochal cyst, polycystic disease, hemangioma, adenomatosis) | | |
| Trauma | Good[j] | None |

[a]very high if HBe-antigen or HBV-DNA positive
[b]if PCR is positive
[c]prognosis depends on how advanced the hepatic osteodystrophy was at the time of transplantation
[d]depends on alcohol-free interval and intensity of pretransplant rehabilitation
[e]depends on etiology and depth of coma at time of transplantation
[f]depends on etiology
[g]hemochromatosis, a disorder of intestinal absorption of iron, is not cured by liver transplantation
[h]longer survival with APUDomas and HES
[i]with post-transplant anticoagulation
[j]if patient survives the surgery
PCR = polymerase chain reaction
From Zakem D, Boyer TD: *Hepatology: A Textbook of Liver Disease.* Philadelphia, W.B. Saunders, 1996. p. 1761. Reprinted with permission.

mor and cause ischemic necrosis and various chemotherapeutic agent combinations.[58]

Although primary liver tumors are most common worldwide, in Western societies metastatic liver tumors are more likely seen. Hepatic metastases frequently develop with primary tumors of the lung, breast, and gastrointestinal tract. Symptoms vary with the primary tumor, and laboratory evaluation may be of little diagnostic value because most liver function tests are not sensitive enough to detect early disease. Liver biopsy is required for a final diagnosis in most cases.

## Liver Transplantation

Liver transplantation has become an effective and accepted treatment for patients with irreversible hepatic failure. The first orthotopic liver transplant in a human was performed by

Dr. Thomas Starzl in 1963. Since that time, dramatic improvements have been made in patient survival and the quality of life for transplant recipients. Recent developments in surgical techniques, better selection of both patients and donors, and the introduction of alternate immunosuppression therapies for transplant patients have improved the overall 1-year survival rate to approximately 90%.[59] The health status of the patient before the transplant, the disease process being corrected by the transplant, and the presence of certain complicating factors will affect the prognosis for each individual undergoing the procedure. Currently, the risk of death from liver failure is much more significant than the mortality risk of the transplant procedure itself or any complications that may arise from it.

The number of transplants being performed in the United States is a function of the availability of acceptable donor organs. Donor selection is based on ABO blood type compatibility between donor and recipient, relative physiologic health of the donor, and an approximate organ and body size match. In general, a patient should be transplanted when it becomes apparent that the degree of liver dysfunction is both severe and irreversible and that failure to transplant will jeopardize the patient's life. Moreover, it should occur before the patient's general condition is so poor that the procedure itself would not be tolerated. Table 16–11 summarizes the disease-specific indications for transplantation.[60]

Although the disease processes and the clinical and laboratory indications for transplantation in a given individual are important, clear contraindications for liver transplantation are even more critical to identify. The list of relative contraindications grows shorter as the transplant procedure becomes more routine and the management of the transplant patient improves.

Liver transplantation is not without risks and complications. The laboratory is able to provide important information in the evaluation of patients for transplantation and in following their progress post-transplantation. Organ rejection is a constant concern, and many transplant recipients develop at least one episode of infection during the recovery period. Symptoms of rejection include malaise, fever, graft tenderness, increasing jaundice, and increasingly abnormal liver function tests that usually develop 5 to 10 days after the procedure.

Currently, over 10% of candidates awaiting transplantation die before an organ becomes available.[61] Because of the shortage of donor organs, several options are being used to increase the number of patients receiving transplants. Reduced size and split liver transplants make more efficient use of donor organs. Reduced size liver transplantation involves reduction of adult livers to fit into pediatric recipients. Although this process increases the number of livers available for children, some liver tissue is discarded as unusable in another patient. Improvements in surgical techniques have resulted in split liver transplants to allow for optimal use of the organ by transplanting the larger right lobe of the donor organ into an adult recipient and the smaller left lobe into a child. Live related liver transplantation is also a relatively new option, whereby a relative of the recipient donates the left lobe of the liver. The livers in both donor and recipient should regenerate to normal size and function within 6 weeks of surgery.

## SUMMARY

The investigation of liver disease is an example of a truly interdisciplinary study. Cooperation among all members of the health care team is mandatory in the gathering of only the most useful data from each discipline and integrating it to obtain the correct diagnosis as well as an effective treatment for the patient.

The versatility of the liver can be demonstrated by the wide variety of information that must be obtained for a complete and accurate diagnosis of a liver malfunction. Any history of exposure to either infectious or toxic agents should be identified and the patient must be evaluated to determine the extent and type of symptoms exhibited. The clinical laboratory is instrumental in gathering the diagnostic data to assess overall functions of the organ. The clinical chemistry laboratory provides the basic information to initiate a differential diagnosis through a routine liver function profile. From that beginning, other laboratory and health care disciplines add specific information to confirm the suspected diagnosis. Special chemistry laboratory determinations and results from the hematology, urinalysis, and immunology laboratory sections are often required to identify a specific liver disease. Even toxicology laboratory results are helpful for toxic hepatitis cases, the blood bank in the identification of hemolytic transfusion reactions and microbiologic studies to identify causes of liver infections. Genetic studies of inheritance patterns for the inborn errors of metabolism that affect liver function are helpful in identifying and counseling persons at risk.

Although the clinical laboratory certainly plays a pivotal role in the evaluation of the liver, information from a variety of sources completes the picture. Histologic examination is important because many times a definitive diagnosis can only be made through information obtained by a liver biopsy. Through the use of radiography, ultrasonography, computed tomography scans, and magnetic resonance imaging, the radiology department provides valuable data in obstructive liver diseases and in the discovery of liver tumors. New surgical techniques and pharmacologic therapies in the treatment of liver diseases expand the current options available to those with liver ailments.

There is still much to be learned about the liver. Identification of additional viral agents causing hepatitis, more effective treatments, and prevention of all forms of hepatitis are ongoing efforts. The effect of liver diseases on other organs and the effect that other diseases have on the liver is also being studied extensively. Other issues being investigated include new and better treatments for hepatocellular carcinoma, methods for early identification of all liver tumors, the expanded use of living donor transplants and the resultant quality of life for transplant recipients.

## REFERENCES

1. Fody EP: Liver function. In Bishop ML, Duben-Engelkirk JL, Fody EP: *Clinical Chemistry: Principles, Procedures, Correlations.* 4th ed. Philadelphia, Lippincott Williams & Wilkins, 2000, p. 354.

2. Price SA, Wilson LM: *Pathophysiology: Clinical Concepts of Disease Processes.* 2nd ed. New York, McGraw-Hill, 1982.

3. McNamara JR, Warnick GR, Wu LL: Lipids and lipoproteins, in Bishop ML, Duben-Engelkirk JL, Fody EP: *Clinical Chemistry: Principles, Procedures, Correlations,* 4th ed., Philadelphia, Lippincott Williams and Wilkins, 2000; p. 233.

4. Roy-Chowdhury J, Jansen PLM: Bilirubin metabolism and its disorders. In Zakim D, Boyer TD: *Hepatology: A Textbook of Liver Disease.* 3rd ed. Philadelphia, WB Saunders, 1996, p 323.

5. Friedman LS, Martin P, Munoz SJ: Liver function tests and the objective evaluation of the patient with liver disease. In Zakim D, Boyer TD: *Hepatology: A Textbook of Liver Disease.* 3rd ed. Philadelphia, WB Saunders, 1996, p 791.

6. Larson AM, Carithers RL Jr.: Management of alcoholic liver disease. In Krawitt EL, ed.: *Medical Management of Liver Disease.* New York, Marcel Dekker, 1999, p 181.

7. Johnston DE: Special considerations in interpreting liver function tests. Am Fam Physician 59:2223–2230, 1999.

8. Rosalki SB, Dooley JS: Liver function profiles and their interpretation. Br J Hosp Med 51(4):181–186, 1994.

9. Cooper AD, Ellsworth JL: Lipoprotein metabolism. In Zakim D, Boyer TD: *Hepatology: A Textbook of Liver Disease.* 3rd ed. Philadelphia, WB Saunders, 1996, p 92.

10. Lauff JJ, Kasper ME, Ambrose RT: Separation of bilirubin species in serum and bile by high-performance reversed-phase liquid chromatography. J Chromatogr 226:391–402, 1981.

11. Total bilirubin test methodology: Publication MP2-39. Rochester, NY, Johnson and Johnson Clinical Diagnostics, Inc., 1996.

12. BuBc bilirubin test methodology: Publication MP2-40. Rochester, NY, Johnson and Johnson Clinical Diagnostics, Inc,. 1996.

13. Sundberg M, Lauff JJ, Weiss J, et al.: Estimation of unconjugated, conjugated, and "delta" bilirubin fractions in serum by use of two coated thin films. Clin Chem 30:1314–1317, 1984.

14. Test methodology information: Publication C-305. Rochester, NY, Eastman Kodak Co., 1985.

15. Gitlin N: Hepatic encephalopathy. In Zakim D, Boyer TD: *Hepatology: A Textbook of Liver Disease.* 3rd ed. Philadelphia, WB Saunders, 1996, p 605.

16. Jay DW: Nonprotein nitrogen. In Bishop ML, Duben-Engelkirk JL, Fody EP: *Clinical Chemistry: Principles,*

*Procedures, Correlations.* 4th ed. Philadelphia, Lippincott Williams & Wilkins, 2000, p 261.

17. Pratt DS, Kaplan MM: Evaluation of abnormal liver-enzyme results in asymptomatic patients. N Engl J Med 342(17):1266–1271, 2000.

18. Schiff L, Schiff ER: *Diseases of the Liver.* 7th ed. Philadelphia, JB Lippincott, 1993, pp 108–109.

19. Blackburn S: Hyperbilirubinemia and neonatal jaundice. Neonatal Netw 14(7):15–25, 1995.

20. Balistreri WF, Grand R, Hoofnagle JH, et al.: Biliary atresia: Current concepts and research directions. Hepatology 23:1682–1692, 1996.

21. Lefkowitch JH: Biliary atresia. Mayo Clin Proc 73:90–95, 1998.

22. Pfeil SA, Lynn DJ: Wilson's disease. J Clin Gastroenterol 29(1):22–31, 1999.

23. Bacon BR, Schilsky ML: New knowledge of genetic pathogenesis of hemochromatosis and Wilson's disease. Adv Intern Med 44:91–116, 1999.

24. Teckman JH, Qu D, Perlmutter DH. Molecular pathogenesis of liver disease in $\alpha$-1-antitrypsin deficiency. Hepatology 24:1504–1516, 1996.

25. Stoller JK: Clinical features and natural history of severe $\alpha$-1-antitrypsin deficiency. Chest 111:123S–128S, 1997.

26. Bacon BR, Tavill AS: Hemochromatosis and the iron overload syndromes. In Zakim D, Boyer TD: *Hepatology: A Textbook of Liver Disease.* 3rd ed. Philadelphia, WB Saunders, 1996, p. 1439.

27. DeHart MA: Hereditary hemochromatosis: Diagnosis and treatment in primary care. Tenn Med Nov: 415–417, 1999.

28. Lynch SR: Iron overload: Prevalence and impact on health. Nutr Rev 53(9):255–260, 1995.

29. Andrews NC: Disorders of iron metabolism. N Engl J Med 341:1986–1995, 1999.

30. Fahey S: The experience of women with primary biliary cirrhosis: A literature review. J Adv Nurs 30:506–512, 1999.

31. Poupon R, Poupon RE. Primary biliary cirrhosis. In Zakim D, Boyer TD: *Hepatology: A Textbook of Liver Disease.* 3rd ed. Philadelphia, WB Saunders, 1996, p 1329.

32. Parikh-Patel A, Gold E, Mackay IR, et al.: The geoepidemiology of primary biliary cirrhosis: Contrasts and comparisons with the spectrum of autoimmune disease. Clin Immunol 91:206–218, 1999.

33. Berk PD, Noyer C. The familial conjugated hyperbilirubinemias: Sem Liver Dis 14:386–394, 1994.

34. Jansen PLM: Diagnosis and management of Crigler-Najjar syndrome. Eur J Pediatr 158(Suppl 2):S89–S94, 1999.

35. Berk PD, Noyer C. The familial unconjugated hyperbilirubinemias: Sem Liver Dis 14:356–385, 1994.

36. Nanji AA, Zakim D. Alcoholic liver disease. In Zakim D, Boyer TD: *Hepatology: A Textbook of Liver Disease.* 3rd ed. Philadelphia, WB Saunders, 1996, p 891.

37. Tung BY, Carithers RL Jr.: Cholestasis and alcoholic liver disease. Clinics in Liver Disease 3(3):585–601, 1999.
38. Diehl AM: Liver disease in the alcoholic: Clinical aspects. In Zakim D, Boyer TD: *Hepatology: A Textbook of Liver Disease.* 3rd ed. Philadelphia, WB Saunders, 1996, p 1050.
39. Samaik AP: Reye's syndrome: Hold the obituary. Crit Care Med 27:1674–1676, 1999.
40. Fried MW: The liver in systemic illness. In Zakim D, Boyer TD: *Hepatology: A Textbook of Liver Disease.* 3rd ed. Philadelphia, WB Saunders, 1996, p 1706.
41. Knox TA, Olans LB: Liver disease in pregnancy. N Engl J Med 335:569–576, 1996.
42. Van Dyke RW: The liver in pregnancy. In Zakim D, Boyer TD: *Hepatology: A Textbook of Liver Disease.* 3rd ed. Philadelphia, WB Saunders, 1996, p 1734.
43. Robinson WS: Biology of human hepatitis viruses. In Zakim D, Boyer TD: *Hepatology: A Textbook of Liver Disease.* 3rd ed. Philadelphia, WB Saunders, 1996, p 1146.
44. CDC: Prevention of hepatitis A through active or passive immunization: Recommendations of the Advisory Committee on Immunization Practices (ACIP). Morb Mortal Wkly Rep: October 1, 1999: 48(RR-12), 1999.
45. CDC Viral hepatitis B fact sheet. Atlanta, GA, Centers for Disease Control and Prevention, p 1, 2000.
46. Fry DE: The ABCs of hepatitis: Adv Surg 33:413–437, 1999.
47. Sacher RA, Peters SM, Byran JA: Testing for viral hepatitis: A practice parameter. Am J Clin Pathol 113:12–17, 2000.
48. Hochman JA, Balistreri WF: Viral hepatitis: Expanding the alphabet. Adv Pediatr 46:207–243. 1999.
49. Al-Saden PC, McPartlin F, Daly-Gawenda D, et al.: Hepatitis C: An emerging dilemma. AAOHN J 47(5):217–222, 1999.
50. Catalina G, Navarro V: Hepatitis C: A challenge for the generalist. Hosp Pract 35(1):97–118, 2000.
51. Labrique AB, Thomas DL, Stoszek SK, et al.: Hepatitis E: An emerging disease. Epidemiol Rev 21:162–177, 1999.
52. Bass NM, Ockner RK: Drug-induced liver disease. In Zakim D, Boyer TD: *Hepatology: A Textbook of Liver Disease.* 3rd ed. Philadelphia, WB Saunders, 1996, p 962.
53. Meyer zum Büschenfelde KH, Gerken G: Immune mechanisms in the production of liver disease. In Zakim D, Boyer TD: *Hepatology: A Textbook of Liver Disease.* 3rd ed. Philadelphia, WB Saunders, 1996, p 1243.
54. Shakil AO, Mazariegos GV, Kramer DJ: Fulminant hepatic failure. Surg Clin North Am 79(1):77–108, 1999.
55. Mas J, Rodes J: Fulminant hepatic failure. Lancet 349: 1081–1085, 1997.
56. McChesney LP, Fagan EA, Rowell DL, et al.: Extracorporeal liver perfusion. Lancet 353:120–121, 1999.
57. Kew MC: Tumors of the liver. In Zakim D, Boyer TD: *Hepatology: A Textbook of Liver Disease.* 3rd ed. Philadelphia, WB Saunders, 1996, p 1513.
58. Bruix J: Treatment of hepatocellular carcinoma. Hepatology 25:259–262, 1997.
59. Pirenne J, Koshiba T: Present status and future prospects in liver transplantation. Int Surg 84:297–304, 1999.
60. Steiber AC, Gordon RD, Galloway JR. Orthotopic liver transplantation. In Zakim D, Boyer TD: *Hepatology: A Textbook of Liver Disease.* 3rd ed. Philadelphia, WB Saunders, 1996, p 1759.
61. Grewal H, Amiri H, Vera S, et al.: In situ split-liver transplantation. Tenn Med Nov: 411–414, 1999.

# CHAPTER 17

# Tumor Markers

*Margot Hall*

Cancer is rapidly becoming the major health issue in the industrialized nations second only to heart disease. Indeed in 1998, the American Cancer Society estimated that there were greater than 1 million new cancer cases and 0.5 million cancer deaths in the United States, exclusive of in situ and skin cancers.[1] Early diagnosis and treatment in combination with improved therapeutic modalities can increase the survival rate significantly. One minimally invasive method for early detection and therapeutic monitoring of cancer involves the measurement of tumor markers. They will be the subject of this chapter.

A **tumor** or **neoplasm** is an abnormal (uncontrolled) proliferation of cells in a eukaryotic organism. A **benign neoplasm** is one that remains confined to its primary site during the life span of the organism. A **malignant neoplasm** is one that is capable of invading surrounding normal tissue and metastasizing through the circulatory and lymphatic systems to distant body sites. **Metastasis** is the process by which the tumor cell spreads to other distant body sites. **Cancer,** from the Latin word for crab, is a malignant neoplasm. The term also refers to a large group of malignant neoplastic diseases. Since benign neoplasia are restricted to their original locations, they can usually be removed surgically. This explains why they are generally not life threatening (an exception to this would be certain benign brain tumors). In contrast, malignant neoplasia are invasive and metastatic, making it more difficult to remove the tumors completely. This explains their increased mortality rate. Additionally, malignant neoplasia usually proliferate more rapidly and become more **anaplastic** (less well differentiated and more primitive) than benign neoplasia, which tend to resemble their normal cell counterparts. This also contributes to the poorer prognosis and higher mortality rate associated with malignancy.[2]

The classification of neoplasia is based on the tissue type and cell type from which they originate. During embryogenesis three germ layers (distinct layers of cells) develop: (1) ectoderm, (2) mesoderm, and (3) endoderm. Skin and nervous tissue are derived from the ectoderm, whereas bone, muscle, and blood come from mesoderm and the internal organs with their linings come from endoderm. Malignant neoplasia are classified as **carcinomas** if they are of epithelial cell origin (derived from the ectoderm or endoderm) and **sarcomas** if they are of mesenchymal origin. Although cancers of the blood and lymph systems are derived from mesoderm and therefore technically sarcomas, they are classified separately and called simply **leukemias** and **lymphomas.** Subclassification of malignant neoplasia depends on the cell type or anatomical site of origin. For example, an adenocarcinoma is a neoplasm of glandular epithelium, whereas an osteosarcoma is a tumor of the bone. Similarly, benign neoplasia are classified according to their tissue of origin and given the suffix "oma." Thus a colon **adenoma** is a benign neoplasm (an exception to this is melanoma, which is a highly malignant skin cancer). The histologic classification of neoplasia is important because it forms the basis for the diagnosis, prognosis, and treatment modality(ies).[3]

Traditionally, the development of malignancy has been thought to be the result of a progression of incremental changes in the cellular DNA with resultant changes in cellular morphology and biochemistry. The malignancy can originate in any cell (at any site in the organism) and initially affects only one cell. There is an **initiation** step that involves a mutation at the level of the nuclear DNA. The mutated cell can die, remain dormant, or proceed to proliferate (cellular division). When it proliferates, a clone of genetically altered cells is produced (**promotion**) that "fixes" the original transformation. As further mutations occur in daughter cells, subsets of the original clone develop, leading to a progressively more malignant neoplasm (**progression**). These changes can be detected through DNA sequencing, karyotyping, histology and cellular morphology, biochemical assays, and a variety of imaging techniques. As the malignancy progresses, the neoplasm synthesizes and secretes chemicals that enhance cellular proliferation, degrade the basement membrane, which permits invasion and metastasis, increase angiogenesis and thereby develop a blood supply for the tumor, increase cellular motility, and mask (protect) the neoplastic cells from the host's immune system. The processes by which these occur have been logical areas of research and have lead to specific types of therapeutic intervention.[4]

The assessment of the extent of tumor growth, invasion, and metastasis (extent of tumor progression) is called tumor staging and has important diagnostic and therapeutic implications. Numerous systems for staging have been developed, but recently a unified system of staging was adopted by the American Joint Committee on Cancer[5] and the International Union Against Cancer.[6] Often referred to as the TNM system, this staging system uses subscripts to describe the presence, size, and degree of invasiveness of the primary tumor (T), regional lymph nodes (N), and distant metastases (M). A unified system of staging has greatly aided in efforts to evaluate different therapies and therapeutic monitoring devices.

If a malignant tumor or neoplasm is allowed to grow unchecked by treatment, it will, in time, be fatal to the organism. The pathogenicity of the disease is largely due to obstruction and destruction of other vital structures in the body, functional activity of a substance produced by the tumor, bleeding, infection, or toxic substances associated with infarction and necrosis. Many of the therapeutic interventions address one or more of these symptoms. However, surgical removal of the tumor is still the major approach to the disease treatment.[7]

The pathogenesis of the disease has been associated historically with (1) chemical carcinogens, (2) radiation, (3) viruses, and (4) heredity. This has led to a unified theory of carcinogenesis. Mechanistically, all of these act by causing DNA mutations, culminating in the loss of growth control with increased cellular proliferation and decreased cellular differentiation. Since neoplastic transformation is associated with altered gene expression, which in turn affects the production of enzymes, hormones, receptors, proteins and metabolites that are released into the circulatory system, measurement of these substances aids in the diagnosis and characterization of the disease. Similarly, the DNA content of a tumor cell can be examined for mutations, the absence of suppressor genes that would prevent tumor formation, and the presence of oncogenes that turn on tumor growth and ploidy, which is an indicator of growth rate and aggressiveness. This group of substances has come to be known as **tumor markers.**[4]

## CHARACTERISTICS OF AN IDEAL TUMOR MARKER

A tumor marker is a substance synthesized by the tumor or by the host in response to a tumor that can be used to detect the presence of the tumor. An ideal tumor marker[8] has the following characteristics:

1. Specificity for cancer. The substance should be produced only by the tumor. No benign condition should cause an elevation and the marker should not be present, or be found only in trace amounts in a normal population. To be completely ideal, the substance should be found in one type of tumor only.
2. Sensitivity for cancer. A very small tumor growth or metastasis produces measurable amounts of marker.
3. The amount of marker produced correlates well with the tumor load.
4. There should be a consistent concentration of the tumor marker in patients with stable disease.
5. The half-life of the marker needs to be short enough so that when production drops, the level of marker falls off rapidly, producing low or undetectable concentrations in patients who are in remission.

6. Levels of the marker (initial and serial) should have prognostic value.
7. The assay for the marker should be analytically sensitive, specific, accurate, precise, easy to perform, inexpensive, and rapid.

Tumor marker research has netted several markers that have some characteristics of the ideal marker. Unfortunately, there are no ideal tumor markers.

## USES OF TUMOR MARKERS

Clinical applications[8] of tumor markers include the following:

1. Screening for disease in asymptomatic population.
2. Diagnosis of disease in symptomatic patients.
3. Aid in clinical staging.
4. Measurement of tumor burden.
5. Therapeutic monitoring and selection.
6. Detection of recurrence of disease (relapse).
7. Prognostic indicator.

Because of low diagnostic specificity and/or low disease prevalence, to date the majority of tumor marker assays have not proved useful as screening tests. An exception to this is prostate-specific antigen (PSA), which has been recommended as a screening tool for prostatic cancer in men over 50 years of age.[9]

Tumor markers have limited use in diagnosis because of the overlap between values obtained in benign and malignant disease. However, in a population at risk, or with some evidence of disease, there are markers that can be used to help make or confirm a diagnosis. Additionally, the use of tumor marker panels (multiple markers) with disease or tissue-specific patterns has greatly improved the diagnostic efficacy of certain markers.[8]

The primary use of tumor markers is to monitor therapy in patients who have been diagnosed as having a malignant tumor. Tumor markers are also useful in detecting recurrence of disease, determining a prognosis, and as an adjunct to tumor staging. At the time diagnosis is made, one or more potential markers should be measured. Elevated markers should be periodically quantitated after surgical resection or following the initiation of other therapeutic measures.

## BIOLOGIC SOURCES

Chemical and cellular moieties that form a part of a neoplastic cell, are produced by that cell, or are produced in response to signals from that cell may be used as tumor markers. In general, these are found and measured in body fluids and tissues. Traditionally, structural molecules and their epitopes, secretion products, enzymes, and markers of cell turnover have been used as tumor markers. Additionally, oncogenes and their products, cellular ploidy (amount of DNA), cell growth cycle markers (both promoters and inhibitors), and the percentage of cells in the proliferative phase of the cycle can be used as tumor markers.[4]

Benign tumors are generally well differentiated. The cells in a benign tumor are similar to the cells of the corresponding normal tissue, and therefore the tumor markers produced are typically the products found in the normal tissue. They may be found in increased amounts in the circulation, depending on the size of the tumor.[3]

Malignant tumors may produce substances associated with a normal cell or they may be different. Each somatic cell of a living organism has the same genetic material. As a zygote is transformed into an embryo, which then evolves into a fetus, the rapidly dividing cells become differentiated into specialized tissues by selective gene expression. The genes expressed are responsible for such things as production of hormones, enzymes, receptors, structural proteins, and cell metabolism. When a normal cell is transformed into a tumor cell, gene expression changes. The affected cell may lose its ability to synthesize some specific cell product, or it may manufacture greatly increased amounts. The cell may be less specialized than the tissue it evolved from and assume the characteristics of the less well-differentiated cells of the embryo, synthesizing proteins (oncofetal) found in the embryo but not in a normal adult. Cell proliferation rates change as the metabolic rate of the cells increases.[3]

Tumors are assumed to be unicellular in origin. After the cell is transformed, it loses growth control and begins to divide rapidly. The cells lose contact inhibition and invade the primary site. They then invade the adjacent organs and blood and lymph systems, which may carry the cells to distant organs. The cells may then lodge in a capillary bed and begin to invade the new site. As this invasion process takes place, new proteins are produced that actively aid in the invasion. These proteins can also be used as markers.[3]

Patterns of commonly measured chemical analytes may serve as possible markers of neoplastic disease and often serve as a clue to the origin of the disease.

## CLASSIFICATION

The classification of tumor markers may be predicated on chemical structure (e.g., protein, DNA, polyamine), function (e.g., enzyme, signal molecule), method of detection (e.g., antigenic property-immunologic assay, enzymatic activity assay) or anatomic source (e.g., placental, salivary). Thus, prostate-specific antigen (PSA) may be listed as an enzyme, an antigen, or a prostatic tumor marker. In one classification scheme, tumor markers are categorized into the following groups:

1. Enzymes and isoenzymes
2. Hormones, neurotransmitters, and their metabolites
3. Receptors (estrogen, progesterone, androgen, and corticosteroid)
4. Proteins (immunoglobulins, glycoproteins, carcinoembryonic proteins, or oncofetal antigens)
5. Genetic markers (oncogenes and suppressor genes)
6. Other markers (sialic acid conjugates, polyamines, and amino acids)

## Enzymes

Enzymes may have been the first markers used in screening for cancer. Although the elevation of an enzyme is never specific for cancer, a routine chemistry profile often includes the enzymes lactate dehydrogenase and alkaline phosphatase and may include creatine kinase, amylase, or gamma-glutamyltransferase. Each of these enzymes may be elevated in one or more forms of cancer. An elevated level of any one of them leads to a more extensive search for disease, although certainly this does not always lead to the discovery of a malignant disease.[4]

Other enzymes are more specific for cancer. These include the collagenases, cathepsin D, and the proteases secreted by malignant cells to break down surrounding tissue being invaded by the tumor.[8] See Table 17–1 for a list of enzymes sometimes used as tumor markers and their associated diseases.

### ACID PHOSPHATASE

Increased levels of acid phosphatase (ACP) have been found in some patients with prostatic adenocarcinoma. ACP is not a reliable screening or early disease diagnostic tool.[10] This enzyme has several isoenzymes, one of which is produced in the prostate. Elevated levels of the prostatic isoenzyme (PAP) of acid phosphatase have been used to diagnose and monitor prostate cancer but may not necessarily be found when malignancy is present, especially in the early stages of disease. Elevated levels of PAP may also be found in patients with benign prostatic hyperplasia, prostatitis, or following prostatic massage.[11] In recent years, the use of PAP has been largely superceded by prostate-specific antigen (PSA) for the detection of prostate tumors. However, it is sometimes used in conjunction with PSA to discriminate between patients who have extracapsular disease and those whose disease is encapsulated.[12]

ACP is quite labile. If it cannot be assayed immediately after collection, it must be stored frozen. There are several assays available for measuring ACP in serum. A monoclonal antibody directed toward the prostatic fraction of ACP has been developed and several radioimmunoassay (RIA) and enzyme-immunoassay (EIA) kits are commercially available using this antibody.[13–15] The phosphatase activity can be measured directly using a low pH buffer and thymolphthalein phosphate. Following hydrolysis and the addition of a base to change the pH, a colored end product is produced.[16] Another method utilizes the substrate alpha-naphthyl phosphate with and without the addition of L-tartrate, which inhibits prostatic isoenzyme of ACP (from which PAP can be calculated). Diazonium then reacts with the product of hydrolysis to form a colored end product.[17]

TABLE  17-1

### Enzymes and Isoenzymes Used as Tumor Markers

| ENZYME | SITE/TUMOR |
|---|---|
| Prostatic acid phosphatase | Prostate |
| Alkaline phosphatase | Metastases to bone, liver, Leukemia Osteogenic sarcoma |
| Placental alkaline phosphatase (Regan isoenzyme) | Ovary, lung, trophoblastic tissue, gastrointestinal tissue, seminoma, Hodgkin's disease |
| Creatine kinase-BB | Prostate, breast, ovary, colon, lung, gastrointestinal tissue |
| Lactate dehydrogenase | Liver, colon, breast, lung, stomach leukemia, lymphoma, germ cell tumors, adenocarcinomas |
| Neuron specific enolase | Neuroblastoma, brain, testes, small cell tumor of lung |
| Amylase | Pancreas |
| Lipase | |
| Trypsin | |
| Ribonuclease | |
| 5'Nucleotidase | Liver |
| Gamma glutamyltransferase | |
| Terminal deoxynucleotidyl Transferase | Leukemia |
| Collagenase | Bone |
| Cathepsin D | Breast cancer |
| Histaminase | Medullary thyroid carcinoma |
| Muramidase (lysozyme) | Leukemia |

## ALKALINE PHOSPHATASE

Quantitation of total alkaline phosphatase (ALP) is useful in the diagnosis of primary bone and hepatic malignancies and metastases to these organs. Organ-specific ALP isoenzymes have been identified (bone, kidney, liver, small intestine, and placenta [Regan isoenzyme]), and often it is necessary to identify which isoenzymes are present before ALP can be used as a tumor marker. Frequently, one needs to differentiate the bone from the liver fraction. This can be done by heat inactivation of the bone fraction, selective adsorption (affinity chromatography), zone electrophoresis, or isoelectric focusing.[18] The isoenzymes may then be quantitated. Alternatively, test results may be confirmed by measuring other liver enzymes such as 5' nucleotidase or gamma-glutamyltransferase. Also, an immunoradiometric assay exists for bone alkaline phosphatase.[19]

Elevations of ALP correlate well with osteoblastic activity and can be used to monitor therapy and look for recurrence in patients with osteosarcoma or metastatic prostate cancer. Osteoclastic activity, as seen in metastatic breast cancer, usually causes only minor elevations of serum ALP.[20] Liver metastases seen in leukemia patients can exhibit marked elevations of ALP and these correlate with the extent of liver involvement. Synthesized by the trophoblast, placental ALP is elevated in the sera of pregnant women and patients with trophoblastic, ovarian, lung, and gastrointestinal cancers, as well as seminomas and Hodgkin's disease.[21] The Regan isoenzyme (placental ALP) is heat-stable, resistant to urea inhibition, and sensitive to L-phenylalanine inhibition.[22]

## CREATINE KINASE

The BB isoenzyme of creatine kinase (CK-BB, CK-1), commonly known as the brain fraction, is normally not observed in serum due to the blood–brain barrier. CK-BB is the fetal form of the enzyme and as such is associated with many malignant diseases, especially those of epithelial cell origin. Malignancy in the lung, prostate, breast, colon, ovary, stomach, kidney, and bladder may show elevations of serum CK-BB. CK-BB measured in cerebrospinal fluid (CSF) may be used in estimating lesion size in brain tumors, although it may also be detected in nonmalignant disease. CK-BB found in the serum is not specific enough to be used in differentiating tumor sites but has been used in conjunction with PAP to monitor prostate cancer patients. CK isoenzymes are identified and quantitated using electrophoresis.[23–24]

## LACTATE DEHYDROGENASE

Lactate dehydrogenase (LD) is a nonspecific marker. Benign and malignant solid tumors show an increased level of serum LD that correlates well with the growth rate of the tumor. Elevations are seen in tumors of the colon, breast, lung, liver, stomach, germ cell tumors, a variety of adenocarcinomas, and in leukemias and lymphomas. There is no consistent isoenzyme pattern associated with malignancy. Elevated serum LD-1 has been described in germ cell tumors (teratoma and testicular seminoma). Similarly, increased serum concentrations of LD-3 are observed in patients with leukemias and lymphomas, whereas the LD-5 isoenzyme is frequently elevated in patients with colon, breast, lung, liver, stomach cancers, and a variety of adenocarcinomas such as prostate.[25–26]

## NEURON-SPECIFIC ENOLASE

Neuron-specific enolase (NSE) is a specific marker for tumors associated with the neuroendocrine system. Serum and/or CSF elevations of this marker are observed in cases of neuroblastoma, neurogenic tumors, small cell carcinoma of the lung, glucagonomas, insulinomas, carcinoid tumors, and malignant pheochromocytomas.[27–33] NSE may be quantitated by RIA and the levels correlate well with the tumor burden.

## AMYLASE, LIPASE, TRYPSIN, AND RIBONUCLEASE

Amylase (AMS), lipase (LPS), trypsin (TPS), and ribonuclease (RNase) are enzymes associated with the pancreas. They may be elevated in patients with pancreatic tumors but are frequently elevated in pancreatitis and other diseases of the pancreas, thus diminishing their utility. Ribonuclease may also be elevated in cancers of the breast, colon, stomach, liver, and lung.[34]

## 5' NUCLEOTIDASE AND GAMMA GLUTAMYLTRANSFERASE

5'Nucleotidase (5'NT) and gamma glutamyltransferase (GGT) are both more sensitive markers for liver cancer than ALP. However, neither of them is specific for cancer. They may both be elevated in cases of cirrhosis and GGT is elevated in a large percentage of pancreatic cancers.[34]

## TERMINAL DEOXYNUCLEOTIDYL TRANSFERASE

Terminal deoxynucleotidyl transferase (TdT) is a marker (antigen) found on immature lymphoid cells. This enzyme is capable of enzymatically synthesizing DNA without a template. It is quantitated using an immunoassay (RIA or EIA) and is used to predict prognosis and responsiveness to drugs as well as to help classify the leukemias.[35] It has also been used occasionally to help classify non-Hodgkin's lymphomas.[36]

## COLLAGENASE AND CATHEPSIN D

Collagenase and cathepsin D are part of a larger class of compounds known as proteases. Synthesized and secreted by malignant cells, these compounds are responsible for degrading the extracellular matrix and thus permitting their invasion and metastasis. Both can be quantitated in extracts from surgically removed solid tumors. The results correlate well with the 5-year survival time for patients and hence are used in developing a prognosis. Collagenase is measured in bone malignancies and cathepsin D is often quantitated in breast cancer patients.[37–38]

## HISTAMINASE

Histaminase or diamine oxidase (DAO) has been used as a tumor marker in cases of medullary thyroid cancer to confirm a high level of calcitonin, which is normally found in this disease. Familial medullary carcinoma of the thyroid can present with microscopic tumors and distant metastases not observed on radiologic examination. The disease can also present as part of a multiple endocrine neoplasia. The enzyme concentration reflects tumor burden.[8,34,39]

## MURAMIDASE

Muramidase or lysozyme is sometimes used in the monitoring of monocytic and myelomonocytic leukemias. Similarly, it has been reported elevated in some forms of colon cancer. The usefulness of the marker is still under review.[8,40]

## Hormones

Hormones may be secreted in abnormally increased concentrations by tumors of the endocrine glands normally responsible for their production (eutopic production) or by tumors of other organs that normally do not produce the hormone (ectopic production). The synthesis and secretion of these hormones can cause severe symptoms and even life-threatening effects. The paraneoplastic endocrine syndromes, which result from the excessive hormonal production, are often the first indication of malignancy and the quantitation of the hormone(s) in question can support or establish a diagnosis. Hormones are regularly employed to monitor a patient following surgery and other therapeutic modalities but they have not been used to screen an asymptomatic population.[41] It is important to note that benign as well as malignant tumors secrete excessive amounts of hormone. A tumor may secrete multiple hormones, some of which may be synergistic and some antagonistic to each other. A tumor may secrete intact hormones, hormone precursors, fragments, and subunits of hormones.[42] Table 17–2 lists hormones most frequently used as tumor markers with their typical presenting endocrinopathy or clinical symptoms.

## HUMAN CHORIONIC GONADOTROPIN

Human chorionic gonadotropin (HCG) or choriogonadotropin is a pregnancy-associated hormone, normally secreted by the syncytiotrophoblastic cells of the placenta. It is commonly measured to confirm pregnancy and to diagnose ectopic pregnancy. In addition, HCG is used extensively as a tumor marker for the diagnosis and clinical management of gestational trophoblastic pathologies (**hydatidiform moles, choriocarcinomas,** and placental trophoblastic tumors). HCG is used in conjunction with alpha-fetoprotein (AFP) in the classification of germ cell tumors of the ovary and testis according to their degree of differentiation. HCG is produced by syncytial trophoblastic cells, whereas AFP is produced by the more differentiated embryonal type cells. Both AFP and HCG are measured and the pattern of elevation or normal value determines which cell types are present. Elevated serum HCG has also been observed in a variety of other neoplastic pathologies, including melanoma, mammary, gastrointestinal, lung, and ovarian carcinomas. Serum HCG concentration correlates well with tumor burden and patient prognosis.[34]

HCG is a dimer composed of an alpha and a beta subunit. The beta subunit confers specificity, and the alpha subunit is found in luteinizing hormone (LH), follicle-stimulating hormone (FSH), and thyroid-stimulating hormone (TSH). Development of monoclonal antibody has eliminated the cross-reactivity problems found in the early assay. The use of monoclonal antibodies allows the measurement of free beta subunits or intact molecules, or both. Tumor production may include free alpha and beta chains, intact molecules, or both in any combination. It is therefore recommended that the assay used for tumor marker testing measure free beta subunits as well as intact molecules.[43] Also available is an assay for urinary gonadotropin peptide (UGP), which is a fragment of the beta subunit of HCG.[44]

## CALCITONIN

Calcitonin (HCT), also called thyrocalcitonin, is synthesized and secreted by the C cells of the thyroid. Its actions are antagonistic to those of parathyroid hormone, inhibiting the release of calcium from bone and increasing the renal excretion of calcium. Serum calcitonin is elevated in cases of medullary thyroid cancer with and without metastases. Calcitonin has

TABLE  17 – 2

**Hormones and Neurotransmitters Used as Tumor Markers**

| HORMONE/NEUROTRANSMITTER | SITE/TUMOR | ENDOCRINOPATHY/CLINICAL SYMPTOM(S) |
|---|---|---|
| Human chorionic gonadotropin | Trophoblastic tumors, choriocarcinoma, germ cell tumor of ovary and testes | Menstrual irregularities |
| Calcitonin | Medullary thyroid cancer | Hypocalcemia |
| Adrenocorticotropic hormone | Adrenals, oat cell carcinoma of lung | Cushing's syndrome |
| Catecholamines and metabolites | Pheochromocytomas, neuroblastoma, ganglioneuroma | Hypertension |
| Serotonin, 5-HIAA | Carcinoid Tumors | Carcinoid syndrome |
| Antidiuretic hormone | Pancreas, prostate, adrenal cortex, oat cell carcinoma of lung | Hyponatremia |
| Gastrin | Gastrinoma | Zollinger-Ellison syndrome |
| Glucagon | Glucagonoma | Glucagonoma syndrome |
| Insulin | Insulinoma | Hypoglycemia |
| Prolactin | Pituitary adenoma, kidney, lung | Abnormal lactation |
| Estrogens | Ovarian tumors, testicular tumors, adrenal cortex, chorioepithelium | Precocious puberty, feminization |
| Androgens | Leydig's cell tumor of testes, adrenal cortex, ovarian tumor | Precocious puberty, masculinization |
| Thyroid-stimulating hormone | Trophoblastic tumors, prostate, bronchogenic carcinoma, blood, pituitary | Hyperthyroidism |
| Human placental lactogen | Trophoblastic tumors | Abnormal lactation |
| Growth hormone | Pituitary adenoma, kidney, lung | Acromegaly, pituitary giantism |
| Parathyroid hormone | Parathyroid, liver, kidney, breast, lung | Hypercalcemia |
| Erythropoietin | Kidney | Erythrocytosis |
| Renin | Kidney | Hypertension, aldosteronism |
| Aldosterone | Adrenal cortex | Conn's syndrome, aldosteronism |

5-HIAA = 5-hydroxyindole-3-acetic acid.

been useful in screening asymptomatic relatives of patients with medullary thyroid carcinoma, diagnosing symptomatic patients with nonpalpable micro tumors not located by imaging techniques, and monitoring patients following therapeutic intervention(s). Serum levels reflect the tumor burden. Immunologic assays exist for this marker.[34]

## ADRENOCORTICOTROPIC HORMONE

Adrenocorticotropic hormone (ACTH) or corticotropin is normally synthesized by the anterior pituitary and regulates the production of steroid hormones (cortisol, aldosterone, and androgens) by the adrenal cortex. Both pituitary and ectopic ACTH-secreting tumors have been reported. These result in hypercortisolism (**Cushing's syndrome**) with its triad of elevated blood glucose, abnormal immunologic reactions, and electrolyte imbalance–induced hypertension. Elevated ACTH

is frequently observed in small cell carcinoma of the lung but can be the result of other ectopic tumors. Moderate elevations of ACTH may represent neurologic (pituitary) origin but high levels usually reflect ectopic disease. Failure of dexamethasone to suppress the production of ACTH, and consequently cortisol, is a good indicator for an ectopic source of ACTH. As expected, serum ACTH is abnormally decreased in patients with primary hypercortisolism (adrenal disease). Immunometric assays exist for ACTH and are useful for the elucidation of the source of hypercortisolism in patients with symptoms of Cushing's syndrome and for patient monitoring following surgery.[34]

## CATECHOLAMINES AND THEIR METABOLITES

The catecholamines, epinephrine (adrenaline), norepinephrine (noradrenaline), and dopamine are normally produced and stored in the brain, adrenal medulla, and in sympathetic neurons. Catecholamines are released into the circulation following sympathetic nerve stimulation and are transported by the blood to their target cells. There they bind to adrenergic receptors initiating metabolic and blood pressure changes. Catecholamines are metabolized fairly rapidly following their release into blood and are normally found in very small concentrations in plasma. The metabolites of catecholamines include metanephrine, normetanephrine, 3-methoxytyramine, vanillylmandelic acid (VMA), and homovanillic acid (HVA). Catecholamines and their metabolites are excreted into the urine.[45]

Two tumors are associated with production of high levels of catecholamines, **pheochromocytomas** in the adult and **neuroblastomas** in infants and children. Pheochromocytomas are tumors of the chromaffin cells. They are most frequently found in the adrenal medulla but are occasionally found along the aorta, in thoracic paravertebral ganglia, and along the wall of the urinary bladder. There is, in some cases, a familial predisposition to development of these tumors. Pheochromocytomas secrete large amounts of catecholamines, predominantly epinephrine and norepinephrine. Release of the catecholamines is intermittent or sustained, and causes hypertension. Diagnosis is usually predicated on the observation of elevated urinary metanephrines. Testing can be performed in combination with assays for urinary VMA and free catecholamines. Plasma catecholamine determination requires precise sampling as many variables can alter the release of catecholamines into the bloodstream.[34]

Neuroblastomas are a common tumor of childhood. There may be a familial tendency toward the development of these tumors. The neuroblastoma develops in the neural crest tissue in the adrenals, paravertebral, or elsewhere. The tumor growth is rapid with metastases occurring before diagnosis is made in many cases. In infants there are documented cases of spontaneous tumor regression. This may be linked to the development of immunity. There are also cases involving the evolution of the tumor to a benign ganglioneuroma. The prognosis after a child has reached the age of 1 year is very poor. Neuroblastomas frequently secrete dopamine and may secrete norepinephrine but not epinephrine. Diagnosis is made on the basis of elevated urinary HVA, VMA, dopamine, and norepinephrine.[2]

The method of choice for measuring catecholamines and their metabolites is high performance liquid chromatography (HPLC). Generally, a 24-hour urine is collected from a patient with suspected pheochromocytoma so that episodal secretion is not missed. In infants and children suspected of having neuroblastoma, episodal secretion is not a problem so a single random collection may be adequate. VMA and HVA can be measured and reported as a ratio to creatinine to compensate for the relative dilution of the urine. Slightly increased levels of catecholamines and their metabolites are usually associated with stress or heavy exercise rather than with a malignant tumor. Catecholamines can also be measured in plasma by HPLC. This may be done to check response to medications

or to help locate the tumor. Small pheochromocytomas secrete high levels of catecholamines and, if the tumor cannot be visualized, a catheter may be threaded into each possible location. Blood samples may be taken from each location and tested to see which has the highest level of catecholamine in an effort to locate the tumor.[45]

## SEROTONIN AND 5-HYDROXYINDOLE-3-ACETIC ACID

Serotonin (5-hydroxytryptamine) (5-HT) is produced in the enterochromaffin cells of the gastrointestinal tract as well as in the brain, and it is metabolized to 5-hydroxyindole-3-acetic acid (5-HIAA) in the lungs. Serotonin is a powerful vasoconstrictor and is carried in high concentration by platelets and released during clotting. Tumors of the enterochromaffin cells, called **carcinoid tumors** or **argentaffinomas,** release increased amounts of serotonin. Most of these tumors are primary to the gastrointestinal (GI) tract but they may also be found in the breast, thymus, liver, gallbladder, lung, and ovary. They grow rather slowly and may also secrete histamine, kallikrein, and prostaglandins. Carcinoid tumors are associated with symptoms such as flushed skin, diarrhea, nausea, hypotension, asthma, dermatitis, and cyanosis. The symptoms depend on the location of the tumors. The associated disease state is called carcinoid syndrome.[34] It should be noted that some patients may present with multiple endocrine tumors (carcinoid plus other tumors) causing elevations of other hormones (e.g., ACTH) as well.

Serotonin is measured in serum or in whole blood as it is found in the circulation concentrated in the platelets. 5-HIAA is measured in urine, although occasionally other body fluids are tested. Before testing, the patient should abstain from foods rich in serotonin such as bananas, avocados, eggplant, tomatoes, plums, pineapple, and walnuts. Some drugs may also cause elevation. Serotonin and 5-HIAA are extracted from body fluids and quantitated using HPLC.[34,40]

## ANTIDIURETIC HORMONE

Antidiuretic hormone (ADH) or vasopressin is synthesized in the hypothalamus, stored and released from the posterior pituitary, and regulates the reabsorption of free water at the Loop of Henle, collecting ducts and distal portion of the distal tubules in the nephron. Increased synthesis and secretion of ADH is observed in patients with a variety of malignancies and is called syndrome of inappropriate ADH secretion **(SIADH).** Very high serum levels of ADH have been reported in cases of small cell carcinoma of the lung. Likewise, pancreatic, duodenal, and adrenal malignancies have been associated with SIADH. Diagnosis is made on the basis of the serum and urine sodium and osmolality (hypoosmolal plasma, hyperosmolal urine, hyponatremia, and inappropriately elevated urinary sodium). This diagnosis is confirmed by quantitating ADH in serum. Immunologic assays for ADH exist and are especially useful in monitoring the patient's status following surgery.[34]

## GASTRIN

Gastrin is synthesized and secreted by G cells of the stomach, and duodenum and the D cells of the pancreas. It stimulates the secretion of gastric acid by the parietal cells and pepsinogens and intrinsic factor by the mucosal cells of the stomach. Likewise, it stimulates the secretion of small intestinal secretin, hepatic bile, and pancreatic digestive enzymes and bicarbonate. Gastrin-secreting duodenal and pancreatic tumors (gastrinomas) are responsible for a condition called **Zollinger-Ellison syndrome.** Symptoms include peptic ulcers, gastric hypersecretion, hypergastrinemia, and diarrhea. Diagnosis is based on markedly elevated serum gastrin levels in the presence of gastric acid hypersecretion. Elevated serum gastrin following intravenous infusion of secretin (secretin challenge test) confirms the diagnosis. Immunoassays for gastrin exist and blood samples should be collected following an overnight fast, separated, and frozen until assayed.[34]

## GLUCAGON

Glucagon is synthesized and secreted by the alpha cells of the islets of Langerhans in the pancreas. It stimulates glycogenolysis in the liver, thereby increasing blood glucose levels. **Glucagonomas** are glucagon-secreting tumors of the pancreas. Symptoms include those of hyperglycemia. Diagnosis is made by demonstrating the presence of elevated serum glucagon and glucose. Immunologic tests for glucagon exist.[2]

## INSULIN

Insulin is synthesized and secreted by the beta cells of the islets of Langerhans in the pancreas. It binds to insulin receptors present on most cells allowing the transport of glucose into the cell and inducing a series of anabolic reactions. **Insulinomas** are insulin-secreting tumors of the pancreas. Hypoglycemia is always present in these patients and can be severe following a prolonged fast. The diagnosis is based on hyperinsulinemia in the presence of hypoglycemia. The endogenous source of the insulin may be confirmed by quantitating the serum C-peptide concentrations. An elevated C-peptide represents de novo synthesis of the insulin (C-peptide is the connecting peptide in proinsulin), whereas low levels of C-peptide represent commercially prepared insulin. Immunologic assays exist for both insulin and C-peptide. Increasing serum concentrations of C-peptide following pancreatectomy in cancer patients suggests the recurrence of the tumor or the presence of metastases.[46]

## PROLACTIN

Prolactin (PRL) is synthesized and secreted by the lactotropic cells of the pituitary. It is under hypothalamic control. Inhibition of PRL secretion by prolactin inhibitory factor (PIF) (dopamine) is its major regulatory mode. Stimulation of PRL secretion by thyrotropin-releasing hormone (TRH) is a minor regulation pathway. Prolactin stimulates lactation by the mammary glands. Pituitary adenomas can cause hyperprolactinemia, which in turn causes galactorrhea. Diagnosis of a prolactin-secreting tumor is made on the basis of elevated serum prolactin in the presence of a pituitary mass observed by imaging techniques (MRI or CAT scan) or in the absence of other explanations such as abnormally decreased dopamine or elevated TRH. Both competitive binding RIAs and immunometric assays exist. Results should be correlated (converted) to international units as the assays do not use the same calibration.[8]

## ESTROGENS AND ANDROGENS

Estrogens (primarily estradiol) are produced by the ovary, and in the gravid female by the placenta. Normally, only very small amounts of estrogen are synthesized by the adrenal cortex and the testis. Estrogen-secreting tumors are typically of ovarian origin. However, estrogen-secreting tumors of the testis, the adrenal cortex, and chorioepithelium have been reported.[47] Symptoms can include precocious puberty of the female and feminization in the male. Estrogen-secreting tumors of the female have been implicated in increased risk of breast cancer.

Androgens (primarily testosterone) are produced by the testis in the male. Smaller amounts of androgens are synthesized by the ovary in females and the adrenal cortex in both males and females. Androgen-secreting tumors of the testis and of the ovaries and adrenals have been reported and are responsible for precocious puberty in the male and virilization in the female.[47]

Immunologic assays exist for both estradiol and total estrogens (estradiol plus estrone) as well as assays for testosterone and epiandrosterone. Alternatively, urinary metabolites can be measured for these hormones.

## THYROID-STIMULATING HORMONE

Thyroid-stimulating hormone (TSH), also known as thyrotropin, is synthesized and secreted by the anterior portion of the pituitary. It is under positive control by increased concentrations of thyrotropin releasing hormone (TRH) from the hypothalamus, and negative control by increased levels of the circulating thyroid hormones thyroxine ($T_4$) and triiodothyronine ($T_3$). In turn, it regulates the synthesis and release of $T_4$ and $T_3$ from the thyroid. Trophoblastic tumors and some tumors of the prostate, lung, blood, and pituitary secrete TSH, causing increased synthesis of the thyroid hormones with symptoms of hyperthyroidism. There are sensitive immunometric assays for TSH. The diagnosis is made on the basis of elevated TSH in the presence of elevated $T_4$ and $T_3$ accompanied by clinical symptoms of hyperthyroidism. Following surgery and other therapeutic interventions the patient should be monitored using the TSH assay.[48]

## HUMAN PLACENTAL LACTOGEN

Human placental lactogen (HPL), also called human chorionic somatomammotropin, is synthesized and secreted by the synctiotrophoblastic cells of the placenta during normal pregnancy. Elevated serum HPL has been reported in cases of gestational, gonadal, and extragonadal trophoblastic cancers. Serum concentrations are typically lower in malignancy than in normal pregnancy, where the concentrations correlate well with the placental weight and hence fetal development. Immunologic assays exist and have been used to monitor therapy and to help discriminate between normal pregnancy and cancer.[49]

## GROWTH HORMONE

Growth hormone (GH, somatotropin) is synthesized and secreted by the somatotropic cells of the anterior pituitary. Its major functions are to stimulate growth of bone, cartilage, and other soft tissue and to increase the synthesis of protein. Growth-hormone-secreting tumors of the pituitary cause **acromegaly** in adults and **pituitary gigantism** in children prior to epiphyseal closure of the long bones. Diagnosis is predicated on elevated levels of serum GH and clinical presentation, including enlarged mandible and hands in adults and abnormal height and general growth in children. Both competitive binding RIAs and immunometric assays for GH exist. Serum samples should be collected from fasted and rested subjects and stored frozen until testing.[34]

## PARATHYROID HORMONE

Parathyroid hormone (PTH) also called parathormone is synthesized and secreted by the chief cells of the parathyroid glands in response to low circulating levels of calcium. PTH regulates blood calcium by binding to bone and kidney receptors, causing increased osteoclastic activity with calcium release and renal calcium retention with phosphate excretion. Additionally, PTH regulates the hydroxylation of cholecalciferol in the kidney to produce active vitamin D, which in turn regulates the absorption of calcium and phosphate at the level of the gut. PTH-secreting tumors of the parathyroids have been reported and are associated with elevated circulating PTH and hypercalcemia. Other malignancies associated with hypercalcemia (e.g., breast cancer) have low or low normal serum PTH concentrations. The hypercalcemia is associated with bone metastases in these cancers. Ectopic production of intact PTH is extremely rare,[50] but there is an ectopically produced PTH–related protein (PTHrP) which contains much of the PTH sequence that binds to bone and kidney PTH receptors, causing hypercalcemia. Immunoassays for PTH and for PTHrP exist. PTHrP does not cross react in PTH immunoassays, which facilitates diagnosis. PTHrP is elevated in a majority of nonparathyroid malignancies associated with hypercalcemia but not in parathyroid malignancy or malignancies that are not associated with hypercalcemia.[51]

## ERYTHROPOIETIN

Erythropoietin is synthesized and secreted by the kidney. Its secretion is regulated by oxygen tension at the level of the kidney. In turn, erythropoietin stimulates the production of erythrocytes by the bone marrow. Certain renal malignancies can cause increased erythropoietin production with consequent erythrocytosis and polycythemia. There is an enzyme-linked immunosorbent assay (ELISA) assay available for erythropoietin, and published reference intervals are correlated with the altitude as this affects the normal blood erythrocyte concentration.[34]

## RENIN AND ALDOSTERONE

Renin is synthesized in the juxtaglomerular cells of the kidney in response to low renal perfusion pressure and/or hyponatremia. In turn, renin controls the conversion of angiotensinogen from the liver to angiotensin I. Angiotensin I is then converted to angiotensin II, which stimulates the synthesis of aldosterone by the adrenal cortex, promotes vasoconstriction, and, to a lesser extent, regulates ADH secretion by the posterior pituitary. Since aldosterone increases renal reabsorption of sodium and water and excretion of potassium and hydrogen ions, the net effect of increased renin and/or aldosterone is to increase the blood pressure. The major stimulator of aldosterone secretion is renin; however, it is also regulated by circulating ACTH levels.[40]

Renin-secreting tumors of the kidney have been reported, and there is an assay for renin. In the assay, the patient's plasma is challenged to convert renin to angiotensin I, which in turn is measured immunologically.[52] Ambulatory versus supine posture, hydration, diet, and a variety of drugs affect the test results and hence the reference intervals used. The diagnosis is made on the basis of extremely elevated renin levels in the presence of the anticipated electrolyte balance. Circulating aldosterone levels would also be elevated.

**Conn's syndrome** is the result of an aldosterone-secreting adrenal adenoma and is characterized by elevated aldosterone, decreased renin, hypernatremia, hypervolemia, hypokalemia, and metabolic alkalosis. Aldosterone-secreting carcinoma of the adrenal gland has been reported and has similar laboratory results. Secondary aldosteronism due to ACTH secreting tumors of the pituitary or renin-secreting tumors of the kidney can be discriminated on the basis of assays for these analytes. Aldosterone can be measured by RIA,[53] or alternatively the diagnosis may be made on the basis of clinical symptoms, inappropriate potassium urinary excretion, hypernatremia, hypokalemia, and low circulating renin.

## Receptors

Cell receptors are protein structures located on external cell membranes and within the cell. The function of the receptor is to recognize and bind a specific ligand such as a hormone or neurotransmitter. The ligand-receptor complex then initiates a biologic response. There are many different receptors. Each binds with high affinity to a specific substance and initiates one particular cellular response. Receptors must function properly for normal regulation of the cell. The production of receptors is regulated in part by ligand concentration. Numbers of cell receptors may increase or decrease or receptors may be inactivated in response to the concentration of the circulating ligand. There are defects in receptor production or function that are inherited, caused by malignant transformation or due to an autoimmune disorder (antibody directed against receptor). Because malignancy causes changes in receptor function and quantity, receptors can be used as tumor markers.[54]

## ESTROGEN AND PROGESTERONE RECEPTORS

Estrogen (ER) and progesterone (PgR) receptors are assayed clinically to determine which breast cancer patients may respond to endocrine therapy. If tumor growth is stimulated by estrogen, an antiestrogen such as tamoxifen may be used to limit the growth of the tumor. Estrogen receptors must be present and functioning for progesterone receptors to be produced. Increased receptor concentration correlates with improved response to therapy. When both are present, there is about an 80% chance that the tumor will respond to endocrine therapy. By contrast, patients who are positive for one receptor (>10 fmol/mg of cytosolic protein) and negative (<10 fmol/mg of cytosolic protein) for the other are less likely to respond to hormone manipulation.[55–56] Estrogen and progesterone receptors have also been used to predict the response of patients with endometrial cancer to hormonal therapy.

There are two basic methods of cell receptor quantitation. The first is the ligand-binding assay and the second is an immunoassay. Cell receptor studies are done on a tissue sample obtained from tumor biopsy or excision. The tissue must be homogenized and centrifuged prior to testing the supernatant.

## OTHER RECEPTORS

Androgen (AR) and progesterone (PgR) receptors have been measured to predict the outcome of antiandrogen therapy in prostate cancer patients.[57] Similarly, glucocorticoid receptors as a prognostic indicator are being evaluated in cases of lymphoblastic leukemia.[58]

Epidermal growth factor receptor (EGFR) is a glycoprotein known to bind epidermal growth factor (EGF) and transforming growth factor alpha (TGF-$\alpha$). The absence of this receptor correlates well with a good response to tamoxifen. High levels of the receptor seem to indicate a poor prognosis in terms of relapse and patient survival.[59]

Laminin receptor is another potential marker for breast cancer. Laminin is a major constituent of basement membrane and binds other important constituents, among them collagen, heparan sulfate, proteoglycan, and entactin. Laminin receptors allow malignant cells to attach to basement membranes, which are then dissolved, and the cells destroyed as cancer invades other tissue. Malignant cells have more unoccupied laminin receptors than do normal cells.[59]

Studies continue to define which receptors may be used as tumor markers. There are increased numbers of other receptors (such as insulin receptors) in tumor tissue, but their significance as markers has not been clearly defined. Table 17–3 lists receptors currently used as tumor markers.

## Proteins

The classification of proteins is somewhat arbitrary. As already noted, prostate-specific antigen (PSA) can be classified as an enzyme or an antigen. Similarly, many glycoproteins can be classified as oncofetal antigens or as carbohydrate markers.

TABLE 17–3

**Receptors Used as Tumor Markers**

| RECEPTOR | SITE/TUMOR |
|---|---|
| Estrogen, progesterone | Breast, endometrium |
| Androgen, progesterone | Prostate |
| Glucocorticoid | Lymphoblastic leukemia |
| Laminin | Measures metastatic potential |
| Epidermal growth factor | Breast |
| Interleukin-2 | Leukemia |

Oncofetal proteins (oncofetal antigens) are proteins that are normally expressed by the fetus but not by the healthy adult. Since these proteins are synthesized in high concentration by tumor cells in cancer patients, they were named oncofetal antigens or proteins. Historically, alpha-fetoprotein and carcinoembryonic antigen were the first of these proteins discovered, and they are usually referred to as oncofetal proteins or antigens. However, many of the protein tumor markers could be similarly classified.[4]

The carbohydrate tumor markers are glycoproteins defined by their antigenic property. They are cell surface antigens or secreted antigens that are expressed by tumor cells, and against which a monoclonal antibody or antibodies has been produced. These cancer antigens or epitopes are generally more specific than natural markers, and are defined by the monoclonal antibody system used to quantitate them. The carbohydrate tumor markers can be subdivided into mucins and blood group antigens. Examples of mucin markers are CA15-3 and CA125, whereas CA19-9 and CA72-4 are examples of blood group antigen markers.[4]

A variety of other proteins such as monoclonal immunoglobulin, beta$_2$-microglobulin, ferritin, and C-peptide have been used as tumor markers.

The advent of monoclonal technology has greatly improved the ability of the laboratory to measure tumor antigens. Immunoassays for these antigens are commercially available using a variety of assay designs. Competitive binding assays are available, but more commonly used are solid phase sandwich designs using radioisotope, enzyme, or chemiluminescent labels. The study of these proteins has provided a more sensitive and specific method for monitoring the progress of disease than was previously available. Many of these antibodies are also used immunocytochemically as tissue stains. The use of monoclonal antibody technology confers improved assay sensitivity and specificity, with little lot-to-lot antibody or assay variation. It should be noted, however, that patients who genetically do not express a particular blood group antigen will test negative for certain tumor antigens even though they have the tumor. Additionally, a given cancer epitope may be present in more than one type of cancer and two or more epitopes may be expressed by a single tumor. For example, CA125, CA15-3, and CA19-9 are expressed in varying quantities by many carcinomas, whereas CA15-3 and CA125 have been co-expressed by a single tumor.[60] The use of mouse monoclonal antibodies in cancer therapy has led to the development of a subset of patients who have **human antimouse antibodies (HAMA),** which interfere with mouse-derived monoclonal antibody immunoassays. Currently, the manufacturers are adding mouse serum to the reagents to correct this problem. Another problem is the **hook effect,** which occurs in sandwich-type assays when a patient has such an extremely high concentration of the antigen that it swamps out the labeled antibody, preventing it from binding to capture antibody-antigen complex and giving a falsely low result. The hook effect can be detected by assaying two dilutions of the sample and is not seen with the competitive binding assays.[61] Some proteins or antigens currently used to detect and monitor tumors are listed in Table 17–4.

## ALPHA-FETOPROTEIN

Alpha-fetoprotein (AFP), so named because it migrates electrophoretically between alpha$_1$ and albumin, is the most abundant protein present during fetal development. Its function is thought to be similar to that of albumin; structurally they are very much alike. AFP is sometimes called fetal albumin. AFP is manufactured mainly by fetal hepatocytes and the yolk sac. It is found in very high levels in the embryo and fetus. The level gradually drops until at the age of about 1 year, AFP is at normal adult levels (0 to 15 ng/mL).[34]

AFP is associated with various germ cell tumors and hepatoma. In patients with yolk-sac tumors (very rare), AFP correlates well with disease activity. Together with HCG, AFP is used to classify germ cell tumors and gestational trophoblastic disease. It is useful in characterization and staging of disease and in monitoring therapy. AFP levels rise before recurrence is detectable by other means.[62]

AFP is a good marker for primary hepatoma because it is elevated in approximately 80% of the cases. Unfortunately, AFP is also elevated in hepatitis, cirrhosis, and several other liver diseases. The level of AFP in these cases may help differentiate benign from malignant conditions. AFP is measured by immunoassay. It is also used extensively as a marker for neural tube defects and it shows potential as a screening tool for Down's syndrome.[62]

## CARCINOEMBRYONIC ANTIGEN

Carcinoembryonic antigen (CEA) is one of the older oncofetal proteins still in use. It was first described in 1965 by Gold and Freedman and was originally thought to be quite specific for colon cancer. It has since been characterized immunologically and by selective adsorption and is now recognized as a family of glycoproteins. The carbohydrate portion varies according to the source and the heterogeneity of tumors. It is not specific for the colon but is found in a variety of malig-

nant and nonmalignant conditions such as breast, GI, lung, ovary, pancreas, and prostate cancers. Additionally, it is elevated in alcoholism, inflammation of the bowel, cystic fibrosis, and in heavy cigarette smokers. Despite the nonspecificity of CEA, it is useful in establishing prognosis and in monitoring therapy. CEA measured in body fluids other than serum (ascitic fluid, fluid from cyst, urine, or lavage from any cavity) may also aid in diagnosis.[63]

### TABLE 17–4

**Proteins Used as Tumor Markers**

| PROTEIN | SITE/TUMOR |
|---|---|
| Alpha-fetoprotein | Liver, ovary, testes, (teratoblastoma) |
| Carcinoembryonic antigen | Colon, breast, lung |
| Prostate-specific antigen | Prostate |
| CA15-3 | Breast |
| CA27.29 | |
| CA549 | |
| BCM | |
| Mucin-like carcinoma-associated antigen | |
| CA19-9 | Pancreas |
| CA195 | |
| CA50 | |
| CA242 | |
| POA | |
| Du-Pan-2 | |
| CA125 | Ovary |
| Ovarian cancer antigen | |
| CA72-4 | Gastric, ovary, colon, breast, lung, pancreas |
| Squamous cell carcinoma antigen | Squamous cell carcinoma, cervix, lung, head, neck |
| Cyfra 21-1 | Lung |
| P-glycoprotein | Drug resistance marker |
| Ferritin | Hodgkin's disease, acute myelocytic leukemia, lung, liver, breast, pancreas, teratoblastoma |
| Beta$_2$-microglobulin | Lymphoma, leukemia, multiple myeloma, Waldenström's macroglobulinemia |
| C-peptide | Insulinoma |
| Immunoglobulins | Multiple myeloma, Waldenström's macroglobulinemia |
| Thyroglobulin | Thyroid |
| Tissue polypeptide antigen | Breast, lung, GI, bladder, ovary, uterus, prostate |

## PROSTATE-SPECIFIC ANTIGEN

Prostate-specific antigen (PSA) is a serine protease produced in the prostate and secreted into the seminal fluid. The function of PSA is to cause liquefaction of seminal coagulum. PSA is the only tissue-specific marker identified so far, but it is not specific for prostate cancer. PSA is found in small amounts in normal prostate and is elevated in benign prostatatic hyperplasia (BPH) and adenocarcinoma of the prostate. It is a more sensitive marker than ACP, and because of its tissue specificity, it became the first tumor marker recommended for screening for prostate cancer in older men. PSA is useful as a diagnostic tool despite overlap between the values seen in BPH and cancer patients. It has proved very useful in staging and monitoring disease. The serum level is roughly proportional to tumor volume and should return to normal within a month after radical prostatectomy. Serum levels are sensitive to recurrence of disease.[64] Two approaches to diagnosis and screening have involved the use of PSA density (serum PSA concentration/prostate volume determined by ultrasound) and the calculation of a slope (PSA velocity) determined by plotting serum PSA concentrations versus time. The first approach is both invasive and expensive, whereas the second approach requires that one restrict preanalytical variability and use the same assay for all data points. Nevertheless, increased PSA density (>0.15) and increased PSA velocity (>0.75 ng/mL/y) correlate better with prostatic cancer than with BPH and help discriminate between those diagnoses in patients with moderately elevated total PSA levels. Another refinement has been the use of age-related reference intervals. This increases the sensitivity of the assay in young men and the specificity in older men.

PSA exists in both free and complexed (PSA complexed to alpha$_1$-antichymotrypsin) form in serum. Although a very small percentage of serum PSA is complexed to alpha$_2$-macroglobulin, it is nonreactive in the currently available assays and therefore will not be included as part of the complexed PSA. Immunologic assays measuring total, free, and complexed PSA are commercially available. Measuring the percentage of free PSA (free PSA/total PSA × 100%) or the amount of complexed PSA may improve the specificity of the assay.[8] The ability to detect prostate cancer is greatly enhanced when measuring free PSA% as compared with total PSA and free PSA assays. One advantage to the free PSA% assay is its lack of age-related variability. By contrast, healthy adult male reference intervals for free PSA and total PSA vary with age and, to some extent, with race (higher values for African American men). A drawback to the free PSA% assay is its lack of correlation with the cancer stage, which in turn is used to select patients for surgical intervention. Since free PSA correlates well with the cancer stage, it is useful in selecting patients who will benefit from surgery. Both complexed PSA and the percentage of complexed PSA (complexed PSA/total PSA × 100%) assays exist and allow one to discriminate between prostatic cancer and BPH. The complexed PSA assay has two advantages over free PSA and total PSA assays. These include: (1) the increased stability of complexed PSA as compared with free PSA, and (2) the improved detection of complexed PSA

(major fraction) over free PSA (minor fraction) when the total PSA concentration is low. The complexed PSA% assay does not exhibit age-related variability for healthy men and has superior assay specificity when compared with free PSA% assays. Since the complexed PSA assay also exhibits superior specificity when compared with the free PSA% assay and does not require the use of a second assay (total PSA), it may prove to be the optimal method for discriminating between prostatic cancer and BPH. At this point, it is clear that both free and complexed PSA assays and their ratios to total PSA are superior to the simple total PSA assay for making the differential diagnosis between prostatic cancer and BPH. In addition, it is imperative that the same assay be consistently used when monitoring a patient and that one apply the appropriate cutoff values for that assay.[8]

### CA15-3

CA15-3 is a glycoprotein mucin present on mammary epithelium. It is detected with an antibody raised against human milk fat globule membrane (115D8) and one raised against a human breast cancer (DF3). Assays for CA15-3 are not specific for breast cancer because they can be elevated in a variety of carcinomas. However, they are sensitive for breast cancer and are currently used to monitor patients following surgery.[65] CA549,[8] CA27.29,[66] breast cancer mucin (BCM),[67] and mucin-like carcinoma-associated antigen (MCA)[68] are newer breast cancer markers that may show similarity to CA15-3 because there appears to be some overlap of the epitopes. All are used for monitoring patients with confirmed breast cancer.

### CA19-9

CA19-9 is a mucin-like oligosaccharide characterized by antibody first developed from mice immunized to a human colon cancer cell line (SW-1116). It has a high specificity for pancreatic cancer but also recognizes other gastrointestinal cancers. CA19-9 is used clinically to monitor therapy and to predict disease recurrence. Because CA19-9 is related to the Lewis substance, Lewis-negative patients will not produce CA19-9.[8] CA19-9 may also be elevated in diseases associated with biliary obstruction and in cystic fibrosis. CA195 CA50, CA242, pancreatic oncofetal antigen (POA), and Du-Pan-2 are other antibody-defined markers that may exhibit similar specificity and sensitivity for pancreatic carcinoma.[69–71] None of these markers is specific for pancreatic cancer. Nevertheless, they all are useful as aids to diagnosis and in monitoring treatment. Both EIA and RIA assays exist for these markers.

### CA125

CA125 is a glycoprotein defined by the monoclonal antibody OC125. It is a good marker for ovarian carcinomas. It has limited use in diagnosis but has been used in conjunction with CEA to characterize ovarian tumors. It has been found to be elevated in nonmalignant conditions such as pregnancy, endometriosis, fibromatosis, pelvic inflammatory disease, pancreatitis, and peritonitis. The highest levels are associated with ovarian cancer but CA125 is elevated in other malignancies, especially those of mullerian ductal origin. It is most useful in monitoring disease in patients with a diagnosis of epithelial ovarian cancers.[72–73] Ovarian cancer antigen (OCA)[8] is thought to be similarly useful. Immunometric assays are commercially available.

## CA72-4

CA72-4 is a marker for gastrointestinal, lung, and ovarian carcinomas, and may exhibit some sensitivity for gastric cancers. Originally purified from a breast cancer TAG-72 (tumor-associated glycoprotein), it was subsequently purified from a colon carcinoma cell line (LS-174T). Immunometric assays for CA72-4 are marketed for use in the detection of all forms of GI cancer, but especially gastric cancer, which does not react especially well with other markers.[34,74]

## SQUAMOUS CELL CARCINOMA ANTIGEN

Squamous cell carcinoma antigen (SCC) is one of 14 subfractions of tumor-associated antigen (TA4). Fifty-eight percent of squamous cell carcinomas (head, neck, lung, esophagus) show elevated levels of SCC, but it can also be elevated with other histologic types and in benign diseases. It is useful in monitoring disease, especially cervical cancer.[75] SCC has been used in combination with CEA and NSE for the detection and monitoring of lung tumors. Immunologic assays are marketed commercially.

## CYFRA 21-1

Cyfra 21-1 is a marker for non-small cell lung cancer. It is a cytokeratin 19 fragment (epithelial cell intermediate filament protein). These filament proteins form a part of the cytoplasmic matrix, are increased during mitosis, and released from necrotic cells. Cyfra 21-1 is especially useful in monitoring squamous cell carcinoma of the lung. Quantitation is by immunoassay.[8]

## P-GLYCOPROTEIN

P-glycoprotein is found in cell membranes of drug-resistant cells. It is normally found in kidney, liver, adrenal, and GI tract cells. Most tumors that develop in these organs are fairly drug resistant. Cells resistant to one drug may also show resistance to other unrelated drugs, a phenomenon given the name multidrug resistance. It is theorized that P-glycoprotein is active in transporting the drugs out of the cells. P-glycoprotein can be measured using a monoclonal antibody, C219. The tumor cells are stained with labeled antibody or are tagged and counted using flow cytometry. This test may predict response to therapy, help identify therapeutic measures to be used, and help establish a treatment schedule.[76]

## FERRITIN

Ferritin is the major iron storage protein and is found in most cells. Only a small percentage of total body ferritin is found in plasma where it binds and transports iron (the major iron transport protein is transferrin). It is frequently assayed as an indicator of iron status since the plasma or serum ferritin level is directly proportional to the body iron stores. Ferritin is elevated in any disease that causes a profound disturbance in iron metabolism and erythropoiesis. It may be elevated in hepatitis and aplastic anemia, but it is also elevated in leukemias, lymphomas, myeloma, neuroblastoma, gastric, colon, pancreatic, lung and breast cancers, and in melanoma. Levels are also affected by secondary complications of cancer such as obstruction and anemia. Ferritin released from malignant tumors has a more acidic isoelectric point than normal ferritin, and thus may be differentiated by isoelectric focusing.[34]

## BETA₂-MICROGLOBULIN

Beta₂-microglobulin (B2M) is an antigen found on the surface of all nucleated cells. It is a subunit of human leukocyte antigen (HLA) and is elevated in all diseases associated with rapid cell turnover. It is used as a marker for leukemias, lymphoma, and multiple myeloma and it correlates well with B lymphocyte activity. It may also be elevated in patients suffering from human immunodeficiency virus (HIV) infection. It is measured by immunoassay.[77]

## C-PEPTIDE

C-peptide is the connecting peptide between the A and B chain of proinsulin. It is dissociated from these chains to produce active insulin. C-peptide is elevated in patients with increased endogenous insulin production, for example, insulinoma. C-peptide is not metabolized by the liver, and does not cross react with anti-insulin antibodies that can interfere with insulin assays. C-peptide is not elevated in patients receiving exogenous insulin. Therefore, assay of C-peptide allows one to reliably measure pancreatic beta cell function. Some patients with beta cell pancreatic tumors produce fluctuating levels of insulin but their C-peptide levels are uniformly high. This permits early diagnosis of recurrent disease following pancreatic surgery, even when insulin levels are within normal reference intervals. A number of commercial immunoassays are on the market but there is considerable variation between their reference intervals, so care should be taken if switching assays.[78]

## IMMUNOGLOBULINS

The immunoglobulins have been used as markers in multiple myeloma and in Waldenström's macroglobulinemia for many years. They are quantitated and characterized using electrophoresis and immunoelectrophoresis (monoclonal bands) and by using turbidimetric methods with specific antisera. Bence Jones protein (urinary free immunoglobulin light chains) are also present in patients with these cancers. The concentrations of serum and urine monoclonal immunoglobulins have been used to aid in diagnosis, develop a prognosis, and monitor treatment of these patients.[34]

## THYROGLOBULIN

Thyroglobulin (Tg) is a large glycoprotein located in the thyroid where it serves as a precursor to thyroxine ($T_4$) and triiodothyronine (T$_3$). Thyroglobulin is elevated in patients with follicular and papillary thyroid carcinoma and thyroid adenoma as well as in a variety of other thyroid conditions. Since thyroglobulin is not elevated in patients with medullary thyroid carcinoma, it serves to help discriminate between this and other hyperthyroid diseases. Endogenous antibodies to thyroglobulin interfere with the RIA assays available, but not to any great extent with the immunometric assays.[34]

## TISSUE POLYPEPTIDE ANTIGEN

Tissue polypeptide antigen (TPA) is an oncofetal protein related to the cytokeratins. It is synthesized during mitosis and therefore is a useful marker of cellular proliferation. It is elevated in a variety of normal health conditions (pregnancy) and abnormal (autoimmune, infectious, and hepatic) conditions. It is also elevated in the sera of patients with breast, lung, gastrointestinal, bladder, ovarian, uterine, and prostatic cancers. Quantitation of this marker has proved useful in monitoring and staging because it correlates well with the tumor burden.[79–80]

## Genetic Markers

Direct analysis of nuclear DNA is useful in determining diagnosis (benign versus malignant), determining prognosis (survival time), monitoring patients for increased aneuplasia, and predicting or evaluating therapeutic response.

Normal nonproliferating cells (in G$_1$ or G$_0$ cell cycle phase) are diploid, whereas DNA doubles during the synthesis phase **(S phase)** of proliferation and remains doubled (cell cycle G$_2$) until mitosis **(M phase).** Cancer cells may have an abnormally increased amount of DNA **(aneuploidy)** owing to increased number of chromosomes, increased DNA per chromosome, and minutes (small pieces of DNA from viruses). Additionally, cancer cells may have an abnormally high percentage of their cells that are in S phase. Both the **ploidy** (DNA amount) and the percentage of cells going through S phase can be determined by flow cell cytometry, giving a measure of tumor aggressiveness.[61]

There are two types of genetic tumor markers: (1) **oncogenes,** and (2) **anti-oncogenes (suppressor genes).** The oncogenes are derived from normal cellular genes (proto-oncogenes), which are involved in regulating cellular growth, proliferation, differentiation, and **apoptosis** (programmed cell death). The oncogenes are activated by mutational events that cause increased transcription of growth and proliferation, promoting protein products or products which antagonize (suppress) normal cellular apoptosis. Mutations include: insertions, deletions, translocations, inversions, and point mutations. Many oncogenes are of viral origin and many human oncogenes are associated with hematologic malignancies but a few are associated with solid tumors. The suppressor genes code for normal protein products that down regulate (control) cellular proliferation. The loss of these genes, and consequently their protein products, allows continuous transcription of growth, proliferation, and metastasis, promoting protein products. Methods of anal-

ysis include: immunohistochemical assays, karyotyping with special staining techniques to view repeated and inverted sequences, fluorescence in situ hybridization **(FISH)** to look for translocations and other genomic anomalies, gene probe technology using Southern and Northern blots, and polymerase chain reaction **(PCR)** technology to detect fusion chromosomal genes.[4] Monoclonal antibody tests specific for the oncogene products have been developed and are being evaluated. Table 17–5 lists some currently used oncogene and suppressor gene markers.

## ONCOGENES

Located on chromosome 1, N-ras is an oncogene that is the result of a single point mutation. It codes for a tyrosine kinase product (p21) that normally functions in signal transduction, and its overexpression is associated with neuroblastoma and acute myeloid leukemia (AML).[4,81]

The c-erbB-2 gene (HER-2/neu) codes for a transmembrane receptor with protein kinase activity. The protein product functions as a growth factor receptor and the overexpression of the gene is strongly associated with breast and ovarian cancer. It has been reported in gastrointestinal cancer. Assays exist for both the gene and the protein product, and results correlate well with prognosis.[4,81]

The c-myc gene codes for a protein product (p62) that binds to DNA and regulates transcription. Overexpression of the gene is associated with small cell carcinoma of the lung, breast carcinoma, gastric and other GI cancers, and promy-

T A B L E   1 7 – 5

**Oncogenes and Suppressor Genes Used as Tumor Markers**

| ONCOGENE | SITE/TUMOR |
| --- | --- |
| N-ras | Acute myeloid leukemia, neuroblastoma |
| c-erb B2 (HER 2 neu) | Breast, ovary, GI |
| c-myc | Lung, lymphoma, GI, brain, colon |
| c-abl/bcr | Chronic myelogenous leukemia |
| N-myc | Neuroendocrine |
| **SUPPRESSOR GENE** | |
| DCC | Colon carcinoma |
| p53 | Colon, breast, lung, brain, bladder |
| NF-1 | Brain |
| RB | Eye, lung, breast, bladder, prostate, retinoblastoma, osteosarcoma |
| WT | Kidney cancer |

elocytic leukemia. Translocation of the gene is seen in Burkitt's lymphoma and a variety of other B and T cell lymphomas.[4,81]

The **Philadelphia chromosome** is the result of a translocation of the abl gene from the distal portion of chromosome 9 to the bcr region of chromosome 22. The result of this abnormal gene splicing is to produce an abl-like tyrosine kinase protein product that reacts faster and with a wider group of substrates. The c-abl/bcr gene is involved in signal transduction and associated with chronic myelogenous leukemia.[4,81]

The N-myc oncogene was first observed in brain cancer. It is the result of abnormal DNA amplification and its protein product functions as a transcription regulator. It is associated with neuroendocrine tumors.[4,81]

### SUPPRESSOR GENES

The DCC gene is located on chromosome 18 and encodes a protein that is similar to cell adhesion proteins. It is responsible for down regulating proliferation in gastrointestinal cells. The loss of this gene causes late stage colon cancer. The gene is of interest because it is useful in discriminating between early and late stage disease in patients with colon cancer, and therefore in staging and prognosis.[4]

The gene for p53, located on chromosome 17, codes for a protein that regulates transition into S phase of the cell cycle. Mutation or loss of this gene leads to continuous cellular proliferation. Abnormal or absent p53 gene and its product are associated with several cancers including breast, colon, and lung carcinomas as well as some sarcomas, leukemias, and neurologic tumors.[4,81]

The NF1 gene is located on chromosome 17 and acts as a ras GTPase activator. The loss of this gene causes neurofibromas, sarcoma, and glioma.[4,34]

The RB gene was first described in patients with inherited retinoblastoma. The gene is located on chromosome 13 and the protein product (pRB) is an important transcription inhibitor and regulates transition from $G_1$ to S phase. Loss of this gene and its product is seen in patients with retinoblastoma, osteosarcomas, rhabdomyosarcomas, and carcinomas of the bladder, breast, and prostate. Two types of retinoblastoma patient presentations are known: inherited and sporadic. The inherited disease first presents in children and usually involves both eyes but always involves more than one clone of abnormal cells. This is because one of the two RB gene alleles is absent in the germ line, and therefore it only takes the loss of one (the other) allele to produce a tumor. The sporadic disease first presents in adults and involves only one clone (in one eye). This is due to the extremely low probability of losing both alleles for the RB gene in the same cell.[4,82]

The WT1 gene is located on chromosome 11 and codes for a nuclear protein that acts as a transcription factor. Loss of this gene causes Wilms' tumor (nephroblastoma), a childhood kidney cancer.[4]

The BRCA1 and BRCA2 suppressor genes are currently under investigation as markers of genetic susceptibility for breast cancer. The majority of familial (inherited) breast cancer patients have a mutation or loss of one of these genes. Monoclonal assays for the protein product are under production and their use should facilitate the analysis of samples from family members of breast cancer patients.[83]

## Other Markers

### LIPID-ASSOCIATED SIALIC ACID

Sialic acid is a family of acylated derivatives of neuraminic acid usually found on the terminal end of the carbohydrate portion of glycoprotein or glycolipid in cell membranes. The carbohydrate portion may influence cell-to-cell interaction, affecting cohesion, adherency, and antigenicity. These characteristics change following malignant transformation of a cell. The level of sialic acid may be altered with the change. Sialic acid, whether the total is measured or the lipid-associated fraction is extracted to be quantitated separately, is a nonspecific marker for malignant neoplasia.[84] It is used for monitoring patient response to therapy and recurrence of disease. The assay is a colorimetric test and uses plasma.

### HYDROXYPROLINE

Hydroxyproline (Hyp) is an amino acid that is elevated in patients with bone metastases. It is a marker of invasion and metastasis and is measured in urine using HPLC.[8]

### POLYAMINES AND ACETYLATED POLYAMINES

Polyamines (putrescine, spermidine and spermine) are stabilizing agents that associate with cell membranes and nucleic acids. The polyamines are metabolic products produced by all proliferating cells and acetylated in the liver. Since their concentration in urine appears to parallel the rate of proliferation, they have been used to monitor therapy and recurrence of disease. They are measured in urine by HPLC or GC.[85]

### BLOOD CELL SURFACE ANTIGENS

Antibodies to lymphoid and myeloid cell surface antigens together with flow cell cytometry can be used to confirm the diagnosis of leukemias and lymphomas and to discriminate between different subtypes. This is an aid in diagnosis and gives reliable prognostic information.[86]

## CLINICAL APPLICATIONS

## Gastrointestinal Cancers

Gastrointestinal cancers are a diverse group that includes cancers of the colon and rectum as well as the esophagus, stomach, and small intestine. Colorectal carcinoma ranks third in new cancer cases in the United States and is second only to lung cancer in mortality.[87] Symptoms of colorectal cancer include bleeding, change in bowel habits, and pain. The high-risk population includes those with a family history and those with a high-fat diet. Diagnosis is usually made after examination with a proctosigmoidoscope. Therapy usually involves surgical resection and radiation because colon tumors tend to be resistant to chemotherapy using cytotoxic drugs. When detected early, the 5-year survival rate is high (87%), but if metastasis has occurred, survival rates drop significantly. The tumor markers commonly used to monitor patients with colon cancer include CEA, CA19-9, and CK-BB. When colorectal cancer has metastasized to the liver, AFP and liver enzyme analysis may also be included. Gastric cancer ranks first among cancers worldwide and is increasing in the United States. It is diagnosed by gastroscopy and a variety of imaging techniques and is treated by surgery with chemotherapy and radiotherapy as adjuvant treatment. The tumor markers usually associated with it are CEA, CA72-4, CA19-9, CA-50, and CK-BB. Tumors of the small intestine are rare. Tumors of the esophagus are most commonly squamous cell carcinomas, but these are not found often in the United States. Carcinoid tumors of the enterochromaffin cells of the gastrointestinal tract have been discussed in this chapter, and there are other tumors associated with the endocrine glands of the gastrointestinal tract, e.g., gastrinoma.[7]

## Breast Cancer

With 182,000 estimated new cases in the year 2000, breast cancer incidence ranks first among U.S. women.[87] Breast cancer affects 1 in 10 women. Warning signs include breast changes such as a lump or thickening, dimpling or change of the nipple, discharge or pain. Women at high risk include those with a family history of breast cancer, age over 50 years, nulliparous women, and obese women. A monthly self-examination is recommended for all women, and it is suggested that all women have a baseline mammogram when they are between the ages of 35 and 40, with a follow-up mammogram every 1 or 2 years thereafter. Therapy usually involves surgical resection, radiation, chemotherapy, or endocrine therapy.[7]

There are more tumor marker options available for use in evaluating breast cancer than for most other cancers. Serum markers include CEA, CA15-3, CA27.29, CA549, BCM, MCA, ferritin, and CK-BB. Tissues can be analyzed for estrogen and progesterone receptors, cathepsin D, epidermal growth factor receptor, laminin receptor, ploidy, c-erbB-2, and collagenase.[88] Choices of therapy depend on the results of these assays. Multiple markers can be used at the time of diagnosis to help establish prognosis. The prognosis is greatly improved if there is minimal or no nodal involvement.

## Bronchogenic Carcinoma

Bronchogenic carcinoma (lung cancer) ranks first in cancer mortality and second (after breast cancer in women and prostate cancer in men) in cancer incidence in the United States.[87] Cigarette smoking and exposure to chemicals are the principal risk factors associated with this disease. Symptoms include a persistent cough, chest pain, infection, and blood-streaked sputum. Lung cancers are classified as squamous cell carcinomas, adenocarcinoma, small cell carcinomas, and large cell carcinomas. Squamous cell carcinomas are the most common, whereas small cell carcinomas are the most aggressive and are sometimes associated with ectopic hormone production. The lungs are a frequent site of metastatic tumor growth. Early detection is difficult because symptoms do not appear early and the 5-year survival rate is very low. Therapeutic measures include surgical resection, radiation, and chemotherapy. In small cell tumors, chemotherapy without surgery is effective.[7] The markers used to monitor this disease include CEA, Cyfra 21-1, CK-BB, AFP, CA72-4 and, especially in the case of small cell tumors, ADH and neuron-specific enolase.[8]

## Pancreatic Cancer

Pancreatic cancer is silent and deadly. The majority of cases occur after age 65 and many are associated with prior pancreatitis, diabetes, or cirrhosis. Diet may be a contributing factor. The 5-year survival rate is <3%. Most pancreatic carcinomas are exocrine rather than endocrine. Insulinoma, an endocrine tumor, is generally a more localized tumor and more treatable with higher survival rates. Radiation and chemotherapy are not highly effective.[7] Tumor markers associated with pancreatic carcinoadenoma include CA19-9, CA195, CA242, CA50, CEA, POA, insulin, amylase, lipase, trypsin, ribonuclease, and ferritin. Many of these are useful in diagnosis and in establishing prognosis.[8]

## Prostate Adenocarcinoma

Prostate adenocarcinoma is the most common cancer in men with risk increasing with age.[87] Symptoms include difficulty with urine flow, pain, and bleeding. In the 60% that are discovered before metastasis, the prognosis is good. The usual therapy includes surgical resection with radiation, chemotherapy, or hormone manipulation. Chemotherapy and hormones may be used to shrink the tumor before surgical excision is attempted. Tumor markers used in establishing the diagnosis, prognosis, staging, and monitoring therapy include PSA, PAP, or ACP, CEA, CK-BB, LD-5, and TPA. ALP may be used if bone metastases are present.[7] PSA may be used rather than surgery to evaluate the risk of disease recurrence.

## Ovarian Cancer

Ovarian cancer is silent and produces more deaths than any other gynecologic cancer. Risks increase with age, family history, and nulliparity or low parity. Benign tumors are common in young women. Symptoms are vague and include enlargement of the abdomen, pain, digestive disturbances, and malaise. Screening can best be done by pelvic examination. Approximately 95% of all ovarian carcinomas are epithelial carcinomas (many are cystic), which are subclassified as serous (filled with fluid), mucinous (composed of mucous-secreting cells), and endometroid tumors. Less common are the germ cell tumors.

They are classified as embryonic carcinoma, teratoma, dysgerminoma, yolk sac tumors and choriocarcinoma which is usually associated with the placenta and may originate from an ectopic pregnancy.[24] Metastasis is likely to occur with malignant tumors often before diagnosis is made. Tumor markers are used to classify tumors, to follow therapy, and to replace surgery for detecting metastasis and recurrence. Tumor markers for ovarian cancer include CA125, OCA, AFP, CEA, HCG, CA72-4, and sialic acid. Examination of the ratio of CA125/CEA may help differentiate ovarian cancer from other abdominal cancers. It is important to emphasize that many ovarian tumors are benign.[88]

## Uterine Cancer

Uterine cancer is treatable if discovered early. Every woman is encouraged to have a Papanicolaou cytological test (PAP smear) done yearly. Symptoms include bleeding and discharge and the populations at high risk include those with multiple sex partners, those who have had sexually transmitted infections, women on estrogen therapy, and smokers. Herpes simplex virus II and human papillomavirus infections are associated with an increased incidence of uterine carcinoma. Endometrial carcinoma is associated with estrogen stimulation. Surgical resection, cryotherapy, or electrocoagulation of the cells on the cervix, along with radiation and progesterone therapy, are the usual therapeutic measures.[7,24] With early detection and in situ disease, survival approaches 100%. Tumor markers include SCC for squamous cell carcinoma, TPA, sialic acid, and histaminase.

## Testicular Tumors

Testicular tumors include a variety of cancers. Most are germ cell tumors, which are highly aggressive neoplasms and are classified as seminoma, spermatocytic seminoma, embryonal carcinoma, yolk sac tumor, polyembryoma, choriocarcinoma, and teratoma or classified as a mixture of the above. In addition to germ cell tumors, there are a small number of stromal tumors, including Leydig's cell tumors, Sertoli's cell tumors, and granulosa cell tumors. These tumors are classified partially by the presence of abnormal levels of the tumor markers HCG and AFP. LD may also be used as a marker in testicular cancer.[7,24]

## Skin Cancers

There are three types of skin cancers. Basal cell and squamous cell carcinomas are highly treatable, but melanoma is very aggressive and dangerous and may metastasize to the lymph nodes and systemically from there. Skin cancer risk is high in fair-skinned people and is increased with sun, radiation, and chemical exposure. Skin cancer diagnosis involves recognition of changes on the skin, pale, waxlike, or red, scaly patches, or changes in a mole. Tumor markers are not used extensively with skin cancers. Diagnosis is made by biopsy and microscopic examination and treatment involves surgical removal or cryotherapy.[7]

## Neuroblastomas and Pheochromocytomas

Neuroblastomas and pheochromocytomas have been discussed earlier in this chapter. Tumors of the brain are associated with symptoms such as headaches, dizziness, blurred or double vision, and nausea. Many of the symptoms are caused by pressure from the tumor growth crowding the brain and nerves. Malignant tumors of the central nervous system are classified according to which cells are affected. Surgical excision of tumors is done quite successfully in some cases, whereas other tumors have a high mortality rate.[7] Tumor markers associated with tumors of the brain and central nervous system include catecholamines and metabolites, CK-BB, CEA, and the polyamines as general markers of proliferation.

## Leukemias and Lymphomas

Leukemias and lymphomas are relatively common malignancies. Lymphomas are cohesive lesions mainly composed of lymphocytes that arise in lymph nodes throughout the body. Leukemias are overgrowths of blast cells that originate in the bone marrow and flood the circulating blood with immature and mature cells. Children are at risk for acute lymphoblastic leukemia and adults for acute myeloblastic leukemia and chronic lymphocytic leukemia. Diagnosis is based on blood and bone marrow testing, but there are markers associated with these diseases. HTLV-I retrovirus exposure should be determined, since this has been isolated as a possible causative agent in T cell leukemias and lymphomas.[7,61]

TdT is a marker associated with acute lymphoblastic leukemia. B2M is associated with several lymphomas and with multiple myeloma. The Philadelphia chromosome is closely associated with chronic myelocytic leukemia and multiple myeloma or plasma cell myeloma is associated with increased amounts of IgG.[8]

## Miscellaneous Tumors

Less common are tumors of the bladder and kidney and primary hepatoma. The marker of choice for bladder tumors is CEA and for kidney tumors, erythropoietin, renin, and PTH. Primary hepatoma may follow hepatitis, cirrhosis, or viral disease. Markers for primary hepatoma include AFP, GGT, LD-5, 5'NT, and the liver isoenzyme of ALP. Metastases to the liver are very common, and the markers associated with primary hepatoma may also be elevated in metastatic disease.[88]

## NEW DIRECTIONS

The development of multiple markers has made it possible to use ratios and patterns of markers assayed in panels to improve the sensitivity and specificity of those markers for cancer testing. Most of the markers discussed are now used clinically in the United States, and others are used domestically in medical research and clinically abroad. New markers are continually being discovered and investigated. A few areas of emerging tumor markers include markers associated with: oncogenes, suppressor genes, angiogenesis, the cell cycle, cell adhesion, nuclear matrix proteins, autoantibodies, growth factors, cytokines, and heat shock proteins.[8]

In addition to use in disease diagnosis, classification, and management of therapy, some markers have possible use as immunotherapeutic agents.[8] For example, if cytotoxic or cytolytic agents can be conjugated to tumor-specific monoclonal antibodies, tumor cell destruction without damage to normal cells will be facilitated. Radiolabeled antibodies can aid in location and visualization of tumors.[89] Likewise, the use of antiangiogenic factors could control the importation of blood vessels by the tumor and hence limit its growth.[90] Continuing advances in the area of tumor markers will help to better understand and even predict malignant disease.

## SUMMARY

Cancer is a disease of uncontrolled cellular proliferation. A tumor marker is any substance synthesized by the tumor or by the host in response to a tumor that can be used to detect the presence of the tumor. An ideal tumor marker would have the following characteristics: diagnostic specificity, diagnostic sensitivity, correlation between marker concentration and tumor burden, stability of marker concentration in the presence of stable disease, reasonably short marker biologic half-life, marker concentrations that have prognostic value, and good analytical performance. Most tumor markers have not proved to be very useful for screening asymptomatic patients (PSA is a possible exception to this rule of thumb). Tumor markers are routinely used as an aid to diagnosis, clinical staging, measurement of tumor burden, therapeutic monitoring, detection of disease recurrence, and as a prognostic indicator. Chemical and cellular moities that form a part of, are produced by, or are produced in response to signals from a tumor cell may be used as tumor markers. Tumor markers may be classified according to their chemical structure, biologic function, method of detection, or anatomic source. One classification scheme divides tumor markers into: (1) enzymes and isoenzymes, (2) hormones, neurotransmitters, and their metabolites, (3) receptors, (4) proteins and antigens, (5) genetic markers, and (6) other markers. Tumor markers currently in clinical use include markers that are relatively specific for a given type of cancer or anatomic origin. For example, serum PSA concentration reflects prostatic disease, whereas CA125 is useful for monitoring ovarian cancer. The detection of some cancers can be improved by using more than one tumor marker (panel of markers). For example, breast cancer detection and monitoring can involve the use of CEA, CA15-3, CA27.29, CA549, and a variety of other markers. Analyte measurement includes chemical tests, kinetic assays, immunoassays, histologic and cytologic techniques, flow cytometry, molecular biology techniques, and karyotyping techniques.

## REFERENCES

1. Landis SH, Murray T, Bolden S, et al.: Cancer statistics, 1998. CA Cancer J Clin 48:6, 1998.
2. Cooper GM: *Elements of Human Cancer.* Boston, Jones and Bartlett Publishers, 1992.
3. Ruddon RW: *Cancer Biology.* 2nd ed. New York, Oxford University Press, 1987.
4. Franks LM, Teich NM: *Introduction to the Cellular and Molecular Biology of Cancer.* 3rd ed. New York, Oxford University Press, 1997.
5. American Joint Committee on Cancer: *Manual for Staging of Cancer.* 3rd ed. Philadelphia, JB Lippincott, 1987.
6. International Union Against Cancer: *TNM Atlas.* 3rd ed. New York, Springer-Verlag, 1990.
7. International Union Against Cancer: *Manual of Clinical Oncology.* 5th ed. New York, Springer-Verlag, 1990.
8. Wu J, Nakamura R: *Human Circulating Tumor Markers, Current Concepts and Clinical Applications.* Chicago, American Society of Clinical Pathologists Press, 1997.
9. Catalona WJ, Smith DS, Ratliff T, et al.: Measurement of prostate specific antigen in serum as a screening test for prostate cancer. N Engl J Med 324:1156, 1991.
10. Heller JE: Prostatic acid phosphatase: its current clinical status. J Urol 137:1091, 1987.
11. Pappas AA, Gadsden RH: Acid phosphatase, clinical utility in detection, assessment and monitoring of prostatic carcinoma. Ann Clin Lab Sci 14:285, 1984.
12. Bahnson RR, Catalona WJ: Adverse implications of acid phosphatase levels in the upper range of normal. J Urol 137:427, 1987.
13. Wu JT: Applications of enzymes: Tumor markers, new enzymes and atypical isoenzymes. J Med Technology 2 #7:438, 1985.
14. Hybritech, Inc., San Diego, CA, PAP Package insert, 1988.
15. Hall M, Johnson JT, Carr J: Assays for serodiagnosis of prostate cancer. Lab Med 23(9):607, 1992.
16. Du Pont Company, Wilmington, Delaware, ACP package insert.
17. Kaplan L, Chen I, Sperling M, et al.: Clinical utility of serum acid phosphatase measurement for detection (screening), diagnosis and therapeutic monitoring of prostatic carcinoma; assessment of monoclonal and polyclonal enzyme and radioimmunoassays. Am J Clin Pathol 84:334, 1985.
18. Narayanan S: Alkaline phosphatase as a tumor marker. Ann Clin Lab Sci 12:133, 1983.
19. Panigraphi K, Delmas PD, Singer F, et al.: Characteristics of a two site immunoradiometric assay for human skeletal alkaline phosphatase in serum. Clin Chem 40:822, 1994.
20. Tatarinov Y: New data on the embryo specific antigen components of human blood serum. Vopr Med Khim 10:584, 1964.

21. Fishman WH, Inglis NR, Stolbach LL, et al.: A serum alkaline phosphatase isoenzyme of human neoplastic cell origin. Cancer Res 28:150, 1968.

22. Fishman WH: Perspectives on alkaline phosphatase isoenzymes. Am J Med 56:617, 1974.

23. Silverman LM, Dermer GB, Zweig MH, et al.: Creatine kinase BB: A new tumor associated marker. Clin Chem 25:1432, 1979.

24. Moossa AR, Robson MC, Schimpff SC: *Comprehensive Textbook of Oncology*. 2nd ed. Baltimore, Williams & Wilkins, 1991.

25. Zondag HA, Klein F: Clinical Applications of lactate dehydrogenase isoenzymes: Alterations in malignancy. Ann N Y Acad Sci 151:578, 1968.

26. Sell S: Cancer markers of the 1990s. Clin Lab Med 10:27, 1990.

27. Schmechel D, Marangos PJ, Brightman M: Neuron specific enolase is a molecular marker for peripheral and central neuroendocrine cells. Nature 276:834, 1978.

28. Zeltzer PM, Marangos PJ, Evans AE, et al.: Serum neuron specific enolase in children with neuroblastoma. Cancer 57:1230, 1986.

29. Carney DN, Ihde DC, Cohen MM, et al.: Serum neuron specific enolase. Lancet 1:583, 1982.

30. Schmechel D, Marangos PJ, Zis PA, et al.: Brain enolases as specific markers of neuronal and glial cells. Science 199:313, 1978.

31. Jorgenson LGM, Hirsch FR, Skov BG, et al.: Occurrence of neuron specific enolase in tumour tissue and serum in small cell lung cancer. Br J Cancer 63:151, 1991.

32. Burghuber OC, Worofka B, Schemthaner G, et al.: Serum neuron specific enolase is a useful tumor marker for small cell lung cancer. Cancer 65:1386, 1990.

33. Tapia FJ, Polak JM, Barbarosa AJ, et al.: Neuron specific enolase is produced by neuroendocrine tumours. Lancet 1:808, 1981.

34. Burtis CA, Ashwood ER: *Tietz Fundamentals of Clinical Chemistry*. 4th ed. Philadelphia, WB Saunders, 1996.

35. Gibco BRL, Gaithersburg, MD, TdT package insert, 1990.

36. Murphy S, Jaffe ES: Terminal transferase activity and lymphoblastic neoplasms. N Engl J Med 311:1373, 1984.

37. Graeff H, Harbeck N, Pache L, et al.: Prognostic impact and clinical relevance of tumor associated proteases in breast cancer. Fibrinolysis 6(Suppl):45, 1992.

38. Schmitt M, Janicke F, Graeff H: Tumor associated proteases. Fibrinolysis 6:3, 1992.

39. Henry JB: *Clinical Diagnosis and Management by Laboratory Methods*. 19th ed. Philadelphia, WB Saunders, 1996.

40. Kaplan LA, Pesce AJ: *Clinical Chemistry, Theory, Analysis, Correlation*. 3rd ed. St Louis, Mosby, 1996.

41. DeWys WD, Killen JY: The paraneoplastic syndromes. In Rubin P, Bakemeier RF, Krachov SK (eds): *Clinical Oncology: a Multidisciplinary Approach*. 6th ed. Chicago, American Cancer Society, 1983, p 112.

42. Braunstein GD: Hormones: New potential for tumor markers. Diagn Med 1:59,1981.

43. Saller B, Clara R, Spottl, G, et al.: Testicular cancer secretes intact human choriogonadotropin (HCG) and its free beta subunit: Evidence that HCG (+HCG-B) assays are the most reliable in diagnosis and follow-up. Clin Chem 36:234, 1990.

44. Triton Biosciences Inc.: Urinary gonadotropin peptide as a marker for the monitoring of ovarian and other gynecological malignancies. Poster presented at the XIV International Congress of Clinical Chemistry, Alameda, CA, 1990.

45. Bakes-Martin, RC: Urine catecholamine assays in suspected pheochromocytoma: A practical approach. Lab Manage June:47, 1987.

46. Threatte GA, Henry JB: Carbohydrates. In Henry JB (ed.): *Clinical Diagnosis and Management by Laboratory Methods*. 19th ed. Philadelphia, WB Saunders, 1996, p 194.

47. Tietz NW: *Clinical Guide to Laboratory Tests*. 3rd ed. Philadelphia, WB Saunders, 1995.

48. Jialal I, Winter WE, Chan DW: *Handbook of Diagnostic Endocrinology*. Washington, DC, American Association for Clinical Chemistry Associated Press, 1999.

49. Rosen SW, Weintraub BD, Vaitukatis JL, et al.: Placental proteins and their subunits as tumor markers. Ann Intern Med 82:71, 1975.

50. Nussbaum SR, Gaz RD, Arnold A: Hypercalcemia and ectopic secretion of parathyroid hormone by an ovarian carcinoma with rearrangement of the gene for parathyroid hormone. N Engl J Med 323:1324, 1990.

51. Burtis WJ, Brady TG, Orloff JJ, et al.: Immunochemical characterization of circulating parathyroid hormone related protein in patients with humoral hypercalcemia of cancer. N Engl J Med 322:1106, 1990.

52. Sealey J, Cambell G, Preibisz J: Hormone assays: Renin, aldosterone, periferal vein, and urinary assays. In Laragh J, Brenner B (eds.): *Hypertension: Pathophysiology, Diagnosis, and Management*. New York, Raven Press, 1990, p 236.

53. Chattorzji SC, Watts NB: Endocrinology. In Tietz, N (ed.): *Textbook of Clinical Chemistry*. Philadelphia, WB Saunders, 1986, p 997.

54. Wu, JT, Knight, JA: Cell receptor assays, basic concepts and clinical applications. ASCP Check Sample CC89-4 (CC202), 1989.

55. Jaing NS: Breast cancer: Estrogen and progesterone receptor assays as a guide to therapy. Mayo Clin Proc 58:64, 1983.

56. Lesser ML, Rosen PP, Senie RT, et al.: Estrogen and progesterone receptors in breast carcinoma: Correlation with epidemiology and pathology. Cancer 48:299, 1981.

57. Geller J: Hormone dependency of prostate cancer. In

Thompson BE, Lippman ME (eds.): *Steroid Receptors and the Management of Cancer.* Boca Raton, CRC Press, 1979, p 113.

58. Young PCM, Ehrlich CE: Progesterone receptors in human endometrial cancer. In Thompson BE, Lippman ME (eds.): *Steroid Receptors and the Management of Cancer.* Boca Raton, CRC Press, 1979, p 135.

59. Brandt-Rauf PW, Luo JC, Carney WP. The detection of increased amounts of the extracellular domain of the c-erbB-2 oncoprotein in serum during pulmonary carcinogenesis in humans. Int J Cancer 56:383, 1994.

60. Yu H, Schlossman DM, Harrison CL, et al.: Coexpression of different antigenic markers on moieties that bear CA 125 determinants. Cancer Res 51:468, 1991.

61. Pannall P, Kotasek D: *Cancer and Clinical Biochemistry.* London, ACB Venture Publications, 1997.

62. Wu JT, Knight JA: The use of alpha-fetoprotein (AFP) in clinical medicine. ASCP Check Sample CC87-5 (CC-183), 1987.

63. Wu JT, Knight JA, Knight D: Carcinoembryonic antigen (CEA) in the diagnosis and management of colorectal cancer. ASCP Check Sample CC86-8 (CC176), 1986.

64. Bostwick D, Brawer M, Oesterling J: Panel discussion, XIV International Congress of Clinical Chemistry, Alameda, CA, 1990.

65. Safi F, Kohler I, Rottinger E, et al.: The value of the tumor marker CA 15-3 in diagnosis and monitoring breast cancer: A comparative study with carcinoembryonic antigen. Cancer 68:574, 1991.

66. Fujirebio Diagnostics Inc (Centocor), Malvern, PA: Truquant BR™ CA27.29 product literature, 2000.

67. Abbott Diagnostic Laboratories, North Chicago, IL: BCM product literature, 1990.

68. DeWit R, Hoek FJ, Bakker PJM, et al.: The value of MCA, CA 15-3, CEA, and CA 125 for discrimination between metastatic breast cancer and adenocarcinoma of other primary sites. J Intern Med 229:463, 1991.

69. Wu JT, Knight JA: Monoclonal immunoassays for tumor markers. ASCP Check Sample CC88-4 (CC192), 1988.

70. Centocor Inc.: Centocor 19-9 blood test. Malvern, PA, 1989.

71. Hybritech Inc.: TANDEM-R CA195 package insert. San Diego, 1988.

72. Bast R, Hunter V, Knapp R: Pros and cons of gynecological tumor markers. Cancer 60:1984, 1987.

73. Atack D, Nisker J, Allen H: CA125 surveillance and second-look laparotomy in ovarian carcinoma. Am J Obstet Gynecol 154:287, 1986.

74. Centocor Inc.: Investigational CA72-4 product literature. Malvern, PA, 1990.

75. Molina R, Filella X, Torres M et al.: SCC antigen measured in malignant and nonmalignant diseases. Clin Chem 36:251, 1990.

76. Centocor Inc.: Investigational P-glycochek C219 product literature. Malvern, PA, 1990.

77. Wu JT, Clayton F, Myers S: A simple radial immunodiffusion method for assay of $\beta_2$-microglobulin in serum. Clin Chem 32:2070, 1986.

78. American Diabetes Association: Clinical practice recommendations 2000. Diabetes Care 23:(Suppl 1):1, 2000.

79. Buccheri G, Ferrigno D: Prognostic value of the tissue polypeptide antigen in lung cancer. Chest 101:1287, 1992.

80. Eskelinen M, Hippelainen M, Kettungen J et al.: Clinical value of serum tumor markers TPA, TPS, TAG 12, CA 15-3, and MCA in breast cancer diagnosis: Results from a prospective study. Anticancer Res 14:699, 1994.

81. Ross DW: *Introduction to Molecular Medicine.* New York, Springer-Verlag, 1992.

82. Knudson AG: Mutation and cancer: statistical study of retinoblastoma. Proc Natl Acad Sci USA 68:820, 1971.

83. Easton DF, Bishop DT, Ford D, et al.: Genetic linkage analysis in familial breast and ovarian cancer: results from 214 families. Am J Hum Genet 52:678, 1993.

84. Erbil K, Jones J, Klee G: Use and limitation of serum total and lipid-bound sialic acid concentrations as markers for colorectal cancer. Cancer 55:404, 1985.

85. Horn Y, Beal SL, Walach N, et al.: Further evidence for the use of polyamines as biochemical markers for malignant tumors. Cancer Res 42:3248, 1982.

86. Bray RA, Landay AL: Identification and functional characterization of mononuclear cells by flow cytometry. Arch Pathol Lab Med 113:579, 1989.

87. Cancer Facts and Figures 2000: Graphical Data. Internet, 2000.

88. Hubbard E: Tumor markers. Diagnostic and Clinical Testing 28:3, 1990.

89. Butch AW, Nassoll NA, Pappas AA: Tumor Markers. In Bishop ML, Duben-Engelkirk JL, Fody EP (eds.): *Clinical Chemistry, Principles, Procedures, Correlations.* 4th ed. Philadelphia, Lippincott Williams & Wilkins, 2000, p 522.

90. Folkman J, Shing Y: Angiogenesis. J Biol Chem 267:10931, 1992.

# C H A P T E R   1 8

# Porphyrins

*Susan Cockayne*

Although the primary (inherited) disorders in porphyrin metabolism are relatively uncommon, several secondary (induced) disorders are very common in some groups of the population. All of these disorders are rather complex metabolic diseases with overlapping clinical and biochemical features. However, with management and therapy becoming increasingly effective, an early and accurate diagnosis assumes added importance. Systematic approaches to diagnoses of porphyrinopathies have now been developed using combinations of newer developed methods for measuring metabolite concentrations and enzyme activities. Many reviews of the biochemical and clinical features of porphyrin disorders and their diagnosis and treatment have been published.[1–4]

**Porphyrins** are derivatives of porphin, a macrocyclic, highly unsaturated molecular structure composed of 4 pyrrole rings bound by four methene bridges (— CH ═). Certain substituted porphins make up the porphyrins; they are differentiated on the basis of the kinds and order of substituents occupying the 8 peripheral positions on the 4 pyrrole rings (Figure 18–1). Many kinds of porphyrins are known; however, very few are found in nature and only 3 of these, **uroporphyrin, coproporphyrin,** and **protoporphyrin** have clinical significance (a few other porphyrins might be rarely mentioned in the medical literature). These metal-free porphyrins have no biologic function in humans; porphyrins are metabolically active only in the form of metal chelates. The iron chelates of porphyrins are **hemes; protoheme** is by far the most common (Figure 18–2). Heme functions only as a prosthetic group of a protein. In mammals, hemoproteins participate in a variety of biochemical processes, all of which are associated with some aspect of oxidative metabolism, such as oxygen transport (hemoglobin) and cellular respiration (cytochromes). Zinc protoporphyrin is found in trace amounts in normal metabolism; it can increase markedly when iron utilization is impaired or iron is deficient in the body such as occurs in iron deficiency anemia.[5] A cobalt chelate, cobalamin or vitamin $B_{12}$, and a magnesium chelate, chlorophyll, are other forms of naturally occurring tetrapyrroles.

Crystalline porphyrins and their concentrated solutions are very dark red or purple. In acid solution, porphyrins are recognized by their intense orange-red fluorescence (620 to 630 nm) on exposure to long-wavelength ultraviolet light (~400 nm), a property that is used in most porphyrin analyses. The intense color and fluorescence of porphyrins are due to the high degree of conjugated unsaturation, or resonance, in the tetrapyrrole ring. In general, metal-free porphyrins tend to be more stable in acid solution and in the dark. Dilute hydrochloric acid solutions of extremely low concentrations of coproporphyrin are stable for a very long time and are most often used as a standard in porphyrin assays by fluorometric techniques.

Water solubility of the porphyrins is influenced by the number of carboxyl groups in the pyrrole substituents. **Uroporphyrin,** having 8 carboxyl groups, is the most water-soluble porphyrin at physiologic pH. **Protoporphyrin,** having only 2 carboxyl groups, is quite insoluble in aqueous media at this pH but is very soluble in lipid solvents. **Coproporphyrin,** with its 4 carboxyl groups, has intermediate solubility in each kind of solvent with the distribution between solvents being influenced by pH. These differing solubility properties often form the basis for the separation and assay of the individual porphyrins. Using suitable analytical procedures, one can also identify and quantitate intermediate porphyrins in the pathway having 7, 6, or 5 carboxyl groups that may occur in trace amounts. For all practical purposes, uroporphyrin is excreted exclusively in the urine, protoporphyrin exclusively in the feces, and coproporphyrin by either route depending on its rate of formation and the pH of the urine, with alkalinity favoring coproporphyrin excretion in the urine.

**Porphyrinogens** are reduced forms of porphyrins containing 6 additional hydrogen atoms, 1 at each of the 4 methene bridge carbons and 1 at each of the 2 nonhydrogenated pyrrole nitrogens (Figure 18–1). Porphyrinogens are colorless, nonfluorescent, and highly unstable, especially in an acid medium where they rapidly oxidize to porphyrins, which makes their analysis somewhat impractical for laboratory diagnosis. The porphyrinogens, but not the porphyrins, undergo alterations in their side-chain substituents during heme biosynthesis. Hence, they are functional precursors of heme. Oxidation of a porphyrinogen to the corresponding porphyrin irreversibly removes that molecule from the heme biosynthetic pathway, with protoporphyrin being the one exception. For these reasons, only porphyrins and their precursors are significant in the diagnosis of porphyrinopathies, since these are measurable in various biologic fluids and correlations with disease have been established.

Few pharmacologic effects of porphyrins are known since they cause subtle, if any, direct alterations in metabolism. On the other hand, porphyrins deposited in skin that is then exposed to long-wavelength ultraviolet light can cause consider-

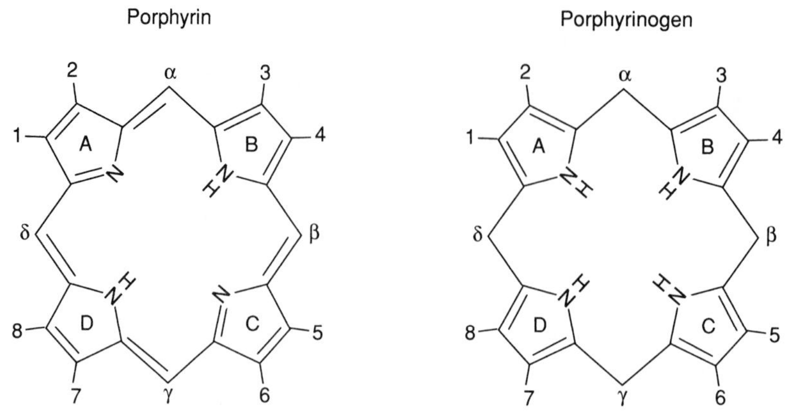

Porphyrin                                         Porphyrinogen

SUBSTITUENTS IDENTIFYING DIFFERENT PORPHYRINS

| Ring | Position | URO | COPRO | PROTO |
|------|----------|-----|-------|-------|
| | | *Porphyrin III or Porphyrinogen III* | | |
| A | 1 | Acetate | Methyl | Methyl |
| | 2 | Propionate | Propionate | Vinyl |
| B | 3 | Acetate | Methyl | Methyl |
| | 4 | Propionate | Propionate | Vinyl |
| C | 5 | Acetate | Methyl | Methyl |
| | 6 | Propionate | Propionate | Propionate |
| D | 7 | Propionate | Propionate | Propionate |
| | 8 | Acetate | Methyl | Methyl |
| | | *Porphyrin I or Porphyrinogen I* | | |
| D | 7 | Acetate | Methyl | Not known to |
| | 8 | Propionate | Propionate | occur in nature |

**FIGURE  18-1**

Structure of porphyrin and porphyrinogen and a listing of the substituents that identify
the different porphyrins.

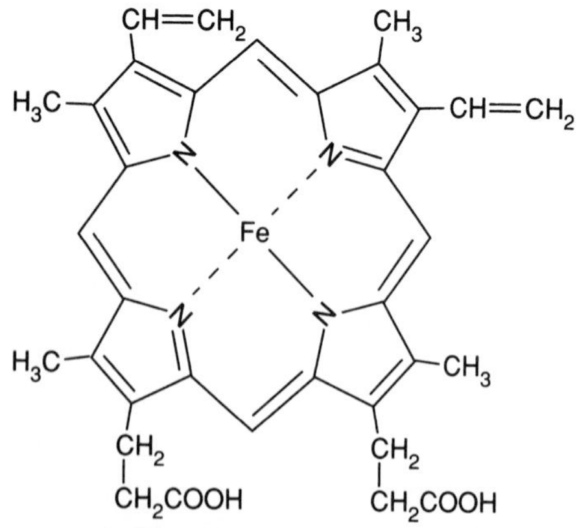

**FIGURE  18-2**

The structural formula of protoheme, a chelate of
ferrous iron and protoporphyrin IX. The vinyl groups
occur in positions 2 and 4 of rings A and B, and the
propionic acid (carboxyethyl) groups occur in positions
6 and 7 of rings C and D.

able tissue damage. The different lesions that are caused by
uroporphyrin, coproporphyrin, or protoporphyrin probably
relate to their respective solubilities. The more lipophilic protoporphyrin accumulates predominantly in cell membranes,
whereas the other porphyrins are confined largely to intercel-
lular and intracellular aqueous fluids. The clinical symptoms
that are characterized by porphyrin deposition in the skin are
related to the photochemical properties, the stabilities, and the
solubilities of the porphyrins. The clinical correlation of these
chemical differences is reflected in the observation that uroporphyrin and coproporphyrin typically cause delayed bullous
lesions but protoporphyrin causes an almost immediate burning sensation and inflammatory reaction in sun-exposed areas
of the skin.

The porphyrin precursors, δ-aminolevulinic acid and porphobilinogen, have very low renal thresholds, which partially
explains their low blood concentrations. These precursors are
considered not to produce pharmacologic effects, at least after

administration to animals or human subjects. On the other hand, the expression of neurologic symptoms is always accompanied by the excessive excretion of porphyrin precursors. Several lines of evidence suggest that this precursor excess is a significant factor in the pathogenesis of neurologic abnormalities. Despite these associations, the correlation between the level of precursor excretion and the severity of neurologic symptoms is poor. Free porphyrins in the skin absorb light in the UV region (400 nm). When activated in this manner, the porphyrins react with molecular oxygen producing activated oxygen and peroxide radicals. These free radicals then damage cellular structures such as lysosomes. Following lysosomal damage, cytotoxic enzymes are released that result in the characteristic cutaneous photosensitivity.

## BIOSYNTHESIS OF PORPHYRINS AND HEME

Porphyrin and heme biosynthetic activity is quantitatively most prominent in bone marrow and liver; however, porphyrins and heme are synthesized in all mammalian cells. The series of heme biosynthetic reactions (Figure 18–3) begins with the condensation of succinyl coenzyme-A and glycine; pyridoxal phosphate is a cofactor. Following the condensation, the glycine moiety is decarboxylated, forming $\delta$-aminolevulinic acid. The enzyme catalyzing the reaction is $\delta$-aminolevulinate synthase. Two molecules of $\delta$-aminolevulinate are then condensed and cyclized

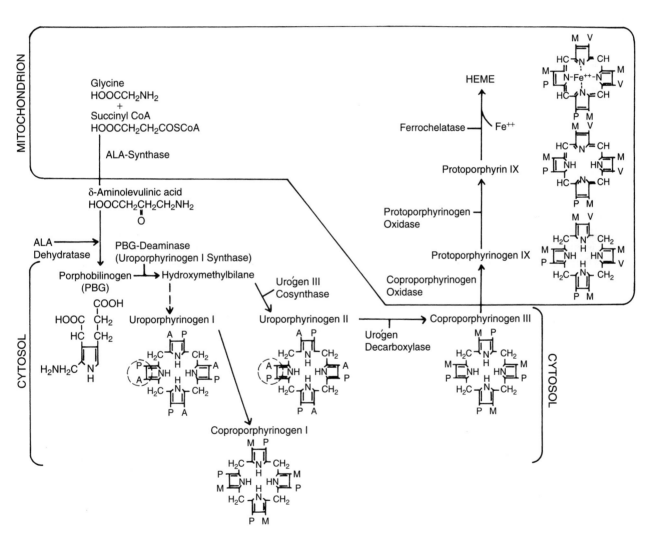

### FIGURE 18-3

The heme biosynthetic pathway showing the distribution of enzymes between the mitochondria and cytoplasm. Between porphobilinogen and uroporphyrinogen III, a complex reaction occurs in which hydroxymethylbilane, designated by (X), has been identified. $B_6PO_4$ = pyridoxal phosphate.

through the action of porphobilinogen synthase (formerly called δ-aminolevulinic acid dehydratase) to form the mono-pyrrole porphobilinogen. This enzyme requires zinc. Porphobilinogen is condensed and cyclized through the concerted action of 2 enzymes, porphobilinogen deaminase (formerly called uroporphyrinogen synthase) and uroporphyrinogen cosynthase, to form uroporphyrinogen. Subsequently, the 4 acetate side chains of uroporphyrinogen are decarboxylated through the action of uroporphyrinogen decarboxylase to form coproporphyrinogen. Next, coproporphyrinogen oxidase decarboxylates and dehydrogenates the propionic acid side chains in positions 2 and 4, converting these to vinyl groups and yielding protoporphyrinogen. Protoporphyrinogen oxidase then oxidizes protoporphyrinogen to protoporphyrin. Finally, ferrochelatase catalyzes the chelation of a ferrous ion by protoporphyrin to form heme. The reactions between δ-aminolevulinate and coproporphyrinogen occur in the cellular cytosol; the remaining reactions occur in the mitochondria. These 4 cytosolic enzymes are retained in erythrocytes during maturation and after loss of the mitochondria.

Free porphyrins that are found in body fluids, tissues, and excreta arise as nonenzymatic oxidation byproducts of porphyrinogens from the heme biosynthetic pathway. Normally, only trace amounts of porphyrins escape the biosynthetic processes because control mechanisms maintain the pathway in a delicate state of balance to meet the requirements of each cell. In erythrocytes, for example, only about 1 molecule of excess protoporphyrin accumulates for each 30,000 molecules of heme that are formed in the process of hemoglobin synthesis and losses of other porphyrins are at least an order of magnitude less than this. However, a number of pathologic conditions cause stimulated or inhibited heme biosynthesis leading to abnormal tissue levels or excretion rates of the porphyrins and their precursors. From a diagnostic purpose, only increased levels of porphyrins and their precursors are clinically significant. No known clinical significance can yet be ascribed to an occurrence of abnormally low concentrations of porphyrins or their precursors.

## CLINICAL APPLICATIONS

The metabolic abnormalities characteristic of each porphyria result from inherited deficiencies of specific enzymes in the heme biosynthetic pathway (Table 18–1). Most classifications of the porphyrias have utilized categorization of the diseases into hepatic and erythropoietic groups. This is an historical concept based on the presumed major sites of excess porphyrin and porphyrin precursor production.

The proposal to describe and classify the porphyrias primarily into broad clinical categories, i.e., neurologic and cutaneous, is an effort to simplify the clinical and chemical correlations in these disorders, with the aim of improving the efficacy of the diagnostic evaluations of porphyria. Although this approach has some limitations, it simplifies the ordering and interpretation of laboratory tests for physicians and laboratories.

## Neurologic Forms of Porphyria

Excess excretion of the porphyrin precursors δ-aminolevulinic acid and porphobilinogen are the characteristic chemical abnormalities in acute intermittent porphyria during symptomatic episodes. In fact, the acute attack or neurologic forms of porphyria may be considered, for purposes of this discussion, as disorders involving porphyrin precursors. Each of the diseases that comprise this group reflects a specific enzyme defect that is inherited as an autosomal dominant trait. They include **acute intermittent porphyria, variegate porphyria,** and **coproporphyria.** The acute attack manifestations of each are identical. Symptomatic illness can be latent for indeterminant periods and those individuals who present with symptomatic disease may experience one or multiple symptomatic episodes. During the acute phase, δ-aminolevulinic acid and porphobilinogen are excreted in the urine in excess, but during asymptomatic intervals these biochemical abnormalities may resolve. Thus, although measurement of δ-aminolevulinic acid and porphobilinogen may be diagnostic at any particular time, their normal excretion during quiescent periods do not rule out a diagnosis. Although each of these disorders has a unique enzyme abnormality, urine and fecal porphyrin excretion *patterns* are generally used in the clinical laboratory for establishing the specific form of porphyria (Table 18–1) or other porphyrin disorder. Two disorders in this class, namely variegate and coproporphyria, often exhibit photosensitivity and may be considered as mixed porphyrias. Neurologic symptoms are usually the more severe types of symptoms.

Symptoms of an acute attack may include abdominal pain, back pain, nausea, paresthesia, weakness, inability to think clearly, and self-destructive thoughts. Signs of acute attacks often include hypertension and tachycardia; constipation or diarrhea may occur, with the former more common; nausea is occasionally accompanied by vomiting. Paralysis, blindness (may be transient), and seizures are less common. Diaphoresis without fever or infection is part of the autonomic neuropathy. The attack may last several days to several weeks. The spectrum of signs and symptoms as well as the duration and intensity of symptoms is quite variable among patients. Unusually severe illness with profound neurologic impairment cannot be anticipated, nor can the inciting agent nor degree of exposure be correlated with the intensity of clinical disease. An acute attack may be precipitated by drugs and other factors including sedatives and anticonvulsants, some steroid hormones, alcohol, and starvation. Therefore, prevention is a primary mode of patient management. This, of course, requires recognition of the illness. For previously unrecognized patients, the diagnosis is often made after a protracted illness. As a result, neurologic disease may develop. The clinical course of an acute attack may include significant morbidity and occasional mortality. The mortality figures for the acute forms of por-

## TABLE 18-1

### Enzyme Defects and Associated Laboratory Findings in Porphyrinopathies

| SPECIFIC ENZYME DEFECT | PORPHYRINOPATHY | DIAGNOSTIC LABORATORY FINDINGS |
|---|---|---|
| $\delta$-Aminolevulinate synthase | None known; probably lethal lesions if primary | Not applicable |
| Porphobilinogen synthase ($\delta$-aminolevulinate dehydratase) | Porphobilinogen synthase deficiency | Decreased enzyme activity (RBCs) |
| Porphobilinogen deaminase (uroporphyrinogen synthase) | Acute intermittent porphyria | ↓ Porphobilinogen deaminase (RBCs)<br>↑ Urinary $\delta$-aminolevulinic acid*<br>↑ Urinary porphobilinogen*<br>↑ Urinary uroporphyrin |
| Uroporphyrinogen III cosynthase | Congenital erythropoietic porphyria | ↑ Urinary uroporphyrin, coproporphyrin<br>↑ Blood porphyrins<br>↑ Fecal porphyrins |
| Uroporphyrinogen decarboxylase | Porphyria cutanea tarda | ↑ Urinary uroporphyrin<br>↑ Urinary 7-COOH porphyrin |
| Coproporphyrinogen oxidase | Coproporphyria† | ↑ Urinary $\delta$-aminolevulinic acid<br>↑ Urinary porphobilinogen*<br>↑ Urinary coproporphyrin<br>↑ Fecal coproporphyrin |
| Protoporphyrinogen oxidase | Porphyria variegata | ↑ Urinary $\delta$-aminolevulinic acid<br>↑ Urinary porphobilinogen*<br>↑ Urinary coproporphyrin<br>↑ Fecal protoporphyrin, coproporphyrin |
| Ferrochelatase | Protoporphyria | ↑ Blood protoporphyrin<br>↑ Fecal protoporphyrin |

*Typical finding during acute neuropathy; may be normal in remission.

†The term *hereditary coproporphyria* is commonly used, but it is redundant because porphyrias by definition are hereditary.

↓ = decreased; ↑ = increased.

phyria, especially acute intermittent porphyria, have decreased over the years. This trend is often attributed to improved physician awareness of porphyria as a diagnostic possibility as well as the avoidance of contraindicated medication or potential precipitating factors in individuals known to have the disease. Considering the importance of prevention and the realization that the most severe clinical problems typically arise in individuals in whom the diagnosis is unsuspected, genetic counseling with appropriate diagnostic studies to identify family members with latent states of porphyria is essential.

Therapy for the acute attack porphyrias consists of intravenous glucose infusion or a high carbohydrate diet and the administration of heme or hematin. Heme and hematin act to repress hepatic ALA synthase activity, which, in turn, results in lower levels of the precursor molecules $\delta$-ALA and PBG.

## Cutaneous Forms of Porphyria

The common feature linking this group of diseases is the characteristic excess porphyrin production and excretion; porphyrin precursors are unaffected. Lesions are usually confined to the dorsum of the hands, face, and ears. However, the di-

rect relationship of sun exposure to the development of skin lesions is frequently not appreciated by affected individuals. A bullous dermatosis is common. Skin fragility and the resulting lesions are probably the most characteristic symptoms of **porphyria cutanea tarda.** Pigment changes, scarring, and milia, which are small subepidermal keratin cysts, accompany chronic skin disease. The skin on the dorsum of the hands may be remarkably thin and delicate in appearance. Excessive hair growth known as hypertrichosis, is frequent. Acute attacks do not occur, and neither neurologic nor psychotic symptoms are present.

Originally, porphyria cutanea tarda was considered an acquired disease. Recently, however, uroporphyrinogen decarboxylase deficiency has been identified in familial clusters that suggest mendelian-dominant inheritance. Further family studies using the measurement of uroporphyrinogen decarboxylase activity have confirmed autosomal dominant transmission of a deficiency of this enzyme in both affected and nonaffected family members. Both familial and acquired forms of this porphyria are now recognized. Excessive alcohol consumption is commonly associated with this disorder. However, iron accumulation is the principal causative factor because of an inhibitory effect of iron on uroporphyrinogen decarboxylase. Estrogen exposure in older men being treated for prostate carcinoma and in younger women using oral contraceptives are other causative factors. Porphyria cutanea tarda is the most common form of porphyria seen in North America. When iron overload is present, treatment consists of repeated phlebotomy of 1 unit of blood twice monthly for a total of 5 to 10 L as indicated by the patient's hematocrit level. Improvement occurs within several months to a year. Equally important is avoidance of sunlight, alcohol, and iron.

**Congenital erythropoietic porphyria** is one of the rarest forms of inherited porphyrin disorders. It is unique among the porphyrias for having an autosomal recessive inheritance. The basic defect is a deficiency of uroporphyrinogen cosynthase in the bone marrow and accumulation of series I isomers of porphyrins. Dark red urine and severe photosensitivity are typically observed in the neonatal period, but patients with onset in adulthood have been reported. Porphyrins stain the bones and teeth (erythrodontia) of these individuals, which results in a bright red-orange fluorescence of the stained areas on exposure to long-wavelength ultraviolet light. Porphyrin deposition in these tissues is a result of the avidity of water-soluble porphyrins for calcium-containing structures. This phenomenon also suggests that excess porphyrin production was occurring in fetal life. Hemolytic anemia, ineffective erythropoiesis, and splenomegaly complicate the clinical course.

**Protoporphyria** is the result of a ferrochelatase deficiency that leads to excessive metal-free protoporphyrin accumulation associated with severe photosensitivity. The cutaneous reaction occurs within 15 to 20 minutes of sun exposure, and this correlation of symptoms with exposure is readily recognized by affected people. The skin reaction begins with burning and itching followed by eventual painful swelling and erythema, which may last for 48 hours or longer. The photosensitivity in protoporphyria can become so disabling that photoprotection is important. A therapeutic advance has been the observation that $\beta$-carotene may afford photosensitivity protection. Of course, $\beta$-carotene is available in carrots and other food, but consumption of protective amounts of the pigment in its biologic form can be very difficult with food alone. A preparation of $\beta$-carotene in capsule form is now marketed (Solatene). Use of $\beta$-carotene must be planned, since several months may be needed to build up adequate tissue levels.

A discussion of the clinical features of protoporphyria would be incomplete without noting the occurrence of hepatobiliary disease in a subgroup of these patients. The major route of protoporphyrin excretion, whether of erythrocyte or hepatic origin, is via the liver. Impaired liver function and bile excretion in this group of patients connote hepatic injury secondary to protoporphyrin accumulation in the liver parenchyma. Often, cholelithiasis occurs in protoporphyria at an unusually early age. In rare instances, protoporphyrin deposition has been documented in stones that were removed surgically.

**Porphobilinogen synthase deficiency** is a recently described disorder with an autosomal dominant inheritance. Het-

erozygous individuals appear to be totally asymptomatic but identification and study of further cases are necessary to elucidate the true clinical significance of this enzyme deficiency. Homozygous neonates experience extreme neurologic deficits.

## Secondary Disorders of Heme Biosynthesis

A variety of clinical conditions besides porphyrias are accompanied by excess accumulation and excretion of porphyrins or porphyrin precursors. Moreover, symptoms in these conditions may be indistinguishable from those of the porphyrias. In such cases, the disturbance of porphyrin metabolism is a result of a superimposed disorder or toxin reaction rather than the result of an inherited defect in the heme biosynthetic pathway. Those disorders, which produce the clinical picture of an acute attack of porphyria, exhibit increased amounts of only $\delta$-aminolevulinic acid in the urine. Porphobilinogen excretion is not usually increased, which demonstrates the specificity of porphobilinogen for acute intermittent porphyria. The two diseases in this category are **lead poisoning** and **hereditary tyrosinemia.** Lead inhibits both the activity of porphobilinogen synthase and the incorporation of iron into heme. In addition to increased urine excretion of $\delta$-aminolevulinic acid, erythrocyte protoporphyrin concentration (as a zinc chelate) is increased. Urine coproporphyrin is elevated as a delayed response. Despite the excess coproporphyrin in the urine and zinc protoporphyrin in erythrocytes, individuals with lead poisoning do not experience photosensitivity. Hereditary tyrosinemia also produces an acute illness similar to porphyria. One of the metabolites accumulating in excess (succinyl acetone) is a potent inhibitor of porphobilinogen synthase. Coproporphyrinuria occurs in this disorder as well. Metals such as mercury, bismuth, copper, gold, silver, and arsenic are not known to cause elevation of urinary $\delta$-aminolevulinic acid or erythrocyte zinc protoporphyrin but may cause coproporphyrinuria.

All conditions that produce an imbalance between rates of protoporphyrin formation and iron availability can lead to accumulation of erythrocyte protoporphyrin or its zinc chelate. This abnormal metabolite is best known for its marked increase in chronic lead exposure. Zinc protoporphyrin also increases in iron deficiency, but this response has received less attention. Zinc protoporphyrin circulates in the erythrocyte attached to a heme site on globin, where it serves no biologic function. Sideroblastic anemia, in which iron is not properly utilized; hemolytic anemia, in which erythropoiesis is greatly accentuated; secondary polycythemia, in which there is a stimulus to erythropoiesis extrinsic to the marrow; excessive erythrocyte destruction, and the commonly seen inflammatory block are all associated with elevated erythrocyte protoporphyrin or its zinc chelate. Anemia accompanying chronic disease also may cause elevated zinc protoporphyrin. The conditions of heme biosynthesis associated with secondary protoporphyrinemia typically have protoporphyrin concentrations below 400 $\mu$g/dL of erythrocytes, whereas erythropoietic protoporphyria typically produces erythrocyte protoporphyrin concentrations in considerable excess of those occurring in these secondary disorders.

Coproporphyrin is most commonly excreted in secondary porphyrinuria, which has many origins. Hexachlorobenzene, alcohol, sedatives, and hypnotics such as chloral hydrate, morphine, ether, and nitrous oxide as well as lead can all cause coproporphyrinuria. Also, neoplasia, liver disease, myocardial infarction, and thalassemia have on occasion been associated with coproporphyrinuria. Infection and fever are common causes of coproporphyrinuria. Clearly, this finding alone has little diagnostic value.

# LABORATORY DIAGNOSIS OF PORPHYRIN DISORDERS

Essentially, the screening or quantitation of 3 different porphyrins and 1 or both precursors comprise the basis for the laboratory diagnosis of most disorders affecting porphyrin metabolism (Table 18–1). These are uroporphyrin, with 8 carboxyl substituents; coproporphyrin, a 4-carboxyl molecule; and protoporphyrin, which has only 2 carboxyl groups (Figure 18–2). Certain other porphyrins can also be identified in the blood, urine, or feces. For example, the heptacarboxyl porphyrin is seen as a major excretion product in porphyria cutanea tarda and identification of this porphyrin in the urine is helpful for the diagnosis of this porphyria. Recent association of partial deficiencies of specific enzymes in the heme biosynthetic pathway that are unique with various types of porphyrias may eventually replace comparative chemical studies of porphyrin excretion and blood levels for the diagnosis of specific porphyrin disorders. When a diagnosis of porphyria is suspected, laboratory tests will continue to include assessment of the excretion of porphyrins (uroporphyrin, coproporphyrin, or protoporphyrin) or porphyrin precursors ($\delta$-aminolevulinic acid and/or porphobilinogen), with the aim of detecting patterns of change.

Because of the variety of clinical disorders that share the term *porphyria* as well as their overlapping clinical and biochemical features, it is often difficult to know which specific laboratory studies are indicated when porphyria is a suspected diagnosis. Therefore, in clinical practice, a classification relating to symptomatology may be more useful (Table 18–2). In outlining a general approach for the clinical laboratory diagnosis of a patient suspected of having a porphyrin disorder, two clinical situations should be considered: First is the presence of a presumptive diagnosis of porphyria, and second is the confirmation and assignment of a specific type of porphyria to the patient in whom a porphyrin abnormality has been clinically identified. Porphyrins, porphyrin screen, or urine porphyrins are typical laboratory requests by physicians. These requests reflect the awareness that a disorder of porphyrin metabolism may be present, but the fact that porphyria is more than one disease must not be overlooked.

TABLE  18 – 2

**Classification of Porphyrinopathies**

*Primary* (inherited)
  **Neurologic** (acute attack)
    Acute intermittent porphyria (porphobilinogen deaminase [uroporphyrinogen synthase] deficiency)
    Porphobilinogen synthase deficiency (symptoms probably in homozygotes only)
  **Cutaneous** (photosensitive)
    Congenital erythropoietic porphyria (uroporphyrinogen cosynthase deficiency)
    Porphyria cutanea tarda (uroporphyrinogen decarboxylase deficiency)
    Protoporphyria (ferrochelatase deficiency)
  **Mixed** (neurologic and/or cutaneous)
    Coproporphyria (coproporphyrinogen oxidase deficiency)
    Porphyria variegata (protoporphyrinogen oxidase deficiency)
*Secondary* (induced)
  **Coproporphyrinuria** (no specific biochemical lesion)
    (Examples: tyrosinemia, lead poisoning, alcoholism)
  **Protoporphyrinemia** (as the zinc chelate)
    (Examples: iron deficiency, lead poisoning, inflammation)

If an acute neurologic porphyria is suspected, the primary screening test is for porphobilinogen. Increased urinary porphobilinogen is the characteristic biochemical abnormality of acute intermittent porphyria, variegate porphyria, and coproporphyria during an acute attack. Since porphobilinogen excretion in the urine is usually increased only during symptomatic periods, screening procedures should be reserved for the specific question of whether a patient's acute symptomatology is a result of a neuropathic porphyria. False negatives are rare and false positives are revealed by assay of porphobilinogen in a 24-hour urine sample. A negative screening test is usually reliable in a symptomatic patient. When porphyria is strongly suspected on clinical grounds and quantitative urine studies are performed, it may be worthwhile to determine both $\delta$-aminolevulinic acid and porphobilinogen concentrations. The two measurements allow a differentiation of lead poisoning and tyrosinemia, 2 disorders that resemble acute porphyria clinically but typically exhibit normal urinary porphobilinogen with an elevated urinary $\delta$-aminolevulinic acid level.

Porphobilinogen deaminase (uroporphyrinogen I synthase) deficiency, unlike increased urine porphobilinogen excretion, can be measured even during asymptomatic periods. Latent cases without clinical or urine abnormalities can also be identified on the basis of decreased porphobilinogen deaminase activity, which is often useful for counseling family members. The 2 other acute attack forms of porphyria may have an identical clinical and chemical picture during the acute phase, but the porphobilinogen deaminase activity will be normal in variegate and coproporphyrias.

The photosensitive porphyrias are best characterized chemically as disorders of porphyrin excess, as opposed to porphyrin precursor excess. In addition to urine porphyrins, erythrocyte protoporphyrin assay is essential to diagnose a photosensitive porphyria because protoporphyrin is not excreted in the urine. Fecal porphyrin assays can be helpful in diagnosing coproporphyria, and are usually considered essential to confirm a diagnosis of porphyria variegata.

Specific enzyme deficiencies along the entire heme biosynthetic pathway have now been described. Demonstration of enzyme deficiencies in erythrocytes, liver, cultured skin fibroblasts, and peripheral blood leukocytes confirms the distribution of enzyme deficiencies among tissues in affected individuals. These new biochemical insights are leading to precise diagnostic capabilities not previously available. However, only the measurement of porphobilinogen deaminase is readily available at this time in service laboratories; tests for the remainder of the heme biosynthetic enzymes remain research laboratory tools.

## ANALYTICAL PROCEDURES

Two porphyrin precursors, δ-aminolevulinic acid and porphobilinogen, accumulate or are overproduced in the neuropathic porphyrin disorders. When used in clinical diagnosis, measures of porphyrin precursors are limited to urine. Both screening tests and assays are used for porphobilinogen but no satisfactory screening test exists for δ-aminolevulinic acid.[3] Serum concentrations can provide clinically useful information but the much lower concentrations of the porphyrin precursors make their analysis somewhat more difficult; hence, serum assays are usually restricted to research laboratories.

### δ-Aminolevulinic Acid

#### PRINCIPLE

δ-Aminolevulinic acid is condensed with ethyl acetoacetate to form a pyrrole. This derivative is purified by extraction into ethyl acetate. The extracted pyrrole derivative in ethyl acetate is then reacted with Ehrlich's reagent to give a cherry-red compound that is measured spectrophotometrically at 555 nm. This procedure obviates the need for commonly recommended ion-exchange chromatography and usually yields results that are adequate for a diagnosis when used in conjunction with other laboratory tests for porphyrins. Chromatographic purification has the advantage, however, in that it gives more accurate results. Furthermore, commercially prepared, easy-to-use columns are now available (Bio-Rad Laboratories, Richmond, CA).

### SPECIMEN HANDLING

A 24-hour urine collection is obtained and the total volume recorded. The urine collection container should be refrigerated and should contain 2 g of barbituric or tartaric acid to preserve the δ-aminolevulinic acid. If porphyrins or porphobilinogen are also to be assayed, substitute 4 to 5 g (1 teaspoon) of sodium bicarbonate for the acid to ensure a near neutral pH.[6]

### SOURCES OF ERROR

Ehrlich's reagent reacts with many different substances that can cause an analytical interference. This can be prevented with careful purification of the δ-aminolevulinic acid.

### REFERENCE RANGE

Note that this is method dependent. For δ-aminolevulinic acid, it is 1.5 to 7.5 mg per 24 hours for the method above.

## Porphobilinogen

### PRINCIPLE

Porphobilinogen condenses with *p*-dimethylaminobenzaldehyde in an acid solution (Ehrlich's aldehyde reagent) to form a magenta-colored product. Since similar reactions can occur with other urinary constituents, the two established screening tests use pH adjustment and solvent extractions to remove interfering substances, thus making the tests reasonably specific. For quantitative analysis, porphobilinogen is purified by adsorption to an ion-exchange resin. Color-producing interfering substances, such as urobilinogen, methyldopa, or chlorpromazine, as well as indole and related compounds that interfere by reacting with the chromophore to produce colorless derivatives, may be removed by repeated washings of the column with water before the elution of porphobilinogen with acetic acid. Commercially prepared columns also are available (Bio-Rad Laboratories, Richmond, CA). A screening test recently described[7] requires more purification and a spectrophotometric measurement, but it is reportedly more sensitive and free of many interferences.

### SPECIMEN HANDLING

Screening tests for porphobilinogen are done preferably on a fresh morning specimen. Quantitative analyses should be performed on 24-h urine collections. If the pH of the urine is adjusted to near neutrality (pH 6 to 8) with sodium bicarbonate, the specimen can be stored for periods up to 2 weeks frozen,[6] although assays should be performed as soon as possible. If only porphobilinogen is to be assayed, sodium carbonate to make the pH distinctly alkaline is the better preservative.

### SCREENING TESTS

The best-known qualitative procedure for the detection of porphobilinogen is the Watson-Schwartz test; a modification, the Hoesch test, has been introduced more recently. Despite modifications to improve the specificity of these tests, an inexperienced person can have difficulties with interpretation of results using either the Watson-Schwartz or Hoesch test. Each of these two screening methods has its unique features and yields useful information, but their clinical value is often enhanced by familiarity with the procedure. An effective solution to the uncertainties of interpretation is the combined use of the Watson-Schwartz and the Hoesch tests, which can be performed simultaneously using similar reagents.

The most common interfering substance is urobilinogen, which produces a color with Ehrlich's reagent similar to porphobilinogen. Importantly, the Hoesch test gives no reaction with urobilinogen, thereby serving primarily as an added means of eliminating this interference and of confirming the results of the Watson-Schwartz test. Other substances sometimes present in urine can give a variety of colors, including yellow, orange, and red. All of these tend to make a positive identification of porphobilinogen difficult. By contrast, indoles and related compounds can act to decolorize the chromophore. Under these circumstances or with any uncertainty in interpretation, the quantitative procedure for porphobilinogen permits its positive identification.

In the Watson-Schwartz test, porphobilinogen and the chromogen that it forms always remain in the aqueous phase. The extractions with chloroform and butanol are essential for removing frequently occurring substances that interfere with the test. If no magenta color is observed in the upper (aqueous) phase following the chloroform extraction, the *n*-butanol extraction may be omitted and the test considered negative. The most common interfering substance is urobilinogen (chloroform soluble), which produces a color with Ehrlich's reagent similar to porphobilinogen.

## QUANTITATIVE ASSAY

The reaction of porphobilinogen with Ehrlich's reagent yields a product whose absorbance follows Beer's law from the lower limits of detection through an absorbance of at least 0.750. If porphobilinogen is present in significant amounts, the color developed by Ehrlich's reagent should be rose to crimson. On addition of Ehrlich's reagent, maximum color develops within 6 minutes. The color remains stable for 2 to 3 minutes and then begins to fade slowly. Within 20 minutes, absorbance decreases by about 10%. The ratio of $A_{525}/A_{555}$ should be near 0.83. A ratio of $A_{525}/A_{555} > 1.00$ is rare and indicates that interfering substances are still present; the result should not be interpreted as an abnormal concentration of porphobilinogen. Alternatively, an Allen correction can be applied by measuring the absorbance at 535, 555, and 575 nm and then utilizing the formula $A_{Corrected} = 2A_{525} - (A_{535} + A_{575})$. Calculating with this corrected absorbance helps to eliminate the effects of interfering chromogens but a chromatographic purification remains essential. With a porphobilinogen concentration 2 to 3 times normal, which is clinically significant, no difficulty is likely to be encountered in its quantitation.

### Reference Ranges

The reference range for porphobilinogen is <1 mg/24 h.

## Porphyrins

### PRINCIPLE

Virtually all porphyrin analyses are based on the isolation of the porphyrins from the specimen, separation of the individual porphyrins by chromatography, and observation or measurement of the porphyrins by fluorometry or spectrophotometry. Porphyrins are usually isolated from body excreta or tissues by extraction into an acidified organic solvent. For screening purposes, minimal purification is required. For quantitation, the individual porphyrins are separated by selective solvent extraction or by chromatography. Their characteristic orange-red fluorescence (620 to 630 nm) on irradiation with long-wavelength ultraviolet light (398 to 408 nm) allows porphyrins in acid solutions to be detected fluorometrically at concentrations below $10^{-8}$ mol/L. Alternatively, when the concentrations of porphyrins are sufficiently high, they can be measured spectrophotometrically.

### SPECIMEN HANDLING

Whole blood specimens are collected using any common anticoagulant. Urine for screening purposes should preferably be a morning specimen, but random specimens can be used. Since the assay of a single urine specimen provides less meaningful data with no reference range, quantitative analyses should be performed on 24-hour collections. In this case, the urine should be collected in a container to which 4 to 5 g of sodium bicarbonate has been added to maintain the specimen at pH 7 or above. If feces are used only for qualitative tests, a small specimen (1 g) is adequate. When porphyrin analyses cannot be performed soon after collection of the specimens, they should be stored in the dark at 4°C, or they should be kept frozen if more than 1 to 2 days elapse before analysis.

### IDENTIFICATION OF PORPHYRINS

When abnormal levels of porphyrins are seen or suspected in a screening test, identification of the specific porphyrin or porphyrins that are elevated can aid in diagnosis. Identification can be accomplished most simply with thin-layer chromatography, although high-pressure liquid chromatography (HPLC) is coming into wider use for porphyrin analysis.

### QUANTITATIVE ASSAY BY HPLC

The importance of urine preparation to good analyses must not be overlooked. Before processing, urine has much fluorescent material that can obscure the uroporphyrin peak, interfere with interpretation of other peaks, and possibly quench porphyrin fluorescence. Unlike original clinical laboratory methods, HPLC separates all porphyrins based on the number of carboxyl groups. Since some techniques still in use measure more than one compound as uroporphyrin or coproporphyrin because of cross-contamination as well as the presence of minor components, an HPLC method gives a more accurate account of each porphyrin present. Results of an HPLC assay may include 7-, 6- and 5-carboxyl porphyrins as well as uroporphyrin and coproporphyrins.

## Reference Ranges

The reference ranges for porphyrins are method dependent, but the following are typical examples:

Uroporphyrin            4 to 20 $\mu$g/24 h
Coproporphyrin        13 to 179 $\mu$g/24 h

## ERYTHROCYTE PROTOPORPHYRIN

### Principle

Several simplified, rapid micromethods for erythrocyte protoporphyrin measurement have been developed. Typically, all red cell porphyrins are first removed from the blood by adsorption or extraction. The simple methods do not discriminate among uroporphyrin, coproporphyrin, or protoporphyrin, but this has little clinical consequence since the predominant analyte is protoporphyrin. The adsorbed porphyrin is further purified and then measured fluorometrically using coproporphyrin as a standard.[8]

### Specimen Handling

Whole blood is anticoagulated with EDTA or heparin. The specimen is stable for several days when stored at 4°C. It should not be frozen since this affects porphyrin extractability.

### Sources of Error

This measurement has utility well beyond the diagnosis of the porphyrias. Both chronic lead poisoning and iron deficiency cause distinct, albeit more moderate, elevation of erythrocyte protoporphyrin concentration. However, these secondary causes of protoporphyrin elevation are not photosensitive conditions as is protoporphyria. This chemical or clinical discrepancy has been reconciled with the observation that zinc chelate of protoporphyrin occurs in erythrocytes of the non-photosensitive conditions, whereas the metal-free protoporphyrin that causes photosensitivity occurs in protoporphyria. In a common blood assay, the zinc chelate is destroyed by the acid extraction solvent. Metal-free porphyrin, which is then liberated, is usually called *free erythrocyte protoporphyrin* or FEP. The distinction between metal-free and zinc protoporphyrin is essential in differentiating the protoporphyrinemias. When the assay is used for diagnosis, any plasma porphyrins that may be present are clinically insignificant.

### Reference Range

The reference range is 17 to 77 $\mu$g of protoporphyrin per deciliter of erythrocytes. These values are highly method dependent. The units and values may also differ depending on whether porphyrin content is expressed per deciliter of whole blood, deciliter of erythrocytes, gram of hemoglobin, or moles of heme.

## ZINC PROTOPORPHYRIN BY HEMATOFLUOROMETER

### Principle

This method is based on the direct fluorometric measurement of zinc protoporphyrin in blood using front-surface fluorometry as originally described by Blumberg et al.[9] In this case, the specimen absorbs essentially all of the incident light within a thin layer of the specimen surface while allowing all of the emitted light to be efficiently detected. In the hematofluorometer, the incident light strikes the bottom of a drop of blood on a glass slide. Emitted light is detected at an acute angle to the incident beam. The emission intensity is related to the ratio of zinc protoporphyrin fluorescence to hemoglobin absorbance.

### Specimen Handling

The test requires 1 drop (approximately 50 $\mu$L) of anticoagulated blood obtained by either venipuncture or skin puncture. The zinc protoporphyrin is stable in a refrigerated specimen for at least 1 week; however, assay by hematofluorometry must be performed before the specimen becomes hemolyzed.

### Sources of Error

Because the spectral properties of hemoglobin are altered by oxygen, complete oxygenation of the blood is an essential requirement for this assay. When the blood is partially deoxygenated, erroneously low results will be obtained. This problem can be avoided using reagents that were developed to stabilize the hemoglobin.[10] Since the results are not influenced by the hematocrit, equal dilution of the blood with isotonic saline can aid in mixing and oxygenation. Positive interference due to abnormally high bilirubin also poses a problem.

### Reference Range

Zinc protoporphyrin results using the hematofluorometer are linear from normal (300 $\mu$g/L) to grossly elevated levels (11,000 $\mu$g/L) and correlate well with results obtained using extraction methods. Precision is ±2%.

Results from the hematofluorometer and from assays involving extraction procedures may correlate, but confusion about interpretation is common because porphyrin content may be expressed in terms of erythrocyte concentration, whole blood concentration, or hemoglobin (or heme) present. Since reference ranges can be greatly influenced by both instrumental and methodologic factors, each laboratory should establish its own range until standardization becomes better established. Low concentrations of protoporphyrin or zinc protoporphyrin have no known clinical significance; therefore, a reference range is important only in terms of the upper limit found in persons having adequate iron status and no lead exposure.

Protoporphyrin concentration is in the range of 17 to 77 $\mu$g/dL of erythrocytes. The zinc protoporphyrin to heme ratio is ≤80 $\mu$mol/mol.

## Heme Biosynthetic Enzymes

The symptomatic classification presented earlier is a useful approach for the initial evaluation of a patient with a suspected porphyrinopathy. Since a unique enzyme deficiency in heme biosynthesis can now be associated with each primary disorder or porphyria (Table 18–1), it is reasonable to expect that a specific diagnosis pertinent to each of the porphyrias may eventually be established on the basis of enzyme data alone. Unfortunately, the assays of most enzymes pose unique technical problems because of specific chemical and biochemical features such as substrate instability, the fluorescence of both substrate and product, and distribution of the enzymes between the cytoplasm and mitochondria.

Assays for all of the enzymes of the heme biosynthetic pathway have been described. However, only porphobilinogen deaminase activity is being measured regularly in the clinical laboratory. This assay is technically easy to perform because of specimen requirement, the ready availability of substrate, and the need for a simple instrument.

### PORPHOBILINOGEN DEAMINASE ACTIVITY

#### Principle

Two features of this enzymatic reaction have allowed for easy adaptability of the assay to the clinical laboratory. First, the enzyme is cytoplasmic and therefore is retained within mature erythrocytes, which provide an excellent specimen for assay. Second, the substrate for the reaction is nonfluorescent but the product (uroporphyrin) is highly fluorescent, which allows for its measurement in picomolar quantities. The enzyme utilizes the monopyrrole precursor, porphobilinogen, as a substrate to form uroporphyrinogen, which is rapidly oxidized to uroporphyrin during acid deproteinization of the incubation mixture. Uroporphyrin fluorescence is then measured directly without further processing.

#### Specimen Handling

A whole blood specimen is collected with either heparin or EDTA. The specimen can be stored at 4°C for 1 week without significant loss of activity.

#### Sources of Error

The erythrocyte porphobilinogen deaminase activity varies with cell age. Therefore, a shift in the erythrocyte population toward younger cells might lead to an enzyme activity that does not accurately represent the true condition. An elevated reticulocyte percentage would indicate that such a condition may be present.

#### Reference Range

The reference range for porphobilinogen is 1.27 to 2.01 mU/g of hemoglobin.

### UROPORPHYRINOGEN COSYNTHASE

The formation of uroporphyrinogen III requires concerted action of both porphobilinogen deaminase and uroporphyrinogen cosynthase. The deaminase is essential for tetrapyrrole formation, and the cosynthase directs the isomer III synthesis in preference to the nonfunctional isomer I. Assay of uroporphyrinogen III cosynthase requires that isomer production, independent of total porphyrin synthesis, be measured. Although erythrocytes are an accessible source of uroporphyrinogen cosynthase, the technical difficulties of assaying enzyme activity and the relative ease of diagnosis by other means tend to obviate the need for an assay suitable for the clinical laboratory.

### UROPORPHYRINOGEN DECARBOXYLASE

The sequential decarboxylation of the 8 carboxyl uroporphyrinogen to the 4 carboxyl coproporphyrinogen is catalyzed by uroporphyrinogen decarboxylase. Considering reported experiences with assays of this activity using either uroporphyrinogen III on pentacarboxylic porphyrinogen III as substitute, one may assume that this enzyme catalyzes the entire cytosolic decarboxylation sequence from uroporphyrinogen to coproporphyrinogen. The substrate must be in the reduced or "-ogen" form and, of course, the measurement of the reaction product must allow discrimination between substrate and product porphyrins.

### COPROPORPHYRINOGEN OXIDASE

This enzyme catalyzes the decarboxylation and dehydrogenation of the propionic acid side chains at positions 2 and 4 of coproporphyrinogen to vinyl groups, resulting in the formation of protoporphyrinogen. Since this is a mitochondrial enzyme, erythrocytes cannot be used for the assay. Substrate selection for the enzyme is particularly important. If unlabeled coproporphyrinogen is used, then the protoporphyrinogen product can be difficult to differentiate from the substrate since they have similar chemical and fluorescence properties. A radioisotope approach uses $^{14}$C-coproporphyrinogen with the label in the carboxyl carbons of the propionic side chains. The decarboxylation can then be followed by $^{14}CO_2$ release.

### FERROCHELATASE

This mitochondrial enzyme catalyzes the chelation of a ferrous ion by protoporphyrin with release of 2 protons. The measurement of $^{59}$Fe incorporation into heme, the decrease in porphyrin fluorescence by iron chelation, and the direct quantitation of heme formed have all been used for the assay.

## SUMMARY

Porphyrin metabolism disorders or porphyrinopathies usually refer to the inherited diseases, i.e., the porphyrias. However, a variety of secondary or induced disorders in porphyrin metabolism also occur, and in diagnostic procedures, these distinctions must be determined. The laboratory diagnosis of porphyrin disorders is complicated and can seldom be achieved with a single test. The symptoms and laboratory findings of the various porphyrin disorders overlap considerably, which can lead to erroneous diagnoses without careful laboratory work. Usually a confirmed diagnosis is dependent on several measures of porphyrin metabolism, with the conclusion being based on the pattern of change that is found.

The effectiveness of treatment for various porphyrin disorders varies widely from individual to individual and among the different kinds of abnormal metabolism that occur. Although these several metabolic disorders occur in a common pathway, i.e., heme biosynthesis, the treatments are totally different from one disorder to another. Therefore, it is imperative that an accurate diagnosis be made, and this is nearly always dependent on supportive laboratory findings.

Zinc protoporphyrin formation is a special case among the porphyrin disorders in that it results from two very common diseases, namely, chronic lead exposure and iron deficiency. Although all of the other porphyrin laboratory work might be done in specialized settings, the assay of zinc protoporphyrin, especially the zinc protoporphyrin/heme ratio, should be commonly used because it is the most cost-effective diagnosis of iron deficiency as well as being a screening test for chronic lead exposure.

## REFERENCES

1. With TK: A short history of porphyrins and the porphyrias. Int J Biochem 11:189–200, 1980.

2. Meyer UA: Porphyrias. In Wilson JD, Braunwald E, Isselbacher KJ, et al., (eds.): *Harrison's Principles of Internal Medicine*. 12th ed. New York, McGraw-Hill, 1991, pp 1829–1834.

3. Nuttall KL: Porphyrins and disorders of porphyrin metabolism. In Burtis CA, Ashwood ER (eds.): *Tietz Fundamentals of Clinical Chemistry*. 4th ed. Philadelphia, WB Saunders, 1987, pp 731–744.

4. Nuttall KL: The porphyrias. In Stanbury JB, Wyngaarden DS, Fredrickson DS (eds.): *The Metabolic Basis of Inherited Disease*. 7th ed. New York, McGraw-Hill, 1995, pp 1711–1732.

5. Labbe RF, Rettmer RL: Zinc protoporphyrin: A product of iron deficient erythropoiesis. Semin Hematol 26:40–46, 1989.

6. Fernandez CP, Labbe RF: Specimen collection for urinary porphyrin studies. Clin Chem Acta 132:317–320, 1983.

7. Schreiber WE, Jamani A, Pudek MR: Screening tests for porphobilinogen are insensitive. Am J Clin Pathol 92: 644–649, 1989.

8. Piomelli S: Free erythrocyte porphyrin in the detection of undue absorption of Pb and of Fe deficiency. Clin Chem 23:264–69, 1977.

9. Blumberg WE, Eisinger J, Lamola AA, Zuckerman DM: Zinc protoporphyrin level in blood determined by a portable hematofluorometer: A screening device for lead poisoning. J Lab Clin Med 89:712–23, 1977.

10. Rettmer RL, Gunter EW, Labbe RF: Overcoming the limitations of hematofluorometry for assaying zinc protoporphyrin. Ann NY Acad Sci 514:345–346, 1987.

# CHAPTER 19

# Renal Anatomy and Physiology

*Nancy A. Brunzel*

## RENAL ANATOMY

### Components of the Urinary System

Human kidneys are paired, bean-shaped organs located on the posterior wall of the abdominal cavity. They are positioned on either side of the spinal column parallel to the last thoracic and first 3 lumbar vertebrae. Each kidney weighs roughly 120 to 170 g and measures approximately 11 cm long, 6 cm wide, and 2.5 cm deep.[1] At the concave medial area of each kidney, which appears macroscopically as an indentation, is a slitlike opening called the **renal hilus.** The renal artery, vein, nerves, and lymphatic vessels pass through the hilus, as does the renal pelvis, which is the topmost, expanded portion of each ureter.

Gross examination of a kidney reveals an outer thin white membrane called the **fibrous capsule.** When a kidney is cut lengthwise, the cortex and medulla are readily apparent (Figure 19–1). The outermost, darker red and granular–appearing area is the **cortex,** which accounts for approximately 70% of the kidney. The remaining 30% is the **medulla,** which appears as a series of tissue **pyramids** arising from the cortex. The renal medulla can be further divided into an outer zone that is adjacent to the cortex and an inner zone where the renal papilla reside. The apex of each medullary pyramid, called a papilla, extends toward the renal pelvis and terminates at a minor **calyx.** Minor calyces, which can be used by more than one papilla, fuse together to form the major calyces. The calyces function simply as funnels; they receive the urine from the papilla and convey it to the renal pelvis. The calyces and renal pelvis are actually considered components of the extrarenal collecting system because the composition of the urine remains unchanged as it passes through these structures.

The renal pelvis of each kidney is actually the expanded end of the ureter, a fibromuscular tube about 25-cm long that extends from the renal hilus to the base of the bladder. Peristaltic activity of the smooth muscle surrounding the ureters propels the urine down the ureters and into the bladder. At the junction between each ureter and the bladder, a one-way valve permits the flow of urine from the ureters into the bladder, but not in the opposite direction. The bladder, a muscular sac, serves as a temporary reservoir for urine to accumulate. When the bladder becomes distended a nerve reflex, the micturition reflex, is initiated. This reflex causes the urinary sphincter to relax and the bladder to contract, resulting in the movement of urine from the bladder through the urethra to the outside of the body. The urethra, a tubelike connection from the bladder to the body exterior, is significantly different in length between men and women, i.e., approximately 24 cm and 4 cm, respectively.

The functional or "urine forming" units of the kidney are the nephrons. They are tubular structures that traverse both the renal cortex and medulla and terminate at the papilla. Each kidney contains approximately 1 million nephrons, and each nephron has arterial blood supplied individually to its glomerulus. The glomeruli, which are capillary beds derived from individual afferent arterioles, reside exclusively in the renal cortex and their presence impart the somewhat granular and dark-red appearance. Besides the glomerulus, a nephron is composed of sequential tubular segments that are structurally and functionally diverse. The passage of plasma ultrafiltrate through the nephrons, a process controlled by renal blood flow, results in the formation of urine and its release from the papilla into the renal calyces.

### Structure of the Nephron

A nephron has 5 morphologically and functionally distinct regions: the glomerulus, proximal convoluted tubule, loop of Henle or nephron loop, distal tubule, and collecting tubule or duct. Despite a common configuration, the morphologic appearance of each nephron varies depending on the location of its glomerulus in the renal cortex. Similarly, the tubular segments of the nephron are also located in specific zones of the kidney. Their location actually plays an important role in the functional processes that occur in each segment.

#### GLOMERULUS

The glomerulus, also called a *renal corpuscle,* is the site of blood plasma filtration that results in the formation of an ultrafiltrate that ultimately becomes urine. A glomerulus consists of 4 anatomic components: (1) the capillary bed derived from an afferent arteriole, (2) the Bowman's capsule, (3) the basement membrane or basal lamina, and (4) the mesangium (Figure 19–2). The mesangium, in contrast to the other glomerular components, has no role in the ultrafiltration process that occurs in the glomerulus. Rather, the mesangial cells provide

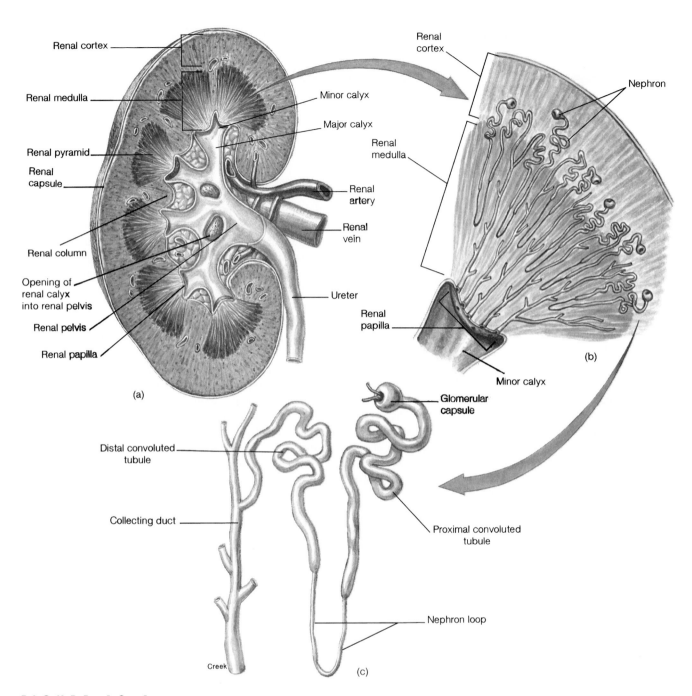

**FIGURE 19-1**

Macroscopic and microscopic features of the kidney. Illustrated are a coronal section of a kidney **(a),** a renal pyramid **(b),** and a single nephron **(c).** (From Van De Graaff KM, Fox IF (eds.): *Concepts of Human Anatomy & Physiology.* 5th ed. Boston, WCB/McGraw-Hill, 1999.)

structural support for the glomerulus and actively remove, by phagocytosis and pinocytosis, molecular entities (e.g., immune complexes) that can become entrapped in the glomerular filtration barrier (GFB). Because mesangial cells have contractile ability, a role in regulating glomerular blood flow is also postulated.

The capillary endothelium of the glomerulus has pores that are the first component of the GFB which must be traversed by the blood plasma. The openings of this fenestrated endothelium are approximately 50 to 100 nm (500 Å to 1000 Å) in diameter.[2] In addition to these pores, a coating rich in polyanionic glycoproteins covers the endothelial surface, im-

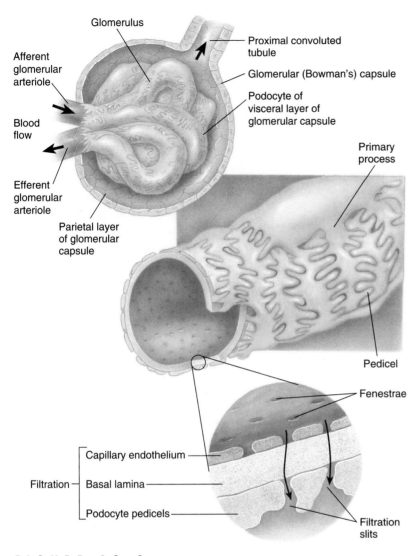

**FIGURE 19-2**

A diagram of a glomerulus illustrating the intimate relationship between the glomerular capillaries, the basal lamina or (basement membrane), and Bowman's capsule. Note that filtered substances leave the bloodstream by way of the capillary fenestrae (or pores), penetrate the basal lamina, and then must pass through the filtration slits of the podocytes into Bowman's space to become the initial ultrafiltrate. The fingerlike processes of the podocytes are called pedicels. (From Van De Graaff KM, Fox IF (eds.): *Concepts of Human Anatomy & Physiology.* 5th ed. Boston, WCB/McGraw-Hill, 1999.)

parting a negative charge that serves to repel anionic molecules in the plasma. Hence, the capillary endothelium plays an initial role in the selectivity of molecules, in both their size and charge, that are able to pass from the plasma into the GFB.

The next anatomic component, the glomerular basement membrane (GBM) or basal lamina, is a trilayer structure composed of type IV and type V collagen, proteoglycans, and glycoproteins. It is actually synthesized by the capillary endothelium on one side and the podocytes (i.e., epithelium) of Bowman's capsule on the other. Visible by transmission elec-

tron microscopy, the outer less dense subepithelial layer is called the lamina rara externa (next to the podocytes); the central electron-dense layer is the lamina densa; and the inner subendothelial layer is the lamina rara interna (next to the capillary endothelium) (Figure 19–3). Numerous proteoglycans, particularly heparan sulfate, are concentrated here imparting an anionic character to the GBM. As with the capillary endothelium, this anionic character influences which molecules are able to pass the GBM from the capillary lumen to Bowman's space.

After a molecule travels from the blood plasma through the capillary endothelium and the GBM, it must pass the epithelium of Bowman's capsule. This thin epithelial layer, composed of cells called podocytes, intimately covers the capillaries of the glomerulus with the GBM sandwiched between.

The podocytes get their name from their footlike shape when observed in cross section (Figure 19–3). When observed by scanning electron microscopy, they resemble octopus-like cells with numerous processes that interdigitate with adjacent cells and completely cover the glomerular capillaries (Figure 19–4). Stretching between the fingerlike processes is the filtration-slit membrane or slit diaphragm, which has rectangular openings $4 \times 14$ nm ($40 \times 140$ Å). These openings allow molecules with an effective molecular radius less than 4 nm to pass. A 12-nm thick protein coat, rich in sialic acid, covers the podocytes.[1] Neutralization of the anionic charge of this sialoprotein coat causes a change in podocyte cell shape that results in an increase in the permeability of the GFB.

In addition to their intimate physical relationship with the glomerular capillaries, this epithelium also forms a space, Bowman's space, into which the filtrate of the blood plasma initially collects. From this space originates the lumen of the proximal tubule for each nephron. As this space becomes the tubular lumen, the epithelium abruptly changes to that characteristic of proximal tubules (Figure 19–5).

In summary, the glomerulus is the site of filtration and formation of the initial plasma ultrafiltrate. Three morphologic components of the glomerulus, collectively called the *glomerular filtration barrier*, are responsible for the composition of this ultrafiltrate. They are (1) the capillary endothelial

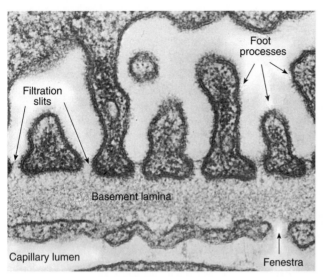

**FIGURE 19-3**

Transmission electron micrograph of a glomerular filtration barrier (GFB). The trilayer structure of the GFB is readily apparent: (1) the fenestrated capillary epithelium, (2) the basal lamina (or basement membrane), and (3) the epithelium of Bowman's capsule, i.e., podocytes. Note the footlike appearance or foot processes of the podocytes and their filtration slits. (From Van De Graaff KM, Fox IF (eds.): *Concepts of Human Anatomy & Physiology.* 5th ed. Boston, WCB/McGraw-Hill, 1999.)

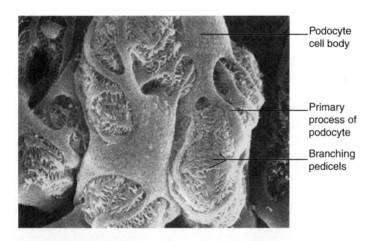

**FIGURE 19-4**

Scanning electron micrograph of podocytes surrounding a glomerular capillary as viewed from Bowman's space. Note the interdigitating foot processes or pedicels of adjacent podocytes. (From Van De Graaff KM, Fox IF (eds.): *Concepts of Human Anatomy & Physiology.* 5th ed. Boston, WCB/McGraw-Hill, 1999.)

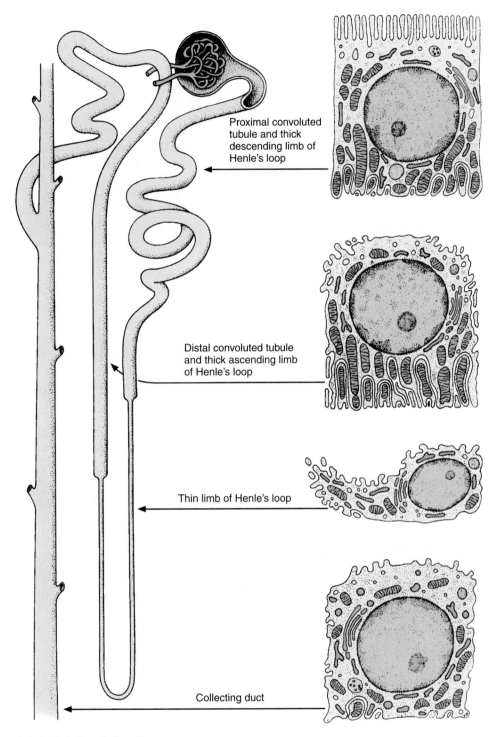

**FIGURE 19-5**

General histologic characteristics of renal tubular epithelium in selected regions of the nephron. Note that the cells of the ascending thick limb of Henle's loop and the distal convoluted tubule appear similar in their ultrastructure but perform significantly different functions. (From Junqueira LC, et al.: *Basic Histology.* New York, McGraw-Hill, 1995.)

Labels within figure:
- Proximal convoluted tubule and thick descending limb of Henle's loop
- Distal convoluted tubule and thick ascending limb of Henle's loop
- Thin limb of Henle's loop
- Collecting duct

pores, (2) the trilayered basement membrane, and (3) the podocytes with the filtration-slit membrane. Together they dictate the molecular size and charge of plasma constituents that can traverse the GFB. Size selectivity is initially screened by the basement membrane but ultimately dictated by the openings of the filtration-slit membrane. Hence, in a healthy glomerulus, passing molecules must have a molecular radius less than 4 nm. Molecular charge is important because of the "shield of negativity" maintained throughout the GFB. Molecules that are neutral readily pass; whereas, positively charged (i.e., cationic) molecules are actually attracted into the GFB. In contrast, anionic molecules, regardless of size, will be repelled. It is worth noting that albumin has a molecular radius of 3.6 nm, small enough to readily pass the GFB. However, owing to its negative charge, only insignificant amounts normally pass the GFB into the ultrafiltrate in Bowman's space. It becomes apparent that if the anionic character of the GFB is compromised or lost (e.g., nephrotic syndrome, untreated type 1 diabetes mellitus), then significantly increased amounts of albumin will readily appear in the ultrafiltrate.

The ultrafiltrate of plasma that initially forms in Bowman's space lacks significant numbers of cellular elements, i.e., red blood cells and white blood cells. Red blood cells (~6–8 $\mu$m in diameter) typically require pores or openings of 500 nm or greater to pass. Similarly, in the healthy individual, significant numbers of white blood cells (~9–15 $\mu$m in diameter) are not present in the ultrafiltrate, despite their ability to penetrate any tissue of the body. In other words, the ultrafiltrate composition resembles plasma with the exclusion of cells and molecules the size of albumin or larger.

## TUBULES

For the purposes of discussion, the nephron can be divided into 4 principal tubular segments: (1) the proximal convoluted tubule, (2) the loop of Henle, (3) the distal convoluted tubule, and (4) the collecting tubule or duct. Keep in mind that each of these segments has been studied extensively and can be subdivided further, from both an anatomical and functional standpoint. However, discussion at that level is beyond the scope and purpose of this text.

From Bowman's space in the glomerulus, the initial ultrafiltrate passes into the **proximal convoluted tubule** (PCT), the first tubular segment of the nephron. The epithelium of this segment is structurally and functionally unique. The cells are large, with well-developed apical microvillus borders (brush borders) and extensive lateral interdigitations with adjacent cells (Figure 19–5). Both of these features serve to significantly increase the cell surface area, providing a large area for the numerous and varied transport processes that take place in this segment. Proximal tubular cells contain numerous large mitochondria, and possess an extensive intracellular digestive system (endocytic apparatus and lysosomes). The convoluted portion of the proximal tubule resides exclusively in the renal cortex. As the tubule straightens and traverses into the medulla, it becomes the straight portion of the proximal tubule.

The next anatomic segment, referred to as the **loop of Henle or nephron loop,** consists of the straight part of the proximal tubule, the thin limb segments, and the straight part of the distal tubule. In the outer zone of the renal medulla (region closest to the cortex), the straight proximal tubule narrows to become a thin limb segment. The total length and segmentation of each loop of Henle differs, depending on the location of its glomerulus in the renal cortex. Those nephrons whose glomeruli reside in the superficial and midcortical regions of the cortex have short loops of Henle dipping only into the outer zone of the medulla. The short-looped nephrons do not have a thin ascending limb; rather, the hairpin turn and ascending limb are a thick tubule. In contrast, juxtamedullary nephrons, those with glomeruli in the cortex regions adjacent to the medulla, have long loops of Henle that reach deep into the inner zone of the medulla. These long-looped nephrons have lengthy ascending and descending thin limbs on either side of their hairpin turn.

The epithelium of the loop of Henle is composed of simple, flat cells. The descending limb cells are noninterdigitating, with tight junctions consistent with a high permeability to water but a low permeability for sodium and chloride. In contrast, the ascending thin limb cells are extensively interdigitating, with cell junctions that are associated with high-ion permeability but low-water permeability.

The thin limb segment gradually transitions to a thick limb at, or shortly before, the hairpin turn in short-looped nephrons or as the thin ascending limb reenters the outer zone of the medulla in long-looped nephrons. This thick segment can be classified as part of the loop of Henle or as the straight portion of the distal tubule. Once in the cortex, the thick ascending limb makes contact with the vascular pole (i.e., site where the afferent and efferent arteriole enter and exit the glomerulus) of the particular nephron from which it was derived (Figure 19–6). This contact region is the site of the **juxtaglomerular apparatus** (JGA); an area composed of morphologically and functionally distinct portions of the afferent and efferent arterioles, the extraglomerular mesangium, and a specialized area of the distal tubule, called the **macula densa.** Compared to the surrounding tubular epithelium, the cells comprising the macula densa that reside immediately adjacent to the arterioles are narrower and smaller, yet have larger nuclei; hence the name, which translates as dense spot or region.

After the macula densa, the tubular segment again becomes circuitous and is termed the **distal convoluted tubule.** Here, the basal two thirds of the tubular epithelial cells have extensive lateral interdigitating processes packed with numerous large and elongated mitochondria. In addition, the type of tight junctions between adjacent cells enables them to maintain a large chemical gradient.

The collecting tubule or duct is the final segment of a nephron. This segment follows the distal convoluted tubule; it begins in the renal cortex but eventually traverses the entire renal medulla until it terminates at a papilla, where the processed filtrate, now urine, is passed into the renal pelvis for

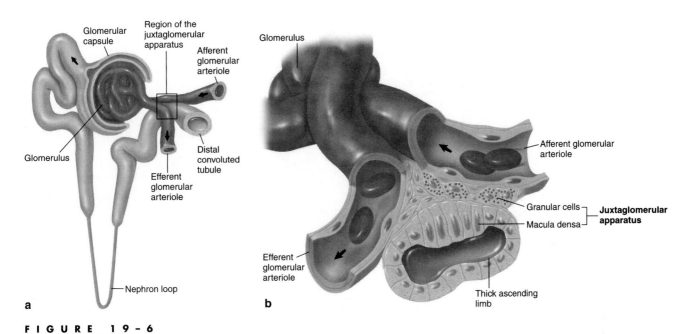

**FIGURE 19-6**

The juxtaglomerular apparatus (JGA). The structure **(a)** includes portions of the afferent arteriole, efferent arteriole, and a specialized region of the distal tubule called the macula densa. At the macula densa, as seen in **(b),** the afferent arteriole has numerous specialized cells called granular cells. The granules in these cells contain large amounts of the enzyme renin. (From Van De Graaff KM, Fox IF (eds.): *Concepts of Human Anatomy & Physiology.* 5th ed. Boston, WCB/McGraw-Hill, 1999.)

conveyance to the bladder. Usually multiple nephrons share a single collecting tubule; hence, these tubules are often referred to as a collecting duct system. The epithelium differs in the cortex and outer medulla collecting ducts, as compared to the deep inner medullary ducts. Initially, in the cortex, the cells are cuboidal with straight lateral borders and nuclei located in the apical half of the cell. As the duct traverses the medulla, the cells become columnar and their nuclei are found closer to the basal surface of the cells. While transitioning through the outer and inner medulla, multiple collecting ducts converge and fuse together to eventually form the large papillary collecting ducts that empty into the renal pelvis.

## RENAL CIRCULATION

The ability of the kidneys to perform their homeostatic functions is directly related to renal blood flow (RBF). Hence, elaborate coordination of intrinsic and extrinsic regulatory mechanisms occur to ensure that 20% to 25% of the cardiac output circulates through the kidneys. Although the kidneys account for only 0.5% of the total body weight (~300 g), they receive blood flow at a rate 5 to 50 times greater than the flow through any other organ. This high degree of renal perfusion enables the filtration of approximately 20% of the plasma, which amounts to an average glomerular filtration rate (GFR) of 120 mL/minute or 170 L per day.[3] Because this remarkably

high perfusion exceeds the renal needs for oxygen or nutrients, it is postulated that the RBF is primarily maintained to sustain adequate glomerular and peritubular pressures, which are compatible with optimum ultrafiltrate formation and processing by the nephrons.

The cardiac output, or blood pressure, actually drives the renal processes. The comparatively wide lumen of the afferent arteriole relative to the efferent arteriole provides a hydrostatic pressure of approximately 55 mm Hg, driving the filtration process in the glomerulus. Two opposing pressures, the oncotic pressure resulting from proteins that remain in the bloodstream and the hydrostatic pressure from the ultrafiltrate already present in Bowman's space, resist the filtration process. However, the sum of these opposing pressures is approximately 45 mm Hg, resulting in a net filtration pressure across the glomerular filtration barrier of approximately 10 mm Hg.

The left and right renal arteries arise from the abdominal aorta, enter the renal hilus, making several subdivisions before becoming the interlobular arteries, which subsequently branch to form the afferent arterioles that supply each glomerulus. Within each glomerulus, the afferent arteriole subdivides to become an anastomosing capillary bed that eventually converges back together to reform another arteriole, the efferent arteriole. After leaving the glomerulus at the vascular pole, the efferent arteriole subdivides again into a capillary network that

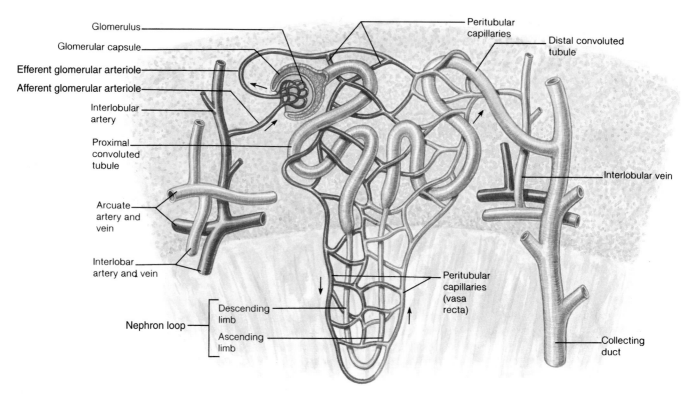

**FIGURE 19-7**

Components of a nephron and its surrounding vasculature. This simplified drawing
shows the flow of blood from the afferent arteriole through a glomerulus to the
peritubular capillaries, the vasa recta, and ultimately into the venous system. (From
Van De Graaff KM, Fox IF (eds.): *Concepts of Human Anatomy & Physiology.*
5th ed. Boston, WCB/McGraw-Hill, 1999.)

surrounds the tubular segments of the nephron (Figure 19–7).
The capillaries surrounding the nephron segments located in
the renal cortex are called **peritubular capillaries,** whereas the
capillary network intimately associated with the segments in
the outer and inner medulla is called the **vasa recta.** This
unique as well as intricate microvasculature enables optimum
renal tubular reabsorption and secretion in addition to tight
regulation of the vascular resistance.

Control of vascular resistance enables the kidney to respond to situations of insufficient or low cardiac output, as well
as excessively high output. The juxtaglomerular apparatus
(JGA) plays a significant role in this regard. The afferent and
efferent arterioles, as well as the extraglomerular mesangium of
the JGA, have contractile ability that enables them to alter
vascular resistance in the glomerulus. In addition, modified
smooth muscle cells of the afferent arterioles produce **renin,**
which is stored in membrane-bound granules. Hence, these cells
are known as *granular cells* (Figure 19–6). The JGA is also richly
supplied with nerves. Together, these features enable regulation
of blood pressure and intravascular fluid balance by the kidney.
Ultimately, a variety of processes work in concert to ensure that
adequate RBF is sustained and, in so doing, ensures that renal
function is maintained.

## RENAL PHYSIOLOGY

### Urine Formation

The ultimate role of the nephrons, the functional units of the
kidney, is to eliminate metabolic wastes (e.g., nitrogenous compounds, organic acids, excess electrolytes), exogenous substances (e.g., radiographic contrast media, drugs), and excess
water. To accomplish this task, approximately 170 L of ultrafiltrate is processed by the nephrons per day, resulting in the
excretion of about 1.2 L of urine. In other words, 99% of
the initial plasma ultrafiltrate is actually reabsorbed by the
nephrons and retained by the body. This ability to selectively
process the blood plasma highlights the kidneys' important
role, not only in the excretion of substances, but also in the
regulation of an optimal chemical composition or balance
throughout the body. In addition, the kidneys play an endocrine function both as a producer of hormones as well as a site
of hormone action.

Each nephron acts independently, yet cooperatively, in
maintaining homeostasis. In diseases characterized by the in-

capacitation or destruction of nephrons, the remaining functional nephrons can actually increase their workload to compensate, thereby maintaining a near-normal GFR. However, this compensatory mechanism cannot sustain itself indefinitely. When 60% to 80% of the nephrons are destroyed, impairment of renal function becomes evident by a decrease in GFR.[4] Despite its large functional reserve, early detection of renal disease is imperative to enable prompt intervention and possible reversal of the renal disease process.

## Urine Volume and Concentration

The principal component of urine is water. To eliminate the solutes from daily metabolic processes, water is required, and additional water that is not currently needed by the body is excreted. Note there is no storage or reserve for water in the body. Therefore, periodic ingestion of water is required to maintain homeostasis. Because the volume of water ingested daily (i.e., state of hydration) can vary dramatically within or between individuals, the concentration of the urine excreted will also vary.

A typical American diet requires the elimination of anywhere from 100 to 1200 milliosmoles (mOsm) of solutes each day; average ~700 mOsm. (A mOsm is 1 millimole [mmol] of particles in a solution and is the term used to express solute number in body fluids.) To eliminate this typical solute load, a minimum volume of approximately 500 mL of water per day is required. In conditions that result in an increased number of solutes in the urine, such as the glucose present in the urine of uncontrolled diabetes mellitus individuals, an increased volume of water is required for excretion. In these individuals, the solute load can be as high as 5000 mOsm per day (mOsm/d) and their urine output often exceeds 3 L/d. The excretion of a urine volume greater than 3 L/d is termed **polyuria.** To sustain this urine output, ingestion of large volumes of water is required, and these individuals experience **polydipsia,** intense and excessive thirst. In healthy individuals, although the volume of urine excreted daily varies depending on their state of hydration, output is usually between 500 and 1800 mL/d. Some clinical conditions (e.g., urinary obstruction, renal tubular dysfunction) can present with **oliguria,** defined as a urine output less than 400 mL/d. When no urine is excreted, the term **anuria** applies and intervention is required to prevent imminent death.

Although the solute composition of urine can be influenced by diet or disease, the predominant solutes in the urine of healthy individuals remain essentially the same. They are, in decreasing millimolar amounts: urea, chloride, sodium, potassium, ammonium, inorganic phosphate, inorganic sulfate, creatinine, and uric acid. Of these solutes, urea and creatinine are characteristically higher in urine compared with any other body fluid; hence, they provide a unique chemical means to specifically identify a fluid as urine.

Solute concentration in urine (i.e., the amount of solutes excreted in a volume of water) is clinically useful in assessing the renal tubular ability to process the plasma ultrafiltrate.

Urine concentration is commonly determined by osmolality or by specific gravity. The measurement principles for these determinations differ. Osmolality, denoted mOsm/kg, measures the number of solute particles per kilogram of solvent. When using freezing-point osmolality, all solutes in the urine are detected and equally contribute to the osmolality result. Because concentration of the urine takes place passively in the collecting ducts as they penetrate deep in the inner renal medulla, the maximum osmolality value possible is dictated by the osmolality of the surrounding interstitial tissue, i.e., 1400 mOsm/kg $H_2O$. A random urine osmolality can range from 50 mOsm/kg $H_2O$ to 1400 mOsm/kg $H_2O$, but more typically resides within 300 to 900 mOsm/kg $H_2O$.

An alternate measurement of urine concentration is specific gravity, which relates the density of urine to that of an equal volume of pure water. The density of a solution is dependent on both solute number and solute weight; hence, all solutes do not contribute equally to this measurement. High-molecular-weight solutes (e.g., glucose, proteins, radiographic contrast media) when present in urine produce a higher specific gravity result than a similar urine containing only typical urine solutes (e.g., urea, creatinine, electrolytes). Also, the presence of glucose, proteins, or radiographic contrast media does not reflect the renal ability to concentrate the urine. Rather, these high-molecular-weight solutes can interfere when trying to evaluate this tubular function. For example, take a urine specimen and divide it into 2 samples, A and B. To sample B, add glucose in an amount typically observed in the urine of diabetic individuals. Determine the osmolality and specific gravity of urine A and B. The osmolality of the samples will be equivalent because the number of glucose molecules is insignificant compared to the total solute number, whereas the specific gravity results will differ, with B producing a higher result because glucose has a high molecular weight.

The effects of high-molecular-weight solutes on specific gravity results differ depending on the method used. Some specific gravity methods measure urine density directly (e.g., urinometer, falling drop, harmonic oscillation densitometry), others indirectly (e.g., refractometry, reagent strip). Of these specific gravity measurements, glucose or proteins do not affect the indirect reagent strip method. Hence, urine specific gravity results using the reagent strip method accurately reflect the renal tubular ability to concentrate the urine, regardless of the presence of glucose or protein.

Because urine can never be as pure as water, a specific gravity of 1.000 is physiologically impossible. In healthy individuals, specific gravity values range from 1.002 to 1.035. Similar to the discussion of osmolality, the maximum value possible for urine specific gravity is 1.035, the same specific gravity as that of the surrounding interstitium deep in the inner medulla where concentration of the urine occurs.

In summary, the initial ultrafiltrate in Bowman's space resembles the composition of the plasma with the exclusion of solutes the size of albumin or larger. At first glance this may not seem possible; however, the number of particles that are excluded from the initial ultrafiltrate (proteins and other high-molecular-weight solutes) is insignificant compared to the large number of small solutes that are present (urea, chloride, sodium, potassium). Hence, the concentration of the initial ultrafiltrate is identical to that of the blood plasma: osmolality ~290 mOsm/kg, specific gravity ~1.010. As the filtrate passes through the tubular segments of the nephron, solutes and water are actively or passively reabsorbed and secreted. If this function is lost, as in end-stage renal disease, then the concentration of the urine will be the same as that of the plasma and initial ultrafiltrate, i.e., 1.010. This condition is called **isosthenuria.**

Remember that the kidney's task is to eliminate any solutes and water not needed by the body, and to retain those substances (including water) that are needed or recognized as beneficial. To accomplish this task, a variety of tubular transport mechanisms determine the final solute concentration of the urine. Also keep in mind that the solute composition of the final urine can vary substantially from that of the initial ultrafiltrate.

## Determination of Urine Composition

Three processes that take place in the nephrons are responsible for the composition of the urine excreted. They are glomerular **filtration,** tubular **reabsorption,** and tubular **secretion.** Filtration can be defined as the process of passing a solution through a filter to separate small molecules or solutes from larger ones. In the kidney, the GFB of the glomeruli act as fil-

ters, and the solution undergoing solute separation is the blood plasma. As previously discussed, hydrostatic pressure from renal blood flow drives the filtration process and an ultrafiltrate collects in Bowman's space. In healthy subjects, the solutes that pass the GFB must fulfill strict stoichiometric, molecular charge, and molecular weight criteria (i.e., molecular radius less than 4 nm, neutral or positive charge, and molecular weight less than ~70,000 daltons). Once past the GFB, the same hydrostatic pressure drives the filtrate into the tubular segments of the nephrons for further processing by the tubular transport mechanisms of reabsorption and secretion.

The tubular transport mechanisms responsible for both solute reabsorption and secretion are identical. It is only the direction of solute movement that differs. Reabsorption refers to the movement of solutes from the tubular lumen fluid into the renal interstitium or bloodstream. In contrast, secretion denotes solute movement from the blood plasma or interstitium into the tubular lumen fluid for excretion in the urine. Secretion enables the elimination of solutes that cannot pass a healthy GFB due to their size or molecular charge, such as numerous substances bound to albumin. It also provides a mechanism to selectively increase the elimination of a solute that readily passes the GFB, such as creatinine. For example, in an attempt to reduce the high plasma creatinine concentration of individuals suffering with renal failure, the nephrons will actually increase the amount of creatinine secreted by the tubules.

The locations in the nephron where reabsorption and secretion occur, as well as the solutes involved, varies (Table 19–1).

TABLE  19–1

**The Tubular Location and Transport Process Used in the Reabsorption and Secretion of Selected Solutes**

|  | PROXIMAL TUBULE | LOOP OF HENLE | DISTAL CONVOLUTED TUBULE | COLLECTING TUBULE |
|---|---|---|---|---|
| Reabsorption | | | | |
| ‡Active | $Na^+$, $HCO_3^-$, glucose, amino acids, proteins, $PO_4$, $SO_4$, $Mg^{++}$, $Ca^{++}$, uric acid | $Na^+$, $Cl-$ (thick ascending limb) | *$Na^+$, $Cl^-$, $SO_4$, uric acid | *$Na^+$ (in cortex) |
| §Passive | $H_2O$, $Cl^-$, $K^+$, urea | $H_2O$, urea (thin descending limb) $Na^+$, $Cl^-$, urea (thin ascending limb) Urea (thick ascending limb) | — | †$H_2O$, $Cl^-$ (in cortex) $H_2O$, urea (in medulla) |
| Secretion | $H^+$, $K^+$, $NH_3$, organic anions and cations | Urea | $H^+$, $NH_3$, $K^+$ | $H^+$, $NH_3$, $K^+$ |

*Sodium reabsorption under aldosterone control.

†Water reabsorption under arginine vasopressin (ADH) control.

‡Active transport processes include primary active transport and secondary active transport.

§Passive transport processes include simple diffusion and facilitated diffusion.

Glomerular filtration together with subsequent processing of the filtrate by selective reabsorption and secretion determine the ultimate composition of the final urine.

## Tubular Transport Mechanisms

### ACTIVE AND PASSIVE TRANSPORT

Numerous studies have been and continue to be performed to elucidate the intricate, diverse, and interrelated transport mechanisms that select and regulate solutes and water in the nephron. The depth and breadth of a thorough discourse is beyond the scope of this text. The following discussion focuses on the principal solutes and primary mechanisms utilized by the tubules.

To discuss tubular transport mechanisms, a basic understanding of solute movement across cell membranes is required. Solute transport can occur by either an active or passive process. **Active transport** occurs against a gradient (uphill), requires energy, and always uses a carrier protein (i.e., specialized proteins of the cell membrane) to move solutes across the cell membrane. Carrier proteins bind specific solutes or classes of solutes and they undergo a conformational change when transporting the solute across the membrane. Because active

transport requires energy and uses carrier proteins, this process is highly specific, competitive, and limited in capacity. In contrast, **passive transport** or diffusion always occurs along a gradient (downhill), requires no energy, and uses either carrier proteins or channel proteins to cross the cell membrane (Figure 19–8). When channel proteins are involved, they assemble to form hydrophilic pores or ion channels through the membrane lipid bilayer that selectively allows the passage of specific ions. In contrast to carrier proteins, solutes do not bind to the channel proteins nor do these proteins undergo a conformational change during ion transport.

Many solute gradients encountered in the nephron are due to concentration differences across a membrane. However, when charged solutes are involved, both a concentration and an electrical gradient can exist. In these cases, the driving force of a charged solute's transport is a combination of both gradients, called an *electrochemical gradient*.

Active transport mechanisms used by the tubular epithelium include primary active transport and secondary active transport. In *primary* active transport, the movement of a solute is coupled directly to an energy (i.e., adenosine triphosphate [ATP])-producing reaction. The classic example of this type of transport is the *sodium pump*, a term used to describe the movement of sodium ions ($Na^+$) out of a cell with the

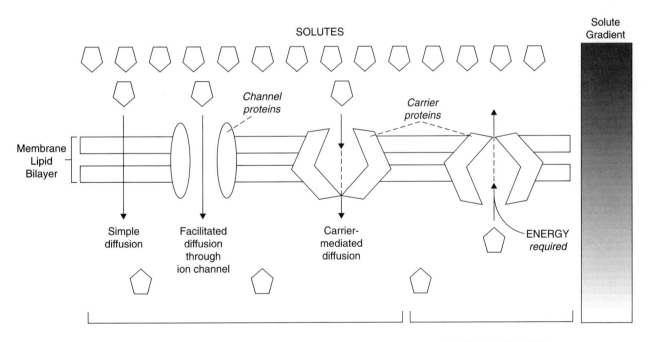

**FIGURE 19-8**

A schematic of active and passive transport mechanisms. Passive transport occurs along a solute gradient (downhill), whereas active transport occurs against a solute gradient (uphill). For active transport, membrane proteins called *carrier* proteins are required. During passive mediated transport, either carrier proteins or channel proteins are used. In contrast, passive transport by simple diffusion does not utilize membrane proteins.

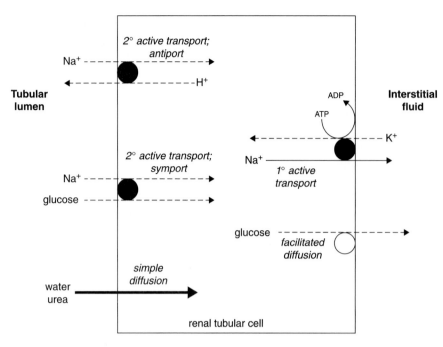

**FIGURE   19-9**

Selected transport mechanisms of renal tubular epithelium. The filled circles indicate
an active transport process, open circles indicate a passive transport process, and an
arrow indicates simple diffusion.

concomitant cellular uptake of potassium ions ($K^+$) (Figure
19–9). The enzyme $Na^+$-$K^+$-ATPase, localized in the basolateral membrane of renal tubular cells, is required to run the sodium pump. Fuel for this pump is the hydrolysis of ATP. Typically, for every ATP molecule hydrolyzed, 3 sodium ions are
driven out of the cell and 2 potassium ions are taken up.[5] This
pump maintains a low intracellular sodium concentration that
in turn establishes a steep sodium gradient; in doing so, this
concentration gradient provides the energy for the sodium-
coupled transport of other solutes (e.g., sodium–glucose,
sodium–amino acid, sodium–hydrogen, sodium–calcium).

*Secondary* active transport involves two solutes; one moving against an electrochemical gradient while the other is moving along an electrochemical gradient. Sodium–glucose coupled transport by renal epithelium is one example of secondary
active transport (Figure 19–9). The energy needed for the
transport of glucose into the cell, against a concentration gradient, is supplied by sodium ions moving down its electrochemical gradient and into the cell. When the transport of
both solutes is in the same direction, it is called *symport*, such
as sodium–glucose and sodium–amino acid transport in the
proximal convoluted tubule (Figure 19–9).

Because the membrane carriers have a high degree of
solute specificity and are limited in number, movement of
solutes by this process can be saturated. In other words, there
is a maximum reabsorptive capacity ($T_m$) for carrier-mediated
solutes. For example, a typical $T_m$ for glucose, which varies

with gender and body surface area, is 350 mg/minute. This
means that the tubules are capable of reabsorbing 350 mg of
glucose from the filtrate in the tubular lumen each minute. If
400 mg of glucose is presented to the tubules each minute, the
additional 50 mg of glucose cannot be reabsorbed and will appear in the final urine.

When transport of 2 solutes is in opposite directions, it
is called *antiport* (or counterport), such as sodium–hydrogen,
and sodium–calcium transport. As previously stated, it is the
steep sodium gradient created by the sodium pump that provides the energy or fuels the active transport of a variety of
solutes into the renal tubular epithelium.

Passive transport used throughout the nephron includes
simple diffusion and facilitated diffusion (Figure 19–8, 19–9),
both of which do not require an expenditure of energy to be
accomplished. Simple diffusion refers to solute movement
along a concentration gradient and is dependent on, or driven
solely by, the gradient itself. In contrast, facilitated or carrier-
mediated diffusion utilizes membrane transport proteins to
move solutes along a gradient. Because carrier proteins are required, it also is a competitive and capacity-limited process.

Another form of facilitated diffusion is the movement of
ions through specialized membrane pathways called ion channels (Figure 19–8). These channels are formed by membrane
proteins orienting in such a manner as to form pores through
which predominantly inorganic ions (e.g., $Na^+$, $K^+$, $Cl^-$) can
move down their electrochemical gradient and into the cell.

Although the transport through these channels is a passive process, when these channels open, ion movement is rapid, highly selective, and tightly regulated.

## TUBULAR FUNCTIONS: REABSORPTION AND SECRETION

Solute reabsorption occurs throughout the nephron; however, the proximal convoluted tubule (PCT) is the primary site for this process (Table 19–1). Electrolytes aside, essentially all other solutes that the body strives to conserve are reabsorbed in this segment (glucose, proteins, amino acids). To osmotically balance the filtrate that remains in the tubular lumen, water is also passively reabsorbed. The end result is that approximately 65% of the ultrafiltrate solutes are reabsorbed in the PCT segment by either an active or passive process. In healthy individuals, the remaining 35% are predominantly ionic solutes, urea, and water.

The PCT epithelium is characteristically and uniquely equipped to perform its function. The cells are endowed with well-developed apical brush borders and lateral interdigitations that provide a large surface area for carrier proteins and solute transport processes. In addition, these cells have numerous large mitochondria to provide the energy needed for the predominantly active transport of solutes into the cells. The PCT cells are also endowed with numerous lysosomes for the digestion and processing of reabsorbed solutes.

The filtrate that enters the loop of Henle has the same osmolality (i.e., number of particles per kilogram of water) as the initial ultrafiltrate despite the significant change in solute composition. In this segment, reabsorption differs dramatically in the descending and ascending limbs. In the descending limb, the simple epithelium is highly permeable to water, a passive reabsorptive process driven by the high osmolality or hypertonicity of the renal medulla. Here, however, the permeability to sodium and chloride is essentially nonexistent. In contrast, the epithelium of the ascending limb is highly permeable to sodium and chloride but not to water. Passive reabsorption and secretion of urea also occurs in the loop of Henle. The net result is that the lumen fluid leaving the loop of Henle is slightly hypoosmotic, i.e., more solute reabsorption has occurred compared to water reabsorption in this segment.

The selective reabsorptive of sodium, chloride and water that occurs in the loops of Henle, in concert with similar processes in the collecting tubules, establishes a **countercurrent multiplier mechanism.** This mechanism, along with the **urea cycle,** establishes and maintains the hypertonicity of the renal medulla, which is ultimately responsible for the concentration of the final urine.

The cells of the distal convoluted tubule (DCT) actively reabsorb solutes, particularly sodium and chloride. Their basolateral borders are rich in $Na^+$-$K^+$-ATPase and they have numerous mitochondria to provide the energy needed for these and other active transport processes. Here, the reabsorption of sodium, against a steep electrochemical gradient, is under the control of the hormone aldosterone. The DCT also plays a role in adding solutes to or exchanging solutes with the lumen

fluid by secretion. Predominantly, hydrogen ions, potassium ions, and ammonia are secreted by the DCT. Note that no water exchange occurs in the DCT; only the solute composition of the lumen fluid is altered.

The lumen fluid that reaches the final segment of the nephron, the collecting tubule (CT) or collecting duct, is reduced significantly in volume; however, it has essentially the same osmolality (i.e., number of particles per kilogram of water) as the initial ultrafiltrate. This highlights the role of the CT in determining the concentration of the final urine as the fluid is processed here. If the body needs water, the CT passively reabsorbs it, under the control of antidiuretic hormone (ADH). In which case, the final urine is more concentrated than the initial ultrafiltrate (i.e., specific gravity > 1.010; osmolality > 290 mOsm/kg). Conversely, if the body needs to eliminate excess water, then water is not reabsorbed and the final urine is more dilute than the initial ultrafiltrate (i.e., specific gravity < 1.010; osmolality < 290 mOsm/kg).

In summary, as the ultrafiltrate of plasma passes through the nephron segments, the total fluid volume is dramatically reduced and the solute composition is significantly altered based on the body's homeostatic needs.

## COUNTERCURRENT MECHANISMS AND UREA CYCLE

The countercurrent multiplier mechanisms and the urea cycle are crucial to the proper functioning of the nephron. Together, these systems are responsible for generating and maintaining the hypertonicity of the renal medulla, the only tissue in the body that is hypertonic with respect to the blood plasma. It is this hypertonicity which produces a massive osmotic force that drives the passive reabsorption of water throughout the nephron. Note that water is never secreted by the nephron; rather, it is passively reabsorbed and only when needed by the body. Hence, the ability to concentrate the urine is dependent on a hypertonic renal medulla.

There are two countercurrent multiplier mechanisms in the renal medulla, one involves the active transport of solutes in the loops of Henle, the other is a passive solute exchange process that occurs in the vasa recta, the capillary network deep in the renal medulla and adjacent to the loops of Henle. Both the loops of Henle and the vasa recta are uniquely configured to perform this solute exchange process. They consist of parallel limbs in close proximity to each other and the lumen fluid in each limb is flowing in opposite directions; hence the name *countercurrent* (Figure 19–10). As the filtrate passes through the descending limb of the loop of Henle, water is passively reabsorbed concentrating the solutes of the lumen fluid, i.e., increasing the fluid osmolality. Later, as the filtrate passes through the ascending limb, water is retained in the lumen while sodium and chloride are actively reabsorbed, resulting in the progressively decreasing osmolality of the lumen fluid. Note that the osmolality of the lumen fluid leaving the ascending limb is actually lower than it was when it entered the descending limb, i.e., the lumen fluid is not concentrated by passage through the loops of Henle. The purpose of this

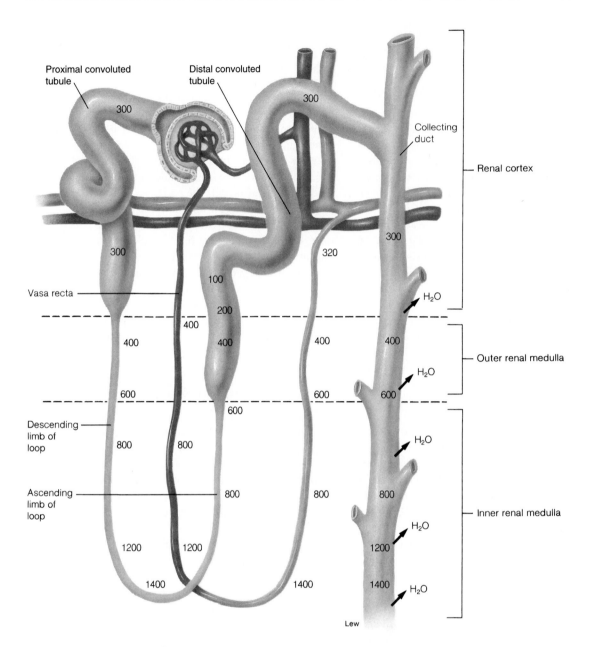

**FIGURE 19-10**

An illustration of the countercurrent multiplier mechanism in the loop of Henle and the countercurrent exchange mechanism in the vasa recta. The osmolality of the lumen fluid in various portions of the nephron and the gradient osmolality of the interstitium are also provided. Note that the osmolality of the final urine can never exceed that of the renal interstitium, i.e., 1400 mOsm/kg $H_2O$. (From Van De Graaff KM, Fox IF (eds.): *Concepts of Human Anatomy & Physiology.* 5th ed. Boston, WCB/McGraw-Hill, 1999.)

selective processing by each limb is to establish and maintain a gradient of hypertonicity in the medullary interstitium; hence the name *countercurrent multiplier mechanism.* The hypertonicity of the medulla is stratified with the osmolality progressively increasing to a maximum of approximately 1400 mOsm/kg $H_2O$ in the deepest regions of the medulla. It is this gradient hypertonicity of the medullary interstitium

that drives the passive reabsorption of water from the lumen fluid to produce a "final" urine that can vary in osmolality from 50 to 1400 mOsm/kg $H_2O$, depending on the body's state of hydration.

This same gradient of hypertonicity drives solute uptake into the blood in the vasa recta. As blood flows down the vasa recta into the medulla, sodium, chloride, urea, and water *passively* diffuse into the capillary from the interstitial fluid. The osmolality in the vessel rises and blood flow slows. Once the blood passes the nadir of the loop, solutes diffuse back into the interstitium and flow increases. Figure 19–10 depicts the medullary gradient and the processing of solutes and water that occurs throughout the loops of Henle and the vasa recta.

The urea cycle refers to the passive reabsorption and secretion of urea in the nephron and vasa recta. This cycle is passive, driven by a concentration gradient between the lumen fluid and the interstitium. Urea is passively reabsorbed from the tubular lumen fluid in the proximal convoluted tubule, the loop of Henle, and the collecting tubules (Table 19–1). It is cycled back into the tubular lumen (secreted) from the interstitium at the loops of Henle located deep in the renal medulla. At the same time, urea reenters the bloodstream through a similar passive process in the vasa recta (Figure 19–10). This cycling of urea in the tubules and the vasa recta establishes a urea concentration gradient throughout the renal medulla that ultimately serves to determine the urea concentration of the final urine. In other words, urea is passively reabsorbed from the lumen fluid in the last segment of the nephron, the collecting tubule, along an established urea concentration gradient. The urea concentration of the final urine will be determined by the equilibrium that is attained as the fluid passes through the CT. Note that it can attain but not exceed the urea concentration of the renal medulla. Because urea cycling is passive, the rate of fluid flow through the tubules directly affects the amount of urea that is cycled, i.e., the amount reabsorbed and secreted. Slow fluid flow through the nephrons results in a larger amount of urea reabsorbed. The urea cycle accounts for approximately 50% of the solutes that maintain the hypertonic renal medulla, whereas the countercurrent multiplier mechanisms account for the remaining 50% of solutes concentrated here.

## Acid-Base Homeostasis

The urinary system plays an integral role in regulating water, electrolytes, and the elimination of waste products to maintain an environment conducive for cell viability, i.e., normal body homeostasis. In concert with the skin and lungs, the kidneys actively and selectively eliminate solutes and excess water.

Renal elimination of hydrogen ion ($H^+$) is critical for maintaining a normal blood pH (pH 7.35 to 7.45). Renal tubular cells throughout the nephron (Table 19–1) eliminate excess $H^+$ by three secretory mechanisms. The mechanisms for $H^+$ elimination in the urine include: Loss in exchange for bicarbonate ($HCO_3^-$) ions, in the form of monobasic phosphates, and in the form of ammonium ions ($NH_4^+$).

In the proximal tubule, $H^+$ secretion is linked to sodium reabsorption and to the recovery of bicarbonate ($HCO_3^-$) (Figure 19–11). Here, as $H^+$ flow out of the renal tubular cells down a concentration gradient and into the tubular lumen, sodium ions are reabsorbed. In the ultrafiltrate, the $H^+$ combine with bicarbonate ions to form carbonic acid, which is rap-

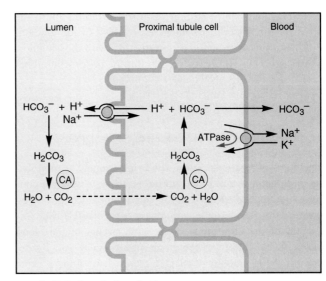

**FIGURE 19-11**

General schematic of bicarbonate ($HCO_3^-$) reabsorption. Begin by looking at the $H^+$ being secreted by countertransport with sodium (sodium is moving into the, $H^+$ is moving out of the cell). The $H_2CO_3$ formed in the tubular lumen is rapidly broken down by carbonic anhydrase (CA) present in the luminal membrane. The resultant $CO_2$ is reabsorbed to regenerate $HCO_3^-$ that returns to the bloodstream, while the $H_2O$ produced is either excreted in the final urine or passively reabsorbed. Note the net result is the reabsorption or recovery of bicarbonate while secreting or eliminating $H^+$. (From Van De Graaff KM, Fox IF (eds.): *Concepts of Human Anatomy & Physiology.* 5th ed. Boston, WCB/McGraw-Hill, 1999.)

idly converted to carbon dioxide and water due to the high concentration of carbonic anhydrase in the proximal tubular brush border and luminal membranes. In tubular lumen:

$$H^+ \text{ (secreted)} + HCO_3^- \text{ (in ultrafiltrate)} \longrightarrow$$

$$H_2CO_3 \xrightarrow{\text{carbonic anhydrase}} CO_2 + H_2O$$

The carbon dioxide and water produced by this reaction is reabsorbed into the renal cells, where the reaction is reversed to once again form $H^+$ and bicarbonate. The intracellular bicarbonate is returned to the peritubular circulation and the $H^+$ ions are once again available for secretion in exchange for sodium ions. In renal cell:

$$CO_2 + H_2O \rightarrow H_2CO_3 \xrightarrow{\text{carbonic anhydrase}}$$

$$H^+ \text{ (available for secretion)} + HCO_3^- \text{ (to blood)}$$

Note that the secretion of $H^+$ in the proximal tubule is a passive process dependent on an electrochemical gradient; hence, if the gradient is disrupted and reversed, the flow of $H^+$ will be reversed, e.g., $H^+$ will flow from the ultrafiltrate into the proximal tubular cells. Maintenance of this $H^+$ ion gradient is achieved by the reaction of secreted $H^+$ with dibasic phosphates (e.g., $Na_2HPO_4$) in the ultrafiltrate to form monobasic phosphates (e.g., $NaH_2PO_4$).

$$Na_2HPO_4 \text{ (filtered)} \rightarrow Na^+ + NaHPO_4^-$$

$$NaHPO_4^- + H^+ \text{ (secreted)} \rightarrow NaH_2PO_4$$

This form of hydrogen ion in the urine, namely as monobasic phosphates, is also called **titratable acids** because the concentration of acid excreted in this form can be determined by titrating the urine sample with a base (e.g., NaOH). The initial pH of the ultrafiltrate is the same as that of the blood plasma being filtered at the glomerulus, namely 7.4. By determining the amount of NaOH required to titrate a urine sample to pH 7.4, the amount of titratable acids secreted is determined. Note that hydrogen ions combined to other solutes (e.g., ammonia) are not measured, only those bound to form monobasic phosphates, i.e., titratable acids.

The third mechanism for $H^+$ elimination requires the secretion of ammonia by renal tubular epithelial cells. This mechanism predominates in the distal convoluted tubules. Ammonia is produced in the renal cells by the action of the enzyme glutaminase on glutamine which is supplied by the plasma. Once formed, ammonia is secreted into the tubular lumen, where it readily combines with free $H^+$ to form ammonium ions ($NH_4^+$).

$$NH_3 \text{ (secreted)} + H^+ \text{ (secreted)} \rightarrow NH_4^+ \text{ (in ultrafiltrate)}$$

$$NH_4^+ + Cl^- \rightarrow NH_4Cl \text{ (excreted)}$$

Because ammonium ions are charged molecules, they cannot diffuse across cell membranes and are retained in the lumen fluid for excretion. In the ultrafiltrate, they combine with a variety of anions to form ammonium salts (e.g., ammonium chloride, ammonium sulfate).

In summary, the kidney regulates the acid-base balance or pH of the body through the elimination $H^+$ in the form of titratable acids and ammonium salts. The hydrogen ions contained in these compounds result from $H^+$ secretion by one of three renal mechanisms. In clinical situations where maximal acid elimination is required (e.g., acidosis), renal tubular cells increase production and secretion of ammonia to compensate. Because this renal process of compensation requires several days to increase ammonia formation, the blood buffers and the respiratory system provide the initial response to acid-base imbalances.

## Hormones and the Kidney

The relationship between the kidney and some hormones is well known and documented, but its involvement with other hormones is only beginning to be elucidated. The kidney plays a variety of important roles that involve hormones. First, it is a site of hormone production. The hormones produced by the kidney may act locally (e.g., renin-angiotensin system) or target other organ systems (e.g., erythropoietin). In this regard, when renal function is compromised due to disease, the function of other organs can also be affected. Second, the kidney is a target for hormone action. Renal hormones (e.g., renin-angiotensin system, prostaglandins), as well as nonrenal hormones (e.g., arginine vasopressin, parathyroid hormone), modulate kidney function. Third, the kidney is a major site for the inactivation and elimination of hormones. If, owing to disease, the kidney is unable to inactivate or remove a hormone from the circulation, the effect of that hormone can be prolonged. For example, a diabetic individual with uremia requires less insulin because their insulin remains in the circulation longer.

Understanding the interactive and diverse roles of the kidney and hormones continues to evolve as technological advances (e.g., molecular biology) enable further elucidation of these relationships. An in-depth discussion of all identified renal hormones and nonrenal hormones that induce major renal actions is beyond the scope of this text. In this chapter, the discussion is limited to the renin-angiotensin system and to two nonrenal hormones that have major renal effects: aldosterone and arginine vasopressin.

## RENIN-ANGIOTENSIN SYSTEM AND ALDOSTERONE

The **renin-angiotensin system** plays an integral role in the regulation of water and electrolyte balance as well as the regulation of arterial blood pressure. Renin, an enzyme, is predominantly produced and stored in the granular cells of the afferent arterioles located near the JGA of each nephron (Figure 19–6). As previously discussed, the JGA includes portions of the afferent and efferent arteriole, the extraglomerular mesangium and specialized cells of the distal tubule called the *macula densa* that are capable of sensing chloride levels in the tubular lumen fluid.[6]

Renin secretion is modulated by numerous factors; the most important include blood pressure, the concentration of sodium chloride (NaCl) in the tubular lumen fluid, the sympathetic nervous system, and circulating angiotensin II. The effect on renin secretion varies with the stimuli. The release of renin from granular cells is inversely related to renal perfusion pressure and to tubular lumen concentrations of NaCl. In other words, a decrease in blood pressure or a decrease in NaCl in the tubular lumen, as sensed by the macula densa, will stimulate renin secretion. Conversely, circulating angiotensin II inhibits renin secretion, whereas, stimulation of sympathetic nerve endings in the JGA directly enhances renin secretion.

Once renin release is initiated, a cascade of events occurs. Angiotensinogen, a glycoprotein produced in the liver is cleaved by renin to form angiotensin I. Angiotensin I, biologically inactive, is converted to angiotensin II by converting enzyme located in vascular endothelium, particularly in the lung. Angiotensin II is biologically active, stimulating vasoconstriction and adrenal cortical secretion of the hormone **aldosterone.** The resultant vasoconstriction increases arterial and glomerular blood pressure, and aldosterone increases the reabsorption of sodium directly and chloride indirectly by the distal and cortical collecting tubules. Similarly, water is also passively reabsorbed. The net result is that the blood volume expands causing an increase in blood pressure. Renin secretion dissipates as the initiating stimuli are resolved and from the negative feedback effect of angiotensin II.

## ARGININE VASOPRESSIN

The major function of **arginine vasopressin** (AVP), also known as antidiuretic hormone (ADH), is the regulation of water balance in the body. AVP, made in the hypothalamus, is stored in the posterior pituitary. It is released from the posterior pituitary in response to either an increase in plasma osmolality or a decrease in blood volume (hypovolemia). For example, when the blood volume decreases, the blood pressure decreases and vascular baroreceptors stimulate the pituitary release of AVP into the bloodstream. As the plasma AVP increases, the permeability of the collecting tubules epithelium changes to enhance reabsorption of water (by osmosis) from the tubular lumen into the renal interstitium. Because of the hypertonicity of the renal medulla, a large osmotic force drives the passive reabsorption of water. As the blood pressure is resolved, signaling from the vascular baroreceptors diminishes and the stimulation for AVP release ceases.

A deficiency of AVP, or the lack of renal response to AVP, causes the clinical disorder termed *diabetes insipidus* (DI). This condition is characterized by the excretion of large volumes of urine (polyuria) with a low osmolality and low specific gravity. Additional discussion of this condition is presented in Chapter 26.

In addition to its antidiuretic effect, AVP also acts as a potent vasoconstrictor by 2 mechanisms. First, it directly induces vascular smooth muscle contraction causing the afferent and efferent arterioles, as well as the mesangial cells in the glomerulus, to constrict. Second, AVP stimulates local production of prostaglandins, potent vasoactive compounds. Together, these mechanisms increase vascular resistance in the glomerulus resulting in the maintenance of optimal renal perfusion and a constant GFR.

## SUMMARY

The structural design of the kidney, as well as its numerous and specialized cell types, enables it to perform many diverse and dynamic functions to maintain normal body homeostasis. The functional unit of the kidney, the nephron, can be divided into 5 principal segments: the glomerulus, the proximal tubule, the loop of Henle, the distal tubule, and the collecting tubules. Together with its surrounding vasculature, the nephrons are responsible for the dynamic reabsorption and secretion processes that conserve vital substances while simultaneously eliminating waste and toxic substances.

Systemic blood pressure drives the initial plasma filtration process in the renal glomeruli as well as fluid movement throughout the nephron segments. Hence, it is a crucial component for the proper functioning of the kidney. At the level of the nephrons, the afferent and efferent arterioles actually fine-tune the glomerular blood flow by dilation or constriction to maintain a constant glomerular filtration rate. This regulation of renal vascular resistance results from the interaction of a variety of neural and hormonal processes.

The formation of urine is required to eliminate waste products of metabolism. These substances are eliminated in the volume of water necessary for the amount of solutes involved as well as any additional water the body does not need. Note that the body is unable to store water. Hence, water intake (i.e. hydration) directly affects the solute concentration and volume of the urine excreted. The urine concentration (of solutes) is expressed in terms of osmolality and specific gravity measurements.

Active and passive transport processes are responsible for the reabsorption and secretion of solutes by the renal tubular epithelial cells. The cellular morphology of the epithelium in each nephron segment is uniquely designed to perform its functions. Hormones, particularly aldosterone and arginine vasopressin, also play an important role in the tubular reabsorption and secretion of selective solutes and water.

Another crucial component for the proper functioning of the nephron is the maintenance of the hypertonicity of the renal medulla. This is achieved through the countercurrent multiplier mechanisms and the urea cycle.

Maintenance of normal body homeostasis, particularly acid-base balance, is achieved through the renal elimination of acid, i.e., hydrogen ions. Three secretory mechanisms are responsible: The loss of hydrogen ions in exchange for bicarbonate ions, the excretion of hydrogen ions as monobasic phosphates (i.e., titratable acids), and the excretion of hydrogen ions as ammonium salts. The initial response to acid-base changes in the body is performed by blood buffers and the respiratory system. However, the renal mechanisms, which take several days to achieve maximal response, are longer lasting and more effective in regulating acid-base elimination.

The kidney performs a variety of functions related to hormones. It produces hormones, is a target for hormone action, and is a major site for hormonal inactivation and elimination. Some hormones produced by the kidney act locally (e.g., renin-angiotensin system), and others target distant organ systems (e.g., erythropoietin). Similarly, some hormones produced elsewhere in the body (e.g., aldosterone, arginine vasopressin) have their major effect on renal processes.

## REFERENCES

1. Hebert SC, Kriz W: Structural-functional relationships in the kidney. In Schrier R, Gottschalk CW (eds.): *Diseases of the Kidney.* 5th ed. Boston, Little, Brown, 1993, p 3.
2. Koushanpour E, Kriz W: *Renal Physiology.* New York, Springer-Verlag, 1986.
3. Arendshorst WJ, Navar LG: Renal circulation and glomerular hemodynamics. In Schrier R, Gottschalk CW (eds.): *Diseases of the Kidney.* 5th ed. Boston, Little, Brown, 1993, p 65.
4. Bourgoignie, JJ, Jacob, AI, et al: Water, electrolytes, and acid-base balance in chronic renal failure. Semin Nephrol 1:2, 91–111, 1981.
5. Vander AJ, Sherman JH, Luciano DS: *Human Physiology: The Mechanisms of Body Function.* New York, McGraw-Hill, 1990.
6. Rabkin R, Dahl DC: Hormones and the kidney. In Schrier R, Gottschalk CW (eds.): *Diseases of the Kidney.* 5th ed. Boston, Little, Brown, 1993, p 303.

## BIBLIOGRAPHY

Vander AJ, Sherman JH, Luciano DS: *Human Physiology: The Mechanisms of Body Function.* New York, McGraw-Hill, 1990.

Brunzel NA: *Fundamentals of Urine and Body Fluid Analysis.* Philadelphia, WB Saunders, 1994.

Cotran RS, Kumar V, Robbins SL: *Robbins Pathological Basis of Disease.* 6th ed. Philadelphia, WB Saunders, 1999.

Schrier R, Gottschalk CW (eds.): *Diseases of the Kidney.* 5th ed. Boston, Little, Brown, 1993.

# C H A P T E R   2 0

# Renal Function: Nonprotein Nitrogen Compounds, Function Tests, and Renal Disease

*Nancy A. Brunzel*

## NONPROTEIN NITROGEN COMPOUNDS

The term *nonprotein nitrogen* (NPN) refers to nitrogen-containing compounds that are not proteins. In the early part of the 20th century, this name was coined to describe those nitrogen-containing compounds that remained in a filtrate after the proteins had been removed by precipitation. At this time, the determination of the total NPN in plasma and other body fluids was recognized as a valuable clinical tool. Analysis was performed using the Kjeldahl method, an accurate although technically challenging and labor-intensive procedure. Currently, the concentration of individual NPN compounds is used to evaluate and monitor renal function as well as other clinical conditions. This is possible because of the development of accurate and precise technical methods for their specific analysis.

In plasma, urea (45%), amino acids (20%), uric acid (20%), creatinine (5%), creatine (1% to 2%), and ammonia (0.2%) account for the majority of NPN compounds. These compounds originate from protein and nucleic acid catabolism (Figure 20–1). When increased amounts of NPN compounds are present in the blood, the term *azotemia* is used. Because the kidney plays an essential role in the elimination of urea, creatinine, and uric acid from the body, causes for alterations in the plasma NPN concentration are often categorized as prerenal, renal, or postrenal in origin. Quantitative testing for the NPN compounds in plasma and urine plays an integral role in the assessment of a patient's renal status.

## Ammonia

Ammonia $NH_3$

### BIOCHEMISTRY

Ammonia arises from the deamination of amino acids. The majority of ammonia in the blood is derived from the gastrointestinal (GI) tract, where it is produced through the action of digestive and bacterial enzymes on proteins. Small amounts of ammonia are also generated during cellular catabolism of amino acids. Note that ammonia is highly toxic to cells; therefore, once in the bloodstream, it is rapidly and ef-

ficiently removed by liver hepatocytes. In the liver ammonia is used to synthesis glutamine, glutamate, and carbamyl phosphate. From carbamyl phosphate, pyrimidines for nucleic acids and urea are synthesized.

### CLINICAL SIGNIFICANCE

Unlike the other NPN compounds, the concentration of ammonia in the plasma is not a useful indicator of renal function. Therefore, ammonia levels are not used in the study of renal disease. However, they are valuable in evaluating liver function because the hepatocytes are the only cells that contain arginase, an enzyme required for the conversion of ammonia into urea.[1]

The most common causes for an increase in the plasma ammonia concentration, *hyperammonemia*, include severe liver disease and several inborn metabolic disorders of the urea cycle. Whether the liver disease is acute (e.g., viral hepatitis, Reye's syndrome) or chronic (e.g., cirrhosis), hepatocyte function is sufficiently impaired to cause an increase in the plasma ammonia concentration.

Central nervous system tissue is particularly susceptible to ammonia and increased levels are associated with encephalopathy. Hence, plasma ammonia determinations are a useful tool in the differential diagnosis of hepatic encephalopathy.

### ANALYTICAL PROCEDURES

Methodology is included in Chapter 16.

## Creatine and Creatinine

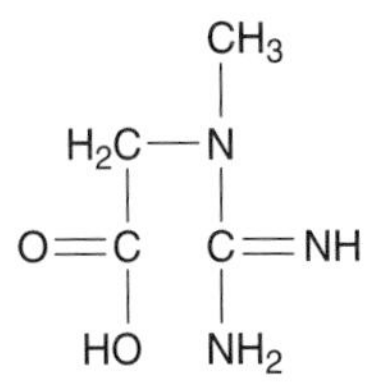

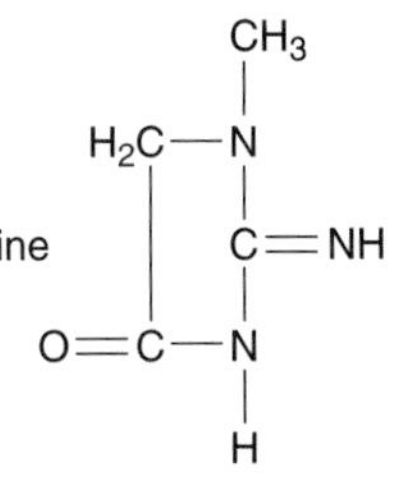

### BIOCHEMISTRY

Creatine is synthesized in the liver and pancreas from 3 amino acids: arginine, glycine, and methionine. Following synthesis, creatine diffuses into the bloodstream and is taken up by

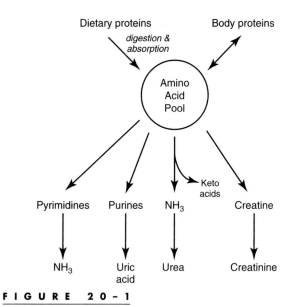

**FIGURE 20-1**

Summary of the relationship of the principal nonprotein nitrogenous compounds and protein metabolism

various tissues, particularly the muscles and brain. There, the enzyme, creatine kinase, catalyzes the conversion of creatine to phosphocreatine that acts as an energy reservoir. When the muscles are at rest, almost all the creatine is phosphorylated. During activity, phosphocreatine spontaneously and nonenzymatically converts to creatinine by cyclizing and splitting out inorganic phosphate ($P_i$). The interrelationship of creatine, creatinine, and phosphocreatine can be depicted as follows:

Creatinine, an anhydride, is a waste product of creatine and phosphocreatine. Conversion of both compounds is spontaneous and nonenzymatic. The amount of creatinine formed daily is proportional to an individual's lean muscle mass (approximately 2% of creatine converts per day) and it is released into the systemic circulation at essentially a constant rate. When the blood passes through the kidneys, both creatine and creatinine readily pass the glomerular filtration barrier and are essentially cleared from the plasma.

Urine contains significantly more creatinine than creatine because of the difference in renal handling. Creatine is reabsorbed by the proximal convoluted tubules, whereas creatinine is not reabsorbed anywhere in the nephron. In fact, a small additional amount of creatinine is also secreted by the tubules into the forming urine. Note that as the plasma creatinine concentration increases (e.g., due to renal disease), the amount of creatinine secreted by the tubules will also increase.

## CLINICAL SIGNIFICANCE

Creatine levels provide no diagnostic information regarding renal dysfunction. However, in conditions characterized by skeletal muscle necrosis or muscle atrophy (e.g., muscular dystrophy, poliomyelitis, trauma), both the plasma creatine and urine creatinine levels are increased. During these disease processes, the enzyme creatine kinase (CK; EC 2.7.3.2) is also released into the systemic circulation. Because plasma creatine assays are not readily available, these conditions are usually monitored using readily available plasma CK methods.

In contrast, creatinine determinations in both plasma and urine play a significant role as an index of renal function, specifically for monitoring the glomerular filtration rate (GFR). Several factors make creatinine an ideal compound for this task: (1) its plasma concentration is maintained at essentially a constant rate, (2) it is completely cleared from the plasma at the glomeruli, and (3) it is *not* reabsorbed by the tubules. Hence, all creatinine cleared is eliminated in the urine. Although a small additional amount of creatinine is secreted, it does not interfere or reduce the usefulness of creatinine determinations in assessing renal function.

Nonrenal factors such as degree of hydration and the level of protein catabolism usually do not affect plasma creatinine values. Although changes in the dietary protein content (i.e., increased ingestion of cooked meat) can abruptly increase creatinine excretion, this effect is rarely encountered and can be avoided by having an individual maintain a typical diet with a consistent protein content. With healthy individuals on a typical diet, plasma creatinine levels can vary 10% to 15% per day.[2]

Unfortunately, plasma creatinine levels alone lack sensitivity in detecting diminishing renal function. Fifty to sixty-seven percent of renal function must be lost before the plasma creatinine value reflects this loss. In some cases, an individual can still have a plasma creatinine value that resides in the normal reference interval. An example of this type of scenario follows:

A small, thin 50-year-old woman has a baseline glomerular filtration rate of 120 mL per minute and a plasma creatinine value of 0.5 mg/dL. Six months later, the patient's GFR decreases to 60 mL per minute, reflecting a 50% loss of function and her plasma creatinine rises to 1.0 mg/dL. The plasma creatinine of 1.0 mg/dL is still within a typical reference interval for this individual (0.8 to 1.2 mg/dL). From this isolated plasma creatinine value, it appears as though the renal function is normal, when in actuality the increase represents a 50% loss of renal function.

A more sensitive indicator of renal function using creatinine determinations is obtained by determining the GFR, initially and periodically thereafter. The GFR can be determined by performing a creatinine clearance test. Despite several drawbacks, the creatinine clearance test remains the most frequently employed clearance test to evaluate the GFR and is discussed later in this chapter.

## ANALYTICAL PROCEDURES

### Specimen Requirements

Creatinine determinations are routinely performed on plasma, serum, and urine. The creatinine method employed has a direct impact on specimen requirements. When using enzymatic methods, fluoride and ammonium heparin anticoagulants should not be used. When using the traditional and popular Jaffe reaction, hemolysis must be avoided due to interference from intracellular noncreatinine chromogens released from erythrocytes. Increased bilirubin concentrations cause a negative bias when the Jaffe reaction or the enzymatic methods are used.[3] Lipemia has been shown to cause a negative bias when using certain enzymatic methods.[3] Although a sporadic heavy protein intake can affect creatinine results, a fasting sample is not required. Plasma and serum samples are stable refrigerated (2 to 8°C) for approximately 1 week, or indefinitely when frozen.

Random and timed urine specimens are acceptable. Timed specimens, especially 24-hour specimens, must be refrigerated during collection or an appropriate preservative added to prevent loss of creatinine from bacterial degradation or conversion to creatine.

Occasionally, other fluid specimens (questionable urine specimens, amniotic fluid) are submitted for creatinine analysis. Although all body fluids contain creatinine, the high concentration in urine is unique. Hence, creatinine determinations provide a means to positively identify or rule out that a fluid is urine or a specimen that has been adulterated (diluted with an agent).

### Analytical Methods

Creatine methods are based on the measurement of creatinine. Because creatine is unstable at both an alkaline or acidic pH, it can be readily converted to creatinine. Determining the creatinine concentration difference, before and after acid condensation, provides the basis for plasma, serum, and urine cre-

atine determinations. The analytical methods employed are the same as those for creatinine quantitation.

Creatinine quantitation dates to 1886 when the Jaffe reaction was developed. In this method, the creatinine in a protein-free filtrate reacts with picrate ion in an alkaline medium to produce an orange-red complex that is measured spectrophotometrically. Note that the actual structure of the colored complex has yet to be definitively elucidated. The Jaffe reaction has been studied extensively, and the importance of reactant concentrations, timing, and the effects of various substances have been evaluated. Important aspects include picrate and hydroxyl ion concentrations, reaction temperature, reading interval when using kinetic methods, and the wavelength used to measure the reaction product. Each of these parameters affects the results obtained and influences whether a particular compound (protein, glucose, acetoacetate, pyruvate, bilirubin) interferes in the reaction. Despite numerous modifications and studies, no single method has proved superior for creatinine quantitation with regard to all testing aspects (specificity, precision, ease of performance, cost). Consequently, methods used to quantitate creatinine today include modifications of the Jaffe reaction, as well as a variety of enzymatic methods. Lente and Suit predict that enzymatic assays will become the methods of choice because they are less susceptible to interference from α-keto–acids and the cephalosporin antibiotics.[4]

### Reference Intervals

Because creatinine production is directly related to lean muscle mass, reference intervals vary with gender and age. In addition, the intervals are assay dependent with enzymatic assays generating lower reference intervals for a group than the Jaffe methods (Table 20–1). Transient increases in creatinine values can be observed following severe exercise or high protein ingestion.

## Urea

$$Urea \quad NH_2-\overset{\overset{\textstyle O}{\|}}{C}-NH_2$$

Historically, urea determinations were performed on whole blood using a testing method that indirectly measured the urea concentration by determining the amount of nitrogen present. Hence, the term *blood urea nitrogen* or BUN was coined. Today, analysis using whole blood is obsolete and the specimens of choice are plasma, serum, or urine. Despite this fact, the use of the acronym BUN persists, whereas the simplified term *urea nitrogen* or UN is more appropriate considering the actual specimen types analyzed.

### BIOCHEMISTRY

Urea, a relatively nontoxic compound, is the major nitrogen–containing waste product of protein catabolism and the

T A B L E   2 0 – 1

**Typical Reference Intervals for Creatinine Values**

| AGE/GENDER | JAFFE METHOD | ENZYMATIC METHODS |
| --- | --- | --- |
| **PLASMA/SERUM** | mg/dL (µmol/L) | mg/dL (µmol/L) |
| Children | 0.5–0.8 (44–27) | 0.2–0.6 (19–52) |
| Adult | | |
| Male | 0.8–1.3 (71–115) | 0.6–1.1 (53–97) |
| Female | 0.6–1.1 (53–97) | 0.4–0.8 (35–71) |
| **URINE, 24-H COLLECTION** | mg/d (mmol/d) | |
| Male | 500–2000 (7.1–17.7) | N/A |
| Female | 600–1800 (5.3–15.9) | N/A |

N/A = not applicable.

principal pathway used to excrete excess nitrogen. As amino acids, the building blocks of proteins, are catabolized within cells by oxidative deamination, ammonia and keto acids are produced. Ammonia is also absorbed from the GI tract. Ammonia, which is highly toxic to cells, is rapidly transferred to the bloodstream. As the blood passes through the liver, ammonia is removed from the plasma by the hepatocytes. Within the hepatocytes, a series of reactions occur to synthesize urea, i.e., 2 molecules of ammonia are joined to a carbon dioxide molecule. Subsequently, the urea enters the bloodstream and is excreted by the kidneys.

In the kidneys, urea readily passes the glomerular filtration barriers into the tubular lumens of the nephrons. Throughout the segments of the nephron, urea is passively reabsorbed. The amount of urea reabsorbed is dependent on 3 factors: the urea concentration of the surrounding renal medulla, the flow rate of the urine through the nephrons, and the body's state of hydration. Note that in healthy individuals, urea is not secreted; however, in individuals with severe renal disease, urea will also be secreted by the tubules.

Because the kidneys are the primary means for urea elimination (90%) from the body, the concentration of urea in plasma is dependent on adequate renal perfusion and function. The remaining 10% is eliminated through the GI tract and skin (i.e., sweat). However, the level of nitrogen metabolism also plays a role in the plasma urea concentration, i.e., changes in the plasma urea concentration can occur despite "normal" renal function. Nonrenal factors that affect the plasma urea concentration include the level of protein catabolism, the protein concentration of the diet, the body's state of hydration, and the functional status of the liver.

## CLINICAL SIGNIFICANCE

Increased plasma levels of urea are specifically referred to as *uremia.* Because most conditions that cause urea to be increased also alter the concentration of other NPN compounds, the

term *azotemia* is often used interchangeably. As previously stated, conditions that increase the plasma urea nitrogen (plasma UN) concentration can be categorized as prerenal, renal, or postrenal in origin (Table 20–2). Prerenal conditions typically affect the plasma UN concentration without a comparable increase in the plasma creatinine level; these include a high-protein intake, dehydration, shock or hemorrhage, and congestive heart failure. Note that several of these prerenal conditions alter the adequacy of renal perfusion, thereby having a direct impact on renal function. Various renal conditions, such as glomerular nephritis, tubular necrosis, chronic and acute renal failure, will increase the plasma UN concentration; however, the concentration is not significantly increased until the GFR decreases to less than 50% of its normal level. In such cases, the plasma UN concentration can rise to as much as 200 mg/dL (71 mmol/L). Similarly, any condition that obstructs the flow of urine through the ureters, bladder, or urethra can cause an increased plasma urea nitrogen concentration, i.e., postrenal azotemia. These include nephrolithiasis (i.e., renal calculi formation), genitourinary tumors, and prostate enlargement.

Historically, urea nitrogen was used to assess the GFR by determining a urea clearance. However, because other factors besides changes in renal function alter the plasma urea concentration (e.g., variations in urine flow, level of nitrogen metabolism), urea clearances are no longer performed.

Despite limitations, the plasma UN concentration serves as a crude indicator of renal function and can be a diagnostic aid in distinguishing various causes of renal insufficiency. Used alone, the plasma UN concentration has limited value; however, when evaluated simultaneously with the plasma creatinine concentration in the UN/creatinine ratio, these analytes can have additional, although limited clinical utility (Table 20–2). In healthy individuals, and assuming a normal diet, the UN/creatinine ratio is usually between 10 and 20. Note, however, that hydration will affect the value of the plasma

**Alterations of Plasma Urea Concentration and the UN/Creatinine Ratio for Selected Conditions**

| PLASMA UREA LEVEL | CONDITION | TYPICAL UN/CREATININE RATIO |
|---|---|---|
| **Increased** | *Prerenal* | |
| | High protein intake | Increased ratio (20–30); urea increase |
| | Dehydration | greater than creatinine increase; |
| | Decreased renal perfusion (shock, | creatinine often "normal" |
| | hemorrhage, congestive heart failure) | |
| | Drugs (corticosteroids, tetracycline) | |
| | *Renal* | |
| | Glomerular diseases | Normal ratio (10–20); proportional |
| | Tubular diseases | increase of urea and creatinine |
| | Acute and chronic renal failure | |
| | Intrinsic renal disorders | |
| | *Postrenal* | |
| | Nephrolithiasis | Increased ratio (>20); disproportional |
| | Genitourinary tumors | increase of urea and creatinine |
| | Prostate enlargement | |
| **Decreased** | Low protein intake | Decreased ratio (<10) |
| | Severe liver disease | |
| | Severe vomiting or diarrhea | |

UN/creatinine ratio. For example, in a healthy, adequately hydrated individual, the urine flow rate is greater than 1 mL/minute, enabling the elimination of about 60% of the urea presented to the nephrons (i.e., ~40% is reabsorbed). In conditions of dehydration and hypovolemia, the urine flow rate is slowed to less than 0.5 mL/minute, enhancing urea absorption and reducing urea elimination to approximately 40% (i.e., ~60% is reabsorbed). Keeping these points in mind, in prerenal azotemia (e.g., dehydration or severe hemorrhage), the plasma UN concentration will increase to a greater extent than the plasma creatinine concentration, causing the UN/creatinine ratio to increase, typically up to 20 to 30. This occurs because all of the creatinine in the tubular lumen is excreted, whereas only 40% of the filtered urea is eliminated (i.e., 60% is reabsorbed). In cases of intrinsic renal disease (i.e., a decrease in functional nephrons), the UN/creatinine ratio is normal despite abnormally increased plasma UN and creatinine results. Postrenal conditions usually present as an increased UN/creatinine ratio with an increased creatinine level. However, this same ratio with an elevated creatinine can be observed in individuals with prerenal azotemia superimposed on an underlying renal disease.

A decreased UN/creatinine ratio (<10) is uncommon but can be obtained from individuals on a low-protein diet, following severe diarrhea or vomiting, with acute tubular necrosis, with severe liver disease, or following renal dialysis (i.e., urea dialyzes more efficiently than creatinine).

Although in theory the UN/creatinine ratio has clinical applicability, in reality, because of the variety of factors that affect urea production and elimination, the UN/creatinine ratio is un-

reliable as the sole indicator. However, combined with other laboratory tests and clinical information, it can assist the clinician in identifying or following disease progression or resolution.

## ANALYTICAL PROCEDURES

### Specimen Requirements

The specimens of choice for urea nitrogen determination are plasma, serum, and urine. Hemolysis should be avoided and the separation of plasma from the cells should occur as soon as possible to prevent an increase in endogenous ammonia (particularly important if an indirect analytical method is employed). Serum and plasma samples are stable at room temperature (22°C) for 24 hours; when refrigerated (2 to 8°C), stability is several days. For indirect methods (that convert urea into ammonia), fluoride and citrate anticoagulants should not be used because they inhibit urease, and ammonium heparin is avoided because it can falsely increase results. Twenty-four-hour urine specimens are preferred; urine should be refrigerated during collection or a preservative added (e.g., thymol) to prevent bacterial growth and the conversion of urea to ammonia.

### Analytical Methods

Two types of methods are available to determine the urea concentration in specimens. Indirect methods involve two steps: (1) the conversion of urea to ammonia by the action of the enzyme urease, and (2) the measurement of the resultant increase in ammonia. For each molecule of urea present, 2 molecules of ammonia are produced. The difference in indirect

TABLE 20-3

**Reference Interval and Interpretation Guidelines for Plasma/Serum Urea Nitrogen Values**

| UREA NITROGEN (mg/dL) | UREA (mmol/L) | INTERPRETATION |
|---|---|---|
| 6–23 | 1.1–8.2 | Reference Interval |
| <6–10 | <1.1–3.6 | Overhydration |
| 50–150 | 17.9–53.6 | Exceeds variations expected due to urine flow rate or nitrogen load, i.e., implies impairment of glomerular filtration rate |
| 150–250 | 53.6–89.3 | Evidence of severe renal impairment |

methods resides in the mode of ammonia detection and quantitation. In contrast, direct methods combine each molecule of urea directly with a reactant (e.g., diacetyl) to form a colored complex or chromophore that is measured spectrophotometrically.

### Reference Interval

In the United States, urea determinations are reported as urea nitrogen in milligrams per deciliter (mg/dL), whereas the SI system reports urea in millimoles per liter (mmol/L). The conversion factor for changing urea nitrogen (in mg/dL) to urea (in mmol/L) is 0.357; the factor for the reverse conversion, from mmol/L of urea to mg/dL of urea nitrogen is 2.80. These factors are based on the fact that for every millimole of urea (60 mg), 28 mg is nitrogen; in addition, the conversion of deciliters to liters is accounted for. For example:

$$\frac{18 \text{ mg Urea N}}{dL} \times \frac{60 \text{ mg Urea}}{28 \text{ mg Urea N}} \times \frac{\text{mmol Urea}}{60 \text{ mg Urea}}$$

$$\times \frac{10 \ dL}{L} = 6.4 \text{ mmol/L Urea}$$

A typical reference interval for plasma and serum urea nitrogen is 6 to 23 mg/dL (or 2.1 to 8.2 mmol/L urea).[5] Note that a value within this range does not guarantee normal renal function. Assuming adequate hydration and protein diet, an individual's urea nitrogen level can double (e.g., from 10 to 20 mg/dL) and still reside in the reference interval, indicating a significant reduction in renal function. Table 20-3 lists general guidelines regarding UN levels and the assessment of renal function.[6]

### Uric Acid

Uric Acid     Urate

### BIOCHEMISTRY

Uric acid is the final end product of purine nucleoside catabolism, specifically adenosine and guanosine, derived from both dietary and endogenous nucleic acids. The conversion of purines to uric acid occurs primarily in the liver, and then it is transferred to the bloodstream. Because the pH of the plasma and tissues is greater than pH 5.57 (the first $pK_a$ of uric acid), uric acid is present in the form of urate ions with approximately 97% associated with sodium as monosodium urate.

As the blood passes through the kidneys, plasma urates are completely filtered by the glomeruli with subsequent proximal tubular reabsorption and distal tubular secretion. The net result is renal excretion of 6% to 12% of the filtered urates (i.e., 88% to 94% is reabsorbed). Although the majority (~75%) of uric acid produced is eventually excreted in the urine, the remainder (25%) is secreted into the GI tract, where it is degraded by bacterial enzymes and excreted in the feces.

### CLINICAL SIGNIFICANCE

Hyperuricemia, defined as plasma uric acid levels that exceed the reference interval, can occur due to a variety of disorders. These conditions can be divided into those that result from altered uric acid production and those characterized by insufficient renal excretion of uric acid (Table 20-4). Deficiencies or defects of the specific enzymes required for uric acid synthesis can result in the accumulation of purine precursors. For example, Lesch-Nyhan syndrome is characterized by the complete lack of hypoxanthine-guanine phosphoribosyltransferase (HGPRT), a major enzyme involved in purine metabolism. Hyperuricemia and hyperuricaciduria are characteristic biochemical features of this disease. Myeloproliferative disorders and the use of chemotherapeutic agents in the treatment of leukemias and lymphomas result in increased cell destruction and the amount of nucleic acids that are processed; hence, uric acid levels are increased. There are also individuals that have asymptomatic hyperuricemia. These individuals are usually identified during a health screening and are routinely monitored thereafter because of their increased risk for the development of renal disease, secondary to hyperuricemia and hyperuricaciduria.

Numerous causes of insufficient renal excretion of uric acid have been identified (Table 20-4). In some cases, intrin-

### TABLE 20-4

**Causes of Hyperuricemia**

| Altered uric acid production | Increased synthesis of purine precursors |
|---|---|
| | Accumulation of purine precursors due to specific enzyme pathway deficiencies or defects (e.g., Lesch-Nyhan syndrome) |
| | Increased turnover of nucleic acids |
| | Myeloproliferative syndromes |
| | Chemotherapy for leukemias and lymphomas |
| Insufficient renal excretion of uric acid | Primary renal disorders |
| | Acute renal failure |
| | Chronic renal failure |
| | Alteration in renal handling |
| | Drug therapy (e.g., diuretics, salicylates) |
| | Organic acidemia (e.g., ketoacidosis, lactic acidosis) |
| | Glycogen storage diseases (e.g., G-6-PD deficiency) |
| | Toxins (lead, alcohol) |
| | Toxemia of pregnancy |

sic renal disease predominates. In others, induced alterations in renal handling (i.e., competition between disease-associated metabolites and urates for renal excretion) is the cause. Included in the latter case are medications, particularly diuretics and salicylates, acidotic states (ketoacidosis, lactic acidosis), glucose-6-phosphate deficiency, toxemia of pregnancy, and toxins. Transient increases in plasma uric acid can occur during dehydration, which stimulates renal reabsorption of uric acid and thereby decreases excretion, and after the ingestion of large quantities of food rich in nucleic acids, i.e., liver, sweetbreads, anchovies, kidneys, and sardines. Acute and chronic renal failure will lead to a progressive increase in the plasma uric acid. This occurs from a reduction in the GFR compounded by alterations in renal tubular reabsorption and secretion.

Gout is a clinical condition characterized by hyperuricemia and the deposition of monosodium urate crystals in the joints and tissues. Because the body fluids are supersaturated with urates, monosodium urate crystals precipitate out as aggregates or tophi in and around joint capsules, tendons, subcutaneous tissues, cartilage, bone, or in the kidney. Most frequently, initial acute attacks involve the metatarsophalangeal joint of the big toe. Following crystal deposition, polymorphonuclear leukocytes and macrophages enter the joint and surrounding tissues to phagocytize the crystals. This process results in lysosomal destruction within the leukocytes and the release of hydrolytic enzymes that ultimately causes localized tissue destruction and inflammation. Pain, swelling, redness, and heat in the affected area are principal signs of gout. Treatment is required to prevent subsequent episodes that can lead to erosive joint disease (i.e., gouty arthritis) or renal damage (e.g., gouty nephropathy, urate nephrolithiasis).

Gout is often classified into two types depending on the cause of the hyperuricemia. Primary gout is inherited, whereas secondary gout encompasses all other causes.[7] Note that many patients with hyperuricemia never develop gout.

Uric acid stones or renal calculi can develop in individuals with or without hyperuricemia. Of the approximate 0.1% of the population that develop renal calculi, only about 6% develop uric acid stones. Of these individuals, only about 1 in 5 has gout.[8] Uric acid is normally excreted in the urine; hence, if the urine pH is less than 5.57 and the ultrafiltrate is supersaturated (e.g., as in dehydration), uric acid crystals can precipitate in vivo and lead to stone formation. Also, note that uric acid crystallization in urine specimens can be induced by storage conditions, i.e., as the urine specimen cools to room temperature or is refrigerated, uric acid crystals can precipitate out of solution. Hence, the finding of uric acid crystals during a routine urinalysis is not unusual and not clinically significant in most individuals.

Hypouricemia, while uncommon, can occur either because of decreased purine synthesis or increased elimination. Reductions in purine synthesis can be observed with severe liver disease or from overtreatment with therapeutic agents that inhibit de novo purine synthesis (e.g., 6-mercaptopurine, azathioprine) or enhance uric acid elimination (e.g., allopurinol). Any condition that reduces renal tubular absorption of urates fosters urate elimination and can cause hypouricemia. Wilson's disease and the Fanconi syndrome are two disorders characterized by defective renal tubular absorption. Chronic exposure to a toxin (e.g., lead, mercury) will also adversely affect proximal tubular function, resulting in an increased elimination of plasma urates. Similarly, an acute yet transient reduction in urate reabsorption can develop after the injection of radioopaque contrast media.

## ANALYTICAL PROCEDURES

### Specimen Requirements

Nonfasting plasma and serum are acceptable specimens for uric acid quantitation. Avoid fluoride and EDTA anticoagulants, which can cause positive interference with analytical methods that employ uricase, whereas oxalate anticoagulants interfere with the phosphotungstic acid (PTA) methods. Plasma and serum samples are stable for 3 to 5 days refrigerated and for 6 months if frozen at −20°C.[5] Twenty-four-hour urine collections should be appropriately preserved during collection.

## Analytical Methods

Historically, analytical methods utilized the ability of uric acid to reduce phosphotungstic acid to form tungsten blue, a blue chromophore.

$$\text{Uric acid} + \text{Phosphotungstic acid} + O_2 \rightarrow$$

$$\text{Allantoin} + CO_2 + \text{Tungsten blue}$$

However, this approach is susceptible to numerous interferences from protein, lipids, and the presence of other reducing substances such as ascorbic acid, glucose, acetaminophen, caffeine, and theophylline. Modifications of PTA methods have not been successful in eliminating these interferences.

Currently, uricase (EC 1.7.3.3) methods predominate due to their increased specificity. Uricase, a bacterial enzyme, is employed in either a single or multistep reaction sequence to catalyze the oxidation of uric acid to allantoin, producing carbon dioxide and hydrogen peroxide. As uric acid is oxidized, the absorbance decreases proportionally. This reaction can be monitored directly at ~290 nm (282 to 292 nm). An alternate and the most popular approach is to couple the hydrogen peroxide generated to an indicator reaction that utilizes peroxidase or catalase to form a chromogen. The colored product is measured at an appropriate wavelength spectrophotometrically or by reflectance photometry in dry slide chemistry systems.

$$\text{Uric acid} \xrightarrow{\text{uricase}} \text{Allantoin} + CO_2 + H_2O_2$$

$$H_2O_2 + \text{Oxygen acceptor} \xrightarrow{\text{peroxidase}} \text{Chromogen}$$

Uric acid can be quantitated using high-performance liquid chromatography (HPLC). These methods employ either ion-exchange or reverse-phase columns to separate and subsequently quantitate uric acid. Despite their specificity, these methods are infrequently performed because they are more time consuming and labor intensive.

### TABLE 20–5

**Typical Plasma/Serum Reference Intervals for Uric Acid, by Gender**

| GENDER | PTA METHOD mg/dL (μmol/L) | URICASE METHOD mg/dL (μmol/L) |
|---|---|---|
| Male | 4.4–7.6 (262–452) | 3.5–7.2 (208–428) |
| Female | 2.3–6.6 (137–393) | 2.6–6.0 (155–357) |

### TABLE 20–6

**Typical Reference Intervals for Uric Acid by 24-Hour Urine Collection**

| DIET | URIC ACID mg/d (mmol/d) |
|---|---|
| Typical | 250–750 (1.48–4.43) |
| Purine free | <420 (2.48) |

## Reference Intervals

Plasma and serum reference intervals differ with gender and are method dependent (Table 20–5). Generally, uricase methods produce lower values than PTA methods. Urinary excretion of uric acid is diet dependent with decreases of 20% to 25% observed from individuals on a purine-free diet (Table 20–6).

# ASSESSMENT OF RENAL FUNCTION

That 25% of the total cardiac output flows through the kidneys is testament to the close relationship of renal function to renal perfusion. Hence, if renal perfusion is compromised, so is renal function. Renal function is a general term that encompasses a variety of dynamic processes that occur in the functional units of the kidney, the nephrons. The net result of these processes is the formation of urine and the elimination of metabolic by-products, foreign substances (e.g., drugs), and excess water. For a substance to be excreted in the urine, it must either freely pass a glomerular filtration barrier into the tubular lumen (glomerular function) or be secreted by the tubular epithelium into the lumen fluid (tubular function). Laboratory tests that assess glomerular and tubular function are useful in evaluating and monitoring not only renal disease but also other disorders that can alter renal function secondarily.

## Assessment of Glomerular Function

### DETERMINATION OF THE GLOMERULAR FILTRATION RATE

Glomerular function is directly dependent on adequate renal blood flow. This flow literally drives the process of glomerular filtration as well as affects the handling of solutes and water by the renal tubules. By definition, the volume of plasma (in mL) processed per minute by the glomeruli is called the glomerular filtration rate (GFR). The GFR is determined by performing a clearance test using either an endogenous or exogenous substance. The substance ($S$) selected is measured in both a plasma specimen and a timed urine specimen and the clearance ($C_S$) determined using the formula:

$$C_S \text{ (mL/min)} = \frac{U_S \times V_{Ur}}{P_S}$$

where $U_S$ is the urine concentration of $S$ in mg/dL; $P_S$ is the plasma concentration of $S$ in mg/dL; and $V_{Ur}$ is the urine flow calculated in mL/minute (determined from the volume of urine excreted during the time interval, e.g., 1800 mL/24 h $\times$ h/60 min = 1.25 mL/min). Note that the units of concentration for the plasma and urine determinations must be the same, thereby canceling out, and the clearance of the substance is in the units of mL/minute.

To accurately measure the GFR, the ideal substance for a clearance test should fulfill the following criteria: (1) the plasma concentration is constant, (2) it readily passes the glomerular filtration barriers, and (3) it is not secreted or reabsorbed by the tubular epithelium. Few endogenous substances fulfill these criteria, with creatinine being the most popular despite its limitations. Conversely, several exogenous substances have been used with the inulin clearance test considered the reference standard. Exogenous substances are not used to routinely assess and monitor GFR because (1) extensive patient preparation is required (intravenous infusion of the substance must begin prior to and be maintained throughout the duration of the test, i.e., more than 24 hours) and (2) the analytical methods for quantitation (e.g., inulin) are more costly and time consuming (and often nonspecific).

In summary, the renal clearance of a substance is the volume of plasma from which the substance is completely cleared and passed into the urine per unit of time. Clearance tests are a useful laboratory tool to assess an individual's renal status because they are more sensitive to changes in functional status than plasma measurements alone.

## Inulin Clearance

Inulin is a fructo-polysaccharide (MW 5200) not normally present in the body. It is an ideal substance for GFR assessment because it readily passes the glomerular filtration barrier and is not reabsorbed or secreted by the tubules. However, because inulin is an exogenous substance, it must be introduced into the body by intravenous (IV) infusion. Additionally, the infusion must progress for an extended period to establish a constant plasma level both initially and throughout the timed test. For this reason, clearances using exogenous substances are rarely performed. Although the inulin clearance remains the reference standard to which other clearance tests are evaluated, research is ongoing to find a substance that accurately determines the GFR and that can be measured in body fluids using a fast, cost-effective analytical method. Other exogenous substances that have been used to determine the GFR include $^{125}$I-isothalamate, $^{131}$I-iodoacetate, $^{131}$I-hippuran, and iohexal, of which only iohexal is nonisotopic.

## Creatinine Clearance

The creatinine clearance test is the most frequently performed test for the evaluation of the GFR. Clinically, the most important information needed regarding an individual's renal status is (1) whether the GFR is normal or abnormal, and

(2) over time, is the GFR changing or remaining stable. The creatinine clearance test can consistently, reliably, and cost effectively provide this information.

Despite its relatively constant plasma concentration and small size (which enables it to freely pass the glomerular filtration barrier), creatinine is not an ideal clearance substance because a small amount is actually secreted by the tubules. A review of studies comparing the inulin and endogenous creatinine clearance tests reveals that some investigators found agreement between the two tests, whereas others found that the creatinine clearance overestimated the GFR by as much as 15%, with an average of 7%.[2] In uremic conditions, several factors have been identified that can result in the overestimation of the GFR. For example, as the plasma creatinine concentration increases, the amount of creatinine removed by tubular secretion increases. In these same patients, studies have shown that creatinine is also degraded and eliminated by the GI tract, which also enhances the overestimation of the GFR.[9] Therefore, in individuals with impaired renal function (e.g., chronic renal failure) alternate modes of creatinine elimination increase (e.g., tubular secretion, creatinine degradation) and the creatinine clearance becomes a less accurate measure of the GFR.

Several medications are known to interfere and, in some cases, completely block tubular secretion of creatinine into the urine, such as cimetidine, trimethoprim, and salicylate. This observation has been used to improve the accuracy of GFR measurements by the creatinine clearance.[10]

The analytical method used to quantitate creatinine is also responsible for some of the variation observed in studies comparing the inulin and creatinine clearance tests. When the Jaffe reaction is used, noncreatinine chromogens, which are present in the plasma but not in urine, falsely increase the plasma creatinine result (i.e., the value of $P$ in the clearance formula). Fortuitously, in most individuals, this plasma increase is counterbalanced by the additional creatinine that is secreted into the urine ($U$) by the tubules. The net result is a creatinine clearance value that approximates the inulin clearance. However, when enzymatic creatinine methods are used, the creatinine clearance is overestimated because the plasma result ($P$) is lower (i.e., noncreatinine chromogens are not measured); whereas, the urine creatinine ($U$) remains unchanged.

Another factor that directly influences the validity of a clearance test is the urine specimen collection and handling. Because of the diurnal variation of the GFR, the urine specimen of choice for a clearance test is a 24-hour collection. In individuals that are periodically monitored, shorter collections (e.g., 12-hour, 4-hour) may be used after the GFR is initially determined using a 24-hour collection. For comparison purposes, when shorter intervals are used, it is important that they occur during the same time of day. The plasma creatinine blood sample can be collected at anytime during the collection as well as within 24 hours preceding or following the urine collection. Patients should be well hydrated during the collection interval to ensure an adequate urine flow. Other precautions include the avoidance of coffee, tea, vigorous exercise, and certain medications during or immediately preceding the testing interval.

Appropriate urine collection during the time interval is also crucial. It is imperative that no urine is discarded, that additional urine is not added, and that the complete collection be adequately mixed before an aliquot is tested. Written as well as verbal instructions given to each patient enhance the likelihood of an appropriately collected urine specimen. Another important aspect is the storage of the urine throughout the duration of the collection. Lack of refrigeration or an appropriate preservative can result in bacterial proliferation and a loss of creatinine due to bacterial degradation. Each of these factors can cause an erroneous clearance result because they directly affect one of the clearance formula parameters: $P$, $U$, or $V$.

Creatinine production and excretion is directly related to lean muscle mass. Therefore, to compare clearance results from patients with differing muscle mass requires that the creatinine clearance test be normalized to an average adult surface area selected to be 1.73 square meters. Determination of surface area (in $m^2$) can be obtained using a standardized nomogram or by calculation using the following formula:

$$SA = W^{0.425} \times H^{0.725} \times 0.007184$$

where $W$ is the weight in kilograms and $H$ is the height in centimeters. If you need to convert the weight and height into pounds and centimeters, convert pounds to kilograms by multiplying by 0.45; convert inches to centimeters by multiplying by 2.54.

With normalization for body surface area, the formula for a creatinine clearance ($C_{cr}$) becomes:

$$C_{Cr} \text{ (mL/min/1.73 m}^2\text{)} = \frac{U_{Cr} \times V_{Ur}}{P_{Cr}} \times \frac{1.73 \text{ m}^2}{SA}$$

where SA is the patient's body surface area in square meters.

Reference intervals for creatinine clearance vary with creatinine methodology and with age and gender, particularly in adults (Table 20–7). The GFR reaches a peak rate during the third decade of life. For each decade thereafter, it decreases by ~6.5 mL/min/1.73 m².[5]

## ASSESSMENT OF GLOMERULAR PERMEABILITY

Permeability of solutes across the glomerular filtration barriers depends on their molecular size and ionic character, as discussed in Chapter 19. In healthy individuals, the glomerular filtration barrier (GFB) allows only minute amounts of albumin to pass (i.e., 0.001 mmol of albumin/24 h urine) and a few blood cells.[11] Therefore, the presence of increased amounts of protein in the urine (proteinuria) as well as increased numbers of blood cells are classic features for a variety of renal disorders and can aid in the identification of a disease process.

**TABLE 20-7**

**Typical Reference Intervals for Creatinine Clearance***

| AGE | MALE (mL/min/1.73 m²) | FEMALE (mL/min/1.73 m²) |
|---|---|---|
| 0–5 y[†] | 45–73 (mean) | |
| 6–8 y[†] | 64–72 (mean) | |
| 9–14 y[†] | 83–109 (mean) | |
| 20–29 y | 88–146 (mean = 117) | 81–134 (mean = 107) |
| 30–39 y | 82–140 (mean = 110) | 75–128 (mean = 102) |

For each decade after 39 years, values decrease ~6.5 mL/min/1.73 m².

*SOURCE: Tietz NW (ed.): *Clinical Guide to Laboratory Tests*, 3rd ed. Philadelphia, WB Saunders, 1995; and Burtis CA, Ashwood ER (eds): *Tietz Textbook of Clinical Chemistry*. Philadelphia, WB Saunders, 1994.

[†]Range of mean clearance values for age interval.

## Proteinuria

In a normal active individual, less than 150 mg of protein is excreted in the urine each day. Stated differently, urine protein concentrations typically range from 1 to 14 mg/dL; excretion of protein in concentrations greater than this indicate proteinuria. Proteinuria can be classified into three types: prerenal, renal, and postrenal. In prerenal conditions, also called overflow proteinuria, excessive amounts of low-molecular-weight proteins in the bloodstream are presented to the kidneys. They can be normal proteins such as acute phase reactants, myoglobin, and hemoglobin or abnormal proteins such as immunoglobulin light chains (i.e., Bence Jones proteins). Because renal tubular absorption of protein is a nonselective, competitive, and threshold-limited ($T_m$) process, the ability to reabsorb all the protein present can be exceeded and any excess protein will be excreted in the urine. Note that in these conditions, the kidneys are functioning normally (i.e., no renal disease is present), simply the tubular ability to reabsorb has been overwhelmed.

Renal proteinuria is often subdivided into glomerular proteinuria and tubular proteinuria. In either case, a normal amount of plasma proteins is presented to the kidneys for processing. In glomerular proteinuria, the problem is a defective GFB such that its selectivity has been compromised. In other words, either the anionic character of the barrier has been lost allowing albumin to freely pass, or the size selectivity has been compromised, i.e., molecules with an effective radius greater than 4 nm can now pass, or a combination of these two processes has occurred. Glomerular proteinuria is seen with the nephritic syndrome, glomerulonephritis and the nephrotic syndrome. It can also occur with infectious diseases, autoimmune disorders, drug therapy, transplant rejection, and preeclampsia.

Transitory hemodynamic changes in the glomeruli due to strenuous exercise, fever, emotional stress, and extreme cold exposure can also induce a glomerular proteinuria. Similarly, postural or orthostatic proteinuria is also considered a glomerular proteinuria. In this condition, the individual excretes additional urine protein only when in the upright or orthostatic position; whereas, urine collected immediately on rising in the morning will contain a normal amount of protein (albumin). Postural proteinuria occurs during the healing phase of many glomerular disorders as well as in individuals with no evidence of renal disease and rarely exceeds 1 g per day. Studies have been mixed regarding the long-term prognosis for individuals with orthostatic proteinuria; however, the majority do not develop renal dysfunction.

The severity of glomerular proteinuria can vary and is often described as mild, moderate, or heavy. In some conditions, the glomeruli retain their selectivity (i.e., their ability to discriminate proteins on the basis of their molecular size); hence, the urinary proteins present are primarily albumin and other proteins of low to moderate molecular weight. In severe cases, the glomeruli become nonselective and all proteins, regardless of size, are present in the urine including large molecular weight proteins (MW > 90,000). When the glomeruli have lost their ability to discriminate, solutes based on their molecular size, for example, plasma lipids (cholesterol, triglycerides), can also pass the glomerular filtration barriers into the urine. These lipids can be present as free-floating fat globules, fat globules incorporated into urinary casts, or fat globules absorbed by cells (i.e., oval fat bodies). The presence of urinary fat is a classic feature of the nephrotic syndrome.

Renal proteinuria can also occur due to defective renal tubular absorption, i.e., tubular proteinuria. In other words, a normal amount of protein is presented to the tubules but they are unable to adequately reabsorb it. The proteins involved in this type of proteinuria are moderate to low molecular weight proteins including albumin, $\beta_2$-microglobulin, retinol-binding protein, and lysozyme. Tubular proteinuria was first identified due to heavy metal poisonings (e.g., cadmium, mercury) but can also be caused by pyelonephritis, renal tuberculosis, the Fanconi syndrome, a variety of drugs (aminoglycosides, sulfonamides, penicillins, cephalosporins), hemolytic conditions (hemoglobin), rhabdomyolysis (myoglobin), transplant rejection, and even strenuous exercise.

Postrenal proteinuria occurs when proteins are added to the urine after it is formed in the kidneys. Inflammatory processes in the renal pelvis, ureters, bladder, prostate, and urethra are the most common causes, i.e., proteins involved in the inflammatory process are added to the urine as it flows through these sites. It is important to note that contamination of the urine with vaginal secretions or blood from hemorrhoids can also cause proteinuria.

In summary, proteinuria can result from (1) increased production and excretion of plasma proteins, (2) renal changes that affect protein handling, (3) inflammation in the urinary system following renal processing, or (4) urine contamination.

Although proteinuria is a hallmark of renal disease, it is important to note that other conditions and situations can cause proteinuria.

Qualitative or semiquantitative protein testing on random urine specimens is one parameter of a routine urinalysis. Hence, screening for increases in urinary protein is frequently performed with a routine urinalysis test. It is also a fast, cost-effective way to monitor proteinuria to determine if a disease process is progressing or regressing. On commercial reagent strips, the protein reaction is based on the protein error of indicators. A buffer in the reaction pad maintains a pH 3; protein present in the urine causes the indicator dye (a derivative of tetrabromphenol blue) to release hydrogen ions, thereby causing the reaction pad to change color. This test is most useful and most sensitive for the detection of albumin. The detection limit, which varies with reagent strip manufacturer, is approximately 15 mg/dL albumin. Technically, other proteins such as mucoproteins, immunoglobulin light chains (Bence Jones proteins), myoglobin, and hemoglobin could produce a positive test. However, the concentration of these proteins is rarely large enough to do so. The one exception is hemoglobin, which if present in a large enough concentration (e.g., greater than 10 mg/dL) can produce a trace protein result; this is extremely rare. Note that this amount of hemoglobin is 250 times the detection limit of the reagent strip (~0.04 mg/dL) and produces a reagent-strip blood result that exceeds the color chart and would be reported as large (4+). Therefore, in a urine sample, if the reagent-strip blood result is less than large, then hemoglobin is not contributing to the protein result. In summary, a negative reagent-strip protein test indicates that either a normal amount of protein is present, or if protein is present, it is not albumin.

Other semiquantitative methods for protein detection in urine are based on the denaturation and precipitation of protein using heat or pH changes. The most common protein precipitation test uses sulfosalicylic acid as the denaturing agent and is sensitive to ~10 mg/dL albumin. When performing the test, the amount of precipitate that forms is measured using turbidimetry or is graded using a plus system, e.g., negative, trace, 1+, 2+, 3+, 4+. One advantage of precipitation methods is their ability to detect any protein, i.e., equally sensitive to all proteins. Before more specific and cost-effective methods were available, these tests (along with a reagent strip protein test) could be used to screen for the presence of immunoglobulin light chains (Bence Jones proteins). For example, in the case of a patient with multiple myeloma excreting immunoglobulin light chains in their urine, a discrepancy between the 2 protein tests would occur, e.g., a negative reagent strip protein test with a 3+ precipitation test. However, a similar discrepancy can also be obtained with other nonprotein substances that precipitate in acidic conditions, such as radiographic contrast media and certain medications (e.g., penicillins).

Today, methods for the quantitation of urine total protein and urine albumin are fast and cost effective. These methods may also be used to evaluate random urine specimens that are highly colored and cannot be accurately assessed using commercial reagent strips.

## Microalbuminuria

The excretion of increased amounts of urine albumin is a sensitive and early marker used to identify individuals with type 1 and type 2 diabetes who are at risk for the development of renal disease. Because very small amounts of albumin are being detected the term *microalbuminuria* was coined. The small increases in urinary albumin are indicative of glomerular permeability changes, described previously. If detected early enough, therapeutic intervention to improve glycemic and hypertensive control can avert the progression to nephropathy or end-stage renal disease (ESRD). Initially, tests for microalbuminuria were used to screen only diabetic individuals. Today, however, microalbuminuria may be used to identify nondiabetic individuals with hypertension that are at an increased risk for the development of cardiovascular disease (e.g., coronary artery disease, stroke, left ventricular hypertrophy, peripheral vascular disease).[12] Various studies indicate potential clinical utility of microalbuminuria in hypertension, pregnancy (preeclamptic states, maternal morbidity, and fetal mortality), nondiabetic renal disease, as well as in assessing the renal effects of various drugs and hormones.

Several rapid semiquantitative and quantitative methods are available to screen urine for low-level increases of albumin and their detection limits vary. Note that the urinalysis reagent strip tests for protein lack the sensitivity required and are unable to detect microalbuminuria. The American Diabetes Association recommends that if a semiquantitative test for microalbuminuria is positive that the results be confirmed by a more specific quantitative method.[13] In individuals with diabetes without microalbuminuria, screening should be performed annually; for those individuals with microalbuminuria, therapeutic intervention is taken and periodic monitoring of the level of albumin excretion should be performed to evaluate the effectiveness of the treatment plan.[13]

Three different urine specimen collections can be used to screen for microalbuminuria: (1) collect a 24-hour urine specimen and simultaneously determine the albumin excretion rate (AER in $\mu$g/min) and the creatinine clearance, (2) collect a timed urine collection (e.g., 4-hour, 12-hour) and simultaneously determine the albumin concentration, the creatinine clearance and the albumin-to-creatinine ratio (ACR), or (3) collect a random urine specimen; simultaneously determine the creatinine and albumin concentrations, then calculate the ACR. The latter option, the collection of a random urine specimen and the calculation of the ACR, is relatively fast, easy, and cost-effective. Consequently, it is the most popular approach and provides reliable clinical information.

Microalbuminuria is defined as an AER between 20 and 200 $\mu$g/minute. Because creatinine excretion varies with gender (due to muscle mass), the ACR discriminator value differs: 1.8 g/mol for men and 2.5 g/mol for women.[14] In other words, if a man excretes more than 1.8 grams of albumin per mole of creatinine, it is indicative of microalbuminuria.

## Hematuria

The presence of an increased number of red blood cells (RBCs) in the urine is termed hematuria. Depending on the analytical conditions for the urinalysis, the normal number of RBCs observed in a concentrated urine sediment vary but is approximately 0 to 3 RBCs per high power field, or 3 to 12 per microliter of urine sediment.[15] All RBCs present in urine came from the vascular system either by passage across compromised glomerular filtration barriers, or by leakage into the urinary system from an area where the integrity of the vascular system has been damaged due to injury or disease.

When changes in glomerular permeability are severe enough to enable RBCs to pass, plasma proteins pass as well. Therefore, in glomerular diseases associated with proteinuria, hematuria is usually present in varying degrees. Passage through the glomeruli or renal epithelium causes RBCs to become distorted or dysmorphic; hence, the presence of numerous dysmorphic RBCs in urine sediment is a classic feature of glomerular disease.

The presence of RBCs and hemoglobin casts is also indicative of glomerular disease or renal parenchymal bleeding. Casts are only formed in the distal and collecting tubules of the nephrons. Therefore, if RBCs are incorporated into a cast, they entered the urinary system at the nephrons either at the glomerulus or along the tubules.

In summary, the presence of hematuria, proteinuria and RBC casts is indicative of glomerular disease. In contrast, hematuria without proteinuria or RBC casts is suggestive of a bleed in the lower urinary tract (i.e., after or below the kidney) or may be due to contamination from hemorrhoids or menstrual blood. It is important to note that transitory changes in glomerular permeability, discussed previously, can also cause a transitory hematuria. These include strenuous exercise, acute febrile episodes, and smoking.[16]

## Assessment of Tubular Function

### TESTS FOR RENAL CONCENTRATION ABILITY

The kidneys are responsible for the overall maintenance of water balance in the body. The nephrons selectively absorb and secrete solutes into the urine, whereas the volume of water excreted is determined by the body's state of hydration (i.e., how much water is available). The collecting tubules under the control of arginine vasopressin (also known as antidiuretic hormone, ADH) regulate the passive reabsorption of water. Note that the amount of water available is dependent on adequate fluid intake, which is regulated by the sensation of thirst. Urine is usually 94% water and 6% solutes; however, the kidneys can alter this composition based on bodily needs. Therefore, evaluating the renal ability to concentrate the urine provides a sensitive indicator of renal function, particularly renal tubular function.

Assuming an adequate renal blood flow and glomerular filtration rate, the changes that occur in the composition of the original ultrafiltrate compared to the final urine are a direct result of the renal tubular absorption and secretory processes. Note that after the urine leaves the nephrons by way of the collecting ducts into the renal pelvis, its composition is unchanged. Renal diseases characterized by the inability to concentrate the urine are usually chronic with impairment progressing slowly and insidiously, e.g., chronic glomerulonephritis, chronic pyelonephritis. Because the tubules are unable to actively reabsorb or secrete the solutes, the concentration of the final urine excreted remains unchanged from the original ultrafiltrate that collected in Bowman's space. This is termed *isosthenuria* and is characterized by the fixation of the urine specific gravity (or osmolality) regardless of hydration at 1.010 (or ~290 mOsm/kg), the same as that of the protein-free plasma that passes through the glomeruli. Clinically, isosthenuria or the impairment of renal concentrating ability is manifested by nocturia, the excessive or increased frequency of urination at night. Normally, the amount of urine excreted during the day is 3 to 4 times greater than that excreted during the night. With nocturia, the volume of urine excreted at night essentially equals that excreted during the day.

Osmolality and specific gravity are two tests that are used to determine the solute concentration of the urine. Osmolality determinations are a more accurate indicator of urine concentration than specific gravity measurements because all solutes contribute equally to the osmolality. However, specific gravity determinations are easier and require less time to perform.

## Osmolality

Osmolality is a colligative property of a solution that depends only on the number of solutes present, either as ions or undissociated molecules. When analyzing body fluids, osmolality is expressed in milliosmoles of solutes per kilogram of water, mOsm/kg $H_2O$. Because the renal regulation of water is based on the body's state of hydration, the urine osmolality can vary greatly. Physiologically, the urine osmolality can be as low as 50 mOsm/kg $H_2O$ to as high as 1400 mOsm/kg $H_2O$ (i.e., the same osmolality as the renal interstitium). A low osmolality (e.g., 50 mOsm/kg $H_2O$) indicates a dilute urine, i.e., a large volume of water with a low number of solutes. In contrast, a high osmolality (greater than 800 mOsm/kg $H_2O$) indicates an attempt by the body to retain water while eliminating solutes in as little water as possible.

Urine osmolality measurements alone have limited usefulness. When compared to the plasma osmolality, the degree to which the kidney has concentrated the glomerular ultrafiltrate becomes evident. The regulation of the plasma osmolality is closely monitored and maintained by the action of ADH within a comparatively narrow window of 275 to 300 mOsm/kg $H_2O$. Typically, the urine osmolality ranges from 275 to 900 mOsm/kg $H_2O$, which is 1 to 3 times that of the plasma. The urine-to-plasma osmolality ratio (U/P), which usually resides between 1.0 and 3.0 in healthy individuals, can be used as a crude indicator of the ability to concentrate or dilute the urine. A ratio greater than 3.0 indicates fluid restriction, whereas a ratio less than 1.0 can indicate excessive fluid intake or diabetes insipidus. Note that an indi-

vidual with chronic renal disease and a fixed urine osmolality could have a normal U/P osmolality ratio.

Of the four colligative properties of a solution—osmotic pressure, boiling point elevation, vapor pressure depression, and freezing point depression—osmolality measurements using freezing point or vapor pressure osmometers predominate. In the clinical laboratory, freezing point osmometers are preferred because the presence of volatile solutes (e.g., methanol, ethanol, and ethylene glycol) is detected. In contrast, vapor pressure osmometers are unable to detect or accurately measure the osmolality in solutions that contain volatile solutes. Compared with specific gravity measurements, osmolality is preferred because of its increased accuracy and lack of interference owing to urine temperature or the presence of glucose, protein, or radiographic contrast media.

## Specific Gravity

By definition, specific gravity (SG) is the ratio of a solution's density compared to an equal volume of pure water at a specified temperature. Hence, SG values are a unitless number, and for urine samples, the ratio always exceeds 1.000 because urine contains solutes (i.e., is never as pure as water). Physiologically possible SG values range from as low as 1.002 to as high as 1.040. However, a typical reference interval for urine SG using a random specimen is 1.002 to 1.030. Note that with extreme fluid restriction, the kidneys can concentrate the urine to the same SG as the hypertonic renal mdeulla, that of 1.040.

In contrast to osmolality, SG is a measure of density that is affected by both the number of solutes present and their mass (size). In other words, two solutions with the same number of solutes (millimoles) will have the same osmolality value but can have different SG values if the mass of the solutes is significantly different. The principal solutes present in urine are: urea, chloride, sodium, potassium, ammonium, inorganic phosphate and sulfate, creatinine, and uric acid. They account for more than 99% of the solutes present. Therefore, when the normal urine solutes are present, the urine osmolality and SG measurements provide similar information regarding renal concentrating ability. In contrast, when solutes not normally present in the urine are increased, such as glucose and protein, the urine osmolality value is unaffected, whereas the SG value will increase significantly. The osmolality value is essentially unchanged because the number of glucose or protein molecules is insignificant compared to the total number of urine solutes. However, the density, i.e., SG, of the solution is affected because of the mass of the glucose and protein molecules.

Specific gravity measurements can be obtained using several analytical approaches. Direct measures of solution density include the urinometer and harmonic oscillation densitometry. The urinometer is no longer recommended for clinical laboratory measurements of SG.[17] Harmonic oscillation densitometry is used by International Remote Imaging Systems (Chatsworth, CA) on the Yellow IRIS, a semiautomated urinalysis workstation. It is based on the frequency attenuation of sound waves by solutes in a solution, which is proportional to the solution's density. Because density measurements are temperature dependent, a thermistor monitors sample temperature at the time of measurement and the result corrected for temperature is obtained. This method requires daily calibration and is linear to SG 1.080.

Indirect SG measurements, which predominate in the clinical laboratory, include refractometry and the reagent-strip method. In refractometry, the refractive index of a solution is measured. The refractive index is a ratio of the velocity of light in air compared to the velocity of light in a solution. It is dependent on the density or concentration of the solution, temperature of the solution, and wavelength of light used for the measurements. By controlling the temperature and wavelength of light (589 nm), the refractive index of a solution is proportional to its density or SG. Advantages of refractometry include the small volume of sample needed and the ability to compensate for temperature if the sample is between 15°C and 37°C. A disadvantage is that SG values by refractometry are also disproportionately affected by high molecular weight solutes such as glucose, protein, and radiographic contrast media, but not as great as direct SG methods. Note that physiologically impossible SG values (greater than 1.040) can be obtained on urine samples that contain radiographic contrast media, whereas SG values obtained on urine with increased amounts of glucose or protein will remain in the physiologically possible range (i.e., 1.002 to 1.040).

The commercial reagent-strip method is an indirect colorimetric estimation of SG based on a $pK_a$ change of a polyelectrolyte impregnated into the test pad. As the $pK_a$ changes, a pH indicator also in the pad undergoes a color change. The SG value is obtained by comparing the reaction pad color to color blocks that range from 1.000 to 1.030 in 0.005 increments. On the reaction pad, the $pK_a$ change is directly related to the number of ionic solutes present in the solution. In other words, nonionic solutes regardless of their molecular weight (e.g., glucose) are undetectable by this method. Because renal tubular function predominantly involves the reabsorption and secretion of ionic solutes, the reagent-strip method provides a means to evaluate renal concentrating ability in urine despite the presence of glucose, proteins, or radiographic contrast media.

## TESTS FOR TUBULAR SECRETORY AND REABSORPTIVE FUNCTION

A variety of substances have been used to elucidate renal secretory and reabsorptive function; however, their clinical utility in routine patient management has yet to be established. A challenge to accurately determining renal secretory and reabsorptive function is finding the ideal substance for the evaluation. Ideally, the substance is maintained at a constant plasma concentration, which, if an exogenous substance is used, requires an intravenous infusion. For secretory function, the challenge is finding a substance that does not filter through the glomeruli and is exclusively secreted by the tubules completely in its first pass through the kidneys. Substances that have been used are exogenous and include phenolsulfonphthalein (PSP)

and *p*-aminohippurate (PAH). For reabsorptive function, the substance used should readily pass the glomeruli and be subsequently extensively reabsorbed. The low-molecular-weight plasma proteins such as $\beta_2$-microglobulin ($\beta_2$-M), retinol-binding protein (RBP), and cystatin C have been utilized. A drawback to several of these proteins is that nonrenal factors can influence their plasma concentrations. A brief discussion of two substances, PSP to evaluate secretory function and $\beta_2$-M to evaluate reabsorptive function, is provided.

### Phenolsulfonphthalein

Phenolsulfonphthalein (PSP) is a pH indicator, is an exogenous substance used to evaluate tubular secretory function. The test requires an intravenous infusion of PSP, after which urine samples are collected at 15-minute intervals. In the bloodstream, PSP binds to plasma albumin and cannot pass the glomerular filtration barriers. The PSP-albumin complex is removed from the plasma in the peritubular capillaries and is eliminated into the urine by tubular secretion (94%). If an individual has normal renal plasma flow, then the amount of PSP excreted in each urine collection is dependent solely on renal tubular secretory function.

With normal renal plasma flow and tubular secretory function, 28% to 51% of the injected PSP is secreted in the first 15 minutes, with an additional 13% to 24% secreted in the second 15 minutes.[18] The first 2 urine collections are considered the most clinically diagnostic. Because an intravenous infusion is required and limited diagnostic information is obtained, this test is not routinely performed.

### Beta₂-Microglobulin

Beta₂-microglobulin ($\beta_2$-M) is a nonglycosylated peptide of 11,800 daltons that is present on the surface of most nucleated cells. It is a portion of the class I major histocompatibility complex antigens present on cell surfaces and is shed at essentially a constant rate from cell membranes into the surrounding body fluid. Consequently, $\beta_2$-M is present in all body fluids and its plasma concentration is essentially constant. Because of its small molecular size, $\beta_2$-M readily passes the glomerular filtration barriers and is reabsorbed (99.9%) by the proximal tubular cells where it is catabolized. Hence, only about 0.1% is excreted in the urine.

Increased excretion of $\beta_2$-M in the urine, without an increased plasma level, is indicative of decreased renal tubular reabsorptive function. This can occur in acute tubular necrosis due to drugs and toxins, such as antibiotics (aminoglycosides), chemotherapeutic agents (cyclosporine), heavy metals (mercury, lead), organic solvents (ethylene glycol), and poisons (mushrooms, pesticides). In contrast, plasma levels of $\beta_2$-M are increased in a variety of conditions characterized by increased cell turnover such as with myeloproliferative and lymphoproliferative disorders as well as with viral infections, amyloidosis, autoimmune disorders, and all types of inflammation. In these conditions and assuming normal renal function, $\beta_2$-M does not appear in the urine unless the renal threshold

$(T_m)$ for protein absorption has been exceeded. Because $\beta_2$-M is not removed from the circulation by dialysis, increased plasma levels are also seen in patients on hemodialysis.

Studies suggest that simultaneous plasma and urine $\beta_2$-M levels are valuable (1) as a predictor of graft rejection following renal transplantation, (2) in the differentiation of glomerular and tubular disease, (3) in differentiating graft rejection and drug nephrotoxicity, and (4) in identifying progression to AIDS in HIV-infected individuals.[19,20,21] In addition, plasma $\beta_2$-M levels have clinical value as a prognostic indicator of disease progression in patients with acute lymphocytic leukemia, lymphoma, and multiple myeloma.[22,23] One disadvantage to measurement of $\beta_2$-M levels in urine is its susceptibility to degradation at a pH less than 6.0, which can occur in vivo in the bladder. Therefore, steps to alkalinize the patient (via diet or medication) should be taken before urine collection, and the collections must be appropriately preserved.

## Urinalysis as an Assessment Tool

### ROUTINE URINALYSIS

Urine is actually a fluid biopsy of the kidneys. Hence, a urinalysis (UA) is a valuable tool to screen for as well as to monitor a variety of renal and metabolic diseases. Another advantage of a UA is that a urine specimen is usually easy to obtain and noninvasive. A routine UA consists of 3 distinct testing phases: (1) a physical examination, which assesses urine color, clarity, and concentration, (2) a chemical examination, which chemically tests for substances that provide information about health and disease, and (3) a microscopic examination, which identifies and counts the type of cells, casts, crystals, and other components (bacteria, mucus) that can be present in urine. For accurate results and subsequent interpretation, the urine specimen for a UA must be appropriately collected and stored. Similarly, standardization of each testing phase must be established and maintained to ensure accurate interpretation of results.

### Physical Examination

Two physical characteristics of urine are its color and clarity, i.e., how clear it is. Urine can be a variety of colors, from very pale or colorless to dark amber, with shades of yellow predominating. Atypical or abnormal urine colors (red, blue, orange, green) can also be observed and are associated with the ingestion of substances (e.g., drugs, foods) or can result from disease processes. At times, differentiation between a pathologic and nonpathologic process may be required. For example, a red-colored urine can indicate the presence of blood or can result from the excretion of a natural pigment following beet ingestion (genetic trait). Note that the chemical and microscopic examinations of the UA will assist in determining the cause for the red color.

The depth of urine color is a crude indicator of urine concentration, i.e., the amount of solutes present in the volume of water excreted. A dilute urine will be pale in color, whereas a concentrated urine will be darker. For example, in a healthy individual the first morning urine (no fluids ingested overnight) is darker in color than a urine collected later in the day following a normal diet and fluid ingestion. Measurements of urine concentration include osmolality (a measure of solute number) and specific gravity (a measure of solution density).

Substances that contaminate the urine can also affect its color. Although not exclusively, this is most often encountered in urine specimens from women. Menstrual blood or blood from hemorrhoids that unintentionally gets into a urine specimen during collection can cause a reddish appearance. Note that this contamination will also cause a positive chemical test for blood. Therefore, the need for patients to follow urine collection instructions (e.g., appropriate cleansing, collect midstream) cannot be overemphasized.

The clarity of urine, assessed by visual inspection of a prescribed volume of urine using adequate lighting, is usually reported as clear, slightly cloudy, cloudy or turbid. The clarity of the urine is not as important as the substance that is causing the urine to be cloudy. Some nonpathologic substances that can cause a urine to be cloudy include mucus, sperm, prostatic fluid, epithelium from the skin, normal urine crystals, and contaminants (e.g., body lotions, powders). Other substances that alter the clarity of urine and indicate a pathologic process include red blood cells, white blood cells, and bacteria.

### Chemical Examination

In most clinical laboratories, the chemical examination is performed using commercial reagent test strips, also known as dipsticks. These narrow plastic strips have several separate reaction pads (up to 10), impregnated with chemicals, adhered to them. Each test pad performs a chemical analysis for a particular substance (glucose) or group of substances (ketones). In a typical UA, the chemical examination includes: SG, pH, protein, glucose, ketones, blood, leukocyte esterase, nitrite, bilirubin, and urobilinogen. Some manufacturers include a reaction pad for ascorbic acid because it is frequently present in the urine and is known to interfere with several of the chemical tests depending on the brand of reagent strips.

When a reagent strip is briefly, but completely, immersed into urine, the urine is absorbed into the test pads and a chemical reaction occurs that results in a color change of the pad. The color change for each reaction pad is compared to a color chart provided with the test strips to determine the result for each test. Note that when performing this relatively simple test, timing is very important. To be accurate, each reaction pad must be evaluated at the appropriate time interval. If too little time or too much time has passed, erroneous results can be obtained. To reduce these potential timing irregularities as well as to eliminate individual differences in color interpretation, instruments are frequently used to assess or read the reaction color of each test pad.

**SPECIFIC GRAVITY**    For a discussion of the reagent strip SG test, see previous section, Tests for Renal Concentrating Ability.

Note that SG is a physical characteristic of the urine; however, it can be determined using a chemical test.

**pH** The reagent strip pH test uses two pH indicators to determine the urine pH. Physiologically possible values for urine range from pH 4.5 to 8.0. The kidneys play an important role in maintaining the acid-base balance of the body. In response to conditions that produce acids or base in the body or to the ingestion of acids or alkalis, the kidneys will excrete these substances in the urine, thereby, directly affecting the urine pH. Urine pH can provide valuable information to assess and manage disorders as well as to determine whether a urine specimen is suitable for chemical testing (i.e., that it has been proper stored, is unadulterated).

Diet directly affects the urine pH. A diet high in protein will result in urine with an acid pH. In contrast, a vegetarian diet, low-carbohydrate diet, or the ingestion of citrus fruits cause a more alkaline urine. The pH of the urine (along with other factors) can induce dissolved urinary solutes to precipitate out in an amorphous or crystalline form. If this occurs while the urine is in vivo (within the nephron, renal pelvis, ureter, or bladder), a renal stone or calculus can form. These are solid aggregates of the solutes that are normally dissolved in the urine. By modifying the urine pH through diet or medications, precipitation of these solutes in vivo can be reduced or eliminated.

After the collection of urine into a specimen container, its temperature decreases from body temperature to room temperature or to refrigerator temperature depending on its storage. This cooling, along with the urine pH, determines which solutes can precipitate out of solution. Because some solutes form similar crystalline or amorphous forms, their specific identification and differentiation requires knowledge of the urine pH.

**PROTEIN** The reagent strip protein test is based on the protein error of indicators and is most sensitive to albumin. Although technically all proteins can be detected by this method, they are rarely encountered in the urine at concentrations high enough to produce a positive test. Early detection of protein by a reagent strip test, such as during a routine urinalysis, aids in the identification, treatment, and prevention of kidney disease. Conditions other than kidney disease that can also result in proteinuria include multiple myeloma, hemolytic conditions, inflammation, malignancies, and injuries of the urinary tract (e.g., bladder, prostate, urethra). Also, transitory proteinuria can occur with strenuous exercise, fever, and stress. Note that vaginal secretions that get into the urine during collection could also cause a positive protein test.

**GLUCOSE** Glucose is normally not present in urine. If present, it results from an excessively high glucose concentration in the blood such that the ability of the kidneys to reabsorb the glucose has been exceeded or a renal tubular dysfunction in which the ability to absorb glucose is diminished or lost. Excessively high plasma glucose concentrations are most often encountered in individuals with diabetes mellitus who have not achieved adequate control with insulin. However, other conditions that can be associated with a high plasma glucose level include hormonal disorders, liver disease, certain medications, and pregnancy. Renal tubular dysfunction that affects glucose reabsorption includes any condition that alters proximal tubular function such as acute tubular necrosis or the Fanconi syndrome. The reagent-strip test for glucose employs the enzyme glucose oxidase; hence, this test is specific for the detection of glucose.

**KETONES** Ketones (acetone, acetoacetate and β-hydroxybutyrate) are normally not detectable in urine nor are they present at an appreciable level in the plasma. They are intermediate products of fat metabolism and are produced when the body turns to fat metabolism to obtain the energy it needs to keep functioning. Consequently, when urine ketones are present they indicate either an inadequate amount of carbohydrate consumption (starvation, certain dietary regimens) or that the carbohydrates consumed cannot be utilized (e.g., diabetes mellitus). Detection of ketones in the urine provides an early indicator of insufficient insulin in a diabetic individual. Note that severe exercise, cold exposure, and loss of carbohydrates (e.g., frequent vomiting) can also increase fat metabolism, resulting in ketonuria.

The reagent-strip ketone tests are variations of the nitroprusside reaction (Legal's test). Depending on the reagent-strip manufacturer, either acetoacetate or both acetoacetate and acetone can be detected. However, this test can be falsely positive if substances that contain a free-sulfhydryl group are also present in the urine. Such substances are common and include cysteine (amino acid), captopril (antihypertensive agent), MESNA (chemotherapeutic rescue agent), N-acetylcysteine (treatment regimen for acetaminophen overdose), and others. Fortunately, the addition of glacial acetic acid directly to the reaction pad can identify these false-positive tests. If the positive purple color fades or disappears, it indicates the presence of a substance with free-sulfhydryl groups. If true ketones are present, the color will not fade or disappear despite acid addition. In fact, with true ketones the purple color will darken with time.

**BLOOD** The reagent-strip blood test should be more appropriately called the reagent-strip *heme moiety* test. It is based on the pseudoperoxidase activity of the heme moiety—protoporphyrin IXa. The two substances with the heme moiety most frequently encountered in urine are hemoglobin and, to a lesser extent, myoglobin.

Normally, a small number of RBCs are present in the urine, and this chemical test is negative. However, when the number of RBCs increases abnormally, a positive test is obtained. Even small increases in the number of RBCs in urine are significant. Numerous diseases of the kidney and urinary tract, as well as trauma, medications, smoking, or strenuous exercise, can result in hematuria or hemoglobinuria.

Myoglobinuria results from muscle injury and muscle diseases such that myoglobin is released from the muscles into the surrounding body fluids. Within muscles, myoglobin is a heme–containing protein involved in oxygen transport. Because of its small molecular size (17,000), myoglobin readily passes the glomerular filtration barriers and is reabsorbed by the proximal tubular cells. Note that both hemoglobin and myoglobin are toxic to tubular cells and if large amounts are absorbed, they can cause acute tubular necrosis.

The reagent-strip blood test provides an early indicator of disease and always requires further investigation. The amount of blood in the urine does not correlate with disease severity nor can the location of the bleed be identified from this test. Contamination of urine with blood from hemorrhoids or vaginal bleeding cannot be distinguished from a bleed in the urinary tract; thereby, highlighting the importance of proper urine collection.

Ascorbic acid (vitamin C) can interfere with the reagent-strip blood test depending on the brand of commercial reagent strips used. If significant amounts of ascorbic acid are present, the test for blood can be falsely low or negative. Hence, laboratories that use reagent strips susceptible to ascorbic acid must be alert for this potential interferent. Most often, the presence of ascorbic acid is intercepted when a discrepancy is encountered, such as the microscopic examination reveals an increased number of RBCs but the reagent-strip blood test is negative.

**LEUKOCYTE ESTERASE**   Leukocyte esterase, an enzyme present in granulocytic white blood cells (WBCs), includes neutrophils, monocytes, and macrophages. This enzyme is not present in lymphocytes. Normally a few WBCs are present in urine and this test is negative. However, when the number of granulocytic WBCs in urine increases significantly, this screening test will become positive. The presence of increased numbers of granulocytic WBCs in urine most often indicates an inflammatory condition somewhere in the urinary tract or kidneys, e.g., bladder infection, pyelonephritis. However, as with the reagent-strip blood test, proper urine collection is important to prevent contamination with vaginal secretions that can also contain WBCs.

The reagent strip test for leukocyte esterase is based on an azo-coupling reaction to form an azo dye. The reaction is not affected by the presence of ascorbic acid.

**NITRITE**   The reagent-strip nitrite test is an important screening tool for the identification of urinary tract infections (UTIs). Normally, nitrite is not present in the urine. However, if bacteria are present in the urinary system (e.g., urethra, bladder or kidney) <u>and</u> they are capable of converting dietary nitrates into nitrite, this test can be positive. The nitrite test is considered a screening test because it can still be negative despite a urinary tract infection. This phenomenon occurs when the infecting bacteria are not capable of converting nitrate to nitrite, when insufficient dietary nitrates are consumed, if in-

sufficient time has elapsed for nitrate to nitrite conversion, or if nitrites are lost due to storage conditions.

The nitrite reaction is based on an azo-coupling reaction to form an azo dye. The reagent strip brands differ with regard to the amine and aromatic compounds impregnated into the pad for the azo-coupling reaction. Substances that produce a highly colored urine, such as phenazopyridine (a urinary analgesic) can mask the pale pink color that indicates a positive test.

**BILIRUBIN**   In healthy individuals, bilirubin is not normally present in the urine. It is a by-product of heme catabolism that is initially unconjugated and bound to albumin in the circulating plasma. Because it is bound to albumin, the kidneys cannot excrete unconjugated bilirubin. It is removed from the circulation by the liver where it is conjugated and normally transferred to the biliary system for excretion into the intestine. However, in certain liver diseases such as biliary obstruction or hepatitis, conjugated bilirubin can leak back into the bloodstream. Because conjugated bilirubin is water soluble and not bound to albumin, it readily passes the glomeruli and is excreted in the urine. The presence of bilirubin in urine is an early indicator of liver disease and can occur before any other clinical symptoms.

The reagent-strip test for bilirubin is also based on an azo-coupling reaction. Bilirubin is an aromatic compound that reacts with a diazonium salt impregnated in the reaction pad. When conjugated bilirubin is present in sufficient quantities ($\sim$0.5 mg/dL), an azo-dye forms and the color of the reaction pad changes.

**UROBILINOGEN**   Urobilinogen is formed in the gastrointestinal tract from bilirubin. A significant amount is absorbed back into the bloodstream ($\sim$20%) and a portion (2–5%) is ultimately excreted in the urine. In healthy subjects, the urobilinogen concentration in a random urine is 1 mg/dL or less.

The chemical reaction for urobilinogen differs depending on the brand of reagent strips. Several brands use a specific azo-coupling reaction, whereas one brand uses a nonspecific modified Ehrlich's reaction. Regardless, these tests are unable to accurately detect decreased amounts or the absence of urobilinogen in urine; rather they are best able to detect normal and increased amounts of urine urobilinogen. As with urine bilirubin, urine urobilinogen aids in the identification and differentiation of liver diseases as well as in identifying conditions associated with increased RBC destruction. Note that this test will have limited clinical utility in cases of hepatic and biliary obstruction where the urine urobilinogen will be decreased or absent.

### Microscopic Examination

The microscopic examination involves pouring a specific volume of well-mixed urine (usually 12 mL) into a conical-bottomed tube and centrifuging it under specified conditions. The particulate matter (cells, bacteria, casts, crystals) in the urine will collect as a sediment in the bottom of the tube.

Typically, most of the supernatant urine (11 mL) is carefully removed and the sediment in the bottom of the tube is resuspended in the remaining 1 mL of urine. A specific volume (~15 $\mu$L) of this urine sediment is then evaluated using a microscope. Standardization of the microscopic examination is important and necessary to ensure accuracy and reproducibility among laboratories and laboratorians.

When performing the microscopic examination, the urine sediment is visualized using both a low power view (LPF; 100×) and a high power view (HPF; 400×). Each entity (cell, crystal, etc.) is counted and reported either as the number observed per field of view or as the number per milliliter of sediment (e.g., 0 to 2 per HPF, or 4400 per mL). If performing the examination at a microscope, this latter reporting format is rarely used because additional calculations are required. With urine workstations or instruments such as the Yellow Iris, where the microscopic examination is automated, this reporting format is readily available. Small entities such as RBCs, WBCs, and bacteria are reported using high power. Large elements such as squamous epithelial cells and casts are reported using low power magnification. In addition, some entities are not enumerated but estimated as few, moderate, or many, such as in estimating epithelial cells, bacteria, and crystals.

**RED BLOOD CELLS**    Normally, a few red blood cells (RBCs) are present in urine sediment, typically 0 to 3 cells per HPF. Inflammation, injury, or disease in the kidneys as well as elsewhere in the urinary tract (e.g., bladder, urethra) can result in the loss of RBCs into the surrounding tissue and into the urine. Differentiation of RBCs that originated in the urinary tract from contamination due to hemorrhoids or menstruation is impossible.

**WHITE BLOOD CELLS**    The number of white blood cells (WBCs) in urine sediment is normally 0 to 8 per HPF. WBCs are an important part of the body's defense and are able to migrate from the bloodstream into any tissue or cavity of the body. When present in increased numbers in the urine sediment, they indicate an infection or inflammation somewhere in the urinary tract. Care must be taken during specimen collection, particularly in women, to prevent vaginal secretions that can have high numbers of WBCs from contaminating the urine.

**EPITHELIAL CELLS**    In the urinary tract, as well as elsewhere in the body, the epithelium is continually sloughed. Normally in men and women, a few epithelial cells from the bladder (transitional epithelial cells) or from the external urethra (squamous epithelial cells) can be found in the urine sediment. In healthy subjects, renal tubular cells originating from the nephrons in the kidney are less commonly observed in the urine sediment. With urinary tract conditions, such as infection, inflammation, and malignancy, increased numbers of epithelial cells can be found. The predominant cells present can help localize the site in the urinary tract where the condition resides. For example, in an individual with a bladder infection, increased numbers of transitional epithelial cells are typically found in the urine sediment.

During the microscopic examination, epithelial cells are classified as squamous, transitional, or renal tubular and each type is individually reported as few, moderate, or many present.

**MICROORGANISMS**    In healthy subjects, the urinary tract is sterile and no microorganisms are present. This environment is maintained by the flushing of urine from the urethra, which aids in preventing external microorganisms from entering the urinary system. When present, microorganisms are usually reported as few, moderate, or many per HPF.

Note that particularly in women, due to their anatomy, bacteria from the surrounding skin could enter the urinary tract at the urethra and move up to the bladder to cause a urinary tract infection (UTI). If left unchecked, this bacterial infection could eventually migrate up into the kidneys and cause pyelonephritis. Therefore, in women in particular, care must be taken during urination to prevent bacteria that normally reside on the skin or in vaginal secretions from either entering the urinary system or from contaminating a urine collection. Also in women (and rarely in men), yeast can be present in the urine. In women, they are most often present because the urine has been contaminated with vaginal secretions (i.e., vaginal yeast infection) during the collection. While a yeast infection in the urinary system is possible, they are rare and occur almost exclusively in immunocompromised patients.

Trichomonads are flagellate parasites that can be observed in the urine from men (rarely) or women. As with yeast, the trichomonads are actually infecting the vaginal mucus membranes and their presence in urine is due to contamination during the urine collection.

**CASTS**    Casts are formed in the tubules of the kidney. They are cylindrical because they form in the distal and collecting tubules of the nephrons. The epithelial cells of the distal tubule (straight portion) secrete Tamm-Horsfall protein, which can subsequently gel in the tubules taking their shape. When this occurs, a hyaline cast is formed. During renal disease processes, elements present in the tubular lumens, for example, RBCs, WBCs, renal epithelial cells, fat, can become trapped in the gel matrix as the cast is being formed. Different types of casts are associated with different kidney diseases. For example, WBC casts are associated with renal inflammation or infection such as acute pyelonephritis or acute interstitial nephritis.

In healthy subjects, a few (0 to 5) hyaline casts or finely granular casts can be present per LPF. With strenuous exercise, the number of hyaline casts can be dramatically increased. In contrast, cellular casts, such as RBC, WBC and renal tubular cell casts, and fatty casts, are considered indicative of disease.

**CRYSTALS**    The numerous solutes dissolved in the urine can precipitate out of solution in amorphous or crystalline forms. The precipitation of solute crystals is dependent on the urine pH, the solute's concentration, and the urine temperature. When present in urine, they are identified on the basis of their shape, color, and the urine pH. Crystals are considered normal if they are from solutes that should be in the urine. If they are from solutes that are not normally present in appreciable amounts in the urine such as amino acids (cystine, tyrosine, leucine, etc.), bilirubin, or cholesterol, they are considered abnormal. Medications (e.g., sulfonamides, ampicillin) and radiographic contrast media can also precipitate in urine. Therefore, it is important that the laboratorian be familiar with and trained in the identification of urine crystals.

When crystals form in the tubules of the kidney, they can coalesce together to form kidney stones or calculi. These stones can become lodged in the kidney itself or in the ureters and cause extreme pain.

**FAT**  When a urine specimen contains a large amount of protein as determined by the chemical examination ($\geq$300 mg/dL), the urine sediment should be screened for the presence of fat during the microscopic examination. Most often, urinary fat originates from the plasma and enters the tubular lumen due to the changes in glomerular permeability; the same changes that allow the increased amount of plasma albumin (protein) in the urine. In these cases, the fat is usually both triglycerides (also known as neutral fat) and cholesterol. Fat stains, such as Sudan III or Oil Red O, can be used to positively identify triglycerides, whereas polarizing microscopy can be used to readily identify cholesterol. Fat can be present in three forms: (1) as free-floating globules; (2) as inclusions within casts, and (3) within cells, called oval fat bodies.

When reporting the microscopic examination results, each form of fat present is reported, e.g., 0 to 2 fatty casts per LPF, 2 to 5 oval fat bodies per HPF, few fat globules per HPF. Note that the type of fat present is not important, rather it is recognizing and reporting its presence in the urine that is important. Lipiduria is a characteristic feature of the nephrotic syndrome and other glomerular disorders. Monitoring the presence and amount of urinary fat in urine sediment can aid the clinician in following the progression or regression of these conditions.

## Cytodiagnostic Urinalysis

Cytodiagnostic urinalysis (CU) is not a routine screening test for urine but is a test used to evaluate and monitor individuals with signs, symptoms, or histories of renal and urinary tract disease. This diagnostic urine test combines the physical and chemical examinations of a UA with a quantitative microscopic examination that utilizes a Papanicolaou (PAP)-stained permanent slide of the urine sediment obtained using cytocentrifugation.

To accurately perform a CU microscopic examination, additional microscopic and cytologic expertise is required. Because a PAP-stained slide of urine sediment is quantitatively evaluated, advantages of a CU include the ability to (1) better discriminate between various mononuclear cells (e.g., lym-

phocytes, plasma cells, eosinophils, macrophages); (2) identify inclusion-bearing cells (viral, drug, and heavy metal-induced); (3) specifically identify certain pathologic casts (e.g., eosinophil, fibrin, fungal, hemoglobin); (4) identify precancerous and malignant cells; (5) distinguish between ischemic and non-ischemic renal tubular injury, and (6) diagnose and monitor diseases characterized by renal parenchymal injury (e.g., acute tubular necrosis, tubulointerstitial inflammation, acute renal graft rejection, glomerular lesions).

CU requires considerable more time and technical expertise; therefore, it is more costly than a routine UA. However, it provides invaluable clinical information that can reduce the number of renal biopsies and other invasive procedures that may be needed to evaluate certain conditions.

# CLINICAL APPLICATIONS

## Renal Disease

Renal diseases can be classified on the basis of the initial or primary morphologic component affected as glomerular, tubular, interstitial, or vascular. However, because of the close structural and functional interactions of these components within the kidney, as a disease progresses, multiple components can become involved. Some renal conditions are transient, and with appropriate treatment, normal renal function can be reestablished, e.g., acute renal failure, nephrotic syndrome. In contrast, others cause permanent, ongoing loss of functional renal tissue that ultimately results in ESRD, e.g., chronic renal failure. The clinical laboratory plays a vital role in the diagnosis of renal disease as well as in monitoring the effectiveness of treatment.

### RENAL FAILURE

#### Acute Renal Failure

Acute renal failure (ARF) refers to a sudden decrease in the GFR and is caused by a diverse group of clinical conditions. Its clinical features are primarily azotemia (markedly elevated plasma UN and creatinine) and oliguria (urine output less than 400 mL), which in some cases evolves to anuria (no urine output). It is important to note that in ARF, despite their inability to function appropriately, the nephrons are morphologically normal. This explains the fact that ARF is usually reversible, in contrast to chronic renal failure (CRF), which is not. However, ARF has a high mortality rate, which is often the result of secondary infections, heart failure, or other treatment-related causes (e.g., potassium intoxication).

Acute renal failure is usually classified according to the underlying cause as prerenal, renal, or postrenal. Prerenal causes are characterized by a sudden decrease in renal blood flow, thereby directly affecting renal function. These include cardiac failure or any condition that suddenly reduces the circulating blood volume, such as hemorrhage, burns, and surgical procedures. When the blood pressure in the afferent arterioles falls below 80 mm Hg, glomerular filtration is dramatically reduced. The kidney's autoregulatory system (increased reabsorption of sodium and water to increase blood volume) works diligently to reestablish an adequate blood flow. If successful, the amount of ischemic tissue damage is minimal and reversible. However, if the ischemic episode is prolonged, severe damage to the renal tubules can result that superimposes a renal type of ARF onto the initial prerenal cause.

In prerenal ARF, the UN/creatinine ratio is increased, usually greater than 20, because of decreased urine flow, which disproportionally increases the reabsorption of urea. A routine UA is unremarkable. In contrast, urine electrolytes are particularly useful in identifying prerenal ARF. The urine sodium will be low, usually less than 15 mmol/L, due to the increased renal tubular reabsorption.

Renal ARF is characterized by renal tissue damage. With acute tubular necrosis responsible for approximately 99% of all renal ARF cases. In contrast to prerenal ARF, the urine sodium concentration increases significantly to 40 to 70 mmol/L or higher in renal ARF. This is due to the loss of tubular reabsorptive function. Additionally, the UN/creatinine ratio is often less than 10.

The cause of postrenal ARF is obstruction to urine flow within the urinary system. The presence of anuria is suggestive of obstruction. Note that any obstruction above the bladder must occur bilaterally (i.e., in both ureters or kidneys) because a single operational kidney is sufficient to perform all renal functions. As a consequence of the obstruction, hydrostatic pressure within the tubules and Bowman's space dramatically increases. This pressure alteration disrupts glomerular flow, significantly reducing the GFR, causing ARF. Obstruction in elderly men is frequently caused by prostatic hypertrophy. Other causes include tumors, as well as the deposition of drug or amino acid crystals (calculi) within the nephrons. A routine UA is usually unremarkable; however, if tumors or calculi are responsible, hematuria and numerous crystals are usually present.

## Chronic Renal Failure

Chronic renal failure (CRF) is characterized by the slow, progressive loss of functional nephrons such that the GFR continuously decreases. Initially, the remaining healthy nephrons are able to compensate for the loss in functional tissue but eventually the loss is too great. Clinically, the decreased GFR does not become evident until it has been reduced to 10 to 20 mL/minute. At this time, the individual will also present with azotemia, acid-base imbalance, electrolyte and water imbalance, hyperphosphatemia, and hypocalcemia. Other clinical manifestations include anemia and bleeding tendencies, hypertension, indigestion, and neurologic dysfunction. The predominant UA findings include a fixed urine SG at ~1.010, proteinuria, hematuria, and numerous casts. In particular, the presence of renal failure casts that indicate significant urinary

stasis in the nephrons, such as waxy casts and broad casts (that form in the large collecting ducts).

Chronic renal failure has been classified according to the amount of renal function that remains. Stage 1 is indicated when 50% to 70% of renal function remains; stage 2 with 25% to 50%; stage 3 with 10% to 25%, and stage 4 with 0% to 10% of renal functions.[24] At each stage, the degree of azotemia (creatinine and urea nitrogen concentrations) also increases. Hence, CRF eventually culminates with stage 4, also known as end-stage renal disease (ESRD). At this stage, in order to sustain life, dialysis or transplantation is required.

Chronic renal disease results from numerous renal and initially nonrenal disorders, with glomerulonephritis and pyelonephritis accounting for 60% to 70% of CRF cases. Other diseases include diabetic nephropathy, chronic hypertension, autoimmune diseases (e.g., systemic lupus erythematosus, amyloidosis), vascular diseases, and congenital abnormalities (e.g., polycystic kidney disease, hereditary nephritis).

## GLOMERULAR DISEASES

Glomerular disease is characterized by damage to the glomeruli, which subsequently affects the GFR and other renal functions. These diseases can a have a sudden onset or be slow and progressive for years. They can cause temporary or permanent, irreversible changes in renal function. The etiology of glomerular disease is diverse and can be categorized as hereditary (e.g., Alport's syndrome), metabolic (e.g., diabetes mellitus), or immunologic (e.g., systemic lupus erythematosus) based.

Glomerular diseases are most often immunologically mediated. In 70% to 80% of glomerulonephritis cases, the deposition of immune complexes within glomeruli can be demonstrated. This process can occur from several mechanisms. One scenario is the entrapment of immune complexes from the bloodstream within the glomeruli. These complexes initiate complement binding and a cascade of immune-response events occurs that causes glomerular damage. Another similar pathway is that of an autoimmune process involving the direct interaction of autoantibodies with glomerular tissue antigens. Circulating antibodies can interact with exogenous antigens that currently or temporarily reside in the glomeruli, such as medications or infectious agents (bacterial, viral). It is important to note that the resultant glomerular damage does not occur from the immune complexes but rather from the chemical mediators and toxic substances that are produced due to immune complex formation.

Glomerular diseases have been categorized by their distinct morphologic changes, which include (1) cellular proliferation within the glomeruli, (2) leukocyte infiltration of the glomeruli, (3) thickening of the basement membrane of the glomeruli, and (4) sclerosis of the glomeruli. The consequence of each of these morphologic changes is alterations in glomerular permeability.

Two syndromes indicative of renal glomerular permeability changes are the nephritic syndrome and the nephrotic syndrome. By definition, a syndrome is a group of findings that occur simultaneously and does not indicate a particular disease, i.e., different diseases can present with the same syndrome. Glomerular damage can result from a primary renal disease or from a systemic disease; consequently, either syndrome can also be manifested with the disease. The **nephritic syndrome** is characterized by variable degrees of hematuria, proteinuria, azotemia, oliguria, edema, and hypertension. In contrast, the **nephrotic syndrome** is characterized by severe proteinuria with lipiduria, hypoproteinemia, hyperlipidemia, and edema. The classic example of the nephritic syndrome is acute glomerulonephritis (AGN); whereas, the nephrotic syndrome occurs with a variety of glomerular diseases as well as systemic diseases such as diabetes mellitus, systemic lupus erythematosus, and amyloidosis.

## Acute Glomerulonephritis

AGN presents with a sudden decrease in the GFR. Consequently, the plasma UN and creatinine (azotemia) increase and oliguria occurs. Fever, malaise, and nausea are additional features. Hypertension is not unusual due to increased sodium and water retention, which in some cases evolves further into congestive heart failure.

Typical urinalysis results from patients with acute glomerulonephritis (AGN) include moderate proteinuria with differing degrees of hematuria. In the urine sediment, two classic microscopic findings are the presence of dysmorphic RBCs and RBC casts. Other typical urine sediment findings include increased WBCs, renal tubular epithelial cells, cellular casts, and granular casts.

One common form of AGN is acute poststreptococcal glomerulonephritis, which occurs a few weeks after a recent infection with group A β-hemolytic streptococci. As with other immune-mediated disorders, the delay in onset of this glomerular disease is directly related to the time needed for antibody formation.

Recovery from AGN is usually followed by the return of normal renal function. However, a small subset of these individuals, particularly adults, go on to develop chronic glomerulonephritis for reasons not clearly elucidated.

## Chronic Glomerulonephritis

It is theorized that all individuals with chronic glomerulonephritis (GN) at some time previously had a form of glomerulonephritis. The timeframe for the development of this disease is slow and silent over many years. Detection usually occurs after significant renal tissue is no longer functional. Morphologic examination of renal biopsies from individuals with chronic glomerulonephritis reveals irreversible damage consisting of hyalinized glomeruli, atrophied tubules, fibrosis in the renal parenchyma, and often lymphocytic infiltrations. Clinical findings include azotemia, proteinuria (>2.5 g per day), isosthenuria, hematuria, hypertension, and edema. Typical urine sediment findings include increased RBCs, WBCs, renal epithelial cells, and all types of casts, particularly granular, waxy, and broad. Because the loss of functional renal tissue is irreversible, these individuals ultimately develop ESRD and require hemodialysis or renal transplantation to sustain life.

## Nephrotic Syndrome

The nephrotic syndrome is characterized by features that are indicative of extreme changes in glomerular permeability, they include severe proteinuria (>3.5 g/day), hypoproteinemia, hyperlipidemia (often serum cholesterol values exceed 350 mg/dL), lipiduria, and edema. Because of glomerular alterations, large amounts of plasma albumin are excreted in the urine, resulting in hypoproteinemia. Simultaneously, the intravascular oncotic pressure associated with albumin is lost, resulting in the movement of plasma water out of the vasculature into the tissues, i.e., edema. In an attempt to compensate for this loss in oncotic pressure, the liver alters lipid metabolism, resulting in hyperlipidemia. It decreases lipid catabolism and increases the production of plasma lipids (e.g., cholesterol, triglycerides, phospholipids, very low-density lipoproteins). Hence, in the nephrotic syndrome, the edema and hyperlipidemia are actually secondary features that result from the profound changes in glomerular permeability and the subsequent loss of plasma albumin.

Lipiduria is indicative and usually pathognomonic of glomerular permeability changes. Because the GFB has been compromised by disease, the size selectivity of the barrier has been lost and plasma lipids pass into the ultrafiltrate in Bowman's space. The ability of the tubules to reabsorb these lipids is exceeded and they appear in the urine. Note that to have lipiduria, proteinuria must also be present. However, it is possible to have proteinuria without lipiduria, i.e., the GFB is not altered enough to permit passage of plasma lipids. Lipiduria is identified during the microscopic examination of urine sediment, where lipids (i.e., cholesterol and triglycerides) can be found as: (1) free-floating fat globules, (2) fat globules entrapped within casts, or (3) fat within cells, called oval fat bodies. Because other microscopic entities can look similar, fat in urine sediment should be confirmed using fat stains or polarizing microscopy. Other urine sediment findings associated with the nephrotic syndrome include an increase in RBCs (usually small), renal epithelial cells, and all types of casts, particularly fatty and waxy.

Numerous renal and systemic diseases can present with the nephrotic syndrome. In children, 90% of nephrotic syndrome cases accompanies a renal glomerular disease compared to 75% in adults. The remaining cases result primarily from systemic disorders such as diabetes mellitus, systemic lupus erythematosus, amyloidosis, or from nephrotoxic agents (e.g., drugs).

## Nephropathy and Systemic Diseases

Nephropathy is a general term that indicates a disease process involving the kidneys. Renal involvement is a well-documented complication of a variety of diverse systemic diseases. Most often, at least initially, the disease affects glomerular function. However, because of the close relationship between glomerular function with peritubular blood flow and tubular function, as a disease progresses, tubular function can also become compromised.

Diabetic nephropathy is a common complication of both type 1 and type 2 diabetes mellitus, with the development of renal disease directly related to hyperglycemia. Therefore, in diabetic individuals, tight control of blood glucose levels and monitoring for microalbuminuria play a key role in the prevention of nephropathy.

Individuals with systemic lupus erythematosus (SLE) will, at some time in the course of their disease, demonstrate renal involvement also called lupus nephritis. Many of the morphologic glomerular changes seen with the different immune-mediated forms of glomerulonephritis are also seen with SLE. Hence, as SLE progresses, these individuals present clinically with either the nephritic and nephrotic syndromes, depending on the extent of renal involvement. It is worth noting that chronic renal failure is a leading case of death for individuals with SLE.

Persistent and ongoing hypertension can cause the development of nephropathy, also known as hypertensive nephropathy. Conversely, renal failure itself can induce hypertension. It is a serious complication that actually accelerates the course of ESRD, in which increases in total body salt and water and the subsequent activation of the renin-angiotensin-aldosterone system are key factors responsible for its development. Regardless of the cause of hypertension, periodic urine testing for microalbuminuria provides a clinically useful tool to identify and monitor individuals with this nephropathy.

By virtue of the fact that renal function is directly dependent on adequate renal perfusion, vascular diseases can also cause renal dysfunction. Any morphologic alterations such as arterial narrowing or occlusion can decrease perfusion to the renal parenchyma, resulting in tissue ischemia. Vascular diseases that can develop a renal component include arteriosclerosis, thrombosis, embolism, and vasculitis.

## TUBULAR DISEASES

A diverse group of disorders can affect renal tubular function, thereby reducing the tubular reabsorption and secretion of solutes and their ability to concentrate the urine. They can be inherited or be induced secondarily, involve a single solute (glucose) or a group of solutes (neutral amino acids), and develop into renal failure or simply cause ongoing, low-level impairment of renal function. Clinically, these alterations in tubular function are manifested by either the presence of a solute in the urine in an increased amount (e.g., glucose), the development of a disorder because the substance is lost (e.g., phosphaturia caused by hypophosphatemic rickets), or renal injury resulting from the solute excretion (e.g., cystine calculi). This includes a vast array of disorders that exceed the scope of this text. Renal tubular disorders are relatively uncommon and include renal tubular acidosis, the Fanconi syndrome, cystinuria, cystinosis, renal phosphaturia, and renal glycosuria. Of these, the most commonly encountered clinically is the *Fanconi syndrome*. This syndrome is characterized by generalized proximal

tubular dysfunction. In other words, essentially all the solutes that are normally reabsorbed from the ultrafiltrate by the proximal tubules appear in the urine (glucose, proteins, amino acids, phosphate, potassium, sodium, bicarbonate, calcium, magnesium, uric acid, etc.). The Fanconi syndrome can be inherited at variable degrees of dysfunction or be induced by heavy-metal poisoning, medications, chemical exposure, malignancies, and other renal diseases.

In contrast, **acute tubular necrosis** (ATN) is a clinical condition characterized by the destruction of renal tubular epithelial cells. It is caused either by the development of renal tissue ischemia or from the processing of toxic substances by the renal tubular epithelium. Causes of ischemic ATN include sepsis, shock, and trauma with postoperative conditions accounting for approximately 50% of all ATN cases.[25] Toxic ATN is caused by myoglobin and hemoglobin as well as by numerous nephrotoxic agents such as drugs (e.g., antibiotics, anesthetics, radiographic contrast media, chemotherapeutic agents) and toxins (e.g., heavy metals, organic solvents, pesticides, poisonous mushroom ingestion). The clinical presentation of ATN is abrupt, developing into renal failure with azotemia, hyperkalemia, metabolic acidosis, and oliguria. The tubular damage from ATN is reversible and usually a full recovery of renal tubular function occurs.

Toxic and ischemic ATN can be differentiated by identification of the type of renal tubular epithelium that is destroyed and sloughed into the urine sediment. A cytodiagnostic urinalysis provides the best means of making this distinction; however, a routine UA microscopic examination performed by an experienced microscopist can also provide the information needed. Renal tubular epithelial cells are sloughed singly or in fragments (3 or more cells with attached borders). The predominant cell types that appear in the urine sediment with toxic ATN are proximal convoluted tubular cells; whereas, with ischemic ATN, collecting duct cells predominate. Both forms of ATN will also have mild proteinuria, hematuria, leukocyturia, and increased pathologic casts, particularly renal cellular, granular, waxy, and broad casts. Because of the reduced tubular function during the acute phase of the disease, the urine specific gravity is usually low. Cytodiagnostic urinalysis or routine urinalysis is also a useful tool for monitoring disease progression and resolution.

## TUBULOINTERSTITIAL DISEASE

Renal diseases that primarily involve the renal interstitium and tubules are often specified as tubulointerstitial diseases. They are frequently subdivided based on their clinical course as acute or chronic. These diseases can be initiated by a variety of events such as bacterial infections, exposure to chemicals, immunologic reactions, congenital anatomic abnormalities, and physical injury or are secondary to another condition (e.g., diabetes mellitus, multiple myeloma, hyperuricemia). Sometimes the cause of tubulointerstitial disease is never elucidated despite numerous tests, including renal biopsy. However, the most common causes for acute onset of disease are pyelonephritis and drug-induced hypersensitivity (also called *interstitial nephritis*).

**Acute pyelonephritis** is an infective process, with sudden onset, that involves the renal interstitium, tubules, and renal pelvis. The infection causes interstitial edema and the infiltration of lymphocytes, neutrophils, and plasma cells to form an inflammatory infiltrate. Several conditions promote the development of a bacterial infection in the kidney, the most common being the migration of bacteria from a bladder infection, up the ureters, into the kidney. There are several predisposing factors that enhance this upward migration and the development of pyelonephritis, which include catheterization, congenital anatomic abnormalities, pregnancy, urinary obstruction, preexisting renal lesions as well as metabolic conditions (e.g., diabetes mellitus).

In contrast, **acute interstitial nephritis** (AIN) is an immune-mediated tubulointerstitial disease that occurs in response to drugs or toxins. With medications, it occurs 3 to 21 days after the initiation of drug therapy. It occurs most often with the use of antibiotics such as the penicillins and sulfonamides; however, furosemide, phenylbutazone, and other types of drugs have also been involved. As these medications are processed by the nephrons of the kidney, they become concentrated in the ultrafiltrate and elicit an immune response. Consequently, an inflammatory infiltrate invades the renal tubules and interstitium, compromising renal function. Clinically, these individuals present with a fever and a skin rash (in ~25% of patients). Two notable features unique to drug-induced AIN are (1) the presence of significant numbers of eosinophils in the renal tissue infiltrate as well as in the urine sediment (observed using special stains), and (2) cessation of the offending drug halts the disease and full renal function usually returns.

**Chronic pyelonephritis** is most often caused by vesicoureteral reflux, metabolic conditions (increased excretion of oxalates and urates), or treatment regimens with analgesics. A common link among these conditions is their long term, low-level insult to renal tissue. This disease develops slowly and is continually sustained, leading to a progressive low-grade inflammatory response in renal tissue. Histologically, this process is characterized by interstitial edema (less than that seen with acute conditions) with infiltrates of primarily lymphocytes and plasma cells. Notably, neutrophils are absent or insignificant in number. In addition, tubular atrophy is present to varying degrees and there is deposition of fibrous tissue in the interstitium between the tubules. With disease progression, extensive irreversible renal parenchyma destruction can occur. In fact, chronic pyelonephritis is responsible for approximately 10% to 15% of the individuals that develop ESRD.

The clinical presentation and prognosis for these tubulointerstitial diseases varies with the degree of impairment, which is directly related to the severity of inflammation and the extent of tissue involvement. In acute conditions with prompt initiation of treatment, renal function usually makes a complete recovery. In chronic conditions, treatment can be delayed simply because a diagnosis is not promptly determined. In these cases, irreversible loss of functional renal tissue occurs.

The clinical presentation of acute pyelonephritis is similar to that of cystitis with a high fever, urination frequency, loin tenderness, dysuria, and back pain. Proteinuria can be present, although it is usually mild (<1 g per day). A urinalysis aids in the differentiation of pyelonephritis from cystitis. A diagnostic feature of pyelonephritis is the presence of WBC casts in the urine sediment. In addition, increased numbers of RBCs, WBCs, renal tubular epithelial cells, and other types of casts (e.g., granular, renal cellular, waxy) are also present. In acute pyelonephritis, bacteria are usually present; however, their numbers can be highly variable from case to case.

In contrast, clinical detection of chronic pyelonephritis usually occurs following a routine urinalysis or the development of renal insufficiency (evidenced by azotemia) and hypertension. A urinalysis reveals proteinuria (more than that seen with acute conditions; <2.5 g per day) and a low specific gravity due to the impaired ability to concentrate the urine. The microscopic examination shows increased numbers of WBCs, macrophages, and several types of casts (i.e., granular, waxy, broad casts and, to a lesser extent, renal cellular and WBC). Bacteria, which are present in variable amounts with acute pyelonephritis, are usually absent in chronic pyelonephritis.

Clinically, AIN patients present with fever, skin rash, and eosinophilia. The renal involvement of AIN is evident with the development of azotemia and from the results of a routine urinalysis. A urinalysis will reveal hematuria, mild proteinuria, and leukocyturia without bacteriuria. The microscopic examination reveals increased numbers of WBCs, predominantly eosinophils (evident only with special staining). Macrophages and increased numbers of renal tubular epithelial cells are also present. Several types of casts, primarily WBC casts (with eosinophils predominating), as well as variable numbers of granular, hyaline, and renal cellular casts can be found. Note that if AIN is drug-induced, drug crystals may be present in the urine sediment.

## Cystitis

Cystitis is defined as an inflammation of the bladder and usually results from a urinary tract infection (UTI). Any bacteria or fungal agent can cause a UTI but most UTIs are caused by gram-negative rods that are normally present in human feces. *Escherichia coli* is the most common pathogen, and other gram-negative rods that are frequently implicated include *Proteus, Klebsiella, Enterobacter*, and *Pseudomonas*. Gram-positive organisms include *Enterococcus faecalis* and *Staphylococcus aureus*.

The clinical features of a UTI include urinary urgency, increased frequency of urination, and pain with urination (dysuria). Suprapubic pain may also be present. Because of anatomical differences it is no surprise that UTIs are 10 times more common in women than men.

With a UTI, a routine UA typically reveals bacteria (or rarely fungi) and increased numbers of WBCs (leukocyturia).

Hematuria and proteinuria may also be present, usually at low levels. In addition, depending on the degree of bladder irritation, increased numbers of transitional epithelial cells may also be sloughed. Diagnosis of a UTI requires a quantitative urine culture and the demonstration of $10^5$ or more colonies per milliliter of urine (assuming a midstream clean-catch urine is used).

## Renal Calculi

Renal calculi or stones are aggregates of urine solutes that have precipitated out of solution while in the renal calyces, pelvis, ureters, or bladder. They are usually a mixture of mineral salts, rarely a single chemical. In 75% of all renal calculi, some form of calcium is present with calcium oxalate the most prevalent combination. At the core of all renal calculi is an organic mucoprotein matrix or nucleus. Several factors that influence renal calculi formation have been identified and include an unchanging urine pH, reduced urine flow, concentrated urine, and a nucleus or "seed" about which solutes initially precipitate. The interaction of these factors initiates solute precipitation and then further enhances calculi formation.

The presence of renal calculi, in addition to causing excruciating pain, can inflict serious renal damage. Hence, hematuria is usually present, although the amount is variable. After renal stones are passed or removed, determining their composition aids in effective patient management. Today in addition to traditional chemical tests, X-ray diffraction, and infrared spectroscopy can be used to accurately determine their chemical composition.

To prevent future nephrolithiasis (stone formation in the kidney), a high fluid intake is recommended regardless of stone composition. Treatment protocols may also include dietary restrictions and medications that enhance solute solubility by altering urine pH or by converting the offending solutes to a more soluble form. A routine UA can provide useful follow-up information regarding the effectiveness of treatment by providing urine pH and urine concentration (specific gravity). In addition, the chemical and microscopic examinations provide an overview of renal health.

## Renal Replacement Therapy

For patients in acute renal failure, hemodialysis or peritoneal dialysis is often employed depending on the severity of azotemia as well as the institutional capabilities. In contrast, patients who have developed ESRD, the irreversible consequence of chronic renal failure, have two options for survival: dialysis or transplantation.

## Hemodialysis

**Hemodialysis** and **peritoneal dialysis** are two treatments that can be used to remove the metabolic waste products that accumulate in the bloodstream due to renal failure. In hemo-dialysis, the patient's bloodstream is shunted through a dialysis instrument or hemodialyzer. The vascular access is established using percutaneous cannulation (IV) of the femoral or subclavian veins or through the insertion of a shunt. As the patient's blood circulates in the hemodialyzer, it encounters a semipermeable membrane with a dialysate flowing on the opposite side of the membrane. Solutes, particularly accumulated waste products, in the bloodstream are removed by simple diffusion down a concentration gradient into the circulating dialysate fluid. The semipermeable membrane determines the size of solutes that can pass, which include water and small molecular weight molecules; blood cells and larger molecular weight solutes are retained in the patient's blood. Several factors affect the efficacy of dialysis, primarily : (1) frequency of dialysis, (2) duration of dialysis, (3) hemodialyzer type and surface area of the semipermeable membrane, (4) composition of the dialysate, and (5) blood and dialysate flow rates. In addition, biocompatibility factors related to the interaction of plasma with the man-made tubing, fittings, and membranes of the hemodialyzer can hamper the effectiveness of dialysis and cause additional problems. Plasma proteins coat and can eventually occlude tubings, membranes, and catheters. As the blood flows through the tubing, complement is activated and the release of cytokines is induced. In addition, the detachment and migration of silicone particles from the tubing into the patient, called *spallation*, can also be a problem as are the generation and movement of microbubbles into the patient.

In contrast to hemodialysis, the membrane employed in peritoneal dialysis is the peritoneum, the thin tissue lining of the abdominal cavity. A catheter is strategically placed into the abdominal cavity by a surgeon or nephrologist. The catheter is subsequently used to infuse 2 L of a hypertonic (2.5% dextrose solution) dialysis solution into the peritoneal cavity. Waste products and other solutes from the bloodstream exchange across the peritoneum by diffusion and convection. In addition to the solute and water exchange with the plasma in the vascular system, the lymphatic system also absorbs the dialysis fluid. After a prescribed period, the dialysate is drained from the abdominal cavity using the same catheter. Primarily 3 factors determine the clearance of solutes during peritoneal dialysis: (1) the peritoneal blood flow, (2) the surface area involved in solute transfer, and (3) the flow rate of the dialysate (when a continuous cycling instrument is attached to the catheter).

Despite the life-saving benefits of dialysis, these patients can develop a variety of clinical conditions that require treatment and the clinical laboratory plays an important role in patient management. Complications of renal dialysis include anemia, bleeding, electrolyte imbalance, hypertension, and malnutrition, and with long-term treatment, the development of dialysis-related cardiovascular disease, amyloidosis, and osteodystrophy.

Hemodialysis and peritoneal dialysis continue to be crucial life-saving therapies for patients in renal failure. In fact, hemodialysis has been able to extend the life of individuals with irreversible renal failure into the their third decade of treatment.[26] One relatively common complication of peritoneal dialysis is the development of peritonitis, which in the long-term limits the clinical utility of this form of dialysis.[27]

## Transplantation

As discussed in this chapter and elsewhere, the kidney plays a multifaceted role in regulating and maintaining normal body hemostasis and in the production of hormones. Despite the effectiveness of dialysis, it is inadequate compared to a functioning kidney. Hence, renal transplantation has become the preferred therapy for patients with ESRD. However, this treatment modality is restricted because of the limited number of available organs for transplantation.

Organs for transplantation are obtained from either a living-related donor or from a cadaver. To determine whether transplantation can be successful, the donor organ and the tissue type of the recipient must be determined. Laboratory tests performed to work up a patient for renal transplant include the determination of ABO blood group, HLA (human leukocyte antigen) compatibility, and preformed HLA antibodies. Additional tests that provide an assessment of the general health of the recipient include electrolytes, complete blood count, clotting profile, liver profile, and renal profile tests as well as those tests that screen for infectious diseases such as cytomegalovirus (CMV), hepatitis, and human immunodeficiency virus (HIV).

Following transplantation, the clinical laboratory's role in patient management is 2-fold: to assess renal function and graft viability, and to monitor immunosuppressant drug therapy (to prevent toxicity). Initially, a successful graft usually produces urine within hours of transplantation. Blood tests used to monitor the postoperative patient include plasma creatinine, urea nitrogen, and electrolytes including calcium and phosphorus. In addition, liver enzyme tests, complete blood counts, and immunosuppressive drug levels are performed.

Immunosuppression is primarily accomplished by the combined use of cyclosporine, corticosteroids, and azathioprine. The common feature of these drugs is that they block T cell proliferation; however, they differ regarding the step at which they produce their effect. During graft rejection, treatment with monoclonal antibodies, such as OKT3, may also be initiated. Of these immunosuppressive agents, cyclosporine, a cyclic polypeptide of fungal origin, dramatically improved graft survival in all transplant recipients when it was introduced in the 1980s. The specific drug combination or regimen for immunosuppression varies with individuals as well as institutions. Regardless, the primary side effect of ineffective treatment is graft rejection. Because excess cyclosporine is nephrotoxic, its concentration in the blood must be monitored to maintain immune suppression while at the same time preventing nephrotoxicity. Today, research continues in the search for new, less toxic immunosuppressive agents with several showing promise including FK-506, rapamycin (structurally related to FK-506), and RS-61443 (a derivative of mycophenolic acid). It is interesting to note that, like cyclosporine, each of these agents is either of fungal origin or related to a fungus in some way.

In long-term transplant recipients, regular monitoring of the plasma creatinine and urea nitrogen levels, as well as a creatinine clearance test, is useful in the evaluation of graft function. However, because creatinine is a relatively insensitive measure of renal function, the search for a more sensitive marker is on-going. Beta$_2$-microglobulin measured simultaneously in plasma and urine is gaining in popularity; however, it too has some drawbacks and is not ideal as was discussed earlier. Other laboratory tests that aid in long-term patient management include routine urinalyses, electrolyte panels, periodic lipid profiles, and liver function tests.

Although some studies claim that hemodialysis, peritoneal dialysis, and cadaveric transplantation have equivalent long-term survival outcomes, the literature varies. Studies do agree, however, that live-related donor recipients have the best rate of survival: up to 95% at 3 years.[26] Despite the successes, challenges for transplantation continue, particularly in the area of overcoming complications that ensue from chronic immunosuppression and in extending the graft survival beyond 5 years for cadaveric transplant recipients.

## SUMMARY

Nonprotein nitrogenous compounds originate from protein and nucleic acid metabolism and include ammonia, creatinine, urea, and uric acid. Because ammonia is toxic to cells, it is quickly removed from the circulation by the liver and metabolized; hence, it provides a useful indicator of liver function. Uric acid is eliminated from the body by the kidney (75%) and the GI (25%) tract. When present at increased levels in the plasma, it can form a salt with plasma cations (i.e., monosodium urate) and precipitate in vivo causing renal and nonrenal disorders such as gout or uric acid calculi. Because the kidney plays a primary and essential role in the elimination of creatinine and urea nitrogen (UN) from the body, tests for creatinine and UN are often used to assess renal status. Because of the differences in renal handling, creatinine and UN can accumulate in the plasma to varying degrees depending on the initiating renal or nonrenal condition. In some cases, determining the plasma UN/creatinine ratio can assist in identifying the disease or following its course.

Renal function is a complex and interdependent process performed by the nephrons of the kidney and is highly dependent on an adequate blood supply. The blood pressure actually drives renal function, which begins with the filtration of the blood plasma by the renal glomeruli. The volume of plasma that is processed by the glomeruli per minute is called the glomerular filtration rate (GFR). Determination of the GFR is a valuable tool for assessing renal function as well as for monitoring the progression or regression of renal diseases. The most commonly employed substance for GFR measurement, although not ideal, is creatinine. The creatinine clearance test determines the amount of creatinine cleared from the plasma per minute. Because of the diurnal variation in GFR, a 24-hour urine collection is preferred; however, periodic monitoring using shorter urine collections can also be effective.

Another glomerular characteristic that can be altered with disease is glomerular permeability, i.e., the size selectivity of the glomerular filtration barrier (GFB). In healthy individuals, molecular size and charge restrict the flow of solutes from the plasma across the GFR into the ultrafiltrate in Bowman's space. The GFB is negatively charged; hence, for molecules to cross they must be neutral or positively charged as well as be equal to or smaller than albumin (MW 69000). With disease, GFB selectivity is compromised initially with loss of the molecular charge restriction, and as the disease progresses, with loss of molecular size discrimination. Consequently, urine albumin determinations serve as a sensitive marker for early minimal changes in glomerular permeability. The monitoring for microalbuminuria has become a valuable clinical tool in the management of diabetic and hypertensive patients. In some renal and initially nonrenal conditions, glomerular permeability can be further compromised and is indicated by varying levels of proteinuria and hematuria. The urine concentration tests, osmolality and specific gravity, are the most frequently employed tests to assess renal tubular function, i.e., the ability to reabsorb and secrete solutes. The use of $\beta_2$-M measurements in simultaneous plasma and urine samples is also increasingly used as an indicator of renal disease as well as in differentiating glomerular and tubular dysfunction.

Urine is essentially a fluid biopsy of the kidney and urinary system. Hence, urine tests can provide valuable information regarding the overall health of the urinary system as well as be used to identify and monitor metabolic disorders that alter the composition of the urine. The most frequently performed urine test is a routine urinalysis, which includes a physical, chemical, and microscopic assessment of the urine. A cytodiagnostic urinalysis, which can provide more cytologic detail and disease-specific information, requires greater technical expertise; hence, its clinical utility is limited. In addition, it is not available in all clinical laboratories.

Renal diseases are diverse in clinical presentation as well as outcome. They can occur suddenly (acute) or result from a process that has been ongoing for years (chronic). Additionally, they can cause temporary (acute renal failure) or permanent loss of functional renal tissue (chronic renal failure). Often renal diseases are differentiated as glomerular, tubular, or tubulointerstitial based on the primary area of the kidney affected. However, all nephron components can become involved if the initial underlying disease is left unchecked. Nonrenal disorders can also cause renal disease. Most notable are diabetes mellitus and autoimmune disorders such as systemic lupus erythematosus and amyloidosis.

Other disorders of the urinary system include cystitis and the formation of renal calculi. Cystitis, the inflammation of the bladder, is most often due to a bacterial infection. In ad-

dition to the clinical presentation, a routine urinalysis test plays an important role in the initial identification of cystitis as well as in the management of these patients. Similarly, a routine urinalysis can be valuable in the management of patients that form renal calculi or nephrolithiasis. Under ideal conditions of pH, solute concentration and tubular fluid flow, solutes can precipitate out of solution in vivo to form renal calculi. Despite being extremely painful, these solute stones or calculi can also cause serious mechanical damage to the urinary system.

When disease has caused permanent irreversible loss of functional renal tissue, survival depends on dialysis or renal transplantation. Both hemodialysis and peritoneal dialysis have proven effective in the removal of metabolic waste products such that survival, in some cases, has been extended up to 3 decades. Although dialysis is life saving, it cannot replace all renal functions (e.g., hormonal, acid-base regulation); nor is it as effective as a functioning kidney. Therefore, renal transplantation is the preferred long-term treatment for ESRD patients. A constant challenge in renal transplant recipients is the management of immunosuppression. Currently, a combination of 3 drugs that block T cell proliferation is frequently used. They are cyclosporine, corticosteroids, and azathioprine.

## REFERENCES

1. Sherwin JE, Sobenes JR: Liver function. In Kaplan LA, Pesce AF (eds.): *Clinical Chemistry Theory, Analysis and Correlation.* 4th ed. St. Louis, CV Mosby, 1996, p 508.

2. Carlson JA, Harrington JT: Laboratory evaluation of renal function. In Schrier RW, Gottschalk CW (eds.): *Diseases of the Kidney.* 5th ed. Boston, Little, Brown, 1993, pp 366–367.

3. Weber JA, van Zanten AP: Interferences in current methods for measurement of creatinine. Clin Chem 37:695, 1991.

4. Lente F, Suit P: Assessment of renal function by serum creatinine and creatinine clearance: Glomerular filtration rate estimated by four procedures. Clin Chem 35:2326–2330, 1989.

5. Tietz NW (ed.): *Clinical Guide to Laboratory Tests.* 3rd ed. Philadelphia, WB Saunders, 1995.

6. Kassirer JP, Gennari FJ: Laboratory evaluation of renal function. In Strauss MB, Welt LG (eds.): *Diseases of the Kidney.* 2nd ed. Boston, Little, Brown, 1979, pp 41–87.

7. Montgomery R, Conway TW, Spector AA: Nucleotide metabolism. In Montgomery R (ed.): *Biochemistry: A Case Oriented Approach.* 5th ed. St. Louis, CV Mosby, 1990, p 579.

8. Whelton A, Watson AJ, Rock RC: Nitrogen metabolites and renal function. In Burtis CA, Ashwood ER (eds): *Tietz Textbook of Clinical Chemistry.* Philadelphia, WB Saunders, 1994.

9. Wyss M, Kaddurah-Daouk R: Creatine and creatinine metabolism. Physiol Rev 80:1107–1182, 2000.

10. Roubenoff R, Drew H, Moyer M, et al.: Oral cimetadine improves the accuracy and precision of creatinine clearance in lupus nephritis. Ann Intern Med 113:501, 1990.

11. Brunzel NA: *Fundamentals of Urine and Body Fluid Analysis.* Philadelphia, WB Saunders, 1994.

12. Agrawal B, Berger A, Wolf K, et al.: Microalbuminuria screening by reagent strip predicts cardiovascular risk in hypertension. J Hypertens 14:223–228, 1996.

13. American Diabetes Association. Standards of medical care for patients with diabetes mellitus. Diabetes Care 21(Suppl 1):S23–S31, 1998.

14. Bakker AJ. Detection of microalbuminuria. Diabetes Care 22:307–313, 1999.

15. Schumann GB, Schweitzer SC: Examination of urine. In Henry JB (ed.): *Clinical Diagnosis and Management by Laboratory Methods.* 18th ed. Philadelphia, WB Saunders, 1991, p 421.

16. Freni SC, Dalderup LM, et al.: Erythrocyturia, smoking and occupation. J Clin Pathol 30:341, 1977.

17. National Committee for Clinical Laboratory Standards: Routine urinalysis. Approved guidelines. NCCLS Document GP 16-A (ISBN 1-56238-282-9), 12(26):5–6, 1995.

18. Painter PC, Cope JY, Smith JL: Appendix. In Burtis CA, Ashwood ER (eds.): *Tietz Textbook of Clinical Chemistry.* 2nd ed. Philadelphia, WB Saunders, 1994, p 2201.

19. Prischl F, Gremmel F, Schwabe M, et al.: Beta$_2$-microglobulin for differentiation between ciclosporin A nephrotoxicity and graft rejection in renal transplant recipients. Nephron 51:330–337, 1989.

20. Lifson AR, Hessol NA, Buchbinder SP, et al.: Serum beta-2-microglobulin and prediction of progression to AIDS in HIV infection. Lancet 339:1436–1440, 1992.

21. Woo J, Floyd M, Cannon DC: Albumin and beta$_2$-microglobulin radioimmunoassays applied to monitoring of renal-allograft function and in differentiating glomerular and tubular diseases. Clin Chem 27:709–713, 1981.

22. Kantarjian HM, Smith T, Estey E, et al.: Prognostic significance of elevated serum beta$_2$-microglobulin levels in adult acute lymphocytic leukemia. Am J Med 93:599–604, 1992.

23. Litam P, Swan F, Cabanillas F, et al.: Prognostic value of serum beta$_2$-microglobulin in low-grade lymphoma. Ann Intern Med 114:855–860, 1991.

24. Newman DJ, Price CP: Renal function. In Burtis CA, Ashwood ER (eds): *Tietz Fundamentals of Clinical Chemistry.* 5th ed. Philadelphia, WB Saunders, 2001, p 706.

25. Anderson RJ, Schrier RW: Acute tubular necrosis. In Schrier RW, Gottschalk CW (eds.): *Diseases of the Kidney.* 5th ed. Boston, Little, Brown, 1993, pp 1287–1318.

26. Friedman EA, Lundin AP: Outcome and complications of chronic hemodialysis. In Schrier RW, Gottschalk CW (eds.): *Diseases of the Kidney.* 5th ed. Boston, Little, Brown, 1993, pp 3069–3095.

27. Khanna R, Oreopoulos DG: Peritoneal dialysis. In Schrier RW, Gottschalk CW (eds.): *Diseases of the Kidney.* 5th ed. Boston, Little, Brown, 1993, pp 2969–3030.

# Electrolytes

*Richard C. Mroz, Jr.*

The internal environment of healthy humans is maintained in a state of homeostasis in which the chemical and physical properties of body fluids exist in a state of relative constancy. Because of the body's attempt to maintain homeostasis, an intricate balance exists between body water and specific chemical constituents of cells, the electrolytes. This homeostatic balance is maintained by tightly controlled regulatory mechanisms that prevent large fluctuations of these substances. Because of this tight control, a change in either the water or electrolyte composition reflects or results in a change in the other constituents. In this chapter, we discuss the water and electrolyte composition of the body, the specific functions of the electrolytes, the regulatory processes that maintain electrolyte and water homeostasis, and disorders that result in electrolyte and water imbalance.

## TOTAL BODY WATER

The total body water constitutes 60% to 65% of body weight in male adults and 50% to 55% of body weight in female adults.[1,2] The lower water content in women is primarily due to a somewhat greater percentage of adipose tissue in women. Nearly all of the biologic molecules in the human body are partially or fully soluble in water, forming an aqueous environment in which all metabolism occurs.

Total body water can be divided into two major compartments: **intracellular fluid** (ICF) and **extracellular fluid** (ECF). The extracellular compartment can be further subdivided into interstitial fluid and intravascular fluid. **Intracellular fluid,** that which is contained within cells, represents about 66% of the total body water and the ECF accounts for the remaining 33%. **Interstitial fluid** immediately surrounds the cells and is separated from intracellular fluid by the cell membrane, whereas the capillary wall separates interstitial fluid from the intravascular compartment. Interstitial fluids account for less than 1% of total body water.

Water molecules can move randomly across a permeable membrane. However, the presence of solutes, primarily electrolytes, in any of these water compartments exerts an **osmotic pressure** that tends to hold water in that compartment. The osmotic pressure is the major determinant of the water distribution between these major compartments. As a result, electrolyte concentrations vary between the different water compartments. However, it is the predominance of $K^+$ in the intracellular fluid and $Na^+$ in the extracellular fluid plus the plasma proteins that are the major contributors to the osmotic pressure. Variations in the concentrations of these solutes result in variations in the water distribution between the compartments.

## OSMOLALITY

Osmolality is a measure of the number of dissolved particles (molecules or ions) in a solution. The major contributors to the serum osmolality are sodium and chloride since these are the major free particles of the ECF. The terms osmolality and osmolarity are often confused. **Osmolality** is measured in osmoles per kilogram of water, whereas **osmolarity** is measured in osmoles per liter of solution. The total volume expressed by osmolality is thus 1 kg of water plus the small volume occupied by the solutes, whereas osmolarity represents a total volume of 1 L. The difference between these two measurements is negligible when dealing with biologic fluids because of the low solute concentration of the ECF. The normal plasma osmolality is expressed in milliosmoles (1/1000 osmole) and ranges from 275 to 295 mOsm/kg. The osmolality of urine ranges from 50 to 1200 mOsm/kg.

In addition to the contributions of sodium and chloride, the concentrations of the low molecular weight organic compounds glucose and urea also contribute to the plasma osmolality level, although their contribution is minor compared to that of the electrolytes. Because these compounds are essentially the only contributors to plasma osmolality, several formulas have been devised to calculate the osmolality from the concentrations of these compounds. The formula that is most commonly used is:

$$P_{osm} = 1.86[Na^+] + \frac{[Glucose]}{18} + \frac{[BUN]}{2.8}$$

where $[Na^+]$, $[Glucose]$, and $[BUN]$ are the plasma concentrations of sodium, glucose, and blood urea nitrogen in mmol/L, mg/dL, and mg/dL, respectively.

Osmotically active particles exert an osmotic pressure that tends to hold fluids in the compartment to which the particles are confined. A solution of higher osmolality will have more particles and less water per unit volume than a solution of lesser osmolality. A decrease in the electrolyte concentration of sodium or chloride will produce a lower than normal osmolality and result in water shifts from the ECF to the ICF to reestablish osmotic equilibrium.

Variations in plasma osmolality of as little as 1% to 2% stimulate control mechanisms that respond to restore normal osmolality. An increase in plasma osmolality stimulates osmoreceptors of the hypothalamus, causing the sensation of thirst, and water is ingested. The posterior pituitary gland also secretes **antidiuretic hormone** (ADH) on stimulation from the hypothalamus. ADH acts on the nephron at the distal convoluted and collecting tubules to increase the amount of water reabsorbed by the kidney. The end result is a tightly controlled system that prevents all but minor deviations in total body water content.

Osmolality can also be measured directly by a variety of methods to be discussed later. Often there are differences between the measured and calculated osmolality. Subtraction of the calculated osmolality from the measured osmolality value yields a value usually less than 10 mOsm/kg, which is known as the **osmolal gap** (Osmolal gap = measured osmolality − calculated osmolality). The difference in these values may be attributed to the presence of other osmotically active compounds other than sodium, glucose, and urea. Metabolic acidosis caused by such nonelectrolytes as lactic acid, keto acids, alcohols, ethylene glycol, and other organic acids may result in differences of 6 to 10 mOsm/kg. A larger osmolal gap is correlated with higher levels of the organic acids and a poorer prognosis. Generally those osmotically active compounds that cause an increased osmolal gap also increase the anion gap, but in the case of ethylene glycol, the anion gap may be increased while the osmolal gap remains within normal limits.[3]

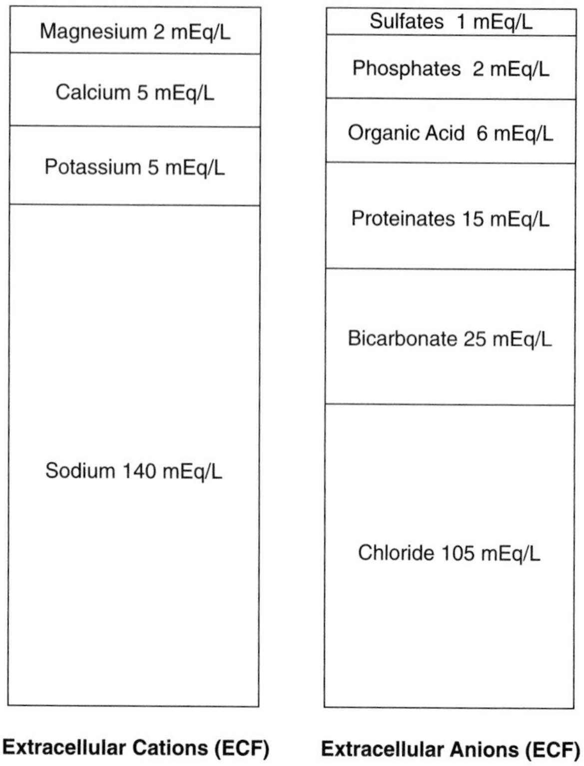

## ELECTROLYTES

**Electrolytes,** by definition, are substances whose molecules dissociate into ions when placed in solution. An ion is an atom or group of atoms with an electrical charge. Those electrolytes with a positive charge are **cations,** and those with a negative charge are **anions.** The major cations of the body are $Na^+$, $K^+$, $Ca^{++}$ and $Mg^{++}$. The major anions include $Cl^-$, $HCO_3^-$, $HPO_4^{--}$, $SO_4^{--}$, plus organic acids (e.g., lactate), and proteins. The electrolyte composition is different in the different water compartments of the body. Some electrolytes are primarily intracellular and some are predominantly extracellular. Regardless of the different concentrations, however, each compartment exists in a state of electroneutrality. The total number of cations is balanced by an equal number of anions. The ECF and ICF electrolyte distributions are illustrated in Figures 21–1 and 21–2.

Electrolyte concentrations are usually expressed in terms of their reactivity as milliequivalents per liter of serum or

| Magnesium 2 mEq/L | Sulfates 1 mEq/L |
| | Phosphates 2 mEq/L |
| Calcium 5 mEq/L | Organic Acid 6 mEq/L |
| Potassium 5 mEq/L | |
| | Proteinates 15 mEq/L |
| Sodium 140 mEq/L | Bicarbonate 25 mEq/L |
| | Chloride 105 mEq/L |

**Extracellular Cations (ECF)**      **Extracellular Anions (ECF)**

**FIGURE 21-1**

Electrolyte distribution of extracellular fluid.

plasma (mEq/L) instead of by weight as mg/dL. The milliequivalent system allows a useful approach to calculating electrolyte balance. One mEq (1/1000 equivalent) of any cation will combine with 1 mEq of any anion. The concentration of all cations in 1 L of plasma is the same as the anion concentration when expressed as milliequivalents. Each liter of plasma has 154 mEq of cations and 154 mEq of anions. This same relationship does not exist if the concentration is expressed as mg/dL. The most widely used unit for electrolyte concentration is millimole/L (mmol/L), which corresponds to the International System of Units.

## Sodium

Sodium is the predominant cation of the extracellular fluid. Its concentration ranges from 136 to 145 mmol/L. Its major function is that of maintaining the normal water distribution and osmotic pressure of the plasma. Because of this osmotic activity, changes in body sodium content reflect or result in changes in plasma volume. If sodium is lost from the plasma, the plasma osmolality decreases, and in an attempt to equalize osmolality between fluid compartments, water tends to flow into cells with a resultant decrease in plasma volume while maintaining appropriate sodium concentration in the plasma.

In contrast, an increased level of plasma sodium causes an increased plasma osmolality. Some water will tend to move out of cells to balance this, but the main response occurs in the

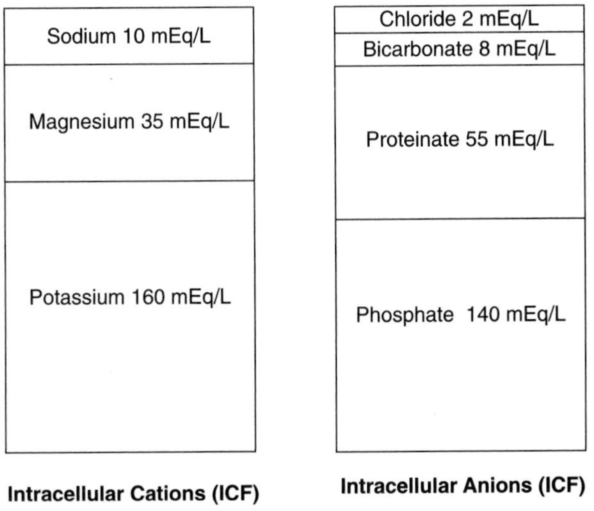

| Sodium 10 mEq/L |
| --- |
| Magnesium 35 mEq/L |
| Potassium 160 mEq/L |

**Intracellular Cations (ICF)**

| Chloride 2 mEq/L |
| --- |
| Bicarbonate 8 mEq/L |
| Proteinate 55 mEq/L |
| Phosphate 140 mEq/L |

**Intracellular Anions (ICF)**

**FIGURE 21-2**

Electrolyte distribution of intracellular fluid.

kidney, where water will be conserved (under the control of ADH) to restore normal plasma osmolality with an expansion of the plasma volume to increase. Thus, it is apparent that total body $Na^+$ content and body water are intricately related. Other functions of sodium include its role in the maintenance of acid-base balance (by the $Na^+$-$H^+$ exchange mechanism in the nephron) and the excitation of nerve and muscle.

## REGULATION OF SODIUM

Dietary intake of sodium is approximately 120 to 260 mmol/d.[4] Sodium is actively absorbed by the small intestine, but the kidneys are the ultimate regulators of sodium content. Sodium is filtered by the glomerulus and most of the reabsorption of the filtered sodium (70%) occurs in the proximal convoluted tubule by active transport processes. The remainder of sodium reabsorption occurs in the ascending loop of Henle and in the distal convoluted tubule (DCT) under the regulation of **aldosterone.** The kidneys have the capacity to reabsorb up to 99% of the filtered sodium. The excreted urine in such extreme cases would essentially contain no sodium.

Aldosterone is a mineralocorticoid hormone secreted from the adrenal cortex and is important in the maintenance of electrolyte balance. In the presence of aldosterone, reabsorption of sodium occurs in the ascending loop of Henle without transport of water since this section of the loop of Henle is refractory to water transport. In the DCT, however, sodium transport occurs along with water, under the influence of ADH. To maintain normal cation-anion balance, as sodium is reabsorbed there is a resultant excretion of $H^+$ and $K^+$ into the urine. When aldosterone is absent or deficient, maximal $Na^+$ reabsorption cannot occur and $Na^+$ is excreted in the urine while $K^+$ and $H^+$ are retained.

Aldosterone secretion is regulated by the renin-angiotensin system. Within the nephron there exists a group of specialized cells collectively called the **juxtaglomerular apparatus** (JGA).

The JGA exists at the point where the distal convoluted tubule and afferent arteriole at the glomerulus come together in close proximity (see Chapter 19). The JGA consists of the juxtaglomerular cells lining the afferent arteriole and the cells of the macula densa that line the early portion of the distal convoluted tubule. These groups of cells activate the renin-angiotensin system by a pressure-sensing mechanism. Changes in pressure of the circulating blood volume or changes in sodium concentration in the afferent arteriole are perceived by the JGA as distortions of the existing stretch or pressure on the arteriolar walls. These varying stretch perceptions then activate the renin-angiotensin system.

Depletion of the extracelluar fluid (ECF) volume, as might occur as a result of bleeding, heart failure, cirrhosis or nephrotic syndrome, results in decreased renal blood flow through the afferent arteriole. This is perceived by the JGA as decreased pressure and renin is secreted. Renin is a proteolytic enzyme that acts on its circulating substrate, angiotensinogen, an alpha$_2$-globulin secreted by the liver. Renin cleaves 10 amino acids from angiotensinogen to form angiotensin I. Angiotensin I is converted into its active form, angiotensin II, by a converting enzyme that splits off 2 more amino acids as the blood circulates through the lung. Angiotensin II is the substance that acts on the adrenal cortex to stimulate the secretion of aldosterone from the adrenal cortex. Angiotensin II is also a powerful vasoconstrictor and acts to increase the blood pressure. Upon secretion, aldosterone exerts its effects on the both the ALOH and DCT by causing $Na^+$ and water retention (DCT) to expand the extracellular fluid volume. This resultant volume expansion is then perceived by the JGA as increased pressure or stretch and further renin production is ceased. The ultimate effect of the renin-angiotensin system has been to restore to normal the sodium concentration and circulating blood volume.[2]

In exchange for $Na^+$ reabsorption, $K^+$ and $H^+$ are secreted into the urine. Aldosterone secretion results in $Na^+$ conservation and $K^+$ and $H^+$ loss. In contrast, an increase in $Na^+$ intake initially expands the ECF, which is perceived as increased pressure by the JGA. This results in reduced secretion of renin and aldosterone, which permits the excretion of excessive sodium and water in the kidneys to restore normal ECF volume and osmolality. Figure 21-3 outlines the renin-angiotensin system.

An additional mechanism that is important in maintaining normal water balance is the action of antidiuretic hormone (ADH), or vasopressin. ADH is a major determinant of renal water excretion. It is a polypeptide hormone synthesized in the hypothalamus and stored in the posterior lobe of the pituitary from where it is secreted upon appropriate stimulation. ADH functions to increase the water permeability in the DCT and collecting tubules of the nephrons leading to increased water reabsorption. The increased retention of water by the kidneys results in a more concentrated (increased osmolality) urine. In the absence of ADH, water reabsorption decreases and large volumes of dilute (low osmolality) urine are produced.

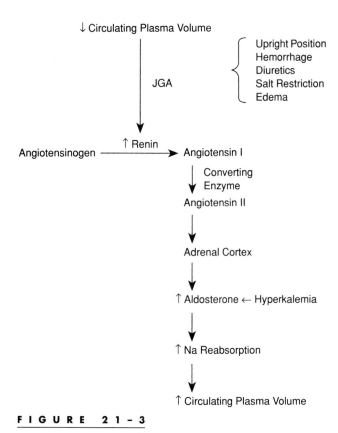

**FIGURE   21 - 3**

Renin-angiotensin-aldosterone system.

ECF volume. There are different schemes for categorizing hyponatremia but one convenient system is presented in Table 21–1 and classifies hyponatremia as depletional, dilutional, or artifactual.

Depletional hyponatremia can be due to either renal or nonrenal losses. Reasons for renal losses include the use of diuretics and hypoaldosteronism. Diuretics, used in the treatment of edema and hypertension, block $Na^+$ or $Cl^-$ reabsorption in the nephron and result in increased urinary excretion (loss) of $Na^+$ and water. Hypoaldosteronism refers to an impairment in the renin-angiotensin-aldosterone axis due to either deficient aldosterone or renin secretion. In primary hypoaldosteronism, there is a deficiency of aldosterone due to some defect in its synthesis within the adrenal cortex. With a deficiency of aldosterone, sodium and its anions are lost in the urine. Secondary hypoaldosteronism refers to deficient aldosterone production due to renin deficiency resulting from damage to the juxtaglomerular apparatus. Without adequate renin secretion, aldosterone production will not be stimulated and $Na^+$ will not be adequately reabsorbed. Addison's disease is the result of an adrenocortical insufficiency of both mineralocorticoid and glucocorticoid hormones. As a result, maximal sodium reabsorption cannot occur.

Sodium can be lost from the body through nonrenal sources such as gastrointestinal losses associated with diarrhea

An increase in the plasma osmolality and a decrease in the circulating blood volume are the two primary stimuli for ADH secretion. An increase in the plasma osmolality of as little as 2 mOsm/kg is sensed by the osmoreceptors in the hypothalamus, which results in increased ADH production and secretion. Figure 21–4 diagrams the effects of ADH on the circulating blood volume.

Other hormones play a role in sodium regulation as well. **Natriuretic peptides** are polypeptide hormones that act on the kidney to promote the excretion of $Na^+$ and water by increasing the GFR and decreasing proximal tubule reabsorption of $Na^+$. The A-form (ANP) and C-form (CNP) originate in the atrium of the heart, whereas the B-form (BNP) originates in the brain and heart. Although the effects of these peptides are minimal, they are released specifically in response to persistent hypervolemia such as might occur in chronic renal failure as a mechanism to promote rapid diuresis and natriuresis.[2]

## HYPONATREMIA

**Hyponatremia** means an abnormally low plasma $Na^+$, usually below 136 mmol/L. This concentration level is actually a reflection of the ratio of $Na^+$ to volume in the plasma and tells nothing directly about the total body $Na^+$ content. Thus, hyponatremia can occur regardless of whether the total body stores of sodium are reduced, normal, or elevated. Hyponatremia can also occur with a reduced, normal, or expanded

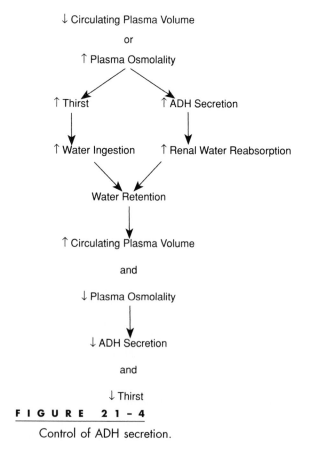

**FIGURE   21 - 4**

Control of ADH secretion.

**TABLE 21-1**

**Causes of Hyponatremia**

| **Depletional**<br>Causes true (absolute) losses of total body sodium | Renal losses | Use of diuretics<br>Hypoaldosteronism<br>   Primary<br>   Secondary Addison's disease |
| | Nonrenal Losses | Gastrointestinal loss<br>   Diarrhea<br>   Vomiting<br>Skin Loss<br>   Burns<br>   Trauma |
| **Dilutional**<br>Causes relative changes due to increased water volume | Syndrome of inappropriate ADH (SIADH) | Excessive water retention |
| | Generalized edema | Congestive heart failure<br>Cirrhosis<br>Nephrotic syndrome |
| | Hyperglycemia | |
| **Artifactual**<br>Falsely low sodium due to analytical errors (pseudohyponatremia) | | Hyperlipidemia<br>Hyperproteinemia |

ADH = antidiuretic hormone.

or vomiting. Sodium can also be lost when the skin is damaged from severe burns or trauma.

Dilutional hyponatremia results from conditions in which there is a greater proportion of water (relative) to sodium than normal so that it appears as if the sodium concentration is low. One cause of dilutional hyponatremia is the syndrome of inappropriate ADH secretion, SIADH. An excessive amount of ADH is produced regardless of the plasma osmolality and water needs of the body. The increased ADH leads to increased water retention, resulting in a mild hypoosmolality and hyponatremia. SIADH may be the result of different clinical disorders, especially malignant tumors with ectopic production of ADH, central nervous system (CNS) disturbances, and head injuries that damage the osmoreceptors in the hypothalamus. Generalized edema occurs in patients who have a markedly increased total body sodium as well as a severe defect in water excretion so that water retention is proportionately greater (relatively) than sodium retention. This often occurs in the late stages of diseases such as congestive heart failure, cirrhosis, and nephrotic syndrome.

Glucose, when present in high concentrations in the plasma, exerts a significant osmotic force that causes a movement of water out of the cells until osmotic equilibrium is restored. The increased ECF water results in a decrease in the sodium concentration. It is estimated that the plasma $Na^+$ decreases by 1.6 mmol/L for each 100 mg/dL increment in blood glucose.[5] However, this correction factor is valid to glucose levels below 400 mg/dL.[6] A new correction factor of 2.4 mmol/L

$Na^+$ for each 100 mg/dL increment in blood glucose provides a better estimate of the relationship of these osmotically active molecules.[6]

Artifactual or pseudohyponatremia occurs in conditions in which the volume of plasma (normally 93% water) contains a significant amount of a nonaqueous component such as triglycerides or proteins that, at high levels, replace a certain amount of water. Since $Na^+$ is confined to the water space, the $Na^+$ content appears low when in actuality it is normal. No signs or symptoms of hyponatremia are present. Pseudohyponatremia due to elevated triglycerides can occur in such diseases as diabetes mellitus, nephrotic syndrome, and some types of cirrhosis of the liver. However, the triglyceride level must be 1500 mg/dL or higher to cause significant displacement of body water. Hyperproteinemia as seen in multiple myeloma and other dysproteinemias may rarely cause pseudohyponatremia.

Hyponatremia rarely causes clinical symptoms until the plasma sodium level is below 125 mmol/L. When symptoms do occur, they are usually the result of the intracellular movement of water to equalize the osmotic pressure between the intracellular and extracellular compartments. Neurologic symptoms appear as water moves into brain cells, causing them to swell and malfunction. Nausea and malaise will also occur. At levels of 110 to 120 mmol/L, headache, lethargy, and obtundation appear. More severe symptoms manifested by seizures and coma may occur at levels below 110 mmol/L. The severity of the neurologic symptoms is directly related to how

TABLE 21-2

**Causes of Hypernatremia**

| | | |
|---|---|---|
| **Water loss** (relative)<br>Sodium is lost less quickly than<br>water, if at all. | Gastrointestinal losses | Vomiting<br>Diarrhea |
| | Excessive sweating | Fever<br>Exercise |
| | Diabetes insipidus | Hypothalamic<br>Nephrogenic |
| **Sodium gain** (absolute) | Ingestion/infusion | |
| | Hyperaldosteronism | Primary (Conn's syndrome)<br>Secondary |
| | Acute renal failure | |

rapidly the $Na^+$ and osmolality decrease. Symptoms almost always resolve with correction of the hyponatremia, but permanent neurologic deficits may occur, especially if the $Na^+$ concentration is below 110 mmol/L. There may also be some muscle weakness because of alterations in the depolarization process. The treatment for hyponatremia is to administer a hypertonic mannitol or NaCl solution to promote an osmotic diuresis.

## HYPERNATREMIA

**Hypernatremia** occurs when the plasma $Na^+$ concentration is greater than 145 mmol/L. Hypernatremia can occur either from water loss or from sodium gain. Table 21–2 outlines the causes of hypernatremia.

Hypernatremia is most commonly the result of water loss (relatively) exceeding that of sodium. The most common means by which relative water loss occurs is through the GI tract from vomiting or diarrhea and from excessive sweating, as might occur from fever and exercise.

A hormonal disorder known as **diabetes insipidus** will also cause a loss of water due to a deficiency of ADH. In this disorder the DCT and collecting ducts are unable to adequately reabsorb water and large quantities of urine are excreted per day. Owing to the water loss, plasma osmolality increases, thereby stimulating the thirst center and water is ingested. If there is inadequate water intake, the patient will develop hypernatremia and hyperosmolality. Diabetes insipidus results from either hypothalamic (absolute) or nephrogenic (relative) causes. The hypothalamic form results from damage to the osmoreceptors with resultant failure of ADH release, whereas nephrogenic diabetes insipidus results from a failure of the kidneys to respond to an adequate production of ADH.

Hypernatremia due to sodium gain can occur with acute ingestion or infusion of hypertonic solutions of NaCl or $NaHCO_3$. Not uncommonly, hypernatremia is produced following infusion of $NaHCO_3$ to counteract metabolic acidosis during cardiac arrest.

Primary hyperaldosteronism, also known as Conn's syndrome, is associated with a hyperfunctioning adrenal gland leading to excess aldosterone production. Aldosterone excess results in increased $Na^+$ reabsorption and $K^+$ excretion.

The symptoms of hypernatremia are primarily neurological and are due to the movement of water out of cells into the plasma to equalize the osmolality. The dehydration of brain cells results in neurologic dysfunction, with symptoms ranging from lethargy and muscle weakness to more severe manifestations of seizures, coma, and death. As with hyponatremia, the severity of symptoms is related to the rapidity and degree of elevation of the $Na^+$ concentration and plasma osmolality. Treatment is aimed at the gradual correction of the hyperosmolal state by oral or intravenous infusion of fluids.

## Potassium

Potassium is the major intracellular cation of the body. Ninety-eight percent of body $K^+$ is located in the intracellular fluids (ICF) with the remaining 2% in the ECF. This results in a major disparity of $K^+$ concentration between the ICF and the ECF. Intracellular $K^+$ concentration is 150 mmol/L compared to a plasma $K^+$ concentration of 3.5 to 5.0 mmol/L. Potassium in red blood cells is approximately 105 mmol/L.[4] The active Na-K-ATPase pump located in the cell membrane pumps $Na^+$ out of the cell and $K^+$ into the cell to maintain the high extracellular $Na^+$ concentration and high intracellular $K^+$ concentration.

Potassium has two major physiologic functions. It has an important role in cell metabolism by participating in the regulation of many cellular processes. When $K^+$ imbalance occurs, a variety of cell functions become impaired. Potassium is also important in neuromuscular excitation. It is not just the serum $K^+$ concentration that is significant, but, more importantly, it is the ratio of the intracellular to the extracellular $K^+$ concentration that is the major determinant of the resting membrane potential across the cell membrane. The resting potential permits the generation of the action potential necessary for normal neural and muscular function. Thus, either increases or decreases in plasma $K^+$ concentration can upset the ratio and lead to cardiac arrhythmias and muscle paralysis.

## REGULATION OF POTASSIUM

Extracellular $K^+$ balance is maintained to a great extent by the kidney. The normal daily intake of $K^+$ is 50 to 150 mmol.[2] Dietary $K^+$ is absorbed by the small intestine and filtered at the glomerulus. Filtered $K^+$ is almost completely reabsorbed in the proximal convoluted tubule. As has been discussed previously, the reabsorption of $Na^+$ in the distal convoluted tubule must be balanced by the excretion of other cations, namely $K^+$ and $H^+$. Thus, urinary $K^+$ excretion depends, in part, on the amount of $Na^+$ available for reabsorption and additionally on the circulating concentration of aldosterone. The kidney is less efficient at conserving $K^+$ than $Na^+$.[2] Even in $K^+$-deficient states, the kidney will continue to excrete a small amount of $K^+$.[1] High $K^+$ levels can directly stimulate the production of aldosterone without activating the renin-angiotensin system (see Figure 21–3). The effect of the increased aldosterone is to enhance urinary excretion of $K^+$ to maintain a normal plasma $K^+$ concentration.

## HYPOKALEMIA

**Hypokalemia** occurs when the plasma $K^+$ level is below 3.5 mmol/L. The major causes of hypokalemia are outlined in Table 21–3.

A decrease of plasma $K^+$ occurs due to elevations of insulin.[2] Excess secretion of insulin can occur with high carbohydrate intake, especially with intravenous hyperalimentation, resulting in transient hypokalemia. In normal cellular metabolism, $H^+$ is exchanged across cell membranes for $K^+$ as cells eliminate the acid. Because there is a deficit of $H^+$ in the ECF in alkalosis, more $H^+$ moves from the cell to the ECF and $K^+$ moves into the cell to maintain cation balance. This intracellular movement of $K^+$ results in hypokalemia. It is estimated that the plasma $K^+$ concentration will decrease 0.6 mmol/L for each 0.1 unit increase in pH during the acid-base disturbance.

Most cases of primary hyperaldosteronism (Conn's syndrome) are caused by a tumor of the adrenal gland, resulting in excessive production of aldosterone. Aldosterone enhances renal $K^+$ excretion by increasing $Na^+$ reabsorption. Secondary hyperaldosteronism results from aldosterone stimulation by the renin-angiotensin system (see discussion under hyponatremia). Renal tubular acidosis results in decreasing $H^+$ excretion and $K^+$ will be excreted to compensate.

Edematous states such as cirrhosis and the nephrotic syndrome are frequently associated with secondary hyperaldosteronism. As edema is forming, there is a resultant decrease in plasma volume. The decreased plasma volume is detected by the JGA as blood flows through the afferent arteriole. This acts to stimulate the renin-angiotensin system with consequent hyperaldosteronism.

Diuretics that act on the PCT increase the flow of the urinary filtrate through the tubule by inhibiting NaCl reabsorption. Potassium secretion and its ultimate excretion are enhanced by the increased flow rate. The chronic ingestion of large amounts of natural licorice causes a pseudohyperaldosterone syndrome. Licorice contains a compound, glycyrrhizinic acid, which acts on the renal tubules in a manner identical to aldosterone. It promotes $K^+$ and $H^+$ secretion and $Na^+$ retention. Some chewing tobaccos are treated with licorice and can also produce this syndrome.

Hypokalemia is a frequent finding in patients with persistent vomiting or nasogastric suction due to $K^+$ lost in the vomitus. Additionally, any condition in which there is prolonged diarrhea may cause hypokalemia. Normally, stool $K^+$ losses are negligible, but they may assume clinical importance in diarrhea and conditions of laxative abuse.

The symptoms induced by hypokalemia are primarily related to the effects of decreased $K^+$ on muscle, renal function, and cardiac conduction. Low $K^+$ concentration increases the resting membrane potential, causing reduced muscle excitability with resultant muscle weakness and paralysis. Symptoms of muscle weakness such as cramps, paresthesia, and tetany may not be manifest until the $K^+$ concentration falls below 2.5 mmol/L.[2,4] However, the appearance of symptoms depends on other factors as well such as the calcium concentration, pH, and the rate at which hypokalemia develops. In more severe cases, death can result from respiratory failure. Hypokalemia can also upset a variety of renal functions including the GFR and the concentrating ability, resulting in symptoms of polyuria.

TABLE 21–3

**Causes of Hypokalemia**

| | | |
|---|---|---|
| **Increased cellular uptake** | Excess insulin | |
| | Alkalosis | |
| **Renal losses** | Hyperaldosteronism | Primary |
| | | Secondary |
| | Renal tubular acidosis | |
| | Diuretics | |
| | Licorice ingestion (pseudohypokalemia) | |
| **Excessive gastrointestinal losses** | Vomiting | |
| | Diarrhea | |
| | Laxative abuse | |

## HYPERKALEMIA

**Hyperkalemia** occurs when the plasma $K^+$ concentration exceeds 5.0 mmol/L. The major causes of hyperkalemia are outlined in Table 21–4.

Increased dietary intake is a rare cause of hyperkalemia and usually does not occur unless there is some other concurrent condition such as renal failure that prevents its excretion. Increased breakdown of tissues with the release of intracellular $K^+$ can cause hyperkalemia. Examples of such tissue destruction would be trauma from motor vehicle accidents or other crush injuries. $K^+$ may also leak from damaged tissues during surgical procedures.

In acidotic conditions, $H^+$ moves into the cells in an attempt to increase the plasma pH, therefore $K^+$ moves out of the cells to maintain an electrochemical balance. Plasma $K^+$ levels may increase approximately 0.6 mmol/L for each 0.1 unit decrease in pH. Renal disorders are a major cause of hyperkalemia since the kidneys are the only significant route of $K^+$ elimination. Hypoaldosteronism and Addison's disease also result in a reduced ability of the kidneys to excrete $K^+$ since $Na^+$ tends to remain in the urinary filtrate. Chronic renal failure is not usually associated with significant hyperkalemia unless the GFR is less than 15 to 20 mL/min.[7]

**Pseudohyperkalemia** is an in vitro phenomenon that occurs when $K^+$ is released from red blood cells, white blood cells, or platelets during coagulation. This phenomenon can be detected by comparing the $K^+$ concentration in both a serum and heparinized plasma sample from the patient. The serum value will usually be 0.2 to 0.4 mmol/L higher than the plasma value due to normal clotting. Patients with extremely high leukocyte and platelet counts may display a pronounced pseudohyperkalemia because of the large numbers of cells that lyse during coagulation after routine venipuncture.[2]

The symptoms of hyperkalemia are associated with muscle weakness and abnormal cardiac conduction. Concentrations of $K^+$ exceeding 7.0 mmol/L constitute a medical emergency. Hyperkalemia decreases the resting membrane potential of cells, resulting in muscle weakness or paralysis. The effects of hyperkalemia are the most severe on cardiac function, where it can result in cardiac arrest.

### TABLE 21–4

**Causes of Hyperkalemia**

| | |
|---|---|
| **Increased intake of $K^+$** | |
| **Increased cell lysis** | Cellular trauma/injury/hemolysis |
| **Altered cellular uptake** | Acidosis |
| | Insulin deficiency |
| **Impaired renal excretion** | Renal insufficiency or failure |
| | Hypoaldosteronism |

## Chloride

Chloride is the major extracellular anion of the body whose concentration ranges from 99 to 109 mmol/L. With few exceptions, the normal metabolism of chloride is closely linked to that of sodium. Because of its association with $Na^+$, the major functions of $Cl^-$ include maintenance of fluid balance and osmotic pressure. Chloride levels usually change proportionately with sodium for any given change in body water content. Any disproportionate change in the $Cl^-$ content relative to that of $Na^+$ can be attributed to alterations of the acid-base balance of the body.

Chloride is also important in the maintenance of normal anion-cation balance as it exchanges with bicarbonate ($HCO_3^-$) in a process known as the chloride shift (Figure 21–5). $CO_2$ accumulates in tissue cells as a product of normal cellular metabolism. It diffuses out of tissue cells into the plasma, where a small amount is dissolved. The majority of $CO_2$, however, diffuses down a concentration gradient into the red blood cell, where it combines with $H_2O$ to form $H_2CO_3$ (carbonic acid). The reaction is catalyzed by the enzyme carbonic anhydrase. $H_2CO_3$ dissociates into $H^+$, which is buffered by hemoglobin and $HCO_3^-$. As the $HCO_3^-$ concentration builds up in the cell, its concentration becomes greater than the extracellular concentration and it diffuses out of the cell. To maintain electroneutrality, $Cl^-$ flows back into the cell in exchange for $HCO_3^-$. This process is known as the chloride shift.

The average daily diet contains 70 to 200 mmol of chloride as the sodium or potassium salt. Dietary chloride is absorbed in the small intestine. Regulation of the chloride concentration is related passively to the $Na^+$ in the PCT with further reabsorption occurring in the loop of Henle.

### HYPOCHLOREMIA

**Hypochloremia** exists when the serum $Cl^-$ level is <99 mmol/L. Causes of hypochloremia are outlined in Table 21–5.

Normally, GI loss of $Cl^-$ is negligible. However, because $Cl^-$ exists in the gastric contents associated with $H^+$ as HCl, loss of gastric contents from prolonged vomiting or nasogastric suction can lead to hypochloremia.

Diuretic use or abuse that promotes the renal excretion of $Na^+$ also promotes the renal excretion of $Cl^-$ because of its association with $Na^+$. In metabolic alkalosis there is an excess of $HCO_3^-$ ions. To offset the accumulation of negative charges due to the $HCO_3^-$ anions, $Cl^-$ is excreted by the renal tubules with a subsequent decrease in the serum $Cl^-$ concentration.

### HYPERCHLOREMIA

**Hyperchloremia** exists when the serum $Cl^-$ level is >109 mmol/L. Causes of hyperchloremia are outlined in Table 21–6.

Generally, those conditions leading to hypernatremia also result in hyperchloremia. However, elevated $Cl^-$ levels with normal $Na^+$ levels may be the result of acid-base disturbances, resulting in a metabolic acidosis in which $HCO_3^-$ is decreased. To maintain a normal anion concentration in such cases, $Cl^-$

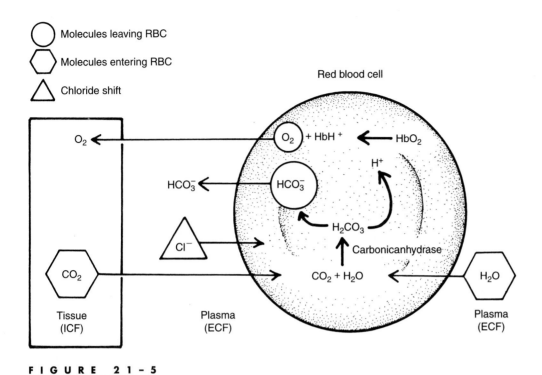

○ Molecules leaving RBC

⬡ Molecules entering RBC

△ Chloride shift

**FIGURE 21-5**

Chloride shift. Chloride ions exchange with bicarbonate as carbon dioxide is transported and buffered in the red blood cell.

is retained by the kidney, resulting in hyperchloremia. Sodium bicarbonate can be lost through the GI tract from prolonged vomiting and from renal tubular acidosis in which there is a decreased reabsorption of bicarbonate by the kidney tubules.

## SWEAT CHLORIDE IN CYSTIC FIBROSIS

One variant of chloride measurement is the analysis of the chloride content of sweat. The sweat chloride test is performed as a screening on newborns and pediatric patients suspected of having cystic fibrosis (CF). CF is a generalized disorder of the exocrine glands characterized by excessive mucus secretions. The mucus is rich in glycoproteins, which precipitate and obstruct organ passages. The main clinical findings of the disease include obstruction of the lungs and upper respiratory tract, leading to eventual respiratory failure, or obstruction of the GI tract, which leads to malnutrition syndrome. CF is inherited as a recessive trait that affects approximately 1 in every 3000 white infants in this country and has a carrier frequency of 1 in 20.[8-10]

One key feature of CF is an abnormal sweat electrolyte pattern manifested by increased $Na^+$ and $Cl^-$ levels. The sweat chloride concentration is considered the most reliable parameter and is the one most often measured. Normal sweat chloride concentrations are below 40 mmol/L. In pediatric CF patients, the sweat chloride ranges from 60 to 160 mmol/L. Various mutations of the CF transmembrane conductance regulator (CFTR) gene have been identified.[11] This has helped to establish a spectrum of CF disease ranging from mild to severe. There are an increasing number of patients with mutations of the CFTR gene with mild lung disease and sweat chloride values that fall into an intermediate range (40 to 60 mmol/L).[11,12]

Sweat is usually collected by a procedure using pilocarpine iontophoresis. Sweating is induced by applying a current gen-

**Causes of Hypochloremia**

| | |
|---|---|
| **Gastrointestinal losses** | Prolonged vomiting |
| | Nasogastric suction |
| **Burns** | |
| **Renal losses** | Diuretics |
| | Metabolic alkalosis |

TABLE 21-6

**Causes of Hyperchloremia**

| | |
|---|---|
| **Dehydration** | |
| **Renal tubular acidosis** | |
| **Metabolic acidosis** | Prolonged diarrhea |
| | Loss of $NaHCO_3$ |
| | Salicylate intoxication |

erated by electrodes on an area of skin such as the forearm. Sweat is collected in a gauze square in which chloride is measured directly by use of an ion-selective electrode placed in the accumulated sweat.

## Bicarbonate

Bicarbonate ($HCO_3^-$) is the second largest anion fraction of the ECF and is the major form of $CO_2$ in the plasma. Its serum concentration ranges from 22 to 28 mmol/L. Bicarbonate functions as a major component of the bicarbonate–carbonic acid buffer system and, as such, it acts promptly to buffer any sudden changes in blood pH. It also serves as a transport form for $CO_2$ produced from metabolic processes in the tissues and delivered to the lungs for exhalation. Bicarbonate concentration is regulated both in the kidneys through increased or decreased tubular reabsorption and in the lungs through exhalation of gaseous $CO_2$ and $H_2O$.

Decreased levels of $HCO_3^-$ in the plasma result in an acid-base disorder known as metabolic acidosis, whereas increased levels result in metabolic alkalosis. The various causes of these acid-base imbalances are further discussed in Chapter 22. However, the $HCO_3^-$ concentration is a necessary part of the complete electrolyte profile inasmuch as $HCO_3^-$ and $Cl^-$ levels tend to vary reciprocally as the body maintains normal electroneutrality.

### ANION GAP

The major body water compartments, intracellular (ICF) and extracellular (ECF), exist in a state of electroneutrality in which the sum of the cations equals the sum of the anions. However, the routine measurement of extracellular electrolytes typically looks only at $Na^+$, $K^+$, $Cl^-$, and $HCO_3^-$ levels. Because all ions are not measured, there exists a mathematical discrepancy between the values of the measured anions and measured cations that is referred to as the **anion gap.** The anion gap is usually calculated from one of two formulas:

$$Na^+ - (Cl^- + HCO_3^-) = 8\text{–}16 \text{ mmol/L}$$

$$(Na^+ + K^+) - (Cl^- + HCO_3^-) = 12\text{–}20 \text{ mmol/L}$$

Because $K^+$ is primarily an intracellular cation, its contribution is small and is frequently omitted from the calculations. The value of 8 to 16 mmol/L represents the contribution of the unmeasured anions such as proteins, sulfate, phosphate, and organic acids. Assuming there are no laboratory errors of the measured electrolytes, any change in the anion gap must necessarily involve a change in the unmeasured anions or cations ($K^+$, $Ca^{++}$, $Mg^{++}$). Calculation of the anion gap is clinically most useful in conditions of acid-base disorders and will be further discussed in that chapter. However, this calculation is also useful as an inexpensive means of laboratory quality control and is performed by many automated electrolyte analyzers.

T A B L E   2 1 - 7

**Causes of an Increased Anion Gap**

| | |
|---|---|
| Decreased unmeasured cations | |
| Increased unmeasured anions | Uremia (phosphate, sulfate) |
| | Lactic acidosis |
| | Ketoacidosis |
| | Ingestion of toxic substances |
| | Methanol |
| | Ethylene glycol |
| | Salicylate |
| Laboratory error | Overestimation of sodium |
| | Underestimation of chloride or bicarbonate |

The most common abnormality is an increased anion gap. The mechanisms responsible for an increased anion gap are outlined in Table 21–7.

An increased anion gap, due to decreased unmeasured cations resulting from hypokalemia, hypocalcemia, or hypomagnesemia is rarely seen clinically because of the relatively low concentrations of these ions compared to sodium. The magnitude of decrease necessary to cause an abnormal anion gap would not be compatible with life unless all three unmeasured cations decreased simultaneously. The anion gap would be increased in these conditions owing to an increase in $Na^+$ or a decrease in a measured anion to offset the loss of the unmeasured cations.

The accumulation of various types of inorganic acids, such as phosphate or sulfate, that occurs in renal failure as well as the accumulation of organic acids from lactic acidosis or ketoacidosis, are the most commonly encountered causes of an increased anion gap. Additionally the ingestion of such toxic substances as methanol, ethylene glycol, and salicylate leads to an accumulation of various anions such as formate and salicylate. When these organic acids are present in large amounts, the measured anions, $Cl^-$ and $HCO_3^-$, will decrease in compensation and produce an increased anion gap.

A decreased anion gap is not as frequently encountered as is an increased gap. The mechanisms responsible for a decreased gap are outlined in Table 21–8.

T A B L E   2 1 - 8

**Causes of a Decreased Anion Gap**

| | |
|---|---|
| Increased unmeasured cations | $K^+$, $Ca^{++}$, $Mg^{++}$ |
| | Paraproteins |
| Decreased unmeasured anions | Hypoalbuminemia |
| | Dilution |
| Laboratory error | Underestimation of sodium |
| | Overestimation of $Cl^-$ or $HCO_3^-$ |

A decreased anion gap due to hyperkalemia, hypercalcemia, or hypermagnesemia is not commonly seen because the extreme values needed to offset the anion gap are life-threatening. Abnormal anions such as IgG, as seen in some gammopathies, assume a positive charge at physiologic pH and behave as cations. Chloride is retained to offset the charge with a consequent decrease in the anion gap.

Decreased anion gap due to hypoalbuminemia is probably the most common cause of this abnormality. The decreased protein anions would be offset by an increase in the measured anions. Although most patients with decreased anion gap have hypoalbuminemia, hypoalbuminemic patients did not necessarily have decreased anion gap.[13] Conditions such as nephrotic syndrome, cirrhosis, or severe hemorrhage are the most likely contributory conditions to the development of hyopalbuminemia. Dilution of the ECF also lowers the gap because of a proportional decrease in the sodium concentration. A laboratory error in the measurement of $Na^+$ or existing conditions that could contribute to pseudohyponatremia also exist as possible causes of a decreased anion gap. Similarly, the overestimation of $Cl^-$, whether due to interferences such as bromide or to laboratory error, also decrease the gap and should be considered carefully as possible causes of the abnormality.

## URINE ELECTROLYTES

The measurement of urine electrolyte levels has limited diagnostic value owing to the number of factors that can influence urinary electrolyte excretion. Variables such as dietary intake, state of hydration, hemodynamic status, posture, acid-base balance, drugs, and disease are all determinants of urine electrolyte concentrations. When proper consideration is given to these variables, however, urine electrolyte levels can provide useful information in certain clinical settings. Reference ranges have been established for 24-hour urine electrolyte measurements but random or spot urine reference ranges have not been established. Urine sodium values range from 40 to 220 mmol/24 hour. Urine potassium values range from 25 to 150 mmol/24 hour.

Urinary $Na^+$ in a spot or random urine is a useful test in the differential diagnosis of hyponatremia when the diagnosis is not otherwise apparent. When the serum $Na^+$ is decreased, the normal renal response is to conserve sodium as manifested by a low urinary $Na^+$ level. Thus, in the presence of normal renal function, a urinary $Na^+$ below 20 mmol/L is generally suggestive of an extrarenal loss, such as through the GI tract, that would account for low urinary sodium. In contrast, a urinary $Na^+$ exceeding 20 mmol/L when accompanied by a low serum $Na^+$ indicates a renal loss of $Na^+$ due to an inability of the kidney to conserve $Na^+$.

Urine potassium levels have more limited usefulness than urine $Na^+$ levels but may be helpful in the evaluation of unexplained hypokalemia. A urine $K^+$ level <10 mmol/L reflects a normal renal response to conserve $K^+$ and is thus suggestive of other losses of $K^+$ including GI losses or inadequate intake. A urine $K^+$ >10 mmol/L indicates renal loss due to such factors as diuretic therapy, alkalosis, aldosterone excess, or renal disease. Urine $K^+$ measurements also provide an indirect indication of mineralocorticoid activity in the form of urine Na:K ratio. The normal urinary Na/K ratio is 2:1, with the urine Na level twice that of urine $K^+$. In hyperaldosteronism, the ratio is reversed and approximates 1:40, indicating increased $Na^+$ reabsorption and $K^+$ excretion. In hypoaldosteronism, the ratio may be as great as 10:1, indicating massive loss of sodium into urine. Urine $K^+$ monitoring is also useful to detect chronic trends toward $K^+$ imbalance before serum $K^+$ levels decrease.

The only common use for urine $Cl^-$ measurement is in the evaluation of persistent metabolic alkalosis. A urine $Cl^-$ <10 mmol/L indicates a gastric or diuretic-induced $Cl^-$ loss, whereas a urine $Cl^-$ >10 mmol/L indicates a renal loss.

## Magnesium

Magnesium is the second most abundant intracellular cation. Approximately 31% of total body magnesium is found intracellularly, 67% is located in bone, and the remaining 1% to 2% is found in extracellular fluid (plasma).[14,15] Plasma concentration ranges from 1.5 to 2.5 mEq/L (0.075 to 0.96 mmol/L). Approximately 35% of plasma magnesium is bound to protein, and the remainder is present as free ions or as small molecular weight complexes.[16] Magnesium has numerous functions in the body. Intracellular magnesium plays a crucial role in cellular physiology and catalyzes numerous enzymatic reactions involved with the transfer, storage, and utilization of energy. Reactions that involve ATP are activated by magnesium. It also plays an important role in the metabolism of carbohydrates, fats, nucleic acids, and proteins.

Many of the factors that regulate magnesium metabolism are unknown. The kidneys are able to conserve magnesium when magnesium deficiency occurs. The renal excretion of magnesium is thought to be controlled by aldosterone in a manner similar to that of potassium.

### HYPOMAGNESEMIA

Hypomagnesemia is present when the magnesium concentration is below 1.5 mEq/L. Symptomatic hypomagnesemia commonly occurs with levels below 1 mEq/L. Causes of hypomagnesmia are outlined in Table 21–9.

It is difficult to produce magnesium deficiency by dietary restriction alone. However, prolonged malnutrition or administration of magnesium-free intravenous fluids can result in hypomagnesemia. Magnesium deficiency is relatively common in hospitalized patients and is frequently present in the general population. In malabsorption syndromes, magnesium is excreted in the feces as magnesium soaps. Diarrhea can also lead to magnesium loss through the GI tract. Alcoholism is also a common cause of hypomagnesemia because of chronic inadequate food consumption.

The usual cause of excessive renal loss of magnesium is diuretic therapy. Renal losses also occur as a result of excessive

TABLE   21 - 9

**Causes of Hypomagnesemia**

| Impaired intake or intestinal | Absorption |
| --- | --- |
| | Malnutrition |
| | Malabsorption syndromes |
| | Diarrhea |
| | Alcoholism |
| Excessive renal losses | Diuretics |
| | Hyperaldosteronism |
| | Primary hyperparathyroidism |

aldosterone production, which enhances magnesium excretion, and from primary hyperparathyroidism, in which the parathyroid hormone (PTH) inhibits magnesium reabsorption in the renal tubule. The symptoms of hypomagnesemia include both psychiatric and neurologic manifestations such as mental depression or confusion, hallucinations, convulsions, and muscle weakness with signs of tetany. Cardiovascular manifestations of magnesium deficiency are of clinical importance because of the occurrence of serious cardiac arrhythmias.[17,18]

The importance of magnesium deficiency is being increasingly noted in the literature. Low plasma magnesium has been linked to onset of diabetes mellitus, increased atherosclerosis, and increased levels of oxidized blood lipids.[19–21] Dietary supplementation of magnesium is being increasingly recommended for the prevention and treatment of cardiovascular disease. Treatment consists of the administration of magnesium salts, the most common being magnesium sulfate. Hypomagnesemia may prevent the action of PTH on bones, causing a concurrent hypocalcemia. When this occurs, calcium supplements must also be administered to correct the deficiencies.

## HYPERMAGNESEMIA

**Hypermagnesemia** may occur when the serum magnesium concentration exceeds 2.5 mEq/L although symptoms do not usually occur until the value exceeds 4 mEq/L. The causes of hypermagnesemia are outlined in Table 21–10.

The most common cause is related to intake of large amounts of magnesium usually in the form of over-the-counter antacids or milk of magnesia, a cathartic agent. Mild hypermagnesemia may be exacerbated by renal failure. More severe hypermagnesemia may occur because of use of magnesium sulfate during surgery.[22]

TABLE   21 - 1 0

**Causes of Hypermagnesemia**

| Magnesium intoxication | Antacids |
| --- | --- |
| | Milk of magnesia |
| Renal failure | |

Symptoms of hypermagnesemia are due to the toxic effects of magnesium on the CNS and on cardiac function. Magnesium levels of 5 to 7 mEq/L cause drowsiness with respiratory center depression and coma occurring at higher levels of 10 to 15 mEq/L. Cardiac arrest occurs at levels of 15 to 20 mEq/L. Increased magnesium levels suppress the release of acetylcholine and block transmission at the neuromuscular junction. Magnesium toxicity can be treated by improving renal function or the use of intravenous calcium.[22]

## Iron

Iron is a trace element that is essential to humans and other living organisms. It functions as an integral part of hemoglobin, myoglobin, cytochrome, and other respiratory enzymes to bind with oxygen and facilitate its transport. The total iron content of the body is approximately 4 to 5 g, of which 66% is found in hemoglobin. An additional 4% is found in myoglobin and the iron-containing enzymes of the cytochrome system. The remaining 30% is found in various storage sites, mainly spleen, liver, and bone marrow. Only 0.1% of total body iron circulates in the plasma bound to the transport protein transferrin, where its concentration ranges from 50 to 130 ug/dL in females and 60 to 150 ug/dL in males.

### REGULATION OF IRON

The average daily intake of iron, in a typical American diet, is about 10 to 20 mg, mostly in the form of heme-containing proteins.[23] Normally, the body absorbs only 5% to 10%, which supplies the daily requirement of 1 to 2 mg from newly absorbed dietary iron.[24] Recycling of iron provides most of the 20 mg required daily for normal erythropoiesis. The amount of iron absorbed, however, varies considerably depending on the composition of the diet and other variables. Iron absorption occurs primarily in the duodenum and can be increased up to 20% in states of iron deficiency and during growth and pregnancy when iron needs are greater.

Dietary iron exists as both heme and nonheme iron pools. Heme iron is found primarily in hemoglobin and myoglobin and can be absorbed directly by the intestinal mucosal cells (Figure 21–6). Nonheme iron is found in food such as vegetables and eggs, where it exists in the form of ferric hydroxide. Dietary iron can only be absorbed in the ferrous ($Fe^{++}$) form. Thus, all dietary iron in the ferric ($Fe^{+++}$) form must first be reduced, mainly by the highly acidic environment of the stomach. Ferrous iron forms complexes with ascorbic acid, amino acids, and sugars to maintain the reduced state of the iron and promote absorption in the somewhat alkaline environment of the jejunum. On the other side of the coin, certain dietary compounds such as oxalates, phytates (cereals and vegetable fiber), phosphates (eggs and dairy), tannins (tea), as well as antacids and antibiotics will decrease iron absorption.

Once reduced to the ferrous form, approximately 5% to 10% of dietary iron enters the mucosal cell. The remainder is lost in the feces. The exact mechanism by which iron is ab-

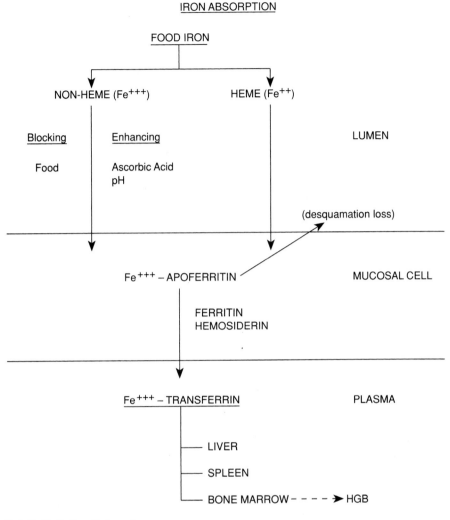

IRON ABSORPTION

**FIGURE  21-6**

Iron absorption.

sorbed is unknown but appears to be carrier mediated. The control of iron absorption resides at the intestinal mucosal level; iron homeostasis is not regulated by excretion.

Upon entering the mucosal cell, iron is oxidized back to the ferric form ($Fe^{+++}$) and is bound to apoferritin, a storage protein. Once iron is bound to apoferritin, it becomes known as **ferritin.** Ferritin is the major iron storage protein found in all cells of the body, especially in the cells of the reticuloendothelial system (RE) system, mainly in bone marrow, spleen, and liver. It is composed of an apoprotein shell surrounding a core of ferric hydroxyphosphate and may contain up to 4500 atoms of iron.[25] Isoforms of ferritin from different tissues can be separated by electrophoretic means on the basis of their differing amino acid composition. Ferritin is a highly soluble protein but may degrade into an insoluble complex called **hemosiderin.** Hemosiderin granules can be observed in tissues using specific iron stains such as the Prussian blue stain. These granules do release iron, albeit more slowly than ferritin-bound iron.

Although most ferritin is found in the tissues, a very small percentage exists in the plasma, where its concentration is proportional to the tissue concentration. Thus, measurement of serum ferritin levels is a direct indication of the amount of storage iron. Serum concentration of ferritin ranges from 20 to 300 ng/mL (or $\mu$g/L) in males and 10 to 120 ng/mL (or $\mu$g/L) in females. Concentrations of less than 10 ng/mL (or $\mu$g/L) are typical in iron deficiency anemia.

When iron is needed by the body for incorporation into the iron-containing molecules, it is released from ferritin, enters the plasma, and is bound to the transport protein, transferrin. Transferrin is a beta globulin synthesized by the liver. Transferrin binds iron in the ferric ($Fe^{+++}$) form and transports it to those tissues with iron requirements, primarily the liver and bone marrow. The transferrin molecule normally is only about 30% saturated with bound iron. The percent transferrin saturation can increase or decrease depending on the iron status of the body. Once transferrin delivers its bound iron to the red cell precursors actively making hemoglobin, it recirculates to transport more iron. Transferrin binds to cells by way of the **transferrin receptor** (TfR). A truncated form of TFRs dissociate from the cell membrane and circulate as serum TfR (sTfR).[25,26]

Senescent red blood cells are engulfed by macrophages in the spleen and other organs, where iron is liberated by catabolism of the hemoglobin molecule. The amount of iron released is approximately 20 mg/day, which is the amount required for daily hemoglobin synthesis. Iron released from hemoglobin remains temporarily in the cells of the RE system. It then slowly leaves these cells and is bound to transferrin, which recirculates it for incorporation into developing cells.

## IRON DEFICIENCY

Iron deficiency occurs when the amount of iron absorbed is inadequate to meet the needs of the body and the serum iron concentration is below 40 $\mu$g/dL. Iron deficiency anemia is considered the most common cause of anemia worldwide.[23] It can affect any person of any age but most frequently occurs in children and women of childbearing age, especially during pregnancy. The common factors that can lead to iron deficiency are outlined in Table 21–11.

Inadequate intake is a rare cause of iron deficiency in adults unless accompanied by another factor. Severe chronic diarrhea and malabsorption syndromes can lead to iron deficiency because of impaired intestinal absorption.

Certain stages of life are associated with increased iron requirements. These stages are most typically the growth phases of infancy, childhood and adolescence, and premenopausal women. Additionally, pregnancy increases iron requirements.

Chronic loss of blood by hemorrhage is the most common causative factor in adults in the development of iron de-

### TABLE 21–11

#### Causes of Iron Deficiency

| | |
|---|---|
| **Decreased availability** | Inadequate intake |
| | Chronic diarrhea |
| | Malabsorption |
| **Increased requirements** | Growth |
| |    Infancy |
| |    Childhood |
| |    Adolescence |
| | Premenopausal women |
| | Pregnancy |
| **Chronic blood loss** | Excessive menstruation |
| | Peptic ulcer |
| | Hemorrhoids |
| | Esophageal varices |
| | Gastritis |
| **Chronic diseases** | Infections |
| | Inflammatory diseases |
| | Malignancies |

ficiency. Typical causes of chronic blood loss include excessive menstruation, peptic ulcer, hemorrhoids, esophageal varices, and gastritis due to salicylate ingestion. In women, menstrual loss is probably the most common cause of iron loss. An average of 20 to 40 mg of iron may be lost during a typical menstrual period. In male adults, however, the discovery of iron deficiency usually suggests an occult source of bleeding, usually from the GI tract.

Iron deficiency is also associated with a wide variety of chronic diseases. These diseases include long-standing infections, inflammatory diseases such as rheumatoid arthritis and other collagen diseases, and malignancies. It is not entirely clear why low serum iron levels occur in such cases but it has been postulated that these disorders alter erythropoietin production, resulting in decreased erythropoiesis. Despite the low serum iron levels, iron stores are increased, in part, because of a block in the transfer of stored iron from RE sources to the plasma.

As iron deficiency develops, iron is released from storage compounds to provide sufficient iron for hemoglobin synthesis and other needs. This process continues until the iron stores are depleted, as indicated by a low ferritin level. Continued iron depletion results in a low serum iron concentration until, ultimately, anemia occurs. The typical biochemical assessment of iron deficiency includes the assay of ferritin levels, serum iron, total iron-binding capacity (TIBC), and % transferrin saturation. The addition of the serum transferrin receptor (sTfR) assay helps distinguish iron deficiency anemia from other forms of microcytic anemia.[25]

The TIBC is an indirect measurement of the amount of transferrin. It is a measure of the iron-binding capacity of transferrin when fully saturated with iron with reference ranges of 250 to 450 $\mu$g/dL (2500 to 4500 $\mu$g/L). The percentage of transferrin saturation measures the degree to which the binding sites of the transferrin molecules are bound by serum iron. Normal saturation ranges from 20% to 50% in males and 15% to 50% in females, with 30% being the most commonly observed value.[23]

TIBC along with % saturation are useful measures in combination with serum iron levels to aid in the differentiation of various causes of iron deficiency. During iron deficiency anemia due to causes other than chronic infections, transferrin levels increase as a result of increased synthesis of the protein in an attempt to transport more iron to the depleted tissues. Because of the increased transferrin but depleted iron stores, the % saturation of transferrin decreases. The % saturation is calculated from the following formula:[23]

$$\% \text{ Transferrin saturation} = \frac{\text{Total Fe}}{\text{TIBC}} \times 100$$

Thus, the classic laboratory findings in iron deficiency anemia are decreased ferritin, decreased serum iron, decreased % saturation with an increased TIBC, and increased sTfR levels.[27,28]

In iron deficiency due to chronic infections, inflammation, and malignancy, the TIBC level is decreased. Transferrin

TABLE 21–12

**Causes of Iron Overload**

| | |
|---|---|
| **Increased absorption** | Primary hemochromatosis |
| | Hemosiderosis |
| | Iron poisoning |
| | Dietary |
| | Medicinal |
| | Transfusional |
| **Increased red blood cell destruction** | |
| **Ineffective erythropoiesis** | Thalassemia |
| | Sideroblastic anemia |

acts as a negative acute-phase reactant protein in such cases; consequently, its synthesis is decreased and its catabolism is increased, contributing to lowered values.

Symptoms of iron deficiency develop in proportion to the degree of the deficiency. Frequently, patients are asymptomatic. As the deficiency becomes more severe, the clinical manifestations include increasing fatigue, headache, and pallor. Many patients exhibit a distorted appetite called pica, with cravings for such substances as earth, clay, or ice. Other abnormalities, including sore tongue or mouth and thinning or spooning of the fingernails (koilonychia), may occur. The Plummer-Vinson syndrome may also be an accompanying abnormality in which the opening to the esophagus may be partially occluded, leading to a sensation of food sticking in the throat.

The administration of iron in the form of ferrous sulfate is the usual treatment for true iron deficiency. However, complete therapy includes an accurate diagnosis of the cause with its subsequent correction.

## IRON OVERLOAD

Increased iron absorption may occur either from an increase in the amount of available dietary iron or through increased intestinal absorption. The most common causes of iron overload are outlined in Table 21–12.

Primary hemochromatosis (PHC) is a genetically determined metabolic disorder resulting in increased iron absorption. There are two known mutations associated with the gene associated with hemochromatosis (HFE).[29,30] The mechanism regulating iron absorption is defective, so that continual iron absorption occurs, although the HFE gene product reduces the affinity of tansferrin bound iron for the cellular transferrin receptors (TfR).[30] Iron accumulates in the tissues with resultant tissue damage and fibrosis leading to organ failure. The classic symptoms of PHC include diabetes mellitus, hyperpigmentation, and hepatic cirrhosis. Because of the combination of these symptoms, the disorder is frequently referred to as "bronze diabetes." The parenchymal cells of the liver, pancreas, and heart are those most affected by excess iron deposition in PHC. The disorder is 10 times more common in men than

in women, and symptoms are not usually manifest until 40 to 60 years of age although the defect is present at birth.

The progressive accumulation of iron results in typical laboratory abnormalities that include increased serum iron level, increased transferrin saturation, often greater than 90%, increased serum ferritin levels, normal or decreased TIBC, and decreased sTfR.[27] The definitive test for the diagnosis of PHC is a liver biopsy from which a histochemical estimation of tissue iron is made.

Many years of excessive iron ingestion may also result in the pathologic features of hemochromatosis in some instances. A condition known as Bantu siderosis occurs in the Bantu population of Africa. Tissue damage resulting from increased iron absorption results from ingestion of food and beverages prepared in iron cooking utensils.

Although rare, hemochromatosis may develop from the prolonged administration of medicinal iron. Ingested doses exceeding 30 mg/kg are toxic, whereas doses over 250 mg/kg may be fatal. Transfusional iron overload results in iron deposition in RE cells rather than parenchymal cells. The resultant overall tissue damage is less severe.

Chronic disorders of erythropoiesis lead to secondary, or acquired, tissue iron deposition. These disorders include defects in hemoglobin synthesis and ineffective erythropoiesis such as thalassemia and sideroblastic anemia.

Treatment for PHC involves removal of excess body iron and treatment of damaged organs. Body iron is best removed by phlebotomy of 500 mL once or twice a week for a 2- to 3-year period. The progress of iron removal can be monitored by periodic serum ferritin levels. Chelating agents such as desferrioxamine are also helpful in lowering iron stores, though less effective than phlebotomy.

A summary of changes of iron parameters in selected disorders is presented in Table 21–13.

TABLE 21–13

**Changes in Serum Fe, TIBC, % Saturation, and Ferritin in Selected Disease States**

| DISEASE STATE | SERUM Fe | TIBC | % SATURATION | SERUM FERRITIN |
|---|---|---|---|---|
| Iron deficiency anemia | ↓ | ↑ | ↓ | ↓ |
| Pregnancy | ↓ | ↑ | ↓ | ↓ |
| Chronic iron deficiency | ↓ | ↓ | ↓ | N, ↓ |
| Primary hemochromatosis | ↑ | N, ↓ | ↑ | ↑ |
| Hemolytic anemia | ↑ | N, ↓ | ↑ | ↑ |
| β-Thalassemia | ↑ | ↓ | ↑ | N, ↑ |

↓ = decreased; ↑ = increased; N = normal.

## ANALYTICAL PROCEDURES

### Sodium and Potassium

The reference methods for measuring $Na^+$ and $K^+$ concentrations is atomic absorption. However, most modern clinical analysis involves use of ion-selective electrodes (ISE).

Ion-selective electrodes are based on the principle of potentiometry, in which there is a voltage change between a reference and indicator electrode proportional to the activity of the ion being measured. ISEs designed to measure sodium incorporate a glass membrane that is permeable to sodium ions and excludes other cations. Potassium ISEs utilize a valinomycin membrane that effectively eliminates interference by $Na^+$ and other ions.

ISE methods are categorized as either direct or indirect. Direct methods require no sample dilution. They determine the activity of an ion in the plasma water where the ions are dissolved rather than in the total volume. Thus, total solids such as lipids and proteins have no effect on electrolyte measurements when their concentration is elevated. Indirect methods require a sample dilution. Since the dilution step is based on the total sample volume, including the volume occupied by total solids, these methods are subject to interference by conditions of hyperlipidemia and hyperproteinemia. Reference ranges for direct ISE methods may be approximately 7% higher than those for indirect ISE methods since only the plasma water compartment is assayed.[23,31] The plasma water represents 93% of the total volume.

Serum, plasma, whole blood, urine, and other body fluids can be analyzed for $Na^+$ and $K^+$. If plasma is used, the anticoagulant should be lithium heparin because sodium heparin invalidates $Na^+$ measurement. Serum and plasma must be separated from cells within 3 hours to avoid leakage of $K^+$ from cells. Any degree of hemolysis causes false elevations of $K^+$ values. Hemolyzed samples should be rejected or noted on the report form if a new sample is unable to be obtained. Serum and plasma samples are stable for at least 1 week at either room or refrigerated temperatures. Reference ranges for the electrolytes are listed in Table 21–14.

### Chloride

A variety of analytical methods are available for chloride analysis including mercurimetric titration, coulometric-amperometric titration, colorimetric methods, and ISEs. The mercurimetric titration methods of Schales and Schales uses $Hg(NO_3)_2$ to titrate a tungstic acid protein-free filtrate (PFF) in the presence of diphenylcarbazone (DPC) as an indicator. The reaction proceeds according to the following equation:

$$2Cl^- + Hg(NO_3)_2 \longrightarrow HgCl_2 + 2(NO_3)^-$$

$$Hg^{++} + DPC \longrightarrow \text{Mercuric diphenylcarbazone}$$

Free mercuric ions combine with $Cl^-$ to form insoluble $HgCl_2$. Following complete titration of $Cl^-$, excess $Hg^{++}$ combines with DPC to form a blue-violet complex indicating the end point of the titration. The major limitation of this method is the difficulty in detecting the end point because this can vary among technologists and can be obscured by the presence of protein, bilirubin, hemolysis, and lipemia.

A frequently used colorimetric method that is adaptable to automation uses mercuric or ferric thiocyanate.

---

TABLE   21 – 14

**Reference Ranges**

| ANALYTE | SERUM | URINE |
|---|---|---|
| Osmolality | 275–295 mOsm/kg | 50–1200 mOsm/kg |
| Sodium | 136–145 mmol/L | 40–220 mmol/24 h |
| Potassium | 3.5–5.0 mmol/L | 25–150 mmol/24 h |
| Chloride | 99–109 mmol/L | |
| Bicarbonate | 22–28 mmol/L | |
| Magnesium | 1.5–2.5 mEq/L | |
| Iron | 50–130 $\mu$g/dL (female) | |
|  | 60–150 $\mu$g/dL (male) | |
| TIBC | 250–450 $\mu$g/dL | |
| % Saturation | 20%–50% | |
| Ferritin | 10–120 ng/mL (female) | |
|  | 20–300 ng/mL (male) | |

$$2Cl^- + Hg(SCN)_2 \longrightarrow HgCl_2 + 2(SCN)^-$$

$$3(SCN)^- + Fe^{+++} \longrightarrow Fe\,(SCN)_3$$

Thiocyanate ions are displaced from Hg by chloride ions. The free thiocyanate then combines with ferric ions to form the ferric thiocyanate, a red complex that can be quantitated spectrophotometrically at 525 nm.

Coulometric-amperometric titration is another method of $Cl^-$ analysis. In this method, two separate electrical circuits are employed. The coulometric circuit generates silver ions ($Ag^{++}$) from a silver electrode that then react with $Cl^-$ to form $AgCl_2$, an insoluble complex. The amperometric indicator circuit employs two additional electrodes that detect an increased current as free $Ag^{++}$ accumulates following complete titration of the $Cl^-$ in solution. The detection of the increased current triggers a relay circuit that stops further generation of $Ag^{++}$ and shuts off a timer. The amount of $Cl^-$ in solution is proportional to the time required to generate sufficient $Ag^{++}$ to titrate the $Cl^-$. The methodologic precision is hampered by dirty electrodes that should be cleaned periodically to prevent buildup of protein residue.

The use of ISEs for chloride analysis is, most likely, the most widely used method since chloride electrodes are now incorporated into many new automated analyzer systems. These electrodes commonly employ a silver chloride-silver sulfide sensing element in the electrode and measure chloride in the same sample used for sodium and potassium determinations, resulting in great economy of time and reagents.

Chloride can be measured in serum, heparinized plasma, urine, or sweat. All methods of $Cl^-$ analysis are subject to interference from other halides such as bromide and iodide. The most clinically significant halide interference is due to bromide, which is found in certain drug preparations. Chloride is stable in serum, plasma, urine, and other fluids for at least 1 week at either room, refrigerator, or freezer temperatures.

## Total Carbon Dioxide

Total carbon dioxide is a measurement of the three principal chemical forms of carbon dioxide ($CO_2$): dissolved (gaseous) $CO_2$, carbamino compounds, and bicarbonate ($HCO_3^-$). Minor contributions are made by carbonic acid ($H_2CO_3$) and carbonate ions ($CO_3^{--}$). $HCO_3^-$ represents the major fraction of total $CO_2$; therefore, the total $CO_2$ measurement is used to indicate $HCO_3^-$ concentration.[32]

In most analytical procedures, all the various forms of $CO_2$ are converted to $CO_2$ gas by acidification of the sample. The amount of gas ($PCO_2$) formed is then measured by various methods. The reference method for total $CO_2$ employs the Natelson microgasometer, which measures the gas pressure as $CO_2$ is liberated by lactic acid. Spectrophotometric methods require the use of a pH indicator, such as cresol red, which produces a color change as the liberated $CO_2$ gas diffuses across a sili-cone membrane, decreasing the pH of the recipient buffer solution.

$$CO_2 + acid \longrightarrow CO_2\ gas$$

$$CO_2\ gas \xrightarrow[\text{membrane}]{\text{silicone}} CO_2\ dissolved,\ \downarrow pH$$

$$H^+ + pH\ indicator \longrightarrow color\ change$$

Some clinical analyzers employ an enzymatic method to photometrically measure $HCO_3^-$ concentration. In this type of reaction, phosphoenolpyruvate carboxylase (PEPC) catalyzes the reaction of $HCO_3^-$ and phosphoenolpyruvate (PEP) to produce oxaloacetate. Oxaloacetate is then reduced to malate by malate dehydrogenase (MDH) with the subsequent oxidation of $NADH \rightarrow NAD^+$. The decrease in absorbance can be measured at 340 nm.

$$HCO_3^- + PEP \longrightarrow Oxaloacetate + Pi$$

$$Oxaloacetate + NADH + H^+ \longrightarrow Malate + NAD^+$$

Ion-selective electrodes have also been adapted to the measurement of total $CO_2$. The pH change is measured by an electrode instead of spectophotometrically as the liberated $CO_2$ gas diffuses across a silicone membrane, resulting in a pH change of the buffer.

Serum or heparinized plasma are suitable samples. Certain precautions must be observed with total $CO_2$ analysis. Concentration of $CO_2$ in serum or plasma samples is much greater than the ambient air. Exposure of the sample to room air results in a rapid decrease of $CO_2$ of approximately 4 to 6 mmol/L after 1 hour. The sample should be handled as anaerobically as possible to prevent loss of $CO_2$. Separated serum or plasma is stable for several days if tightly capped and refrigerated.

## Magnesium

Magnesium is measured by a variety of methods. However, the reference method for magnesium analysis is atomic absorption. Lanthanum and strontium are contained in the diluent to bind with phosphate to prevent the formation of magnesium-phosphate compounds that are not measured. A commonly used method involves calmagite, which forms a reddish-violet complex with magnesium. This complex is then measured spectrophotometrically at 532 nm. The calmagite method does not require pretreatment to remove protein, a distinct advantage for use in automated clinical analyzers. Other methods include use of methylthymol blue (which requires concurrent use of EGTA to eliminate calcium interference) or chlorophosphonazo III (CPZ), which selectively binds magnesium.[33]

An unhemolyzed serum sample is the specimen of choice. In general, plasma samples are unacceptable because of the chelating action of the anticoagulants. Since magnesium is present in erythrocytes in greater concentration, hemolysis will falsely elevate the magnesium level. Serum should be separated from the cells immediately to prevent leakage of magnesium into the serum.

## Osmolality

Certain properties of solutions, known as colligative properties, are related to the number of total particles in that solution. When the osmolality of a solution changes, the colligative properties also change in relationship to the osmolality. For example, an increased osmolality results in an increased osmotic pressure and boiling point of the solution, whereas other colligative properties, such as freezing point and vapor pressure of the solution, are decreased.

One mole of an undissociated solute such as glucose will depress the freezing point of 1 kg of water by 1.858°C. The vapor pressure will correspondingly be decreased by 0.3 mm Hg, whereas the boiling point will be increased by 0.52°C.[34,35] This amount of undissociated solute results in a 1 molal solution, or 1 osmole. In contrast, 1 mole of an electrolyte such as NaCl will dissociate into 2 particles ($Na^+$ and $Cl^-$) when placed in 1 kg of water and will change the colligative properties by a factor equal to the number of dissociated particles, 2 in the case of NaCl. Thus, 1 mole of NaCl when dissolved in 1 kg of water results in a 2 osmole solution. The conventional unit of measurement of osmolality is milliosmole (mOsm/kg) since physiologic fluids have a relatively low osmolality.

The laboratory measurement of osmolality makes use of the colligative properties of biologic fluids. In most clinical chemistry laboratories, osmolality is calculated based on the concentration of sodium, glucose, and urea. The formula for this calculation is found in this chapter in the section on osmolality.

Vapor pressure depression osmometry is the most commonly used method for plasma or urine osmolality because of the simplicity of the instrumentation required. The presence of solute in an aqueous solution reduces the evaporation of the water (solvent) and exhibits an inverse relationship of concentration (osmolality) and vapor pressure. Changes in vapor pressure are determined by placing a small sample of the solution, usually saturated in a paper disk, in a heated and hermetically sealed chamber. The instrument measures the temperature, using a thermocouple to generate an electrical current, when the atmosphere in the chamber is saturated with water. The thermocouple will then cool the chamber and determine the temperature at which the water vapor condenses. By establishing a plateau temperature between the vaporization and condensation phases, an electrical current is generated that is proportional to the concentration of solute in the sample.

Freezing-point depression osmometry uses serum or urine

placed into a controlled cooling bath that supercools the sample below its freezing point to −7°C. The sample is then vibrated rapidly to release the heat of fusion that has been trapped during the rapid cooling. As the heat of fusion is released, the sample reaches its freezing point and the temperature is measured by a thermistor probe inserted into the sample. The degree of freezing-point depression below that of pure water is directly proportional to the total number of particles in the solution or the osmolality.[34] This method requires a large volume of sample, often 2 mL or more. Freezing-point depression is the preferred method when dealing with suspected methanol or ethylene glycol poisoning.[36,37]

## Iron and TIBC

Several methods are available for measuring serum iron and TIBC levels. However, certain reactions are common to each procedure with variations due to different reagents used in each reaction. The following is an outline of the common reactions with examples of reagents used.

1.  Iron ($Fe^{+++}$) must be split from the transferrin complex by exposure to various acids (HCl, $H_2SO_4$, or TCA). Some methods may require that the protein be removed.
2.  Reduction of $Fe^{+++}$ (ferric) to $Fe^{++}$ (ferrous) state using reducing agents such as ascorbic acid, hydrazine, thioglycollic acid, or hydroxylamine. This step is crucial since only ferrous iron will react with the chromagen.
3.  Reaction of $Fe^{++}$ with a chromagen such as bathophenanthroline sulfate, diphenylphenanthroline, ferrozine, or tripyridyltriazine (TPZ). Each of these chromagens will produce a characteristically colored compound that is then measured spectrophotometrically.

The TIBC method uses the same basic reactions as those used to measure serum iron with one important difference: the serum transferrin will first be saturated by addition of excess iron ($Fe^{+++}$), such as ferric ammonium citrate or ferric chloride. The excess (unbound) $Fe^{+++}$ is removed via an ion-exchange resin or chelated by $MgCO_3$. The now saturated transferrin will be assayed by the method used to measure serum iron. The TIBC demonstrates the maximum amount of iron which that protein can bind. Unsaturated iron-binding capacity (UIBC) is the reserve capacity of transferrin to bind iron. Generally, the serum iron level will be about one third of the TIBC; therefore, normal saturation of the serum iron-binding proteins is about 30%. Transferrin saturation may be calculated using [Serum Fe]/[TIBC] × 100 = % saturation.[23]

The specimen of choice for iron and TIBC analyses is serum, preferably collected in an amber-topped tube that has been specifically treated to remove any trace of iron contamination. A fasting, morning sample allows the most accurate assessment of iron status since iron levels are subject to diurnal variation, which causes afternoon samples to be decreased by as much as 30%. Hemolyzed samples are unsuitable because of the iron content of erythrocytes. Glassware used for iron analyses should be acid washed to remove trace contamination of iron and double-distilled water should be used in reagent preparation. Separated serum is stable for 1 week at refrigerated temperatures for both iron and TIBC analyses.

## Ferritin

Methods for measurement of serum ferritin are based on antigen-antibody reactions and incorporate immunoradiometric assays (IRMA) or ELISA techniques. Serum is the preferred specimen. Modern immunochemical methods provide the necessary sensitivity and specificity to accurately detect the small quantity of ferritin in the serum.

## SUMMARY

Electrolytes are important determinants of the state of hydration of the body and play an integral role in fluid homeostasis, neuromuscular function, and acid-base balance. Individual electrolyte concentrations vary between intracellular and extracellular fluid compartments, but total anion concentration within a compartment is equal to the total cation concentration. Thus, a state of electroneutrality exists within the fluid compartments.

Some electrolytes, primarily sodium, are regulated by tight hormonal control. The renin-angiotensin-aldosterone system in conjunction with ADH are the major regulatory mechanisms of fluid (water) homeostasis. Disorders of these systems as well as organ function impairment result in electrolyte disorders with associated symptoms.

Laboratory tests used to assess electrolyte balance include measurement of serum $Na^+$, $K^+$, $Cl^-$, and $HCO_3^-$. Occasionally, urine $Na^+$, $K^+$, and $Cl^-$ measurements are performed. The measurement of serum and urine osmolality frequently accompanies electrolyte measurement to better assess fluid homeostasis. Sweat chloride measurement is performed on infants as a diagnostic aid in the detection of cystic fibrosis.

Electrolyte disorders are frequently accompanied by a mathematical discrepancy in the concentration of measured anions and cations known as the anion gap. Calculation of the anion gap is useful as an inexpensive means of laboratory quality control as well as aiding in the detection and classification of various electrolyte abnormalities.

Iron is a trace element that is a major determinant of the oxygen-carrying capacity of hemoglobin. Its concentration is primarily controlled by a transport mechanism that regulates the amount of iron absorption of the intestinal mucosal cells. Laboratory tests used to assess iron status include serum iron, TIBC, % transferrin saturation, and ferritin.

## REFERENCES

1. Marshall WJ: Water, sodium and potassium. In Marshall WF (ed.): *Clinical Chemistry*. 3rd ed. London, CV Mosby, 1995, pp 11–33.
2. Kleinman LI, Lorenz JM: Physiology and pathophysiology of body water and electrolytes. In Kaplan LA, Pesce AJ (eds.): *Clinical Chemistry: Theory, Analysis and Correlation*. 3rd ed. St. Louis, CV Mosby, 1996; pp 439–463.
3. Eder AF, McGrath CM, Dowdy YG, Tomaszewski JE, et al.: Ethylene glycol poisoning: toxicokinetic and analytical factors affecting laboratory diagnosis. Clin Chem 44:168–177, 1998.
4. Tietz MW, Pruden EL, Siggard-Anderson O: Electrolytes. In Burtis CA, Ashwood ER: *Tietz Fundamentals of Clinical Chemistry*. 4th ed. Philadelphia, WB Saunders, 1996, pp 497–505.
5. Goldberg M: Hyponatremia. Med Clin North Am 65(2):247–451, 1981.
6. Hillier TA, Abbott RD, Barrett EJ: Hyponatremia: Evaluating the correction factor for hyperglycemia. Am J Med 106:399–403, 1999.
7. DeFronzo RA, Bia M, Smith D: Clinical disorders of hyperkalemia. Ann Rev Med 33:521–554, 1982.
8. Rowley PT, Loader S, Levenkron JC: Cystic fibrosis carrier population screening: A review. Genet Test 1(1):53–59, 1997.
9. LeGrys VA: Sweat testing for the diagnosis of cystic fibrosis: Practical considerations. J Pediatr 129:892–897, 1996.
10. Friedman KJ, Silverman LM: Cystic fibrosis syndrome: A new paradigm for inherited disorders and implications for molecular diagnostics. Clin Chem 45:929–931, 1999.
11. Highsmith WE Jr, Burch LH, Zhou Z, Olsen JC, et al.: A novel mutation in the cystic fibrosis gene in patients with pulmonary disease but normal sweat chloride concentrations. N Engl J Med 331:974–980, 1994.
12. Gan K-H, Veeze H, van den Ouwelan AMW, Halley DJJ et al.: A cystic fibrosis mutation associated with mild lung disease. N Engl J Med 333:95–99, 1995.
13. Lolekha PH, Lolekha S: Value of the anion gap in clinical diagnosis and laboratory evaluation. Clin Chem 29:279–283, 1983.
14. Endres DB, Rude R: Mineral and bone metabolism. In Burtis CA, Ashwood ER, (eds.): *Tietz Fundamentals of Clinical Chemistry*. 4th ed. Philadelphia, WB Saunders, 1996, p 690.
15. Elin RJ: Assessment of magnesium status. Clin Chem 33:1965–1970, 1987.
16. Thienpont LM, Dewitte K, Stöckl D: Serum complexed magnesium—a cautionary note on its estimation and its relevance for standardizing serum ionized magnesium. Clin Chem 45:154a–155a, 1999.
17. Dacey MJ: Hypomagnesemic disorders. Crit Care Clin 17(1):155–173, viii, 2001.
18. Agus MS, Agus ZS: Cardiovascular actions of magnesium. Crit Care Clin 17(1):175–186, 2001.

19. Liao F, Folsom AR, Brancati FL: Is low magnesium concentration a risk factor for coronary heart disease? The Atherosclerosis Risk in Communities (ARIC) study. Am Heart J 136:480–490, 1998.

20. Guerrero-Romero F, Rodriguez-Moran M: Hypomagnesemia is linked to low serum HDL-cholesterol irrespective of serum glucose values. J Diabet Complications 14(5):272–276, 2000.

21. Sanders GT, Huijgen HJ, Sanders R: Magnesium in disease: a review with special emphasis on the serum ionized magnesium. Clin Chem Lab Med 37(11–12):1011–1133, 1999.

22. Harker HE, Majcher TA: Hypermagnesemia in a pediatric patient. Anesth Analg 91:1160–1162, 2000.

23. Fairbanks VF, Klee GG: Biochemical Aspects of Hematology. In Burtis CA, Ashwood ER (eds.): *Tietz Fundamentals of Clinical Chemistry*. 4th ed. Philadelphia, WB Saunders, 1996, pp 727–730.

24. Schreiber WE: Iron, porphyrin and bilirubin metabolism. In Kaplan LA, Pesce AJ (eds.): *Clinical Chemistry: Theory, Analysis and Correlation*. 3rd ed. St. Louis, CV Mosby, 1996, pp 697–702.

25. Skikne BS: Circulating transferrin receptor assay—coming of age. Clin Chem 44:7, 1998.

26. Shih YJ, Baynes RD, Hudson BG, et al.: Serum transferrin receptor is a truncated form of tissue receptor. J Biol Chem 265:19077–19081, 1990.

27. Mast AE, Morey A, Blinder AM, et al.: Clinical utility of the soluble transferrin receptor and comparison with serum ferritin in several populations. Clin Chem 44:45–51, 1998.

28. Looker AC, Loyevsky M, Gordeuk VR: Increased serum transferrin saturation is associated with lower serum transferrin receptor concentration. Clin Chem 45:2191–2199, 1999.

29. Powell LW, Yapp TR: Hemochromatosis. Clin Liver Dis 4(1):211–228, viii, 2000.

30. Gochee PA, Powell LW: What's new in hemochromatosis. Curr Opin Hematol 8(2):98–104, 2001.

31. Korzun WJ, Miller WG: Sodium and potassium. In Kaplan LA, Pesce AJ, (eds.): *Clinical Chemistry: Theory, Analysis and Correlation*. 3rd ed. St. Louis, CV Mosby, 1996, pp 461–463.

32. Korzun WJ, Miller WG: Carbon dioxide. In Kaplan LA, Pesce AJ, (eds.): *Clinical Chemistry: Theory, Analysis and Correlation*. 3rd ed. St. Louis, CV Mosby, 1996, pp 480–481, 461–463.

33. Kazmierczak S: Magnesium. In Kaplan LA, Pesce AJ, (eds.): *Clinical Chemistry: Theory, Analysis and Correlation*. 3rd ed. St. Louis, CV Mosby, 1996, pp 550–551.

34. Freier E: Osmometry. In Burtis CA, Ashwood ER (eds.): *Tietz Fundamentals of Clinical Chemistry*. 4th ed. Philadelphia, WB Saunders, 1996, pp 94–97.

35. Kaplan LA: Measurement of colligative properties. In Kaplan LA, Pesce AJ (eds.): *Clinical Chemistry: Theory, Analysis and Correlation*. 3rd ed. St. Louis, CV Mosby, 1996, pp 270–276.

36. Eisen TF, Lacouture PG, Woolf A: Serum osmolality in alcohol ingestions: Differences in availability among laboratories of teaching hospital, nonteaching hospital, and commercial facilities. Am J Emerg Med 7:256–259, 1989.

37. Glaser DS: Utility of the serum osmol gap in the diagnosis of methanol or ethylene glycol ingestion. Ann Emerg Med 27:343–346, 1996.

# C H A P T E R  2 2
# Acid-Base and Blood Gas Physiology

*Lisa J. Johnson*

Over the past several decades, advances in knowledge and technology have revolutionized health care delivery. Patients in critical care units have been the primary beneficiaries of technological advances in the clinical laboratory because results of pH, blood gas, and electrolyte tests, the main urgently needed determinations to assess the critically ill, can be provided quickly and efficiently.

Laboratory services are projected to account for an average of 5% of hospital budgets in the United States.[1] However, laboratory results are estimated to influence 60% to 70% of all critical health care decisions made.[1] Moreover, it has been estimated that of the total cost of critical care, the laboratory evaluation accounts for 25% of the expenditures, with arterial blood gases being the most frequently ordered tests in these units.[2]

Arterial blood gases have been the indisputable reference standard for the assessment of oxygenation status. Other indications for the measurement of arterial blood gases include establishment of the diagnosis and severity of respiratory failure, management of patients in critical care units, guidance in therapeutic decisions, determination of the prognosis of critically ill patients, and monitoring of patients undergoing cardiopulmonary surgery or exercise testing. The measurement of blood pH is typically included in arterial blood gas assessments. The control of hydrogen ion levels is of utmost importance in the body, since changes in pH affect the structure and function of such macromolecules as proteins, nucleic acids, and lipids.

## CLINICALLY IMPORTANT GASES

### Gas Distribution in the Blood

Gas distribution in the blood is governed by physical principles or laws. Boyle's law and Charles' law correlate the volume of an ideal gas to temperature and pressure. **Boyle's law** states that gas volume varies inversely with pressure at constant absolute temperature, whereas **Charles' law** states that volume varies directly with temperature when at constant pressure. These two principles are often combined into one general gas equation:

$$P = (nRT)/V \text{ or } PV = nRT$$

where  $P$ = pressure in units of millimeters of mercury (mm Hg), also called torr,
 $V$ = volume in liters in which the ideal gas is contained,
 $T$ = temperature in degrees Kelvin,
 $N$ = number of moles of the gas, and
 $R$ = gas constant.

The more commonly used unit of mm Hg is derived from the fact that 1 torr of pressure, which is 1/760 of normal atmospheric pressure, supports a column of mercury 1 mm high at 0°C at standard gravity. The SI unit of pressure is the pascal (Pa). One mm Hg is equal to 133.3224 Pa. It is sometimes more advantageous to use the SI unit because 1 atmosphere (atm), which is equal to 760 mm Hg, is approximately equal to 100 kPa. Thus, partial pressures expressed in kilopascals provide close estimates of the percentages of the gases present in one atm.

**Dalton's law** states that the total pressure exerted by a mixture of ideal gases is equal to the sum of the partial pressures of the individual gases in the mixture. For room air, this principle is expressed as

$$P(\text{ambient}) = PO_2 + PCO_2 + PN_2 + PH_2O + PX \cdots$$

where $PH_2O$ is the partial pressure of water vapor and $PX$ is that of the minute amount of remaining gases in the air. The partial pressure of any one gas present in a given volume is dependent on the number of moles of the gas and on the temperature. However, the partial pressure of the gas is independent of the presence or absence of other gases in the same volume. The air we breathe consists of approximately 20.95% oxygen, 0.03% carbon dioxide, 78.1% nitrogen, and 0.1% other inert gases. Thus, at a pressure of 1 atm (760 mm Hg), the partial pressures exerted by the dry gases oxygen and carbon dioxide are 160 mm Hg and 0.25 mm Hg, respectively. Physiologically, however, water vapor pressure must be accounted for in inspired air. At the barometric pressure of 1 atm and body temperature of 37°C, the water vapor pressure of moist inspired gas is 47 mm Hg. Therefore, the partial pressure of oxygen of inspired air is actually (20.95 ÷ 100) × (760 − 47), or 149 mm Hg. The concept of partial pressure is extremely important in regard to blood gas physiology since the actions of a gas depend on the pressure exerted by the gas. Dalton's law is applied only to gases in a gaseous phase. It does not apply to gases dissolved in a liquid. **Henry's law** predicts the amount of dissolved gas in a liquid that is in contact with the gas. More definitively stated, this law defines that the amount of a sparingly soluble gas dissolved in a liquid is proportional to the partial pressure of the gas over the liquid. This principle is of extreme importance since oxygen from the air we breathe is primarily delivered to the tissues through the blood.

## Oxygen

### OXIDATIVE METABOLISM

The oxygen derived from the air that we breathe is required by mammals for life processes. It is dissolved molecular oxygen that fuels cellular metabolism to manufacture the essential bioenergy storage compound, adenosine triphosphate (ATP). On inhalation from the air, oxygen moves down a partial pressure gradient through the respiratory tract, alveolar gas, arterial blood, systemic capillaries, and tissues until it finally reaches the cell. On entry into the cell, oxygen easily moves into the mitochondria, which are the lowest pressure level. In the mitochondria, which are distributed throughout the cell, oxygen is consumed through the process of oxidative metabolism.

Energy production and deployment in the body is derived from the oxidation of food fuels, the principal source being glucose. Quantitatively, each glucose molecule combines with 6 oxygen molecules to produce 6 carbon dioxide molecules, 6 molecules of water, and energy. Consequently, 12 molecules of hydrogen are produced from the oxidation of each molecule of glucose. Each of these hydrogen molecules enters oxidative phosphorylation to yield 3 ATP molecules. Thus, in combination with 2 ATP molecules generated through glycolysis, oxidative metabolism generates a total of 38 ATP molecules.

In spite of oxygen's crucial role in metabolism, the body is unable to maintain physical oxygen stores. Moreover, the amount of oxygen typically circulating in the blood is barely sufficient for 3 minutes of metabolism in the resting state. The physiologic state of abnormally low oxygen pressure is called tissue **hypoxia.**

### FORMS OF OXYGEN IN THE BLOOD

Oxygen is carried in the blood in the physically dissolved state and bound to transport proteins, primarily hemoglobin. In spite of its importance, oxygen is poorly soluble in the blood. Only a small fraction of inspired oxygen is dissolved in the blood; most is delivered to the tissues bound to hemoglobin. Under normal conditions, hemoglobin is typically 95% saturated with oxygen. It has been projected that without hemoglobin the amount of oxygen carried in the blood would be so small that cardiac output would need to be increased by a factor of 20 to provide adequate delivery of oxygen to the tissues.[3] Overall, the amount of oxygen that the blood can carry is dependent on three major factors: (1) the amount of nor-

mal, effective hemoglobin present in the red cells, (2) the partial pressure of oxygen, which indicates how much oxygen is dissolved in the blood, and (3) the affinity of the available hemoglobin for oxygen.

## OXYGEN TRANSPORT

The ability of hemoglobin to efficiently transport and release oxygen is based on its structural characteristics. Hemoglobin, a tetramer, evolved from monomeric myoglobin. The tetrameric structure allows hemoglobin to bind 4 oxygen molecules as opposed to the 1 bound by myoglobin. Though the binding of oxygen is reversible in both proteins, the strength of the bond and ease of detachment is vastly different. On the initial binding of the first oxygen, the 4 polypeptide chains of hemoglobin begin a communication with each other, resulting in the cooperative binding of the remaining oxygen molecules. This cooperative binding is due to allosteric effects, in which the uptake of 1 oxygen molecule influences the affinities of the remaining unfilled binding sites. Thus, the oxygen affinity of each heme-polypeptide subunit of hemoglobin depends on whether oxygen is bound to the neighboring subunits. Upon binding oxygen, conformational changes actually occur in the subunits, creating the language of communication between subunits. Consequently, hemoglobin has two states of quaternary structure, a deoxy form and an oxy form. The switch from the deoxy to the oxy form, which has the higher affinity for oxygen, accounts for the cooperativity in binding. As an aside, it is noteworthy that the tetrapyrrole ring of hemoglobin is also a constituent of chlorophyll and the cytochromes that function in cellular oxidative metabolism.

The degree of association or dissociation between oxygen and hemoglobin is contingent on the partial pressure of oxygen and the affinity of hemoglobin for oxygen. If these two variables are plotted on a graph, oxygen saturation of hemoglobin versus the partial pressure of oxygen, a sigmoidal curve is produced as shown in Figure 22–1. This curve is referred to as the **oxygen dissociation curve.** The sigmoidal shape of the curve is significant because it graphically demonstrates the notion of cooperativity or the increasing efficiency with which hemoglobin binds more oxygen once an initial oxygen molecule is bound. Note that at a $PO_2$ of approximately 100 mm Hg, oxygen saturation of hemoglobin is 100%, whereas at the lower $PO_2$ of 20 mm Hg, which approximates that of the tissues, oxygen saturation drops and ultimately reaches zero. Actually, hemoglobin retains oxygen until the $PO_2$ is reduced to approximately 60 mm Hg. Below this level, hemoglobin rapidly releases its oxygen. Physiologically, this is an ideal system for the transport and delivery of oxygen from the lungs to the tissues. Conversely, the shape of the dissociation curve for myoglobin is hyperbolic, indicating that myoglobin binds oxygen at the $PO_2$ found in the lungs but does not release it efficiently at the $PO_2$ of the tissues.

The location of the oxygen dissociation curve relative to the $PO_2$ necessary to achieve a given level of oxygen saturation in the blood is dependent on the affinity of hemoglobin

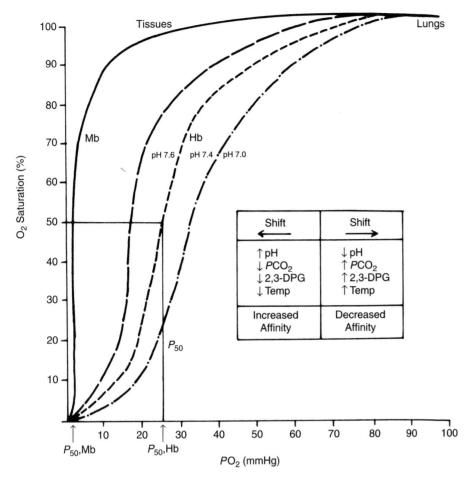

### FIGURE 22-1

Oxygen dissociation curves. Curve Mb represents the association/dissociation of oxygen and myoglobin. Curves Hb, denoted by the dotted lines, represent the association/dissociation of oxygen and hemoglobin at 3 different pH ranges. Factors causing a shift to the left or right in the oxygen dissociation curve for hemoglobin are given in the inset table.

for oxygen. The affinity of hemoglobin for oxygen is dependent on 5 factors: temperature, pH, the partial pressure of carbon dioxide, the concentration of 2,3-diphosphoglycerate (2,3-DPG), and the presence of other hemoglobin species that are nonfunctional. Figure 22–1 illustrates the effect of plasma pH on the location of the curve and is referred to as the **Bohr effect.** Observe that with increasing blood pH, the curve shifts to the left and vice versa. A shift to the left can also be caused by a decrease in the partial pressure of carbon dioxide, 2,3-DPG, or temperature. 2,3-DPG is an intermediate metabolite in the red cell that binds to the $\beta$ chains within the central cavity of hemoglobin, causing a decrease in oxygen affinity. Physiologically, a leftward shift of the dissociation curve means that there is an increased affinity of hemoglobin for oxygen, indicating that oxygen is released at the tissues less efficiently. Conversely, a rightward shift of the curve, indicating a decrease in affinity, may be caused by a decrease in pH or an increase

in the partial pressure of $CO_2$, 2,3-DPG, or temperature. In general, the body tolerates this rightward shift of the dissociation curve much better than the leftward shift. For example, increasing temperature causes an increase in the metabolic rate, which in turn increases the demand for oxygen. The increased oxygen delivery resulting from the rightward shift of the dissociation curve in this situation helps to meet the increased need for oxygen in the tissues.

Another parameter that is sometimes useful to describe the location dissociation curve is the $P_{50}$. The $P_{50}$ is defined as the $PO_2$ at which hemoglobin is half saturated with oxygen; thus, $P_{50}$ is expressed in mm Hg. Increased values for $P_{50}$ indicate displacement of the dissociation curve to the right, whereas decreased values indicate displacement to the left. Causes of a low $P_{50}$ include hypothermia, acute alkalemia (increase in blood pH), hypocapnia (decreased carbon dioxide), low 2,3-DPG, or the presence of an abnormal hemoglobin.

High $P_{50}$ values may be due to hyperthermia, acidemia or decreased blood pH, hypercapnia (increased carbon dioxide), high 2,3-DPG, or the presence of an abnormal hemoglobin having a decreased oxygen affinity. Under normal conditions, the $P_{50}$ is typically about 25 mm Hg. Note in Figure 22–1 the extremely low $P_{50}$ for myoglobin (about 2 mm Hg). This low $P_{50}$ is yet another indicator of myoglobin's high affinity for oxygen and inefficient release at the $PO_2$ found in the tissues.

Thus far, hemoglobin has been described in relation to its normal state, whether it is oxygenated or not. However, other abnormal or dysfunctional hemoglobins may also be present. Both oxyhemoglobin and deoxyhemoglobin are normal functional hemoglobins that are capable of binding and releasing oxygen efficiently. Dysfunctional forms of hemoglobin are not capable of the same reversible association with oxygen as the functional hemoglobins. The most commonly encountered dysfunctional hemoglobins include methemoglobin (MetHb), carboxyhemoglobin (COHb), and sulfhemoglobin (SulfHb). Methemoglobin molecules contain iron in the ferric ($+3$) state, as opposed to the ferrous ($+2$) state found in the functional hemoglobins. Carboxyhemoglobin is formed when carbon monoxide binds with hemoglobin. Carbon monoxide poisoning is of particular danger since this gas has an affinity for hemoglobin that is more than 200 times that of oxygen. Sulfhemoglobin is abnormal because of a genetically determined variant in the globin chain that alters the allosteric binding properties of hemoglobin.

## Carbon Dioxide

### METABOLIC PRODUCTION

The end product of most aerobic metabolic processes is carbon dioxide. Recall that for every glucose molecule metabolized, 6 molecules of $CO_2$ are produced. Thus, upon production in the mitochondria of the tissue cells, $CO_2$ passes through the cytoplasm exiting the cells and entering the extracellular fluid. Since very little $CO_2$ is produced in the red blood cells where metabolism is accomplished anaerobically, it easily diffuses into the red cells and plasma of the surrounding capillaries. In the red cells, $CO_2$ combines with water to form carbonic acid. This reaction is facilitated by the enzyme carbonic anhydrase, which is located in the red cell membrane. The carbonic acid formed, in turn, quickly dissociates into hydrogen ion and bicarbonate. Combined, these reactions are written:

$$CO_2 + H_2O \leftrightarrow H_2CO_3 \leftrightarrow H^+ + HCO_3^-.$$

Though these reactions are reversible, the forward progression predominates under the physiologic conditions found in the red blood cell.

The $CO_2$ produced as a product of oxidative metabolism has been projected to result in carbonic acid generation at a rate of 10 to 15 mmol per minute.[4] Moreover, the oxidation of carbon-containing fuels, such as glucose, results in the tremendous production of 16,000 to 20,000 mmol of volatile

acid ($CO_2$) per day.[5] Hence, the body is constantly challenged by the metabolic production of acids.

## FORMS OF CARBON DIOXIDE IN THE BLOOD

Carbon dioxide exists in three different forms in the blood with approximately 90% existing as bicarbonate ions, 5% as carbamino compounds, and the remaining 5% being physically dissolved. Bicarbonate is the second largest fraction of plasma anions behind chloride. As the bicarbonate concentration increases in the red cell upon ionization of carbonic acid, it diffuses across the cell membrane into the plasma where it circulates bound to sodium. The remaining hydrogen ion produced from the carbonic acid dissociation, however, is unable to exit the cell and enter the plasma because the cell membrane is relatively impermeable to cations. Consequently, to maintain electroneutrality, chloride ions move into the cell to fill the anionic deficit created by the lost bicarbonate ions. This exchange of chloride and bicarbonate ions in the red cell is called the **chloride shift.**

Carbamino compounds are formed when $CO_2$ combines with the N-terminal amino acid residues of blood proteins, primarily hemoglobin. When $CO_2$ binds to hemoglobin, the accessibility of the heme groups to oxygen is altered. Therefore, formation of carbamino compounds has the effect of weakening oxygen's binding affinity to hemoglobin. Conversely, carbamino formation falls with increasing oxygenation. The formation of reduced or deoxygenated hemoglobin, as occurs in the tissues, helps with the loading of $CO_2$, whereas the increased $PO_2$ in the lungs results in the unloading of $CO_2$. The impact of oxygen on carbon dioxide in the form of carbamino compounds is referred to as the **Haldane effect.**

Carbon dioxide is also found in the physically dissolved state in the blood since it belongs to a group of gases having moderate solubility in water. In comparison to oxygen, carbon dioxide has about 24 times greater solubility in water. Thus, more $CO_2$ is found in the physically dissolved form than $O_2$. Through application of Henry's law of gas solubility,

$$dCO_2 = PCO_2 \times \alpha$$

where $dCO_2$ = the concentration of dissolved $CO_2$ in the blood,
$PCO_2$ = partial pressure of $CO_2$, and
$\alpha$ = solubility coefficient for $CO_2$.

When $PCO_2$ is in units of torr or mm Hg and $dCO_2$ is in units of mmol/L, $\alpha = 0.0301$.

## Respiration

The physical activity of respiration is regulated by the medulla of the brain. Certain chemoreceptors respond to the levels of oxygen and carbon dioxide, as well as pH, of the blood and cerebrospinal fluid and initiate signals to the medulla. The medulla then controls the rate and depth of respiration. During inspiration, the thoracic cavity expands creating a temporary vacuum and air moves into the lungs. As the atmospheric air moves in, it fills the numerous tracheal branches ultimately ending up in the alveoli. These small saclike chambers are highly vascularized by capillary beds. Except for the heart, the lung is the only other organ that receives the entire blood circulation. The exchange of gases in the air occurs across the thin alveolar membranes and pulmonary capillaries. During exhalation, air is released as the elastic tissues of the lungs recoil and force air outward as intrathoracic volume is decreased. Many pathologic states involving the lungs are caused by loss of elasticity of the lungs and the destruction of the alveolar membranes.

## GAS EXCHANGE IN THE LUNGS

The diffusion of oxygen and carbon dioxide across the alveolar membranes is governed by gradients in the partial pressures of the gases. As shown in Figure 22–2, oxygen moves down its gradient from the alveolus, where the $PO_2$ is approximately 110 mm Hg, to the pulmonary capillaries, where the $PO_2$ is ~40 mm Hg. The $PO_2$ in the alveoli is lower than that of dry atmospheric air since it is diluted with residual air that remains from the last expiration and saturated with water vapor. The actual alveolar $PO_2$ is determined by a balance between the rate of oxygen removal from the blood, as set by the metabolic demands in the tissues and the rate of oxygen replenishment by ventilation.

Upon inspiration into the alveoli, oxygen is warmed to the body's temperature of 37°C and bound to hemoglobin for delivery to the tissues. If the tissues cannot obtain the oxygen necessary for metabolism, hypoxia occurs, which may lead to cell death. Conditions affecting the uptake and delivery of oxygen to the tissues include those where (1) alveoli are destroyed, such as occurs with emphysema, (2) a barrier to diffusion is created, as occurs with the accumulation of fluid in states of pulmonary edema, (3) airways are blocked, as with asthma or bronchitis, or (4) the blood supply is inadequate, as occurs with a weakened heart or in cases of pulmonary embolism.

Carbon dioxide follows its gradient by diffusing from the capillaries where the $PCO_2$ is ~46 mm Hg to the alveoli where the $PCO_2$ approximates 40 mm Hg. The solubility of $CO_2$ in the blood facilitates this diffusion especially in light of the small pressure gradient. Moreover, $CO_2$ gas exchange is greatly enhanced by carbonic anhydrase, which is present on the surface of endothelial cells lining the pulmonary capillaries. Recall that carbonic anhydrase catalyzes reaction 1:

$$CO_2 + H_2O \overset{1}{\leftrightarrow} H_2CO_3 \overset{2}{\leftrightarrow} H^+ + HCO_3^-.$$

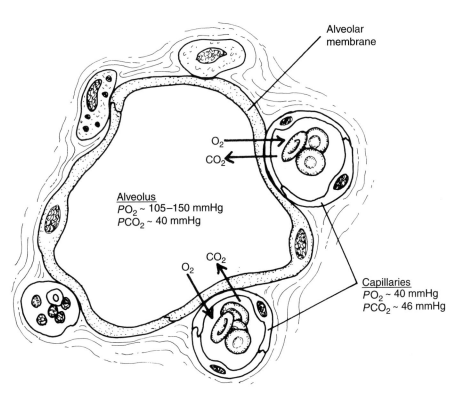

Alveolar membrane

$O_2$

$CO_2$

Alveolus
$PO_2$ ~ 105–150 mmHg
$PCO_2$ ~ 40 mmHg

$CO_2$

$O_2$

Capillaries
$PO_2$ ~ 40 mmHg
$PCO_2$ ~ 46 mmHg

**FIGURE  22-2**

Gas exchange in the lungs. Gas exchange follows the tension gradient, as demonstrated by arrows, denoting gas flow into or out of the alveolus. Thus, oxygen flows out of the alveoli into the capillaries, while carbon dioxide diffuses from the capillaries into the alveoli for final expiration.

Thus, the lower $PCO_2$ of the alveoli pulls the reaction to the left, mobilizing $CO_2$ for elimination through expired air. **Hypercapnia**, $CO_2$ accumulation, occurs as a result of inadequate ventilation. This results in an increased hydrogen ion concentration or decreased blood pH since the increase in $CO_2$ favors the forward direction of the reactions above. Blood pH or hydrogen ion concentration may also be driven in the opposite direction if $CO_2$ removal is faster than that of production. Consequently, the most important factor in the control of ventilation under normal conditions is the $PCO_2$. It has been estimated that in the course of daily activity, the arterial $PCO_2$ is held to within 3 mm Hg.[6]

### GAS EXCHANGE IN THE TISSUES

Just as in the lungs, the diffusion of gases across the membranes of the tissue cells and capillaries is governed by pressure gradients. As shown in Figure 22–3, the $PO_2$ at the surface of the tissue cells is ~20 mm Hg, which is substantially lower than the $PO_2$ in the capillaries (80 to 90 mm Hg). In truth, tissue $PO_2$ probably varies considerably throughout the body with some cells having a $PO_2$ as low as 1 mm Hg. A gradient exists for $PCO_2$, with the difference being 50 to 70 mm Hg in tissue cells and 40 mm Hg in the capillaries. Consequently, in the tissues, the gradient for oxygen is toward the tissue cell and for carbon dioxide it is toward the capillary blood. The increased $H^+$ concentration and $PCO_2$ that are produced during metabolism facilitate oxygen release from hemoglobin at the tissues by changing the structural configuration of hemoglobin to favor the deoxyhemoglobin state.

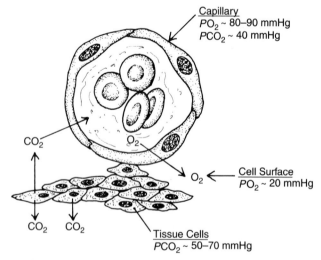

**F I G U R E   2 2 – 3**

Gas exchange in the tissues. Gas exchange follows the tension gradient, as demonstrated by arrows, denoting gas flow into and out of the tissue capillaries. In the tissues, oxygen is released from the capillaries, while cellular carbon dioxide waste is picked up for disposal by the blood.

## MAINTENANCE OF ACID-BASE BALANCE

### Generation of Metabolic Acids

In the chapter section that addresses the metabolic production of carbon dioxide, acid production as a consequence of oxidative metabolism was explained. Recall that the combustion of most carbon-containing fuels, such as glucose, generates $CO_2$ that is converted to carbonic acid. The production rate of this acid has been estimated to be 10 to 15 mmol per minute.[4] The metabolism of certain other body constituents, such as proteins, nucleic acids, and some lipids and carbohydrates, generates specific organic acids that cannot be fully metabolized to $CO_2$. Hence, instead of carbonic acid production, other acids are formed including acetic acid, uric acid, oxalic acid, glucuronic acid, hippuric acid, and others. In addition, inorganic acids such as sulfuric and phosphoric acids are also produced. The normal human diet is almost neutral in pH but provides the foodstuffs from which these volatile and nonvolatile acids are generated. In addition to this dietary source, intestinal bacteria produce approximately 300 mEq of organic acids including acetic, propionic, and butyric acids per day.[5] Bacteria produce these acids anaerobically as they metabolize foodstuffs in the intestinal lumen. After production in the lumen, the acids are quite completely reabsorbed.

In total, it is estimated that the body produces some 15 to 20 moles of hydrogen ions ($H^+$) per day.[7] Normally, the body excretes the acid produced through the lungs or kidneys without allowing any appreciable change in blood pH. In fact, the normal $H^+$ concentration in the extracellular body fluids ranges from only 36 to 44 nmol/L. Accumulation of acids in the body can have devastating effects since the rates of cellular biochemical reactions can be altered causing changes in metabolic processes. Physiologically, acid accumulation in the body fluids may alter the state of consciousness and lead to coma and possibly death. Thus, it is clear that under normal conditions, the acids produced in the body are very effectively buffered.

### Acids, Bases, and Buffers

#### A REVIEW OF BASIC DEFINITIONS

An **acid** is a compound that is capable of donating a $H^+$ and a **base** is a compound that is capable of accepting a $H^+$. When an acid (HA) dissociates, it produces a $H^+$ and its conjugate base ($A^-$) as shown:

$$HA \rightarrow H^+ + A^-$$

The anion ($A^-$) in this reaction is referred to as the **conjugate base** because of its ability to accept hydrogen ions and act as a base. When placed in water, all acids dissociate into the ion forms shown. The difference, however, lies in the degree of dissociation. A **strong acid** completely dissociates into the component ions when placed in water, whereas a **weak acid** separates into the component ions less readily. The concentration or activity of hydrogen ions in a solution determines the acidity of the solution. Hydrogen ion activity of a solution determines the **pH** of the solution as shown below:

$$pH = \log 1/[H^+] \text{ or } -\log [H^+]$$

where pH is a dimensionless quantity that is reciprocally related to hydrogen ion concentration. Thus, pH decreases as $[H^+]$ increases and, conversely, pH increases as $[H^+]$ decreases. Since this relationship is also logarithmic in nature, the correlation between pH and $[H^+]$ is not linear. As illustration of this point, a decrease of 1 pH unit represents a 10-fold increase in the hydrogen ion activity.

A **buffer,** composed of a weak acid or weak base and its corresponding salt, is a system that resists change in pH. The law of mass action applies to the dissociation reaction and an equilibrium is established between the weak acid and its dissociated ions. The degree of ionization is defined by a constant, K, which characterizes the strength of the acid. The larger the K, the stronger the acid and the greater the tendency for it to dissociate.

## BUFFERING AND THE HENDERSON-HASSELBALCH EQUATION

According to the reversible buffer reaction shown below, when an acid is added to a buffer solution (HA), the conjugate base $(A^-)$ of the buffer pair binds the $H^+$ from the acid to form more of the weak acid (HA). In this way, changes in pH are minimized.

$$HA \leftrightarrow H^+ + A^-$$

In compliance with the law of mass action, the equilibrium between a weak acid (HA) and its dissociated ions ($H^+$ and $A^-$) may be written as:

$$K = [H^+][A^-]/[HA]$$

Rearranged to determine the hydrogen ion concentration, the same reaction may be stated as:

$$[H^+] = K\{[HA]/[A^-]\}$$

If the negative log is taken on both sides of the equation, then:

$$-\log [H^+] = -\log K - \log\{[HA]/[A^-]\}$$

Since $-\log [H^+] = pH$, $-\log K = K$. Thus, by substitution the equation may be written as:

$$pH = pK + \log [A^-]/[HA]$$

In this form, the equation is known as the **Henderson-Hasselbalch equation.**

Optimum buffering occurs when the ratio of acid to its conjugate base is ~1. This state is reached when the pH is near the pK, ideally within the interval of ±1 pH unit of its pK. (Figure 22–4**a.**) The pK of an acid indicates the point at which the acid is 50% dissociated. Consequently, when the pH is equal to the pK, a buffer exists in equal proportions of its acid and conjugate base. For acids, raising the pH above the pK causes the acid to dissociate. The lower the value of the pK, the stronger the acid; likewise, the higher the pK, the weaker the acid.

## Clinically Important Buffers

There are four clinically important buffer systems that maintain the normal pH balance in the body between the narrow range of 7.35 and 7.45. These buffers (Figure 22–4**b.**), in order of decreasing physiologic importance, are the bicarbonate-carbonic acid buffer system, hemoglobin, plasma proteins, and phosphates. Although not considered to be the most important physiologically, hemoglobin accounts for the majority (80%) of the chemical buffering capacity of the blood. Plasma proteins are the next most abundant buffer, representing approximately 14% of the chemical buffering capacity of the blood. The remainder of the buffering capacity is represented by the bicarbonate–carbonic acid system (~5%) and inorganic phosphates (~1%). In the body, most buffering takes place inside the cell, where all of the four major buffer systems are found. Outside of the cell, plasma buffers include bicarbonate, proteins, and inorganic phosphates.

### BICARBONATE–CARBONIC ACID BUFFER SYSTEM

Carbonic acid ($H_2CO_3$) is a weak acid with bicarbonate ($HCO_3^-$) serving as its conjugate base. When acid is added to this system, the hydrogen ions react with bicarbonate to form more carbonic acid and thus minimize changes in pH. At body temperature, the pK of this buffer pair is 6.1, more than 1 pH unit away from the normal body pH of 7.4. Consequently, this buffer system would not be expected to be effective from a purely chemical viewpoint. In fact, in vitro, this buffer is not effective at maintaining a pH of 7.4 upon the addition of acid or base. The difference in vivo is that this system is able to react quickly to change the concentration of either carbonic acid or bicarbonate. This reaction is based on the immediate response of the lungs in controlling ventilation and thus $CO_2$, and the additional reaction of the kidneys, which regulate bicarbonate regeneration and acid excretion. Recall that the $PCO_2$ multiplied by the solubility coefficient, $\alpha$, is equal to the concentration of dissolved carbon dioxide. It is more practical to speak in terms of dissolved $CO_2$ or $PCO_2$ since the amount of actual carbonic acid present is negligible. The concentration of dissolved $CO_2$ in plasma is approximately 1000 times greater than that of carbonic acid.

**a.**

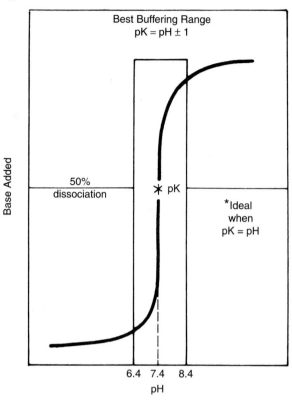

**b.**

| | Buffer | pK |
|---|---|---|
| Most | Biocarbonate Carbonic Acid | 6.1 |
| | Hemoglobin | 6.8–7.3 |
| | Plasma Proteins | 6.8–7.3 |
| Least | Phosphates | 6.8 |

(Physiologic Importance, arrow Most→Least)

**FIGURE 22-4**

Physiologic buffers. **a.** Curve A depicts the titration of base into a buffer and the subsequent change in pH. **b.** Chart B identifies buffers of physiologic importance.

Applying the Henderson-Hasselbalch equation to the bicarbonate–carbonic acid buffer system, the following equation is obtained:

$$pH = 6.1 + \log [HCO_3^-]/[H_2CO_3]$$

Substituting $PCO_2$ for $H_2CO_3$, the equation is written:

$$pH = 6.1 + \log [HCO_3^-]/[PCO_2 \times \alpha]$$

If the desired pH of 7.4 is plugged into the equation, the ratio of bicarbonate to acid may be derived as shown below.

$$7.4 = 6.1 + \log \text{Ratio}$$

Subtracting 6.1 from both sides of the equation, the following is obtained:

$$1.3 = \log \text{Ratio}$$

Finally, by taking the antilog of both sides of the equation, the ratio is determined:

$$20 = \text{Ratio}$$

Therefore, at the normal pH of 7.4, the ratio of bicarbonate to carbonic acid, or $PCO_2$, is 20:1. Figure 22–5 provides a summary of the steps taken in the derivation of the 20:1 ratio. As long as this ratio is maintained, the pH will remain unchanged. Any change in either bicarbonate or dissolved carbon dioxide results in a pH change. The direction of the change in pH follows the same direction as the change in the ratio. For example, if the bicarbonate is increased, the ratio is increased, thus resulting in an increase in pH. If the $PCO_2$ is increased, the ratio would be decreased as would the pH. Another way of stating this relationship is that pH follows change in bicarbonate directly and change in $PCO_2$ indirectly. The overriding principle, however, is that the actual concentration of bicarbonate or $PCO_2$ is not the most important factor in maintaining a normal pH; it is the ratio between these two variables that matters.

## HEMOGLOBIN AS A BUFFER

Intracellularly, hemoglobin is the most important buffer. As carbon dioxide is produced through cellular metabolism, it is picked up by hemoglobin in the red cells. Recall that most of the $CO_2$ produced ultimately combines with water to form carbonic acid that ionizes into $H^+$ and $HCO_3^-$. Transient buffering occurs as the $CO_2$ binds with free uncharged R-NH2

**Step 1**

$$pH = pK + log \frac{[HCO]}{[PCO]} = pK + log\ Ratio$$

**Step 2**

$7.4 = 6.1 + log\ Ratio$

**Step 3**

$1.3 = log\ Ratio$

**Step 4**

$antilog\ 1.3 = log\ Ratio$

**Step 5**

$20 = Ratio$

**Summary**

At a normal pH of 7.4, the ratio of bicarbonate to carbonic acid is 20:1 in the absence of disease.

**FIGURE 22-5**

Derivation of the 20:1 ratio in the bicarbonate:carbonic acid buffer system *Ratio* through the Henderson-Hasselbalch equation.

groups of the hemoglobin chains forming carbamino compounds. As the hydrogen ions are formed from the dissociation of carbonic acid, they too are buffered by hemoglobin. Hemoglobin binding to either $CO_2$ or $H^+$ occurs at the N-terminus and at amino acid side chains containing free uncharged amino groups. As hemoglobin travels through the capillary beds of the tissues, oxygen is lost and hemoglobin is reduced. Thus, the proportion of hemoglobin in this form increases. It is while in this reduced or deoxygenated state that hemoglobin is the more powerful buffer. The hydrogen ion carried on the reduced hemoglobin in the venous blood is released in the pulmonary circulation to recombine with bicarbonate to form carbonic acid. The carbonic acid formed then dissociates into water and carbon dioxide. Hence, the hemoglobin molecule effectively buffered the acid produced in the tissues and is now ready for pickup of more oxygen in the lungs.

## PROTEIN BUFFERS

Proteins account for the greatest portion of the nonbicarbonate buffering in plasma. The primary protein buffer is albumin. At the normal plasma pH of 7.4, most proteins are negatively charged and act as polyanions, meaning that they can bind excess hydrogen ions. The most important buffer groups of proteins at physiologic pH are the imidazole groups of histidines. Each albumin molecule contains 16 imidazole groups for buffering.

## PHOSPHATE BUFFERS

Phosphate buffers account for a minor percentage of the nonbicarbonate buffering in erythrocytes and plasma. The phosphate buffer system, composed of $HPO_4^=$ and $HPO_4^-$, plays an important role in the urine. Phosphate buffers neutralize the hydrogen ions present in the urine filtrate and thus help control urine acidity.

## Regulation of Acid-Base Balance

Maintenance of acid-base homeostasis is carried out in the lungs and the kidneys. These two organs act to ensure that the body's pH is constant within the narrow range of 7.35 to 7.45. The lungs are concerned with the excretion of carbon dioxide, which results from the capture of hydrogen ions by bicarbonate and subsequent conversion to water as shown in Figure 22-6. Thus, the lungs act to move the general equation from left to right. The kidneys, which serve as the site of acid excretion and regeneration of bicarbonate, direct the movement of the equation from right to left. Instead of directly opposing one another as it might appear, these two organ systems act together through application of the Henderson-Hasselbalch equation to maintain acid-base balance. By way of the Henderson-Hasselbalch equation, the lungs and kidneys are linked together since pH is expressed in terms of the $PCO_2$ (lung) and bicarbonate (kidney).

### RENAL CONTROL OF ACID-BASE STATUS

The kidneys serve as the final defense mechanism against changes in body pH. This is accomplished through the reclamation and regeneration of bicarbonate and through acid excretion in the urine. The main role of the kidneys in maintaining acid-base homeostasis is to reclaim the bicarbonate

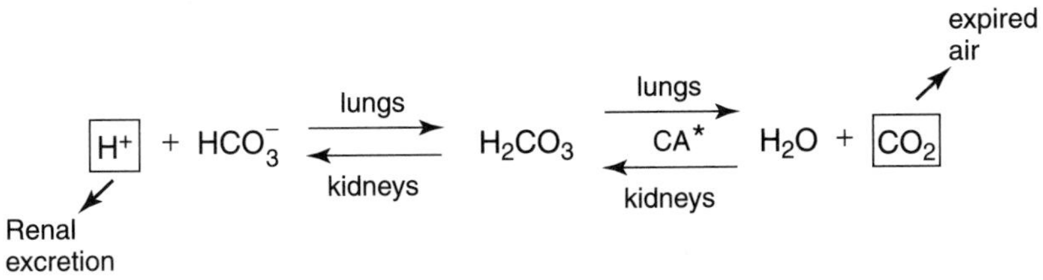

**FIGURE 22-6**

Role of the lungs and kidneys in the management of $H^+$ load.
*Reaction catalyzed by carbonic anhydrase (CA).

from the glomerular filtrate and return it to the circulation. The glomerular filtrate contains roughly the same concentration of bicarbonate ions as found in the plasma. Without the reabsorption of this bicarbonate, large quantities would be lost in the urine, which would then cripple the body's buffering capacity and lead to acid accumulation. Consequently, in health and at normal plasma bicarbonate concentration, virtually all of the filtered bicarbonate is reabsorbed.

At a normal glomerular filtration rate, approximately 4500 mmol of bicarbonate is filtered daily with ~ 90% reabsorbed in an indirect manner in the proximal convoluted tubule. The reclamation process does not occur directly since the luminal surface of the tubular cells is impermeable to bicarbonate. As shown in Figure 22–7, the reclamation of bicarbonate is in fact the diffusion of carbon dioxide from the glomerular filtrate into the tubular cells where it is converted to bicarbonate. Once inside the tubular cell, carbon dioxide is converted to carbonic acid through the reaction catalyzed by carbonic anhydrase. The carbonic acid formed ionizes into bicarbonate and hydrogen ions. The bicarbonate is now able to pass across the tubular cell membrane into the extracellular fluid where it combines with sodium. For each mole of bicarbonate reclaimed, 1 mole of hydrogen ion is formed. These hydrogen ions are exchanged across the cell membrane into the tubular lumen through the $Na^+/H^+$ antiporter located in the luminal membrane. Therefore, for each hydrogen ion secreted into the tubular fluid, 1 sodium ion and 1 bicarbonate

ion enter the tubular cell and ultimately return to the general circulation. Moreover, the reclamation of bicarbonate parallels that of sodium reabsorption.

The process of renal bicarbonate reclamation does not add new bicarbonate to the circulation, it merely prevents the loss of filtered bicarbonate in the urine. However, even if 100% of the filtered bicarbonate is reclaimed, a bicarbonate deficit cannot be corrected by this process alone. Thus, the body must have a mechanism for the generation of new bicarbonate. In essence, this is accomplished through a reversal of the process that occurs in the lungs during respiration. As shown in Figure 22–7, carbon dioxide diffuses into the renal tubular cells and combines with water to form carbonic acid which readily ionizes. The bicarbonate formed from this ionization is secreted into the plasma to maintain adequate bicarbonate concentration for the buffering needs of the body. Once again, however, 1 mole of hydrogen ions is generated for each mole of bicarbonate made. The hydrogen ions produced are primarily neutralized through the creation and excretion of ammonium ions (Figure 22–8). Renal ammonium ion excretion can be equated with bicarbonate generation on a 1:1 basis.

Deamination of proteins, as occurs in the urea cycle, produces ammonia. In the renal tubular cells, ammonia is formed from the oxidation of glutamine and some other amino acids. Free ammonia is a highly diffusible substance. Once it is produced in the tubular cells, it rapidly diffuses across the cell membrane into the tubular lumen. In the lumen, the un-

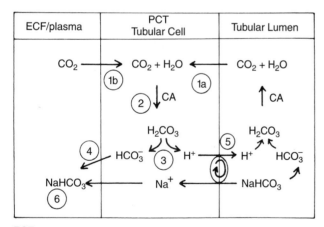

ECF = extracellular fluid; PCT = proximal convoluted tubule; CA = carbonic anhydrase.

**FIGURE 22–7**

Reclamation and regeneration of bicarbonate. *Step 1a*: $CO_2$ produced in the tubular lumen diffuses into tubular cells of the PCT. *Step 1b*: $CO_2$ in the ECF and plasma diffuses into tubular cells of the PCT. *Step 2*: $CO_2$ in the PCT reacts with water to form carbonic acid; reaction catalyzed by carbonic anhydrase. *Step 3*. Carbonic acid dissociates into bicarbonate and hydrogen ions. *Step 4*. Bicarbonate crosses the tubular cell membrane and enters the ECF and plasma. *Step 5*. Hydrogen ions from the tubular cells are secreted into the tubular lumen in exchange for sodium ions through the Na/H antiporter. *Step 6*. Sodium combines with bicarbonate in the ECF/plasma to form sodium bicarbonate.

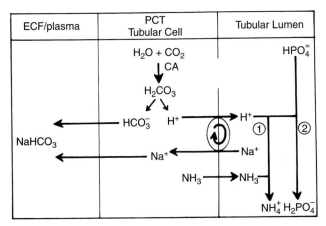

| ECF/plasma | PCT Tubular Cell | Tubular Lumen |
|---|---|---|

**FIGURE 22-8**

Hydrogen ion excretion. Step ①: Hydrogen ions secreted into the tubular lumen through the Na/H antiporter combine with ammonia to form ammonium ions. Ammonium ions are trapped in the tubular lumen and are ultimately excreted in the urine. Step ②: Hydrogen ions are also neutralized by phosphate buffers. As phosphates are filtered into the urine they combine with the hydrogen ions that have been secreted into the tubular lumen through the Na/H antiporter. The resulting dihydrogen phosphate is excreted in the urine.

charged ammonia combines with the free hydrogen ions forming ammonium ions. The ammonium ions are unable to move back into the tubular cells because of their charge; therefore, they remain in the lumen and are excreted in the urine. The ability of the renal tubular cells to generate ammonia provides an important defense mechanism in response to decreases in blood pH.

Another mechanism for neutralizing the hydrogen ions excreted in the urine is through buffering. Quantitatively speaking, phosphate is the most important urinary buffer. As demonstrated in Figure 22-8 phosphates are filtered from the glomerulus into the urine. Here, dibasic phosphate ($HPO_4^=$) combines with free hydrogen ions to form dihydrogen phosphate, ($H_2PO_4^-$) which is excreted in the urine.

## RESPIRATORY CONTROL OF ACID-BASE STATUS

Over 10,000 mEq of carbonic acid are excreted by the lungs daily, as compared with the less than 100 mEq of fixed acids processed by the kidney. This is accomplished through alterations in alveolar ventilation that control the elimination of carbon dioxide. If the lungs are healthy, they react quickly in response to disturbances in acid-base balance. It is the immediate response of the lungs that makes the bicarbonate–carbonic acid buffer system so effective. Accumulation of hydrogen ions, or drops in levels of blood pH, stimulates the respiratory mechanism of hyperventilation. This reaction low-

ers the $PCO_2$, which thereby results in a higher pH. This reaction is carried out until the blood pH has returned to normal. Alternatively, in cases where the blood pH is abnormally high, the respiratory center directs the lungs to hypoventilate or slow respiration. Hypoventilation results in the retention of carbon dioxide by the lungs, thus lowering the pH. Although the respiratory response is immediate, it is generally short term and often incomplete. The renal response, on the other hand, is much slower, taking 2 to 4 days to be effective, but is more long term and potentially more complete. Both systems are necessary to maintain acid-base homeostasis in the body.

## DISTURBANCES OF ACID-BASE BALANCE

### Terminology

When the body's arterial pH falls below 7.35, an **acidemia** is present. Likewise, when the pH rises above 7.45, an **alkalemia** is present. The terms **acidosis** and **alkalosis** refer to the pathologic states that can lead to acidemia or alkalemia. When the primary disturbance is due to an imbalance of bicarbonate, the disorder is referred to as being a **metabolic** disorder. On the other hand, when the primary disturbance is caused by an imbalance in the $PCO_2$, the condition is referred to as a **respiratory** disorder. The adaptive mechanisms that function to restore the normal 20:1 bicarbonate:carbonic acid ratio are referred to as **compensatory** mechanisms. Compensation attempts to return the body's pH to normal. A patient's acid-base status is considered to be **fully compensated** when the blood pH is returned to normal. Note that these compensatory mechanisms never overshoot the return to a normal pH. However, although compensation acts to restore a desirable pH, it does not mean that the primary abnormality is being corrected. Table 22-1 provides a listing of the expected physiologic compensations (renal and respiratory) for the primary disturbances of acid-base homeostasis. Table 22-2 denotes some of the causes of acid-base disorders. Figure 22-9 illustrates the relationship between pH, $HCO_3^-$, $PCO_2$, and the ratio ($HCO_3^- : PCO_2$).

### Metabolic Acidosis

Metabolic acidosis, also known as *primary bicarbonate deficit*, is the most common acid-base disorder. The primary bicarbonate deficit refers to the loss of bicarbonate that occurs either through an increased loss of base directly or loss through the buffering of excess acid. Accordingly, as defined by the Henderson-Hasselbalch equation, loss of bicarbonate corresponds to a decreased ratio (bicarbonate:carbonic acid) and a lowered pH.

In general, there are two types of metabolic acidosis: those associated with an increased anion gap and those with a normal anion gap. The presence of an increased anion gap is

TABLE 22-1

**Expected Compensations in Acid-Base Disorders**

| ACID-BASE DISORDER | COMPENSATION* | |
| | LUNGS | KIDNEYS |
| --- | --- | --- |
| Metabolic acidosis | Hyperventilation—excretion of $CO_2$ | Increased urinary acidity and $NH_3$ (if possible) |
| Respiratory acidosis | Typically, not possible | Retention of $HCO_3^-$; increased $H^+$ secretion |
| Metabolic alkalosis | Hypoventilation—retention of $CO_2$ | Typically, not possible |
| Respiratory alkalosis | Hyperventilation—excretion of $CO_2$ (if possible) | Excretion[†] of $HCO_3^-$; decreased $H^+$ secretion |

*Complete compensation = normal pH; partial compensation = pH not yet returned to normal.

[†]Most respiratory alkalosis is acute; thus, compensation seldom occurs.

frequently the first sign of a metabolic acidosis. As explained in Chapter 21 on electrolytes, the anion gap represents the concentration of unmeasured anions present in the blood. Most anion gap acidoses results from the endogenous production of anionic metabolic products such as ketoacids and lactic acid and from products of congenital disorders of amino-acid metabolism. A small percentage of this type of acidosis is due to the addition of exogenous products such as ethylene glycol, methanol, salicylate, and paraldehyde that can be metabolized to acids. Addition of such acids to the blood results in the replacement of bicarbonate by the acid anion, hence creating the bicarbonate deficit. The amount of acid added to the blood is reflected by the change from baseline of the anion gap.

Of the anion gap acidoses, lactic acidosis is the most serious and also the most common type. Lactic acid, the end product of anaerobic metabolism, is derived from muscle cells and erythrocytes. Normally, lactate is metabolized by the liver; however, in situations of tissue hypoxia, the concentration accumulates in the blood leading to acidosis. Consequently, blood lactate concentration is determined by the rate of production and the rate of metabolism, both of which depend on adequate tissue oxygenation. Lactic acidosis is most often seen in cases of tissue hypoxia such as occurs in severe anemia, shock, pulmonary insufficiency, and cardiac decompensation.

Another endogenously derived metabolic acidosis is that of diabetic ketoacidosis. The hallmark of diabetes is the absolute or relative insufficiency of the hormone insulin, which directs glucose from the blood into the cells for energy. Without insulin, cells are forced to utilize other sources of energy such as fats and proteins. It is during the breakdown of fats that the ketoacids are produced. The buildup of the ketone

TABLE 22-2

**Causes of Acid-Base Disorders**

| | ACIDOSIS | ALKALOSIS |
| --- | --- | --- |
| Metabolic | • Diabetic ketoacidosis<br>• Lactic acidosis<br>• Methanol poisoning<br>• Ethylene glycol poisoning<br>• Renal failure<br>• Diarrhea | • Prolonged vomiting<br>• Diuretic therapy<br>• Hyperadrenocortical disease<br>• Exogenous base (antacids, bicarbonate IV, citrate toxicity after massive transfusion) |
| Respiratory | • Emphysema<br>• Pneumonia<br>• Pulmonary fibrosis<br>• Chronic obstructive pulmonary disease | • Hysteria<br>• Fever<br>• Salicylate poisoning*<br>• Asthma |

*Also results in a metabolic acidosis since salicylate is an acid itself.

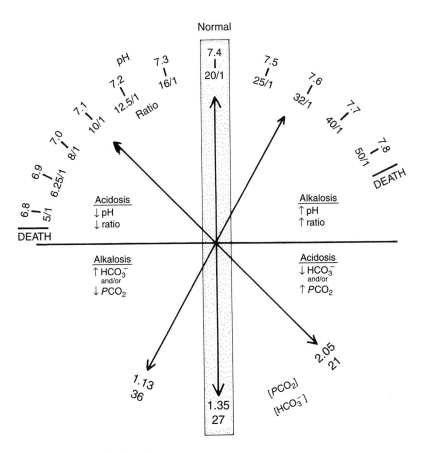

**FIGURE 22-9**

Relationship between pH, ratio, bicarbonate, and dissolved $CO_2$.

bodies acetone, acetoacetic acid, and $\beta$-hydroxybutyric acid leads to an increase in the anion gap. Diabetic ketoacidosis is one of the complications of diabetes mellitus and can lead to coma and death in its most severe form.

Ketoacidosis is also associated with chronic alcohol abusers. This group typically presents with an anion-gap acidosis and ketonemia without significant hyperglycemia. Presentation to the health care institution is usually delayed as the individual progresses through the alcoholic binge period. Consequently, alcohol levels may be unmeasureable or present in only nonintoxicating concentration at the time of presentation.

In addition to ethanol, other alcohols when ingested also cause an anion-gap acidosis. Since methanol is relatively inexpensive, it has been used as an illegal adulterant to ethanol. Although methanol itself is not toxic, it is metabolized in the liver to formaldehyde and formic acid, which can be deadly. Ingestion of as little as 30 mL of methanol can be fatal. Lesser quantities may lead to blindness because formic acid attacks the retina. Similar to methanol, ethylene glycol ingestion can also cause an anion-gap acidosis. This alcohol is commonly used as antifreeze. Again, it is the toxic metabolites that cause the damage. Ethylene glycol is metabolized to glycolic and oxalic acids, which are far more toxic than the parent compound itself.

Because of the ready availability of salicylate, salicylate toxicity remains a source of toxin-induced metabolic acidosis. Salicylate, itself an unmeasured anion, is metabolized in the liver to form a variety of organic acids including acetic and salicylic acid. The accumulation of these acids initially results in a metabolic acidosis with an accompanying high anion gap. Salicylate is also a stimulant for the respiratory center and thus causes an increase in the rate and depth of respiration. Consequently, depending on when the patient is evaluated, the acid-base disturbance may demonstrate acidosis or alkalosis.

Renal failure may also lead to an anion-gap metabolic acidosis. Massive loss of functional renal tubules leads to decreased ammonia formation, decreased filtration, and decreased exchange of sodium and hydrogen. All of these contribute to a decrease in acid excretion in the urine. As with the previously described processes, the resulting acid accumulation results in an increase in unmeasured anions and thus a higher anion gap. The acidosis associated with renal failure, however, typically tends to be milder.

In contrast to the anion-gap acidoses that deplete bicarbonate through the buffering of acid accumulation, acidosis with a normal anion gap is caused by the actual loss of bicarbonate through the kidney or gastrointestinal tract. Bicarbonate may be lost from the gastrointestinal tract during diarrhea or through the kidneys in some forms of renal tubular acidosis. Generally speaking, in renal tubular acidosis bicarbonate is not regenerated. This occurs as a consequence of the failure of the kidney to exchange hydrogen for sodium. As a result, there is a decreased secretion of hydrogen and a net reduction in acid excretion.

Correction of a metabolic acidosis necessitates the reversal of the underlying cause. The adjustment of bicarbonate and $PCO_2$ to return the ratio to the normal 20:1 balance does not correct the pathologic condition. Whether it be rehydration and insulin administration as for diabetic ketoacidosis, or removal of a toxin as in salicylate toxicity, treatment of the acid-base disorder must target the root of the disturbance.

## Metabolic Alkalosis

Metabolic alkalosis, also referred to as primary bicarbonate excess, is the most common type of acid-base disturbance in critically ill hospitalized patients. In such patients, the presence of a metabolic alkalosis delays recovery and prolongs the weaning process from mechanical ventilation devices. Moreover, evidence shows that the more severe the alkalosis, the higher the mortality.[8] In critically ill patients with severe sepsis and trauma, large quantities of citrated blood or lactated Ringer's solution are often administered to correct for the conditions of shock and hypotension. The citrate used as an anticoagulant in blood collected for transfusion is metabolized to bicarbonate in the body. Similarly, lactate solutions are also converted to bicarbonate. Consequently, under these circumstances, bicarbonate accumulates and results in the development of an alkalosis.

Clinically, metabolic alkaloses are divided into two groups: those responsive and those resistant to chloride treatment. The chloride-responsive form is accompanied by a contraction of the extracellular fluid volume. Causes of this type include severe vomiting and diarrhea and, though less frequent, nasogastric suctioning. In each of these conditions, chloride-rich fluid is lost. As in the case of vomiting, chloride is lost in the gastric contents as hydrochloric acid. As the body responds to the acid-base imbalance created by retaining more acid, bicarbonate is also retained in the process. This is often referred to as the *alkaline tide*.

Chloride-resistant metabolic alkalosis is much less common than the chloride-responsive type and is usually associated with the presence of an underlying disease or with excess addition of an exogenous base. Underlying diseases such as primary aldosteronism and Cushing's syndrome cause an alkalosis due to the excessive production of mineralocorticoid hormones, which direct sodium retention with concomitant loss of potassium and hydrogen in the distal tubules. Examples of exogenous base include the citrate toxicity that occurs with massive blood transfusion, aggressive intravenous therapies that contain bicarbonate, and the ingestion of large amounts of milk and antacids. Excessive alkali intake, as occurs with antacid ingestion, typically produces only a mild increase in blood bicarbonate since the kidneys are able to excrete most

of the excess. In contrast to the chloride-responsive metabolic alkalosis, the chloride-resistant form is associated with a normal or expanded extracellular fluid volume.

The clinical signs of metabolic alkalosis are nonspecific in nature. Dehydration may be a prominent feature. In addition, there may be apathy, confusion, stupor, and occasionally coma. If the increase in pH is high enough, increased neuromuscular activity may occur. In fact, tetany may develop in such cases due to a reduction of ionized calcium. This occurs because calcium is bound by proteins and other anions to compensate for the lack of available hydrogen ions.

## Respiratory Acidosis

Respiratory acidosis is due to an accumulation of carbon dioxide in the blood. Any condition that diminishes the elimination of carbon dioxide through the lungs results in an increased $PCO_2$, which causes a decrease in the ratio ($HCO_3$: $PCO_2$) and a lower blood pH. Conditions may be acute or chronic in nature, although most persist as chronic disorders. The most common cause of respiratory acidosis is chronic obstructive pulmonary disease. Other causes of chronic imbalance include asthma, emphysema, pneumonia, pulmonary fibrosis, and cardiac disease. Acute respiratory acidosis is due to disorders of the neuromuscular system, depression of the respiratory chemoreceptors, and acute pulmonary edema. Depression of the respiratory chemoreceptors may occur in trauma to the central nervous system, administration of general anesthesia during surgery, or ingestion of drugs such as morphine, barbiturates, and alcohol. Symptoms of respiratory acidosis are primarily related to the decreased ventilation, which causes the increase in carbon dioxide and decrease in oxygen. Thus, patients often suffer from cyanosis and tachycardia.

## Respiratory Alkalosis

Respiratory alkalosis occurs as the result of a primary deficit of carbon dioxide. The deficit occurs when there is an increase in the rate and/or depth of respiration. Consequently, there is excessive elimination of acid through the respiratory route due to the increase in ventilation. The decrease in $PCO_2$ causes an increase in the ratio ($HCO_3$: $PCO_2$) and the pH. Respiratory alkalosis most commonly occurs as the result of anxiety or hysteria where there is hyperventilation. The imbalance may also occur when the respiratory chemoreceptors are stimulated in hypoxic conditions such as asthma, pneumonia, pulmonary embolism, and pulmonary fibrosis. Thus, respiratory disease may result in an acidosis or alkalosis. If hypercapnia is present due to depressed ventilation, an acidosis develops. Conversely, if hypoxia is present, the body responds through hyperventilation to increase oxygen intake causing an alkalosis. Other causes of respiratory stimulation include high altitude, fever, congestive heart failure, thyrotoxicosis, and ingestion of certain drugs such as salicylates. In the acute form, symptoms of respiratory alkalosis include breathlessness, dizziness, nervousness, choking, and possibly an altered level of consciousness.

## Mixed Acid-Base Disorders

Most disturbances of acid-base homeostasis result from the presence of more than one acid-base disorder. When more than one type of disease process exists, a mixed disorder may result in which the pH can be elevated, decreased, or normal. The actual value of the pH is dependent on the severity of each individual disorder and on the degree of compensation. As a result, blood pH serves as more of a therapeutic guide in mixed disorders, indicating whether the alkalosis or the acidosis should be treated first. By contrast, in single disorders pH is a direct reflection of the extent of acidosis or alkalosis. Thus, pH alone is a poor test for detecting the presence of mixed acid-base disturbances. The anion gap, however, is unaffected by mixed disorders and is therefore a useful test to assess such disturbances. Mixed disorders are detected by comparing the change in bicarbonate with the change in the anion gap. Normally, the decrease in bicarbonate follows the magnitude of the increase in the anion gap. If the change in bicarbonate is greater than that of the anion gap by more than 5 mmol/L, a mixed disturbance is likely to be present.[9] Moreover, an increased anion gap may be the only piece of information indicating the presence of a metabolic acidosis in a mixed disorder. A common example of a mixed disorder is when diabetic ketoacidosis is accompanied by severe vomiting. Although acid production increases in diabetic acidosis, vomiting results in an increased loss of acid. Thus, in such cases, a metabolic acidosis and metabolic alkalosis coexist.

## LABORATORY EVALUATION

### Specimen Collection and Handling

As with any laboratory test result, the quality of the result depends on the control of preanalytical, analytical, and postanalytical factors. Since most errors occur during the preanalytical phase of testing, a clear understanding of recommended protocols for sample collection and handling is necessary. Samples collected for acid-base and blood gas analysis are particularly vulnerable to preanalytical factors. Table 22–3 identifies some of the effects on pH, $PCO_2$, and $PO_2$ due to preanalytical variables.

Acid-base and blood gas determinations are carried out on whole blood specimens that may be venous or arterial collections. Although venous samples may be used if the assessment of oxygenation status is not needed, arterial blood is the preferred specimen. The composition of venous blood is more variable since it is reflective of the metabolic activity of the tissue at which it drains. The greatest difference in venous and arterial blood, of course, is oxygen content. However, other parameters also vary. Some of the other variables include pH, carbon dioxide, lactic acid, ammonium, glucose, and chloride. These differences between venous and arterial blood are even more exaggerated when perfusion is not adequate. If a venous sample is analyzed, the $PO_2$ is approximately 60 to 70 mm Hg lower than that of arterial blood because of the delivery of oxygen to the tissues. The $PCO_2$ is slightly higher, ranging from 2 to 8 mm Hg above that of arterial blood and the pH is lower, on the order of 0.02 to 0.05 units below arterial levels.[10]

Arterial blood samples are usually taken from the radial or brachial artery of the nondominant hand. A local anaesthetic may be administered to minimize the pain and reduce anxiety. This is of particular importance since anxiety or excitement causes the patient to alter his or her breathing pattern. Such a change in ventilation can alter gas tensions within less than a minute.[11] Samples should be collected anaerobically using a short-beveled needle and a sterile syringe that contains lyophilized heparin. Although glass syringes provide an impermeable barrier to the diffusion of gases, plastic syringes are more commonly used. Today, plastic syringes have widely replaced glass syringes because of the ease of disposal and reduction of infection hazard associated with plastic. Furthermore, plastic syringes are no longer as permeable to gases as they once were. As an anticoagulant, lyophilized heparin is preferred over the liquid form because the liquid, which is often acidic, dilutes the sample. This dilutional effect is most prominent when the syringe is not completely filled. Regardless of whether liquid or lyophilized heparin is used, samples must be mixed before analysis by vigorous rolling of the syringe

TABLE 22-3

**Preanalytical Effects on Blood Gas Parameters**

| BLOOD GAS PARAMETER | PREANALYTICAL FACTOR | | | | |
|---|---|---|---|---|---|
| | AIR EXPOSURE | DELAY IN TESTING | HIGH ALTITUDE | LIQUID HEPARIN | ANXIETY/PAIN DURING COLLECTION |
| pH | ↑ | ↓ | ↑ | ↓ | ↑ |
| $PCO_2$ | ↓ | ↑ | ↓ | ↑ | ↓ |
| $PO_2$ | ↑ * | ↓ | ↓ | — | ↓ |

*May be ↓ if patient is on oxygen therapy.

between the palms. Mixing serves to ensure the desired homogeneity of the anticoagulant in the sample as well as proper distribution of the gases. To obtain a sample in a steady respiratory state, it is recommended that the syringe be filled slowly over 1 to 2 minutes.[12]

After the sample is collected, it is important to expel any bubbles or air in the syringe tip to ensure anaerobic conditions. In most cases, samples that are not maintained under anaerobic conditions reflect an increase in $PO_2$. Since the $PO_2$ of atmospheric air is approximately 60 mm Hg higher than that of arterial blood, the blood from patients breathing room air gains oxygen. Those patients on oxygen therapy and having a $PO_2$ greater than 150 mm Hg lose oxygen upon exposure to atmospheric air. Another source of oxygen loss is from continued metabolism in the cellular constituents of the sample. For this reason, many choose to place samples on ice until analysis to reduce cellular metabolism. Under aerobic conditions, cells utilize oxygen as they continue metabolism. Two of the more metabolically active aerobic cells in the blood are leukocytes and platelets. Patients with severe leukocytosis or thrombocytosis have been shown to exhibit spurious hypoxemia. Blood cell metabolism, particularly that of red blood cells, also includes anaerobic pathways. Even though oxygen is not consumed in the anaerobic pathways, the end product of carbon dioxide is the same. Consequently, continued cellular metabolism, whether aerobic or anaerobic, results in an increase in the $PCO_2$ and a decrease in pH. Some studies have shown that the magnitude of change in $PO_2$ and pH for samples collected and maintained at room temperature was 3 times that of those maintained on ice.[13] Also, the lower temperature conditions of the ice generate a slight influx of exogenous oxygen into the cells because ice water has a very high oxygen content. Furthermore, when blood samples at the normal body temperature of 37°C are cooled to 4°C, there is an increase in the oxygen affinity of hemoglobin. Consequently, exogenous oxygen binds to deoxyhemoglobin, thus favoring a greater influx of oxygen. On analysis, when the sample is re-warmed to 37°C, the $P_{50}$ of hemoglobin returns to normal and oxygen is released, resulting in a falsely increased $PO_2$. Other studies have concluded that it is unnecessary to place samples on ice if analysis is performed soon after collection. The protocol outlined by the National Committee for Clinical Laboratory Standards (NCCLS) recommends that plastic syringes containing blood for blood gas analysis be kept at room temperature and analyzed within 30 minutes of collection.[11]

Despite the preference for arterial blood samples, certain hazards are associated with such collections. During collection, some patients can have a vasovagal response that can cause a loss of consciousness. An arteriospasm, a reflex constriction of the artery in response to stimuli such as pain, may also be experienced. As with all punctures, arterial or venous, there is risk of hematoma and thrombosis. Consequently, some have performed capillary sample collections in place of the arterial puncture. Capillary collections are also preferred when blood loss must be minimized. Common sites for capillary collection include the heel, particularly for neonates, finger, toe, or earlobe. Before the puncture, the collection site must be warmed for 10 minutes to create adequate blood flow through the local capillaries. Once the puncture is made, the first drop of blood is wiped away and all subsequent free-forming drops are collected in capillary collection tubes containing lyophilized heparin. One of the difficulties associated with this technique is the oxygenation status of the sample. Capillary blood samples are difficult to obtain anaerobically. Collection of the blood drops as they form helps to minimize exposure to atmospheric air. However, the potential for poor agreement between capillary arterial $PO_2$ and arterial $PO_2$ raises important considerations regarding the usefulness of the technique.

## Arterial Blood Gas Analysis

In the classic method, arterial blood gas analysis is performed on a blood gas analyzer that measures pH, $PCO_2$, and $PO_2$. Some analyzers also include a unit called a cooximeter that measures oxygen saturation ($SO_2$). These measurements remain among the most unique in the clinical laboratory today, since no other test results have more immediate impact on patient care. Although new technologies such as transcutaneous monitoring, pulse oximetry, intraarterial monitoring, fluorescent optical monitors, and point-of-care testing have revolutionized the traditional methods of testing, the laboratory determination of arterial blood gases and pH remain the reference standard for the assessment of oxygenation and acid-base status.

### BLOOD GAS ANALYZERS

The measurement principles of blood gas analyzers are based on the electrochemical techniques of potentiometry and amperometry. Potentiometric analysis, which measures the potential or voltage difference between 2 electrodes under equilibrium conditions, is used for the measurement of pH and $PCO_2$. In a potentiometric system, one electrode having an established electrical potential serves as the reference, whereas the other electrode functions as an indicator electrode by measuring the activity or energy potential of the ion of interest. The composition of the indicator electrode is such that it is selective for the ion of interest. In the measurement of pH, the indicator electrode is a glass membrane that is selective for hydrogen ions in the test solution. $PCO_2$ electrodes, called **Severinghaus electrodes,** incorporate a gas-permeable membrane that allows the carbon dioxide present in the sample to diffuse across the membrane. Reference electrodes are most commonly composed of mercury/mercuric chloride (Hg/HgCl$_2$, **calomel**) or silver/silver chloride (Ag/AgCl$_2$). A voltmeter registers the potential difference between the reference and indicator electrodes. The voltage difference, which represents the activity of the ion of interest, is correlated to concentration through the Nernst equation, which states:

$$\Delta E = \Delta E^{\circ}_{ox,red} + \{RT/nF \times \log [ox]/[red]\}$$

where        E = the electrode potential,

$E^o$ = the standard reduction potential at 25°C,

R = the gas constant (8.316 volt coulombs/ mol × degree Kelvin),

T = absolute temperature (298°K),

n = number of electrons involved,

F = Faraday's constant (96,490 coulombs/ mol), and

[ox] and [red] = the activities for the oxidized and reduced forms of the ions.

The condensed form of the equation states

$$\Delta E = \Delta E^o + 0.059/n + \log a_i,$$

where $a_i$ is the activity of the ion of interest. Molar concentration and activity are assumed to be equal. Thus, the potential difference between the electrodes is directly proportional to ion activity or ion concentration. As with pH, since the relationship between hydrogen ion concentration of pH is inverse, the higher the concentration of hydrogen ions, the less the potential difference between the electrodes.

The second electrochemical application used in blood gas analysis is amperometry. This technique is used to determine $PO_2$. Amperometric measurements monitor the current that flows through an electrochemical cell when a constant potential is applied to the system. In regard to $PO_2$, a gas-permeable membrane allows oxygen present in the sample to diffuse across the membrane into an electrolyte solution and come in contact with a platinum cathode. A small current is constantly applied to the electrodes causing a polarizing potential to be created. As oxygen comes in contact with the cathode, it is reduced and electrons are generated. The current produced is therefore directly related to the amount of oxygen present at the electrode. Another name for the $PO_2$ electrode is the **Clarke electrode.**

The most common source of error associated with electrode measurements is protein buildup on the membrane. The accumulation of protein or other material from clinical samples impedes the diffusion of ions across the membrane and slows electrode response. Manufacturers' protocols for maintenance of blood gas analyzers include routine cleaning and flushing of electrodes to remove proteins and ensure free ion movement. Most other sources of analytical error are related to incorrect or faulty calibration. Today's instruments, however, are typically self-calibrating and are programmed to flag calibration errors based on set limits for electronic signals.

Temperature is another important factor in electrochemical measurements. Gas solubility in a liquid medium is temperature dependent. As the temperature decreases, the solubility of the gas in the liquid increases. Oxygen, a poorly soluble gas, is particularly sensitive to temperature. Furthermore, changes in temperature of the measurement system changes result in voltage. Consequently, potentiometric measurements are also temperature dependent. Blood gas analyzers by con-

vention perform all measurements at the normal body temperature of 37°C. Thus, reference intervals are based on measurements taken at this temperature. For individuals whose body temperature is different from 37°C, temperature correction algorithms are available to modify the results to correlate to actual in vivo conditions at the time of sampling.[14] This practice, however, is controversial.

## COOXIMETRY

The measurement of $SO_2$, or the fraction of hemoglobin that is saturated with oxygen, is an important determinant in the assessment of oxygenation status. The percentage of oxyhemoglobin is most often measured spectrophotometrically using a cooximeter. Because each hemoglobin species has its own characteristic absorption spectra that is known, differential spectrophotometric analysis and the principle of Beer's law can be applied to determine the concentration of each (see Chapter 6 for a more in-depth description of spectrophotometry). The number of hemoglobin species detected depends on the number of wavelengths analyzed by the instrument. At a minimum, cooximeters should measure the 4 wavelengths that correspond to oxyhemoglobin and deoxyhemoglobin and carboxyglobin and methemoglobin, which are the two most common dysfunctional hemoglobins encountered. Instruments that measure at more than these 4 wavelengths have the ability to recognize the presence of sulfhemoglobin, dyes and pigments, turbidity, and abnormal proteins.

## CALCULATED PARAMETERS

Blood gas analyzers are able to make certain measurements indirectly through the use of computerized algorithms. Calculations based on the Henderson-Hasselbalch equation use the measurement data of pH and $PCO_2$ to determine such parameters as bicarbonate, carbonic acid, and total $CO_2$. The calculation of bicarbonate concentration assumes a pK of 6.1 for the bicarbonate:carbonic acid buffer system at normal body temperature. Likewise, the calculation for carbonic acid concentration assumes a normal body temperature. Error results when temperatures other than 37°C exist since the solubility constant for the conversion of $PCO_2$ to $H_2CO_3$ concentration is temperature dependent. Total $CO_2$ is estimated by the addition of the calculated bicarbonate and carbonic acid concentrations.

Oxygen saturation can be calculated from the $PO_2$ through the use of computer algorithms that are based on the predicted shape and location of the oxygen dissociation curve. Since the assumption is made for a specific shape and location of the curve, deviations in shape and location can result in significant error. It is therefore recommended that the calculation of $SO_2$ be clearly identified as an estimation of oxygen saturation as opposed to the more accurate direct measurement.

The fractional or percentage of oxyhemoglobin ($FO_2Hb$) is calculated by expression of the ratio between the concentration of oxyhemoglobin and total hemoglobin. Total hemoglobin includes all forms, both functional and dysfunctional, of hemoglobin. Thus, the accuracy of the calculation is dependent on the measurement of each of the various hemoglobin species by cooximetry. Calculation of $FO_2Hb$, however, is more commonly used as an estimation of oxygen saturation in the absence or unavailability of cooximetry so that the possibility of error is significant. In most healthy individuals, $SO_2$ and $FO_2Hb$ are very close; however, in some cases (e.g., smokers where the concentration of carboxyhemoglobin is high), values can deviate significantly.

## THE EXTENDED LABORATORY

In critical care medicine, real-time clinical laboratory data are of utmost importance for the effective management of acutely ill patients. In the past, this expectation has been compromised by the often long turnaround times and preanalytical variables that affect the accurate and timely reporting of laboratory data. It has been estimated that the turnaround times for results originating out of the main clinical laboratory do not meet physicians' expectations 70% to 90% of the time.[1] Today, point-of-care devices are available for most laboratory tests, including blood gas and acid-base measurements, that are commonly ordered stat. Many advantages have been associated with point-of-care testing (POCT) regarding the assessment of acid-base and oxygenation status.[15] First, turnaround time of result reporting is significantly reduced, allowing physicians to use immediate or real-time laboratory data to guide patient management decisions. Second, the use of real-time information supplements clinical decision making and allows physicians to evaluate patient status and intervene more quickly and effectively. This is of particular importance in cases in which more rapid weaning of patients from mechanical ventilatory support is necessary. In addition, provision of real-time results allows the laboratory to contribute to a more integrated approach to patient care. A third advantage of POCT is the cost savings associated with bedside testing. Depending on the analyzer used and the operating expenses of the device, costs may be significantly lower than those associated with testing in the main laboratory. Fourth, POCT minimizes preanalytic error. As compared to traditional methods, the chance of mislabeling, mishandling, or losing the sample is reduced. In addition, since the time before analysis is lessened, sample degradation is reduced. A final advantage of POCT is that of decreased iatrogenic blood loss. The issue of blood conservation is especially crucial in the critically ill since many of these patients often require multiple blood transfusions. It has been estimated that the average daily blood loss in critically ill patients resulting from delays in laboratory testing is 25 to 125 mL per day.[1]

Although these advantages are substantial, certain disadvantages do exist. The primary disadvantages are associated with cost, personnel, regulatory matters, quality assurance and quality control, documentation, constraints imposed by the ex-

isting laboratory service structure, and the specific patient population served by the institution.[15] Thus, it is important for a facility to determine the efficacy of POCT in each setting before actual implementation.

The evolution of noninvasive technologies has allowed both patients and health care personnel to perform in vivo testing. The benefits of such testing have been identified and discussed in the previous section on point-of-care testing. Intravenous, intraarterial, and subcutaneous and transcutaneous techniques are emerging for the measurement of $PO_2$, pH, and $PCO_2$. Blood gas monitors have been developed to measure these parameters without removal of blood from the patient. These monitors are based on the use of fluorescent optical biosensors called optodes. Optode systems have been miniaturized so that they fit through an arterial catheter. Moreover, they have been found to be stable, provide a rapid response to changes in substrate concentration, and are not consumed in the measurement process.[2] Some, however, have noted occasional discrepancies between blood gas monitors and the traditional blood gas analyzers.[2]

Arterial $PO_2$ and $PCO_2$ can also be monitored transcutaneously through the use of electrodes fixed to the skin surface. Such electrodes first warm the skin and then depend on the diffusion of gases across the skin into the electrode for measurement. Consequently, decreased cardiac output and reduced tissue perfusion significantly affect transcutaneous monitoring. This technology was originally developed for use in neonates; however, modifications have been applied for use in the adult population.

Since the introduction of pulse oximetry, transcutaneous monitoring has actually declined. Pulse oximetry is based on the same principle as cooximetry in that it spectrophotometrically measures the absorbance of light by hemoglobin. It does this, however, directly through the skin. Thus, pulse oximetry requires a pulsating vascular bed for the accurate assessment of oxygenation. Like transcutaneous monitoring, under conditions of low blood flow, pulse oximetry becomes unreliable. The accuracy of pulse oximetry and transcutaneous monitoring is also compromised by the presence of dysfunctional hemoglobins since only oxyhemoglobins and deoxyhemoglobins are detected.

## REFERENCES

1. Harvey MA: Point-of-care laboratory testing in critical care. Am J Crit Care 8(2):72–82, 1999.
2. Hess D: Detection and monitoring of hypoxemia and oxygen therapy. Resp Care 45(1):65–80, 2000.
3. Lumb AB: *Nunn's Applied Respiratory Physiology.* 5th ed. Oxford, England, Butterworth Heinemann, 2000.
4. Schnermann JB, Sayegh SI: *Kidney Physiology.* Philadelphia, Lippincott-Raven, 1998.
5. Cohen RM, Feldman GM, Fernandez PC: The balance

of acid, base and charge in health and disease. Kidney Int 52:287–293, 1997.

6. West JB: *Respiratory Physiology—The Essentials.* 6th ed. Baltimore, Lippincott Williams & Wilkins, 2000.

7. Ehrmeyer SS, Fallon KD: Blood gases, pH, and buffer systems. In Bishop ML, Duben-Engelkirk JL, Fody EP (eds.): *Clinical Chemistry—Principles, Procedures, Correlations.* 4th ed. Philadelphia, Lippincott Williams & Wilkins, 2000, pp 334–351.

8. Webster NR, Kulkarni V: Metabolic alkalosis in the critically ill. Crit Rev Clin Lab Sci 36:497–510, 1999.

9. Halperin ML: *Fluid, Electrolyte, and Acid-Base Physiology: A Problem-Based Approach.* Philadelphia, WB Saunders, 1999.

10. Heusel JW, Siggard-Anderson O, Scott MG: Physiology and disorders of water, electrolyte, and acid-base metabolism. In Burtis CA, Ashwood ER (eds): *Tietz Textbook of Clinical Chemistry.* 3rd ed. Philadelphia, WB Saunders, 1999, pp 1095–1124.

11. Blonshine S, Alberti R, Olesinski RL: *Procedures for the Collection of Arterial Blood Specimens* (H11-A3). Wayne, PA, National Committee for Clinical Laboratory Standards, 1999.

12. Syabbalo N: Measurement and interpretation of arterial blood gases. Br J Clin Pract 1(3):173–176, 1997.

13. Beaulieu M, Lapointe Y, Vinet B: Stability of $PO_2$, $PCO_2$, and pH in fresh blood samples stored in a plastic syringe with low heparin in relation to various blood-gas and hematological parameters. Clin Biochem 32(2):101–107,1999.

14. Burnett RW, Ehrmeyer SS, Moran RF, et al.: *Blood Gas and pH Analysis and Related Measurements* (C46-P).

Wayne, PA, National Committee for Clinical Laboratory Standards, 2000.

15. Kost GJ, Ehrmeyer SS, Chernow B, et al.: The laboratory interface—point-of-care testing. Chest 115:1140–1154, 1999.

## BIBLIOGRAPHY

Dufour, DR: Acid base disorders. In Dufour, DR (ed.): *Course Notes—Professional Practice in Clinical Chemistry: A Companion Text.* Washington DC, AACC Press, 1999, pp 24-1–24-19.

Dufour, DR: Laboratory recognition and testing in acid-base disorders. Lab Med 30(12):776–781, 1999.

Marshall WJ: Hydrogen ion homeostasis and blood gases. In Marshall WJ (ed.): *Clinical Chemistry.* 4th ed. London, Mosby, 1995, pp 37–55.

Ishihara K, Szerlip HM: Anion gap acidosis. Sem Nephrol 18:83–97, 1998.

Smith EKM: *Fluids and Electrolytes—A Conceptual Approach.* 2nd ed. New York, Churchill-Livingstone, 1991.

Tremper KK: Pulse oximetry's final frontier. Crit Care Med 28:1684–1685, 2000.

St. John RE, Thomson PD. Noninvasive respiratory monitoring. Crit Care Nurs Clin North Am 11(4):423–435, 1999.

Galley HF, Webster NR. Acidosis and tissue hypoxia in the critically ill: how to measure it and what does it mean? Crit Rev Clin Lab Sci 36(1):35–60, 1999.

Hlastala MP, Berger AJ. *Physiology of Respiration.* New York, Oxford University Press, 1996.

# CHAPTER 23

# Therapeutic Drug Monitoring

*Susan Cockayne*

By dissecting the phrase "therapeutic drug monitoring," one can learn a great deal about both the content and scope of this chapter. A **drug** can be defined as a chemical used to selectively perturb specific tissues or specific functions of these tissues in an organism. Since not all chemicals are drugs, what makes a particular chemical a drug? A chemical is considered a drug if it has (1) selectivity as to its site of action or target, (2) reversibility in its action, and (3) production of a beneficial, or therapeutic, effect.[1]

The word **therapeutic** is an adjective that describes the drug. A therapeutic drug produces a healing or curative effect when an undesirable physiological or psychological condition is present. For example, if an individual has a headache and takes 2 aspirin tablets for relief, the aspirin is classified as a therapeutic drug. If, however, 100 aspirin tablets are consumed, the therapeutic drug becomes a drug of abuse. The drugs discussed in the chapter are those used under controlled circumstances to produce a specific, curative effect.

**Monitoring** implies a constant process of determining the quantity of drug required to produce a predetermined desirable effect. In the preceding example, when aspirin is taken for a headache, the desirable effect is cessation of pain. However, if the pain does not completely subside within an hour, should more aspirin be taken? No, because aspirin in high concentrations in the body can be toxic, not therapeutic. Likewise, all drugs at some concentration cease to be therapeutic and become toxic. Monitoring, or analyzing a tissue or fluid to determine the concentration of drug in the body, is of utmost importance, especially when trying to maintain the fine line between production of therapeutic versus toxic effects. Therapeutic drug monitoring can therefore be defined as the science of analyzing tissues or body fluids to determine the concentration of a prescribed drug present at a particular time and correlating the concentration of drug in that compartment with its effect on the patient.

Therapeutic drug monitoring is often used to determine when changes in the therapeutic regimen need to be made because of either failure to respond to treatment or symptoms of toxicity. Prime candidates for therapeutic drug monitoring include patients who are at the extremes of age (neonates and geriatric patients), patients with other mitigating medical conditions, and patients undergoing multiple drug therapy.

Therapeutic drugs may be monitored for patient compliance to determine if the patient is actually taking the prescribed drug in the prescribed dosage. This may be pertinent when there are no overt symptoms of which the patient may be aware, for example, in the treatment of hypertension.

Therapeutic drug monitoring is sometimes incorrectly classified under the subject heading of toxicology. Toxicology and therapeutic drug monitoring share the feature of drug monitoring. The clinical toxicology laboratory, however, monitors substances that have no curative effects, either by the nature of the chemical itself or by the higher than normal level of exposure of the individual to the chemical. Thus, toxicology may be considered nontherapeutic drug monitoring. The status of the patient being monitored by the toxicology laboratory and therapeutic drug monitoring laboratory also differs. The former patients may be confused, disoriented, or unconscious and therefore unreliable in providing a complete history. In contrast, patients being monitored for therapeutic drugs are more likely to be amenable to treatment, have a known history, and be on a carefully controlled drug regimen.

## DRUG ACTION

Every drug has a **mechanism of action,** which is the sum of biochemical and/or physical processes that occur to elicit a biologic result. The **response** a drug produces is dependent on the **dose** administered, but only to a certain point. A **dose-response curve** (Figure 23–1), a plot of the intensity of drug response as a function of the dose of drug, illustrates this concept. At some point, increasing the drug dose will not increase the biologic response. Monitoring drug concentration in blood is useful since changes in blood concentration over time may parallel changes in the biologically effective dose, that is, the amount of drug reaching the target site. Measurement of the plasma drug concentration gives a better indication of this relationship than attempting to correlate drug dose with drug action[2] and is the basis by which therapeutic and toxic drug concentration ranges are established.

In discussions of therapeutic drug monitoring, some terms are commonly encountered. The **minimum effective concentration (MEC)** is the lowest concentration of drug in the blood that will produce the desired response. The **minimum toxic concentration (MTC)** is the lowest concentration of drug in the blood that will produce an adverse response. The **therapeutic index** is the ratio of the MTC to the MEC and varies from drug to drug and even from patient to patient (see

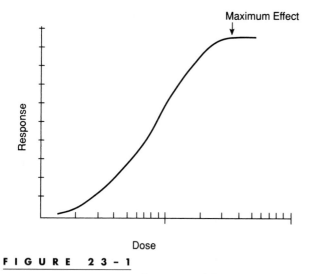

Dose-response curve. The nature of the response varies with different drugs. The plateau on the curve represents the maximum effect of the particular drug.

section on Variables Affecting Drug Disposition). The **trough** is the lowest concentration of drug measured in the blood, and the **peak** is the highest concentration of drug measured in the blood. The trough should be reached immediately before the next dose of drug and should not fall below the MEC. Likewise, the peak should not be higher than the MTC. These con-

cepts are illustrated in Figure 23–2. It is clear that monitoring of therapeutic drugs is necessary to achieve and maintain this delicate balance between therapy and toxicity, especially with drugs having a low therapeutic index.

## DRUG DISPOSITION

What is the route that a drug follows from its initial exposure to the body to production of its pharmacologic response? A drug must undergo a series of steps for it to be removed from the body. These steps represent the rate processes of pharmacokinetics, which are **absorption, distribution, biotransformation,** and **excretion.** They are outlined in Figure 23–3 and are discussed in detail in the following sections. The specific sites at which drugs produce their pharmacologic response are also addressed.

### Absorption

Absorption is the process whereby a drug taken into the body enters the blood. Drugs may be **formulated** to be available for absorption at sites different from the site of administration. Aspirin (acetylsalicylic acid) is absorbed from the gastrointestinal tract. In some formulations, aspirin is coated to prevent it from dissolving in the acid pH of the stomach; the tablet remains intact until reaching the alkaline pH of the in-

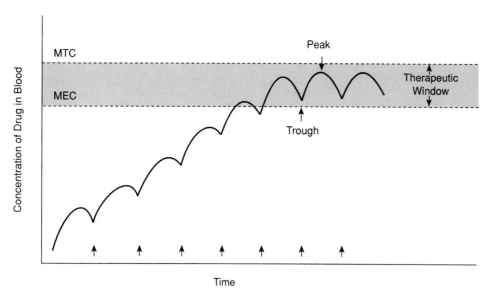

Achievement of therapeutic concentration of drug in blood. After each dose of drug (represented by arrows), the blood concentration rises until dose 7, when no further increase is seen. This steady-state area falls above the minimum effective concentration (MEC) and below the minimum toxic concentration (MTC) within the therapeutic window. Therapy is maintained and toxicity is avoided. The trough and peak are defined at the steady state.

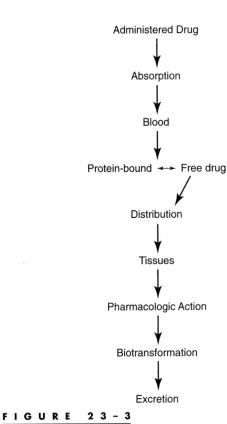

**F I G U R E   2 3 - 3**

Processes of pharmacokinetics.

testine. Salicylic acid, the active component of aspirin, is also therapeutic when absorbed through the skin, but holding an aspirin tablet against the skin will not produce the desired response. Salicylic acid can, however, be formulated as an emulsion, which penetrates the lipid barrier of the skin and permits absorption. The appropriate formulation of a drug is an early step in ensuring drug absorption.

Drugs that are administered by oral, rectal, or sublingual routes are absorbed in the gastrointestinal tract. When drugs are absorbed from the intestine, they are immediately transported to the liver by the hepatic portal vein. In the liver, certain drugs undergo a **first-pass effect.** The drug, on its first pass through the liver, is substantially metabolized even before reaching the systemic circulation. For some drugs that undergo a first-pass effect, the blood concentration of active drug is decreased because of the production of many inactive metabolites. However, other drugs are metabolized to compounds that themselves have pharmacologic activity, causing an increased therapeutic response in the patient. First-pass effects of particular drugs may always be taken into account when determining the dose of drug required to produce a desired response.

Oral administration is not the only route of administration. Drugs that are injected are said to be administered **parenterally.** Parenteral administration includes injection of drug into veins (intravenous), muscles (intramuscular), skin (intradermal), or spinal fluid (intrathecal), and injection beneath

the skin (subcutaneous). Other routes of administration are inhalation of gaseous drugs (respiratory) and administration through the skin (percutaneous).

## Distribution

Unless a drug's site of administration coincides with its site of action, a drug must be translocated to its site of action. This pharmacokinetic process is known as distribution. Blood is the vehicle by which drugs are distributed to all organs and fluid compartments. There are factors that affect the degree of distribution. These include the pH of the physiologic environment and the degree to which the drug binds to plasma proteins. Depending on the pH of the physiologic environment, drugs may exist in both ionized and nonionized forms. When the ionized and nonionized forms are present in equilibrium, an equation may be written and a dissociation constant, **K,** may be assigned:

$$[\text{ionized}] \Leftrightarrow [\text{nonionized}]$$

$$K = \frac{[\text{nonionized}]}{[\text{ionized}]}$$

Each drug has a particular **pK,** which is defined as the pH at which there is an equal concentration of ionized and nonionized forms. For acidic drugs (represented as HA), when the pH of the environment exceeds the pK, the drug will not be completely protonated and thus will exist in the ionized form:

$$pH > pK$$

HA exists mainly as A⁻ (ionized form).

When the pH of the environment is less than the pK, the drug is completely protonated and thus exists in the nonionized form:

$$pH < pK$$

HA is completely protonated and exists as HA (nonionized form).

The pK of an acidic drug is obtained by using the Henderson-Hasselbalch equation, which is

$$pH = pK + \log \frac{[\text{proton acceptor}]}{[\text{proton donor}]}$$

When this is rearranged and the appropriate values are entered, the pK of an acidic drug is obtained:

$$pK = pH + \log \frac{[\text{nonionized form}]}{[\text{ionized form}]}$$

For basic drugs (represented as BOH), when the pH of the environment exceeds the pK, the drug is only partially protonated and thus exists in the nonionized form:

$$pH > pK$$

BOH exists mainly as BOH (nonionized form).

When the pH of the environment is less than pK, the drug is completely protonated and thus exists in the ionized form:

$$pH < pK$$

BOH is completely protonated and exists as $B^+$ (ionized form).

The pK of a basic drug is also obtained by entering the appropriate values into the rearranged Henderson-Hasselbalch equation:

$$pK = pH + \log \frac{[\text{ionized form}]}{[\text{nonionized form}]}$$

Only the nonionized forms of drugs are lipid soluble and can penetrate the lipid cellular membrane. Thus, the pH of the environment determines if a drug can even enter a particular cell. For example, acetylsalicylic acid is an acidic drug with a pK of 3.5. In the stomach, which has a pH of approximately 1.0, the equation is

$$3.5 = 1.0 + \log \frac{[\text{nonionized form}]}{[\text{ionized form}]}$$

The ratio of nonionized form to ionized form is 316:1. Because there is much more nonionized drug than ionized drug, the majority of acetylsalicylic acid will be absorbed.

Depending on the individual drug and the concentration of serum proteins, a drug may distribute in a protein-bound form. Albumin and $\alpha_1$-acid glycoprotein are the usual, although not the exclusive, drug-binding proteins. A protein-bound drug is pharmacologically inactive. Only non-protein–bound (or free form) drugs are pharmacologically active. The extent of protein binding is a factor unique to each drug and most drugs exist in equilibrium between bound and free forms. Drugs may have high affinity (>85% bound), low affinity (<10% bound), or intermediate affinity for proteins. Conditions or disease states that decrease the serum protein concentration, such as hepatic disease or hypoalbuminemic renal failure, may cause increased serum drug concentration with concomitant toxicity. The toxicity results from less protein available for binding and an increased concentration of the free, pharmacologically active drug. Complications may also arise when a second drug is added to a patient's treatment regimen. If the first drug has an intermediate or low affinity for protein binding and the second drug has a higher affinity for protein binding, the first drug can be competitively displaced

from protein-binding sites by the second drug. The amount of the unbound, pharmacologically active form of the first drug then increases and toxicity can result even though the administered dose of the first drug was unchanged. Most laboratories quantitate only total drug concentrations. However, the technology does exist for determination of the concentration of free drugs by methods such as equilibrium dialysis and ultrafiltration. Providing this clinically useful information is among the future trends in the therapeutic drug-monitoring laboratory.

## Biotransformation

The third pharmacokinetic process is biotransformation, or metabolism. The major site of drug biotransformation is the liver. Secondary sites include lungs, kidneys, skin, brain, and gastrointestinal tract. The unmetabolized drug is often referred to as the parent compound and the products of metabolism are referred to as metabolites.

Metabolism may affect a drug in one of three ways. It may increase its activity (activation), decrease its activity (inactivation or detoxification), or have no effect on its activity.

There are two major metabolic pathways, described as phase I and phase II reactions. Phase I reactions metabolize lipophilic drugs to more polar forms to facilitate renal excretion. This is accomplished by oxidative or reductive processes such as hydroxylation, deamination, sulfoxidation, or dealkylation, in which small chemical groups are added to or removed from the drug. One important contributor to phase I biotransformation is a group of enzymes of the smooth endoplasmic reticulum called monooxygenases or mixed-function oxidases. In a series of electron transfer reactions, an oxidized form of the drug is produced that is more polar than the parent compound. Cytochrome P-450, a heme-containing protein, is involved in the final reaction and therefore this metabolic pathway is sometimes termed the cytochrome P-450 system. It is noteworthy that phase I reactions may produce metabolites that have an increased pharmacologic activity relative to the parent drug. Since these metabolic products are pharmacologically active, they must also be quantitated when parent drug concentration is assayed.

Polar drugs, or drugs rendered polar by phase I reactions, may undergo phase II reactions. These reactions involve the conjugation of drugs with compounds such as glutathione, sulfonic acid, glucuronic acid, or amino acids, particularly glycine, to facilitate their elimination. Specific enzymes catalyze each conjugation reaction, depending on the substrate used. The conjugates produced are water-soluble entities and can be readily excreted by the kidneys.

Since metabolism involves enzymatic reactions, the parameters that characterize enzyme-catalyzed reactions apply to drug metabolism. Most drugs are metabolized according to **first-order kinetics,** in which the rate of metabolism is dependent on the concentration of the substrate, in this case, the drug. As the concentration of drug increases, the rate of metabolism increases to keep pace with the amount of substrate (drug) present. Some drugs are not metabolized according to first-order kinetics. For these drugs, at a particular concentration, metabolism fails to increase as the concentration of substrate (drug) increases. Because a constant amount of drug is metabolized per unit of time regardless of the amount of drug in the body, these drugs are said to follow **zero-order kinetics**. The terms **capacity-limited kinetics** and **nonlinear kinetics** are also used to describe biotransformation of these drugs.

## Excretion

If drugs are water soluble or can be rendered water soluble through metabolism, they are eliminated from the body in the urine. An acidic urine facilitates elimination of basic drugs, and an alkaline urine facilitates elimination of acidic drugs by extraction from the plasma. The kidney is the primary organ in drug excretion and both the glomeruli and the tubules must be functioning optimally for optimal drug elimination. Decreased kidney function may lead to decreased excretion and increased blood levels of drugs and hence increased pharmacologic activity. Drugs and their metabolites may also be excreted by bile, feces, saliva, expired air, and breast milk, but urine is most frequently assayed to indicate previous drug exposure.

## Sites of Drug Action

For a drug to produce an effect, it must enter cells; drugs in the blood are, for the most part, pharmacologically ineffective. Therefore, the measurement of the concentration of a drug in the blood is only an estimate of the concentration of the drug available at its target site. Many drugs enter cells via **receptors**. Receptors are usually proteins, located on the cellular membrane or in the cytoplasm, with which the drug binds. There are more than 1 million receptors per cell. Some drugs are structurally similar to endogenous substances, competing for these receptor-binding sites and blocking the action of endogenous substances. Drugs may have affinity for receptors (that is, the drug may bind to the receptor), but if they do not possess intrinsic activity (the ability of a drug to change the conformation of the receptor and elicit a series of biochemical reactions), the drug will not produce a pharmacologic effect. The interaction of drug with its receptor is reversible; it is only desirable that the effect produced by the drug last for a limited time.

## PHARMACOKINETICS

Therapeutic drug monitoring may be thought of as applied pharmacology[3] because in therapeutic drug monitoring it is important to control for variables that affect the plasma drug concentration and therefore affect the pharmacologic response of the drug. To do this, the concentration of a drug at all stages of disposition and the time required for conversion from one stage to the next must be taken into account. Pharmacokinetics measures the **rates** of absorption, distribution, biotransformation, and excretion and is a necessary component of therapeutic drug monitoring.

The **half-life** ($t_{1/2}$) of a drug indicates the time required for elimination. It is defined as the time required for the concentration of a drug to be decreased by one half. For example, if a drug had a half-life of 1 hour and the plasma drug concentration was 100 ng/mL at one time point, 1 hour later the plasma concentration would be expected to be 50 ng/mL. During each half-life, one half of the drug is eliminated. Information on drug half-life is important to determine if therapeutic levels have been achieved and maintained and also to schedule optimal dosing intervals. For drugs following first-order kinetics (that is, where the rate of metabolism is dependent on the concentration of drug), the formula for calculation of half-life is

$$t_{1/2} = \frac{0.693}{K_{elimination}}$$

where 0.693 is derived from the formula $2.303 \log_{10} \frac{1}{2} = -K_{elimination} \, t_{1/2}$, which can be rearranged to $2.303 \log_{10} 2 = K_{elimination} \, t_{1/2}$, and 2.303 is the factor used to convert common logarithms to natural logarithms.

Half-life can be determined by plotting drug concentrations versus time on semilogarithmic paper and drawing a straight line through the points (Figure 23–4). The time required for any concentration to decrease by one half can be easily determined and is the half-life of the drug.

The **volume of distribution** ($V_d$) relates the absolute amount of drug in the body to a relative amount, that is, to a volume; blood volume is usually used. Because the presence of drug in nonblood compartments is not considered, a more descriptive term is the **apparent volume of distribution**. $V_d$ is calculated by

$$V_d = \frac{\text{Dose of drug administered}}{\text{Plasma concentration at zero time}}$$

$V_d$ is usually expressed in units of liters per kilogram of body mass. It is a parameter used to contrast the degrees to which different types of drugs distribute; for example, polar hydrophilic drugs would have a smaller volume of distribution than nonpolar lipophilic drugs, because polar drugs would be more soluble in body fluids.

**Total plasma clearance** ($Cl_T$) is the sum of all processes by which a drug is cleared from the body per unit time. It indicates the volume of plasma that must be completely cleared of a drug, frequently expressed in liters per hour, to account for drug elimination. $Cl_T$ provides a measurement of the

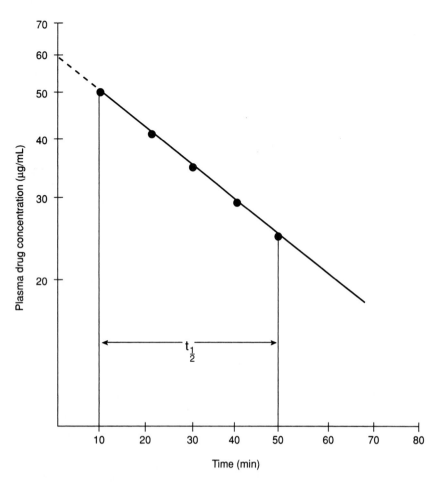

**F I G U R E   2 3 - 4**

Determination of drug half-life. For a drug following first-order kinetics, the plasma concentration versus time is plotted and a straight line is drawn. The time required for the concentration of drug to decrease by one half can be estimated from the graph and is the half-life of the drug. In this example, $t_{1/2}$ = 40 minutes.

body's ability to eliminate a drug and to convert a pharmacologically active drug to a pharmacologically inactive drug. The relationship between $V_d$ and $Cl_T$ can be expressed as

$$Cl_T = V_d K_{elimination}$$

for a drug distribution only in the plasma. A better equation for $Cl_T$ that allows for a drug distribution in many body compartments is

$$Cl_T = \frac{\text{Dose administered}}{\text{AUC}_{0 \to \infty}}$$

where AUC is the area under the plasma concentration of a drug versus time curve. As a method of assessing how rapidly a drug will be cleared from the body, $Cl_T$ is a predictor of toxicity. For example, neonates normally have decreased clearance

as a result of incomplete kidney function. Drugs that are eliminated slowly would thus be more toxic to a newborn than to an adult.

The following example illustrates how these parameters may be used: If a 70-kg patient is treated with a drug that has a half-life of 8 hours and the plasma concentration is 10 $\mu$g/mL immediately after an intravenous injection of 350 mg, the total body clearance can be calculated using the following equations:

1. $Cl_T = V_d K_{elimination}$

2. Find $K_{elimination}$ by $t_{1/2} = \dfrac{0.693}{K_{elimination}}$

$$8 \text{ hours} = \frac{0.693}{K_{elimination}}$$

$$K_{elimination} = 0.087/\text{hour}$$

3. Find $V_d$ by

$$V_d = \frac{\text{Dose of drug administration}}{\text{Plasma concentration at zero time}}$$

$$V_d = \frac{350,000 \ \mu g}{10 \ \mu g/mL} \text{ per 70 kg}$$

$$V_d = 35,000 \text{ mL} = 35 \text{ L}$$

4. $Cl_T = V_d K_{\text{elimination}}$

$Cl_T = (35 \text{ L}) (0.087/\text{hour})$

$Cl_T = 3 \text{ L/hour for 70 kg}$

A **steady-state** level of the drug is achieved when the amount of drug metabolized and distributed equals the amount of the drug entering and leaving the body. Since drug levels are usually expressed as plasma concentrations, the steady state is defined by measuring plasma drug concentrations. When drug elimination follows first-order kinetics, the drug approaches steady-state levels after 5 to 7 half-lives. Steady-state levels for the drug depicted in Figure 23–2 occur after 6 half-lives; subsequent doses do not produce further increases in plasma drug concentration, indicating drug input is balanced by drug elimination.

## VARIABLES AFFECTING DRUG DISPOSITION

There are many reasons why a particular drug dose may not produce the expected therapeutic response. These factors, including physiologic variables, genetic heterogeneity, the presence of pathologic conditions, and drug interactions, are discussed as follows. More detailed information can be found in other sources.[4–7]

The physiologic factors that differentiate one person from another affect how the administration dose of drug affects a particular individual. Age is a variable that must be considered when determining dose. Pharmacokinetic studies of drugs are usually performed on adults. Thus, drug absorption, distribution, biotransformation, and elimination are well defined for this age group. These parameters are less well understood for very young and elderly patients, which is a significant gap considering that the elderly population consumes a disproportionate share of prescription and nonprescription drugs. Neonates and geriatric patients share some age-related differences: decreased gastric acid secretion, which would affect drug absorption; decreased protein binding, which would affect drug distribution; decreased liver function, which would affect drug metabolism; and decreased kidney functions, which would affect drug elimination. There are also differences unique to a particular age group. For example, neonates have decreased lipid stores relative to adults, and the elderly are frequently treated with a combination of drugs (a condition

known as polypharmacy). Because of these variations, dosing must be individualized and monitoring must be more frequent than required for the average adult. Other physiologic factors affecting drug dosage and drug effects are gender, body size, and composition, pregnancy, nutritional status, activity, emotional mood, and body temperature.

Genetic factors cause variability in drug disposition. An entire discipline, pharmacoanthropology, has emerged to compare drug action among different populations. For example, certain individuals inherit a trait that causes them to metabolize some drugs by acetylation more slowly than others (slow acetylators); only 2% of blacks but 10% of whites are slow acetylators. Therapeutic doses of drugs biotransformed by acetylation may produce toxicity in these individuals owing to an increased plasma concentration of drug resulting from decreased metabolism.

Pathologic conditions, different from the one for which treatment is initiated, may affect the disposition of the administered drug. Examples are cardiac disease, causing decreased perfusion of organs; gastrointestinal disease, causing decreased absorption; hepatic disease, causing decreased metabolism; and renal disease, causing decreased elimination of drugs.

Drug interactions may be another variable. For patients treated with more than one drug, the possibility of drug-drug interactions must be considered. The effect of drugs competing for a limited number of protein-binding sites and subsequent alterations in the plasma concentration of a free drug have already been discussed. However, other drug interactions might also be considered in cases of toxicity or therapeutic inadequacies, such as drug-diet and drug-disease interactions.

## SAMPLE COLLECTION AND DATA REPORTING

Errors in collection of blood samples impede, if not prevent, proper drug monitoring. Timing is an important consideration. For a patient receiving the initial dose of a drug, blood should not be drawn before a steady-state concentration of drug has been achieved, which usually requires 5 to 7 half-lives (see Figure 23–2). Thus, to ensure accuracy of results, the time of collection must be noted. A general rule for many drugs is that blood may be drawn 1 hour after the last dose; however, drugs with long half-lives may require many hours to reach equilibrium and this rule would not apply. Another consideration is whether a peak or trough drug level is desired. Peak drug levels are a check on drug toxicity and are drawn immediately on attainment of steady-state levels. Peak drug levels should not exceed the MTC. Trough drug levels check for subtherapeutic effects of the drug and are drawn immediately before administration of the subsequent dose. Trough levels must be above the MEC for the patient to receive the desired therapeutic effect.

The report form should contain the following information: What drug or drugs are being monitored? When was the last dose administered? When is the next dose scheduled? Is a peak or trough level desired? Is the patient on any other drugs? When was the sample collected? What is the clinical status of the patient? Additional information such as the dosage, route of administration, and name of the analyst should be included. Ensuring correct specimen collection and laboratory results requires frequent and open communication between the therapeutic drug monitoring laboratory and nurses, physicians, and pharmacists.

## THERAPEUTIC DRUG MONITORING

### Analytical Techniques

Therapeutic drug monitoring (TDM) has become an important and indispensable laboratory aid in the treatment of disease largely due to the development of sensitive and specific analytical techniques. Additionally, these techniques provide rapid results while requiring only a small sample volume.

Chromatographic techniques such as gas-liquid chromatography (GLC) and high-pressure liquid chromatography (HPLC) have the advantage of analyzing several different drugs simultaneously as well as separating closely related compounds and parent drugs and metabolites. However, few clinical laboratories routinely use these techniques because of the high cost and labor-intensive nature of the instrumentation.

A major advancement in TDM occurred with the development of immunoassays that can be automated. They, too, provide rapid results using small sample volumes. Clinical laboratory scientists, however, must be familiar with factors that may affect results to provide the most accurate data.

Chromatographic and immunoassay techniques measure total drug concentration in the serum, which includes both protein bound and free-drug concentrations even though the free drug is the pharmacologically active form and is most clinically significant. Free drug concentrations can be determined after performing ultrafiltration of the patient sample. Free drug is separated from bound drug by a size-exclusion filter. The free drug levels of phenytoin and valproic acid are of particular clinical importance for patient monitoring.

The type of specimen is also an important consideration in TDM. Serum is the specimen of choice to prevent anticoagulant interference. Additionally, separation gels may adsorb some drugs causing falsely lowered results.

### Specific Drug Classification

Table 23–1 lists the classification, generic names, and proprietary names of some of the commonly encountered drugs requested for therapeutic drug monitoring.

TABLE 23-1

**Classification and Names of Selected Therapeutic Drugs**

| CLASSIFICATION | GENERIC NAME | PROPRIETARY NAME(S) |
|---|---|---|
| Cardiac | Propranolol | Inderal |
| | Digoxin | Lanoxin |
| | Digitoxin | Crystodigin, Purodigin |
| | Lidocaine | Xylocaine |
| | Quinidine | Cardioquin, Quinaglute |
| | Disopyramide | Norpace |
| | Procainamide | Pronestyl |
| Anticonvulsant | Phenobarbital | Luminal |
| | Phenytoin | Dilantin |
| | Valproic acid | Depakene |
| | Primidone | Mysoline |
| | Carbamazepine | Tegretol |
| | Ethosuximide | Zarontin |
| Bronchodilator | Theophylline | Elixophyllin |
| Antimicrobial | Streptomycin | Streptomycin |
| | Gentamicin | Garamycin |
| | Kanamycin | Kantrex |
| | Tobramycin | Nebcin |
| | Neomycin | Mydifradin, Neobiotic |
| | Chloramphenicol | Chloromycetin |
| | Vancomycin | Vancocin |
| Psychotropic | Imipramine | Imavate, Tofranil, Presamine |
| | Desipramine | Norpramin, Pertofrane |
| | Amitriptyline | Elavil, Endep |
| | Nortriptyline | Aventyl, Pamelor |
| | Doxepin | Adapin, Sinequan |
| | Maprotiline | Ludiomil |
| | Lithium | Eskalith, Lithane, Lithobid, Lithonate |
| Antipsychotic | Chlorpromazine | Thorazine |
| | Triflupromazine | Vesprin |
| | Promethazine | Phenergan |
| | Haloperidol | Haldol |
| Antineoplastic | Methotrexate | Mexate |
| | Cisplatin | CPDD, Platinol |
| | Cyclophosphamide | Cytoxan |

## Cardiac Drugs

**Propranolol** is classified as an antiadrenergic drug, meaning that its effects oppose normal adrenergic effects. Adrenergic drugs, such as epinephrine, act on the sympathetic nervous system, which controls the classic fight or flight response. Physiologic responses to adrenergic drugs include rapid heartbeat, increased blood pressure, bronchodilation, increased alertness, and increased blood glucose levels. Propranolol is an antiadrenergic drug that inhibits these effects by blocking beta-adrenergic receptors and is referred to as a beta-blocker. The physiologic effects produced by propranolol are the opposite of those produced by adrenergic drugs and include decreased heart rate, decreased blood pressure, bronchoconstriction, and low doses as an antihypertensive drug and intravenously in high doses as an antidysrhythmic drug (one that controls abnormal heart rhythms). Its therapeutic range for antidysrhythmic effects is 50 to 100 ng/mL and its half-life is 2 to 6 hours. Because it also produces bronchoconstriction, it should not be administered to asthmatic individuals, and it must be used with caution in patients with diabetes because of its hypoglycemic effect.

**Digoxin and digitoxin** are two drugs classified as cardiac glycosides, because their structural formulas contain carbohydrates. They are naturally occurring compounds, extracted from the leaves of the foxglove plant (*Digitalis lanata* or *Digitalis purpurea*). The physiologic effects of both digoxin and digitoxin are to increase the force of the heart's contraction but decrease its rate, that is, to slow and strengthen the contraction. They are used in the treatment of congestive heart failure. Both affect cellular potassium transport, and since decreased potassium levels potentiate cardiac glycoside toxicity, potassium is monitored and is often supplemented when patients are treated with these drugs. Both drugs have a low therapeutic index, and frequent monitoring of plasma levels is required. These drugs concentrate in cardiac tissue at levels 15 to 30 times those found in the blood. Therapeutic levels are determined at the time of peak tissue concentration, which oc-

curs 8 hours after dosing. Signs of toxicity are bradycardia (a slower than normal heart rate) followed by arrhythmia, coma, and death. The interaction of quinidine, another cardiac drug, with digoxin or digitoxin may result in cardiac glycoside toxicity. Digoxin and digitoxin differ in several pharmacokinetic parameters and in other aspects, as described in Table 23–2.

Antidysrhythmic drugs, ones that induce and regulate normal cardiac rhythm, include lidocaine, quinidine, procainamide, and disopyramide. **Lidocaine** is used to treat cardiac dysrhythmias because of its anesthetic effect. It decreases local abnormal initiation of nerve impulses in the heart and is widely used in the treatment of premature ventricular contractions. Because the orally administered drug undergoes extensive first-pass metabolism, parenteral administration is required. The usual administration procedure is a bolus intravenous dose followed by slow infusion, but intramuscular injection is also acceptable. The therapeutic range of lidocaine is 2 to 5 μg/mL, and its half-life is 1 to 2 hours. Active metabolites of lidocaine are monoethylglycinexylidide (MEGX) and glycinexylidide (GX). Signs of toxicity are related to the central nervous system. The first manifestations are dizziness, excitement, or drowsiness and disorientation. These are followed by more severe symptoms, including convulsions, coma, and respiratory arrest.

**Quinidine** is an alkaloid (a naturally occurring physiologically active nitrogen-containing organic compound), derived from the bark of the cinchona tree. It is an isomer of quinine, a commonly used antimalarial drug. Quinidine has long been used in the treatment of rapid and irregular heartbeats by blocking abnormal electrical impulses, decreasing blood pressure and decreasing contraction force. Besides its antidysrhythmic effects, it has antimalarial, antipyretic, and oxytocic effects. Oral administration is most common because intravenous administration may cause a precipitous decrease in blood pressure. The therapeutic range of quinidine is 2 to 5 μg/mL and its half-life is 6 to 7 hours. Cinchonism, a group of central nervous system symptoms including headache, deafness, tinnitus, lightheadedness, and giddiness, and hematologic abnormalities such as leukopenia, thrombocytopenia, and

TABLE   23-2

**Contrasts between Digoxin and Digitoxin**

|  | DIGOXIN | DIGITOXIN |
|---|---|---|
| **Use** | Frequently prescribed | Infrequently prescribed |
| **Plasma half-life** | 1–2 days | 4–6 days |
| **Protein binding** | 25% | 96% |
| **Therapeutic plasma concentration** | 0.8–2 ng/mL | 15–25 ng/mL |
| **Oral absorption** | 65%–80% | 90%–100% |
| **Hepatic metabolism** | None or glucuronide conjugates | Inactive metabolites |
| **Patients treated** | Reduced hepatic function | Reduced renal function |
| **Excretion** | Renal | Renal, hepatic |

anemia are manifestations of toxicity. Quinidine participates in many drug-drug interactions, such as toxicity enhancement of the cardiac glycosides, and is slowly being replaced by cardiac drugs without such untoward effects.

**Procainamide** is used to decrease heart rate and blood pressure. It may be administered orally or parenterally. Its therapeutic range is 4 to 8 $\mu$g/mL and its half-life is 3 to 4 hours. It is metabolized by acetylation to the pharmacologically active compound N-acetylprocainamide (NAPA). In fast acetylators, the concentration of metabolite may exceed that of the parent drug. Since NAPA has antidysrhythmic activity similar to that of the parent drug as well as a longer half-life (8 hours) than the parent drug, coanalysis of NAPA is necessary for complete assessment of procainamide therapy. The therapeutic range for the combination of parent compound and metabolite is 30 $\mu$g/mL. Procainamide toxicity causes severe hypotension, agranulocytosis, and the development of systemic lupus erythematosus. The last is related not to drug concentration but to the acetylator status of the patient, with slow acetylators being more susceptible to development of lupus.

**Disopyramide** is an antidysrhythmic drug used in the treatment of premature ventricular contractions and in the prophylactic prevention of sudden death after myocardial infarctions. The therapeutic range is 2 to 5 $\mu$g/mL and a half-life is 5 to 8 hours. Disopyramide has anticholinergic (prevention of normal digestive function) activity, which produces the unpleasant side effects of dry mouth, urinary hesitance, and constipation. Toxicity results in cardiac abnormalities.

## Anticonvulsant and Antiepileptic Drugs

The anticonvulsant and antiepileptic drugs can be used alone or in combination therapy for treatment of seizures. All are absorbed from the gastrointestinal tract and undergo hepatic metabolism and renal excretion.

**Phenobarbital** is used to treat all seizures except absent seizures. It has a relatively long half-life of 4 days. Because of this, specimens for peak drug concentration should not be collected until 8 hours after phenobarbital administration. The therapeutic range of phenobarbital is 15 to 40 $\mu$g/mL. Concentrations greater than 40 $\mu$g/mL cause sedation and concentrations greater than 60 $\mu$g/mL cause toxicity. Phenobarbital is known to induce the microsomal mixed-function oxidase system involved in metabolism. Therapeutic administration of phenobarbital may therefore cause increased drug metabolism, leading to a decreased plasma concentration of concomitantly administered drugs.

**Phenytoin** not only is the most widely prescribed antiepileptic drug but also is used in the treatment of cardiac dysrhythmias. The therapeutic concentration is 10 to 20 $\mu$g/mL. Concentrations greater than 35 $\mu$g/mL precipitate, rather than alleviate, seizure activity, although other signs of toxicity such as ataxia and nystagmus occur at lower concentrations. Long-term use of phenytoin leads to gum hyperplasia, which is reversible upon withdrawal of the drug. Phenytoin is 90% to

95% protein bound; this high-protein binding results in its participation in many drug displacement interactions. Phenytoin does not obey first-order kinetics and therefore has a saturable hepatic metabolism, leading to a variable half-life. At concentrations less than 10 $\mu$g/mL, the half-life is 1 day, but as drug concentrations increase, the half-life also increases. Because of this, frequent monitoring is necessary since small increases in dose may result in large increases in the plasma concentration.

**Valproic acid** is notable because it is structurally unlike the other anticonvulsant drugs, being a simple 8-carbon, branched-chain fatty acid. Its therapeutic concentration is 50 to 100 $\mu$g/mL, its half-life is 15 hours, and it is highly protein bound (93%). Valproic acid has metabolic effects opposite those produced by phenobarbital; it inhibits the microsomal mixed-function oxidase system, thereby decreasing metabolism and increasing plasma levels of other drugs.

**Primidone** is metabolized by oxidation to phenobarbital; therefore, phenobarbital concentrations must be assayed when therapeutic primidone concentrations are assayed. Another metabolite is phenylethylmalonamide, which also has anticonvulsant activity. The therapeutic concentration of primidone is 8 to 10 $\mu$g/mL and its half-life is 8 hours. Side effects include ataxia and sedation.

**Carbamazepine** is rarely the first choice among anticonvulsant drugs and is usually prescribed only for individuals who have not responded satisfactorily to treatment for other drugs. Carbamazepine therapy requires frequent monitoring for hematologic, hepatic, and renal functions because its use is associated with aplastic anemia, hepatic injury, hypertension, and acute urinary retention. Its therapeutic concentration is 8 to 12 $\mu$g/mL, and its half-life is 27 hours.

**Ethosuximide** is used only in the treatment of absence seizures, also called petit mal seizures. These seizures begin in early childhood but usually do not persist after the age of 20. They are characterized by 5 to 30 seconds of "absence," in which the individual is not fully conscious but not unconscious and can keep from falling but may exhibit minor motor movements. The therapeutic concentration of ethosuximide is 40 to 100 $\mu$g/mL and the half-life is 60 hours in adults and 30 hours in children.

## Bronchodilators

**Theophylline** is chemically classified as a methylxanthine (xanthine is dioxypurine, and theophylline has two methyl groups on the dioxypurine ring). The drug has several pharmacologic activities. It is a central nervous system and respiratory stimulant and a cardiac stimulant. It causes smooth muscle relaxation and diuresis. Its effect on smooth muscle, particularly bronchial muscle, makes it important in the treatment of asthma, chronic obstructive pulmonary disease, and apnea of the premature newborn. Theophylline administration may be by oral, rectal, or parenteral routes. Aminophylline, a mixture of theophylline and ethylenediamine, is often administered in place of theophylline alone, since the solubility of theophylline itself is poor but increases upon the addition of ethylenediamine. In adults, the therapeutic range of theophylline is 10 to 20 $\mu$g/mL. Its half-life may vary, depending on such factors as age and smoking status, but normally is 8 hours. In neonates, the therapeutic range is 5 to 10 $\mu$g/mL and the half-life is 30 hours. Because removal of blood for drug analysis may be difficult and dangerous in premature babies, the measurement of theophylline levels in the saliva of neonates has been evaluated.[8] Some laboratories may also quantitate caffeine, an active metabolite of theophylline, when determining theophylline levels since caffeine itself may be helpful in the treatment of apnea. However, the validity of this remains controversial.[8] Symptoms of theophylline toxicity are nausea, vomiting, diarrhea, irritability, and insomnia. Because of its cardiac effect, high levels of theophylline may be fatal.

## Antimicrobial Agents

**Streptomycin, gentamicin, kanamycin, tobramycin,** and **neomycin** are classified as **aminoglycosides** because they contain amino sugars in glycosidic linkages. They are used for the treatment of infections by gram-negative bacteria. Aminoglycosides are bactericidal because they bind to the bacterial ribosome, causing inhibition of bacterial protein synthesis. These antibiotics are not well absorbed when administered orally and are usually administered by intravenous or intramuscular injection. Because they are polar compounds, they do not cross cellular membranes and are rapidly excreted by the normal kidney. In patients with renal disease, however, half-lives are greatly prolonged and dose adjustments must be made. Since these drugs are toxic to both bacteria and humans, the goal of therapy is production of bacterial toxicity before human toxicity. Ototoxicity, involving both auditory (hearing) and vestibular (balance) functions, may be permanent. Nephrotoxicity is also a major concern. Because of these problems, aminoglycoside use is generally reserved for cases in which other antibiotics have not been effective or for the treatment of severe infections.

**Chloramphenicol,** like the aminoglycoside antibiotics, acts on gram-negative bacteria by inhibition of protein synthesis, primarily by binding the bacterial ribosome. Unlike the aminoglycosides, it has 70% to 90% absorption from the gastrointestinal tract and can be administered either orally or parenterally. The therapeutic range of chloramphenicol is 15 to 25 $\mu$g/mL and its half-life is 2 to 3 hours. A severe problem unrelated to drug dose is bone marrow depression leading to pancytopenia. This condition may occur in patients who are taking prolonged chloramphenicol therapy or who have been treated with repeated courses of the new drug. Although the incidence of pancytopenia is low, fatality rates approach 100%. Therefore, chloramphenicol use is indicated only in carefully controlled and specialized circumstances. Neonates treated with chloramphenicol may develop a fatal toxicity because of problems in metabolism and excretion of the drug. The first

manifestations of this "gray baby" syndrome are vomiting, irregular and rapid respiration, diarrhea, and cyanosis, followed by development of flaccidity, an ashen-gray color, and hypothermia. Death occurs in 40% of these neonates.

**Vancomycin** is an antibiotic that is bactericidal because of its inhibitory effect on synthesis of the bacterial cell wall and cytoplasmic membrane. It is used in the treatment of infections caused by gram-positive bacteria. Because of poor absorption from the gastrointestinal tract, it is usually administered intravenously. Its therapeutic range is 6 to 10 $\mu$g/mL and its half-life is 6 hours. Vancomycin is primarily excreted by the kidney; thus patients with renal disease receiving vancomycin therapy must be frequently monitored. Ototoxicity and nephrotoxicity are the most significant problems.

## Psychotropic Drugs

The psychotropic drugs are used to treat affective disorders, that is, mania and depression. Since these disorders are characterized by changes in mood, antidepressant drugs produce a psychological rather than a physical response. One theory for the cause of depression is an absolute or relative deficiency in the concentration of neurotransmitters at central synapses. Selected drugs may be useful therapeutic agents by potentiating the effects of neurotransmitters such as norepinephrine and serotonin. Because these drugs also block neurotransmitter reuptake into presynaptic neurons, the amount of neurotransmitter available for interaction at the synapse is increased, thus alleviating the biochemical deficiency that resulted in clinical depression.

**Imipramine, desipramine, amitriptyline, nortriptyline,** and **doxepin** are classified as **tricyclic antidepressants.** These drugs have a related 3-ring structure, as their classification implies, and are widely used in the treatment of depression. Desipramine and nortriptyline are actually metabolites of imipramine and amitriptyline, respectively. **Maprotiline** is classified as a **tetracyclic antidepressant** because of its 4-ring structure. All are absorbed by the gastrointestinal tract and are administered orally, but they undergo an extensive first-pass biotransformation, which makes their bioavailability variable among different patients. Because of different patient responses to these drugs, monitoring is performed mainly to ensure an adequate initial dose. Side effects for most of the antidepressants include some degree of sedation, anticholinergic effects (dry mouth, urinary retention, constipation) and cardiac effects, including palpitation, tachycardia (an abnormally rapid heartbeat), and orthostatic hypotension. Toxic effects include cardiac dysrhythmias and precipitation of other cardiac abnormalities.

**Lithium** is used in the treatment of bipolar personality disorder (also called manic-depressive illness). Therapeutic action is thought to involve its ability both to substitute for sodium or potassium ions in cellular transport and to decrease catecholamine activity. Because lithium can decrease sodium and potassium levels, patients treated concomitantly with lithium and other drugs effecting ion loss, such as diuretics, must be frequently dosed, receive ion supplementation, and be carefully monitored. Lithium is orally administered as the carbonate salt (lithium carbonate) and partitions between blood and tissues. Plasma lithium concentrations reflect the amount of lithium in the body and are measured in millimoles per liter (mmol/L) of blood. The therapeutic range is 0.5 to 1.5 mmol/L. Because of its tissue distribution, it is eliminated in two phases; the half-life for the first phase is 4 to 6 hours, and for the second phase, 7 to 20 hours. Lithium monitoring must be performed 8 to 10 hours after the last dose and should be consistent for a particular patient. Side effects of lithium therapy include gastrointestinal, neuromuscular, central nervous system, mental, and cardiovascular disorders. Toxic effects include muscle twitching and rigidity, a hyperactive deep tendon reflex, and epileptic seizures.

## Antipsychotic Drugs

Psychoses are psychiatric illnesses characterized by dissociation from reality and inability to function in society. These drugs are used in the symptomatic treatment of psychoses to produce emotional calmness and mental relaxation.

Because of their structures, **chlorpromazine, triflupromazine,** and **promethazine** are members of the phenothiazine group of antipsychotic drugs. Their mechanism of action is blockage of dopamine receptors in the central nervous system. Besides their behavioral effect, they have antiemetic action, effects on central skeletal muscle mechanisms, alteration of temperature regulation, endocrine actions, and peripheral nervous system effects. The phenothiazines may be administered orally but are slowly absorbed, producing a wide variability in the plasma levels achieved among different patients. Other routes of administration are by suppository or intramuscular injection. The half-life of chlorpromazine is 16 to 30 hours. Metabolites may be found in the urine for several weeks after administration. Side effects include tachycardia, hypothermia, lethargy, orthostatic hypotension, and dryness of the mouth. Phenothiazines show many drug-drug interactions, necessitating a complete patient history and careful monitoring.

**Haloperidol** is a member of the butyrophenone derivatives of antipsychotic drugs. Haloperidol has a similar mechanism of action and produces similar pharmacologic properties to those of the phenothiazines but has a different chemical structure. Its half-life is 13 to 35 hours.

## Antineoplastic Drugs

Antineoplastic drugs are active against some malignant cells and, to an extent, against nonmalignant cells. In therapy, drugs are frequently combined to enhance the activities of other drugs or to provide synergistic action with the other drugs. Monitoring is required for the establishment of clinical protocols and for evaluation of the effectiveness of new multidrug regimens.

**Methotrexate** is classified as an antimetabolite because it interferes with normal cellular metabolism. It is a cell cycle-specific drug (one that inhibits cell replication during a specific phase of the cell cycle) that inhibits the synthesis of DNA. It accomplishes this by inhibition of dihydrofolate reductase, an enzyme needed for the formation of tetrahydrofolate, an essential compound in DNA, RNA, and amino acid synthesis. Malignant cells, which divide more rapidly and therefore synthesize more DNA than nonmalignant cells, are particularly susceptible to the drug's effect, which is the goal of methotrexate therapy. Methotrexate can be administered orally or parenterally. Therapeutic dosing is individualized and depends on the body size of the patient. Half-life varies with an administered dose and ranges from 2 hours at high doses to more than 10 hours at lower doses. Side effects include myelosuppression, nausea, and vomiting. On high-dose therapy, hepatotoxicity may occur. Methotrexate binds the plasma protein; therefore, coadministration of drugs that may compete for protein binding is likely to cause toxicity, with symptoms of diarrhea and bone marrow aplasia.

**Cisplatin** and **cyclophosphamide** are classified as alkylating agents because they replace normal atoms with alkyl groups. When this replacement occurs in DNA, the alkylated DNA cannot undergo correction replication or transcription leading to cell death. Alkylating agents are cell cycle-nonspecific drugs and act on either actively dividing or resting cells. Therapeutic dosing is individualized and depends on the body size of the patient. Cyclophosphamide requires hepatic biotransformation by the microsomal mixed-function oxidase system to produce its active metabolites, 4-hydroxycyclophosphamide and aldophosphamide, which in turn produce the alkylating cyclophosphoramide mustard. Side effects of cyclophosphamide therapy include hematologic suppression, nausea, vomiting, and reproductive dysfunction. Cisplatin, a platinum-containing compound, has additional nephrotoxic and ototoxic effects.

## Immunosuppressive Drugs

Immunosuppressive drugs are administered to prevent or minimize the risk of organ transplant rejection. Even though these drugs are candidates for TDM because of the highly variable nature of the pharmacokinetic processes, especially in the early post-transplant period, they are used in limited populations. These drugs include cyclosporine, tacrolimus (FK-506), and mycophenolic acid. The specimen of choice for monitoring cyclosporine and tacrolimus is EDTA anticoagulated whole blood since the drugs associate with red blood cells.

## SUMMARY

The role of therapeutic drug monitoring is likely to expand in several directions.[9] Clinical pharmacokinetic consulting services to interpret and integrate laboratory data will become routine. Quality assurance with follow-up of all inquiries and complaints related to the use of laboratory data in patient care will expand. Assay of major metabolites of all drugs to classify metabolic profiles of patients will occur. Technology will allow indwelling catheters and sensory monitors to continuously monitor the concentration of drug in a patient's blood. Bedside and physician office testing of drugs will become commonplace. Robotics will perform routine manipulations. The outcome of these advances will be the "freeing [of] technologists to engage in activities that require intellectual and cognitive functions."[9]

The clinical laboratory scientist with initiative, one who seeks professional growth, will find the therapeutic drug-monitoring laboratory an exciting place. A future trend in clinical laboratory science is the establishment of therapeutic drug-monitoring programs. In such programs, clinical laboratory scientists must interact with pharmacists, nurses, and physicians to analyze, advise, teach, and interpret data rather than merely provide a plasma concentration of drug on a report form. A prototype for such a program exists[10]; clinical laboratory scientists receive intensive specialized training, enabling them to handle all routine and some consultation requests related to therapeutic drug monitoring. The benefit to the patient is more complete and individualized care. The benefit to the physician is the interpretation rather than the mere reporting of drug concentrations. The benefit to the clinical laboratory scientist is intellectual stimulation and growth, thus preventing "excellent people from leaving [clinical laboratory science] for other jobs."[10]

## REFERENCES

1. Loomis TA, Hayes AW: *Loomis's Essentials of Toxicology.* 4th ed. Philadelphia, Lea & Febiger, 1996.

2. Woosley RL: Role of plasma concentration monitoring in the evaluation of response to antiarrhythmic drugs. Am J Cardiol 62:9H–17H, 1988.

3. Spector R, Park GD, Johnson GF, et al.: Therapeutic drug monitoring. Clin Pharmacol Ther 43:345–353, 1988.

4. Boeckx RL: Therapeutic drug monitoring: The hidden factors. Lab Manage 21:29–34, 1983.

5. Annesley TM: Special considerations for geriatric therapeutic drug monitoring. Clin Chem 35:1337–1341, 1989.

6. Warner A: Neonatal pharmacokinetics. Clin Lab Sci 3: 98–99, 1990.

7. Koch-Weser J: Serum drug concentrations in clinical perspective. Ther Drug Monit 3:3–16, 1981.

8. Toback JW, Gal P, Erkan NV, et al.: Usefulness of theophylline saliva levels in neonates. Ther Drug Monit 5:185–189, 1983.

9. Pippenger CE: Commentary: Therapeutic drug monitoring in the 1990s. Clin Chem 35:1348–1351, 1989.

10. Cox S, Walson PD: Providing effective therapeutic drug monitoring services. Ther Drug Monit 11:310–322, 1989.

# CHAPTER 24

# Toxicology

*Joan Radtke*

Toxicology is the study of poisonous substances, their actions on the living organism, their detection by laboratory and other methods, and measures taken to counteract their biologic effects. A comprehensive treatment of such a vast body of knowledge is beyond the scope of a single chapter in a textbook of clinical chemistry. This chapter focuses on clinical laboratory analyses that are commonly provided to support the diagnosis and treatment of the poisoned patient, to monitor exposure of individuals to common environmental toxins, or to screen selected populations for evidence of substance abuse. Emphasis is on clinical laboratory toxicology: identification, and in some cases quantitation, of toxic substances in body fluids.

The modern clinical laboratory provides toxicology services that can assist in providing answers to three questions pertinent to the care of the suspected poisoned patient.

1. What toxic substances, if any, are present in the specimen submitted for testing?
2. Are the laboratory results for toxic substances related to the patient's presenting signs and symptoms?
3. What treatment or intervention, if any, should be provided on the basis of the clinical and laboratory findings?

If an individual ingests or is otherwise exposed to almost any substance in sufficient quantity, that substance, in theory, can have a damaging effect on health. However, for economic and other practical purposes, the clinical toxicology laboratory must limit its available testing services to those substances that are most commonly encountered in the population served, and for which testing methods exist that can produce valid and useful results in a timely manner.

To derive a "menu" of testing services that a clinical toxicology laboratory should be prepared to provide, it is necessary to consider the actions or intentions that lead to poisoning and the common classes of poisons. Human actions that lead to toxic episodes may be classified as intentional or unintentional on the part of the victim (patient). Intentional exposures include suicidal gestures, suicidal attempts, and recreational use of substances. Unintentional exposures include those in which the victim is unaware of the effects, unaware of the exposure, and/or unwillingly exposed, as in a pediatric or geriatric patient; an occupational, industrial or environmental exposure; or a homicide or homicidal attempt.

Each toxic substance that is commonly implicated in an exposure may be described as representative of one of 6 classes of poisons: gases, volatiles, corrosives, metals, nonmetals, and nonvolatile organics. The toxic substances commonly tested in the clinical laboratory, grouped according to class and usual types of exposure, are listed in Table 24–1. Four of the 6 classes are represented in this table. Exposure to corrosives such as strong acids and bases (e.g., household cleaning agents) may occur as accidents, homicides, suicides, or pediatric cases, but the clinical laboratory is usually not directly involved in diagnosis or treatment. Nonmetals such as boron and the halogens (chlorine, fluorine, or bromine) may also be implicated in toxic episodes, but are sufficiently uncommon in most clinical situations as to render routine availability of testing impractical. Each class is, of course, represented by a vast array of potentially toxic substances, but the emphasis here is on those substances listed in Table 24–1 that meet the criteria of commonly encountered toxic substances for which the clinical laboratory should be prepared to provide timely and accurate testing services.

## CLASSES OF TOXIC SUBSTANCES

### Gases (Carbon Monoxide)

**Carbon monoxide** (CO) is a tasteless, odorless, and colorless gas that is produced by incomplete combustion of organic matter. Atmospheric sources commonly implicated in poisoning include automobile exhaust, improperly vented gas heating systems, and fires. CO has an affinity for the hemoglobin molecule about 250 times greater than that of oxygen.[1] Upon exposure to CO, **oxyhemoglobin** is converted to **carboxyhemoglobin,** reducing the delivery of oxygen to the tissues and resulting in tissue hypoxia and anoxia. Annually, many deaths result from both accidental and intentional exposure to toxic levels of CO. Exposure to CO is a common toxic condition that must be recognized and treated in a timely manner, usually aided by a series of laboratory tests. If rescued in time, patients usually recover with no complications, unless brain damage has occurred during prolonged exposure.

CO in small quantities is normally produced in the body during the catabolism of heme. This endogenous source plus variable environmental sources, such as cigarette smoke and automobile exhaust, result in the **reference levels** for carboxyhemoglobin, % of total hemoglobin, differing from about

TABLE 24-1

**Common Toxic Substances Tested in the Clinical Laboratory**

| SUBSTANCE | CLASS | USUAL EXPOSURE |
|---|---|---|
| Carbon monoxide | Gases | U,S |
| Ethanol | Volatiles | R |
| Other alcohols | Volatiles | U,R |
| Methanol | | |
| Isopropanol | | |
| Ethylene glycol | | |
| Lead | Metals | U,O,P |
| Pesticides | Nonvolatile | U,O,P |
| Organophosphates | Organics | |
| Carbamates | | |
| Drugs of Abuse | Nonvolatile | |
| Acetaminophen* | Organics | U,P,S |
| Amphetamines | | R,S |
| Barbiturates* | | R,S |
| Benzodiazepines* | | R,S |
| Cannabinoids* | | R,S |
| Cocaine | | R,S |
| Hallucinogens | | R,S |
| Opioids* | | R,S |
| Salicylates* | | U,P,S |
| Steroids (anabolic)* | | R |
| Tricyclic antidepressants* | | R,S |

U = unintentional; S = suicidal; O = occupational;

R = recreational; P = pediatric.

*May also be classified as therapeutic drugs in overdose.

including oxyhemoglobin, reduced hemoglobin, methemoglobin, and carboxyhemoglobin.

Several automated instruments for point of care and benchtop applications are available that measure the various hemoglobin species and calculate the concentration of carboxyhemoglobin. These instruments take spectrophotometric measurements at 4 to 7 wavelengths, and the % carboxyhemoglobin as well as % oxyhemoglobin, deoxyhemoglobin, methemoglobin, and total hemoglobin are calculated using a series of equations. Results obtained using these instruments generally compare well with gas chromatography procedures at concentrations greater than 2% to 3%. The specimen of choice for carboxyhemoglobin measurement is whole blood that is anticoagulated with heparin or EDTA.

A manual method, based on the work of Tietz and Fiereck, utilizes the spectral differences of the various hemoglobin species after a hemolysate of whole blood is treated with sodium hydrosulfite. Sodium hydrosulfite reduces oxyhemoglobin and methemoglobin, but does not react with carboxyhemoglobin, thus leaving only carboxyhemoglobin and reduced hemoglobin in the specimen. These two species have similar absorbances at a wavelength of 555 nm, but carboxyhemoglobin has a greater absorbance than reduced hemoglobin at 541 nm (Figure 24–1). Absorbance of the hemolysate is measured at these 2 wavelengths and the ratio ($A_{541}/A_{555}$) exhibits a linear relationship to the relative concentration of carboxyhemoglobin.

0.5% in rural-dwelling nonsmokers to 5% to 6% in urban smokers. At whole blood carboxyhemoglobin levels of 10% to 20%, subtle symptoms such as shortness of breath and a slight headache are seen, progressing to irritability, fainting, confusion, and impairment of judgment at 40% to 50% and coma, respiratory failure, and death when carboxyhemoglobin levels reach 70% to 80%.[1]

Toxic levels of CO are assessed by the measurement of CO released from hemoglobin or the determination of carboxyhemoglobin. The direct measurement of CO is performed using **gas chromatography,** which is considered to be the reference procedure. This method is accurate and precise at all levels but requires special equipment and highly trained personnel.

In emergency medical settings, CO in whole blood is most commonly measured as **carboxyhemoglobin** using **differential spectroscopy.** The results are expressed as percentage of total hemoglobin. Measurement depends on differences in the absorption spectra of the hemoglobin species found in blood

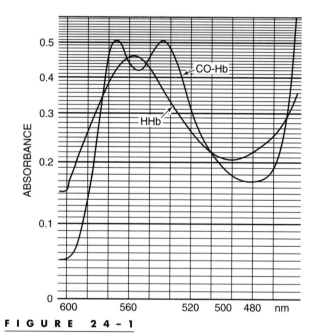

**FIGURE 24-1**

Absorbance spectra of carboxyhemoglobin (COHb) and reduced hemoglobin (HHb). In the COHb method of Tietz and Fiereck, measurements are taken at 555 nm, where the two species have similar absorbances, and at 541 nm, where COHb has a greater absorbance.

When a case of CO toxicity is encountered, the first step in treatment is removal of the patient from the source of exposure. The half-life of CO (time needed to reduce the blood concentration by 50%) in adults breathing room air is 5 to 6 hours. This may be reduced to about 1.5 hours by administration of 100% oxygen and further reduced by administration of pure oxygen at increased pressure using a hyperbaric chamber. Hyperbaric treatment is not without risk and is therefore reserved for the most severe cases.[1]

## Volatiles

### ETHANOL

**Ethanol** is the most readily available and widely used of all toxic substances and one of the most lethal. The 1999 National Household Survey on Drug Abuse[2] revealed the following estimates:

- 105 million Americans aged 12 years and older (47.3%) used alcohol at least once during the 30 days before being interviewed.
- 45 million people (20.2%) engaged in binge drinking, meaning they drank 5 or more drinks on one occasion during the 30 days before being interviewed. Of these, 12.4 million had 5 or more drinks on one occasion 5 or more days during the same period.
- 18.6% of adolescents aged 12 to 17 years used alcohol in the month before the survey and 10.9% were binge drinkers.

Alcoholism is a serious socioeconomic and health problem throughout the world. In the United States, liver disease and related health problems, particularly cancer and heart disease, and birth defects are associated with alcohol consumption. In 1997 the proportion of traffic crash fatalities that were alcohol-related was 30.6%.[3]

Ethanol is readily absorbed through the gastric and intestinal mucosa with a peak blood level appearing about 1 hour after ingestion. Absorption rates for alcohol depend on the amount and type of food in the stomach, body weight, and gender. Alcohol consumed after a meal containing fat, protein, and carbohydrates is absorbed three times more slowly than alcohol consumed on an empty stomach. Women absorb and metabolize alcohol differently than men and are more susceptible to developing alcohol-related diseases. The liver metabolizes most of the ingested alcohol. A small amount is excreted unchanged by the lungs and kidneys. Until all the alcohol has been metabolized, it is distributed throughout the body, affecting the brain and other tissues.[4]

The toxic effects of ethanol ingestion on the liver and central nervous system are believed to be the result of either the alcohol itself or its chief metabolite **acetaldehyde.** The principal pathway for ethanol metabolism utilizes **alcohol dehydrogenase,** which converts ethanol to acetaldehyde. Acetaldehyde is highly reactive. Most of it is quickly converted to acetic acid, which enters the Krebs cycle as acetyl CoA, where final metabolism occurs. Acetaldehyde is the chief causative agent of liver damage, including liver fibrosis and collagen formation. The metabolite readily attaches to components of the cell membrane forming destructive adducts that damage cells directly or create new antigenic stimulants. Organ damage resulting from ethanol consumption may be immunologically based. The causative agent for fetal alcohol syndrome appears to be ethanol, independent of acetaldehyde.[5,6]

Ethanol affects the metabolism of many medications, increasing the drug's effect for some and decreasing the activity of others. Acetaminophen (Tylenol™), a commonly available analgesic, is particularly dangerous if taken after a binge by heavy drinkers. Chronic heavy drinking appears to increase utilization of an alternative metabolic pathway for alcohol metabolism involving the enzyme cytochrome P450IIE1 (CYP2E1). The enzyme may be involved in the transformation of acetaminophen and other drugs into hepatotoxic chemicals.[4]

Serum concentrations ranging from 0.05% (g/dL) to 0.10% (500 to 1000 mg/L) are achieved in the average-sized adult (male, 170 lb; female, 137 lb) after 2 to 5 drinks, where drink is defined as 0.54 oz of alcohol (approximately 1 shot of distilled spirits, 1 can of beer, or 1 glass of wine). In most states, a blood alcohol concentration (BAC) of 0.10% (g/dL) is defined by law as being too intoxicated to operate a motor vehicle. Many consider this level to be too high since drivers with a BAC one half that level (0.05%) exhibit impairment in eye movement, glare resistance, visual perception, reaction time, certain types of steering tasks, and information processing. Seventeen states have adopted a BAC limit of 0.08% and the American Medical Association in 1986 endorsed lowering the legal limit to 0.05%.[7] Blood concentrations of 2.0% to 2.5% are generally correlated with gross intoxication, decreased alertness, slurred speech, lethargy, and loss of coordination. Stupor to coma and death may occur at 3.0% to 5.0%, although there is a great deal of individual biologic variation in these clinical correlations.[5]

As a result of its high use and abuse, the measurement of ethanol is one of the most frequently performed toxicology tests. Whole blood, plasma, serum, urine, or saliva may be used in a laboratory setting for the determination of ethanol. Since blood collection is an invasive procedure requiring the assistance of medical personnel, law enforcement personnel perform **breath analyses** for ethanol on individuals suspected to be driving under the influence of alcohol. If blood is used, the venipuncture site should be cleansed with a disinfectant, such as aqueous benzalkonium chloride (Zephiran), that does not contain any type of alcohol. Serum, plasma, and saliva have higher concentrations of ethanol than corresponding whole blood specimens because alcohol distributes into the aqueous compartments of the blood. Sodium fluoride is the anticoagulant of choice because it inhibits fermentation. Specimens for analysis of all volatiles should be analyzed immediately or kept stoppered and refrigerated until tested to avoid evaporation.

The two most common quantitative methods of analysis for ethanol are **gas-liquid chromatography** (GLC) and **enzymatic** analysis using alcohol dehydrogenase (ADH). A GLC method for the measurement of common serum volatiles is described in the following section. General principles of GLC analysis are described in the final section of this chapter.

The ADH reaction previously described for the metabolism of ethanol also forms the basis for the most commonly used chemical method for measurement of ethanol in serum, plasma, or whole blood. Whole blood is used directly in some methods, whereas others require the preparation of a trichloroacetic acid filtrate.

$$CH_3CH_2OH + NAD^+ \xrightarrow{ADH} CH_3CHO + NADH + H^+$$

Reagent ADH from yeast catalyzes the dehydrogenation of ethanol to acetaldehyde and the concomitant reduction of $NAD^+$ to NADH. The increase in absorbance at 340 nm with the formation of NADH is directly proportional to the concentration of ethanol in the specimen. This reaction is selective, but not entirely specific, for most ADH methods. Interference from related toxins, relative to ethanol, is around 7% for isopropanol, 3% for methanol, and 4% for ethylene glycol. Some manufacturers claim to have better specificity. In the absence of other low-molecular-weight alcohols, the method may be considered relatively specific for ethanol. Ethanol assays utilizing ADH have been adapted for use on most automated analyzers and are convenient for laboratories that do not have gas chromatographic equipment.[1]

Breath concentrations of ethanol have been shown to reflect the whole blood ethanol concentrations. Alcohol present in alveolar capillary blood rapidly equilibrates with alveolar air in a ratio of 2100: 1 (blood:breath). The most common devices for breath alcohol measurements utilize infrared absorption spectroscopy.[1]

## TOXIC ALCOHOLS

Other low-molecular-weight alcohols that are occasionally involved in acute toxic episodes are **methanol, isopropanol,** and **ethylene glycol.** Methanol, or wood alcohol, is a common solvent used in paint products and window cleaning fluids and an accidental contaminant in illegal whiskey. Isopropanol is sold over the counter as rubbing alcohol and ethylene glycol is used as antifreeze in automobile cooling systems. Ingestion of these compounds is usually unintentional, or by alcoholics as a substitute for ethanol, since each of them produces an initial effect somewhat similar to ethanol intoxication.[8] Children may be attracted to ethylene glycol and methanol-based window washing solvents because of their attractive colors and acceptable taste. In a metabolic pathway analogous to the one for ethanol, **methanol** is converted to **formaldehyde** and **formic acid.**

$$Methanol \xrightarrow{ADH} Formaldehyde \longrightarrow Formic\ Acid \longrightarrow Formate\ (toxic)$$

The metabolites are extremely toxic to the central nervous system (CNS) and gastrointestinal (GI) tract. Symptoms include visual and GI disturbances, with metabolic acidosis that is often delayed. The blurring of vision may progress to temporary or permanent blindness. Associated laboratory findings are a severe metabolic acidosis (low pH and extremely low total $CO_2$, with $PCO_2$ lowered in compensation) with an increased anion gap due to the formate produced.[8]

**Isopropanol** is converted to acetone by ADH and produces a ketosis, confirmed by a positive nitroprusside tablet test with serum or urine, but no marked metabolic acidosis develops. Associated clinical findings are CNS depression, fruity breath, hypotension, and cardiovascular complications and coma. Unlike the symptoms associated with the other toxic alcohols, isopropanol intoxication usually does **not** lead to blindness, renal failure, or an acidosis. Since isopropanol (rubbing alcohol) is commonly available, children are at increased risk for unintentional exposure.

**Ethylene glycol** is metabolized to **formic acid** and **oxalic acid.** The toxic metabolites produce a severe metabolic acidosis and increased anion gap, which is often accompanied by the appearance of **oxalate crystals** in the urine.

$$Ethylene\ glycol \xrightarrow{ADH} Glycolaldehyde \longrightarrow Glycolic\ acid \longrightarrow$$
$$Glyoxylic\ acid \longrightarrow Oxalic\ acid$$

After ingestion, ethylene glycol is rapidly absorbed from the GI tract and symptoms appear early. Toxic sequelae include CNS depression, hypertension, and renal failure.

The presence of toxic alcohols in body fluids represents abnormal findings requiring medical attention. Whereas ethanol overdose usually requires only supportive treatment or observation, toxic episodes involving methanol, isopropanol, or ethylene glycol require more aggressive medical intervention. The toxic alcohols by themselves are relatively nontoxic; harmful effects of intoxication are due to their metabolites and the conditions (e.g., metabolic acidosis) that they produce.

The goals of treatment for **methanol** and **ethylene glycol** intoxication are to prevent metabolism of the alcohols and facilitate their removal from the body. Both alcohols are initially broken down by the action of ADH. Treatment is based on the strong preference that ADH has for ethanol. The affinity of ADH for ethanol is 10 times greater than its affinity for methanol and for ethylene glycol it is 100 times greater. The severely toxic patient is given intravenous ethanol and either undergoes dialysis or is treated with diuretic agents; the ethanol saturates ADH binding sites while the dialysis or diuresis removes methanol or ethylene glycol before they are converted to toxic metabolites. An antidote for ethylene glycol, 4-methylpyrozole (4-MP), is available and it has fewer side effects than ethanol. Hemodialysis, rather than ethanol therapy, is used for severe **isopropanol** intoxication because the conversion of isopropanol to acetone occurs rapidly.[8]

Methanol and isopropanol, as well as ethanol, lend themselves to measurement by gas-liquid chromatography (GLC),

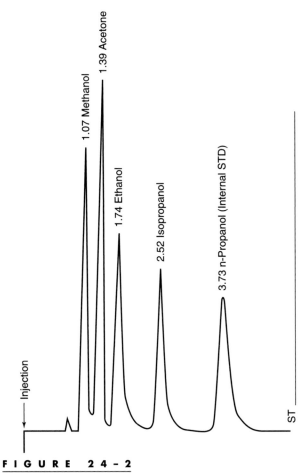

**FIGURE 24-2**

Gas-liquid chromatogram of serum volatiles with n-propanol as internal standard, using a flame ionization detector. Numbers above peaks are retention times in minutes.

which is considered the reference method. Because these substances are volatile at a temperature below the boiling point of water, serum and urine can be injected directly onto a GLC column at relatively low temperature, around 80 to 85°C. No chemical derivatization or extraction of the specimen is necessary and good separation of methanol, ethanol, isopropanol, and acetone (a metabolite of isopropanol) is obtained.

A typical chromatogram of serum volatiles, obtained by GLC with a flame ionization detector, is shown in Figure 24–2. Volatiles in an unknown specimen are **identified** by their retention times on the GLC column as compared with the retention times of pure volatile standards. Substances identified are **quantitated** by comparing the peak size (area or height) in the unknown with peak sizes (areas or heights) of standards of known concentration.

To improve the accuracy and precision of GLC measurement of volatiles, the methods may be modified to include the use of n-propanol as an internal standard. Unknowns and volatile standards are diluted with the internal standard, which is a volatile not readily available to the public and not likely

to be encountered in a patient specimen. The n-propanol peak has a longer retention time than the other volatiles, as shown in Figure 24–2. The ratio of the peak size of the unknown is compared to that of n-propanol. Similarly, the ratios of peak sizes of volatile standards to that of the n-propanol standard are also determined. Concentrations of volatiles in unknowns are then obtained by comparing unknown:internal standard ratios with volatile standard:internal standard ratios.

**Headspace analysis** is an alternative sample injection method used for GLC alcohol analysis. The sample is extremely clean, which extends the performance of the column and avoids problems such as clogged syringe needles. Volatile alcohols and acetone are present in measurable concentrations in the air space (headspace) above the sealed liquid specimen. Blood or serum is first pretreated by diluting the sample with a saturated sodium chloride solution containing the internal standard. The mixture is covered and allowed to reach equilibrium. A portion of the headspace gas mixture is then injected onto the chromatographic column for analysis. Headspace analysis is the preferred method for determination of methanol. A modification of the method is used to measure formate.[1]

**Ethylene glycol** is a dihydric alcohol and not a volatile by definition because its boiling point (197°C) is well above that of water. It is usually grouped with the volatiles in discussions of clinical toxicology because there are similarities between ethylene glycol and monohydric alcohols in terms of symptoms and treatment of toxicity. Because it is not a volatile, GLC analysis of ethylene glycol requires that the specimen be pretreated with a derivitizing agent. A GLC method is available that simultaneously measures ethylene glycol and its metabolite, **glycolic acid.** The method is rapid, relatively simple, and not subject to interference. A rapid estimate of ethylene glycol concentration may be determined using a method based on the inhibition of glycerol dehydrogenase, the enzyme that functions as the indictor enzyme in kinetic triglyceride procedures. The method is subject to interference from glycerol and other molecules.[1]

Accurate identification of ethanol and individual toxic alcohols is important to clinicians who must quickly institute treatment strategies. GLC is a reliable method for this purpose given a well-maintained instrument and an experienced laboratory scientist, but this combination may not always be available in the emergency situation. The presence of volatiles should always be confirmed by correlation among laboratory results as shown in Table 24–2.[8]

Osmolal gap, or Δ osmolality, is the difference between the measured serum osmolality, as determined with a freezing point osmometer, and the calculated serum osmolality. For toxicology purposes, the osmolality is estimated using a formula based on the concentrations of serum electrolytes (sodium), glucose, and BUN, which, for normal individuals, are the major contributors to serum osmolality.

$$\text{Calculated osmolality} = 2\,\text{Na}^+ + \frac{\text{Glucose}}{20} + \frac{\text{BUN}}{3} + \frac{\text{ETOH}}{5}$$

TABLE    24 - 2

## Clinical Laboratory Correlations in Toxicity with Ethanol and Other Alcohols

| ALCOHOL | OSMOLAR GAP | METABOLIC ACIDOSIS WITH ANION GAP | SERUM ACETONE | URINARY OXALATE | URINE KETONES |
|---|---|---|---|---|---|
| Ethanol | + | o/+ | o/+ | o | o/+ |
| Isopropanol | + | o | + | o | + |
| Ethylene glycol | + | + | o | o/+ | o |
| Methanol | + | + | o | o | o |

+ = increased or abnormal; o = negative or no change.

The calculated osmolality is based on the contributions to serum osmolality of these analytes only, whereas the measured osmolality is based on the contributions to freezing point depression of all particles in serum. Normal osmolal gap is less than 10 mOsm/kg $H_2O$. Alcohols, when present, contribute significantly to increases in osmolality and can account for a serum osmolality that is considerably higher than the calculated osmolality. This difference between measured and calculated osmolality is found whenever any alcohol is present in serum. An elevated osmolar gap does not differentiate among alcohols, but is always present when one or more alcohols are seen in serum. Ethanol is included in the equation because in emergency toxicology, ethanol is commonly seen in combination with other toxic alcohols or drugs.[8]

## Heavy Metals

Metals of physiologic importance include aluminum, arsenic, cadmium, chromium, cobalt, copper, fluoride, iron, iodine, lead, manganese, mercury, molybdenum, nickel, selenium, silica, silver, thallium, and zinc. Some of the metals such as iron, copper, and zinc are micronutrients that are essential at trace levels and are fully discussed in the chapter covering nutritional assessment. Others, like lead, mercury, arsenic and cadmium, are always considered toxic even at very low levels of exposure. This section discusses the heavy metals that, when present in excessive amounts, exert effects ranging from subtle CNS disturbances to overt disease or death.

Heavy metal environmental and industrial sources are monitored and studied by the U.S. Environmental Protection Agency (EPA), the National Institute for Occupational Safety and Health (NIOSH), the Occupational Safety and Health Administration (OSHA), and health care specialists practicing in urban and industrial settings. Clinical laboratory scientists, who know of the hazardous effects of heavy metals, should support efforts to minimize contamination of workplaces and, indeed, all segments of our fragile environment. Also, consumption of mega doses of trace elements in an effort to improve one's health status has heightened warnings of overdoses from various over-the-counter vitamin formulations and drinks.

Analysis of biologic fluids for heavy metals is performed using atomic absorption spectrometry, inductively coupled plasma-emission spectroscopy, inductively coupled plasma-mass spectrometry, and high-performance liquid chromatography-mass spectroscopy (HPLC-MS). Some of these techniques offer simultaneous determinations of multiple elements, so their usefulness for screening and improved operational efficiency is enhanced. Since these techniques require specialized instrumentation and sophisticated operator training, heavy metal analysis is typically performed in referral or specialized laboratories.[9]

## ALUMINUM

Aluminum is present in trace amounts in our diets and is normally filtered by the kidney and eliminated in the urine. Toxic levels of aluminum may result from industrial sources but most are iatrogenic in nature. Patients with poor renal function, especially those undergoing dialysis, are most susceptible to aluminum toxicity. Aluminum that is not excreted accumulates in the brain and the bones. In the brain, the aluminum causes a type of encephalopathy or dialysis dementia. Renal dialysis patients may be exposed to high levels of aluminum from dialysis water and medications. Dialysis is not as effective as a healthy kidney for the removal of aluminum so the metal accumulates. The encephalopathy that results can lead to abnormal speech, jerks, and convulsions. Aluminum can also replace calcium in the bone and interfere with calcium regulation by the parathyroid hormone. Workers in aluminum smelting industries in the mid 1980s began to exhibit abnormal neurologic behaviors similar to patients with Alzeimer disease. In fact, aluminum does accumulate in the CNS tissue of Alzeimer patients, but the association is controversial.[9,10]

Aluminum is measured by atomic absorption spectroscopy using electrothermal atomization. Blood samples must be collected using special aluminum-free evacuated collection tubes. Standard evacuated tubes have rubber stoppers made with aluminum silicate that will cause falsely elevate results.[9]

## ARSENIC

Arsenic's history as a "romantic" poison is well known. Besides expeditiously doing away with foes, it was also used to treat syphilis. When taken chronically in low doses, arsenic served as an antidote against acute poisoning. Today, toxic forms of arsenic are a common component of insecticides. It is also considered a carcinogen. Arsenic binds to enzymes, and in doing so, it inhibits key metabolic processes.[9]

The metal exists in several forms. The inorganic forms, As III and As V, are toxic and form the partially detoxified metabolites monomethylarsine (MMA) and dimethylarsine (DMA). Nontoxic forms of arsenic form organic molecules that are present in many foods, particularly fish. Since the commonly used methods cannot distinguish toxic arsenic from nontoxic forms, obtaining a blood specimen from a patient shortly after consuming seafood would likely result in a false-positive result.

Serum is the least useful specimen to establish exposure to arsenic since the half-life in blood is only 4 to 6 hours. Therefore, serum arsenic levels would apply only to recently (less than 4 hours) exposed patients. Urine is the specimen of choice for recent exposure, since the metal is excreted by the kidney and gets concentrated in the process. Hair is the best specimen to determine time of arsenic exposure or exposure occurring over a long period. The concentration of arsenic is higher in hair and nails than in any other tissue because the metal is strongly attracted to the keratin that forms hair and nails.[9]

## CADMIUM

Cadmium (Cd) has no known biologic function, so it is considered toxic at any level. The metal's primary target organ is the kidney, but the metal also damages liver and lung tissue. Cadmium is a product of industrial processes such as zinc and lead smelting and is used in electroplating, the production of rechargeable batteries, and as a pigment in paint.[10]

Chronic exposure to Cd has been associated with the development of renal disease with proteinuria of slow onset due to renal tubule damage and Cd-induced lesions. Painters who spray organic cadmium–containing paint without protective gear are at risk of developing kidney disease and emphysema. Cadmium is also present in tobacco products so smokers have similar risks. In 1992, NIOSH mandated that workers in industries known to have high Cd exposure be periodically monitored to protect their health. Urine Cd and creatinine levels are measured and the results are reported in terms of urine cadmium per gram of creatinine. Workers having greater than 3 μg Cd/g of creatinine are considered to have had significant exposure.[9]

## CHROMIUM AND COBALT

Chromium, necessary for insulin activity, and cobalt, a cofactor of vitamin $B_{12}$, are both essential trace metals. Yet, both metals can reach toxic exposure levels in some industrial processes. Chromium is used for stainless-steel manufacturing, chrome plating, leather tanning, and textile manufacturing and as a corrosive in cooling systems. The toxic form of chromium is $Cr^{6+}$, which rarely occurs except in the manufacturing processes noted. Inhalation of $Cr^{6+}$ causes squamous cell carcinoma of the lung. After the metal is inhaled, it is converted to the common form, $Cr^{3+}$. Measurements of chromium in body fluids therefore do not provide information on exposure

to the toxic chromium ion. To safeguard workers from dangerous $Cr^{6+}$ levels, the air quality is checked by monitoring $Cr^{6+}$ concentration.

Cobalt is used in the production and machining of metal alloys. Toxic levels of exposure can produce interstitial lung disease. Acute cobalt levels are known to produce cardiomyopathy and renal failure. Urinary cobalt levels can detect excessive exposure.[9]

## LEAD

Lead is a bluish-gray metal found in trace amounts throughout our environment. It has no special taste or smell. High concentrations of lead originate from human activities such as mining, manufacturing, and the burning of fossil fuels. Lead poisoning has been a health problem in advanced civilizations since ancient times. During the era of the Roman Empire, environmental lead exposure originated in plumbing and utensils used for cooking and eating. The major source of lead exposure in modern times is breathing in contaminated air or ingesting contaminated dust, food, or water. Workers in industries that use lead, along with stained-glass and ceramic hobbyists, need to be concerned about air quality. Children can be exposed to lead by playing in contaminated soil, by living in old homes that are poorly maintained or undergoing rehabilitation, or by eating foods grown in lead-contaminated soil.[11]

Lead-based paint and auto emissions from leaded fuel are major sources of lead toxicity. Since the mid 1970s, public health agencies in the United States have directed much attention to the screening of children for lead exposure and removing lead from the environment. Some states require that physicians and persons in charge of lead-screening programs report cases of lead toxicity to an appropriate agency so that abatement of the source of lead, patient education, and treatment can be monitored. Federal legislation passed in 1976 and 1984 removed lead from gasoline and leaded paint was finally phased out for residential use in 1978. Even so, it is estimated that more than one half of the entire U.S. housing stock and 75% of units built before 1978 contain some lead-based paint. Removing lead from gasoline and food cans has served to lower the average blood lead level in the general population. Efforts are now being focused on control of lead from deteriorated lead-based paint.[11]

All children, regardless of income or racial subgroup are at risk of having unsafe blood lead levels. The prevalence of children with elevated levels, however, is highest among inner-city underprivileged minority children who live in old deteriorating housing. In 1997, it was estimated that some 890,000 U.S. children have blood lead levels high enough to affect their ability to learn.[12] Furthermore, over 1 million U.S. workers in many occupations, including lead smelting, battery manufacturing and demolition, are exposed to lead. Lead dust can be carried home from the workplace on skin, hair, and clothing. The children of parents who work with lead, or who live near lead-related industrial sites, are at increased risk of lead toxicity.[13] Sources of lead exposure are listed in Table 24–3.

TABLE   2 4 - 3

**Sources of Lead Exposure***

| OCCUPATIONAL | ENVIRONMENTAL | HOBBIES | SUBSTANCE USE |
|---|---|---|---|
| Plumbers and pipe fitters | Lead-containing paint | Glazed pottery making | Folk remedies: azarcon and greta |
| Lead miners | Soil/dust near lead industries, | Target shooting | Health foods |
| Auto mechanics | roadways, | Lead soldering | Cosmetics, primarily |
| Glass, plastic, rubber, or battery manufacturers | lead-painted homes | Painting | from Asian and |
| Printers | Plumbing leachate | Preparing fishing sinkers | Middle Eastern |
| Construction workers | Ceramicware | Stained-glass making | communities |
| Lead smelters and refiners | Leaded gasoline | Car or boat repair | Moonshine whiskey |
| Firing range instructors | Burning painted wood | Home remodeling | Gasoline "huffing" |
| Steel welders or cutters | | Refinishing furniture | |
| Gas station attendants | | | |
| Bridge reconstruction | | | |
| Police officers | | | |
| Shipbuilders | | | |

*Based on data from the U.S. Department of Housing and Urban Development,[11] and Royce SE, Neddleman HL.[13]

Ingestion of lead is an even greater problem for unborn and young children who are more sensitive to the effects of lead toxicity. Crawling and the natural exploratory behavior of small children, sometimes combined with **pica** (compulsive eating of nonfood materials such as paint chips and dirt), increases the amount of lead ingested. Overall absorption of lead from the GI tract is estimated to be 10% to 15% in adults and as high as 50% in children and pregnant women.[13] Once absorbed into the blood, the lead is distributed to the blood, soft tissue (kidney, bone marrow, liver and brain), and to mineralizing tissue (bone and teeth). Most of it, 95%, is transferred to the mineralizing tissue. The lead stored in the teeth and bone serves as an inert pool of lead that can be mobilized in periods of physiologic stress such as pregnancy, lactation, or chronic disease. The mobilized lead moves into the blood and soft tissue compartments where the damaging effects occur. A higher rate of bone turnover in children makes lead more available to blood and soft tissues. Lead has a **half-life** of 25 days in blood, 40 days in soft tissue, and 25 years in the inert portion of the mineralized tissue. Chronic low-dose exposure can therefore lead to lead poisoning because the body can accumulate the metal over a lifetime and release it slowly into the circulation.[13]

Most of the manifestations of lead toxicity are related to its effects on red blood cells, the gastrointestinal tract, the kidneys, and the central and peripheral nervous systems. The tissue most sensitive to the effects of lead is the nervous system. Indeed, the first signs of lead toxicity in children may be behavioral changes such as decreased attention span, irritability, hyperactivity, and learning disabilities. Symptoms are extremely generalized and include loss of appetite, nausea, muscle weakness, fatigue, pallor, and headache. The hematologic picture of lead toxicity includes an increased reticulocyte count and basophilic stippling of red blood cells. Basophilic stippling occurs in patients who have sustained moderately high blood lead levels over a prolonged period. The most serious effects of chronic lead exposure are permanent CNS damage, severe anemia, and renal disease. Lead encephalopathy is usually associated with blood lead concentrations of 100 $\mu$g/dL or greater and is an acute medical emergency requiring aggressive treatment.[13]

The toxic effects of lead are due to its ability to noncompetitively inhibit many enzyme systems. Lead inhibits the activity of several enzymes in the biosynthetic pathway for heme including delta-aminolevulinic acid dehydrase and ferrochelatase (Figure 24–3). The substrates of these enzymes, delta-aminolevulinic acid (ALA) and protoporphyrin IX, accumulate in red blood cells. When ferrochelatase is inhibited or when iron is not available, excess protoporphyrin IX combines with zinc in the erythrocyte to produce zinc protoporphyrin (ZPP). Elevated urinary ALA and EP concentrations in red blood cells are related to lead toxicity and were used historically as screening tests.[14]

Because of lead's relatively high incidence and widespread distribution in the pediatric population, the Centers for Disease Control (CDC) in 1991 issued recommendations calling for universal screening of all children 12 to 72 months of age for lead exposure. A whole blood lead level of 10 $\mu$g/dL (100 $\mu$g/L) was established as the **safety threshold level** since even at this very low level, there was evidence that learning was impaired.[12]

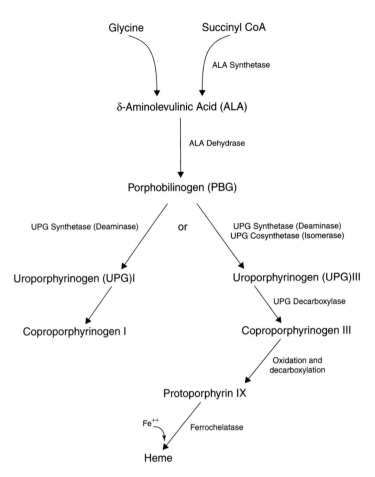

Glycine          Succinyl CoA

ALA Synthetase

δ-Aminolevulinic Acid (ALA)

ALA Dehydrase

Porphobilinogen (PBG)

UPG Synthetase (Deaminase)          or          UPG Synthetase (Deaminase)
                                                 UPG Cosynthetase (Isomerase)

Uroporphyrinogen (UPG)I                     Uroporphyrinogen (UPG)III

UPG Decarboxylase

Coproporphyrinogen I                         Coproporphyrinogen III

Oxidation and
decarboxylation

Protoporphyrin IX

Fe⁺⁺          Ferrochelatase

Heme

**F I G U R E   2 4 - 3**

Heme synthetic pathway. Aminolevulinic acid (ALA) dehydrase and ferrochelatase are inhibited by lead, leading to accumulation of ALA and fluorescent protoporphyrin IX in red cells. The latter is combined with zinc to form zinc protoporphyrin, which is measured by hematofluorometry.

Treatment of toxic lead exposure includes separation of the patient from the source of lead, and depending on symptoms and blood lead concentrations, treatment of severely exposed patients with one or more chelating agents such as British anti-Lewisite (BAL) and calcium EDTA (Ca-EDTA). These agents act by combining with lead in extracellular fluids (both agents) and intracellular fluids (BAL only). Used together, they draw lead from the soft tissues and combine with it in the extracellular fluids, promoting excretion in the urine and the bile. Chelating agents may be toxic themselves and are administered under careful medical attention.[13]

Lead levels in **whole blood** most accurately reflect exposure to lead and is the CDC recommended test for initial screening and diagnostic evaluation. Serial **blood lead levels (BLL)** are recommended for treatment management. EDTA and heparin are the anticoagulants of choice for BLL. Capillary and filter paper collections are used for lead screenings but potential contamination is a major concern.[15,16]

Lead levels in **serum** are of limited value since lead de-

creases soon after exposure. **Urine lead** screening has little clinical value but is nonetheless used to monitor workers who may be exposed to lead compounds. Proteins in tissues that have been exposed to lead will have lead bound to them. **Hair analysis** for lead concentration is an alternative marker for exposure but specimen contamination is difficult to control.[9,17]

Since lead is a ubiquitous pollutant, special precautions need to be taken to prevent specimen contamination and the false-positive results that may occur. All collection materials and testing supplies must be checked for lead contamination. Air-quality checks and dust-control measures are also recommended. Blood collection tubes are available specifically for trace metal analysis (royal blue caps) or certified lead-free tubes for blood lead level determination (tan/brown caps).[17]

Before 1991, **erythrocyte protoporphyrin (EP),** commonly assayed as **zinc protoporphyrin (ZPP)** levels, was widely used to screen for lead exposure because the test was inexpensive, easy to perform, and not subject to environmental contamination. Currently, the CDC recommends that

EP no longer be used to screen for lead exposure because many studies demonstrated poor sensitivity and specificity at the 10 $\mu$g/dL decision level.[15] EP levels, together with BLLs, are of value for the management of children with confirmed elevated lead levels. EP is also used as a screening test for iron deficiency anemia. Acid extraction and hematofluorometry are two methods used to measure ZPP in whole blood specimens.[12]

Whole blood lead determinations are most commonly performed using graphite furnace atomic absorption spectrometry (GRAAS) or anodic stripping voltammetry (ASV). Variations on atomic absorption spectrophotometry (AAS) such as methylisobutylketone (MIBK)–extraction flame AAS, Delves-cup microsampling flame AAS, and an inductively coupled plasma interfaced to a quadraple mass spectrometer (ICP-MS) are also used.[12]

**Atomic absorption spectrophotometry** employs the absorption of light by activated atoms. Each atomic species or element is capable of absorbing light at a very narrow bandwidth that corresponds to the specific line spectrum for the element. In the atomic absorption spectrophotometer, a hollow cathode lamp (HCL) with a filament made of the material to be analyzed (in this case, lead) is used to produce light of a wavelength that corresponds to the line spectrum of lead in the specimen. Standard methods of atomic absorption spectrophotometry are modified for blood lead determinations to increase the sensitivity and precision of the assay. Figure 24–4 displays a functional diagram of an atomic absorption spectrometer as used for measurement of blood lead.

The specimen is placed in a carbon rod or "graphite furnace," which is positioned within the instrument so that light from the HCL passes through it. In the middle of the cylindrical furnace is an opening through which the pretreated specimen is pipetted into the furnace. An electrical current is passed through the furnace, which dries, chars, and finally atomizes the sample to an energy level at which the atoms of lead are capable of absorbing the specific wavelength of light from the HCL.

When light from the HCL passes through the atomized specimen in the furnace, the lead atoms in the specimen absorb the emitted light. Light not absorbed by the lead atoms passes through the furnace to strike a detector. The difference in the quantity of specific light leaving the HCL and the quantity striking the detector is proportional to the concentration of lead in the specimen.[18]

The measurement of BLL using **anodic stripping voltammetry (ASV)** requires that whole blood lead be completely dissociated from other molecules in preparation for plating as the free +2 aqueous cation ($Pb^{+2}$). After specimen pretreatment, the $Pb^{+2}$ in solution makes contact with an electrode that consists of a thin film of mercury on an inert graphite surface. The electrode is initially introduced into the unknown and standard solutions at a negative electrical potential that causes the $Pb^{+2}$ to plate out or dissolve into the mercury coat. After coating has taken place, the electrode potential changes to the positive or anodic direction. At a specific and characteristic voltage for Pb, the metal will "strip" from the electrode and go back into solution. At this critical moment, a current is generated and measured. The rate of current flow is related to the concentration of lead in solution. Besides lead, ASV can be used to measure several other metals.[12,19]

## MERCURY AND THALLIUM

Mercury is naturally released from the earth into our environment. Unnatural sources of contamination include fossil fuel combustion, waste from metal smelting processes, and waste incineration. The heavy metal is used as a fungicide, as a part in electrical switches and pressure regulators, and a component of dental fillings (amalgams).[10] Elemental mercury, Hg°, is essentially nontoxic. If ingested, the body does not absorb it. Mercury vapor, on the other hand, is efficiently absorbed into the lungs with approximately 80% being retained by the body. The more toxic forms of mercury are ionized mercury ($Hg^{2+}$) and methyl mercury ($CH_3Hg^+$). They inhibit the activity of proteins by binding to sulfhydryl groups and modifying the tertiary structure of the molecule. Mercury targets the kidney and central nervous system (CNS). CNS effects include tremors, irritability, and depression. Congenital abnormalities, including mental retardation, occur through transplacental transfer of methyl mercury.

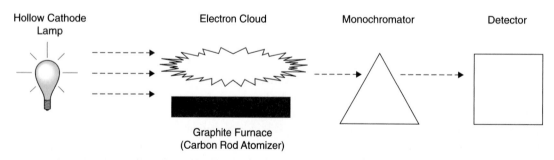

**F I G U R E   2 4 - 4**

Principle of flameless atomic absorption spectrometry using a graphite furnace for determination of lead in blood.

When present in food, mercury usually has the more toxic structure and is easily absorbed when digested. Fish exposed to lake or ocean sediments containing elemental mercury can have high concentrations of toxic mercury, thereby threatening the safety of our food supply. Elemental mercury enters the ocean's food chain through the action of microorganisms that have the ability to convert it to the more toxic alkyl form. To add perspective to this information, individuals who eat moderate amounts of fish, have well-maintained dental fillings, and are not occupationally exposed to mercury are unlikely candidates for mercury toxicity. However, for those who are occupationally exposed, mercury levels in blood and urine should be periodically checked to ensure that they do not reach unhealthy levels.[9,10]

Mercury exposure is assessed by analyzing Hg levels in blood, urine, or hair specimens. Blood and urine are used to evaluate the degree of toxicity, whereas hair samples can indicate peak exposure during the length of time that the hair was growing.

Thallium is used as a rodenticide and is also a heavy metal by-product of lead smelting. Accidental exposure to the thallium containing rat poison is the usual cause of toxic thallium exposure. Thallium has the same level of toxicity as mercury and lead and produces similar effects.[9]

## SILICON

Silicon is the most abundant element on earth. Asbestos is an amorphous oxide of silicon and the causative agent of asbestosis, a debilitating lung disease. If asbestos-containing dust is inhaled, it deposits in the alveoli of the lungs. The needle-shaped spicules are initially surrounded by macrophages, followed by protein and mucopolysaccharide to form asbestos bodies. Direct examination of lung tissue for silicon is not helpful. The diagnosis is made by X-ray analysis of the lung and the presence of asbestos bodies in lung tissue or sputum.[9]

## Nonvolative Organics

### PESTICIDES

Pesticides are compounds whose purpose is to kill specific animal pests, such as insects and rodents. Most pesticides are potentially harmful to humans as well. Toxic exposures are usually acute poisonings of adults using pesticides for their intended purpose, but without proper safety precautions, or unintentional ingestions by children.

Organophosphates and carbamates are the largest groups of pesticides currently in use, and together cause many of the pesticide poisonings that present in clinical settings. Organophosphates are active ingredients in malathion, parathion, diazinon, and Dursban; whereas, carbamates are found in Sevin and Furadan. Both types of pesticides act by inhibiting the actions of acetylcholinesterases, which function to neutralize acetylcholine, an essential neurotransmitter present in nervous tissue. Buildup of acetylcholine causes a cholinergic response

characterized by symptoms that are generally related to the stimulation of smooth muscle and inhibition of skeletal muscle including vomiting, diarrhea, slowed heart rate, involuntary urination and defecation, skeletal muscle weakness, twitching and cramps, restlessness, and insomnia. In acute cases, death results from weakness of the respiratory muscles leading to respiratory failure.[1]

Testing for exposure to organophosphate and carbamate pesticides is based on determining the degree of inhibition of acetylcholinesterase by the toxin. Since the acetylcholinesterase, located within neuromuscular junctions, is not accessible for testing, laboratory assessment is limited to measuring cholinesterase activity in serum or red cells. Red cells contain acetylcholinesterases that are similar to those found in nervous tissue and seem to be similarly inhibited by pesticides. The enzymes found in nerves and red cells are known as "true" cholinesterases and designated as AChE. Most clinical laboratories are not prepared to determine red cell acetylcholinesterase (AChE) on a routine basis and therefore offer measurement of the cholinesterase found in serum, which is commonly designated pseudocholinesterase or ChE. The measurement in body fluids of the pesticides themselves, although methods are available, is not practical in most clinical laboratories.

Pseudocholinesterase activity (ChE) in serum represents a group of enzymes capable of hydrolyzing a number of choline esters other than acetylcholine. The physiologic role of these enzymes is not known, but their activities in serum decline and return to normal more rapidly than red cell cholinesterases following acute exposure to organophosphate and carbamate pesticides. However, measurement of ChE is not entirely specific for toxic pesticide exposure. Pseudocholinesterase, synthesized by the liver, is decreased in liver disease and other acute and chronic disorders. Also, there are inherited forms of pseudocholinesterase characterized by decreased ChE activity. Clinical presentations, however, usually include some information regarding use or ingestion of a pesticide and this combined with decreased ChE activity may be taken as presumptive evidence of pesticide exposure.[1]

Methods for measurement of serum ChE activity are commonly based on hydrolysis of a synthetic substrate, a thiocholine ester, to release thiocholine, which reacts with a color reagent to produce a detectable product. ChE levels may be used to screen for pesticide exposure. Symptoms generally begin when ChE falls to about 50% of normal, but interpretation is complicated by variable normal levels. Treatment for pesticide exposure includes administration of atropine sulfate and, in acute cases, pralidoxime, which restores cholinesterase activity.[1]

### DRUGS OF ABUSE AND OVERDOSE

The substances classified as drugs of abuse are structurally nonvolatile organics. Since the topic is so complex, the next section covers the toxicology and analysis of this important group of toxic substances.

## DRUGS OF ABUSE AND OVERDOSE

In 1999, it was estimated that 6.7% of Americans over 12 years old (14.8 million) were current users of illicit drugs (used at least once during the 30 days before being interviewed). Annually, abuse of drugs and alcohol kills more than 120,000 Americans. Indeed, American taxpayers pay nearly $276 billion a year in preventable health care costs, extra law enforcement, auto crashes, crime, and lost productivity related to alcohol and drug abuse.[2] Clinical laboratory scientists identify and measure drugs of abuse, thereby playing a significant role in prevention and treatment. Laboratorians need to know the federal and private agency guidelines that regulate drug testing and have a practical understanding of the analytical principles that differentiate screening from confirmatory methods. This section serves as a basic introduction to the complex toxicology of drugs of abuse. In addition to texts and journals covering the topic, the U.S. government provides statistics and a wealth of information on drugs of abuse and drug usage that can be found on web sites sponsored by the National Institute on Drug Abuse (NIDA), National Institutes of Health (NIH), and the Substance Abuse and Mental Health Services Administration (SAMHSA).

Drugs found in overdose cases fall within one of 5 classifications: (1) depressants, (2) stimulants, (3) hallucinogenics, (4) analgesics, and (5) antidepressants. The depressants include alcohol, sedative/hypnotics, narcotics, and tranquilizers. Stimulants include cocaine, amphetamines, and amphetamine-like substances that are found in many over-the-counter medications, such as appetite suppressants and cold medicines. Phencyclidine (PCP), LSD, mescaline, and MMDA are in the hallucinogenics group. The analgesics and antidepressants categories represent over-the-counter medications such as salicylate and acetaminophen and prescription drugs such as tricyclic antidepressants. Many of the drugs listed in Table 24–4 are legally available and, when taken as prescribed, do not fall under the drugs of abuse classification. However, when intentionally or unintentionally taken in high doses, they can reach toxic levels and are therefore considered in this section of the text.

Although the number of drugs with potential for abuse is enormous, the actual drugs or groups of drugs encountered in an overdosed patient, in a particular laboratory setting, is limited. Screening tests are performed in medical emergencies to diagnose and treat the poisoned patient or to investigate accident-related injuries. The major drugs or drug classes commonly detected include ethanol, cocaine, opioids, acetaminophen, cannabinoids, antidepressants, and benzodiazepines. Use of more than one drug, particularly ethanol, in combination is also a common finding. Depending on preference and availability, the types of drugs prevalent in one geographic location may differ from those found in another. Also, screenings performed for medical emergencies should be available on an urgent basis. Therefore, to provide cost-effective and timely emergency toxicology services, a laboratory must concentrate on identifying drugs or drug groups that are likely to be found in the patient population it serves.[18]

Screening selected populations for substance abuse is common today because clinical laboratories can economically and practically **screen** for drugs of abuse and accurately **confirm** their presence. In 1986, legislation was enacted that required federal employees working in safety sensitive positions, such as those operating heavy equipment, trucks, and airplanes, to undergo drug testing.[20] Screening of employees and prospective employees for drugs of abuse is now common practice in both public and private business, particularly where the actions of an employee may pose harm to the general public. Minors and pregnant women in which drug abuse is suspected may also be screened to allow intervention by public health agencies, and most major sporting events, such as the international Olympic competition, require that athletes be screened to rule out use of performance-enhancing drugs.

### Analgesics

**Acetaminophen,** one of the most commonly used over-the-counter medications in the United States, is similar to salicylate in its **analgesic** and **antipyretic** properties. Although acetaminophen does not possess the anti-inflammatory properties of salicylate, it also does not cause stomach irritation or decrease platelet function when ingested in therapeutic doses. Although safe when ingested as prescribed, toxic amounts of acetaminophen causes severe liver toxicity. The parent compound is metabolized to a highly reactive intermediate metabolite, N-acetylbenzoquinoneimine, that accumulates in the liver and is responsible for damaging the organ.[1]

An acute overdose of acetaminophen is not readily apparent. A patient who has ingested a toxic amount of acetaminophen may appear asymptomatic or may develop nonspecific gastrointestinal symptoms such as nausea or vomiting for the first 24 hours. Even though clinical symptoms may not increase in severity until as long as 72 hours, hepatic necrosis begins at 24 to 48 hours with hepatic enzymes, bilirubin, and prothrombin time rising. At 3 to 4 days after ingestion, symptoms resembling viral hepatitis caused by hepatic necrosis become apparent. In addition to liver enzyme determinations, **quantitative** serum acetaminophen determinations are important in assessing the probability of hepatic damage. For this purpose, an acetaminophen level should be drawn no sooner than 4 hours after ingestion (the usual peak level). A nomogram developed by Rumack and Matthew can be used to predict toxicity in the case of an acute overdose.[21] Quantitative acetaminophen methods are available using immunologic (EMIT and FPIA) and chromatographic (HPLC) methods. A spot test using orthocresol to produce an indophenol blue complex is available for qualitative assessment.[18]

Management of acetaminophen toxicity includes methods to remove the drug, such as gastric lavage and administration of activated charcoal to remove any undigested drug

**Common Drugs of Abuse and Overdose**

| DRUG/DRUG GROUP | CLASSIFICATION | GENERIC NAME(S) | TRADE OR SLANG NAME(S) |
|---|---|---|---|
| • Acetaminophen/ salicylates | Analgesic | Acetaminophen Acetylsalicylic acid | Aspirin, Anacin, Excedrin, Tylenol |
| • Amphetamines | Stimulant | Amphetamine | Dexedrine |
| | | Methamphetamine | Desoxyn, speed, ice, meth, chalk, fire, crystal, crank, glass |
| • Amphetamine-like | Stimulant | Ephedrine | Primatene |
| | | Pseudoephedrine | Actifed, Sudafed, Drixoral |
| | | Phenylpropanolamine | Dexatrim, Triaminic |
| | | Phentermine | Fastin |
| | | l-methamphetamine | Vicks™ inhaler |
| • Barbiturates | Depressant (sedative/hypnotic) | | |
| | Long-acting | Phenobarbital | Luminal |
| | Intermediate-acting | Amobarbital | Amytal |
| | | Butabarbital | Butisol |
| | | Butalbital | |
| | Short-acting | Pentobarbital | Nembutal |
| | | Secobarbital | Seconal |
| • Benzodiazepines | Depressant (tranquilizer) | Diazepam | Valium |
| | | Chlordiazepoxide | Librium |
| | | Oxazepam | Serax |
| | | Flurazepam | Dalmane |
| | | Lorazepam | Ativan |
| | | Alprazolam | Xanax |
| • Cocaine | Stimulant | Cocaine | Crack, coke, snow, blow |
| • Cannabinoids | Hallucinogen | Tetrahydrocannabinol | Marijuana, hashish, pot, reefer, grass |
| • LSD | Hallucinogen | Lysergic acid Diethylamide | Acid, boomers, yellow sunshines |
| • MDMA | Stimulant/ Hallucinogen | Methylenedioxymethamphetamine | Ecstasy, XTC, X, Adam, clarity, lover's speed |
| • Opioids | Narcotic (opiate) | Heroin | Diacetylmorphine, smack, horse, skag |
| | | Morphine | Duramorph |
| | | Codeine | Methylmorphine, Robitussin A-C |
| | Narcotic | Propoxyphene | Darvon, Darvocet-N |
| | | Methadone | Dolophine |
| • PCP | Hallucinogen | Phencyclidine | PCP, angel dust |
| • Steroids (anabolic) | Muscle builder | Testosterone analogs | Dianabol, Nandrolone |
| • Tricyclic antidepressants | Antidepressant | Amitriptyline | Elavil, Endep |
| | | Nortriptyline | Pamelor, Aventyl |
| | | Imipramine | Tofranil |
| | | Desipramine | Norpramine |

from the stomach. Unlike most other drugs, acetaminophen has a specific antidote that is used in severe overdose cases. **N-acetylcysteine** (Mucomyst) replenishes glutathione stores in the liver, effectively reducing the accumulation of the toxic acetaminophen metabolite. Because a specific antidote is available and because acetaminophen toxicity may be difficult to diagnose initially, all emergency room toxicology screens should include a test for acetaminophen in either serum or urine.

**Salicylates** are classified as **anti-inflammatory, antipyretic analgesics** and are used to reduce inflammation, fever, and pain. Aspirin (acetylsalicylic acid) is metabolized to salicylic acid, which exerts the primary pharmacologic effects. Side effects of salicylate ingestion, even in therapeutic doses, include stomach irritation and decreased platelet function. Salicylate administration is contraindicated in children and adolescents because there is an association between its use during viral infections and the development of Reye's syndrome.

Salicylate toxicity is common in children as well as adults. Acute overdoses may occur unintentionally in pediatric cases or intentionally in suicidal gestures or attempts. Initially, salicylate toxicity causes respiratory alkalosis because the drug stimulates the respiratory center of the central nervous system causing hyperventilation. Salicylates also inhibit enzymes in the Krebs' cycle, causing pyruvate to be converted to lactic acid; lipid metabolism is increased and amino acid metabolism is decreased, and accumulation of organic acids eventually leads to metabolic acidosis.[1]

Clinical symptoms of salicylate toxicity include tinnitus (ringing in the ear), hyperventilation, sweating, lethargy, vomiting and possibly coma, convulsions, and hyperthermia in severe cases.[21] Severity of the overdose is assessed by arterial blood gas and electrolyte results. Respiratory alkalosis is apparent in the early stages of toxicity, and metabolic acidosis with an increased anion gap may be apparent in later stages of very severe cases. No specific antidote exists for salicylates, therefore treatment consists of treating acid-base and electrolyte imbalances and removing any drug that has not been absorbed.[1]

In contrast to many of the drugs of abuse, assessment of salicylate poisoning requires **quantitative** serum levels. A commonly used spectrophotometric method is that of Trinder, in which salicylates react with ferric nitrate to form a colored complex. Salicylate methods are also available using immunologic (EMIT and FPIA) and chromatographic (GLC and HPLC) methods.[1,18] Severity of acute toxicity, for patients who have ingested a single toxic dose of salicylate, is assessed by plotting the serum salicylate level against the time since ingestion on a nomogram developed by Done. The nomogram is not useful for assessment of toxicity resulting from chronic overdosing with salicylates.[1]

## Amphetamines

Amphetamine and methamphetamine are addictive CNS stimulants or "uppers" that have limited medical use. Methamphetamine, the more effective of the 2 drugs, is easily synthesized and is the most common illicitly produced controlled substance in the United States. The drugs release high levels of catecholamines, mainly dopamine and norepinephrine, which stimulate brain and CNS cells producing an initial euphoria, increased self-esteem, and heightened mental and physical capacity. Symptoms of amphetamine use include loss of appetite, insomnia, fatigue, irritability, anxiety, dilated pupils, and excessive speech and motor activity. Amphetamines cause hyperthermia, irregular heartbeat, and increased heart rate and blood pressure that can result in strokes and cardiovascular collapse. No specific antidote for amphetamine overdose is available and treatment is usually limited to supportive therapy.[1,22] Immunoassay methods are used for initial screening for amphetamines and confirmed using GC-MS.[1]

Other less harmful sympathomimetic amines include ephedrine, pseudoephedrine, *l*-methamphetamine, and phenylpropanolamine. These amphetamine-like drugs are available in over-the-counter medications as diet aids and nasal decongestants in cold medications. Clinical laboratory scientists need to consider the potential for these compounds to interfere in methods for the detection of amphetamine and methamphetamine, producing a false-positive result.[22]

## Barbiturates

Barbiturates (depressants) are classified according to duration of pharmacologic effect. The short-acting to intermediate-acting barbiturates (amobarbital, butabarbital, butalbital, pentobarbital, and secobarbital) have sedative-hypnotic properties and are commonly abused, whereas the longer-acting barbiturates (phenobarbital) are rarely abused and have anticonvulsant properties. Long-term users develop a tolerance to the drugs and so increasingly larger doses are needed to maintain the drug's effect. Because of the high potential for barbiturate abuse, the benzodiazepines, which have similar properties and are considered safer, are prescribed more frequently when a depressant is indicated. Symptoms of barbiturate abuse include slurred speech, slowing of mental functions, constricted pupils, and CNS depression. Respiratory depression and cardiac insufficiency from CNS depression are usually the causes of death in overdose cases. Treatment of barbiturate overdose includes supportive therapy and urinary alkalinization to promote ionization of the drugs. Ionization prevents tubular reabsorption and enhances excretion.[1] Immunoassay methods or TLC are used for initial screening for barbiturates and confirmed using GC-MS.[1]

## Benzodiazepines

The **benzodiazepines** group includes a long list of drugs that have sedative-hypnotic, muscle relaxant, and anticonvulsant properties. Some examples of drugs in this group include diazepam, oxazepam, flurazepam, lorazepam, alprazolam, and chlordiazepoxide. The benzodiazepines exert their effect on the CNS by potentiating the effect of gamma-aminobutyric acid

(GABA), a major endogenous inhibitory neurotransmitter whose function is to diminish neural electrical discharge. Benzodiazepines are used to treat insomnia, anxiety, seizure disorders, and for preanesthetic sedation. The demand for sedative and anxiety-reducing drugs in our society is very high. Benzodiazepines are used by more Americans than any other prescribed drug because they are considered safe, have few side effects, and have a low addictive potential. Symptoms of benzodiazepine ingestion are similar to those of the barbiturates but less intense. Because these drugs usually do not induce prolonged or serious CNS depression, treatment of an overdose consists of supportive therapy. Few deaths have been attributed to benzodiazepine overdose alone.[1] Rohypnol, another benzodiazepine, with the street name of "rophies" and the "date rape" pill, is not approved for legal use in the United States. Besides its sedative effects, the drug can cause its user to not remember events they experience while under its influence and has been reportedly used in sexual assaults.[23] Immunoassay methods are used for initial screening for benzodiazepines and confirmed using GC-MS. HPLC is generally used when quantitation is required.[1]

## Cannabinoids

The cannabinoids are a group of substances, classified as hallucinogens, found in the *Cannabis sativa* plant species. The most active ingredient and the main psychoactive agent in marijuana is delta-9-tetrahydrocannabinol (THC). Common names for the cannabinoids include marijuana, pot, and reefer. **Marijuana** is the most frequently used illegal substance in the United States. It is usually smoked in cigarette form or pipes, but may also be ingested orally. Hashish or hash is the dried resins of the plant, which has a higher concentration of THC than marijuana and may be smoked. Although marijuana is usually classified as a hallucinogen, typical doses do not produce hallucinations. Reported effects of cannabinoid use include a sense of relaxation and well-being and mild euphoria. Because THC is lipid soluble, it has a tendency to accumulate in body fat where it has a half-life of 1 day in casual users and 3 to 5 days in chronic users. The principal urinary metabolite, 11-nor-$\Delta^9$-tetrahydrocannabinal-9-carboxylic acid (THC-COOH), may remain detectable in urine for several days to 1 week after exposure by an infrequent smoker. In a chronic long-term user, THC that has accumulated in fatty tissue is gradually released into the circulation; therefore, the metabolite remains detectable for 21 to 30 days or longer after the last dose.[1,24]

Associated with marijuana use is loss of short-term memory, concentration, and other intellectual performance skills and impairment of psychomotor skills such as those required to drive a vehicle. Its use may cause problems for heavy long-term users because marijuana contains more carcinogenic hydrocarbons than tobacco. A synthetic THC (drobinolol) is legally prescribed to treat anorexia and nausea in patients with AIDS and those undergoing chemotherapy.[1] Immunoassay

methods are used to screen for cannabinoids and confirmation is performed using GC-MS.[1]

## Cocaine

**Cocaine** is a potent CNS stimulant that promotes a state of euphoria and increased alertness. The drug is extracted from the leaves of the coca plant that grows in South America. Its medical use is limited to that of a topical anesthetic for nasal surgery and emergency nasotracheal intubation. Despite government efforts to curb its abuse, cocaine continues to dominate the U.S. illicit drug problem.[25] Cocaine use during pregnancy has been shown to contribute to increased incidence of premature deliveries, medical problems at birth and in early life, and effects on the cognitive abilities of the child.[26] Cocaine may be administered as the hydrochloride salt by nasal insufflation ("snorting") or less frequently by intravenous injection. Cocaine can also be inhaled or smoked by converting the salt to the more volatile freebase form known as **crack.** The crack form of cocaine produces a more rapid onset of symptoms.[22] Cocaine is the only naturally occurring anesthetic and the most potent naturally occurring CNS stimulant. Symptoms of cocaine abuse are similar to those of the amphetamines. In addition to the stimulant effects, cocaine may also have a direct cardiotoxic effect that is believed to be a factor in cocaine-related deaths. Cocaine is rapidly metabolized by separate liver esterases to benzoylecgonine and ecgonine methyl ester. **Benzoylecgonine** is the metabolite that is measured by screening methods for cocaine use. Immunoassay methods are used to screen initially for benzoylecgonine. Cocaine use is confirmed using GC-MS.[1]

## Hallucinogenics

Hallucinogens are drugs that alter and distort visual and auditory perceptions, thoughts, and feelings. **Lysergic acid diethylamide (LSD),** structurally similar to serotonin, binds to serotonin receptors located in the CNS. LSD produces perceptual distortions of color, sound, distance, and shape. Under the influence of the drug, emotions are said to change rapidly from ecstasy to depression or paranoia. Psychological effects begin 30 to 60 minutes after ingestion and peak 3 to 5 hours later. The most common adverse effects of LSD are panic attacks and unpredictable flashbacks of hallucinations. Ingestion is the main route of administration and it is commonly prepared as a dried liquid on blotter paper, tiny tablets, or gelatin squares. The clinical effects of LSD usually require no medical intervention, but the psychological effects may be severe enough to require treatment with a tranquilizer such as diazepam.[1,24] Immunoassay methods are used to screen for LSD and confirmation is performed using GC-MS.[1]

**Phencyclidine (PCP)** causes hallucinations but may also act as both a CNS stimulant and depressant. PCP was originally developed as a surgical anesthetic for humans but its sale and manufacture was eventually stopped. The drug may be ingested or more commonly sprinkled on tobacco, marijuana, or parsley and smoked. When smoked in the form of a joint, the user has more control over the dosage and bad trips are said to occur less frequently. The effects of an overdose are unpredictable and variable. PCP may cause the user to experience a sense of superhuman strength but may also lead to coma. Fatalities are most often caused by accidental or intentional trauma consequential to the user's bizarre behaviors. Other symptoms of a PCP overdose include generalized muscle rigidity, seizures, tachycardia, and hypertension. Treatment of an overdose is limited to supportive medical and psychiatric care.[1] Immunoassay methods are used to screen for PCP and confirmation is performed using GC-MS. In some locations, low use of the drug may limit the availability of routine testing.[1]

**Methylenedioxymethamphetamine (MDMA)** is a synthetic drug, structurally related and derived from amphetamine, with additional psychoactive properties. Street names for this "designer" hallucinogenic-stimulant drug include **ecstasy,** Adam, and XTC. MDMA is popular among young adults who attend all-night dance clubs. Users claim that the drug produces a feeling of euphoria, heightens sexuality, and expands consciousness without loss of control. MDMA can be extremely dangerous in high doses causing fatal malignant hyperthermia, seizures, tachycardia, and DIC, which leads to kidney and cardiovascular system failure. Methylenedioxyamphetamine (MDA) and methylenedioxyethamphetamine (MDEA) are designer drugs with properties similar to MDMA.[22]

## Opioids

**Opioid** is a general term applied to drugs that have properties similar to morphine, whereas **opiate** describes natural or semisynthetic drugs that are derived from the opium plant. Drugs included in this group are considered narcotics. Naturally occurring substances isolated from *Papaver somniferum,* the opium poppy, include opium, morphine, and codeine. Heroin, hydromorphone (Dilaudid), and oxycodone (ingredient in Percodan) are semisynthetic opiates. Examples of synthetic opioids are meperidine (Demerol), methadone (Dolophine), propoxyphene (Darvon), pentazocine (Talwin), and fentanyl (Sublimaze). Opioids are used clinically for their analgesic properties including relief of intense pain in burn, orthopedic, and the terminally ill patients, cough suppression, and preoperative anesthesia. Opioids also produce a state of euphoria and so lend themselves to abuse.[1,27]

Heroin, hydromorphone, and methadone are frequently abused opioids that produce intense euphoria. Heroin may be taken intravenously, intranasally, or orally. Symptoms of opiate use include CNS depression, depressed mental status, decreased respiratory rate, pinpoint pupils, needle track marks on skin, and hypothermia. Symptoms associated with withdrawal include agitation, muscle cramps, hypertension, tachycardia, and vomiting. The opioids are one of the few drug groups that have a specific antidote. **Naloxone** is a specific opioid antagonist that reverses CNS depression.[1,27] Immunoassay methods are used to screen for opiates and confirmation is performed using GC-MS.[1]

**Methadone,** or Dolophine, is an opioid that produces many of the same, but less intense, effects as morphine. The synthetic drug is used for relief of pain and for detoxification and maintenance of heroin addicts. When used for heroin addiction control, methadone, a long-acting opioid, replaces the shorter-acting heroin molecule. The high degree of protein binding observed with methadone causes it to be eliminated very slowly. Heroin addicts are given high methadone maintenance doses to prevent their use of the illegal drug. If the addict uses the illegal drug, a methadone overdose may result and unpleasant symptoms, similar to a heroin overdose appear, that last for a long time. Symptoms and treatment of overdose are the same as those described below for opiates.[1,27] Immunoassay methods are used to screen for methadone and confirmation or quantification is performed using GC-MS.[1]

**Propoxyphene** (Darvon) is a widely prescribed narcotic analgesic, which is structurally similar to methadone. Propoxyphene can be lethal in overdoses with its metabolite, **norpropoxyphene,** believed to be a contributor. Propoxyphene is prescribed most often in combination with acetaminophen or aspirin. Therefore, when a propoxyphene overdose occurs, quantitative measurements of salicylates and acetaminophen may also be indicated. Symptoms of propoxyphene overdose, depending on severity, can range from drowsiness, nausea or vomiting to coma, respiratory depression, and cardiovascular collapse in severe cases. Naloxone is used to reverse the CNS and respiratory depressant actions of propoxyphene but has little effect on cardiotoxicity.[1,27] Immunoassay methods are used to screen for propoxyphene. A positive screen is confirmed using GC-MS to detect norpropoxyphene, a major metabolite.[1]

## Steroids (Anabolic)

Synthetic steroids, related to androgens, are used to build muscle and boost athletic performance. Steroid abuse disrupts normal hormone regulation and can cause changes, some of which are irreversible, that affect secondary sex characteristics, the cardiovascular system, the musculoskeletal system, and the liver. Steroids, developed for legitimate medical purposes, can be taken orally or injected. Many formulations are available but all must be prescribed. Most steroids that are used illegally are smuggled in from other countries, stolen from U.S. pharmacies, or synthesized in clandestine laboratories. As with all illegal drugs, users risk exposure to nonsterile or impure drug preparations.[28] Gas chromatography and high-performance liquid chromatography methods are used to detect steroid abuse.[6]

## Tricyclic Antidepressants

The **tricyclic antidepressant** group represents a class of drugs prescribed to treat major endogenous depression. Some of the more common drugs within this class include imipramine, amitriptyline, and their N-demethylated derivatives, desipramine and nortriptyline. Other cyclic antidepressant drugs, although not technically tricyclic compounds, may be included in this group. These drugs include doxepin, trazodone, amoxapine, fluoxetine, and maprotiline.[1]

Tricyclics appear to reduce depressive disorders by inhibiting the uptake of norepinephrine, serotonin, and other amines in the brain. These drugs have a narrow therapeutic range and may produce toxic effects at relatively low doses. Unfortunately, the patient populations that are prescribed tricyclics, such as adults suffering from major depression, are prone to intentional or unintentional overdoses that may prove fatal. Clinical features of an overdose include tachycardia, altered mental status, respiratory depression, and seizures. Cardiac arrest is the most life-threatening aspect of tricyclic overdose. Treatment of an overdose consists of eliminating any drug not yet absorbed, supportive therapy, and monitoring of vital signs. Although qualitative methods may be used to confirm a diagnosis of tricyclic toxicity, quantitative determinations of tricyclic levels are of limited value in treating an overdose. Tricyclics are highly protein-bound, so hemodialysis or hemoperfusion are not effective means of removing drug already absorbed.[1] Immunoassay methods are available for screening and quantitation of tricyclics (EMIT and FPIA). HPLC is the most commonly used chromatographic method.[1]

## ANALYTICAL PROCEDURES

**Qualitative** and **quantitative** laboratory methods are available for measuring drugs of abuse and those found in overdose. Qualitative measurements predominate since, for most drugs, there is little added clinical value in determining the drug's concentration in a body fluid like urine, so the additional cost is not justified.

### Screening Methods

**Screening methods** use techniques that are fast, economical, and technically simple to perform. **Immunoassays** are the methods of choice for initial screening. However, some laboratories use chromatographic methods, particularly **thin-layer chromatography** (TLC), for mass screenings. Chromatographic methods are capable of detecting a large number of drugs quickly and accurately but require specialized equipment and highly trained personnel. The primary goal of a screening test is to rule out specimens that do not contain drugs of abuse above an established drug-level threshold and provide preliminary information about drugs that are present in positive specimens. Specificity is commonly sacrificed so false-positive results must be a recognized shortcoming of screening tests. Laboratories performing screening tests need to establish policies for dealing with positive screening results to prevent false accusations of drug usage.

**Confirmatory methods** further evaluate specimens that demonstrate a positive screening test result. **Gas chromatography with mass spectrometry** (GC-MS) detection is the most widely used method for confirmation and quantitation of drugs of abuse and overdose. Confirmatory methods are highly specific by design to produce no false positives and require more time and sophisticated instrumentation to perform than screening methods. Since GC-MS instrumentation and expertise is not always available, confirmatory testing may be accomplished by using a screening test in conjunction with a second independent method, such as a spot test or TLC. However, identification of drugs in a patient specimen by any single method other than chromatography with mass spectrometry must be considered presumptive.

Drug screening and confirmation protocols for nonemergency purposes such as preemployment and preathletic drug usage assessments may be the only evidence gathered to deny an individual valued activities and rights. Therefore, all aspects of testing (preanalytical, analytical, and postanalytical) require the highest standards of practice. To ensure this, laboratories offering to test for drugs of abuse should follow the guidelines and be certified by the Substance Abuse and Mental Health Service Administration (SAMHSA) of the U.S. Department of Health and Human Services or the Forensic Urine Drug Testing program cosponsored by the American Association for Clinical Chemistry (AACC) and the College of American Pathologists (CAP).[1]

### TYPES OF SPECIMENS

Screenings for drugs of abuse are usually performed on **random urine specimens.** Urine contains a high concentration of drugs or drug metabolites and is easy to obtain. Drugs are readily extracted from urine and can be concentrated to improve the method's sensitivity. It is important for clinical laboratory scientists to know the average length of time that drugs or their metabolites remain positive in a specimen. For most drugs, the window of detectability in urine is only a few days. Urine drug screening can only detect recent exposure and cannot differentiate chronic and heavy users from those who rarely take a drug.

Since urine samples may be **adulterated** (diluted or chemically treated) or **switched** to prevent detection of drug usage, the collection may require some invasion of privacy and loss of dignity, including direct observation, to validate the integrity of a urine sample. To detect urine that was altered by addition of water or other chemicals, temperature is commonly checked immediately after collection and later analyzed for pH, specific gravity, or creatinine.[1]

In utero drug exposure is best detected using **meconium,** the first fecal material excreted by the newborn. Meconium represents the intestinal contents of the fetus before birth and serves as a depository for drugs during fetal development. Although urine represents exposure to drugs of abuse over the last 2 to 3 days, a positive meconium represents maternal drug usage during the last half of the gestational period. Meconium has a complex matrix, which requires pretreatment before drug analysis is performed.[26]

Hair, sweat, and saliva are used as alternative specimens to urine for the detection of drugs of abuse. As methods are perfected, use of these types of specimens will likely increase.

## SPOT TESTS

Methods used to detect drugs in urine vary greatly in terms of the technical expertise and the instrumentation required. Easiest and least complex are the so-called spot tests, in which reagents are added to an aliquot of the specimen and a colored complex is formed in the presence of a particular drug. Commonly used spot tests include tests for acetaminophen, salicylates, tricyclic antidepressants, phenothiazines, and ethchlorvynol.[1] Spot tests are rapid and inexpensive, and require little technical expertise but they are often less sensitive and specific than other readily available methods.

## IMMUNOASSAYS

The immunoassays are the most common screening method for drugs of abuse since they are easy to perform, require no sample pretreatment, are sensitive, provide rapid turnaround time, and have been adapted for use on both automated analyzers and point-of-care (POC) instruments. For these reasons, most health care settings are able to have access to drug screening, if warranted, on a 24-hour emergency basis.

In immunoassay screening procedures, a drug present in a patient's specimen competes with a labeled drug for a limited number of binding sites on antibodies that are specific for the drug being measured. The reader is advised to read the chapter covering immunoassay and related principles for more information. There are two disadvantages to immunoassay drug-screening methods. First, some immunoassay tests are specific for **one drug** (e.g., for LSD or propoxyphene), whereas others detect **drug groups** (e.g., amphetamines, opiates, or barbiturates) and immunologic methods are not available for all drugs of abuse. Second, some of the immunoassays have poor specificity and therefore **cross-react** with other structurally similar drugs or drug metabolites. Immunoassays for amphetamines, for example, may give false-positive results with amphetamine-like drugs (see Table 24–3) commonly found in over-the-counter medicines.[1]

Different immunoassay techniques have been used for drug-screening protocols and many have been adapted for use on high throughput automated systems. Most frequently used are enzyme-multiplied immunoassay technique (EMIT), fluorescence polarization immunoassay (FPIA), cloned enzyme donor immunoassay (CEDIA), and kinetic interaction of microparticles in solution (KIMS).[18] Immunoassays are also utilized on POC drug screening devices.[1]

## CHROMATOGRAPHIC METHODS

Chromatographic techniques have traditionally been the cornerstone for drug analysis and are useful for drug screening and confirmation. Drug identification is based on the attraction a particular drug has for the stationary phase over the mobile phase, a process that uniquely separates one drug from another. The degree to which a drug in the mobile phase interacts with the stationary phase is determined by the physical and chemical properties of the two phases. Methods include thin-layer chromatography (TLC), gas-liquid chromatography (GLC), gas chromatography with mass spectrometry detection (GC–MS), and high-performance liquid chromatography (HPLC). Quantitative measurement of drugs is also performed using all types of chromatography except TLC. Chromatography requires a high degree of technical expertise, and methods such as GLC, GC–MS, and HPLC require expensive instrumentation and maintenance as well. Chromatography is generally not suitable for emergency drug-screening use since the turnaround time is too long. Spot tests and immunoassays are preferred when screening is ordered to guide therapy of a potential overdose patient.

### Thin-Layer Chromatography

Thin-layer chromatography (TLC) is commonly used to **screen** for drugs of abuse in urine and does not require expensive instrumentation. It does, however, require a well-trained analyst and is the most subjective of the chromatographic methods. As with other chromatographic methods, sample pretreatment is required. The drugs must be extracted from the body fluids and concentrated. Drugs such as barbiturates require an acid extraction, whereas most other drugs such as amphetamines and methadone require an alkaline extraction.[1] Following the acidification or alkalinization of the specimen, the specimen is shaken with an organic solvent to extract the drugs. The organic phase is removed and evaporated to near dryness and the residue is then applied to a plate (stationary phase), which consists of a thin layer of dried inorganic material such as silicate on a solid support. The end of the plate, containing the concentrated drugs, is placed into an organic solvent (mobile phase). As the solvent moves up the plate over the point-of-sample application, the drugs are dissolved and carried along in the solvent. Separation of drugs occurs because some of the drugs move up the plate faster than others because of a lesser degree of attraction to the stationary phase. To visualize the drugs, the plate is either dipped into or sprayed with a series of reagents and viewed with ultraviolet light. Multiple drugs and their metabolites can be identified by their relative migration (Rf) and color patterns on the plate, as compared to the Rf and color reactions of a standard solution of known drug content applied to the same plate. Interpretation of the chromatogram is subjective and results are strictly qualitative. TLC is not appropriate for urgent requests, since it may take as long as 3 hours to perform. A commercially available TLC system to detect drugs of abuse is available from Toxi-Lab (Irvine, CA). Figure 24–5 illustrates the principle of TLC.

### Gas-Liquid Chromatography

For gas-liquid chromatography (GLC) separation, sample pretreatment, extraction and concentration, similar to the TLC extraction, is commonly required. Derivatization of some drugs to a less polar or volatile form may be needed as well. Following injection of sample, the volatilized substances are

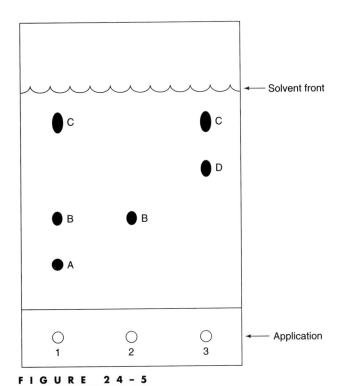

**F I G U R E   2 4 - 5**

A thin layer chromatogram after migration and visualization of spots with color reagents. Sample 1 is a standard containing drugs A, B, and C. Sample 2 is an unknown containing a spot consistent with drug B. Sample 3 is an unknown containing a spot consistent with drug C, and a second spot (D) not seen in the standard.

then carried by a carrier gas, usually nitrogen or helium, through a capillary column coated with a liquid stationary phase. The drugs and metabolites move through the column at different rates depending on their solubility and interaction with the liquid phase on the column. After being separated, the substances are detected as they elute from the column. Figure 24–6 displays a functional diagram of a GLC system. Two types of detectors commonly used for drug analysis are the flame ionization detector (FID) and the thermionic-selective detector (TSD), also known as nitrogen-phosphorus detector. The TSD is a modification of the FID and is more sensitive to organics containing phosphorus and nitrogen.[29] The FID consists of a small hydrogen-air flame at the end of a jet with an electrode above the flame. When organic compounds are introduced into the flame by the carrier gas, ions are formed. Applying a voltage across the flame collects the ions. The resulting current is amplified by an electrometer and a chart recorder produces a chromatogram. The length of time each substance requires to pass through the column, the retention time, is characteristic for a specific drug and allows them to be identified. The peak sizes (area or height) may be used for quantitation of the drugs.

## High-Performance Liquid Chromatography

High-performance liquid chromatography (HPLC) is similar to GLC, except that the mobile phase is a liquid rather than a gas and the detector is usually a spectrophotometer. The technique is particularly useful for identification of nonpolar drugs. After a sample has been extracted and concentrated, it is injected into the mobile phase of the HPLC system that carries the sample through a column. Most HPLC for drug analysis is performed using a C 18 type, reverse-phase (nonpolar) column. As the mobile phase passes through the column, drugs are separated by their interaction with the column material and are identified by the time required for them to elute from the column (retention time). To detect the eluting drugs, the mobile phase passes through a spectrophotometer, which is set at a wavelength at which the drugs of interest will absorb. A diode array detector may also be used. As the drugs pass through the detector a chromatogram is produced. HPLC, like GLC and GC–MS, can be used for qualitative as well as quantitative drug identifications. A commercial, completely automated HPLC system (REMEDI; BioRad Laboratories, Hercules, CA) is available for drug screening. The system is capable of identifying about 300 drugs and drug metabolites and may also be used for drug quantitation.[1]

## Gas Chromatography–Mass Spectrophotometry

Gas chromatography–mass spectrophotometry (GC–MS) involves the use of a gas chromatograph with a mass spectrometer as the detector. In the mass spectrometer, drugs are bombarded with electrons as they elute from the GC portion of the instrument. Ions are produced that are fragments of the bombarded drugs. These ions are separated electrically and electromagnetically by their mass to charge ratio. Then, the separated ions are detected by an electrically charged detector and amplified to boost sensitivity. The composite tracing of all

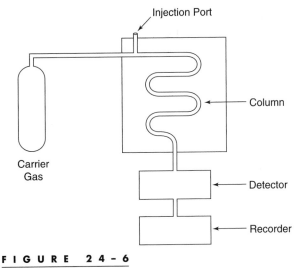

**F I G U R E   2 4 - 6**

Functional diagram of a gas-liquid chromatograph.

ions of an analyte, its mass spectra, constitutes a distinctive fingerprint that can be used to unequivocally identify an analyte. The mass spectra produced are highly specific for a given substance and can be used for definitive identification of a drug or drug metabolite.[29] Of all the chromatographic methods, GC–MS is the most specific technique and is capable of quantitation as well as definitive drug identification.

## SUMMARY

Clinical laboratory toxicology is the identification, and in some cases quantitation, of toxic substances in body fluids for purposes of health care. Although the variety of potentially toxic substances is almost limitless, the clinical laboratory must limit its testing services to those substances among the common classes of poisons that are available to and used by the population served.

Common toxic substances discussed in this chapter include carbon monoxide, ethanol, other volatiles, lead and other toxic heavy metals, pesticides, drugs of abuse, and therapeutic drugs commonly found in overdose. The drugs of abuse commonly encountered in the toxicology laboratory include cannabinoids, cocaine, amphetamines, hallucinogens, opioids, and benzodiazepines. Toxic exposures may be unintentional (e.g., pediatric and geriatric populations), in connection with a suicide or homicide, occupational, environmental, or recreational. In this chapter, each of these substances is discussed in terms of prevalence, mechanisms of toxicity, symptoms, and associated laboratory findings, specimen collection and handling, principles of common methods of analysis, and a description of treatment.

Methods of analysis discussed include spectrophotometry for carboxyhemoglobin; enzymatic analysis for ethanol; gas-liquid chromatography for volatiles; atomic absorption spectrometry and anodic stripping voltometry for lead, atomic absorption spectrometry for heavy metals, and colorimetric assay of pseudocholinesterase activity for pesticide exposure. Methods of analysis for drugs of abuse include spot tests, immunoassays, thin layer chromatography (TLC), gas-liquid chromatography (GLC), high-performance liquid chromatography (HPLC), and gas chromatography–mass spectrometry (GC–MS).

### REFERENCES

1. Porter WH: Clinical toxicology. In Burtis CA, Ashwood ER (eds.): *Tietz Textbook of Clinical Chemistry.* 3rd ed. Philadelphia, WB Saunders, 1999, p 906.
2. SAMHSA. 1999 *National Household Survey on Drug Abuse.* Substance Abuse and Mental Health Services Administration, National Clearinghouse for Alcohol and Drug Information (NCADI), Rockville, MD. Available electronically at samhsa.gov
3. NIAAA: *Surveillance Report #4: Trends in Alcohol-Related Fatal Traffic Crashes, United States, 1975–97.* National Institute on Alcohol Abuse and Alcoholism, Division of Biometry and Epidemiology, Bethesda, MD, December, 1999.
4. NIAAA: *Alcohol Alert No. 35: Alcohol Metabolism:* National Institute on Alcohol Abuse and Alcoholism, Bethesda, MD, January, 1997. Available electronically at silk.nih.gov/silk/niaaa1/publication/aa35.htm
5. Mendell CL, Weesner RE: Alcoholism. In Kaplan LA, Pesce AJ (eds.): *Clinical Chemistry: Theory, Analysis and Correlation.* 3rd ed. St. Louis, MO, Mosby–Year Book, 1996, p 682.
6. Thorne DP: Toxicology. In Bishop JL, Duben-Engelkirk JL, Fody, EP (eds.): *Clinical Chemistry: Principles, Procedures and Correlations.* 4th ed. Philadelphia, Lippincott Williams & Wilkins, 2000, p 506.
7. Hingson RW, Heeren T, Winter MR: Preventing impaired driving. Alcohol Res Health 23:31, 1999.
8. Williams RH, Erickson TE: Evaluating toxic alcohol poisoning in the emergency setting. Lab Med 29:102, 1998.
9. Moyer, TP: Toxic metals. In Burtis CA, Ashwood ER (eds.): *Tietz Textbook of Clinical Chemistry.* 3rd ed. Philadelphia, WB Saunders, 1999, p 982.
10. Ash, KO: Trace elements: When essential nutrients become poisonous. Lab Med 26:266, 1995.
11. US Department of Housing and Urban Development. *Putting the Pieces Together: Controlling Lead Hazards in the Nation's Housing.* Summary Lead-Based Paint Hazard Reduction and Financing Task Force, HUD-1542-LBP(1), 1995.
12. Centers for Disease Control. Screening young children for lead poisoning: guidance for state and local public health officials [Report]. Atlanta, GA, US Department of Health and Human Services, 1997.
13. Royce SE, Neddleman HL (eds.): *Case Studies in Environmental Medicine: Lead Toxicity.* US Public Health Service, ATSDR, revised 9/92. National Lead Information Center DOC#700, 1998.
14. Scheiber WE: Iron, porphyrin, and bilirubin metabolism. In Kaplan LA, Pesce AJ (eds.): *Clinical Chemistry: Theory, Analysis and Correlation.* 3rd ed. St. Louis, MO, Mosby, 1996, p 705.
15. Parsons JP, Reilly AA, Esernio-Jenssen D: Screening children exposed to lead: An assessment of the capillary blood lead fingerstick test. Clin Chem 43:302, 1997.
16. Stanton NV, Maney JM, Jones R: Evaluation of filter paper blood lead methods: Result of a pilot proficiency testing program, Clin Chem 45:2229, 1999.
17. Centers for Disease Control and Prevention. Update: Blood lead levels–United States, 1991–94. Morbid Mortal Wkly Rep 46:141, 1997.
18. Poklis A, Wong J, Pesce AJ: Toxicology. In Kaplan LA, Pesce AJ (eds.): *Clinical Chemistry: Theory, Analysis and Correlation.* 3rd ed. St. Louis, MO, Mosby, 1996, p 1017.

19. Kaselis T: *The Pocket Guide to Clinical Laboratory Instrumentation.* Philadelphia, FA Davis, 1994.

20. Pelehach L: How the drugs of abuse industry evolved. Lab Med 27:162, 1996.

21. Williams RH, Erickson TE: Evaluating acetaminophen and salicylate poisoning in an emergency setting. Lab Med: 29:33, 1998.

22. Williams RH, Erickson TE: Evaluating sympathomimetic intoxication in an emergency setting. Lab Med 31:497, 2000.

23. NIDA: Rohypnol and GHD, *INFOFAX.* National Institute on Drug Abuse, National Institute of Health, last updated 11/5/99. Available electronically at nida.nih.gov/Infofax/RohypnolGHB.html

24. Williams RH, Erickson TE: Evaluating hallucinogenic or psychedelic drug intoxication in an emergency setting. Lab Med 31:394, 2000.

25. NIDA. Nationwide Trends 13567, INFOFAX. National Institute on Drug Abuse, National Institute of Health, last updated 3/29/2000. Available electronically at nida.nih.gov/Infofax/nationtrends.html

26. Moore CM, Negrusz A: Drugs of abuse in meconium. Forensic Sci Rev 7:104, 1995.

27. Williams RH, Erickson TE: Emergency diagnosis of opioid intoxication. Lab Med 31:334, 2000.

28. NIDA: Anabolic Steroid Abuse. National Institute on Drug Abuse, National Institutes of Health, Research Report Series, 00-3721, revised April, 2000. Available electronically at nida.nih.gov/ResearchReports/Steroids/AnabolicSteroids.html

29. Ullman MD, Bowers LD, Burtis CA: Chromatography. In Burtis CA, Ashwood ER (eds.): *Tietz Fundmentals of Clinical Chemistry.* 4th ed. Philadelphia, WB Saunders, 1996, p 105.

# Introduction to Hormones and Endocrinology

*Jocelyn J. Hulsebus*

The endocrine system consists of a series of glands that produce chemical messengers called **hormones.** These messengers cause changes in physiologic and chemical processes that help to maintain body equilibrium or homeostasis.

Most of the glands in the human body are categorized as either **endocrine** or **exocrine.** The endocrine glands are ductless glands interspersed with many blood capillaries. The products (hormones) that the endocrine glands produce are released from the cell, pass directly into the circulation, and are carried by the blood to other body tissues. The exocrine cells also produce a product for export (often an enzyme) that must pass out of the cell and away from the gland by means of a single duct into a lumenal area such as the oral cavity or the intestine. Products from the exocrine glands do not directly enter the circulation.

Hormones are the chemical messengers produced by the endocrine cells that travel through the circulation to specific body cells where they are utilized. The body cells that contain **receptors** for specific hormones are called **target cells.** Only those cells containing receptors will bind hormones. The binding of a hormone to its receptor is very specific, concentration dependent, and reversible. Historically the interaction of a hormone with its receptor on a distant and distinct target cell (**endocrine action**) is changing to include both **autocrine** and **paracrine** action. Autocrine is the interaction of a secreted chemical messenger with a receptor on the cell that synthesized it. Paracrine is the interaction of a secreted chemical messenger with receptors on adjacent cells.

## CLASSIFICATION OF HORMONES

### Protein Hormones

Hormones are classified into two main groups, protein and steroid. The protein hormones are composed of **amino acids.** Included in this group are peptides, chains of 8 amino acids or less, amines, and modified amines. The protein and peptide hormones are synthesized in the endocrine glands as larger precursor molecules called **preprohormones.**[1] The preprohor-

mone contains a leader sequence of amino acids called a signal sequence. The signal sequence is cleaved from the molecule after insertion into the endoplasmic reticulum (ER) (Figure 25–1). The resulting molecule is now called a **prohormone.**[1] The prohormones are enzymatically cleaved to smaller molecules and additional molecular modifications such as molecular folding or addition of carbohydrate moieties are made within the ER, if necessary. Finally the finished active hormones (Figure 25–1) are packaged into secretory vesicles. The secretory vesicles can either migrate to the plasma membrane, fuse and release their hormones, or remain in the cytoplasm of the cell as storage vesicles. The storage vesicles provide the body immediate access to the hormone in time of increased demand. In general, this group of hormones does not attach to plasma proteins and circulates in the blood as free hormone. However, the thyroid hormones (modified amines) circulate bound to thyroid-binding globulin (TBG) and are an exception. The response of protein hormones to stimuli is rapidly initiated and often the reaction is not sustained. In addition, the **half-life** of protein, peptide, and amine hormones is considered to be short and can be measured in minutes. The half-life of a hormone is the time it takes to remove half of the secreted hormone from circulation.

### Steroid Hormones

The **steroid** hormones are synthesized in the cytoplasm by multienzyme processes. All steroid hormones are derived from **cholesterol** (Figure 25–2a.) and have the basic perhydrocyclopentanophenanthrene ring structure (Figure 25–2b.). The steroid hormones are separated into groups based on the number of carbons present; C-18 is estrogens, C-19 is androgens, and C-21 is glucocorticoids, mineralocorticoids, and progestins. Unlike the protein hormones, the steroids are not packaged into secretory vesicles and no reserve hormones are stored in the cell. Steroid hormones can freely diffuse across the plasma membrane and into the bloodstream. Within the circulation, most of the steroids bind to specific plasma proteins, which allows them to remain in circulation for longer than the unbound or free form of the hormone. Only free hormone is considered the active form, and only the active form can bind to its receptor. Steroid hormones take longer to initiate their

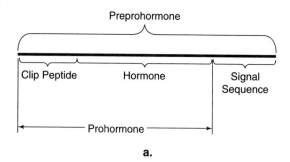

Preprohormone

| Clip Peptide | Hormone | Signal Sequence |

Prohormone

**a.**

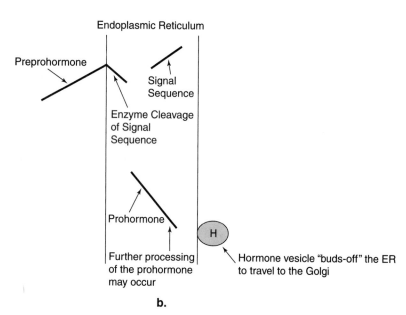

Endoplasmic Reticulum

Preprohormone

Signal Sequence

Enzyme Cleavage of Signal Sequence

Prohormone

Further processing of the prohormone may occur

H

Hormone vesicle "buds-off" the ER to travel to the Golgi

**b.**

**Golgi Apparatus**

H

H    *cis*    H

H

Vesicle from ER containing hormone

*medial*    H

H

Hormone passes in and out of the Golgi Apparatus, further processing may occur

*trans*    H

H

Active form of the hormone is packaged into a secretion vesicle and is now ready for release or storage

**c.**

**F I G U R E    2 5 – 1**

Protein hormones are synthesized as large precursor molecule called preprohormone. **a.** The prehormone molecule is inserted into the endoplasmic reticulum (ER). **b.** In the ER, a portion of the molecule called the signal sequence is enzymatically cleaved from the molecule. The resulting molecule is now called a prohormone. The prohormone travels through the ER to the Golgi apparatus. **c.** Here the final enzyme cleavage takes place to produce the final hormone. The hormones are then packaged into secretion granules.

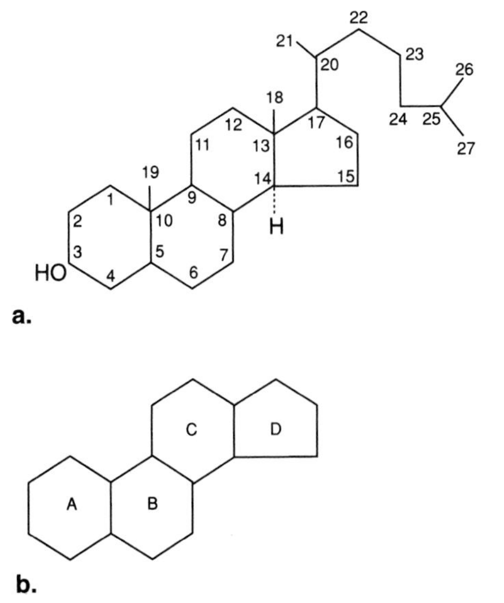

a.

b.

**FIGURE 25-2**

Molecular structure of **a.** cholesterol and **b.** perhydro-cyclopentanophenanthrene nucleus.

action and once started, the action is sustained for a prolonged period. In general, steroid hormones have long half-lives because of their binding to the plasma protein carriers. Table 25–1 is a list of the major endocrine glands and the hormones present in each gland.

## Growth Factors and Neurotransmitters

As new discoveries are made on the structure and function of chemical messengers, it is important to expand our definition of a hormone to include **growth factors** and possibly **neurotransmitters.** Growth factors are composed of amino acids and share many of the same characteristics as the protein hormones. Growth factors do not come from organized endocrine glands but from individual cells or groups of cells. Each growth factor has its own specific extracellular receptor since they cannot cross the plasma membrane. In addition, the separation between hormones and neurotransmitters is increasingly a gray area. A single messenger (epinephrine or norepinephrine) may serve as either a hormone or a neurotransmitter, the primary difference being the site of synthesis and action.

**TABLE 25-1**

**Major Endocrine Glands and Their Hormones**

| GLAND | HORMONES PRESENT | TYPE OF HORMONE |
| --- | --- | --- |
| • Pineal | Melatonin | Protein |
| • Anterior pituitary | Follicle-stimulating hormone (FSH) | Protein |
| | Luteinizing hormone (LH) | Protein |
| | Growth hormone (GH) | Protein |
| | Prolactin (PRL) | Protein |
| | Adrenocorticotropic hormone (ACTH) | Protein |
| | Thyroid-stimulating hormone (TSH) | Protein |
| • Posterior pituitary | Oxytocin | Protein |
| | Antidiuretic hormone (ADH) | Protein |
| • Thyroid | Calcitonin | Protein |
| | Thyroxine (T4) | Protein |
| | Triiodothyronine (T3) | Protein |
| • Parathyroid | Parathormone (PTH) | Protein |
| • Pancreas islets of Langerhans | Insulin | Protein |
| | Glucagon | Protein |
| | Pancreatic polypeptide | Protein |
| | Somatostatin | Protein |
| • Adrenal medulla | Epinephrine | Protein |
| | Norepinephrine | Protein |
| • Adrenal cortex | Cortisol | Steroid |
| | Aldosterone | Steroid |
| • Ovary | Estrogen | Steroid |
| | Progesterone | Steroid |
| • Testis | Testosterone | Steroid |

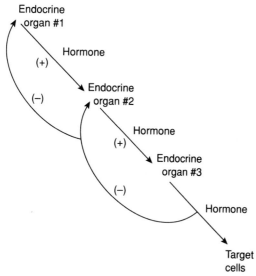

**F I G U R E   2 5 – 3**

Example of negative feedback hormonal regulation (stimulation [+], inhibition [−]).

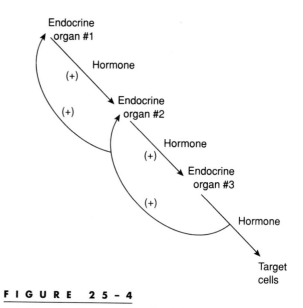

**F I G U R E   2 5 – 4**

Example of positive feedback hormonal regulation (stimulation [+]).

## REGULATION OF HORMONE SECRETION

Many hormones are secreted in a cascade manner. The regulation of this secretion pattern is often through a process called **negative feedback.** In negative feedback, the final hormone produced regulates its own secretion by inhibiting the secretion of 1 or more of the precursor hormones (Figure 25–3). This process is concentration dependent, meaning that if the end product is in high plasma concentration, it will inhibit the cascade. If it is in low plasma concentration, the inhibition will be removed and the cascade will once again be initiated.

In rare circumstances, hormone secretion is regulated through **positive feedback.** Here, the final hormone produced actually enhances or induces the initial hormone and causes its own production to be increased (Figure 25–4).

## MECHANISMS OF ACTION

### Protein Hormone Action

Protein (peptide and amines) hormones and growth factors cannot cross the plasma membrane and enter the cell. Therefore, their receptors must be located on the extracellular side of the plasma membrane so that the hormone can bind to it. One exception is the thyroid hormones, triiodothyronine ($T_3$) and thyroxine ($T_4$).[2] These hydrophobic hormones can readily diffuse through the cell membrane to attach to their high-affinity intracellular receptors. After a protein hormone binds to an extracellular receptor, there must be a means of transmitting the signal from the hormone into the cell.[3,4] The transduction of the signal is frequently done by a system composed of an intramembrane protein (called a G protein)[5,6] with several subunits (alpha, beta and gamma) and an enzyme (adenylyl cyclase) that is attached to the intracellular side of the plasma membrane (Figure 25–5). The G proteins are actually a group of different intramembrane proteins. These proteins bind and hydrolyze[2] GTP and are required for the activation ($G_s$) or inhibition ($G_i$) of the adenylyl cyclase enzyme.[6] The activated $G_s$ stimulates the enzyme adenylyl cyclase to produce a molecule **(cAMP)** that is called a **second messenger.**[5] The second messenger (cAMP) proceeds inside the cell to either activate or inhibit one or more enzymes to modify intracellular metabolic processes. Although cAMP is a common second messenger for many of the protein hormones, it is not the only one known. Inositol triphosphate is a second messenger generally associated with the growth factors. Generation of this second messenger includes a G protein ($G_p$) and an enzyme, phospholipase C.[6] Phospholipase C cleaves inositol triphosphate from a membrane lipid, phosphotidylinositol. Inositol triphosphate does not interact with any cellular enzymes[6] but will induce large increases in the concentration of intracellular free calcium. The increase in the free calcium appears to come from release of intracellular storage in the endoplasmic reticulum and an increased influx of calcium into the cell. It is actually the increase in calcium that stimulates a variety of intracellular actions. One way that calcium may influence intracellular mechanisms is through calmodulin, a calcium-binding protein. Calmodulin will combine with calcium and in turn can activate some cellular enzymes.

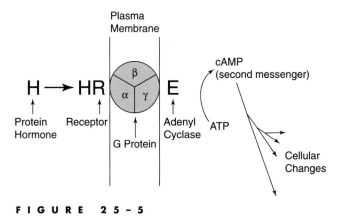

**FIGURE 25-5**

Mechanism of protein hormone action. Protein hormones bind to extracellular receptors. This in turn activates an intramembrane protein (G) to transduce the signal to an enzyme (adenylyl cyclase) to produce a second messenger (cAMP). The second messenger will cause intracellular changes.

## Steroid Hormone Action

Steroid hormones can diffuse across the plasma membrane and enter the cell.[3,4] All receptors for these hormones are located intracellularly.[7] A model has been proposed for the steroid receptor.[2] The proposed receptor has hormone binding sites, DNA binding sites, and is associated with a heat shock protein that disassociates after hormone binding occurs. It appears that the heat shock protein probably disassociates to expose the DNA binding site.[2] Once a steroid hormone binds to its receptor, 2 hormone-receptor complexes associate to form a dimer and the dimer migrates to the DNA (Figure 25–6) binding[8] with a specific region. The DNA binding site is rich in cysteine residues and appears to need the presence of zinc ions for optimal binding to the DNA.[2] The binding of the complex initiates mRNA synthesis and eventually the synthesis of a protein. It appears that the thyroid hormone receptor is similar in structure to the steroid receptor and may indicate a similarity in regulating gene expression between the 2 classes of hormones.[2]

## DISORDERS OF THE ENDOCRINE SYSTEM

Most disorders of the endocrine system can be separated into two main categories, primary and secondary. **Primary disorders** involve some problem with the gland that produces the hormone (either hypersecretion or hyposecretion) even though the outside stimulating agents are normal. With **secondary disorders,** the gland that produces the hormone is capable of normal function. The outside stimulating agents are either in excess (resulting in glandular hypersecretion) or are deficient (resulting in glandular hyposecretion). Either abnormality will

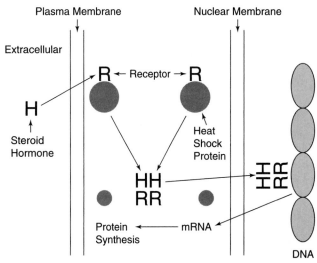

**FIGURE 25-6**

Mechanism of steroid hormone action. Steroid hormones (H) diffuse across the cellular membrane to bind with their intracellular receptors (R). A heat shock protein disassociates from the receptor after binding. The hormone-receptor complex (HR) migrates into the nucleus and binds with a specific region on the DNA. A mRNA is produced and a protein is synthesized.

cause clinical features that may be identified with the endocrine disorder.

Hypersecretion of a hormone is often more difficult to correct than hyposecretion. In **hypersecretion,** the gland must be inhibited, which may lead to destruction of the endocrine tissue. Many times the end result from treating hypersecretion is inducing hyposecretion. **Hyposecretion** is often not detected until approximately 80% to 90% of the gland is nonfunctional. The treatment for hyposecretion usually involves hormone replacement therapy.

## SUMMARY

The endocrine system is composed of glands that produce chemical messengers called hormones. These hormones help cells to communicate with one another so that they can maintain a body equilibrium or homeostasis. Hormones only interact with specific cells called target cells. For a hormone to cause an action in a target cell that cell must contain a receptor. Every hormone has its own individual receptor.

Hormones are divided into two main groups, protein and steroid. The protein hormones are composed of amino acids, are stored in secretory vesicles, do not circulate bound to plasma proteins, and have short half-lives. In addition, protein hormones cannot enter the target cells and bind to extracellular receptors. Once binding occurs, a signal is transmitted into the cell and a second messenger is produced. The second messenger is responsible for causing changes inside the target cell. The exception is the thyroid hormones. These modified amines bind to a plasma protein, diffuse into the cell, and bind with an intracellular receptor that appears to be similar in structure to the steroid hormone receptor.

The steroid hormones are derived from cholesterol, are not stored in the endocrine cells, often circulate bound to plasma proteins, and have longer half-lives. Steroid hormones can freely diffuse across the plasma membrane to bind with intracellular receptors. Once bound to the receptor, the hormone-receptor dimer binds to specific areas of the cellular DNA, stimulates the production of mRNA, and finally causes protein synthesis.

## REFERENCES

1. Brownstein HJ, Russel JT, Grainer H: Synthesis, transport and release of posterior pituitary hormones. Science 207:373–378, 1980.

2. Gardner DG: Mechanisms of hormone action. In Greenspan F (ed): *Basic and Clinical Endocrinology.* 5th ed. Stamford, CT, Appleton & Lange, 1997, p 58.

3. Sutherland EW: Studies on the mechanism of hormone action. Science 177:401–408, 1972.

4. O'Malley B, Birnbaumer L (eds.): *Receptors and Hormone Action.* New York, Academic Press, 1978.

5. Gilman AG: G protein and dual control of adenylate cyclase. Cell 36:577–579, 1984.

6. Hanle RM, Steiner AL: The second-messenger system for peptide hormones. Hosp Pract August:59–70, 1989.

7. Walters MR: Steroid hormone receptors and the nucleus. Endocr Rev 6:512–543, 1985.

8. Ringold, GM: Steroid hormone regulation of gene expression. Ann Rev Pharmacol Toxicol 25:259–266, 1985.

# C H A P T E R   2 6

# Hypothalamus and Pituitary Endocrinology

*Jocelyn J. Hulsebus*

## HYPOTHALAMUS

The **hypothalamus** is the part of the brain that is located under the third ventricle and directly above the pituitary. The pituitary is physically connected to the hypothalamus by the infundibulum, or pituitary stalk. Within the hypothalamus are specialized neurons called neurosecretory cells that produce stimulating and inhibiting neuropeptides[1] (hormones). The primary function of these neuropeptides is to modify the secretion of hormones from the anterior pituitary. Table 26–1[1,2] lists the neuropeptides that are produced within the hypothalamus and their primary function.

## PINEAL GLAND

The **pineal gland** is located on the posterior wall of the third ventricle of the cerebrum (Figure 26–1). The exact function of this gland is unknown. It does produce a hormone called melatonin (synthesized from serotonin) that is responsible for inhibiting gonadotropic hormones in lower vertebrates.[3] Melatonin may or may not inhibit gonadotropic hormones in humans. Other hormones present in the pineal are thyrotropin-stimulating hormone (TRH), somatostatin, gonadotropin-stimulating hormone (GnRH) and norepinephrine. How these hormones participate in physiologic function is unknown. The pineal gland appears to play a role in controlling circadian rhythms.

## PITUITARY (HYPOPHYSIS) GLAND

The infundibulum, or pituitary stalk, is the connection between the pituitary and the hypothalamus.[4] It is through this structure that the neuropeptides migrate from the hypothalamus to the pituitary via the hypothalamo–hypophyseal portal circulation.[1]

The **pituitary,** or **hypophysis,** protrudes from the inferior surface of the brain and resides in a depression of the sphenoid bone called the sella tursica (Figure 26–2). In humans, the pituitary is divided into 2 main lobes, the **anterior pitu-**

itary, or **adenohypophysis,** and the **posterior pituitary,** or **neurohypophysis.** The intermediate lobe is present in the human fetus but is rudimentary in the adult human.

The posterior pituitary **stores** 2 hormones, oxytocin and antidiuretic hormone (ADH), often called arginine vasopressin (AVP).[5] Although these two hormones are stored and secreted from the posterior pituitary, they are actually synthesized by neurosecretory cells in the hypothalamus. The neurosecretory cells have long axonal processes that pass through the pituitary stalk and terminate within the posterior pituitary (Figure 26–3). After synthesis, the hormones travel down the axonal processes and are released into the posterior pituitary for storage.[5]

The anterior pituitary synthesizes and secretes numerous hormones including corticotropin (ACTH) and related peptides (beta-lipotropin, endorphins, and enkephalins), gonadotropins (follicle-stimulating hormone, FSH, and luteinizing hormone, LH), prolactin (PRL), growth hormone (GH), and thyrotropin (TSH).[4] Most of these hormones are responsible for initiating synthesis and secretion of hormones from other endocrine glands located throughout the body. Exceptions are GH and PRL. GH can directly stimulate growth in many different cells throughout the body and stimulate the production of a growth factor (somatomedin-C) from the liver. PRL can directly stimulate breast tissue but no hormone is released in response to this stimulation. Hormones (see Table 26–1) from the hypothalamus act on the various types of cells (acidophils, basophils, or chromophobes, based on their staining properties using hematoxylin-eosin) in the anterior pituitary and modify their synthesis and secretion of the anterior pituitary hormones. The acidophils stain red and are the somatotrophs (GH) and the lactotrophs or mammotrophs (PRL). The basophils stain blue and are the thyrotrophs (TSH) and gonadotrophs (FSH and LH). The chromophobes do not stain and are the corticotrophs (ACTH). The anterior pituitary hormones help to regulate their own secretion by a negative feedback mechanism to the hypothalamus, thus inhibiting the release of the hypothalamic hormones or factors. This is called short-loop negative feedback (Figure 26–4).

### Posterior Pituitary Hormones

#### ANTIDIURETIC HORMONE

**Antidiuretic hormone** (ADH) is a posterior pituitary peptide that stimulates the cells of the distal convoluted tubules and

TABLE 26-1

**Hypothalamic Hormones**

| HORMONE | MAJOR FUNCTION |
|---|---|
| Corticotropin-releasing hormone (CRH) | Increases ACTH and other hormones (beta-lipotropin and beta-endorphin) |
| Thyrotropin-releasing hormone (TRH) | Increases TSH |
| Gonadotropin-releasing hormone (GnRH) | Increases follicle-stimulating hormone (FSH), luteinizing hormone (LH) |
| Prolactin-inhibiting factor (PIF) (PIF = dopamine) | Decreases prolactin PRL |
| Prolactin-releasing factor (PRF) (undetermined, may be TRH) | Increases PRL |
| Growth hormone–releasing hormone (GRH, somatocrinin) | Increases growth hormone (GH) |
| Growth hormone–inhibiting hormone (Somatostatin, SS) | Decreases GH |
| Melanocyte-inhibiting factor (MIF) | Decreases melanocyte-stimulating hormone (MSH) |
| Antidiuretic hormone (ADH, AVP) | Increases reabsorption of water from glomerular filtrate and urine, vasoconstriction of smooth muscle |
| Oxytocin | Stimulates uterine muscle contraction |

ACTH = adrenocorticotropic hormone; AVP = arginine vasopressin.

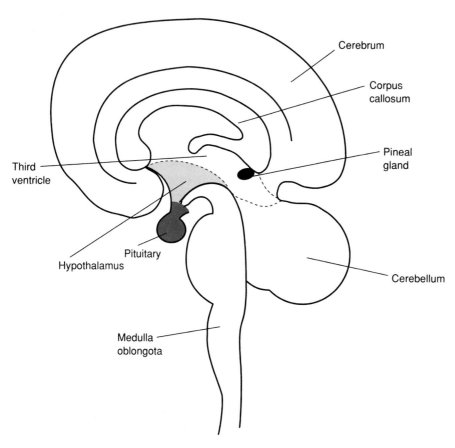

FIGURE 26-1

Anatomy of the brain and pineal gland.

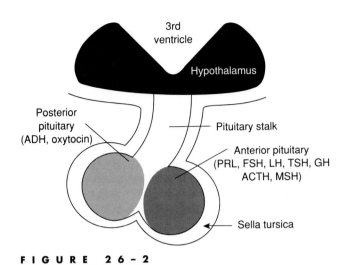

**FIGURE 26-2**

Anatomy of the pituitary gland and the hypothalamus.

collecting ducts of the nephron to increase the reabsorption of water. ADH stimulation starts with its binding to the $V_2$ receptor located on the distal convoluted tubules and collecting ducts. Adenylyl cyclase is activated and cAMP is generated. The second messenger (cAMP) probably initiates the phosphorylation of a membrane protein or proteins, causing an increase in the luminal membrane permeability to water. In addition to regulating water balance in the body, the action of ADH has a concentrating effect on the urine. The primary stimulus for ADH secretion is an increase in the plasma osmolality as detected by the osmoreceptors in the brain. Patients with an ADH deficiency have polydipsia (increased thirst) and polyuria (increased urine output). The name arginine vasopressin (AVP) is also applied to this hormone, since it can cause generalized vasoconstriction and may help in maintaining blood pressure during traumatic injuries.

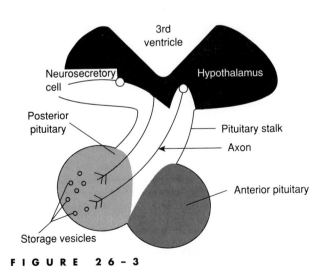

**FIGURE 26-3**

Posterior pituitary storage of hypothalamic hormones, ADH and oxytocin.

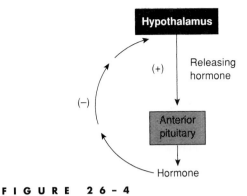

**FIGURE 26-4**

Short-loop negative feedback of anterior pituitary hormones [+ (stimulation), − (inhibition)].

Analysis of ADH is generally performed by radioimmunoassay (RIA). The specimen of choice for this analysis is plasma anticoagulated with EDTA in prechilled tubes.[6] The blood specimen should be centrifuged as soon as possible after drawing and the plasma quickly removed from the cells.[6] The plasma can be frozen until used for analysis. It should be noted that ADH levels deteriorate with prolonged storage. Concentrations for plasma ADH are reported in conjunction with the patient's plasma osmolality. Table 26-2 lists the reference ranges[6] for ADH. Low concentrations of ADH are often misinterpreted because low normal and the absence of hormone cannot be distinguished.

An indirect measure of the ADH content can be obtained by doing an overnight water deprivation test.[6] Water is withheld from the patient for 8 hours. A series of timed blood and urine samples is obtained as well as the weight of the patient. The osmolality of each urine and serum sample is determined. Patients with ADH deficiency should show increasing serum osmolality and decreasing urine osmolality over the time tested. These changes in osmolality occur because as the plasma is filtered through the kidney, a higher percentage of the water remains in the glomerular filtrate and urine instead of being reabsorbed, as would normally occur with the action of ADH. This causes a concentrating effect on the plasma and a dilutional effect on the urine. Patients with normal ADH responses should not have weight losses greater than 3%, and the de-

TABLE 26-2

**Reference Ranges for Antidiuretic Hormone (ADH)**

| OSMOLALITY (mOsm/kg) | ADH (pg/mL) |
|---|---|
| 270–280 | <1.5 |
| 280–285 | <2.5 |
| 285–290 | 1–5 |
| 290–295 | 2–7 |
| 295–300 | 4–12 |

crease in water intake should stimulate the release of ADH.[6] The increased ADH causes normalizing adjustments in the serum osmolalities (by increasing the amount of water reabsorbed from the urine) and values remain within the reference range (275 to 295 mOsmol/kg).[6]

## OXYTOCIN

**Oxytocin** is a small peptide stored and secreted from the posterior pituitary and appears to be most active in pregnant women.[4] The two strongest stimuli for oxytocin release are distention of the uterus and neonatal suckling of the nipple. At term, oxytocin induces uterine contractions and is sometimes used to hasten labor. In the mammary glands, oxytocin induces lactation by stimulating contractions of the myoepithelial cells. Basal levels of oxytocin can be measured in nonpregnant women and men. The actual role of oxytocin in these individuals has not been determined.[4]

The preferred method of analysis for oxytocin is radioimmunoassay (RIA).[6] Plasma anticoagulated with EDTA in prechilled tubes appears to be the specimen of choice. The plasma can be frozen until used for the analysis. The reference range for oxytocin is 1 to 5 pg/mL.[6]

## Anterior Pituitary Hormones

### PROLACTIN

Prolactin (PRL) is a protein hormone produced by the lactotroph (mammotroph) cells in the anterior pituitary. Growth hormone and prolactin appear to be closely related since there is some structural and sequence homology between the two hormones.[7] PRL, in conjunction with a number of other hormones, helps stimulate development of the breast tissue needed for lactation.[7] In postpartum women, prolactin induces synthesis of milk in the mammary gland. PRL is present in nonlactating women, men, and children, but the serum levels in these individuals (<20 ng/mL) are lower than those seen in pregnant women (first trimester <80 ng/mL, second trimester <169 ng/mL, third trimester <400 ng/mL).[6] The actual function of prolactin in nonlactating women, men, and children is not fully understood, although hypersecretion of prolactin is associated with hypogonadism in both men and women.[7] Secretion of prolactin appears to be under the control of a prolactin-inhibitory factor (PIF), known as dopamine, which comes from the hypothalamus.[7] If dopamine levels decline, prolactin will be secreted. If dopamine levels increase, prolactin secretion will be inhibited. No specific prolactin-releasing factor has ever been identified, but thyrotropin-releasing hormone (TRH) has been shown to induce increases in prolactin levels.[6] The actual role that TRH plays in regulating prolactin secretion has not been established.[6]

The method of choice for analysis of prolactin is RIA. The preferred specimen is fresh, nonhemolyzed serum. The serum should be frozen as soon as possible after drawing if it is not analyzed immediately.[6] The time that the specimen was drawn must be carefully recorded, since prolactin levels are highest in the morning. In addition, prolactin increases if the patient is under stress. There is an immunoradiometric assay (IRMA) available for measuring PRL, but it appears not to recognize all the forms of PRL found in circulation.[11]

## GROWTH HORMONE

**Growth hormone** (GH) is a protein hormone produced by the somatotroph cells in the anterior pituitary. Of all the hormones present in the cells of the anterior pituitary, GH is found to be in the highest concentration. Overall, GH is anabolic in most tissues and stimulates the synthesis of new proteins.[7] An exception to this anabolic action occurs in adipocytes where GH induces lipolysis. GH is required for the growth and development of cartilage and bone, but the action is indirect. First, the liver is stimulated by GH to produce proteins called somatomedins (growth factors).[8] Two somatomedins are found in human plasma, insulinlike growth factor II, or IGF-II (somatomedin-A), and insulinlike growth factor I, IGF-I (somatomedin-C).[9] The compound that was known as somatomedin-B is actually an acidic glial cell growth factor and not one of the somatomedins.[9] GH stimulates IGF-I (somatomedin-C) to be produced by the liver. Second, IGF-I binds to receptors on the cartilage and bone cells to stimulate DNA synthesis and cell growth.[8] The regulation of GH secretion appears to be multifaceted. The hypothalamus contains growth hormone-releasing hormone (GRH), also called somatocrinin,[2] a small peptide that induces the secretion of GH. Also present in the hypothalamus is growth hormone-inhibiting hormone (GHIH or GIH), also called somatostatin. These two hormones act together to cause increases and decreases in the concentration of circulating GH. In addition, hypoglycemia will induce the secretion of growth hormone as well as many physiologic, pharmacologic, and pathologic conditions.[10]

The specimen of choice for the analysis of GH is fresh serum, but heparinized plasma may be used.[6] EDTA plasma may result in lower values with some methods. The method of choice is RIA. There are a number of excellent kits available for GH analysis. The approximate reference ranges for GH are 0 to 18 ng/mL for females and 0 to 4 ng/mL for males.[11]

### GONADOTROPINS

The gonadotropins, **follicle-stimulating hormone** (FSH) and **luteinizing hormone** (LH), are produced by the same gonadotroph cell in the anterior pituitary. They are involved in regulating the sex cells and sex hormones from the gonads in both sexes. The major stimulus for secretion of these hormones is GnRH from the hypothalamus.[12] The gonadotrophs are discussed briefly here and in more detail in Chapter 31.

FSH, LH, and thyroid-stimulating hormone (TSH) are similar in structure and comprise a group called the glycoprotein hormones.[12] These large hormones are composed of two chains (alpha and beta) held together by disulfide bonds with attached carbohydrate side groups. The alpha chains of the glycoproteins are nearly identical in sequence, but the beta chains are unique in sequence and lend specificity to the molecule.[12] Another closely related glycoprotein hormone is human chorionic gonadotropin (hCG) that is produced by the placenta.

In women, FSH and LH are released in varying amounts during the menstrual cycle. The highest levels of both hormones are obtained just prior to ovulation on about day 14 of the cycle.[12] FSH stimulates follicle growth as well as growth and maturation of the ovum. As the cells of the follicle grow, they produce estrogen. Estrogen has a positive feedback effect on the secretion of GnRH. After ovulation, LH stimulates the follicle to become a corpus luteum. Once formed, the corpus luteum will produce progesterone.

In men, FSH aids in spermatogenesis in the seminiferous tubules of the testes. The Leydig or interstitial cells respond to LH and produce testosterone. The LH and FSH in the men are not secreted in a cyclic pattern as seen in women.[12]

The preferred method of analysis for FSH is RIA. The preferred method of analysis for LH is an IRMA assay, since there appears to be a high degree to cross-reactivity with hCG in most RIA tests.[11] Analysis can be done on serum or plasma. In women, interpretation of results may be difficult unless the time of the menstrual cycle is also included.

## THYROID-STIMULATING HORMONE

Thyroid-stimulating hormone (TSH) is produced by the anterior pituitary and stimulates the thyroid gland to produce thyroxine ($T_4$) and triiodothyronine ($T_3$). Secretion of TSH is controlled in part by TRH from the hypothalamus. TSH function and analysis are discussed in more detail in Chapter 27.

## ADRENOCORTICOTROPIC HORMONE

Adrenocorticotropic hormone (ACTH) is an anterior pituitary hormone that is cleaved from a large precursor molecule called proopiomelanocortin. The primary target tissue for ACTH is the adrenal cortex. After binding to its receptor, ACTH initiates steroidogenesis with cortisol as the final product synthesized. The regulation of the secretion of ACTH is primarily through the action of corticotropin-releasing hormone (CRH) and the negative feedback action of cortisol.[10,13,14]

The method of choice for analysis of ACTH is RIA,[6] although there are a number of good IRMA kits on the market. The specimen of choice is either EDTA or heparinized plasma. ACTH is unstable in whole blood and adheres onto the sides of the glass tube.[6] For proper separation of the plasma, the specimen should be spun the first time in a refrigerated centrifuge, removed, and then centrifuged again. This removes additional formed elements that may include proteolytic enzymes that could break down ACTH during the freeze and thawing process.[6] The specimen should be frozen if it is not analyzed immediately. ACTH levels are at their lowest concentration at approximately midnight and their highest concentration at approximately 8 A.M. For proper interpretation of results, the time the specimen was drawn must be noted. The reference ranges for ACTH at 8:00 A.M. are 25 to 100 pg/mL and at 6:00 P.M. <50 pg/mL.[6]

## Clinical Applications

### DIABETES INSIPIDUS

Diabetes insipidus (DI) is caused by a deficiency of ADH (neurogenic DI) or the failure of the kidney to respond to the ADH (nephrogenic DI).[13,15] Patients with this disorder produce large amounts of urine (polyuria) with a low specific gravity (<1.005) and urine osmolality (<400 mOsm/kg). These findings are similar to those seen in patients with uncontrolled diabetes mellitus. If water intake is restricted in any way, the plasma osmolality (>320 mOsm/kg) and plasma sodium (>150 mmol/L) become elevated and patients may lose more than 3% of their body weight.[11,15] In addition, patient symptoms may include fatigue, severe dehydration, hypothermia, and shock. Polydipsia (increased water intake) is a common side effect of this disorder.

In neurogenic DI, the cause of the ADH deficiency may be a pituitary tumor, traumatic injury, surgical injury, genetic, autoimmune, or idiopathic. Nephrogenic DI patients have normal to elevated plasma concentrations of ADH, but the kidney is unable to respond to the hormone. Some causes of nephrogenic DI are chronic renal disease such as chronic pyelonephritis, protein starvation, hypokalemia, sickle cell anemia, drugs (lithium carbonate, fluoride, methoxyflurane anesthesia, colchicine, propoxyphene), multiple myeloma, amyloidosis, and congenital defects in the receptor in the kidney or defects in the structure of the kidney tubule.[14] The most valuable diagnostic tests for diabetes insipidus are plasma and urine osmolality.[11,13] The urine osmolality is usually low (<400 mOsm/kg) and the urine volume for 24 hours (>3000 mL) is increased. The plasma osmolality will be normal (275 to 295 mOsm/kg) if water intake has not been restricted. A water deprivation test can also be used to aid in the diagnosis. Plasma ADH levels determined by RIA are often misleading, since low normal values may not be accurate and can be interpreted as absence of hormone.[6,11] The patient may be given exogenous ADH to test their response to the hormone. Normal patients respond by decreasing their urine output and increasing their urine osmolality. Nephrogenic DI patients will show no response to the ADH injection and neurogenic DI patients should show an increase of >10% in their urine osmolality.[11]

### SYNDROME OF INAPPROPRIATE ANTIDIURETIC HORMONE

Hypersecretion of ADH induces excess water retention, causing a dilutional effect on the plasma components, and hypoosmolality (<275 mOsm/kg) occur,[11] causing a condition known as syndrome of inappropriate ADH (SIADH). Analysis for plasma sodium may result in low values (<135 mmol/L), but the total body sodium is often increased and urine osmolalities may be 300 to 400 mOsm/kg. The hyponatremia (low sodium) can induce generalized weakness, mental confusion, coma, and convulsions.[6] The RIA for ADH is of value and can be used to detect the actual amount of ADH present. The cause of the hypersecretion may be a pituitary tumor or some type of carcinoma not located within the pituitary. Most often, carcinomas that secrete ADH occur in the lung.

## GROWTH HORMONE DEFICIENCY

Deficiencies of GH may be caused by pituitary tumors, traumatic injury, congenital disorders, or be idiopathic.[6,8,14] Children that are deficient in GH will fail to grow and be short in stature. If the failure to grow is due to GH deficiency and not the inability of the body to utilize the GH, such as a receptor abnormality, the patient may be treated with replacement GH. The major problem with giving exogenous GH to the patient is that the human body only responds to human GH. Recently, this problem has been overcome by being able to produce human GH by genetic engineering and recombinant methods. Children with true GH deficiencies usually respond and grow following injections of GH. Adults who are deficient in GH rarely show any clinical symptoms. Random measurements of GH are rarely of value since normal individuals often have low basal levels of GH.[6] To prove GH deficiency, a patient must fail to respond to two different stimulation tests (GH levels <5 ng/mL). One of the oldest stimulation tests uses an injection of exogenous insulin to induce severe hypoglycemia, which in turn stimulates an increase in plasma GH. This test is dangerous because of the degree of hypoglycemia that may be induced. A physician should be present at all times during this test.[6] Currently, an injection of CRH is substituted to stimulate an increase in GH secretion. This test is safer for the patient since hypoglycemia is not induced. Another test used to increase plasma GH involves strenuous exercise. The patient is asked to exercise for 20 minutes. A blood specimen is drawn immediately and assayed for GH. Levels >6 ng/dL are considered normal.[6,11] Increases in plasma GH can also be induced with injections of arginine hydrochloride. Normal patients will show increases in GH that may be 3 times the patient's basal level within 1 to 2 hours after the initial injection.[6]

## GROWTH HORMONE HYPERSECRETION

If overproduction of growth hormone begins in childhood before the epiphyseal plates of the bones are closed, the disorder is known as gigantism. The principal manifestation is a rapid increase in height without distortion of body proportions.

Hypersecretion of growth hormone in adults is most often caused by a pituitary adenoma. This primary disorder is a disfiguring condition called acromegaly. The majority of the disfiguring physical features (excessive bone growth) is caused by the increased amounts of IFG-I (somatomedin C) from the liver. In addition, there is increased growth of most body soft tissues. Patients with acromegaly can be either male or female, are about 40 years of age, and often go undiagnosed for at least 5 years.[10] The first symptoms seen are usually increases in the size of the hands and feet with coarsening of the facial features, especially development of bony ridges over the eyes.[10] Patients may have high levels of insulin, increased postprandial glucose, elevated phosphorus and calcium, joint pain,

weight gain, goiter, heat intolerance, and increased sweating.[10] Confirmation of the diagnosis of acromegaly is done with serial measurements of the serum GH. Serial measurements of GH are necessary since secretion of the hormone is episodic throughout the day. Acromegaly patients average GH levels of 50 ng/mL or higher (normal reference range of basal GH, 1–5 ng/mL).[10] Treatment for the most common type of acromegaly is transsphenoidal surgical removal of the pituitary adenoma. Serum GH levels decrease in 30% to 80% of the patients. Usually the smaller the tumor, the more likely the patient sees a large reduction in the amount of serum GH. Patients with smaller reductions in the serum GH levels may also need radiation therapy.

## PANHYPOPITUITARISM

**Panhypopituitarism** is a generalized hypofunction of the pituitary gland with resulting decreases in all pituitary hormone levels. Generally, panhypopituitarism is seen after severe damage has occurred in the pituitary. These patients have thyroid and adrenal insufficiency as well as absence of gonadal function. Most often, the treatment for this syndrome is replacement of the deficient hormones.

Simmonds' disease is a form of panhypopituitarism that develops after destruction of the pituitary by surgery, infection, injury, or tumor.[14,16,17] The symptoms may vary in intensity and include extreme weight loss, general debility, dry skin, bradycardia, hypotension, atrophy of the genitalia and breasts, and progress to premature senility.

Sheehan's syndrome is another form of panhypopituitarism, often with an insidious onset. This syndrome is caused by a pituitary infarction following complications of postpartum hemorrhage.[14,16,17] It is thought that the infarction may be caused by vascular spasms of the hypophyseal arteries, resulting in decreased blood flow to the pituitary, tissue hypoxia, and necrosis.[17] During pregnancy, the pituitary is slightly enlarged from an increased demand for hormones, causing an increased need for nutrients and oxygen to the pituitary cells. This may make it more susceptible to the hypoxia induced by the vascular spasm.[17] The first symptoms of Sheehan's syndrome are failure of lactation (decreased PRL) and postpartum amenorrhea (decreased FSH and LH).[16] The number of symptoms and the severity depend on the actual amount of pituitary tissue destroyed. Decreased TSH results in hypothyroidism (dry skin, hair becomes coarse, bradycardia, hypotension). Mineralocorticoids from the adrenal cortex are usually not affected by decreases in ACTH, so plasma sodium is generally normal. If the posterior as well as the anterior pituitary is damaged, the patient may also have diabetes insipidus. Women with poor prenatal care are more likely to develop Sheehan's syndrome. This syndrome is becoming a rare disorder largely because of improved prenatal care.

## HYPERPROLACTINEMIA

Excess secretion of PRL (>125 ng/mL) from the pituitary is often caused by a pituitary tumor. Although tumors are associated with hyperprolactinemia, other diseases such as acromegaly, hypothyroidism, and chronic renal failure can also induce it.[16] In women, hyperprolactinemia is associated with decreased concentrations of gonadotropins and estradiol. In these women, the PRL increase can cause continuous milk flow (galactorrhea) from the breast even though there is no nursing infant.[14] Along with the galactorrhea, the patient generally stops menstruating (amenorrhea). Transient high levels of PRL can be detected in normal women following vigorous exercise.[16]

Men who develop hyperprolactinemia may show enlargement of the breast tissue (gynecomastia). In addition, decreased function of the gonads (hypogonadism) may occur, leading to a decrease in testosterone production with atrophy of the testes.[16]

## SUMMARY

The hypothalamus is physically connected to the pituitary by means of the infundibulum. The neurosecretory cells of the hypothalamus produce a series of stimulating and inhibiting hormones and factors that act on the anterior pituitary to induce secretion of its hormones.

The pituitary is divided into two main lobes, the anterior pituitary and the posterior pituitary. The posterior pituitary produces no hormones but stores and releases two hormones produced by cells in the hypothalamus. The two hormones that are found in the posterior pituitary are oxytocin and ADH. Oxytocin is most active in pregnant women and induces contractions in the uterus and myoepithelial breast cells for milk release. ADH acts on the nephron tubules to increase reabsorption of water.

The anterior pituitary produces the hormones ACTH, FSH, PRL, GH, LH, TSH, and MSH. These hormones act on other endocrine glands throughout the body to cause many varied physiologic actions. PRL is involved in breast tissue growth and lactation. GH is structurally related to PRL and, as the name implies, is involved in total body growth. The action of GH on bone and cartilage is indirect and mediated by means of the somatomedins. FSH, LH, and TSH are the large glycoprotein hormones that are both similar and unique in structure. FSH and LH are called the gonadotropins and actively stimulate both the ovary and testes. TSH stimulates the thyroid gland to synthesize and secrete $T_3$ and $T_4$. ACTH is cleaved from a large precursor molecule. Its primary target tissue is the adrenal cortex, and it acts to stimulate the production of cortisol.

The endocrine disorders of the pituitary may involve the excess or deficiency of one hormone or multiple hormones. The cause of the disorder may be in the pituitary itself or the hypothalamus. Stimulation and inhibition tests are necessary to diagnose the actual site of the problem.

## REFERENCES

1. Guillemin R and Burgus R: The hormones of the hypothalamus. Sci Am 227:24–33, 1972.
2. Guillemin R: Physiological studies with somatocrinin, a growth hormone-releasing factor. Ann Rev Pharmacol Toxicol 25:463–485, 1985.
3. Ebels I, Benson B: A survey of the evidence that unidentified pineal substances affect the reproductive system in mammals. Prog Reprod Biol 4:51–89, 1978.
4. Holmes RL, Ball JN: The Pituitary Gland. Cambridge, England, Cambrige University Press, 1974.
5. Brownstein MJ, Russel JT, Gainer H: Synthesis, transport and release of posterior pituitary hormones. Science 207:273–278, 1980.
6. Whitlet R, Meikle AW, Watts NB: Endocrinology. In Burtis CA, Ashwood ER (eds.): Tietz Textbook of Clinical Chemistry. 2nd ed. Philadelphia, WB Saunders, 1994, p 1645.
7. Nicoll CS, Mayer GL, Russel SM: Structural features of prolactins and growth hormones that can be related to their biological activity. Endocr Rev 7:169–203, 1986.
8. Van Wyk JJ, Underwood LE: Growth hormone, somatomedins, and growth failure. In Kreiger DT, Hughes JC (eds.): Neuroendocrinology. Sunderland, MA, Sinauer Associates, 1980, p 299–309.
9. Spencer EM: Somatomedins. In Greenspan F (ed.): Basic and Clinical Endocrinology. 4th ed. Norwalk, CT, Appleton & Lange, 1991, p 133.
10. Aron DC, Findling JW, Tyrrell JB: Hypothalamus and pituitary. In Greenspan F, Gardner D (eds.): Basic and Clinical Endocrinology. 6th ed. Norwalk, CT, Appleton & Lange, 2001, p 100.
11. Escolas KM: Endocrinology. In Lehmann CA (ed.): Saunders Manual of Clinical Laboratory Science. Philadelphia, WB Saunders, 1998, pp 181–190.
12. Pierce JG, Parsons TF: Glycoprotein hormones: structure and function. Ann Rev Biochem 50:465–495, 1981.
13. Bondy PK: Disorders of the adrenal cortex. In Wilson JD, Foster DW (eds.): Williams Textbook of Endocrinology. 3rd ed. Philadelphia, WB Saunders, 1985, p 816.
14. Gornall AG, Luxton AW, Bhavnani BR: Endocrine disorders. In Gornall AG (ed.): Applied Biochemistry of Clinical Disorders. 2nd ed. Philadelphia, JB Lippincott, 1986, p 285.
15. Ramsey DJ: Posterior pituitary gland. In Greenspan F (ed.): Basic and Clinical Endocrinology. 4th ed. Norwalk, CT, Appleton & Lange, 1991, p 177.
16. Daughaday WH: The anterior pituitary. In Wilson JD, Foster DW (eds.): Williams Textbook of Endocrinology. 3rd ed. Philadelphia, WB Saunders, 1985, p 568.
17. Finding JW, Tyrrell JB: Anterior pituitary gland. In Greenspan F (ed.): Basic and Clincal Endocrinology. 4th ed. Norwalk, CT, Appleton & Lange, 1991, p 79.

# CHAPTER 27
# Thyroid Endocrinology

*Marcia H. Hicks*

The thyroid gland is an integral part of the body's endocrine system. Through the hormones it secretes, the thyroid exerts an effect on most organ systems and numerous metabolic processes.[1] The laboratory plays a major role in managing the patient with thyroid disease by providing methods for measuring thyroid hormone levels and other related analytes. Physicians rely heavily on the information derived from laboratory tests in both diagnosing and treating thyroid disease.

The contents of this chapter include basic thyroid anatomy, synthesis and release of thyroid hormones, and current testing methods. Also included are descriptions of the various disorders of the thyroid gland, their causes and symptoms, and the clinical applications of the information provided by the laboratory.

## THYROID ANATOMY

The thyroid gland is centered around the trachea at the level of the second and third cartilage rings and is held in position by loose connective tissue. It has a bilobular butterfly shape and is connected in the center by an isthmus. Often the right lobe is slightly larger than the left. In the adult, the thyroid gland weighs 15 to 25 g, is 3 to 5 cm long, and is reddish brown (Figure 27–1).

Microscopically, the thyroid consists of two types of cells, follicular and parafollicular. Follicular cells are arranged in spheres that average about 200 $\mu$m in diameter. Each sphere or follicle consists of a single layer of epithelial cells that have a more narrow apical end facing the interior of the follicle and a broader basal end facing the interstitium (Figure 27–2).[1,2]

The follicle is the fundamental structural unit of the thyroid gland. The follicular epithelial cells produce thyroglobulin, a glycoprotein with a molecular weight of about 660,000 daltons, which is then secreted into the interior of the spherical follicle. The central portion of each follicle is filled with a proteinaceous material known as colloid, which receives and stores thyroglobulin. It is within the follicular cells and the colloid that the thyroid hormones are formed.[1,2]

The area between the follicles, the interstitium, contains the blood supply and the parafollicular cells or C cells. The C cells are so named because they are responsible for secreting the hormone calcitonin, which is involved in calcium and phosphorus metabolism.[1]

## THYROID PHYSIOLOGY

### Physiologic Effects of Thyroid Hormones

The thyroid gland exerts influence over many organs and metabolic processes, including heat production and energy expenditure and most aspects of carbohydrate and lipid metabolism. Thyroid hormones also play a major role in growth, maturation, and sexual development. Some organ-specific effects include increased heart rate and increased gastrointestinal motility.[1–4] For a more extensive list of the effects of thyroid hormone, refer to Table 27–1.

### Synthesis of Thyroid Hormones

The thyroid regulates metabolism through the synthesis and secretion of triiodothyronine ($T_3$) and tetraiodothyronine ($T_4$) (Figure 27–3). The initial step leading to thyroid hormone synthesis is the trapping of iodide from the circulating blood. Iodine in the diet is essential and a deficiency will limit the rate of hormone formed and result in hypothyroidism. The iodide trap is an energy-dependent, active transport mechanism that removes iodide from the blood and pumps it into the cells of the thyroid follicle. The concentration of iodide within the follicle is about 25 times greater than in blood and can actually be much higher during maximum thyroid activity.[4,5]

Iodide is oxidized in the thyroid cells to iodine and attaches to the tyrosine residues of thyroglobulin. In this way, monoiodotyrosine (MIT) and diiodotyrosine (DIT) are formed. MIT and DIT are then enzymatically coupled to form $T_3$ and $T_4$.[2] These steps of thyroid synthesis take place primarily at the

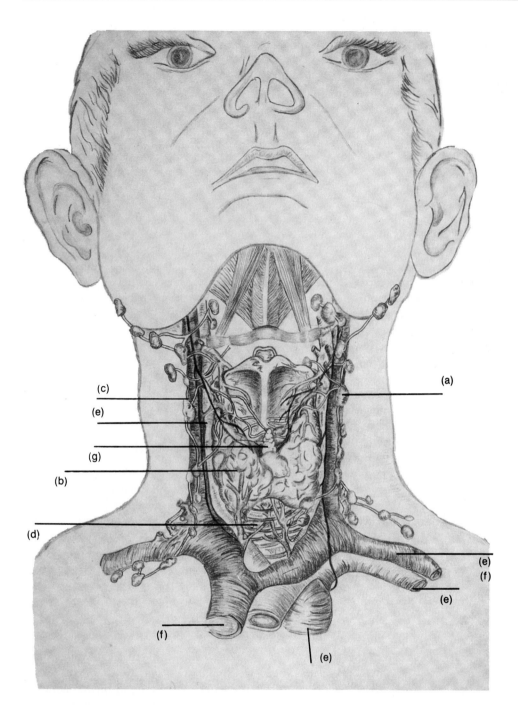

**FIGURE 27-1**

Anterior view of the thyroid gland and surrounding structures: **a.** lymphatic node, **b.** thyroid gland, **c.** nerves, **d.** trachea, **e.** arterial blood supply, **f.** venous blood supply, and **g.** pyramidal lobe.

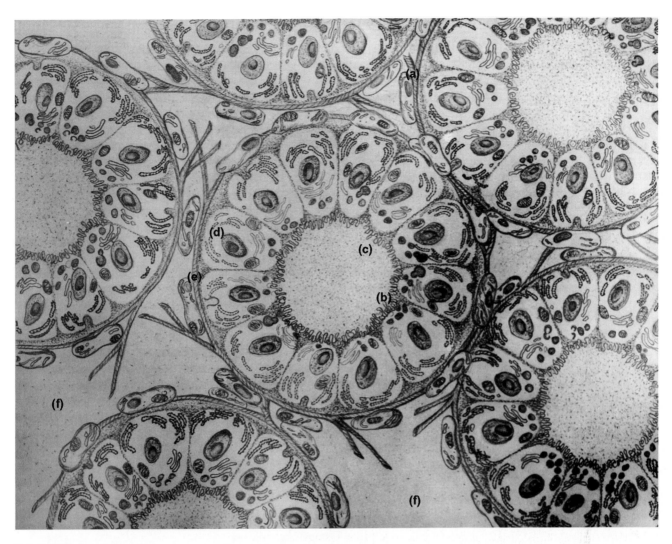

**FIGURE 27-2**

Thyroid gland structure: **a.** thyroid follicle; **b.** follicular cell, apical side; colloid-filled lumen; **d.** follicular cell, basal side; **e.** capillary plexus; **f.** interfollicular spaces.

interface between the follicular cell membrane and the colloid. Thyroglobulin not only serves as a contributor to thyroid hormone synthesis but also provides a storage mechanism, since the newly formed $T_3$ and $T_4$ remain attached to the thyroglobulin molecule and are stored in the colloid until they are ready for release into the blood.[2-5] Figure 27–4 is a schematic depiction of this thyroid hormone synthesis.

## Release and Transport

In response to stimulation by the pituitary, the peptide bonds between the tyrosine residues of thyroglobulin are enzymatically cleaved. $T_3$ and $T_4$ are released from the thyroglobulin and diffuse back through the follicular cell into the circulation as needed. MIT and DIT remain in the follicle, are broken down, and become an endogenous source of iodine for future hormone synthesis.[4,5]

$T_4$, also commonly known as thyroxine, is the major hormonal product of the thyroid gland. It is released in an amount 10 times greater than is $T_3$. However, once $T_4$ enters the blood and reaches peripheral tissues, a portion deiodinates to become $T_3$. The primary site for deiodination is the liver, and to a lesser extent, other tissues as well. Most of the circulating $T_3$ is produced by this process rather than through thyroid synthesis. Of the two hormones, $T_3$ is the more biologically potent, 3 to 5 times more active than $T_4$, although the functions of both

**TABLE 27–1**

**Basic Physiologic Effects of Thyroid Hormones and Their Relationship with Syndromes of Thyroid Dysfunction\***

| | | USUAL SYMPTOMS | |
| SYSTEM | THYROID HORMONE EFFECTS | HYPERTHYROIDISM | HYPOTHYROIDISM |
| --- | --- | --- | --- |
| Metabolic | Increased calorigenesis and O$_2$ consumption<br>Increased heat dissipation<br>Increased protein catabolism<br>Increased glucose absorption and production (gluconeogenesis)<br>Increased glucose use | Heat intolerance<br>Flushed skin<br>Increased perspiration<br>Increased appetite and food ingestion<br>Muscle wasting, proximal weakness<br>Weight loss<br>Onycholysis (nail disease)<br>Lid lag<br>Proptosis (exophthalmos) | Cold intolerance<br>Dry, pale skin<br>Coarse skin<br>Lethargy<br>Generalized weakness<br>Weight gain<br>Voice coarsening, slow speech<br>Myxedema |
| Cardiovascular | Increased adrenergic activity and sensitivity<br>Increased heart rate<br>Increased myocardial contractility (inotropy)<br>Increased cardiac output<br>Increased blood volume<br>Decreased peripheral vascular resistance | Palpitations<br>Tachycardia<br>Bouncy, hyperdynamic arterial pulses<br><br>Shortness of breath<br>Atrial fibrillation<br>Widened pulse pressure | Bradycardia<br>Low blood pressure<br>Heart failure<br>Heart enlargement |
| Central nervous | Increased adrenergic activity and sensitivity | Restlessness, hypermotility<br><br>Nervousness<br>Emotional lability<br>Fatigue<br>Exaggerated reflexes<br>Tremor | Apathy<br>Mental sluggishness<br>Depressed reflexes<br>Mental retardation |
| Gastrointestinal | Increased motility | Hyperdefecation | Constipation |

\*From Lucas MH, Fernadez-Ulloa M: Thyroid. In Kaplan LA, Pesce AA (eds.): *Clinical Chemistry, Theory, Analysis, Correlation.* 3rd ed. St Louis, MO, Mosby, 1996, p 878.

hormones seem to be identical. Deiodination of T$_4$ can also result in the formation of reverse T$_3$ (rT$_3$), a biologically inactive stereoisomer of T$_3$ (Figure 27–5).[4,5]

Once the thyroid hormones are released into the circulation, they immediately become bound to transport proteins. These proteins include thyroxine-binding globulin (TBG), thyroxine-binding prealbumin (TBPA), and albumin. So strong is the affinity between the hormone and the carrier protein that over 99% of T$_3$ and T$_4$ (99.7% and 99.97%, respectively) are bound, leaving only a minute amount of free hormone that can participate in biologic activity. This tight binding allows for a very slow rate of release of hormone to target tissues.[4,5]

## Regulation and Feedback

The synthesis and release of thyroid hormones is very tightly controlled by a complex feedback mechanism involving the hypothalamus, the pituitary, and the thyroid. Thyrotropin-releasing hormone (TRH) is produced by the hypothalamus and stimulates the pituitary to release thyroid-stimulating hormone (TSH), also known as thyrotropin. As the concentration of free hormone in the blood decreases, TRH responds by increasing pituitary release of TSH, which in turn acts to stimulate the thyroid to increase the synthesis of T$_3$ and T$_4$. Increased levels of thyroid hormones depress the release of TSH. This feedback system, known as the hypothalamic-

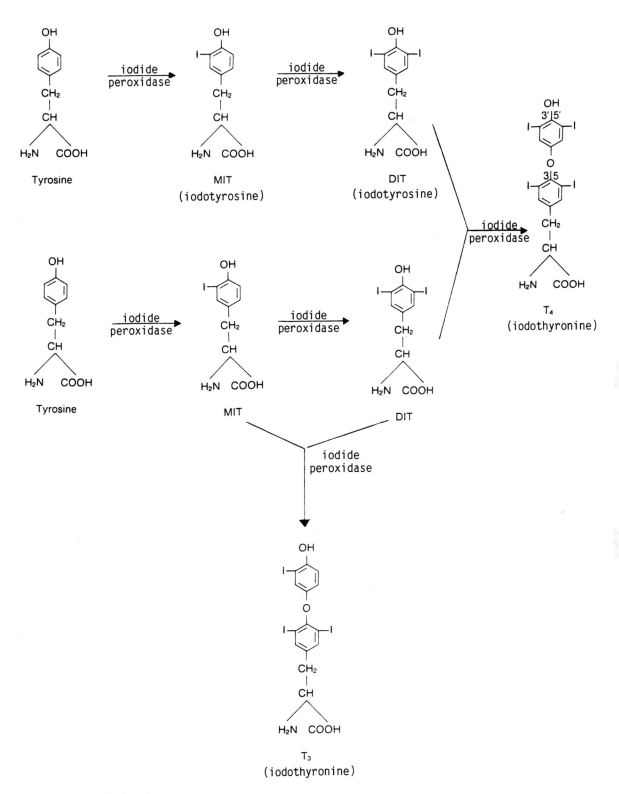

**FIGURE 27-3**

The formation of iodotyrosine and iodothyronine. Sequential iodination of tyrosine forming monoiodotyrosine (MIT) and diiodotyrosine (DIT) is catalyzed by thyroid peroxidase. Coupling iodotyrosines forming iodothyronines, T₃ and T₄ are also catalyzed by thyroid peroxidase.

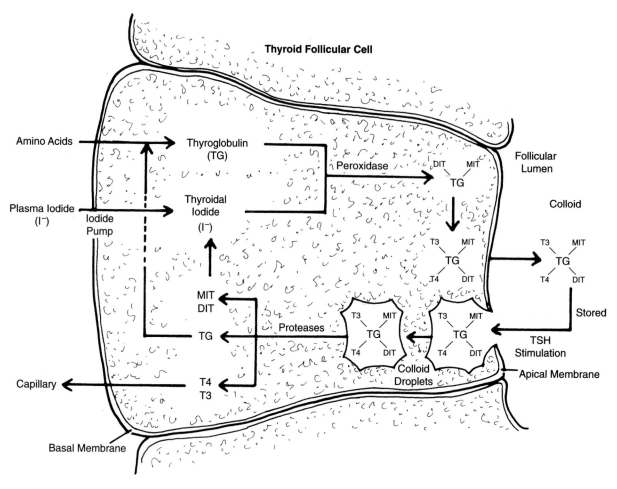

**FIGURE 27-4**

Pathway of thyroid hormone synthesis and storage within and release from the follicle.

pituitary-thyroid axis, helps to ensure that circulating levels of thyroid hormone are adequate at all times (Figure 27–6).[3–5]

TSH, a glycoprotein hormone secreted by the anterior pituitary, is the chief regulator of thyroid hormone synthesis. It increases all known activities of the thyroid gland. It causes an increase in the size and number of follicular cells so they can trap more iodide to synthesize more hormone, and it accelerates breakdown of thyroglobulin, thereby increasing the release of thyroid hormone into the circulation. If TSH levels remain elevated for various reasons over an extended period, the results are increased vascularity and hypertrophy of the thyroid tissue, a condition known as goiter.[4,5]

## THYROID FUNCTION TESTING

The many thyroid function tests available today make selection and interpretation of these assays confusing and often difficult. The rapidly advancing technological developments are chang-

ing the rationale for evaluating thyroid status. Ideally, thyroid function tests should accurately reflect thyroid peripheral hormone concentration. However, the interrelationships between thyroid hormone synthesis, secretion, and protein binding and other conditions such as pregnancy, malnutrition, and chronic illness, complicate the laboratory diagnosis of thyroid disease.

## Thyroid-Stimulating Hormone

Synthesis and release of thyroid hormone from thyroglobulin in the thyroid gland is regulated by thyroid-stimulating hormone (TSH), which is produced in the pituitary. The pituitary is under positive stimulation by TRH, which is produced in the hypothalamus and under negative feedback by circulating thyroid hormone. The effect of TSH on the thyroid is to increase the production and release of $T_4$ from thyroglobulin, which in turn is converted to $T_3$ at the peripheral tissue.

Blood levels of TSH are significantly elevated in primary hypothyroidism and $T_4$ and $T_3$ levels are low. If the TSH remains low or low normal in the presence of decreased thyroid

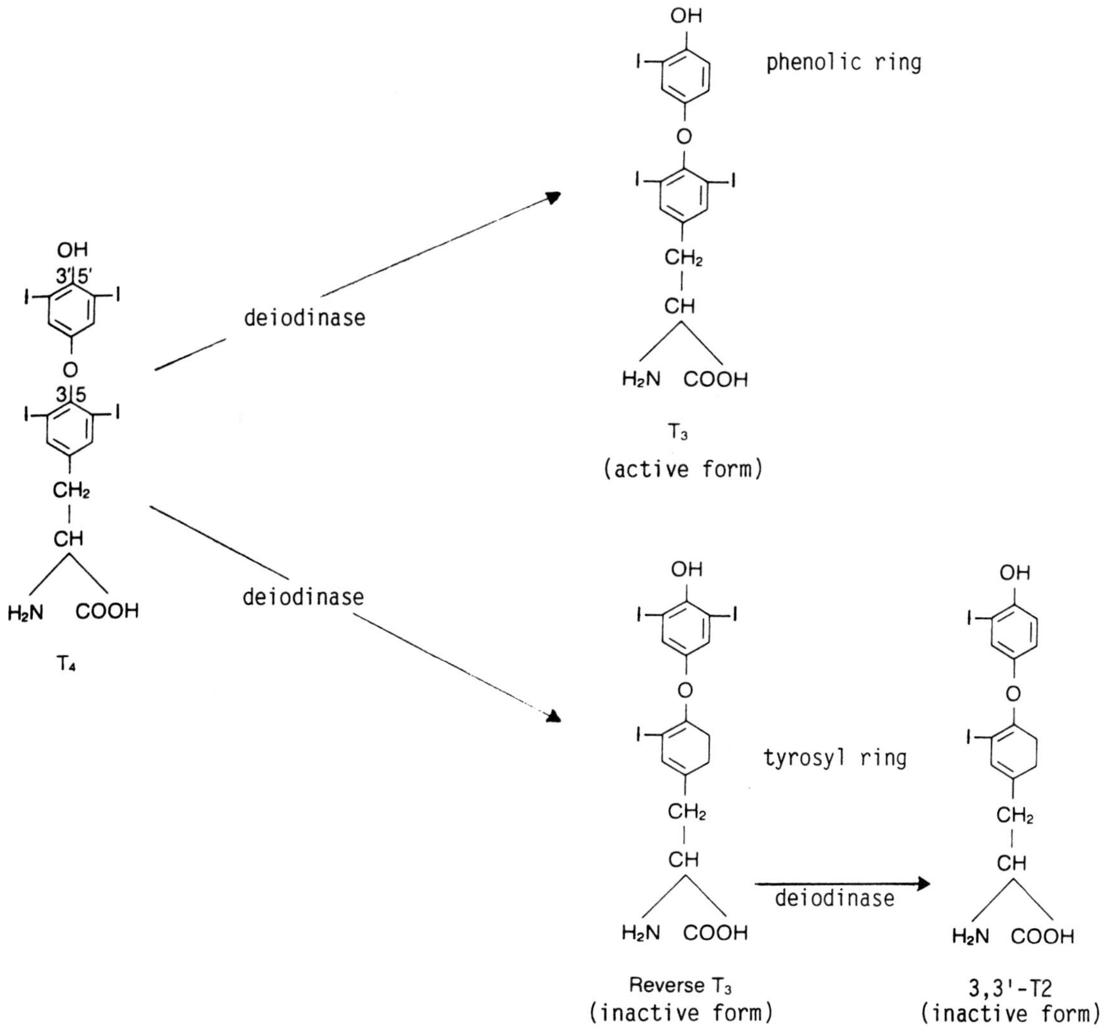

**FIGURE 27-5**

Deiodination of $T_4$ by deiodinases forming $T_3$ (phenolic ring) or $rT_3$ (tyrosyl ring) with further deiodination of $rT_3$ to 3,3'-$T_2$.

hormone, a pituitary malfunction is usually suspected. This condition is known as secondary hypothyroidism. Increased TRH fails to stimulate the production of TSH and thyroid hormone secretion is suppressed. Conversely, the elevated $T_4$ and $T_3$ of hyperthyroidism suppress pituitary production of TSH and blood levels become decreased.[6]

The advent of immunoassay technology made it possible to measure TSH levels in the blood, and immunoassays remain the standard for TSH testing in the laboratory. Older radioimmunoassay (RIA) methods were able to detect TSH in normal to elevated ranges but lacked sufficient sensitivity to accurately quantitate this hormone at the abnormally low levels associated with hyperthyroidism. With hormone testing in general, there has been a shift away from RIA toward nonisotopic immunoassay methods such as enzyme immunoassays and chemiluminescence.[3,7] These newer technologies allow for rapid, sensitive analyses that are easily automated. The devel-

opment of such nonisotopic tests for TSH has greatly improved sensitivity in the lower ranges. With each generation of TSH testing, accuracy at lower and lower levels is achieved. RIA represents the first generation of methods that have a detection limit of between 1 and 2 mU/L. Second-generation assays are referred to as immunometric immunoassays and have an improved sensitivity with a detection limit of 0.1 to 0.2 mU/L. TSH methods with such low detection limits are called sensitive TSH or sTSH assays. Further advances in technology have resulted in the development of third- and fourth-generation TSH testing. They employ chemiluminescence and time-resolved fluorescence and have a detection limit of 0.01 to 0.02 mU/L.[3,4,6,8]

Immunometric assays of later generation tests use a double-antibody sandwich technique. The first antibody binds to a portion of the beta subunit of the TSH molecule and the second antibody binds to a different site, often on the alpha

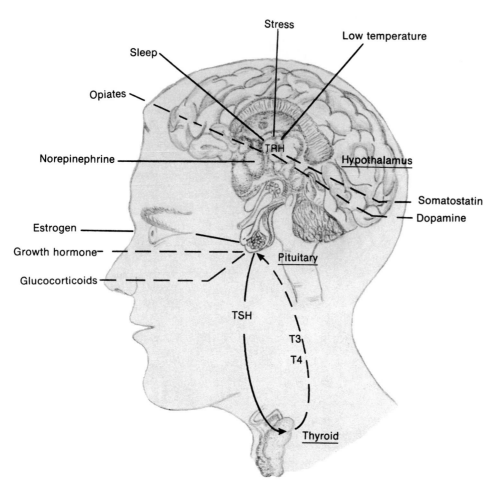

**FIGURE   27-6**

Compounds affecting feedback regulation of the hypothalamic-pituitary-thyroid axis.
Solid arrows show stimulation; dashed lines indicate inhibition.

subunit portion. The result is an extremely sensitive and specific method (Figure 27–7).[9]

Because of the increase in sensitivity at very low levels, sTSH has revolutionized the diagnosis of hyperthyroidism and has become the test of choice for initial diagnosis of thyroid dysfunction.[10,11] TSH levels are also useful for monitoring patients who are receiving levothyroxine ($T_4$) or levotriiodothyronine ($T_3$) for hypothyroidism.[3,6]

## Thyroxine

Measuring the amount of circulating thyroid hormone, particularly thyroxine ($T_4$), has for many years been used to help diagnose thyroid disease. Typically, $T_4$ is elevated in overt hyperthyroidism and depressed in overt hypothyroidism. The difficulty in using $T_4$ to accurately assess thyroid function is that approximately 99.97% is bound to transport proteins. Until recently, the most practical way to measure thyroxine was to perform a **total $T_4$** (TT$_4$). Total $T_4$ assays detect both the $T_4$ bound to protein and the free, biologically active $T_4$. Thyroid-binding globulin (TBG) and other thyroid-binding proteins

can vary greatly in their concentration. Total $T_4$ measurements reflect TBG concentrations, and thereby often provide incorrect information regarding actual thyroid status[2,12] (Table 27–2). However, $T_4$ abnormalities attributed to alterations in binding proteins are, for the most part, mild,[11] and TT$_4$ is still used extensively in many laboratories as an aid to thyroid function assessment.

Assays for TT$_4$ employ nonisotopic immunoassays such as fluorescence polarization immunoassay (FPIA) and chemiluminescence.[8,12,13] A typical reference range for TT$_4$ is 5 to 12 $\mu$g/dL.

Although **free thyroxine** (FT$_4$) is present as a very small fraction of total $T_4$ (only 0.02% of total), it is a much better indicator of thyroid status than is total $T_4$. It is the free $T_4$ that can enter cells and undergo conversion to the metabolically potent $T_3$. Serum free $T_4$ concentration is elevated in approximately 95% of ambulatory hyperthyroid patients. A clinically suspected diagnosis of thyrotoxicosis can be confirmed by an elevated FT$_4$ with a suppressed sTSH result.

Until recently, there were no simple methods for the assay of FT$_4$. Typically, laboratories would (and still do) measure a

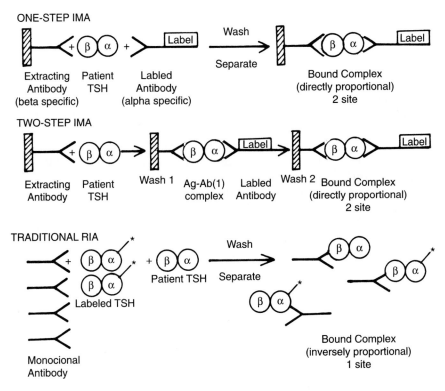

ONE-STEP IMA

Extracting Antibody (beta specific) + Patient TSH + Labled Antibody (alpha specific) → Wash / Separate → Bound Complex (directly proportional) 2 site

TWO-STEP IMA

Extracting Antibody + Patient TSH → Wash 1 → Ag-Ab(1) complex + Labled Antibody → Wash 2 → Bound Complex (directly proportional) 2 site

TRADITIONAL RIA

Monoclonal Antibody + Labeled TSH + Patient TSH → Wash / Separate → Bound Complex (inversely proportional) 1 site

**FIGURE 27-7**

Immunometric assay (IMA) and radioimmunoassay (RIA) for TSH. (From: Taylor CS, Brandt DR: Developments in thyroid-stimulating hormone testing: the pursuit of improved sensitivity. Lab Med 24:337, 1994.)

TABLE 27-2

**Factors That Alter Thyroxine-Binding-Globulin (TBG) Levels***

| INCREASE | DECREASE |
|---|---|
| Pregnancy | Cushing's syndrome |
| Neonatal period | Corticosteroids |
| Estrogen replacement therapy | Androgens |
| Oral contraceptives | Anabolic steroids |
| Chronic active hepatitis | Acromegaly |
| Porphyria | Nephrotic syndrome |
| Hydatidiform mole | Cirrhosis |
| Heroin or methadone abuse | Malnutrition |
| Clofibrate | L-asparaginase therapy |

*Based on data from Kaplan LA, Pesce AJ (eds.): *Clinical Chemistry: Theory, Analysis, Correlation.* 3rd ed. St. Louis, MO, 1996, pp 1108–1123; Madeddu G et al: Clinical and laboratory assessment of subclinical thyroid disease. Rays 24:229–242, 1999, Camacho PM, Dwarkanathan AA: Sick euthyroid syndrome. What to do when thyroid function tests are abnormal in critically ill patients. Postgrad Med 105:215–219, 1999.

total $T_4$ and a T-uptake, and combine these numbers in a calculation known as a free thyroxine index, or $FT_4I$ (see expanded description in section on estimation of free thyroid hormone), which would normalize the $T_4$ to account for alterations in TBG concentration.[14] Equilibrium dialysis, a complex and impractical method, was the first used to measure free thyroxine. It is still considered to be the reference method for this analyte, even though it is not routinely used in the laboratory.[3]

Newer assays have been developed for the measurement of $FT_4$ that are faster and easier and offer a sensitive indication of true thyroxine levels that are free from the effects of variations in TBG concentration. More and more physicians have begun using these determinations as a replacement for older methods that are actually estimations of free $T_4$ based on calculated values.[11] These new assays employ nonisotopic immunoassays such as microparticle enzyme immunoassay (MEIA) and chemiluminescence. Reference ranges for $FT_4$ differ slightly among laboratories, but typically fall between 0.8 and 1.8 ng/dL.[13–15]

## Triiodothyronine ($T_3$)

**Total $T_3$** is primarily useful in evaluating suspected thyrotoxicosis in which the $FT_4$ is normal. Elevated $T_3$, in this case, in the absence of increased TBG, is diagnostic of $T_3$ thyrotoxicosis.

$T_3$ is useful in diagnosing mild hyperthyroidism because $T_3$ rises earlier and more markedly than does $T_4$ in all common forms of hyperthyroidism. Clinicians typically use $T_3$ to monitor patients receiving sodium liothyronine. This assay is of little clinical usefulness in evaluating hypothyroidism.

Methods for measuring $TT_3$ are similar to those used for $TT_4$ and include enzyme immunoassays (MEIA) and chemiluminescence. Reference ranges are approximately 80 to 180 ng/dL[16,17]

The measurement of **free $T_3$** ($FT_3$) is of limited value in the evaluation of hypothyroidism; it is primarily used as a confirmation test in hyperthyroidism, especially in $T_3$ thyrotoxicosis. Free $T_3$, correlating well with total $T_3$, may offer the advantage of not being affected by changes in TBG, but it depends on the methodology of the assay. Methods of measurement include RIA and chemiluminescence and the reference range is 1.4 to 4.4 pg/mL.

**Reverse $T_3$** ($rT_3$) is a metabolically inactive isomer of $T_3$ and is present in serum almost entirely as a result of generation from $T_4$ in peripheral tissues. Removal of iodide from an inner phenyl ring of thyroxine produces $rT_3$, whereas iodide removal from an outer ring produces the metabolically active $T_3$. Elevated $rT_3$ levels are seen in patients with severe systemic illness as a result of decreased conversion of $T_4$ to $T_3$ as well as inhibition of $T_3$ degradation. Because the amount of $T_4$ is a major factor in $rT_3$ concentration, $rT_3$ is elevated in hyperthyroidism and low in hypothyroidism. Reverse $T_3$ can be measured in serum using radioimmunoassay.[13] In clinical practice, however, rT is seldom used.

## Estimation of Free Thyroid Hormone

The free thyroid hormones are present in serum in relatively constant concentrations that are independent of variations in thyroxine-binding proteins (TBPs). The free and bound portions of these hormones exist in a reversible equilibrium. Diagnostically, it is important to determine whether changes in the total hormone levels are a result of alterations in the free hormone secretion or alterations in TBPs.[4]

The **thyroid hormone-binding ratio** (THBR) is the test formerly known as the resin $T_3$ uptake. As a result of confusion between this and the $T_3$ (total triiodothyronine) assay, the Committee on Nomenclature of the American Thyroid Association recommended in May 1987 that assays such as the resin $T_3$ uptake test be termed *thyroid hormone-binding ratio assays*. The test was originally named for one of the reagents used, radiolabeled $T_3$. It was designed to reflect the unsaturated binding capacity of the thyroid hormone carrier proteins, primarily TBG. This assay is a correction method designed to more accurately reflect thyroid function in conditions in which there are variations in the level of TBG. The THBR value varies inversely with changes in TBG.

The resin $T_3$ uptake test has been replaced by the more recent (nonisotopic) T uptake. T uptake is a fluorescence polarization immunoassay method that utilizes a fluorescein-label $T_4$ tracer, which binds to the serum thyroxine-binding proteins. The Abbott T-uptake assay shows a linear relationship between T-uptake units and unsaturated thyroxine-binding protein concentrations. Serum with high unsaturated TBP concentration takes up more $T_4$ tracer, resulting in increased net polarization. Patients with either increased serum thyroxine or low serum TBG levels have lower T-uptake levels than normal.[18]

The **free thyroxine index ($FT_4I$)** is a calculation used for the purpose of normalizing the total $T_4$ and the THBR values in the presence of protein alterations. Multiplication of the total $T_4$ by the THBR provides an index of effective free $T_4$ concentrations independent of changes in protein binding. Note that it is not a true $FT_4$ value but that it is only an index of this measurement.

$$FT_4I = TT_4 \times THBR/100$$

This method for the indirect estimate of free thyroxine levels provides results that are fairly comparable to those produced by more direct measurements in most patients, the exception being those with severe alterations in binding proteins.[4] A free $T_3$ index can also be calculated to estimate circulating free $T_3$.

## Thyroid Hormone-Binding Proteins

Alterations in thyroid hormone-binding proteins affect total but not free concentrations of $T_4$ and $T_3$. Use of the estimation method, $FT_4I$, together with a free $T_4$ determination, demonstrates this effect. However, in patients with large changes in TBG because of such conditions as acute liver disease or congenital abnormalities, it may be necessary to directly measure the binding protein by RIA or immunoenzymatic assay. Electrophoresis is useful in studying aberrant binding proteins such as abnormal forms of albumin and prealbumin. This methodology is particularly useful in diagnosing familial dysalbuminemic hyperthyroxinemia. This syndrome is characterized by elevations in serum thyroxine and $FT_4I$. These elevations are from an albumin that has an abnormal binding site with a much greater affinity for thyroxine compared to triiodothyronine. It is important to differentiate this syndrome, a euthyroid (normal) state, from hyperthyroidism with which it is confused.

## Thyroglobuin

Thyroglobulin (Tg), the storage form of the thyroid hormone precursors, is measured primarily in the monitoring of patients with follicular or papillary thyroid cancer. Injury to the thyroid gland, as occurs in these malignancies, results in leakage of thyroglobulin from the follicle into the patient's serum. It is a useful tumor marker, if present, and reflects recurrence or remission of the primary disease.

Thyroglobulin levels are increased with stimulation by TSH, thyroid-stimulating immunoglobulin (TSI$_g$), TRH, or human chorionic gonadotropin (hCG). Tg is the last parameter to normalize after thyrotoxicosis, and is therefore useful in resolving thyroid history in the presence of normal T$_4$ and T$_3$ with clinical symptoms consistent with recent thyrotoxicosis. Tg may also be useful in differentiating subacute thyroiditis, in which elevated levels of Tg are present, from thyrotoxicosis factitia, which is characterized by low Tg.

Before a thyroglobulin assay is performed on a patient's serum, the sample must be screened for the presence of anti-thyroglobulin antibodies, which can interfere with the method and yield inaccurate results. If the antibody screen is positive, the Tg analysis should not be performed. Patients who are to receive a thyroglobulin test and are taking thyroid hormone replacement therapy should discontinue their medication for approximately 6 weeks prior to the testing. The time interval should be long enough to produce an elevated TSH. Measurements of thyroglobulin are most sensitive for detecting recurrent thyroid cancer if patients are free of the effects of thyroid hormone replacement therapy. Thyroglobulin can be measured by chemiluminescence. A typical reference range is 10 to 40 ng/mL; athyroidic patients are usually <10 ng/mL.[4,13]

## Thyroid Antibodies

Detecting the presence of thyroid antibodies in sera is important both for the purpose of confirming or ruling out autoimmune disease as well as evaluating their possible interference in assays of their respective antigens. T$_4$ and T$_3$ autoantibodies are particularly useful in explaining FT$_4$, T$_4$, and T$_3$ results that are conflicting with clinical evaluation. Thyroid microsomal antibodies (TMAb) are present in about 95% of patients with Hashimoto's thyroiditis and in 85% of those with Graves' disease. Antithyroglobulin antibodies (TgAb) are found in 60% of patients with Hashimoto's thyroiditis and in 30% of patients with Graves' disease. The presence of antithyroid antibodies, however, does not give exact information about thyroid function. Titers of these antibodies are usually low in subacute thyroiditis. The presence of both TMAb and TgAb may be of value as a predictor of outcome of antithyroid drug therapy in patients with Graves' disease because patients with both antibodies were found least likely to relapse. TSH receptor antibodies (TRAb), also known as thyroid-stimulating immunoglobulins (TSIg), are of limited clinical use, although they have clarified the pathophysiology of Graves' disease substantially. Methods for detecting TMAb and TgAb are hemagglutination tests in which erythrocytes that have been coated with either Tg or microsomes agglutinate when the respective antibody is present. Commercial kits are available that provide a more sensitive measurement and include RIA and enzyme-linked immunosorbent assays (ELISA).[5,13]

More recently, tests for antithyroid peroxidase antibodies have been developed. These tests take advantage of the discovery that thyroid peroxidase (TPO) is the main autoantigenic component of microsomes. Anti-TPO test methods are much more sensitive and specific than the hemagglutination assays and lend themselves better to high-volume testing. They include RIA, ELISA, and more recently chemiluminescence.[5,13]

## TRH Stimulation Test

The TRH stimulation test takes advantage of the extreme sensitivity of TSH secretion to the feedback mechanism of the hypothalamus-pituitary-thyroid axis. This test can detect abnormalities before thyroid hormone concentrations are outside their reference ranges. It is useful in distinguishing between pituitary and hypothalamic hypothyroidism and in confirming mild hyperthyroidism in patients whose free T$_3$ and T$_4$ results are equivocal and yet whose other clinical findings are suggestive of thyrotoxicosis.

The TRH stimulation test is performed by injecting 200 to 500 $\mu$g of synthetic TRH after determining a baseline TSH level. Typical serum drawing times for TSH determination are 15, 30, and 60 minutes. A flat response is seen in hyperthyroidism because elevated levels of T$_4$ and T$_3$ override additional stimulation of the pituitary by TRH. A flat response differentiates hypothyroidism secondary to hypopituitarism from hypothalamic hypothyroidism in which a delayed peak is seen. The augmented response seen in primary hypothyroidism provides little additional information from that derived from the combination of an elevated sTSH and decreased FT$_4$. The sTSH, which can discriminate the undetectable levels of TSH found in overt and subclinical hyperthyroidism from those found in euthyroid individuals, makes the TRH stimulation test redundant for this evaluation. The test is invasive with side effects such as headache, nausea, chest tightness, and mild hypotension. It is also time consuming.

## Specimen Requirements

Serum is the specimen of choice for the thyroid tests mentioned in this section. The patient need not be fasting. The analytes are stable at refrigerator temperature for up to 4 days. If testing is delayed for longer periods, freezing is required to ensure stability. Upon thawing, specimens should be mixed well; repeated cycles of freezing and thawing should be avoided.[13]

## CLINICAL APPLICATIONS

## Hyperthyroidism

Hyperthyroidism refers to a variety of conditions characterized by an increase in circulating thyroid hormone, both free and total. Hyperthyroidism can be overt, with clinical symptoms that are readily apparent, or subclinical. Subclinical hyperthyroidism is asymptomatic and can be detected by performing serum thyroid function testing. Such testing typically shows normal thyroid hormone levels with a decreased sTSH. Identifying subclinical hyperthyroidism is important because patients with this condition are at increased risk for atrial fibrillation, osteoporosis and eventual development of overt disease. At particular risk are women older than age 50. sTSH has a very high negative predictive value and therefore is the test of choice when screening for subclinical thyroid disease. Thyroid screening, however, is not recommended for the general population. Exceptions include those populations considered to be at risk for developing thyroid disease, including older women and newborns. The causes of subclinical hyperthyroidism are the same as for overt disease.[3,19–21]

Overt hyperthyroidism is associated with elevated free and total $T_4$ and $T_3$ accompanied by a markedly decreased sTSH. **Thyrotoxicosis** is the term used to describe the condition that occurs when excessive amounts of thyroid hormones in circulation affect peripheral tissue. Hyperthyroidism has several known causes and the symptoms include decreased weight with normal appetite, nervousness, sweating, palpitations, heat intolerance, and muscle weakness. The patient may also have clinical signs such as enlarged thyroid (goiter), eyelid retraction, and tremor.[3,8]

**Thyroid storm** is the term used to describe the state of thyroid crises that a patient with thyrotoxicosis may experience that requires emergency treatment. Thyroid storm may occur following an infection, childbirth, diabetic ketoacidosis, the withdrawal of antithyroid drugs, the therapeutic use of radioiodine [131]I, or surgical treatment in the thyrotoxic patient. The effects of a sudden increase in circulating thyroid hormones result in a spectrum of metabolic responses. Symptoms include tachycardia, heart failure, high fever, nausea and vomiting, neurologic and psychiatric disorders, and coma. If left untreated, thyroid storm can be fatal in 70% to 80% of cases.[8,22]

Diagnosis of hyperthyroidism depends both on clinical and laboratory evaluations. Figure 27–8 represents a pathway for diagnosis of hyperthyroidism using laboratory testing. A significantly subnormal sTSH and elevated $FT_4$ are confirmatory. Thyroid antibody testing can aid in differentiation between various conditions. A $T_3$ or $FT_3$ determination may be necessary to follow up a subnormal sTSH found in conjunction with a normal $FT_4$. An elevated $T_3$ or $FT_3$ value in this case would suggest $T_3$ thyrotoxicosis.

Once a diagnosis of hyperthyroidism is made, it then becomes necessary to determine the cause. The causative factors

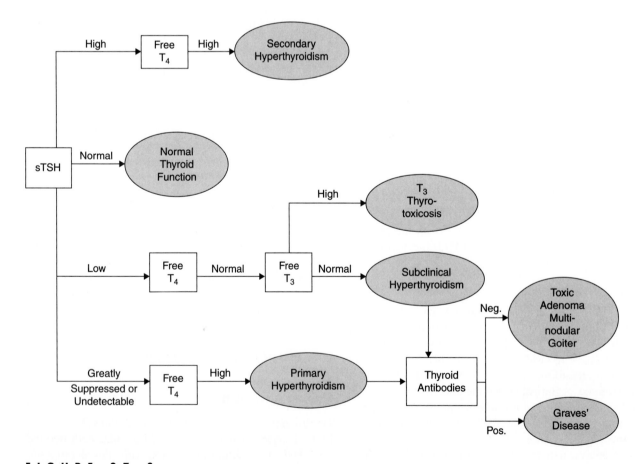

**FIGURE 27-8**

Pathway for laboratory diagnosis of hyperthyroidism, starting with sTSH.

of hyperthyroidism may be divided into three general categories: diseases caused by excess thyroid stimulators, primary thyroid disease, and disorders that result from iatrogenic and factitious causes.[11,22,23]

## EXCESS THYROID STIMULATORS

Graves' disease is the most common cause of hyperthyroidism and occurs 10 times more often in women than in men. All ages and racial groups are affected but the typical age of onset is between 30 and 50 years. Diagnosis of Graves' disease is based on a combination of laboratory test results and physical signs and symptoms. There is a classic triad of symptoms associated with Graves' disease: hyperthyroidism, goiter, and exophthalmos (bulging eyes) that is unique to this condition, and the presence of these signs aids in diagnosis. However, the symptoms are not always present and may vary with the severity of the disease, so a definite diagnosis may be difficult to make. To further complicate matters, there are other disorders that may mimic some of the manifestations of Graves' disease. They include anxiety neurosis, menopause, pheochromocytoma, drug abuse, or other forms of thyrotoxicosis.[11]

Graves' disease, also called toxic diffuse goiter, is an autoimmune disorder with a strong hereditary component. T lymphocytes respond to certain antigens within the thyroid and in turn stimulate the production of thyroid-stimulating immunoglobulin (TSIg) by the B lymphocytes. TSIg (formerly called long-acting thyroid stimulator, LATS) is an IgG that binds tightly to TSH receptors on the follicular cell membranes. TSIg mimics TSH and causes the thyroid to increase the synthesis and release of $T_4$. However, it is not regulated by normal feedback mechanisms, and therefore is not inhibited by increased circulating thyroid hormone. The result is constant thyroid activity and excessive production of hormone, growth in size and number of thyroid follicles, increased blood supply, and enlarged gland (goiter).[5,23] It is possible that numerous tissues (thyroid, eye muscles, and skin) have similar antigenic properties and are therefore subject to the same autoimmune response. This could account for the eye and skin changes that typically accompany Graves' disease.[23]

Exophthalmos is a condition frequently seen in Graves' disease (Figure 27–9). Because of the infiltration by leukocytes of the eye muscles, the eyeballs bulge forward and may actually protrude from the socket. Exophthalmos can be present in varying degrees of severity, or may be absent.[11,22,23] Other eye signs (over 23 have been documented) can also be found in Graves' disease.

Diagnostic confirmation in patients without typical symptoms can be made by the detection of antithyroid antibodies in the serum. Elevated TSIg or thyroid peroxidase antibodies (TPOAb) titers are suggestive of Graves' disease.[5,11] Treatments include medication that inhibits TSH, destruction of thyroid tissue with radiation, and surgical removal of the gland.

Two types of Graves' disease of the newborn may occur in infants born to mothers who have Graves' disease. The first form results from high levels of maternal TSIg that are passed

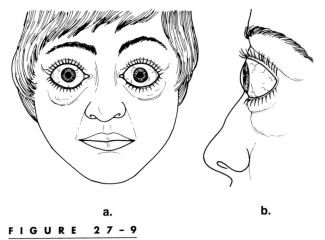

**a.**                                          **b.**

**FIGURE 27-9**

Exophthalmos in patient with Graves' disease.
**a.** frontal, **b.** lateral.

to the infant across the placenta. In contrast to normally elevated levels of TSH at birth, infants with Graves' disease have suppressed levels. This disease is self-limited, and the infant gradually becomes euthyroid as the TSIg levels subside.[24]

The second form of Graves' disease of the newborn is characterized by slower onset of symptoms and persistent brain dysfunction. This form, requiring prolonged therapy, may be caused by genetic inheritance of endogenous TSIg production.[24]

Excessive stimulation of the thyroid by TSH or by hormones similar in structure to TSH is another cause of hyperthyroidism. TSH-producing pituitary adenoma is a very rare cause of endogenous excess thyroid stimulation. Trophoblastic tumors such as hydatidiform mole and choriocarcinoma secrete excessive HCG. Because such high circulating levels are present, HCG, which is a weak thyroid stimulator because of the alpha subunit similarity, can cause hyperstimulation of the thyroid, resulting in thyrotoxicosis.

## PRIMARY THYROID DISEASE

Although Graves' disease is the most frequent cause of hyperthyroidism, the second most common cause is toxic nodular goiter, which involves hypersecretion of thyroid hormones from one or more nodules within the thyroid gland. This autonomous activity of the nodules causes suppression of pituitary TSH. Symptoms include those that are typical for hyperthyroidism, generally milder than with Graves' disease; ophthalmopathy is rare in this condition.[5] Laboratory findings include elevated $T_3$ and somewhat elevated $T_4$. Toxic adenoma (Plummer's disease) falls under this category and generally affects individuals older than age 40.

Hyperthyroid phases occur in both subacute thyroiditis and painless lymphocytic thyroiditis. In subacute thyroiditis, hyperthyroidism results from follicular rupture and leakage of large amounts of stored hormone into the circulation. (Refer to the thyroiditis section for more information.) In rare cases, thyroid carcinoma of the follicular type with widespread metastases can cause thyrotoxicosis. (See section on neoplasms, follicular.)

## IATROGENIC AND FACTITIOUS CAUSES

Exogenous hyperthyroidism is usually caused by iatrogenic administration of replacement hormones in doses that exceed the amount needed for normalization. Replacement dosage of levothyroxine sodium should be monitored to avoid "chemical hyperthyroidism." Drugs such as amphetamines can also cause a mild hyperthyroidism by stimulating the hypothalamic release of TRH.[2]

# Hypothyroidism

Hypothyroidism occurs when there is a deficiency of thyroid hormones. Like hyperthyroidism, it can be overt or subclinical, the latter being asymptomatic with thyroid hormone levels remaining in the normal range. TSH is so sensitive to changes in circulating $T_4$ and $T_3$ that even minor decreases can cause the TSH to rise in response. Slightly elevated sTSH and low normal levels of thyroid hormones are the test results usually associated with primary subclinical hypothyroidism. Women older than 60 years are more likely to have this condition, and are at increased risk for hypercholesterolemia and development of overt hypothyroidism, especially if their sTSH is >10 mU/mL or if high antithyroid antibody titers are detected.[19,21]

The symptoms of overt hypothyroidism result from a general slowing down of metabolic processes and include fatigue, cold intolerance, weight gain, constipation, dry skin, and mental changes. **Myxedema** is a syndrome found in patients with severe hypothyroidism. The skin on the face, hands, and feet thickens as do the tongue and vocal cords. The patient experiences mild hypothermia and progressive physical and mental lethargy.[5,8]

**Myxedema coma** is a severe manifestation of long-standing hypothyroidism. Occurring primarily in elderly patients, this rare condition is characterized by the gradual onset of lethargy, progressing to stupor or coma with alveolar hypoventilation, hypoxia, hypotension, shock, and seizures. Myxedema coma is usually precipitated by another stressful factor such as trauma or infection (especially pneumonia). Even with the best treatment, mortality is greater than 50%. The survival rate is poorest for myxedema patients who demonstrate hypothermia with a temperature less than 90°F.

Causes of hypothyroidism are numerous and can be congenital or acquired later in life.

## CONGENITAL

Congenital causes of hypothyroidism include thyroid dysgenesis (deficiency in amount of thyroid tissue), inborn defects in thyroid hormone synthesis, and pituitary or hypothalamic disorders. A transient form of primary neonatal hypothyroidism results from the placental transfer of thyrotropin receptor-blocking antibodies from a mother with autoimmune thyroid disease. This condition is self-limiting and is usually resolved in 3 to 6 months as the maternal antibodies are gradually broken down and eliminated.[25] An ectopic thyroid that functions poorly may be the result of a fetal thyroid gland that fails to descend during embryonic development. Symptoms that are observed in neonatal hypothyroidism include respiratory distress in the presence of increased birth weight, delayed skeletal maturation, hypothermia, persistence of physiologic jaundice beyond 3 days, hoarse cry, and edema. If left untreated, congenital hypothyroidism will result in stunted growth and mental retardation, a condition known as cretinism.[5]

The mental retardation associated with congenital hypothyroidism is highly preventable, but early detection and treatment are essential. Thyroid testing was added to existing newborn screening panels in the mid 1970s, and is performed on blood spots collected on filter paper from a heelstick. In North America, $T_4$ is measured, followed up by a TSH determination if the $T_4$ result is below a designated cutoff level. A $T_4$ below the 10th percentile and a TSH greater than 20 $\mu$U/L indicate hypothyroidism. Confirmation tests on serum should follow. However, newborns normally have higher levels of $T_4$ than do adults, so results must be referred to age-related ranges.[25]

## ACQUIRED

Acquired primary hypothyroidism can result from several conditions. Radiologic destruction or surgical removal of the thyroid gland to treat Graves' disease, atrophy associated with aging, and autoimmune thyroiditis are common causes.[5,8] Interference from drugs such as lithium carbonate or ingestion of excessive iodide may also cause hypothyroidism. Secondary hypothyroidism can result from hypopituitarism due to a pituitary adenoma associated with an underproduction of TSH. Hypothalamic dysfunction as a cause of hypothyroidism is rare. The possibility of peripheral resistance to thyroid hormones exists in patients who appear to be clinically hypothyroid and yet have normal values on currently available thyroid function tests. Figure 27–10 shows a diagnostic pathway that can be helpful in differentiating between various causes of hypothyroidism using laboratory tests.

# Thyroiditis

Thyroiditis is not a single disorder but is a term used to describe a group of inflammatory diseases that affect the thyroid gland. For the purpose of discussion, it is useful to divide these diseases into acute, subacute, and chronic thyroiditis.

## ACUTE THYROIDITIS

Acute thyroiditis, also known as acute suppurative thyroiditis, is an uncommon inflammatory disease that results from an infection of the thyroid gland by a gram-positive microorganism such as *Streptococcus pyogenes*, *Staphylococcus aureus*, or *Streptococcus pneumoniae*. Frequently affected are patients with preexisting thyroid disease such as nodular goiter. Clinical symptoms include painful goiter, high fever, sore throat, and skin

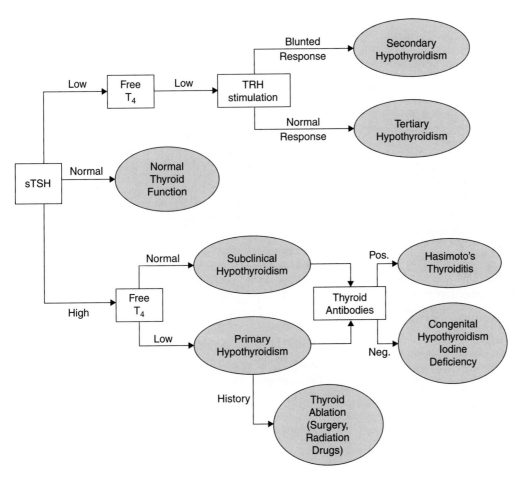

**FIGURE 27-10**

Pathway for laboratory diagnosis of hypothyroidism, starting with sTSH.

rash.[26] Laboratory findings show neutrophilic leukocytosis and an elevated sedimentation rate. Thyroid function tests are usually normal. Confirmatory diagnosis is made by needle aspiration and culture revealing a pathogenic organism.

## SUBACUTE THYROIDITIS

Subacute granulomatous thyroiditis, also known as DeQuervain's thyroiditis, is an inflammatory disorder of the thyroid gland that is most likely due to a virus. The patient is usually a woman between the ages of 20 and 50 years who has firm, tender goiter. An upper respiratory infection generally precedes infiltration with inflammatory cells. In the early stages of this illness, symptoms are those usually associated with hyperthyroidism. Goiter and neck pain are also present. Laboratory findings at this time demonstrate elevated $T_4$ and $T_3$ with a low sTSH. A significant elevation of the sedimentation rate is a classic laboratory finding. Because serum thyroglobulin levels are significantly elevated in subacute thyroiditis, a normal thyroglobulin level in a patient with anterior neck pain virtually excludes this diagnosis. Thyroid antibodies appear in low titers, if present at all, and are probably the result and not the cause of the disease. As the disease pro-

gresses, the $T_4$ and $T_3$ decrease and TSH rises, resulting in symptoms of hypothyroidism. Anti-inflammatory agents are used to treat the symptoms. Usually recovery is spontaneous in 2 to 6 months, at which time the antibodies, if present, disappear.

Subacute lymphocytic thyroiditis (or painless thyroiditis) may occur either sporadically or during the postpartum period. Histologic evidence of lymphocytic infiltration, in addition to the presence of antithyroid antibodies, characterize this disorder. Thyroid microsomal antibodies are present in up to 50% of patients, and antithyroid peroxidase antibodies are found in almost all patients with subacute lymphocytic thyroiditis.[26] The clinical course of painless thyroiditis parallels the phases observed with subacute thyroiditis—hyperthyroidism, hypothyroidism, and finally resolution to euthyroidism.

## CHRONIC THYROIDITIS

Chronic lymphocytic thyroiditis, also called Hashimoto's thyroiditis, is the most frequent cause of hypothyroidism in the United States. It is three times more common in women than in men. A genetic predisposition for this disorder has been found and is inherited as a dominant trait. Hashimoto's thyroiditis is characterized by infiltration of thyroid tissue by lymphocytes and plasma cells. Although most patients have goiter, nearly three fourths are euthyroid, one fourth are hypothyroid, and a small portion are hyperthyroid. Euthyroid disease generally progresses to hypothyroidism at a rate of 5% per year.[26]

Hashimoto's thyroiditis is an autoimmune disease in which thyroglobulin autoantibodies are present in high levels in the early phase, contrasting with the later stage in which thyroid peroxidase antibodies (TPOAb) predominate. Laboratory findings include a decreased $T_4$ and $T_3$ as a result of the destruction of the thyroid structure. As the circulating levels of these thyroid hormones decline, pituitary TSH rises as a response of the negative feedback system. This form of thyroiditis is usually permanent and requires treatment with replacement thyroid hormone, which decreases goiter size by inhibiting TSH secretion. The sTSH is useful in monitoring replacement therapy, which is administered to normalize $T_4$ and TSH levels without producing excessive TSH suppression. However, even after treatment, thyroid antibodies generally persist. In rare cases, Hashimoto's can progress to thyroid lymphoma, which is malignant.[26]

## Neoplasms

Although the presence of thyroid nodules is common, thyroid cancer is rare in the United States, with an incidence of 7 deaths per year per 1 million population. Exposure to ionizing radiation during childhood greatly increases the risk of developing thyroid malignancies. Others at risk include women, persons with goiter, or individuals with a family history of multiple endocrine neoplasia.[5] Among the diagnostic procedures used are fine-needle aspiration biopsy and radiologic studies.

Among the thyroid neoplasms, papillary carcinoma occurs with the greatest frequency (more than 60%), compared to follicular (about 25%), medullary (about 5%), and undifferentiated tumors (less than 10%).

### PAPILLARY CARCINOMA

Papillary carcinoma, which usually affects young patients and especially women,[5] is characterized by a firm, solitary nodule that is clearly different from the rest of the gland. Papillary cancers do not have the ability to synthesize thyroid hormone and do not cause thyroid dysfunction. Thyroglobulin, which is secreted by many papillary carcinomas, can be used as a tumor marker for recurrence or metastasis of the cancer. The primary treatment is surgical resection followed by [131]I thyroid ablation and replacement thyroxine administration.

### FOLLICULAR CARCINOMA

Follicular cancer, which usually affects individuals of middle age, is more invasive than papillary cancer and can spread to the lymph nodes of blood vessels, with metastases to bone, lung, and other tissues. Malignant follicular tissue retains some ability to produce thyroid hormones and may, though rarely, cause thyrotoxicosis as a result of widespread follicular metastatic disease. Total thyroidectomy, followed by radioactive iodine ablation, is indicated for patients with thyroid cancer of follicular cell origin. This treatment thereby increases the sensitivity of serum thyroglobulin for detecting persistent or recurring tumor.

### MEDULLARY CARCINOMA

Medullary carcinoma arises from the C or parafollicular cells of the thyroid gland, which have an endocrine function. The parafollicular cells all produce excess calcitonin, and some may produce excess adenocorticotropic hormone (ACTH), prostaglandin, serotonin, and other amines, which indicate this condition to be a multiple endocrine neoplasia. Following total thyroidectomy, calcitonin levels should be determined by provocative testing with pentagastrin or calcium to be sure that all malignant tissue has been removed. Medullary carcinoma occurs in a sporadic form (80%) or as an autosomal dominant familial form (20%).

### UNDIFFERENTIATED THYROID CARCINOMA

This group of tumors includes small cell, giant cell, and spindle carcinomas. They usually occur in older patients with long histories of goiter that shows a sudden change in growth. Because it is resistant to therapy, undifferentiated thyroid carcinoma usually causes death within 1 year. Total thyroid hormone levels are normal with these tumors, and no thyroid antibodies are detected.

## Selected Medical Conditions

### NONTHYROIDAL ILLNESS

Thyroid function assays, which are reliable indicators of thyroid status for otherwise healthy patients, may become misleading and difficult to interpret in the chronically or acutely ill hospitalized patient. Additionally, the effects of certain drugs administered to these patients make interpretation of thyroid tests even more confusing. Clinicians must understand the complex ways in which serious illnesses and medications influence thyroid function tests when they evaluate the thyroid status of patients with nonthyroidal illness.

Sick euthyroid syndrome is the term used when thyroid functions tests become abnormal in patients who are seriously ill with causes other than primary or secondary thyroid dysfunction. Some of the diseases resulting in sick euthyroid syndrome include cardiac failure, renal failure, trauma, febrile infectious processes, liver disease, and surgical procedures. Low $T_3$ syndrome refers to the most common alteration in thyroid testing seen in nonthyroidal illness. Following the onset of such illness, $T_3$ levels decline quickly (within 30 minutes to 24 hours). There is a concurrent rise in $rT_3$ while TSH and free and total $T_4$ remain normal. These results help to rule out true hypothyroidism, where findings would include decreased levels of thyroid hormones with an increased TSH. It is thought that low $T_3$ syndrome reflects a decrease in peripheral conversion of $T_4$ to $T_3$. There is also an increased conversion of $T_4$ to $rT_3$.[27]

Severely ill patients will often have low levels of total thyroid hormones with the free fraction remaining in the normal range. This is generally a consequence of altered TBG such as is found in cirrhosis of the liver (decreased synthesis) or nephrotic syndrome (increased urinary loss). Lowered values of $T_4$, $T_3$, and TSH in the most severely ill patients seem to indicate a decreased pituitary or hypothalamic responsiveness to serum thyroid hormone and a suppressed release of TSH. The abnormality of thyroid function tests seems to be related to the severity of the illness and may, in some cases, help to predict the outcome.[27] Diagnosis and treatment of true underlying thyroid disease is difficult in hospitalized patients, and in the absence of overt symptoms, intervention other than close monitoring is not recommended. The patient can be retested once recovery from nonthyroidal illness is complete.[10,27]

## DRUGS

Many drugs can have an effect on thyroid hormone levels. They may compete for binding sites on TBG, inhibit conversion of $T_4$ to $T_3$, or cause alterations in the production of thyroid-binding proteins. Table 27–3 is a list of drugs and their effects on thyroid hormone levels. The American Thyroid Association recommends that sTSH be used for detection of hyperthyroidism or hypothyroidism in patients who are taking such drugs.

## DEPRESSION

Abnormalities of the hypothalamic-pituitary-thyroid axis are frequently investigated in search for evidence of biologic causes of depression. Serum $T_4$ and $T_3$ are usually reported to be in the reference range. However, elevated basal serum concentrations of TSH, blunted response of TSH to TRH stimulation, and the presence of antithyroid antibodies occur with greater than expected frequency in depressed patients. A persistently blunted TRH response after clinical improvement of depression appears to be related to a higher incidence of relapse. A low norepinephrine activity could underlie the blunted TSH response.

Normally, TSH demonstrates circadian variation, which is characterized by a nocturnal surge that antecedes onset of sleep. There may be a correlation between major endogenous depression and loss of nocturnal TSH surge.

## PREGNANCY

Hormonal changes and metabolic demands during pregnancy result in complex alterations of thyroid function. TBG levels approximately double during pregnancy. A new equilibrium is reached between bound and free thyroid hormones but free levels remain normal. There is an increased demand for iodide because of increased renal iodide clearance and increased utilization by the fetus. The size of the thyroid gland may also increase.

TABLE 27-3

**Drugs That Affect Thyroid Function Tests***

**Drugs that increase TSH secretion**
 Amiodarone
 Lithium
 Phenytoin
 Morphine
 Valproic acid
 Phenobarbital
**Drugs that decrease TSH secretion**
 Dopamine
 Cortisone compounds
**Drugs that increase free $T_4$**
 Amiodarone
 Cortisone compounds
 Propranolol
**Drugs that decrease free $T_4$**
 Phenytoin
 Carbamazepine
 Lithium
 Phenobarbital
 Dopamine

*Based on data from Kaplan LA, Pesce AJ (eds.): *Clinical Chemistry: Theory, Analysis, Correlation.* 3rd ed. St. Louis, MO, 1996, pp 1108–1123; Hammett-Stabler C: Update on thyroid testing. Adv Med Lab Professionals 7:10–16, 1998; Madeddu G et al: Clinical and laboratory assessment of subclinical thyroid disease. Rays 24:229–242, 1999; Camacho PM, Dwarkanathan AA: Sick euthyroid syndrome. What to do when thyroid function tests are abnormal in critically ill patients. Postgrad Med 105:215–219, 1999.

In euthyroid nonpregnant women, most of the $T_3$ arises from the peripheral conversion of $T_4$ to $T_3$ by the liver and kidneys. During pregnancy, the placenta is an additional site for this conversion, which may be a contributing factor in the decrease in the ratio of $T_4:T_3$ that occurs between the first and third trimesters. The increased level of free $T_4$ observed in early pregnancy is probably the result of thyroid stimulation by hCG, which is structurally similar to TSH and has a similar but milder effect on the thyroid when present in greatly elevated concentrations.

The regulation of the maternal thyroid results from both elevated hCG (mainly in the first half of gestation) and increased TSH (mainly in the second half of gestation). Serum thyroglobulin levels increase in pregnancy, especially in the last trimester. The rise in TSH levels in late pregnancy can be interpreted as an appropriate feedback response to lower free hormone levels from the reduced hCG stimulation.[28]

Postpartum thyroiditis is a fairly common (5%) autoimmune disease that occurs in the first year following childbirth and is caused by a transient rebound of the autoimmune process. It is characterized by antimicrosomal antibodies and lymphocytic infiltration of the thyroid. The most common course of the disease is a period of transient hyperthyroidism, followed by hypothyroidism, resolving spontaneously in several months.[28]

## EATING DISORDERS

A complex interrelationship exists between the thyroid gland and the physiologic effects observed in self-induced malnutrition states of anorexia nervosa and bulimia. Most major studies report the presence of the low $T_3$ or sick euthyroid syndrome in patients with anorexia nervosa. Laboratory findings include low $T_3$, low or normal $T_4$, and increased $rT_3$, a pattern that indicates impaired peripheral conversion of thyroid hormones. Another factor contributing to the low $T_3$ may be decreased $T_3$ secretion by the thyroid gland in response to TSH, which reflects hypothalamic-pituitary-thyroid dysfunction before and after weight recovery. Although TSH response to TRH improves after refeeding, $T_3$ response to TSH remains lower than the controls. The occurrence of this low $T_3$ response to TRH after refeeding suggests a possibility that TSH of lower biologic activity is secreted after a period of TRH deficiency. It is also possible that after extended periods of low TSH stimulation, the thyroid undergoes relative atrophy.

A delayed TSH response to TRH is seen in patients with anorexia nervosa as well as those with bulimia nervosa. However, bulimic patients have a nonblunted response, in contrast to those with anorexia who demonstrate a blunted response.

The clinical similarities between anorexia nervosa and hypothyroidism are adaptations of the body to prolonged starvation. Symptoms observed in patients with food eating disorders include cardiovascular abnormalities such as bradycardia, dysrhythmias, and marked orthostatic pulse and blood pressure instability. The hypothermia commonly observed may be related to the body's need to conserve its meager energy stores. It is probably associated with the down-regulation in the thyroid function, or possibly with hypothalamic dysfunction. Hypercholesterolemia occurs as a consequence of the markedly decreased $T_3$ levels. Results of case studies demonstrate the need for clinicians to become familiar with the medical complications of eating disorders and their complex relationships with the hypothalamic-pituitary-thyroid axis.

## SUMMARY

The thyroid gland is located in the neck, centered around the trachea. The follicle is the functional structural unit and is responsible for the biosynthesis of the thyroid hormones.

Regulation of the thyroid gland begins with the hypothalamus, which releases TRH. TRH in turn stimulates the pituitary to secrete TSH. TSH acts directly on the follicular cells to increase the production and release of thyroid hormones.

Free $T_3$ and $T_4$ are involved in the negative feedback control mechanism.

Today's technological developments allow for more reliable diagnosis and monitoring of treatment in the management of thyroid disease. Sensitive immunoassays for $T_4$, $T_3$, and TSH as well as assays for the detection of the thyroid antibodies have had a major impact on the evaluation of thyroid function. These rapid advances in methodology demand that medical clinicians keep informed of the current rationales for thyroid testing and diagnostic interpretation. The complex endocrinologic patterns present in such diverse conditions as pregnancy and anorexia nervosa emphasize the need for integration of knowledge from many perspectives. The future technologies based in molecular biology can increase our understanding of complex processes and interactions at the cellular level. Results of this increased understanding may include gene transfer therapies as treatment for genetic defects, new therapeutic agents engineered through the use of recombinant DNA techniques, and enhanced knowledge of the pathogenesis of the autoimmune mechanisms as expressed in Hashimoto's thyroiditis and in Graves' disease. Through the use of these advances in technology, new means for diagnosis and treatment of thyroid disorders are sure to emerge.

## REFERENCES

1. Rubin E, Farber JL: The endocrine system. In Rubin E, Farber JL (eds.): *Pathology.* 2nd ed. Philadelphia, Lippincott, 1994, pp 1108–1123.

2. Lucas MH, Fernandez-Ulloa M: Thyroid. In Kaplan LA, Pesce AJ (eds.): *Clinical Chemistry: Theory, Analysis, Correlation.* 3rd ed. St Louis, MO, Mosby, 1996, pp 867–891.

3. Hammett-Stabler C: Update on thyroid testing. Adv Med Lab Professionals 7:10–16, 1998.

4. Whitley RJ, Mielke AW, Watts NB: Endocrinology part III: thyroid function. In Burtis CA, Ashwood EA (eds.): *Tietz Fundamentals of Clinical Chemistry.* 4th ed. Philadelphia, WB Saunders, 1996, pp 617–648.

5. Stern C: Thyroid and parathyroid functions and alterations. In Bullock BL (ed): *Pathophysiology.* 4th ed. Philadelphia, Lippincott-Raven, 1996, pp 708–720.

6. Abbott Laboratories Diagnostics Division: *Architect Systems: TSH.* Abbott Park, IL, 1998.

7. Mayo Medical Laboratories: *Mayo 2000 Test Catalog.* Mayo Medical Laboratories, Rochester, NY, 1999, pp 463–478.

8. Escolas KM: Endocrinology. In Lehman CA (ed.): *Saunders Manual of Clinical Laboratory Science.* Philadelphia, WB Saunders, 1998, pp 191–200.

9. Taylor CS, Brandt DR: Developments in thyroid-stimulating hormone testing. The pursuit of improved sensitivity. Lab Med 24:337, 1994.

10. Attia JM, Margetts P, Guyatt G: Diagnosis of thyroid disease in hospitalized patients. Arch Intern Med 159: 658–665, 1999.
11. Felz MW, Stein PP: The many faces of Graves' disease. Part 2. Practical diagnosic testing and management options. Postgrad Med 106:45–52, 1999.
12. Abbott Laboratories, Diagnostics Division: *Architect Systems: Total T₄.* Abbott Park, IL, 1998.
13. Mayo Medical Laboratories: *Mayo 2000 Test Catalog.* Mayo Medical Laboratories, Rochester, NY, 1999, p 18.
14. Abbott Laboratories Diagnostics Division: *Architect systems: Free T₄.* Abbott Park, IL, 1999.
15. Abbott Laboratories Diagnostics Division: *Axsym Systems: Free T₄.* Abbott Park, IL, 1995.
16. Abbott Laboratories Diagnostics Division: *Axsym Systems: T₃.* Abbott Park, IL, 1994.
17. Abbott Laboratories Diagnostics Division: *Architect Systems: T₃.* Abbott Park, IL, 1998.
18. Abbott Laboratories Diagnostics Division: *Axsym Systems: T-uptake.* Abbott Park, IL, 1998.
19. Madeddu G, Spanu A, Falchi A, et al.: Clinical and laboratory assessment of subclinical thyroid disease. Rays 24:229–242, 1999.
20. Kaplan MM: Clinical perspectives in the diagnosis of thyroid disease. Clin Chem 45:1377–1383, 1999.
21. Woeber KA: The year in review: the thyroid. Ann Intern Med 131:959–962, 1999.
22. Maussier ML, D'Errico G, Putignano P, et al.: Thyrotoxicosis: Clinical and laboratory assessment. Rays 24:263–272, 1999.
23. Felz MW, Stein PP: The many faces of Graves' disease. Part 1. Eyes, pulse, skin and neck provide important clues to diagnosis. Postgrad Med 106:57–64, 1999.
24. Zimmerman D: Fetal and neonatal hyperthyroidism. Thyroid 9:727–733, 1999.
25. La Franchi S. Congenital hypothyroidism. Etiologies, diagnosis, and management. Thyroid 9:735–740, 1999.
26. Slatosky J, Shipton B, Wahba H: Thyroiditis. Differential diagnosis and management. *Am Fam Physician* 61:1047–1052, 2000.
27. Camacho PM, Dwarkanathan AA: Sick euthyroid syndrome. What to do when thyroid function tests are abnormal in critically ill patients. Postgrad Med 105:215–219, 1999.
28. Fantz CR et al: Thyroid function during pregnancy. Clin Chem 45:2250–2258, 1999.

# Parathyroid Glands and Calcium-Phosphate Metabolism

*Susan Cockayne and Shauna C. Anderson*

## ANATOMY

The parathyroid glands are embedded in the thyroid gland. Two are located in the superior pole and two are located in the inferior pole of the thyroid. The location can, however, vary in different individuals, and parathyroid tissue may also be found in other parts of the neck and in the mediastinum.

Microscopically, the parathyroid glands consist of two distinct cell types. The chief cells have a clear cytoplasm and are the most abundant cell type. These cells secrete parathyroid hormone (PTH). The oxyphil cells are larger, less abundant, have a pyknotic nucleus, have an affinity for acidic dyes, and are believed to be senescent chief cells.

## PARATHYROID HORMONE

### Biosynthesis and Metabolism

PTH is synthesized as a preprohormone consisting of 115 amino acids. It is immediately cleaved to produce a prohormone of 90 amino acids. The pro-PTH is packaged into secretory vesicles where 6 more amino acids are cleaved off to produce the form of PTH that is secreted into the circulation. The half-life of circulating PTH is 15 to 20 minutes. The liver and kidneys produce at least two major fragments from the circulating PTH. Therefore, three species of PTH exist in the circulation: (1) intact PTH molecule, (2) a carboxyl-terminal fragment, and (3) an amino-terminal fragment. Only the intact molecule and the amino-terminal fragment have biologic activity.

The ionized calcium concentration in the circulation is the major regulatory mechanism for the synthesis and secretion of PTH. High calcium levels inhibit PTH, whereas low levels stimulate PTH secretion. Other mechanisms may have the same influence on PTH levels. A low serum magnesium level can stimulate PTH secretion if it occurs rapidly; however, a low level may impair the release and tissue response to PTH. High serum phosphorus levels also stimulate PTH se-

cretion. This is actually an indirect mechanism because the high phosphorus depresses the serum calcium. Since a receptor for vitamin D metabolites has been identified, it is now also possible that these metabolites have the direct ability to suppress PTH release.[1]

### Mechanisms of Action

PTH can produce an effect on three tissues: bone, kidney, and intestine. The mechanisms of action occur by binding to a cell membrane receptor and activating adenyl cyclase or facilitating a cellular influx of calcium.[2]

The bone consists of metabolically active cells: osteoblasts, osteocytes, and osteoclasts. These cells control the formation and resorptive processes of the bone. Osteoclasts normally resorb bone, delivering calcium into the extracellular fluid. Osteoblasts, on the other hand, synthesize unmineralized bone. Although the exact mechanism of PTH action on bone has not been fully described, under the influence of PTH, bone resorption occurs, immediately followed by an increase in bone formation.

Of the amount of calcium that is filtered at the glomerulus, about 10% is delivered to the distal tubules, where reabsorption is regulated by PTH. PTH causes an increased calcium reabsorption and reduced calcium excretion. PTH also promotes the reabsorption of hydrogen ions, magnesium, and ammonia. In contrast, phosphate, sodium, potassium, and bicarbonate ion excretion is enhanced with the effects of PTH.

PTH stimulation of cAMP content and calcium influx have not been demonstrated in the intestine. PTH does, however, stimulate the intestinal transport of calcium and phosphorus. This is probably an indirect mechanism involving the circulating levels of the vitamin D metabolite 1,25 dihydroxyvitamin D (1,25-$(OH)_2$ $D_3$).

## REGULATION OF CALCIUM AND PHOSPHORUS

Calcium is the most abundant electrolyte in the human body mainly because of its high concentration in the skeleton.

Ninety-nine percent of total body calcium is bound in the skeleton. Calcium is a divalent, predominantly extracellular ion that is essential to many physiologic functions. It is important for proper neuromuscular activity, blood coagulation, bone metabolism, and maintenance of the functional integrity of cell membranes. Calcium also serves as an intracellular second messenger similar to cAMP.

In bone, calcium combines with phosphorus to form the crystalline structure of hydroxyapatite, a complex calcium phosphate salt with the general formula $Ca_{10} (PO_4)_6 (OH)_2$. Both bone resorption and formation occur in the bone. Bone resorption is mediated by osteoclastic cells that break down the hydroxyapatite crystal to release calcium and phosphorus into the extracellular fluid (ECF). Bone formation is mediated by osteoblastic cells and occurs in response to stress and strain whenever bone is needed. Only 0.03% of total body calcium is found in the plasma, where its concentration ranges from 8.5 to 10.5 mg/dL (2.25 to 2.60 mmol/L).

Total serum calcium is found in three forms: protein-bound, (46%), complexed with citrate, phosphate, lactate, and sulfate (7%) and free, or ionized, calcium (47%). Albumin accounts for about 80% of protein binding, and globulins account for the remaining 20%. The only physiologically active form is ionized $Ca^{++}$, whose serum concentration is maintained by a tight regulatory mechanism. Variations in serum protein levels alter the concentration of the protein-bound fraction and hence total calcium levels. However, the ionized fraction remains normal and the patient will be asymptomatic. Because of the effect of protein on total calcium levels, serum protein levels must be considered for the proper interpretation of total serum calcium levels. A rough estimate of the ionized calcium level can be calculated by considering that 1 g of serum albumin binds approximately 0.8 mg of calcium. The serum calcium can be adjusted to correct for a decreased albumin by utilizing the following formula:

Adjusted calcium (mg/dL) = Calcium total (mg/dL)

$$- \text{Albumin (g/dL)} + 4.0$$

The acid-base status of the body also influences the binding of $Ca^{++}$ to albumin. The effect is to decrease the concentration of ionized $Ca^{++}$, which may produce symptomatic hypocalcemia. A change in pH of 0.1 unit will alter the ionized $Ca^{++}$ fraction by 0.16 mg/dL.[3] In acidosis, the excess $H^+$ binds to albumin, freeing the protein-bound calcium with a resultant increase in the ionized fraction. These significant changes in the ionized fraction due to acid-base abnormalities can occur without corresponding changes in the total calcium.[4]

Phosphorus is abundant in the body as both an intracellular and extracellular anion. Intracellularly, it exists as organic phosphate in combination with lipids and proteins. As phospholipids and phosphoproteins, phosphorus is essential for the structural integrity of cell membranes and is an important component of nucleic acids and high-energy nucleotides such as adenosine triphosphate (ATP). The majority of extracellular phosphate (85%) is found in bone combined with calcium to form hydroxyapatite. Approximately 85% of serum phosphate exists as inorganic mono ($HPO_4^{--}$) or dihydrogen phosphate ($H_2PO_4^-$). The ratio of $HPO_4^{--}/H_2PO_4^-$ at a normal body pH of 7.4 is 4:1. In these forms, it acts as a principal buffer of the urinary system to facilitate excretion of $H^+$. The remaining 12% to 15% is bound to proteins. Serum inorganic phosphorus is present in a concentration of 2.8 to 4.0 mg/dL.

A balanced daily diet provides from 600 to 1000 mg of calcium, which is sufficient for normal calcium needs. Calcium requirements are increased during the normal physiologic growth process, pregnancy, and lactation. Dietary calcium is absorbed from the small intestine by both passive and active mechanisms. The intestinal absorption of calcium becomes more efficient when calcium intake is low.[5] In the kidneys, the diffusible fractions of calcium, which include both the ionized and complexed forms, are filtered by the glomerulus. Most filtered calcium is reabsorbed in the tubules. The urinary calcium excretion of normal adults ranges between 100 and 400 mg/day. Seventy to ninety percent of ingested phosphorus is absorbed by the intestine. Phosphorus filtered by the glomerulus is mostly reabsorbed in the proximal convoluted tubule and distal convoluted tubule. Urinary excretion depends on adequate renal function.

The serum concentrations of ionized calcium and, to a lesser extent, inorganic phosphorus are maintained within narrow limits by homeostatic mechanisms involving an interaction of three hormones: PTH, vitamin D, and calcitonin. This hormonal regulation involves responses from three target organs: bone, kidney, and intestine. Table 28–1 outlines the actions of these hormones.

PTH synthesis is stimulated by a decreased concentration of ionized calcium through a negative feedback mechanism. Conversely, high ionized calcium levels inhibit its release. PTH has numerous functions that help to increase serum calcium levels when needed. Owing to the reciprocal relationship between calcium and phosphorus, PTH also has a phosphorus lowering effect. It activates the osteoclastic cells of the body, causing bone resorption with the release of calcium and phosphorus from bone into the ECF. In addition to activating the osteoclasts, PTH may also increase the number of osteoclasts. PTH enhances distal renal tubular reabsorption of calcium, resulting in increased serum calcium levels while decreasing the amount of calcium excreted in the urine. The hormone also inhibits proximal renal tubular reabsorption of phosphorus with consequent lowering of the serum phosphorus level while increasing its urinary excretion. PTH stimulates the synthesis in the kidneys of 1,25-$(OH)_2 D_3$, the active form of vitamin D. This action of PTH indirectly enhances calcium and phosphorus absorption from the intestine.[6] Both the intact PTH molecule and the amino-terminal fragments bind to receptors on the major target organs. Binding of hormone and receptor activates the enzyme adenylate cyclase to produce cAMP, which mobilizes calcium from the bone. Urinary cAMP levels can be assayed as an indication of PTH activity.

TABLE 28-1

**Effects of Calcium Regulating Hormones**

| HORMONE | BONE | KIDNEY | INTESTINE |
|---------|------|--------|-----------|
| PTH | ↑ Ca resorption<br>↑ PO$_4$ resorption | ↑ Ca reabsorption<br>↓ PO$_4$ reabsorption | ↑ Ca absorption (indirect)<br>↑ PO$_4$ absorption (indirect) |
| Vitamin D | ↑ Ca resorption<br>↑ PO$_4$ resorption | ↑ Ca reabsorption<br>↑ PO$_4$ reabsorption | ↑ Ca absorption (direct)<br>↑ PO$_4$ absorption |
| Calcitonin | ↓ Ca resorption<br>↓ PO$_4$ resorption | ↓ Ca reabsorption<br>↓ PO$_4$ reabsorption | None |

↑ = increased; ↓ = decreased.

Vitamin D is also essential for maintenance of normal calcium levels. It can either be absorbed from the gastrointestinal tract or formed in the skin by the action of ultraviolet radiation. Vitamin D must undergo two hydroxylation steps to become biologically active. In the liver, hydroxylation occurs at C-25 to produce 25-hydroxyvitamin D (25-OH D$_3$). The second hydroxylation step occurs in the proximal convoluted tubule of the kidney, where another hydroxyl group is attached at C-1 to produce 1,25-dihydroxyvitamin D, the active form of vitamin D. This step is tightly regulated, with PTH serving as the primary regulator. Vitamin D exerts its hormonal influence on calcium levels by stimulating osteoclastic bone resorption, increasing intestinal calcium and phosphorus absorption and, less importantly, by increasing renal tubular reabsorption of calcium.

In contrast to the calcium-elevating effects of PTH and 1,25-(OH)$_2$ D$_3$, calcitonin acts to lower serum calcium levels. Calcitonin is a peptide hormone secreted from the C cells of the thyroid gland. It acts on both bone and kidney to inhibit osteoclastic bone resorption and tubular reabsorption of calcium. The latter effect enhances renal excretion of calcium. Calcitonin exerts its effects by activating adenyl cyclase upon binding to specific membrane receptors. High serum levels of ionized calcium stimulate the release of calcitonin, whereas low ionized calcium levels inhibit its release. The precise role of calcitonin in calcium homeostasis is not entirely clear, however, since deficiencies of calcitonin do not lead to hypercalcemia.[7]

## SPECIFIC ANALYTES

## Calcium

### METHODOLOGY

The reference method for calcium analysis is atomic absorption. However, clinical analysis most commonly employs methods based on calcium precipitation, fluorescence, or color-complex formation. Ion-selective electrodes for measuring the ionized fraction of calcium are available in some analytical instruments.

In the classic precipitation methods of Clark and Collip, calcium is precipitated as calcium oxalate. Acidification redissolves the calcium oxalate, freeing oxalic acid, which is then mixed with potassium permanganate. The purple $Mn_2O_7^{--}$ is reduced to $Mn^{++}$, a colorless compound. This procedure is tedious and time-consuming and is not widely used.

$$Ca^{++} + oxalate \rightarrow Calcium\ oxalate\ (ppt)$$

$$Calcium\ oxalate\ (ppt) + H_2SO_4 \rightarrow Oxalate + CaSO_4$$

$$2KMnO_4 + 5\ Oxalate + 3H_2SO_4 \rightarrow$$
$$K_2SO_4 + 2MnSO_4 + 10\ CO_2 + 8\ H_2O$$

Another precipitation method uses chloranilic acid, which reacts with calcium to form a calcium-chloranilate complex. The precipitate is redissolved with EDTA, thereby liberating chloranilic acid whose red-purple color can be measured spectrophotometrically.[8]

$$Ca^{++} + Chloranilate \rightarrow Ca\text{-}chloranilate\ (ppt)$$

$$Ca\text{-}chloranilate\ (ppt) + EDTA \rightarrow Ca\text{-}EDTA + Chloranilic\ acid$$

Fluorescent methods with good sensitivity are available. In one method, calcium is added to an alkaline solution of calcein, forming a fluorescent calcium-calcein complex. Subsequent EGTA titration binds calcium, causing a decreasing fluorescence. The amount of EGTA used in the titration is proportional to the calcium concentration.

$$Ca^{++} + Calcein \rightarrow Ca\text{-}calcein\ (fluorescent)$$

$$EGTA + Ca\text{-}calcein \rightarrow Ca\text{-}EGTA + calcein$$

A common direct spectrophotometric method incorporates the metal-complexing dye o-cresolphthalein complexone

(CPC). This dye forms a red complex with calcium in alkaline solution:

$$Ca^{++} + o\text{-}CPC \rightarrow Ca^{++}\text{-}o\text{-}CPC \text{ (red)}$$

8-Hydroxyquinoline is added to the reagent to eliminate interference from cations, most specifically magnesium. Other indicator dyes are available such as arsenazo III.

The measurement of ionized calcium activity is available with some commercial analytical instruments. Measurement is analogous to the principle of the pH glass electrode used to measure hydrogen ions. Organophosphate or other organic ion-exchanger compounds are used for selective measurement of calcium.

### SPECIMEN COLLECTION AND HANDLING

Suitable specimens for calcium analysis include serum, heparinized plasma, and urine. Serum and urine samples are stable at refrigerated temperatures for several months. Stored heparinized plasma may result in the loss of calcium since calcium may coprecipitate with fibrin and be removed by centrifugation.[9] Plasma with oxalate or EDTA anticoagulants is not acceptable because of the calcium chelation effect. The calcium level may also be affected by postural changes, with a recumbent position decreasing the level 4%.[8] A 24-hour urine specimen should be preserved with 5 to 10 mL of 6-M HCl. Glassware used for calcium analysis should be acid-washed to eliminate calcium contamination.

Serum or heparinized whole blood can be used with ion-selective electrodes for measurement of ionized calcium. When results are needed immediately, the use of heparinized whole blood eliminates clotting and centrifugation time. However, excessive amounts of sodium heparin can lower the ionized fraction 3% to 5%.[8] Sample collection should be controlled to minimize loss of $CO_2$. The resultant increase in pH would contribute to lower ionized calcium levels. Ionized calcium in clotted or heparinized whole blood is stable for at least 6 hours at refrigeration temperatures.[8]

## Inorganic Phosphate

### METHODOLOGY

Most methods for the analysis of inorganic phosphate are modifications of the original method of Fiske and Subbarow. The principle is based on the formation of a complex of phosphate ions and molybdate. A trichloroacetic acid protein-free filtrate is reacted with ammonium molybdate at an acid pH to form phosphomolybdate. Phosphomolybdate is then reduced to molybdenum blue and measured spectrophotometrically at 660 nm. Several reducing agents have been employed in the reduction step. One such agent is a stannous chloride-hydrazine sulfate complex. The general reaction is:

$$PO_4 + H_2SO_4 + (NH_4) \; 6 \; Mo_7O_{24} \cdot 4H_2O \rightarrow$$

$$Mo{:}PO_4 \text{ complex}$$

Several automated analyzers measure the unreduced phosphorus-molybdate complex at a wavelength of 340 nm.[8]

### SPECIMEN COLLECTION AND HANDLING

Serum or heparinized plasma are acceptable samples. Other anticoagulants inhibit formation of the phosphomolybdate complex.[9] Fasting samples should be obtained since phosphorus values are lower following meals. Serum must be separated from the cells promptly to avoid leakage of intracellular phosphorus into the serum. Hemolyzed samples are unacceptable because of the presence of phosphorus in red blood cells. Urine samples must be acidified with HCl.

## Parathyroid Hormone

Parathyroid hormone (PTH) exists in three forms in the circulation: intact PTH, the amino-terminal fragment (N-terminal), and the carboxyl fragment (C-terminal). The biologically active forms are the intact molecule and the N-terminal fragment. C-terminal fragments normally circulate at a concentration 10 times greater than intact PTH, and levels are increased disproportionately when renal function is impaired because of their longer circulating half-life. Biologically active intact PTH is rapidly metabolized, releasing the biologically active N-terminal fragment and the inactive C-terminal fragment. Older methods of PTH measurement incorporated competitive binding assays such as radioimmunoassay (RIA). But, because they detected various circulating PTH fragments, they produced conflicting results and poor disease correlation.

Newer, two-site immunometric assays for intact PTH provide a much more accurate assessment of PTH levels by excluding the inactive C-terminal fragment. These newer assay methods are based primarily on two-site immunometric assays such as IRMA or chemiluminescence, depending on which type of labeled antibody is used (see Chapter 7). Serum is the preferred sample type. The reference range for normal adults is 10–55 pg/mL.

### PARATHYROID HORMONE-RELATED PEPTIDE

Humoral hypercalcemia of malignancy (HHM) is associated with solid tumors such as those found in the lung, kidney, and breast. PTH-related peptide has been identified as the major causative factor for the hypercalcemia produced by these cancers. HHM accounts for about 75% to 80% of patients with hypercalcemia-associated malignancy. Parathyroid hormone-related peptide (PTH-rP), after being secreted by tumors, acts as an endocrine hormone on its target tissues causing hypercalcemia. Though not routinely performed, IRMA assays have been developed with a reported range in normal individuals from 0 to 5 pmol/L.

## Biochemical Markers of Bone Metabolism

Recently, various serum and urinary markers have been investigated as useful indicators of calcium balance, bone turnover, and bone fragility largely because of the interest in the development and prevention of osteoporosis. Analytes providing early clues to bone status include urinary hydroxyproline, serum alkaline phosphate, tartrate-resistant acid phosphatase, osteocalcin levels, and calculation of the urinary calcium-creatinine ratio. However, these tests have not found much clinical utility because of the inability to halt or prevent the development of osteoporosis. New advances in this area have stimulated the development of newer, more sensitive and specific biochemical tests as markers of bone metabolism. These can be divided into markers of bone formation and markers of bone resorption.

Markers of bone formation include bone-specific proteins such as osteocalcin, bone-specific alkaline phosphatase, and procollagen-I extension peptide. Synthesized by mature osteoblasts, they eventually enter the circulation where they can be measured by RIA or enzyme-linked immunosorbent assay (ELISA) techniques. Other markers enter the circulation as a result of osteoclastic activity. Collagen cross-links, which assist in collagen synthesis, are hydrolyzed during bone resorption. Several different cross-links can be identified in the urine. They include free pyridinoline and deoxypyridinoline, N-telopeptides, and C-telopeptides.

## CLINICAL APPLICATIONS

### Hypocalcemia

#### CAUSES

Hypocalcemia occurs when the serum calcium level is <8.5 mg/dL. However, calcium levels must be interpreted in light of the variables that can affect the physiologically active ionized calcium. The total calcium level must be evaluated in conjunction with the albumin level and the acid-base status, as previously discussed, to ensure that it is an accurate reflection of the ionized fraction since only alterations in the ionized fraction lead to clinical symptoms. Table 28–2 outlines the common causes of hypocalcemia.

#### Hypoparathyroidism

Several factors contribute to the development of hypoparathyroidism. Most commonly, the condition is due to removal

TABLE 28 – 2

**Causes of Hypocalcemia**

Hypoparathyroidism
Pseudohypoparathyroidism
Vitamin D deficiency
   Rickets
   Osteomalacia
Chronic renal failure (renal osteodystrophy)

of or damage to the parathyroid glands during thyroid surgery. Some cases may have an autoimmune component. There may be defects in the parathyroid gland so that there is deficient production of PTH. Additionally, although not commonly encountered, the circulating PTH may be sufficient in quantity but physiologically inactive as a result of impaired production. Finally, one or more target organs may be resistant to the action of PTH. The end result of hypoparathyroidism is reduced concentration or ability of PTH to maintain normal serum calcium levels. The circulating concentration of $1,25\text{-}(OH)_2$ $D_3$ is also reduced in hypoparathyroidism in part because of the inability of PTH to facilitate its conversion in the kidney to the active form.

The typical laboratory findings in hypoparathyroidism are decreased calcium, decreased PTH, and elevated phosphorus. Table 28–3 summarizes analyte levels in hypocalcemic disorders. The phosphorus level is elevated primarily because of its decreased renal clearance caused by inadequate PTH action on the renal tubules. If bone disease accompanies hypoparathyroidism, alkaline phosphatase levels may also be increased inasmuch as the enzyme is present in high concentration in the osteoblasts. In addition to these typical laboratory abnormalities, the measurement of urinary cAMP excretion following the administration of PTH is helpful in the differential diagnosis. Upon administration of PTH in hypoparathyroid patients, there is an increase in urinary cAMP excretion since the effects of PTH are mediated through cAMP.

### Pseudohypoparathyroidism

Pseudohypoparathyroidism is a rare hereditary disorder. It is characterized by symptoms of hypoparathyroidism with hypocalcemia, but serum levels of PTH are elevated instead of decreased. The common causative factor is target organ resistance (bone and kidney) to the action of PTH because of a receptor defect. In addition to symptoms of hypocalcemia, characteristic skeletal abnormalities are seen. These include a round face, short stature, and shortening of the fourth and fifth metacarpals and metatarsals. Some degree of mental retardation may also occur. In pseudohypoparathyroidism, administration of PTH does not result in increased urinary cAMP excretion because of the target organ resistance to PTH. Thus, the PTH infusion test is useful in the differential diagnosis. In another rare condition, pseudopseudohypoparathyroidism, similar skeletal abnormalities are present but the serum calcium concentration is normal; thus, hypocalcemic symptoms are not observed.

### Vitamin D Deficiency

Vitamin D deficiency may be due to inadequate dietary intake, malabsorption, or inadequate exposure to ultraviolet sunlight. Whatever the cause, the end result is a decreased amount of 25-OH $D_3$, the substrate necessary for synthesis of the active form of the vitamin, $1,25\text{-}(OH)_2$ $D_3$. Since $1,25\text{-}(OH)_2$ $D_3$ facilitates intestinal absorption of calcium and phosphorus, its deficiency leads to their decreased absorption and, hence, decreased serum levels. Secondary hyperparathyroidism

T A B L E   2 8 - 3

**Analyte Levels in Hypocalcemic Disorders**

| | SERUM Ca | SERUM PO$_4$ | PTH | URINE Ca | URINE PO$_4$ | cAMP |
|---|---|---|---|---|---|---|
| Hypoparathyroidism | ↓ | ↑ | ↓ | ↓ | ↓ | ↓ |
| Pseudohypoparathyroidism | ↓ | ↑ | ↑ | ↓ | ↓ | ↓ |
| Vitamin D deficiency | ↓ | ↓ | ↑ | ↓ | ↑ | |
| Chronic renal failure | ↓ | ↑ | ↑ | ↓ | ↓ | |

↓ = decreased; ↑ = increased.

results from increased PTH secretion stimulated by the hypocalcemia. In late stages of the vitamin deficiency, PTH is unable to restore calcium levels to normal, but its hypophosphatemic effects are noticeable.

Without adequate calcium and phosphorus levels, the tendency toward bone mineralization does not occur. The bone involvement characteristic of vitamin D deficiency is age-related. In children, the condition is known as rickets and in adults it is called osteomalacia. In both conditions, there is a defective mineralization of bone so that the bones become soft, bend easily, and are prone to deformities. In rickets, the growing skeleton is involved and defective mineralization occurs in the epiphyseal cartilage as well as in the bone. The bones are incapable of withstanding normal mechanical stresses and tend to undergo bowing deformities during growth. Frequent fractures occur because of the inadequate skeletal structure.

In adult osteomalacia, the skeletal deformities are not as prominent. The major symptoms are varying degrees of skeletal pain and tenderness. However, minor trauma may cause bone fractures.

**Chronic Renal Failure**

Serum PTH levels are elevated in many patients with chronic renal failure. Renal disease is associated with decreased synthesis of 1,25-(OH)$_2$ D$_3$ which leads to hypocalcemia. The body responds to the low calcium levels by increasing the secretion of PTH. Hypocalcemia associated with increased PTH levels is also known as secondary hyperparathyroidism and may occur in conditions other than chronic renal failure. The increase in PTH, however, may not be able to restore normal calcium homeostasis as the renal failure progresses. Because of the absence of sufficient 1,25-(OH)$_2$ D$_3$, the bone is resistant to the calcium-mobilizing effect of PTH. Elevated serum phosphorus levels are also present in renal disease. The hyperphosphatemia is due, in part, to renal phosphate retention from the reduced filtered load of phosphate. The hyperphosphatemia also plays an important role in producing hypocalcemia. Skeletal lesions also occur in chronic renal failure owing to defective bone mineralization from the altered calcium:phosphorus concentration. The condition is referred to as renal osteodystrophy when bone involvement is present.

**SYMPTOMS**

The symptoms of hypocalcemia are manifested by increased excitability of neuromuscular function. The most characteristic sign is tetany. A typical attack of tetany begins with sensations of tingling in the fingertips and around the mouth. The lower extremities may also be involved. These paresthesias gradually become more severe and spread along the limbs. The muscles of the extremities and facial muscles may then go into painful spasm. The spasm may appear as a cramp or stiffness. Tetany may also be accompanied by hyperventilation as a result of anxiety.

Lesser degrees of neuromuscular excitability, or latent tetany, may be recognized by certain signs. Twitching of muscles supplied by the facial nerve, known as Chvostek's sign, may be elicited by tapping the facial nerve just below and in front of the ear lobe or between the zygomatic arch and the corner of the mouth. Trousseau's sign is elicited by inflating a blood pressure cuff to above the systolic pressure. A typical attack of carpal spasm will occur within 2 to 3 minutes.

Hypocalcemia may also affect the central nervous system, causing seizures resembling epilepsy. Psychiatric symptoms including emotional depression, memory impairment, and confusion and hallucinations may also be apparent.

Tetany can be treated by intravenous administration of calcium gluconate to raise the serum calcium concentration. Calcium salts may also be given orally. Hypoparathyroidism is treated with calcium salts and vitamin D.

**Hypercalcemia**

**CAUSES**

Hypercalcemia occurs when the total serum calcium level is >10.5 mg/dL. The causes of hypercalcemia are numerous. However, over 90% of hypercalcemic cases are due to either primary hyperparathyroidism or malignancy. Table 28–4 outlines the causes of hypercalcemia.

**Primary Hyperparathyroidism**

Caused by a single benign adenoma of the parathyroid glands in 80% of patients. The remaining 15% to 20% of cases are

### Causes of Hypercalcemia

Primary hyperparathyroidism
Malignancy
Toxicity
    Vitamin D
    Milk-alkali syndrome
Miscellaneous
    Sarcoidosis
    Immobilization

due to hyperplasia of two or more parathyroid glands. Parathyroid carcinoma occurs in <1% of cases. The incidence of primary hyperparathyroidism ranges from 1 in 500 to 1 in 1000. It occurs at all ages with a peak incidence in the sixth decade of life.[10] The condition is readily diagnosed by the presence of both hypercalcemia and elevated levels of PTH. Additional laboratory findings include decreased serum phosphorus and increased urinary excretion of calcium, phosphorus, and cAMP. The increased urinary calcium excretion can be explained by considering that there is a greater filtered load of calcium due to the increased activity of PTH, which exceeds the normal reabsorptive capacity of the kidney; thus the excess is excreted in the urine. Table 28–5 summarizes analyte levels in hypercalcemic disorders.

Most commonly, primary hyperparathyroidism is an asymptomatic disorder with mild but persistent hypercalcemia. The major sites of involvement in symptomatic cases are the skeleton or the kidneys. The most common complications are renal manifestations such as nephrolithiasis and nephrocalcinosis. The classic symptom of skeletal involvement is osteitis fibrosa cystica, an erosive bone disease.

In primary hyperparathyroidism due to adenomas, PTH secretion is independent of the negative feedback mechanism. Its secretion, therefore, continues despite the elevated serum calcium levels.

### Malignancy

Hypercalcemia of malignancy is frequently due to direct invasion of bone by the tumor. The invasive tumors of multiple myeloma and breast carcinoma, for example, activate the osteoclasts, causing bone resorption with resultant hypercalcemia. The assay of PTH is an important laboratory aid in differentiating malignancy-associated hypercalcemia from primary hyperparathyroidism. Activity of the parathyroid glands is inhibited in malignancy; thus an elevated PTH, which is typical of primary hyperparathyroidism, would not be expected in malignancy.[10]

### Vitamin D Toxicity

Hypercalcemia may be associated with vitamin D toxicity. Such toxicity can occur in conjunction with therapy for hypoparathyroid states or can result from excessive ingestion of vitamin D. However, an excess of 50,000 IU of vitamin D consumed over a period of several months is required to produce hypercalcemia.[11]

Excessive calcium ingestion (3 to 6 g/day) in association with the use of absorbable antacids for the treatment of peptic ulcer can lead to a form of hypercalcemia known as the milk-alkali syndrome. Although not currently a common finding, this syndrome may be more frequently encountered as a result of the use of calcium carbonate as a supplemental nutrient.[10]

### Miscellaneous

Many granulomatous diseases are associated with hypercalcemia. In sarcoidosis, the mechanism responsible for the elevated calcium levels is presumably the production of 1,25-$(OH)_2$ $D_3$ by the granulomatous tissue. This extrarenal production of 1,25-$(OH)_2$ $D_3$ is probably not subject to the tight regulatory control found in the kidney.

Immobilization may cause hypercalcemia in children and adolescents but is rarely associated with hypercalcemia in adults. The hypercalcemia appears to be a result of disproportionate rate of bone formation and resorption due to the sudden loss of weight bearing. The calcium levels usually return to normal on resumption of activity.

### SYMPTOMS

Generally, calcium levels <12 mg/dL are not associated with symptoms, whereas higher levels are most often symptomatic.[10] The severity of symptoms is also related to how rapidly the calcium level rises. Hypercalcemia leads to a decrease in activity of nerve and muscle cells; thus the manifestations

### Analyte Levels in Hypercalcemic Disorders

| | SERUM Ca | SERUM PO$_4$ | PTH | URINE Ca | URINE PO$_4$ | cAMP |
|---|---|---|---|---|---|---|
| Primary hyperparathyroidism | ↑ | N,↓ | ↑ | ↑ | ↑ | ↑ |
| Malignancy | ↑ | ↓,↑,N | N,↓ | ↑ | ↑ | N,↑ |
| Vitamin D toxicity | ↑ | ↑ or N | ↓ or N | ↑ | ↓ | |

↑ = increased; N = normal; ↓ = decreased.

are multisystemic. General symptoms include weakness, anorexia, nausea, and constipation due, in part, to skeletal and intestinal smooth muscle hypofunction. Central nervous system involvement is manifested by impaired concentration and degrees of mental confusion, ranging from lethargy to stupor and coma. Renal involvement is accompanied by polyuria due to the calcification of the tubules with loss of concentrating ability. Prolonged deposition of calcium salts can lead to nephrolithiasis, the formation of renal stones. Hypercalcemia may also affect the cardiovascular system, causing hypertension and changes in the electrocardiogram. Skeletal system involvement results in bone pain, cysts, and fractures. Continued hypercalcemia may lead to calcium deposits in soft tissues such as kidney, vessels, and joints. Additionally, calcium salts may be deposited in the cornea of the eye, a manifestation known as band keratopathy.

Treatment of hypercalcemia is dependent on the cause and the degree of elevation. Rehydration promotes calcium excretion and may be the only treatment necessary for mild hypercalcemia with few accompanying symptoms. More severe symptoms require prompt therapy that may include the use of drugs such as furosemide or ethacrynic acid to promote renal calcium excretion.

## Metabolic Bone Diseases

### PAGET'S DISEASE

Paget's disease, also known as osteitis deformans, is a bone disorder characterized by excessive bone resorption due to increased osteoclastic activity. This event is followed by an increase in bone formation as the osteoblasts attempt to compensate. The deposition of new bone is often haphazard and irregular. The incidence of Paget's disease is estimated to be about 3% in individuals older than the age of 40. The cause is unknown.

The increased bone resorption causes calcium and phosphate ions to be released from bone. However, since these ions are reutilized for new bone formation, their plasma levels are commonly within the normal reference range. Hypercalcemia and hypercalciuria may rarely occur if the rate of bone resorption is markedly greater than bone formation. High levels of alkaline phosphatase are observed because of the increased osteoblastic activity.

Many patients with Paget's disease are asymptomatic, with the disorder being discovered during the course of examination for unrelated complaints. Other individuals may detect swelling or deformity of long bones with associated pain. Therapy ranges from treatment with mild analgesics or nonsteroidal anti-inflammatory drugs for pain relief to orthopedic procedures in more severe cases.

### OSTEOPOROSIS

Osteoporosis is a term used to describe disease from numerous causes in which the bone mass is reduced to a level below

that required to maintain adequate mechanical support. There is no known abnormality in the mineral structure of organic matrix of the bone. The reduction in bone mass indicates that the rate of bone resorption is greater than that of bone formation.

The major clinical manifestations are due to vertebral fractures in addition to fractures of other bones such as wrist, hip, humerus, and tibia. The major accompanying symptoms are pain, fractures, and spinal deformity.

Loss of bone mass with advancing age is a universal finding. However, it begins early and advances more rapidly in women than in men. The perimenopausal years are associated with a tendency toward accelerated bone loss. Numerous factors have been implicated in the acceleration of bone loss, including decreased estrogen availability, decreased calcium intake and intestinal calcium absorption, cigarette smoking, and the inability to synthesize adequate amounts of $1,25(OH)_2 D_3$.

The plasma levels of calcium and phosphorus are usually normal in patients with osteoporosis. Postmenopausal women may develop a slight hyperphosphatemia, and about 20% may have a significant hypercalciuria. Alkaline phosphatase levels are usually normal but may be increased following fractures.

The course of treatment depends on the underlying disorder leading to the development of osteoporosis. The use of estrogens tends to decrease the rate of bone resorption but does not restore skeletal mass. The major role of estrogen therapy is prevention rather than treatment. Oral calcium preparations also tend to decrease bone resorption in some patients but do not cure the osteoporosis. Oral administration of vitamin D may also be helpful in some cases.

## Hypophosphatemia

Hypophosphatemia is common laboratory finding and occurs when the serum phosphorus level is <2.4 mg/dL. Severe hypophosphatemia occurs when the serum concentration is less than 1.0 mg/dL.[12] Table 28–6 outlines the causative factors.

An increased renal excretion of phosphate ions occurs in both primary and secondary hyperparathyroidism. The action of elevated PTH on the renal tubules accounts for the excessive loss in primary hyperparathyroidism. During the recovery phase of diabetic ketoacidosis, hypophosphatemia occurs be-

TABLE 28–6

**Causes of Hypophosphatemia**

Renal excretion
  Primary hyperparathyroidism
  Secondary hyperparathyroidism
  Diabetic ketoacidosis (recovery phase)
Decreased intestinal absorption
  Vitamin D deficiency
  Malabsorption

TABLE 28-7

**Causes of Hyperphosphatemia**

Renal insufficiency
Hypoparathyroidism
Vitamin D toxicity

cause of the increased uptake of phosphate ions into the depleted tissues. Because of the importance of vitamin D for intestinal absorption of both calcium and phosphorus, its deficiency eventually results in inadequate phosphate absorption. Malabsorption syndromes impair intestinal absorption as well.

Since phosphate is present in all cells, numerous organ systems are involved when phosphate levels are depleted. Central nervous system involvement is manifested by symptoms such as irritability, malaise, confusion, seizures, or coma. Muscle weakness may be present as well as bone pain and joint stiffness. Chronic hypophosphatemia will eventually result in rickets and osteomalacia. Treatment includes intravenous or oral administration of phosphate salts while attempting to eliminate the causative factors.

## Hyperphosphatemia

An excess of phosphate ions occurs when the serum phosphorus concentration >4.7 mg/dL. The causative factors are outlined in Table 28-7.

Hyperphosphatemia is most commonly a consequence of renal insufficiency due, in part, to a reduction in the filtered load of phosphate. Hyperphosphatemia is a consequence of both hypoparathyroidism and pseudohypoparathyroidism. The deficient secretion of PTH in hypoparathyroidism results in decreased renal phosphate clearance. In pseudohypoparathyroidism, the target organs do not respond adequately to the secretion of PTH; hence phosphate clearance is similarly reduced.

The symptoms associated with hyperphosphatemia are mainly those associated with altered calcium metabolism, since it is usually accompanied by some degree of hypocalcemia. However, when prolonged elevations occur, there is a driving force for mineralization. Calcium phosphate deposits tend to occur in soft tissues such as vessels, connective tissue around joints and renal tubules, and other areas of the kidney.

## SUMMARY

There are usually four parathyroid glands embedded in the thyroid gland. The chief cells produce PTH, which is initially produced as a larger precursor molecule. The ionized calcium level is the major regulatory mechanism for the synthesis and secretion of PTH.

Calcium is the most abundant electrolyte in the human body. It is important in neuromuscular activity, blood coagulation, bone metabolism, and maintenance of the functional integrity of cell membranes. It also serves as an intracellular second messenger. Intracellularly, phosphorus is found in combination with lipids and proteins. Most of the extracellular phosphorus is found in hydroxyapatite. Serum calcium levels are regulated by PTH, vitamin D and calcitonin. Phosphorus has a reciprocal relationship with calcium.

There are several causes of hypocalcemia. The symptoms observed in these patients include tetany, seizures, and psychiatric manifestations. Patients with hypercalcemia manifest with a variety of symptoms including weakness, anorexia, nausea, constipation, mental impairment, and nephrolithiasis.

Laboratory data can provide valuable information in the diagnosis of several metabolic bone diseases. These include Paget's disease, osteomalacia, and rickets. The most common laboratory procedures performed in these instances are serum calcium, phosphorus, and alkaline phosphatase.

## REFERENCES

1. Altenahr E, Kietel M, Dorn G, Montz R: The effect of 1,25-dihydroxycholecalciferol on the parathyroid hormone secretion of porcine parathyroid glands and human parathyroid adenomas in vitro. Acta Endocrinol (Copenh) 86:533, 1977.
2. Rasmussen H: Ionic and hormonal control of calcium homeostasis. Am J Med 50:567, 1971.
3. Schrier RW: *Renal and Electrolyte Disorders*. 3rd ed. Boston, Little Brown, 1986.
4. Levine MM, Kleeman CR: Hypercalcemia: Pathophysiology and treatment. Hosp Pract 22:93–110, 1987.
5. Klee GG: Parathyroid hormone. Clinical Chemistry News 15(2):5–6, 1989.
6. Kokko JP, Tannen RL: *Fluids and Electrolytes*. Philadelphia, WB Saunders, 1986.
7. Toffaletti J: Calcitonin. Clinical Chemistry News 10(7):20–21, 1984.
8. Pesce AJ, Kaplan LA: *Methods in Clinical Chemistry*. St. Louis, MO, C.V. Mosby, 1987.
9. Tietz NW: *Fundamentals of Clinical Chemistry*. 4th ed. Philadelphia, WB Saunders, 1996.
10. Bilezikian JP: Hypercalcemia. Dis Month 34:771–775, 1988.
11. O'Dorisio TM, Cataland S: Hypercalcemia: Etiology and management. Hosp Med 19(6)197–226, 1984.
12. Harrison TR: *Principles of Internal Medicine*, 12th ed. New York, McGraw-Hill, 1991.

# CHAPTER 29

# Adrenocortical Endocrinology

*Jocelyn J. Hulsebus*

## ANATOMY

The two adrenal glands are located one above each kidney (Figure 29–1). These glands are divided into two portions, each producing its own hormones. The outer portion, called the cortex, is discussed in this chapter. The **cortex** has a high lipid content and produces steroid hormones. The inner portion is called the **medulla** and is discussed in Chapter 30.

The cortical region of the adrenal gland produces a variety of steroid hormones. Most of the steroid hormones produced fit into two categories, the glucocorticoids that influence glucose metabolism and the mineralocorticoids that influence sodium regulation. The cortex can be roughly separated into three layers (Figure 29–2), each producing different hormones.[1,2] The outermost layer is called the **zona glomerulosa** and produces the mineralocorticoid aldosterone. The middle layer is called the **zona fasciculata** and produces the glucocorticoids, primarily cortisol.[1,2] The innermost layer that is closest to the adrenal medulla is the **zona reticularis** and produces small quantities of androgens and minute quantities of estrogen. The androgens produced are primarily androstendione and dehydroepiandosterone (DHEA).[1,2] The amount of estrogen produced is so small that it is usually considered insignificant.

## ADRENAL HORMONES

### Biosynthesis

The biosynthesis of the adrenal steroids is a multienzyme (cytochrome P-450 oxygenases[1]) process that takes place in the cytoplasm and mitochondria of the cortex endocrine cells. Synthesis of the various steroid hormones starts in the mitochondria with the conversion of cholesterol, primarily from the plasma lipoproteins, to pregnenolone.[3,4] The pregnenolone must be transported out of the mitochondria and to the various intracellular sites for the process of hormone synthesis to continue. In addition, this is the rate-limiting step in the synthesis of the adrenal steroids and is primarily under the control of adrenocorticotropic hormone (ACTH). It is at this point that the pathways[3] diverge to produce the different hormones (Figure 29–3). The individual layers of the adrenal cortex contain the enzymes necessary for each of the respective hormones produced there. For example, the zona glomerulosa has the enzyme 18-hydroxysteroid dehydrogenase[5] that is necessary for the production of aldosterone but lacks the enzyme 11-$\beta$-hydoxylase necessary for cortisol synthesis. This layer also lacks the enzyme 17-$\alpha$-hydroxylase that is required for the production of androgens.[1] Figure 29–3 diagrams the pathway of the various steroid hormones.

### Metabolism

The major site of metabolism for the steroid hormones is the liver.[5] The rate of metabolism by the liver is dependent on whether the hormone is bound to a protein carrier. A higher percentage of aldosterone is not protein bound and is removed from circulation and metabolized by the liver more rapidly than cortisol, which is mostly bound to a protein carrier, transcortin (also called corticosteroid-binding globulin, CBG). Most steroids that are excreted in urine must be conjugated by the liver to either glucuronic acid or sulfates to form soluble compounds.[3,5] The metabolism of cortisol begins in the liver with a $\Delta$ reductase enzyme[4] and dehydrocortisol is produced. Dehydrocortisol is not excreted in urine and is further metabolized by 3-$\alpha$-hydroxysteroid dehydrogenase. The metabolites formed from this reaction are the major (50%) excretory compounds of cortisol (tetrahydrocortisol, tetrahydrocortisone).[5] Approximately 30% of the urinary metabolites of cortisol are cortol and cortolone and are formed by the hydrogenation of the C-20 ketone group. Cortisol is also metabolized in the kidney by the action of 11-$\beta$-hydroxysteroid dehydrogenase to cortisone.[6] In normal patients, very little urinary-free cortisol is found. Conversely, relatively large amounts of urinary-free cortisol are seen in patients with Cushing's syndrome.

### Specific Analytes

#### CORTISOL

ACTH from the anterior pituitary is responsible for stimulating the release and synthesis of glucocorticoids from the zona fasciculata. The conversion of cholesterol to pregnenolone (the

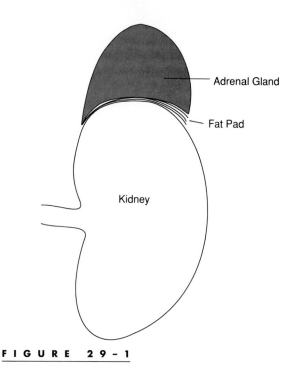

**FIGURE 29-1**

Anatomic location of the adrenal gland.

rate-limiting step) is under the control of ACTH as well as subsequent reactions that produce cortisol.[3] Cortisol is the most potent and clinically significant glucocorticoid. Most (90%) of the cortisol released into the blood circulates attached to CBG or albumin and has a half-life of approximately 90 minutes.[5] The secretion of cortisol is diurnal and is associated with a person's sleep–wake cycle. A peak level of cortisol is usually observed between 6:00 and 8:00 A.M. and a low level between 6:00 P.M. and 12:00 A.M. The concentration of cortisol in the plasma at 8:00 P.M. is approximately 50% of the level at 8 A.M.[5] Changes in sleeping patterns or stress levels cause alterations in the secretion of ACTH and cortisol.

Cortisol stimulates both gluconeogenesis and glycogenesis in the liver, resulting in increases in the plasma glucose. The

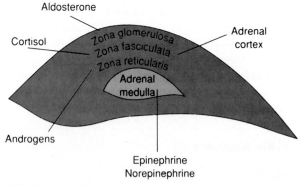

**FIGURE 29-2**

The anatomy of the adrenal gland and location of hormone production.

stimulation of gluconeogenesis in the liver occurs in the fasting state and, in conjunction with cortisol's inhibition of glucose uptake in peripheral tissues, causes the increase in plasma glucose.[3] Since many amino acids are being used for gluconeogenesis in the liver, muscle uptake of amino acids is inhibited. In addition, protein synthesis in muscle is inhibited and protein catabolism increases, usually causing a loss of muscle tissue. Excess cortisol has been shown to decrease the amount of calcium that is absorbed from the intestine, initiating a decrease in plasma calcium. Plasma calcium concentrations are maintained by the body by removing calcium from storage in the bone tissue. Cortisol will stimulate lipolysis in adipose tissue so that the plasma concentration of glycerol and free-fatty acids will increase.[1] Cortisol in high concentrations causes both anti-inflammatory and immunosuppressive actions. These actions of cortisol make it a valuable therapeutic agent in some types of diseases such as rheumatoid arthritis, systemic lupus erythematosis, and multiple sclerosis.[2]

Blood and urine samples are used for analysis of cortisol and its metabolites. Serum or plasma may be used with most cortisol assays and may be frozen if not analyzed immediately. Cortisol is generally measured by immunologic assays in the clinical laboratory. In addition, a free-cortisol concentration can be measured reliably in saliva by high-performance liquid chromatography (HPLC).[7] Radioimmunoassay (RIA) is the method of choice for serum and urinary-free cortisol although testing by HPLC is increasing.[5,7] Serum cortisol can be measured directly but urinary-free cortisol usually requires an extraction step to remove cross-reacting metabolites before analysis. Because of the diurnal (circadian) variation of cortisol levels, serum cortisol is usually measured at both 8:00 A.M. and 4:00 P.M. Another popular way to measure cortisol is on the TDx analyzer (Abbott Laboratories).[5] This immunologic assay uses fluorescent tags and fluorescence polarization to measure cortisol. The approximate reference ranges for plasma cortisol are 8:00 A.M., 5 to 23 μg/dL and 4:00 P.M., 3 to 15 μg/dL.[5]

**The following tests for urinary steroids are considered antiquated, and have been replaced by plasma and urine assays (most commonly HPLC) for specific steroids.** They are discussed here since they are available at some reference laboratories and may be ordered by physicians. A 24-hour urine must be collected for the analysis of urinary steroids by the following methods. The four general steps used for urinary steroid analysis are hydrolysis of conjugates, extraction of the compound to be measured, purification of the compound from interfering substances, and quantitation.[2,5] The urinary metabolites of cortisol that are measured are 17-hydroxycorticosteroids and 17-ketogenic steroids.[5] The 17-hydroxycorticosteroids have hydroxyl groups at C-21 and C-17 and a keto group at C-20; this configuration is known as the dihydroxy acetone side chain. These compounds are measured by the Porter-Silber[5] method (Figure 29–4). 17-hydroxycorticosteroids and phenylhydrazine are incubated at 60°C for 30 minutes. A characteristic yellow pigment is formed that can be measured in a spectrophotometer at 410 nm.

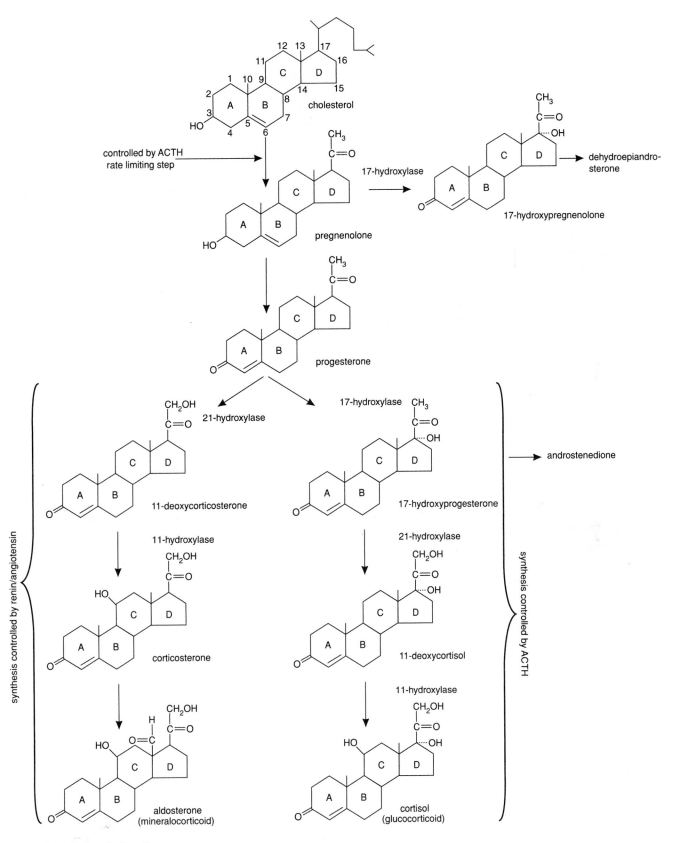

**FIGURE  29-3**

Synthesis of aldosterone and cortisol.

The Porter-Silber reaction for the determination of 17-hydroxycorticosteroids.

The measurement of 17-ketogenic steroids can be done with the Appleby[5] method that incorporates the Zimmerman reaction.[5] There are four groups of 17-ketogenic steroids: group I (cortisol, cortisone, 11-deoxycortisol, tetrahydro S); group II (cortols and cortolones); group III (pregnanetriol and 11-oxygenated derivatives); and group IV (17-hydroxyprogesterone, 17-hydroxypregnenolone).[5] Before the oxidation step, a sodium borohydrate reduction is done so that all C-21 17-hydroxycorticosteroids are measured. Next, the 17-ketogenic steroids are oxidized to 17-ketosteroids after chemical treatment with sodium bismuthate or sodium *m*-periodate to break the 17-hydroxy bond and replace it with a keto group at position 17. The 17-ketosteroids are then quantitated by producing a color reaction with *m*-dinitrobenzene in the presence of alcohol and potassium hydroxide (KOH). This color reaction is known as the Zimmermann reaction. A reddish-purple pigment is formed and readings are taken in a spectrophotometer at 480, 520, and 580 nm[5] (Figure 29–5). Any 17-ketosteroids present in the original specimen will be reduced by the sodium bismuthate to 17-hydroxysteroids and will not react in the Zimmermann reaction.

## ALDOSTERONE

Aldosterone is produced by the zona glomerulosa layer of the adrenal cortex. Aldosterone is a C-21 steroid that helps regulate body sodium and potassium by stimulating cells of the distal convoluted tubule and collecting duct in the nephron to reabsorb more sodium from the filtrate. It also stimulates the tubular cells to secrete potassium and hydrogen into the urine. The initial steps of aldosterone synthesis (cholesterol to pregnenolone) are under control of ACTH, but the steps following pregnenolone synthesis are controlled by the renin-angiotensin system and the fluid volume.[6] If the sodium concentration and/or plasma volume decreases, the proteolytic enzyme renin is released from the juxtaglomerular cells of the nephron into the plasma. Baroreceptors in the juxtaglomerular cells respond to changes in blood pressure, and possibly

cells in the macula densa (specialized cells of the descending loop of Henle)[6] respond to decreases in chloride and sodium. If the baroreceptors are stretched because of an increase in blood pressure, renin secretion is inhibited, whereas a decrease in blood pressure stimulates renin secretion.[1] A circulating protein called *angiotensinogen* is cleaved by the renin to form angiotensin I. Angiotensin I is modified by converting enzymes in the plasma and lung tissue to become angiotensin II.[8] Angiotensin II stimulates the cells in the adrenal cortex to synthesize and release aldosterone. In addition, angiotensin II causes constriction of the peripheral arteries, resulting in an increase in the blood pressure and an increased filtration rate in the kidney.[8] Aldosterone can be analyzed in serum, plasma, or urine by RIA.[5] This method of choice is readily available in a number of commercial kits. Since steroid hormones are stable compounds, no special precautions are needed during the drawing stage. The position of the patient, either lying down (supine) or upright, must be noted for proper interpretation of the results (there is some overlap in normal and aldosterone insufficiency levels).[5] The blood specimen must be centrifuged and the serum or plasma removed as soon as possible. The specimen can be frozen if it is not analyzed immediately. The approximate references ranges for aldosterone are upright, 5 to 30 ng/dL, and supine, 3 to 10 ng/dL.[5]

The activity of renin is measured rather than the concentration of the enzyme itself and is based on the amount of angiotensin I produced from angiotensinogen. The measurement of angiotensin I is available using RIA kit methods. The renin activity is expressed in nanograms of angiotensin I /h/mL.[5] The specimen of choice for the analysis of renin activity is EDTA plasma. The patient's position, either supine or standing, must be noted and great attention to detail must be followed when drawing a specimen for renin analysis. The whole blood specimen should be centrifuged immediately. The plasma is then removed and frozen[5] at −20°C until needed. The approximate reference ranges for renin are supine, 0.1 to 3.1 ng/h/mL, and standing, 1.6 to 7.4 ng/h/mL.[5]

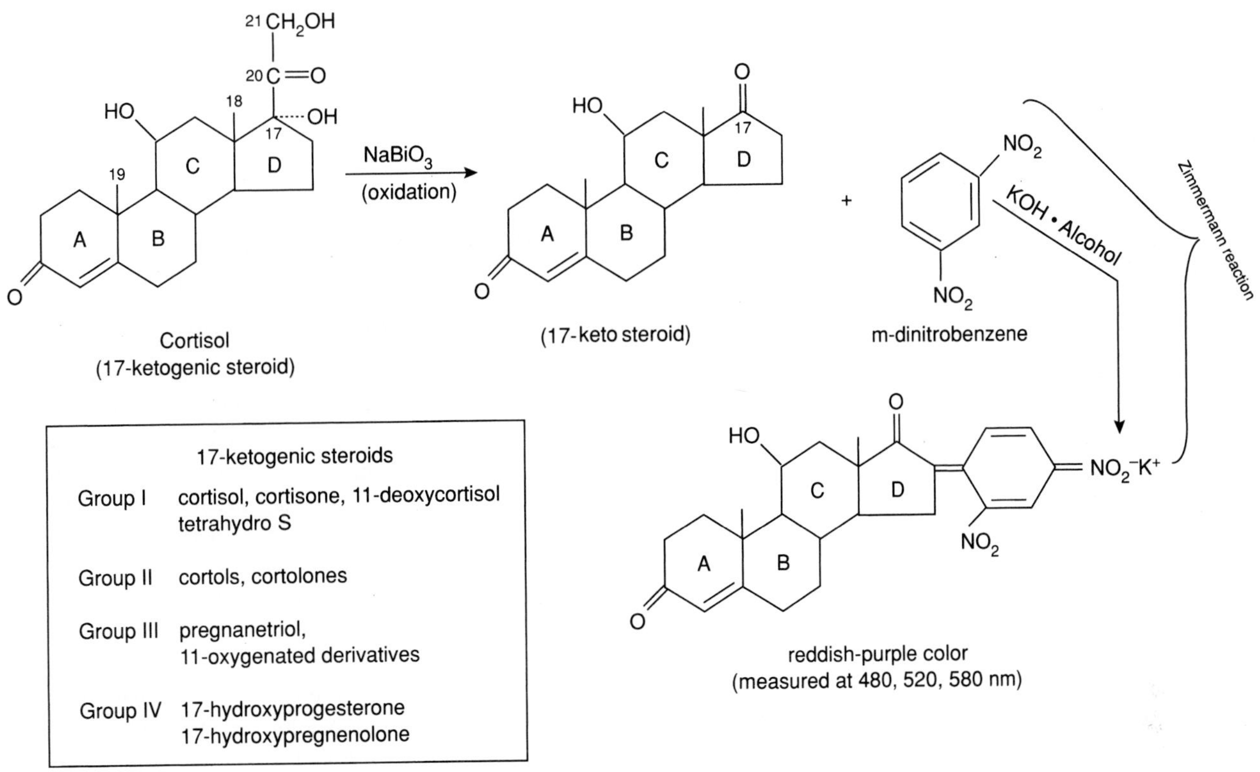

**17-ketogenic steroids**

Group I    cortisol, cortisone, 11-deoxycortisol
           tetrahydro S

Group II   cortols, cortolones

Group III  pregnanetriol,
           11-oxygenated derivatives

Group IV   17-hydroxyprogesterone
           17-hydroxypregnenolone

**FIGURE 29-5**

The Appleby method using the Zimmerman reaction for the determination of 17-ketogenic steroids.

## SEX STEROID HORMONES

The sex steroids (androgens, estrogens, progesterone) are normally produced in small amounts by the adrenal cortex. These hormones become clinically significant when an adrenal cortex tumor occurs, resulting in excess hormone production. The action and analysis of the sex steroid hormones are discussed in detail in Chapter 31.

## ADRENAL FUNCTION TESTS

### ACTH Stimulation Tests

When decreased concentrations of cortisol are detected, it is necessary to determine if the problem lies in the adrenal gland's inability to produce hormone (primary disorder) or in the absence of stimulating hormones to induce cortisol synthesis and secretion (secondary disorder). The starting point for this determination is to perform an ACTH stimulation screening test. The patient receives an intravenous (IV) injection of 250 μg of synthetic ACTH.[2] Timed blood specimens are drawn at 30-minute intervals and assayed for cortisol. An increased cortisol concentration suggests that the disorder is secondary and

that the problem is probably due to the absence of adrenal stimulation by ACTH. An increase of about 70 μg/L is expected before it is considered a positive stimulation test.[2,5] Cortisol concentrations that remain unchanged suggest that the disorder is primary and that the adrenal gland is unable to produce cortisol.

If the preceding screening test is positive, a longer ACTH stimulation test should be performed. Baseline values for cortisol are obtained before the ACTH stimulation. Patients receive an IV injection of synthetic ACTH for 3 consecutive days.[5] Cortisol levels should increase approximately 2.5 times over the baseline values. If primary adrenal insufficiency is present, there will be little or no increase in the cortisol concentrations.[5] Patients that are deficient in ACTH because of a primary pituitary or hypothalamic problem (secondary adrenal insufficiency) will show increasing levels of cortisol over the 3-day injection period.

### Dexamethasone Suppression Tests

#### OVERNIGHT DEXAMETHASONE SUPPRESSION TEST

Dexamethasone is an analog of cortisol that suppresses the secretion of ACTH from the pituitary. This analog is given to patients who have increased levels of cortisol and are suspected of having Cushing's syndrome (discussed later). A screening test consists of giving the patient a single dose (1 mg of dexamethasone, orally) at 11:00 P.M.[2] A blood sample is drawn for cortisol analysis at 8:00 A.M. the next morning. Reference values are $<5$ $\mu$g/dL ($<50$ $\mu$g/L) and elevated levels (suspected Cushing's) are $>10$ $\mu$g/dL ($>100$ $\mu$g/L).[2] Increased cortisol levels ($>5$ $\mu$g/dL) may be seen in other conditions such as during stress and endogenous depression. A longer confirming dexamethasone suppression test should follow all positive screening tests.

### LOW-DOSE DEXAMETHASONE SUPPRESSION TEST

The procedure may be performed on patients having a positive overnight dexamethasone screening test. The patient receives 0.5 mg of dexamethasone orally every 6 hours for 2 consecutive days. Normal subjects respond to the dexamethasone with a low plasma cortisol and urinary-free cortisol. Patients with hypercortisolism (Cushing's syndrome) will show an elevation of cortisol.

### HIGH-DOSE DEXAMETHASONE SUPPRESSION TEST

The high-dose dexamethasone procedure was designed to provide for a differential diagnosis of Cushing's syndrome. The test is performed by administering a 2.0-mg dose of dexamethasone for 2 consecutive days. The plasma cortisol and urinary-free cortisol levels are determined. Patients with an ACTH-producing tumor of the pituitary gland (Cushing's disease) will usually exhibit a suppression of cortisol. Patients with Cushing's syndrome due to other causes (adrenal cortical tumors or ACTH-producing ectopic tumors) usually do not exhibit a change in the cortisol levels.

## Metyrapone Stimulation Test

Metyrapone will inhibit the enzyme ll-$\beta$-hydroxylase that is necessary for the synthesis of cortisol.[2] By decreasing the amount of cortisol, ACTH concentrations increase in normal patients. The increased ACTH causes an increased level of 11-deoxycortisol (compound S), the compound produced immediately preceding the metabolic block.

This test can be used to help evaluate pituitary function and secondary adrenal insufficiency. Patients receive 3 g of metyrapone at 11 P.M. A blood sample is then drawn at 8:00 A.M. and analyzed for cortisol. In normal patients, this cortisol value should be decreased and can serve as a control for proving that the patient did receive the dose of metyrapone. In addition, ACTH should be measured in this sample. In normal patients, a value of 100 ng/L or greater should be obtained for the ACTH concentration.[2] In patients with a secondary adrenocortical insufficiency, there is no increase in the 11-deoxycortisol level because there is no increase in ACTH levels since the pituitary is incapable of producing ACTH. On the other hand, patients with primary adrenal insufficiency

demonstrate no increase in 11-deoxycortisol since the adrenal gland is incapable of producing cortisol but would have an increased ACTH level.

## CLINICAL APPLICATIONS

### Congenital Adrenal Hyperplasia

Congenital adrenal hyperplasia, also called **adrenogenital syndrome,** is characterized by the decrease or absence of an enzyme necessary for the synthesis of one or more of the adrenal steroid hormones. The decreased production of cortisol leads to an increase in the plasma concentration of ACTH[2] and hyperplasia of the adrenal cortex. A block in the metabolic pathway may cause an increased production of androgens, which results in the virilizing syndrome. If a female fetus is exposed to excessive quantities of circulating testosterone, the child may exhibit ambiguous external genitalia at birth. In males, manifestation of the disorder may be difficult to detect at birth. However, virilization continues and may be manifest by increased somatic growth and premature signs of puberty.

The most common enzyme deficiency reported is that of 21-hydroxylase. This deficiency results in the accumulation of progesterone, 17-hydroxyprogesterone, and 11,17-dehydroxyprogesterone in the blood and therefore excessive excretion of pregnanediol, pregnanetriol, and 11-hydroxypregnanetriol in the urine. The disorder is transmitted as an autosomal recessive condition. In mild cases, a female patient demonstrates excess hirsutism (excessive hairiness) and reduced breast development and fails to menstruate at puberty. In severe cases, the female child demonstrates excess masculinization at birth with ambiguous genitalia and hirsutism. About one half of these patients tend to be hypotensive because of the decreased production of the mineralocorticoids. These patients consequently lose sodium and retain potassium.

The second most frequent enzymatic defect is the absence of 11-hydroxylase. This condition leads to the overproduction of 11-deoxycorticosterone (DOC), which is a potent sodium retainer. The sodium retention leads to hypertension, potassium depletion, increased extracellular volume, and the inhibition of renin production. Laboratory findings include decreased cortisol and increased ACTH levels in the serum and increased 17-ketosteroids and decreased aldosterone levels in the urine.

If deficiencies of one or more hormones are detected soon after birth, the prognosis is often grave. Children who do not demonstrate symptoms until their teenaged years have a milder form of the disease and can be treated successfully. In all of the enzyme deficiencies, there is a decrease in cortisol. Therefore, the treatment for all the enzyme deficiencies is the administration of cortisol.

## Adult Adrenogenital Syndrome

Adrenal hyperplasia caused by increased ACTH levels is the most common condition associated with the adrenogenital syndrome. If this occurs in adults, it is most often caused by an adrenal adenoma or carcinoma and is known as the **adult adrenogenital syndrome,** although tumors may occur from early infancy to late in life. The overproduction of androgens in the female patient causes a development of a masculine habitus with hirsutism, receding hairline, and clitoral enlargement. Menstruation and ovulation cease and the breasts and uterus atrophy. These virilizing tumors usually produce excessive amounts of dehydroepiandrosterone, which can be detected in the plasma or increased excretion of 17-ketosteroids in the urine.

## Hypercortisolism

**Cushing's syndrome** is a term referring to a complex of clinical signs and symptoms that result from exposure to high levels of cortisol. The hypercortisolism may be due to excessive production of ACTH such as occurs when a basophilic adenoma is present in the pituitary gland. The increased ACTH production causes hyperplasia of the adrenal glands and the term applied to this condition is **Cushing's disease.** There are other causes of hypercortisolism, and thus Cushing's syndrome. These include (1) adenoma, carcinoma, or nodular hyperplasia of the adrenal gland, (2) exogenous administration of glucocorticoids or ACTH, and (3) ectopic ACTH-secreting tumors.

Patients with Cushing's syndrome may have obvious physical symptoms such as a "moon face," truncal obesity with a "buffalo hump," and occasionally hirsutism.[2,3] Other clinical symptoms include hypertension, which may be due to increased mineralocorticoid secretion or the weak mineralocorticoid activity produced by the large amounts of cortisol; menstrual disturbances secondary to increased adrenal androgens; osteoporosis, and emotional disorders.[3] The catabolic effect of high levels of cortisol may also result in capillary fragility, resulting in easy bruisability and muscle weakness. Generally, not all of the preceding symptoms are present and a wide variety of combinations may occur.

Routine laboratory data may reveal several abnormalities. Glucose intolerance may be indicated with an increased serum glucose, glycosuria, and abnormal glucose tolerance test. The serum sodium may be increased and serum potassium decreased. The diurnal pattern of cortisol secretion is absent and early morning cortisol levels may be 2 to 3 times the reference range (5 to 25 $\mu$g/dL)[5]. In patients with Cushing's syndrome due to adrenal neoplasms, ACTH levels will be decreased because of the negative feedback action of cortisol. Patients with Cushing's disease (pituitary Cushing's syndrome) will have increased levels of ACTH owing to its production by the pituitary tumor. Increased levels of ACTH can also be found in patients with ectopic production of ACTH such as in a lung carcinoma (ectopic ACTH) and who have developed Cushing's syndrome. The high-dose dexamethasone suppression test may be of value in differentiating the cause of Cushing's syndrome.

## Hypocortisolism

There are two types of adrenal insufficiency, primary and secondary. In **primary adrenal insufficiency** there is a marked increase in plasma ACTH levels, whereas in **secondary adrenal insufficiency,** there is a decreased plasma ACTH. Both conditions result in a decreased production of cortisol and thus hypocortisolism.

There are two manifestations of primary adrenal insufficiency, acute and chronic. Acute adrenal insufficiency is a life-threatening condition that arises from a sudden decrease of cortisol.[7] The destruction of the adrenal cortex may be caused by trauma, hemorrhage, thrombosis, or infection. It may also follow surgery or acute stress in patients whose cortisol reserve has been diminished. The Waterhouse-Friderichsen syndrome is a specific type of acute primary adrenal insufficiency due to a meningococcal meningitis and septicemia.[2] Patients with acute primary adrenal insufficiency may present with a fever, headache, abdominal pain, hypotension, and cyanosis. Laboratory findings include elevated levels of potassium, urea nitrogen, calcium, and ACTH (>250 pg/mL). Decreased levels of sodium, glucose, and cortisol are also be observed.

Chronic primary adrenal insufficiency is also know as Addison's disease and is characterized as gradual decline of adrenal steroids, primarily cortisol.[2,9] The cause of this deficiency may be an autoimmune disease, but most often it is considered to be of idiopathic origin. The major clinical symptoms of the chronic disorder include weakness and easy fatigability. These symptoms may be the result of the hypoglycemia, although the pathophysiologic mechanism has not been fully elucidated. Nausea, vomiting, diarrhea, and abdominal pain may also be frequently occurring symptoms. The hyperpigmentation of the skin and mucous membrane that is seen in some patients is the result of the increased ACTH levels produced in response to the hypocortisolism. An aldosterone deficiency results in the loss of sodium in the urine and a block in the renal secretion of hydrogen ions and potassium. The net result is a decrease in total body sodium, plasma volume, cardiac output, hyperkalemia, and metabolic acidosis. Thus, hypotension is a frequent finding in these patients. The laboratory findings are similar to those seen in acute adrenal insufficiency. The diagnosis, however, is based on the demonstration of decreased cortisol levels. Since the onset of this condition is slow, it may be well advanced, with 90% of adrenal glandular function destroyed before it is diagnosed. Immediate replacement treatment may be required and be lifelong.

Secondary adrenal insufficiency may be due to a deficiency of ACTH secretion (0 to 50 pg/mL) from the pituitary. Patients develop what appears to be Addison's disease without the hyperpigmentation.[2] Differential diagnosis is based on the ability of the adrenal gland to release cortisol when challenged with exogenous ACTH (ACTH stimulation test) and the presence of low plasma concentrations of ACTH.

## Hypoaldosteronism

Primary hypoaldosteronism is sometimes seen in conjunction with deficiencies of other adrenal steroids when there is nonspecific destruction of the adrenal tissue. It can be found in Addison's disease, bilateral adrenalectomy, adrenal gland hemorrhage, and 21-hydroxylase deficiency. These patients show a marked inability to respond or adjust to stress. Because of the lack of aldosterone, plasma sodium concentration is low and potassium is high.[3] Patients become dehydrated and hypotensive. Kidney function is decreased, resulting in an increased urea nitrogen and creatinine in the plasma. Renin concentrations in the plasma are increased due to the deficiency of aldosterone.[3]

Congenital primary hypoaldosteronism is a rare genetic disease. This disease is due to the absence of the enzyme methyloxidase that is required for the synthesis of aldosterone. Secondary hypoaldosteronism can occur in patients with renal disease. The kidney's inability to produce and release renin results in decreased plasma concentrations of aldosterone. Patients with severe diabetes often develop decreases in aldosterone because of renal disease associated with their diabetes.

## Hyperaldosteronism

Adrenal adenoma or hyperplasia may lead to primary hyperaldosteronism or **Conn's disease**.[2,3] These patients develop a benign hypertension, muscle weakness, polyuria, and polydipsia. Plasma concentration of aldosterone increase, causing an increase of sodium reabsorption in the kidney and also an increase of potassium secretion into the urine. The resulting hypernatremia induces a slight hypertension. It is not unusual for the patient to develop disturbances in acid-base balance that lead to alkalosis. Potassium depletion results in muscle weakness and fatigue. Potassium depletion may also cause a defect in the ability to concentrate urine. Patients frequently have nocturnal polyuria. The decreased potassium may also impair the insulin release from the pancreatic beta cells. The patients may demonstrate a glucose intolerance. Diagnosis is based on the inability of the patient to suppress aldosterone when given high doses of sodium and to have decreased plasma renin concentrations. Laboratory findings include an increased serum sodium and urine aldosterone, decreased serum potassium, low to normal plasma renin, and tendency toward metabolic alkalosis.

Secondary hyperaldosteronism results with some types of kidney lesions. Renin levels increase dramatically, causing excess stimulation of aldosterone synthesis and release. It is the high plasma renin levels that distinguish secondary from primary hyperaldosteronism.

## SUMMARY

The adrenal cortex produces glucocorticoids (cortisol), mineralocorticoids (aldosterone), and small amounts of sex steroid hormones. These steroid hormones are produced by multienzyme processes from cholesterol. The steroid hormones from the adrenal cortex are primarily metabolized in the liver, where they may be chemically modified or conjugated with glucuronic acid or sulfates. These metabolites are then excreted in the urine.

Cortisol is the most potent and clinically significant glucocorticoid. This hormone (90%) circulates in blood bound to CBG. Cortisol has a characteristic diurnal secretion pattern with a peak level between 6:00 and 8:00 A.M. and a trough level between 6:00 P.M. and 12:00 A.M. Cortisol can stimulate gluconeogenesis in the liver and cause a glucose-sparing action in the peripheral tissues. In addition, cortisol can be used as a therapeutic agent because of its anti-inflammatory and immunosuppressive actions. Excess amounts of cortisol can induce Cushing's syndrome. Inadequate production of cortisol may be due to primary or secondary adrenal insufficiency. Chronic primary adrenal insufficiency is known as Addison's disease. The mineralocorticoid aldosterone helps with the regulation of body sodium and potassium by acting on the cells of the kidney tubules to reabsorb more sodium and secrete potassium into the urine. The synthesis and secretion of aldosterone is primarily controlled by the renin-angiotensin system and the blood volume. Low levels of aldosterone cause dehydration with increases in the plasma potassium, creatinine, and BUN and decrease in the plasma sodium. Hypersecretion of aldosterone (Conn's disease) leads to increased plasma sodium, benign hypertension, and muscle weakness. To test adrenal cortex function, there are several stimulation and inhibition tests that help with the diagnosis of the endocrine disorder. Included in the list of tests are ACTH stimulation, water deprivation, dexamethasone suppression, and metyrapone stimulation.

### REFERENCES

1. Tyrrell BJ, Aron DC, Forsham PH: Glucocorticoids and adrenal androgens. In Greenspan F (ed.): *Basic and Clinical Endocrinology*. 4th ed. Norwalk, CT, Appleton & Lange, 1991, p 323.
2. Gornal AG, Luxton AW, Bhavnani BR: Endocrine disorders. In Fornall AG (ed.): *Applied Biochemistry of Clinical Disorders*. 2nd ed. Philadelphia, JB Lippincott Co., 1986, p 285.
3. Bondy PK: Disorders of the adrenal cortex. In Wilson JD, Foster DW (eds.): *Williams Textbook of Endocrinology*. 3rd ed. Philadelphia, WB Saunders, 1985, p 816.
4. Brown MS, Kovanin PT, Goldstein JL: Receptor mediated uptake of lipoprotein-cholesterol and its utilization

for steroid synthesis in the adrenal cortex. Rec Prog Horm Res 35:215–257, 1979.

5. Whitlet RJ, Meikle AW, Watts NB: Endocrinology. In Burtis CA, Ashwood Ed (eds.): *Tietz Textbook of Clinical Chemistry*. 2nd ed. Philadelphia, WB Saunders, 1994, p 1645.

6. Findling JW, Aron DC, Tyrrell JB: Glucocorticoids and adrenal androgens. In Greenspan F (ed.): *Basic and Clinical Endocrinology*. 5th ed. Norwalk, CT, Appleton & Lange, 1997, p 317.

7. Aron DC, Findling JW, Tyrrell JB: Glucocorticoids and adrenal androgens. In Greenspan F, Gardner D (eds.): *Basic and Clinical Endocrinology*. 6th ed. New York, McGraw-Hill, 2001, p 348.

8. Carey RM, Sen S: Recent progress in the control of aldosterone secretion. Rec Prog Horm Res 42:251–291, 1986.

9. Angeli A, Frairi R: Simultaneous diagnosis and treatment of acute adrenocortical insufficiency. Lancet 2:1217–1218, 1975.

# Adrenal Medullary Endocrinology

*Jocelyn J. Hulsebus*

## ANATOMY

The middle region of the adrenal gland is called the **medulla.** This area is composed primarily of **chromaffin cells** that originate from the same part of the neural crest as the sympathetic nervous system. Neural crest cells are embryonic cells that separate from the neuroectoderm to become peripheral and autonomic nerves of the central nervous system. The **catecholamine hormones,** epinephrine and norepinephrine, are modified amines that are produced in the medulla, with epinephrine being produced in the highest quantity, approximately 90% of all catecholamines produced.[1] The reason for the high production of epinephrine is the presence of the enzyme phenylethanolamine-*N*-methyltransferase (PNMT) that is necessary to convert norepinephrine to epinephrine and found only in tissues that produce epinephrine. In addition, PNMT is induced by the high concentrations of glucocorticoids found in the medulla. The adrenal medulla is a highly innervated tissue with many neurons that appear to be in direct contact with the chromaffin cells. Catecholamine hormone release can be stimulated by the action of these neurons.

## ADRENAL MEDULLARY HORMONES

### Synthesis

The catecholamine hormones are synthesized from the amino acid L-tyrosine by enzymatic processes, which are diagrammed in Figure 30–1. The first step in the biosynthetic pathway is the hydroxylation of L-tyrosine to L-dopa by the enzyme tyrosine hydroxylase.[1,2] Since this is the rate-limiting step in catecholamine synthesis, the body can regulate the synthesis of catecholamine hormones by influencing the activity of this enzyme. Next, L-dopa is decarboxylated by L-aromatic amino acid decarboxylase, a nonspecific decarboxylase found in most tissues, to dopamine. Dopamine-$\beta$-hydroxylase (DBH) adds a hydroxyl group to dopamine to form norepinephrine. In the final step of catecholamine synthesis, the enzyme PNMT adds a methyl group to norepinephrine to form epinephrine.[1] Once synthesized, the hormones can either be secreted or stored within the chromaffin cells in storage granules.

## Metabolism

Catecholamines that are secreted into the plasma have a short half-life of about 1 to 2 minutes. They are rapidly removed from the circulation by the liver and kidneys or are taken up by sympathetic neurons. Two enzyme systems are responsible for the breakdown or inactivation of the catecholamine hormones. Monoamine oxidase (MAO)[1] deaminates the catecholamines and is present in many tissues throughout the body (Figure 30–2). The second enzyme, catechol-o-methyltransferase (COMT),[1] methylates a hydroxyl group on the aromatic ring structure of the catecholamine molecule (Figure 30–2). COMT is found in highest concentration in the kidneys and liver. The methylation reaction of this enzyme produces **metanephrine** from epinephrine and **normetanephrine** from norepinephrine. Both metanephrine and normetanephrine can be conjugated with sulfate or glucuronide and excreted in the urine. The final metabolite of both epinephrine and norepinephrine is **vanillylmandelic acid** (VMA).

## Receptors

The action of the catecholamine hormones is mediated through adrenergic receptors.[1,3] There are two **alpha receptors** and two **beta receptors.** These receptors are found throughout the body in most tissues. Some tissues have both alpha and beta receptors present, whereas other tissues may have only one type. Both epinephrine and norepinephrine interact with these receptors, although the receptor affinity for the two hormones may be different. The alpha$_1$-adrenergic receptor uses calcium and phosphatidylinositol for its second messengers.[1] Both epinephrine and norepinephrine are strong stimulants for the $\alpha_1$-adrenergic receptor.[4] The $\alpha_2$-, $\beta_1$-, and $\beta_2$-adrenergic receptors use cAMP as their second messenger.[1] Many $\beta_1$-adrenergic receptors are found on myocardial cells. Blocking these receptors with drugs (beta blockers) to decrease the strength of the contraction is currently a valuable treatment for patients with heart disease.

## Specific Analytes

### DOPAMINE

**Dopamine** is a catecholamine that appears in the highest concentration in the central nervous system (CNS), where it

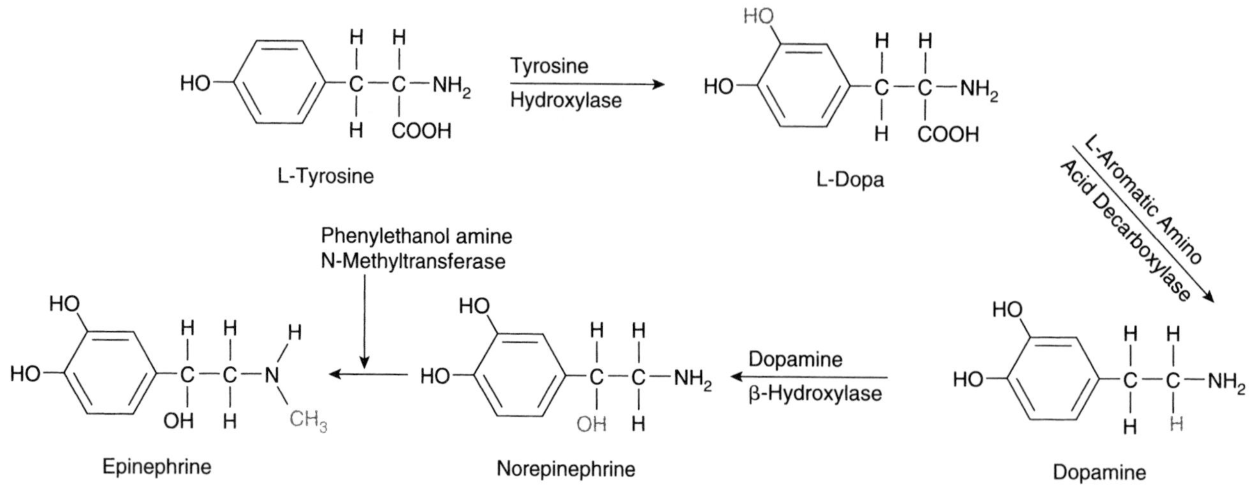

Synthesis of the catecholamines.

functions primarily as a neurotransmitter. In addition, dopamine from the hypothalamus helps to control the synthesis and secretion of prolactin from the pituitary. When dopamine is present, prolactin is inhibited, and when dopamine is absent, prolactin is freely secreted.[1]

Most dopamine is synthesized in the CNS, but there may be a small amount synthesized in the adrenal medulla.[5] As with all catecholamines, dopamine is synthesized from the amino acid L-tyrosine (see Figure 30–1). The enzymatic metabolism of dopamine can be catalyzed by either COMT or MAO. The final metabolite of dopamine is **homovanillic acid** (HMV).[1]

Methods for measuring dopamine in plasma are at best difficult. The first problem encountered when doing an assay for dopamine is obtaining a good specimen for analysis. It is best to draw blood for any catecholamine analysis from an indwelling catheter, since a venipuncture may cause catecholamine levels to increase.[2] In addition, the patient should be lying down for at least 30 minutes because levels will be 2 to 3 times higher in a patient who is sitting upright.[6] Patients should be fasting for at least 4 hours and should not have consumed coffee or tea and not have used tobacco within that time. Aldomet, a medication for hypertension, should be discontinued for at least 1 week before testing.[2] In addition, the blood drawing tubes should be prechilled and contain sodium thiosulfite (antioxidant) and EDTA.[2] Blood samples must be placed on ice immediately after drawing. The blood should be separated using a refrigerated centrifuge as soon as possible after drawing and the plasma frozen at −70°C until the analysis is performed.

Analysis of dopamine in plasma can be performed using a radioenzymatic kit method.[2] This method uses the enzyme COMT to transfer a $^3$H-methyl group to the catecholamines. All catecholamines present in the sample are $^3$H-methylated. The catecholamines are extracted from the sample and sepa-

rated by thin-layer chromatography. The amount of radioactivity in each of the chromatography spots can be measured and the individual catecholamines can be quantitated. The approximate reference range for dopamine using this procedure is 0 to 83 pg/dL.[2]

HVA is the major urinary metabolite of dopamine. This compound is relatively stable in urine. It may be easier or more convenient to analyze for HVA in urine than for dopamine in plasma. A 24-hour urine specimen is collected and 10 mL of concentrated HCl is added as a preservative.[2] During the collection time, the urine container should be kept in a refrigerator. Once the 24-hour urine specimen is returned to the laboratory, the total volume should be recorded. Any aliquots for testing should be adjusted to about pH 3 to 4 using 6-M HCl.

HVA can be extracted from the urine specimen and quantitated by either gas chromatography (GC) or high-performance liquid chromatography (HPLC). Both methods have a high amount of preparative work and require a certain degree of expertise by the technologist performing the assay. The method of gas chromatography analysis for free catecholamines and urinary metabolites has been described in detail by Williams and Greer.[7] The HPLC technique for separation of urinary catecholamines and metabolites has been described by Shoup and Kissinger.[8] The approximate reference range for HVA in urine for an adult is <15 mg/24 h.[2]

## NOREPINEPHRINE

The highest concentration of norepinephrine is found in the brain (CNS) and to a lesser degree in the sympathetic nervous system (SNS).[5] The primary function of **norepinephrine** is to act as a neurotransmitter in both the CNS and SNS. Neurons that produce norepinephrine can be found in the hypothalamus and help to regulate some hypothalamic functions. The adrenal medulla also produces norepinephrine but it represents

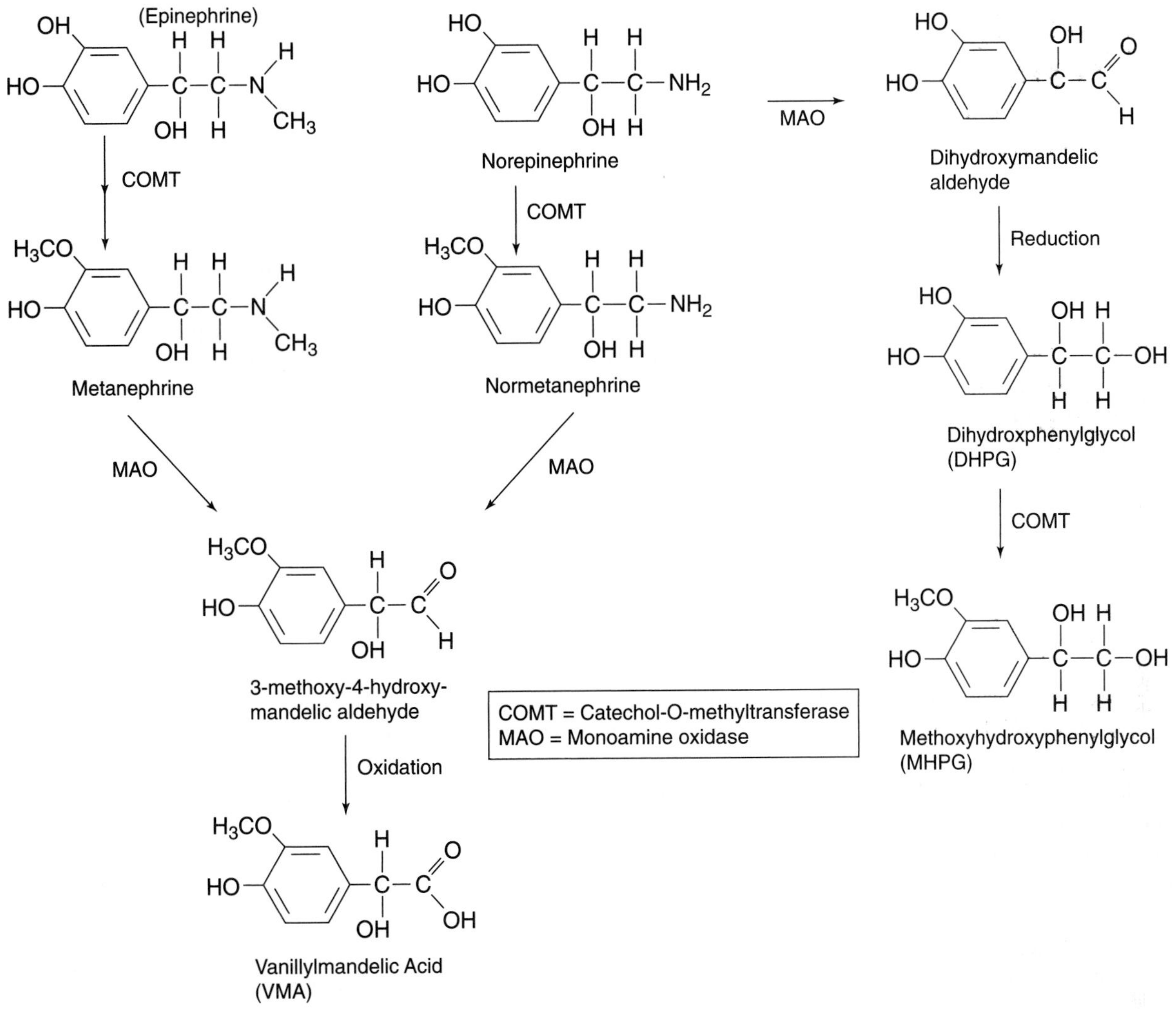

**F I G U R E   3 0 - 2**

Metabolism of epinephrine and norepinephrine.

only about 10% of the total amount of catecholamine produced there. Acting through primarily the **alpha**-adrenergic receptors, norepinephrine can cause many varied responses. These responses include such physiologic actions as vasoconstriction of the small vessels in the skin or relaxation of the smooth muscle in the gastrointestinal tract.

The synthesis of norepinephrine is shown in Figure 30–1. As with all catecholamines, norepinephrine synthesis starts with L-tyrosine. Metabolism of norepinephrine begins with either of the two enzymes COMT or MAO.[1] The action of COMT produces the metabolite normetanephrine that is secreted into the urine and can be further metabolized to VMA. The action of MAO will deaminate norepinephrine and start the metabolic breakdown that ultimately leads to the formation of VMA. Norepinephrine, normetanephrine, and VMA can be measured in urine.[2]

## EPINEPHRINE

**Epinephrine** is the major catecholamine produced by the chromaffin cells of the adrenal medulla. It is the final catecholamine produced in the synthesis cascade that starts with L-tyrosine (Figure 30–1). This hormone has widespread physiologic actions that are mediated through both the $\alpha$- and $\beta$-adrenergic receptors.[3] Epinephrine is often called the "flight or fight" hormone since it is released in response to physiologic (injuries) or psychological (stress, anxiety) threats. Epinephrine secretion causes increases in heart rate, blood pressure, respiration, and metabolic rate. In addition, it stimulates glycogenolysis in the liver and skeletal muscle that will lead to increases in the plasma glucose level.[1]

The metabolism of epinephrine also begins with either of the two major enzymes, COMT or MAO. COMT causes the formation of the metabolite, metanephrine, that can be excreted in the urine. MAO deaminates epinephrine, initiating its metabolism. The final end product for epinephrine metabolism is VMA. Both VMA and metanephrine can be measured in the urine.

The method of obtaining a suitable specimen for the analysis of plasma epinephrine and norepinephrine is as described previously with dopamine.[2] Specimens that are kept frozen for long periods before analysis tend to have lower values. Specimens should not be thawed and refrozen.

Weil-Malherbe[9] describe an ethylenediamine (EDA) fluorometric method for the analysis of plasma epinephrine and norepinephrine. This analysis involves extracting the catecholamines from the plasma first with an alumina column followed by an Amberlite CG-50 column. EDA is added to the collected eluate, where it combines with the catecholamines. Three fluorescent products are obtained from norepinephrine and one from epinephrine. These products are measured in a fluorometer at 2 different wavelengths (emission 510 and 580, activation 420) and concentrations of the hormones are calculated. The approximate reference range for norepinephrine using this method is 360 to 800 pg/mL and epinephrine is 140 to 300 pg/mL.[2] Some common drugs (ampicillin) and beverages (coffee, tea) may interfere with this fluorometric method.

The radioenzymatic method[2] described above for dopamine, using COMT and $^3$H-methylation of the catecholamines followed by thin-layer chromatography, can also be used for plasma epinephrine and norepinephrine analysis. The approximate reference range for norepinephrine using this method is 111 to 603 pg/mL and epinephrine is 0 to 62 pg/mL.[2]

The measurement of urinary catecholamines and their metabolites can be done on a 24-hour urine specimen by using HPLC.[8] The 24-hour urine specimen must be collected with an acid preservative such as HCl as in the previously described method for HVA. The urine specimen should be divided into aliquots for the various catecholamine assays. Catecholamines must be extracted from the urine specimen, usually by various kinds of column chromatography. The catecholamines in the column eluate are separated on a reverse-phase HPLC with an amperometric detector. The individual catecholamines can be quantitated from the recorded printout. The approximate reference ranges for adults are epinephrine 0.5 to 20 $\mu$g/24 h and norepinephrine 14 to 80 $\mu$g/24 h.[2]

Metanephrine and normetanephrine can be measured together as total metanephrines by a colorimetric method.[2] First the urine is acid hydrolyzed. Next, the metanephrines are removed from solution using an Amberlite CG-50 column. Periodate is added to oxidize the metanephrines to vanillin. The absorbance of each solution is measured in a spectrophotometer at 360 nm. The approximate reference range for total metanephrines (since normetanephrine and metanephrine cannot be separated with this procedure) is 0.3 to 0.9 mg/24 h.[2]

The final metabolite of epinephrine and norepinephrine is VMA. The measurement of VMA in urine can be done with a relatively easy kit method. The VMA is removed from the urine by means of a resin column.[2] This column binds the VMA and not other phenolic acids present in the urine (found in coffee, vanilla, chocolate, bananas, citrus fruits) that can interfere with the VMA measurement.[2] The VMA is then eluted from the column and periodate is added to the eluate to oxidize the VMA to vanillin. The solutions containing the vanillin are measured in a spectrophotometer at 360 nm. The approximate reference range for VMA in an adult is 2 to 7 mg/24 h.[2] Since the parent catecholamines and metabolites can be measured more precisely with HPLC, the previously described methods for VMA and metanephrines are being replaced. They may still be available in some reference laboratories.

## CLINICAL APPLICATIONS

### Pheochromocytoma

**Pheochromocytoma** is a rare tumor of the chromaffin cells.[10] Adrenal chromaffin cell tumors make up about 90% of all pheochromocytomas. The adrenal tumors may secrete large amounts of epinephrine, norepinephrine, or varying combinations of both. Pheochromocytomas found in areas other than the adrenal medulla secrete mostly norepinephrine. Most of the pheochromocytomas occur in adults and in either sex about equally.

Patients with pheochromocytoma are usually hypertensive and have episodes of sweating, tachycardia, and headaches.[10,11] The clinical findings in a pheochromocytoma can be explained by the pharmacologic actions of epinephrine and norepinephrine. The hypertension seen in connection with a pheochromocytoma is an alpha-receptor effect related to the excess norepinephrine produced. The hypertension can be sustained or paroxysmal. The hypermetabolic features seen in a pheochromocytoma resemble those seen in a patient with hyperthyroidism. These include heat intolerance, tremor, weight loss, palpitations, and an increased basal metabolic rate. In contrast to hyperthyroidism, where the patient often experiences hyperdefecation, patients with pheochromocytoma experience constipation. The increased levels of catecholamines reduce gastrointestinal motility and increase sphincter tone, which also leads to nausea, abdominal pain, and possibly intestinal obstruction. Pheochromocytomas may be misdiagnosed since the symptoms are similar to several other disorders. When diagnosed correctly, they are easily treated surgically. If left untreated, the patient usually dies.

Catecholamines have a tendency to block insulin release, increase gluconeogenesis, and cause fatty-acid mobilization. These actions can elevate serum glucose levels. Some patients will have a hypokalemia resulting from their diuretic therapy or an elevation of plasma renin and aldosterone. The diagnosis of pheochromocytoma requires the demonstration of increased concentrations of catecholamines and metabolites in either plasma or urine. Measuring one or more of the following, plasma epinephrine, norepinephrine, urinary metanephrines, or VMA, is considered appropriate for diagnosing pheochromocytoma.[10,11]

## Neuroblastoma

**Neuroblastoma** is a rare form of malignant tumor of cells that are neuron precursors found in infants and children[10,12] The primary tumor often is in or near the adrenal gland and is not found until after the tumor has metastasized to another site such as the liver. Neuroblastomas secrete sporadic increases in catecholamine hormones. The symptoms from the catecholamines may be transient hypertension, sweating, tachycardia, and headaches. Generally the most persistent symptoms are due to tissue damage from the secondary metastatic sites, i.e., liver or lymph nodes. Urinary measurement of VMA, or possibly HVA, may be helpful in the diagnosis of neuroblastoma.[10,12] Several problems are involved with these measurements. The first difficulty is in obtaining a 24-hour urine specimen from infants and small children. Second, about 70% to 80% of the children show increases in urinary VMA, but the increases vary from just slightly increased to about 10 times the normal level. A much smaller number of patients with neuroblastoma have increases in urinary HVA.[10,12]

## SUMMARY

The adrenal medulla produces the catecholamine hormones epinephrine, norepinephrine, and probably a small amount of dopamine. All catecholamine hormones are synthesized by enzymes using L-tyrosine as the starting compound. Dopamine is found primarily in the brain, where it functions as a neurotransmitter. Norepinephrine can function either as a neurotransmitter in the brain and sympathetic nervous system or as a hormone from the adrenal medulla by interacting with the adrenergic receptors. Only about 10% of the total catecholamines produced by the adrenal medulla are norepinephrine. Epinephrine is the primary hormone produced by the adrenal medulla. It has widespread physiologic actions that are mediated through the $\alpha$- and $\beta$-adrenergic receptors. Two enzyme systems are responsible for the metabolism of the catecholamines, COMT and MAO. The final metabolite for dopamine is HVA, whereas the final metabolite for both epinephrine and norepinephrine is VMA. The half-life of the catecholamines in plasma is only about 1 to 2 minutes. Since the half-life is so short it makes it relatively difficult to accurately measure these hormones in plasma. Special care must be taken when drawing a specimen for catecholamine analysis to

preserve the hormones as much as possible. Probably the best method to analyze plasma catecholamines is an HPLC or radioenzymatic assay using COMT. With problems incurred in obtaining an acceptable sample for plasma analysis of catecholamines, it may be easier and less time consuming to analyze for the parent compound or the urinary metabolite metanephrines, VMA or HVA.

## REFERENCES

1. Landberg L, Young J: Catecholamines and the adrenal medulla. In Wilson JD, Foster DW (eds.): *Williams Textbook of Endocrinology.* 3rd ed. Philadelphia, WB Saunders, 1985, p 891.
2. Chattoraji SC, Watts NB: Endocrinology. In Tietz N (ed.): *Textbook of Clinical Chemistry.* Philadelphia, WB Saunders, 1986, p 997.
3. Hoffman BB, Leftkowitz RJ: Alpha-adrenergic receptor subtypes. New Eng J Med 302:1390–1396, 1980.
4. Axelrod J: Neurotransmitters. Sci Am 230:58–71, 1974.
5. Williams CM, Greer M: Estimation by gas chromatography of urinary homovanillic acid and vanillylmandelic acid in neuroblastoma. Methods Med Res 12:106–114, 1970.
6. Shoup RE, Kissinger PT: Determination of urinary normetanephrine and metanephrine by liquid chromatography with amperometric detection. Clin Chem 23: 1268–1274, 1977.
7. Weil-Malherbe H: The chemical estimation of catecholamines and their metabolites in body fluids and tissue extracts. In Glick D (ed.): *Methods of Biochemical Analysis.* New York, Interscience Publishers, 1971, p 119.
8. Gornall AG, Luxton AW, Bhavnani BR: Endocrine disorders. In Gornall AG (ed.): *Applied Biochemistry of Clinical Disorders.* 2nd ed. Philadelphia, JB Lippincott, 1986, p 285.
9. Keiser HK, Doppman JL, Robertson CN, et al.: Diagnosis, localization and management of pheochromocytoma. In Lack EE (ed.): *Pathology of the Adrenal Glands.* New York, Churchill Livingstone, 1990, p 237.
10. Kretschmar CS: Childhood neuroblastoma: Clinical and prognostic features. In Lack EE (ed.): *Pathology of the Adrenal Glands.* New York, Churchill Livingstone, 1990, p 257.
11. Goldfien GD: Adrenal medulla. In Greenspan F, Gardner D (eds.): *Basic and Clinical Endocrinology.* 6th ed. New York, McGraw-Hill, 2001, p 405.
12. Escolas KM: Endocrinology, Lehmann CA (ed.): *Saunders Manual of Clinical Laboratory Science.* Philadelphia, WB Saunders, 1998, p 205.

# Reproductive Endocrinology

*George B. Kudolo*

## MALE REPRODUCTIVE SYSTEM

The male reproductive system is made up of a pair of gonads called the testicles (or testes), the vas deferens, the seminal vesicles, the prostate gland, and the penis (Figure 31–1). The testis is anatomically and biochemically equipped to perform two basic functions: **spermatogenesis** and **androgen** (male steroid) biosynthesis. The testis, composed of loops of convoluted seminiferous tubules, is located in the scrotum, which is suspended outside the abdominal cavity. Along the inside walls of the seminiferous tubules are two basic cell types: Sertoli and Leydig. Cells of the germinal epithelial layer (the **spermatogonia**) line the seminiferous tubules, which are eventually transformed into spermatozoa. The Sertoli cells, also found inside the seminiferous tubules, are involved with the maturation of the spermatozoa. Outside the seminiferous tubules are located the Leydig cells, in which androgen synthesis takes place. Both ends of the convoluted tubules drain into the epididymis, where further maturation of the spermatozoa takes place. From here the spermatozoa pass into the vas deferens before they enter the body of the prostate gland. A pair of seminal vesicles, one located on each side of the prostate gland, produce a mucus-like nutritive secretion that is rich in fructose and other chemicals. Prostatic ducts carrying a thin, milky, alkaline secretion from the prostate gland and secretions from other accessory glands, such as the Cowper's gland, are added and this suspension of spermatozoa (now known as **semen**) are emptied into the ejaculatory duct. A summary of the composition of semen is shown in Table 31–1. At ejaculation, the semen is propelled through the urethra, which ends in the penis, to the exterior.

## Spermatogenesis

The hypothalamus produces a decapeptide called gonadotropin-releasing hormone (GnRH), which travels through the hypophyseal–portal venous system to the adenohypophysis (anterior pituitary gland), where it enhances the release of two polypeptide hormones, luteinizing hormone (LH) and follicle-stimulating hormone (FSH).[1–4] Beginning in early adolescence, the spermatogonia develop into primary spermatocytes, which

undergo meiotic cell division to reduce the chromosome number from a diploid to a haploid number. Further division of the primary spermatocytes into secondary spermatocytes and then into spermatids is under the control of testosterone, the predominant androgen synthesized in the testis. Further maturation of the spermatids into spermatozoa, which takes place in the deep folds of the cytoplasm of the Sertoli cells, is under control of FSH. Both FSH and testosterone stimulate the synthesis of androgen-binding protein (ABP) in the Sertoli cells. ABP is responsible for the transport of testosterone in the Sertoli cells and to the epididymis. The Sertoli cells mediate the first mitotic division of the spermatocytes. The epididymal cells produce nutrients and factors necessary for the final maturation process of the spermatozoa, which includes the ability to fertilize an ovum. This phenomenon is termed **capacitation.** Peak levels of spermatogenesis takes place about 2°C lower than the temperature of the body. Hence the location of the testes outside the body. Wearing tight nylon underpants, which hold the testes too close to the body, is a significant cause of sterility. Spermatogenesis does not follow a cyclic hormonal pattern. The whole process of spermatogenesis takes approximately 6 weeks, and at completion, the spermatozoa are released from the Sertoli cells into the lumen of the seminiferous tubules.

## Hormonal Control of the Male Reproductive Function

There are three levels of control of the reproductive system. In the male, the testis, the anterior pituitary gland, and the hypothalamus represent the primary, secondary, and tertiary levels of control, respectively (Figure 31–2). There are two specific primary target cells in the testis that respond to two specific pituitary gonadotropins. The development of the glycogen-containing Sertoli cells, located inside the seminiferous tubules, is stimulated by the pituitary gonadotropin FSH. The Sertoli cells provide nourishment to the dividing cells during spermatogenesis. It is believed that these cells possess the enzymes to convert small amount of testosterone to estrogens under the influence of FSH, which activates adenylate cyclase in the Sertoli cells and consequently causes the aromatization of testosterone to estradiol. Sertoli cells cannot synthesize significant amounts of testosterone from cholesterol since they

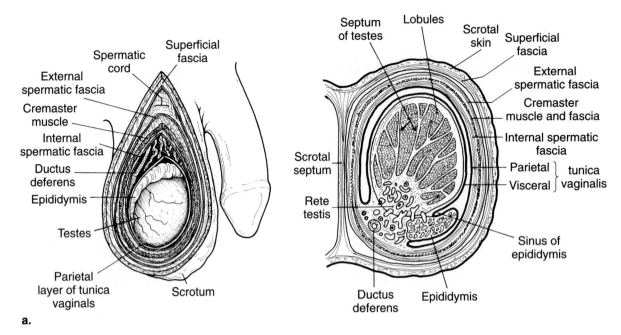

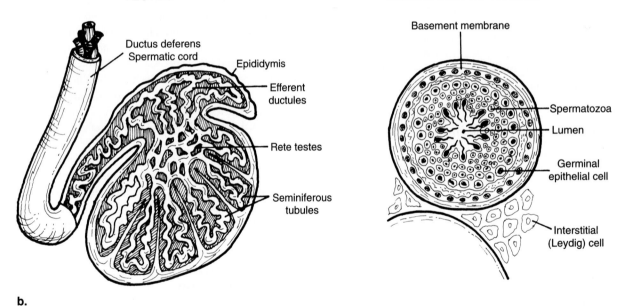

### FIGURE 31-1

**a.** Diagram of the organs that make up the male reproductive system. Note that the testis is outside the body so as to maintain its temperature about 2°C below body temperature. **b.** A sagittal section of the testis showing the position of the epididymis and a transverse section of a seminiferous tubule. *(continued)*

do not possess the necessary enzymes. The testosterone found in these cells is the result of diffusion from the Leydig cells. FSH also appears to be necessary only for the initial wave of spermatogenesis that occurs during puberty and may not be necessary in the maintenance of spermatogenesis in later years. Inhibin is a peptide that is synthesized within the Sertoli cells

that, together with testosterone from the testis and GnRH from the hypothalamus, appears to participate via a negative feedback mechanism to control FSH release from the pituitary gland.

The Leydig cell, located outside the seminiferous tubules and formerly called the interstitial cell, is the second target cell

Spermatogonia (46 chromosomes)

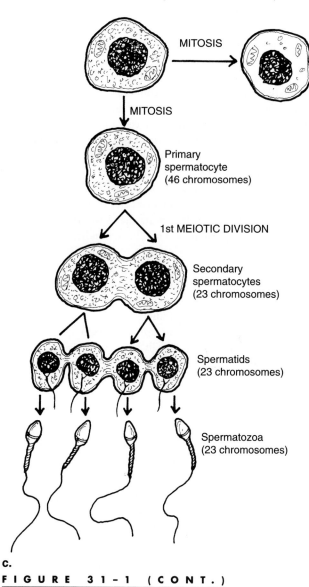

**c.**

**FIGURE 31-1 (CONT.)**

**c.** Schematic representation of spermatogenesis. (From Van De Graaff KM, Fox SI: *Concepts of Human Anatomy & Physiology.* Boston, WCB McGraw-Hill, 1999.)

in the testis. These cells are stimulated by the gonadotropin LH to produce testosterone, the principal androgen in the male. Some of the testosterone that is produced is delivered to the seminiferous tubules, where it acts on Sertoli cells to stimulate spermatogenesis, and the rest enters the peripheral circulation to promote secondary sexual differentiation of the male. Testosterone and its biologically active metabolites inhibit the release of GnRH from the hypothalamus and its actions at the anterior pituitary level via a negative feedback mechanism. These sites have high-affinity receptors for testosterone and its metabolites.

TABLE 31-1

**Composition of Human Semen**

General characteristics
  Color: White, opalescent
  Specific gravity: 1.028
  pH: 7.35–7.50
  Sperm count: 100 million/mL; >50% viable
  Buffers: Phosphate and bicarbonate
Major components
Seminal vesicles (60% of total volume)
  Fructose (1.5–6.5 mg/mL)
  Phosphorylcholine
  Ascorbic acid
  Prostaglandins
Prostate gland (20% of total volume)
  Acid phosphatase
  Cholesterol
  Citric acid
  Hyaluronidase
  Phospholipids
  Spermine

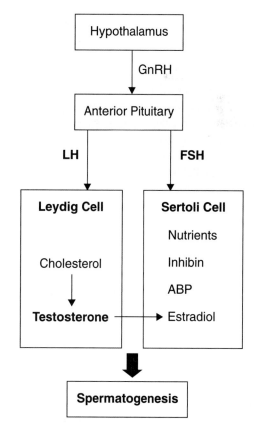

**FIGURE 31-2**

Schematic representation of the two-gonadotropin, two-cell, two-steroid hormonal control of spermatogenesis.

## FEMALE REPRODUCTIVE SYSTEM

The female reproductive system consists of a pair of gonads (ovaries) and oviducts (Fallopian tubes), the vaginal tract, and the uterus. The ovaries are the germinal reproductive organs. These are situated on the lateral wall of the upper pelvic cavity and attached to the uterus by a ligament. As with the testis, the ovary serves two basic functions: the production of eggs (ova) during the process of ovulation and the synthesis of estrogens for the development of secondary sexual characteristics and endometrial preparation for pregnancy and progestins for the maintenance of pregnancy.[1,2]

The Fallopian tubes are slender cylindrical structures that extend from the ovaries to the uterus, not only for the purpose of transporting ova but also it is the site of fertilization and the transport of the zygotes (Figure 31–3). The tentacle-like structures (fimbriae) sweep across the surface of the ovaries capturing the ovulated ova. The sweeping actions of tiny fingerlike projections in the lumen of the Fallopian tubes called **cilia** facilitate the transport of the zygotes into the uterus for implantation. The uterus is a thick-walled muscular organ consisting of the cervix, the fundus, and the body of the organ itself. The cervix is the lower portion of the uterus, which serves as the passageway and the connection between the vaginal canal and the interior of the uterus. The mucosal lining of the uterus is called the **endometrium** and the second layer, made up of smooth muscle cells, is called the **myometrium.** Even though both layers respond to sex steroid hormones, it is the endometrium that is most sensitive to the hormones produced by the ovary. Because ovarian development is cyclic, the endometrial changes are also cyclic, creating a synchronized distinctive phenomenon called the **ovarian/menstrual cycle** (Figure 31–4). The menstrual cycle refers to the sloughing of the endometrial lining of the uterus in the absence of pregnancy. During the reproductive years, the endometrium thickens each month in preparation for possible pregnancy. If pregnancy does not occur, the mucous lining sloughs off and is discharged in the process of menstruation.

## Ovarian Cycle

Events in the ovarian cycle accomplish the two basic functions of the ovary. A section through the ovary reveals a complex organ consisting primarily of the primary **oocytes** organized into follicles at different stages of growth and maturation (Figure 31–5). It is estimated that the human female is born with approximately 2 million eggs, 50% of which are already in the degenerative state. Each of these eggs is surrounded by a single layer of granulosa cells forming the primordial follicles. Some of these primordial follicles may eventually degenerate in the process called **atresia,** which continues throughout the life of the female.[3] At the age of

puberty, the remaining follicles, which is estimated to be about 300,000 in both ovaries, begin development in cohorts. At the beginning of each ovarian cycle, a cohort of about 400 to 500 follicles are recruited to begin development through the different stages of follicular development, with a noticeable increase in the layers of granulosa cells (Figure 31–5). In the matured graafian follicle, connective tissue surrounding the follicle can be seen to have clearly differentiated into theca cells. The theca and the granulosa cells have separate and distinct hormone synthetic assignments. On average, only one graafian follicle is selected for ovulation and the rest of the cohort undergoes atresia. It is estimated that at 35 years of age, each ovary contains about 30,000 follicles (from 150,000 at puberty) and this number decreases to fewer than 1000 follicles at **menopause.** It appears that a woman may expect to ovulate approximately 360 to 420 eggs in her lifetime. The time required for the development of the graafian follicle is approximately 14 days, and this constitutes the follicular phase of the cycle. The phenomenon of the rupture of the graafian follicle to expel the ovum is known as ovulation. After ovulation, the residual follicle remains in the ovary becoming transformed into the corpus luteum (yellow body) and the theca and granulosa cells are transformed into lutein cells. If pregnancy does not occur, the corpus luteum becomes nonfunctional without steroid synthetic capacity and is known as the corpus albicans (white body). The period from ovulation to the end of the ovarian cycle is called the **luteal phase** and may last from 10 to 14 days. If pregnancy occurs during this period, the lifespan of the corpus luteum is extended so that it may continue progesterone production to sustain the pregnancy until the placenta develops to supplement this role.

## Menstrual Cycle

The menstrual cycle refers to the cyclic physical and hormonal changes that take place in the endometrial layer of the uterus in concert with the changes taking place in the ovary (see Figure 31–4). The structural changes in the endometrial cells are mediated by the steroids produced by the maturing follicles and the corpus luteum. The first menstrual cycle **(menarche)** begins at the age of puberty with the first recruitment of follicles. The age of menarche is gradually getting younger. In 1865, menarche was around 16 years, and in 1994, it was estimated to be 12.5 years.[2,4] The release of FSH by the anterior pituitary gland triggers the beginning of the menstrual cycle and the early growth of the primary follicle (FSH stimulates the proliferation of the granulosa cells of the primordial follicles leading to the formation of the primary [pre-antral] follicles). LH, on the other hand, stimulates the formation of testosterone from cholesterol molecules in the theca cells, which diffuses into the granulosa cell fraction of the follicle. Under the influence of FSH, the androgen is then converted

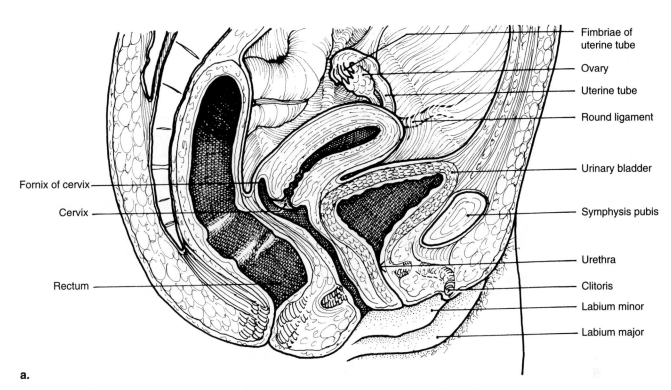

Fimbriae of
uterine tube

Ovary

Uterine tube

Round ligament

Urinary bladder

Symphysis pubis

Urethra

Clitoris

Labium minor

Labium major

Fornix of cervix

Cervix

Rectum

a.

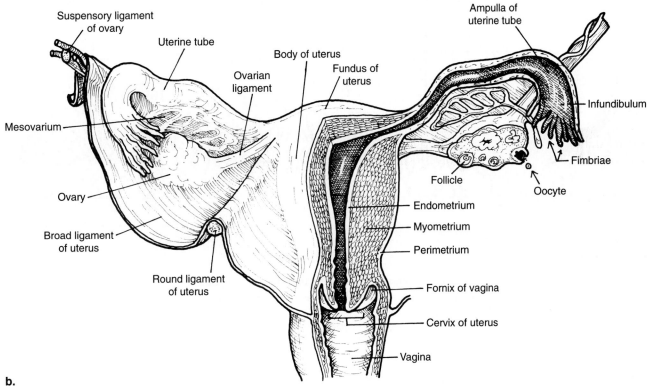

Suspensory ligament
of ovary

Uterine tube

Body of uterus

Fundus of
uterus

Ovarian
ligament

Ampulla of
uterine tube

Infundibulum

Fimbriae

Oocyte

Follicle

Endometrium

Myometrium

Perimetrium

Fornix of vagina

Cervix of uterus

Vagina

Mesovarium

Ovary

Broad ligament
of uterus

Round ligament
of uterus

b.

## FIGURE 31-3

**a.** Diagram showing organs that make up the female reproductive system. **b.** Note
the physical connection between the Fallopian tubes and the uterine cavity (right
portion of the figure) at the proximal end and the loose connection between the
fimbriae and the surface of the ovaries at the distal end. (From Van De Graaff KM,
Fox SI: *Concepts of Human Anatomy & Physiology.* Boston, WCB McGraw-Hill,
1999.)

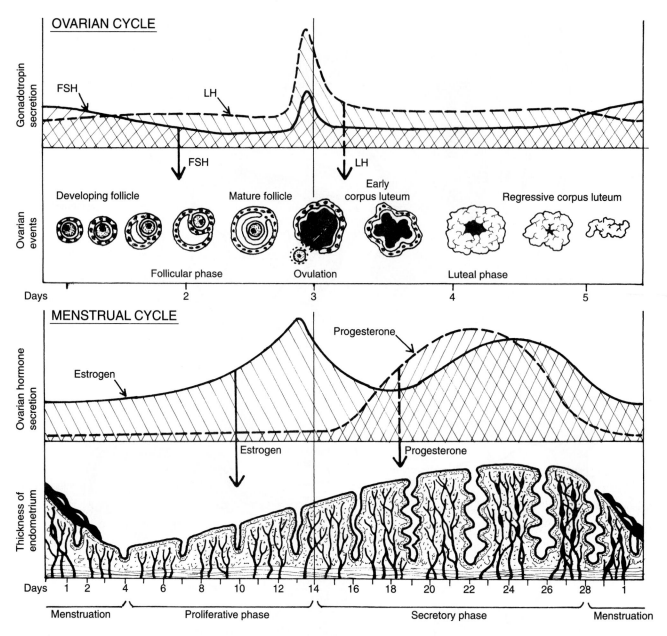

**FIGURE 31-4**

Schematic drawing of the synchronized events of the ovarian and menstrual cycles. The downward pointing arrows indicate the stage of the cycles in which the respective hormones act. (From Van De Graaff KM, Fox SI: *Concepts of Human Anatomy & Physiology.* Boston, WCB McGraw-Hill, 1999.)

to estradiol by the aromatase enzyme (Figure 31–6). Estradiol causes the granulosa cells to form more FSH receptors, making them more sensitive to FSH, which leads to the synthesis of more estradiol. The rising estradiol levels during the follicular phase of the ovarian cycle leads to growth and thickness of the endometrial layer, which contains estrogen receptors. One of the significant consequences of the action of estradiol during this part of the cycle is the synthesis of the progesterone receptor in the endometrial lining as part of the endome-

trial maturation process. It is via these progesterone receptors that progesterone from the corpus luteum works during the **secretory** phase of the menstrual cycle.

The rising level of estradiol that occurs in the early to mid-follicular phase inhibits the production of pituitary FSH through a negative feedback mechanism. Since FSH supports estradiol production, this produces a sharp drop in peripheral estradiol levels, which in turn stimulates the pituitary gland to release LH. Additionally, the drop in peripheral estradiol lev-

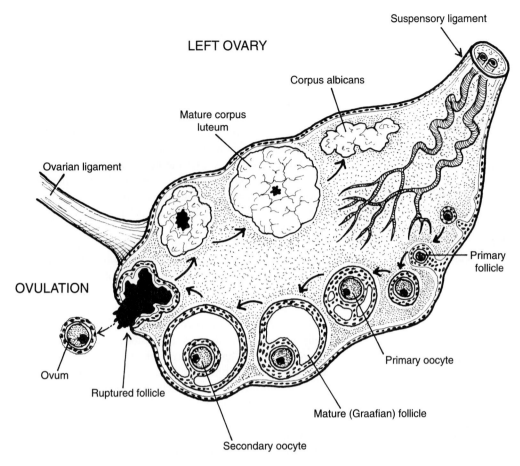

LEFT OVARY

Suspensory ligament

Corpus albicans

Mature corpus
luteum

Ovarian ligament

Primary
follicle

OVULATION

Primary oocyte

Ovum

Ruptured follicle

Mature (Graafian) follicle

Secondary oocyte

**FIGURE 31-5**

A drawing of an ovarian section showing the organization of oocytes into primordial follicles and the different stages of follicular maturation from the primary follicle to post-ovulation events (from left to right in the figure). (From Van De Graaff KM, Fox SI: *Concepts of Human Anatomy & Physiology.* Boston, WCB McGraw-Hill, 1999.)

els is a consequence of the selection of one dominant graafian follicle for ovulation and the concomitant degeneration of the rest of the cohort.[5] The resultant surge of LH leads to ovulation with follicular rupture and corpus luteum development. It is still unclear what cue leads to the selection of only one follicle (out of about 500) for ovulation. All that is known is that LH is necessary for the final follicular growth and influences the transformation of the follicular cells into lutein cells. The corpus luteum produces progesterone, which inhibits gonadotropin release by the pituitary gland and causes the endometrium to cease proliferating and mature to a secretory glandular-type of mucosa. This constitutes the luteal or secretory phase of the menstrual cycle, which may last about 10 to 14 days. The endometrial layer responds to the changes in the ovarian hormones and is the source of menstrual discharge if pregnancy does not occur. If a fertilized ovum implants in the **secretory** endometrium, the placental tissue that develops produces human chorionic gonadotropin (hCG), which maintains the corpus luteum throughout the pregnancy as a source of estrogen and progesterone.

As a woman approaches 50 years of age, the menstrual cycle becomes shorter and irregular and is usually accompanied by **oligomenorrhea.** Eventually, the menstrual cycle ends when ovulation stops. This is the age-acquired physiologic condition called **menopause.** The normal range of the age of a woman at menopause in the United States is 45 to 52 years.[2] The causes of menopause include changes in GnRH pulsatile secretion pattern, insensitivity of the ovaries to respond to pituitary gonadotropins, and the inability of the ovaries to produce sufficient steroids (because the stock of ovarian follicles have all become atretic). In the absence of significant estrogen production from the ovaries, adrenal androgens may overwhelm the woman's physiology. Hence, the tendency to develop deep voice and facial hair growth after menopause. The major laboratory finding during menopause is the increased gonadotropin production (FSH is about 10 times and LH is about 4 times the levels found in younger, menstruating women). This gonadotropin-rich urine extract from postmenopausal women is available clinically as human menopausal gonadotropin (hMG).

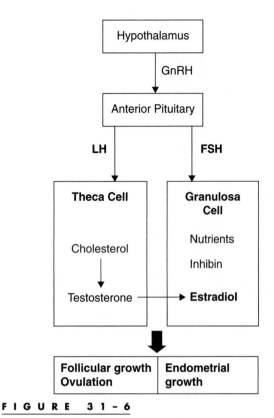

**F I G U R E    3 1 - 6**

The two-gonadotropin, two-cell, two-steroid hormonal control of the female reproductive system.

Although not fully elucidated, an inhibin-mediated mechanism may be present in the regulation of female reproduction as well. It is thought that the granulosa cells produce inhibin and subsequently decrease release of FSH. The measurement of inhibin is currently of research laboratory practice only.

## STRUCTURE AND FUNCTION OF GONADAL STEROIDS

This chapter focuses primarily on ovarian estrogens and progesterone and testicular androgens. The principal sites of sex steroid hormone production for the control of reproduction are the testes and the ovaries (in the nonpregnant female). In the pregnant female, the placenta plays a major role in steroid synthesis. Cholesterol molecules, either extracted directly from the peripheral circulation or synthesized by the ovaries and the testes themselves, are precursors of all steroid hormones (Figure 31–7). The rate-limiting step for the biosynthetic pathway is the conversion of cholesterol to pregnenolone in both gonads. The end product of the biosynthesis pathway, however, depends on the type of gonad. The hypothalamus in both males and females produces the same GnRH, which stimu-

lates the anterior pituitary gland to produce the gonadotropins, FSH and LH. The testis produces predominantly the androgen testosterone and the ovary produces the estrogens and progestins (predominantly progesterone and, to a lesser extent, 17-hydroxyprogesterone). In the female, the adrenal gland supplies about 60% of the androgens found in the peripheral circulation, which serves as a substrate for estrogen production. The presence of the placenta in the pregnant female leads to an extensive metabolism of estradiol to estriol.

Structurally, the sex steroid hormones, like other steroids found in the body, are characterized by the presence of the **perhydrocyclopentanophenanthrene nucleus**. It is the side-chain substitutions that confer special properties on specific steroid hormones.

The **androgens** are synthesized in the Leydig (or interstitial) cells of the testis. As shown in Figure 31–7, there are two possible pathways for the conversion of 17–hydroxypregnenolone to testosterone. The first route is the 5-ene pathway that leads to the production of dehydroepiandrosterone (DHEA), which is further converted to androstenediol and finally testosterone. Alternatively, testosterone could be produced via the 4-ene pathway, where the 17-hydroxypregnenolone is first converted to 17-hydroxyprogesterone and then to androstenedione, which may then be converted to testosterone. The enzymes for both of these pathways are located in the smooth endoplasmic reticulum of the cells. Once synthesized, the lipid-soluble testosterone is secreted into the bloodstream, where it is transported bound to several nonspecific plasma-binding proteins such as albumin and the specific binding protein, sex hormone–binding globulin (SHBG), formerly called the testosterone-estradiol binding globulin (TeBG). As the name suggests, SHBG binds to both estradiol and testosterone, rendering these steroids biologically inactive as they travel in the peripheral circulation. The estradiol and testosterone binding to SHBG has a relatively high affinity (the dissociation constant [Kd] is in the nanomolar range with a low binding capacity). Compared to albumin with Kd in the micromolar ($\mu$M) range, it is estimated that approximately 56% of circulating testosterone is bound to SHBG. Only low amounts of testosterone (3%) circulate unbound (free) and because of its relative ease in entering target cells (low molecular weight and lipophilic character), it is the only fraction responsible for its biologic responses. Once testosterone enters the target cell, such as the skeletal muscle or the liver, it is converted into 5$\alpha$-dihydrotestosterone (DHT), which is biologically more potent than testosterone itself (Figure 31–8).

The catabolism of these androgens, as it is with all drugs and chemicals, occurs in the liver, where conjugation with sulfuric acid or glucuronic acid converts the lipid-soluble steroid molecules into water-soluble sulfates and glucuronides, which are then capable of being excreted by the kidney. The major urinary metabolites of androgens are androsterone, a weak androgen, and etiocholanolone, an isomer of androsterone that lacks androgenic activity. Together with dehydroepiandrosterone sulfate (DHEAS), they comprise the principal steroids referred to

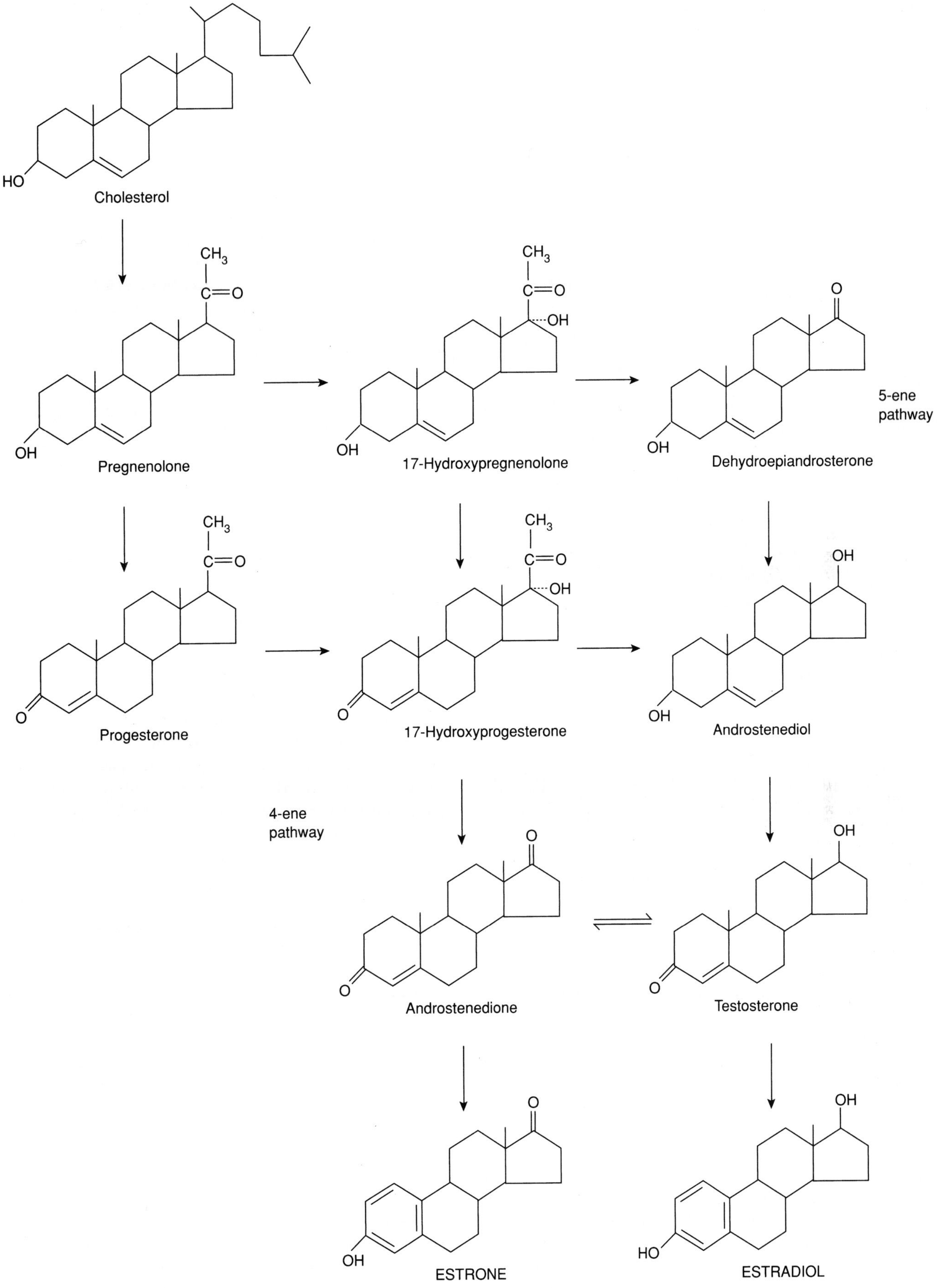

**FIGURE 31-7**

The synthetic pathways for the production of androgens and estrogens.

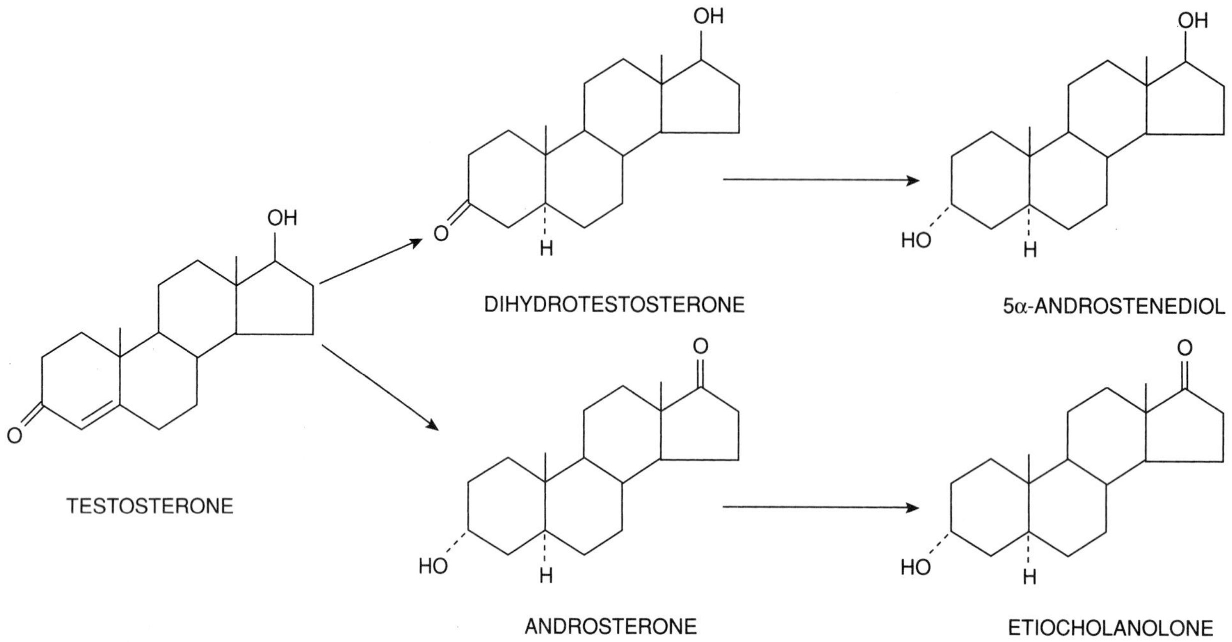

OH

DIHYDROTESTOSTERONE

5α-ANDROSTENEDIOL

OH

TESTOSTERONE

ANDROSTERONE

ETIOCHOLANOLONE

**F I G U R E   3 1 – 8**

The principal products of testosterone metabolism. Note that dihydrotestosterone is
the most potent androgen in the body. Etiocholanolone, a biologically inactive
androgen, is one of the major components of urinary 17-ketosteroids.

collectively as 17-ketosteroids (17-KS) (Figure 31–8). However, androgens derived from the adrenal gland are also precursors for 17-KS and so clinical interpretation of urinary 17-KS output must take into account the gender of the patient and also must be done with caution. In females, in particular, increased urinary 17-KS may be indicative of a testicular feminization, the androgenital syndrome or primary hypoadrenalism (Addison's disease) accompanied by hirsutism. Decreased urinary excretion of 17-KS in the male may be suggestive of primary hypogonadism (Klinefelter's syndrome) or secondary hypogonadism (panhypopituitarism). The virilizing character of testosterone or DHT is due to the presence of the carbon 19 (C-19) substitution on the steroid nucleus. These androgens are responsible for the growth of the external genitalia at puberty and the deepening of the voice and masculine pattern of development of skeletal muscle. Other secondary male sex characteristics such as acne, body and facial hair, and recession of the scalp hairline are also dependent on DHT. Tissues in the seminal vesicles and prostate glands also respond to DHT for their growth and secretory capabilities. Hence the high frequency of prostate hyperplasia in men with increasing age.

The **estrogens** are classified as C-18 steroid hormones derived principally from androgens in the ovarian follicle and the adrenal gland. In fact, about 60% of the androgens found in the peripheral circulation in the female are derived from the adrenal gland. In the ovarian follicular tissue, particularly in the theca cells, cholesterol is converted to androstenedione

through pregnenolone in virtually identical pathways as described for the male. The androgens androstenedione and testosterone then diffuse into the granulosa cell compartment, where aromatization of the androgens takes place to produce the estrogens (Figure 31–7 and Figure 31–9). **Aromatization** is a term that refers to the conversion of the A-ring of the steroid nucleus to a benzene or phenolic A-ring by placing a

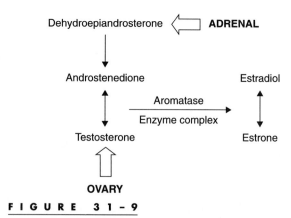

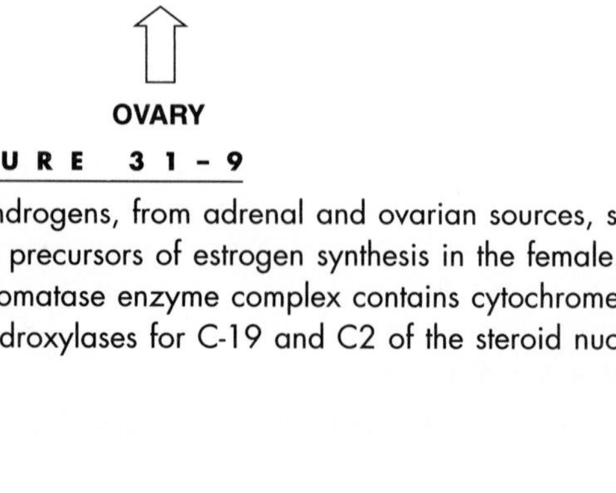

**F I G U R E   3 1 – 9**

Androgens, from adrenal and ovarian sources, serve
as precursors of estrogen synthesis in the female. The
aromatase enzyme complex contains cytochrome P450
hydroxylases for C-19 and C2 of the steroid nucleus.

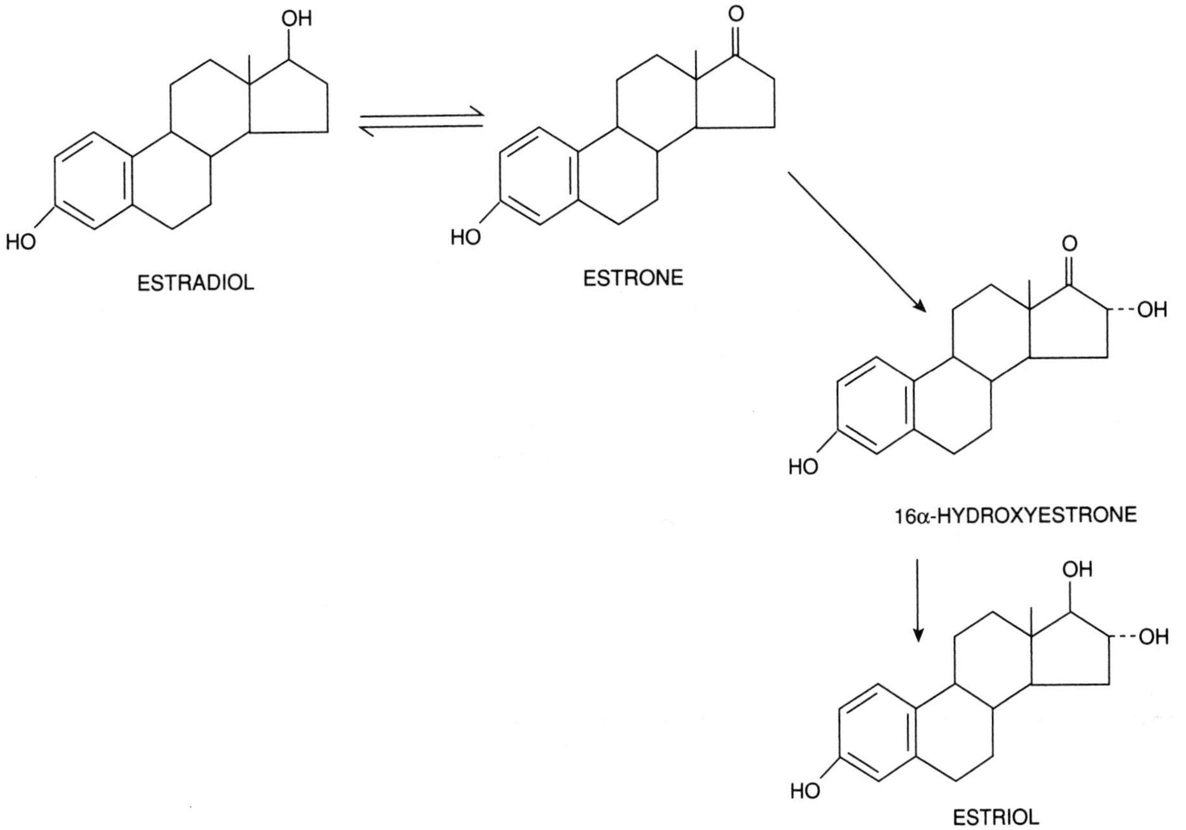

ESTRADIOL

ESTRONE

16α-HYDROXYESTRONE

ESTRIOL

**F I G U R E   3 1 - 1 0**

Interactions of the three principal biologically active estrogens. Estradiol is the most potent, with potency ascribed to the hydroxyl group on C19. Estradiol conversion to estriol takes place predominantly in the placenta.

hydroxyl group on carbon 3. Aromatization of androstenedione yields predominantly estrone whereas aromatization of testosterone leads to estrogen production (Figure 31–9). These processes involve enzymatic as well as nonenzymatic steps and the result is that estrogens lose the C-19 carbon atom and therefore lose the virilizing effect associated with androgens. Instead, the estrogens acquire unique substitutions on the aromatic ring (A), which promote the development of female secondary sexual characteristics. When secreted into the bloodstream, estradiol and estrone are bound (>97%) to albumin and SHBG to be transported to target tissues. The synthesis and secretion of estradiol exceeds that of estrone but both are metabolized to form estriol (Figure 31–10) in the liver. After conjugation with sulfuric acid or glucuronic acid, the water-soluble sulfates and glucuronides are excreted by the kidney.

**Progesterone** is a C-21 steroid hormone and is produced primarily by the ovary of the nonpregnant female. In the corpus luteum, pregnenolone is converted to progesterone and 17-hydroxyprogesterone (collectively designated progestogens or progestins), which are secreted as the principal end prod-

ucts. Progesterone is transported in the peripheral circulation bound primarily to cortisol specific binding protein **transcortin** and the nonspecific binding protein albumin. Again, only the free unbound fractions are biologically active. The catabolism of progesterone results in the formation of pregnanediol and the catabolism of 17-hydroxyprogesterone results in the formation of pregnanetriol (Figure 31–11). These compounds are then conjugated in the liver, principally with glucuronic acid to form water-soluble pregnanediol and pregnanetriol glucuronides to facilitate excretion by the kidney in the urine.

## MECHANISM OF HORMONE ACTION

The reproductive hormones fall into two main groups on the basis of their structure and the cellular location of their specific receptors. The hypothalamic hormone GnRH, a decapeptide, and the pituitary glycoprotein hormones FSH and LH (and hCG) are protein (polypeptide) hormones. The

Cholesterol

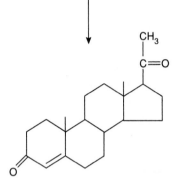

Pregnenolone

17 Hydroxy-
pregnenolone

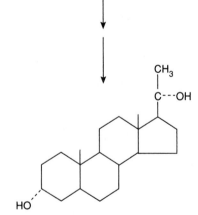

Progesterone

17-Hydroxyprogesterone

Pregnanediol

Pregnanetriol

**F I G U R E   3 1 - 1 1**

The biosynthesis and metabolism of progestins. These metabolites have both extensive
enterohepatic circulation and urinary excretion (as glucuronide complexes).

pituitary hormones in particular are similarly structured, consisting of 2 subunits, $\alpha$ and $\beta$, joined by noncovalent bonding. The $\alpha$ subunits are all identical within each species. The specific biologic effects of these hormones are determined by the $\beta$ subunit, which is highly conserved between the different hormones. FSH and LH, as well as GnRH, bind to specific receptors located on the plasma membranes of target cells. This results in the activation of the adenylate cyclase and increased cAMP production, which mediate the responses specific for each target tissue.

As shown above, the steroid hormones are also similar in structure. Unlike the polypeptide hormones, steroid hormone receptors are intracellularly located. Target tissues with these receptors accumulate the steroids from the peripheral circulation against a concentration gradient (or locally in the cells). The interaction of the steroids with their receptors in the cytoplasm leads to the formation of a steroid-receptor complex, which becomes activated and transformed to a species with increased affinity for the nuclear sites. The steroid-receptor complex therefore translocates into the nucleus, where it is found associated with components of the chromatin and DNA sites that are specific for each steroid. The interaction of the steroid-receptor complex with the nuclear chromatin acceptors leads to the synthesis of specific mRNAs, which code for specific proteins involved in the cellular functions. For example, one of the proteins synthesized as a result of estrogen action is the progesterone receptor. This explains why estrogen action in the follicular phase of the ovarian cycle is important for progesterone action in the subsequent luteal or secretory phase of the menstrual cycle. One of the major actions of both estrogens and progesterone is the change of the uterine endometrium during the menstrual cycle. These changes are mediated through the ovary and corpus luteum. Estrogens generally increase the number of glandular cells, whereas the progestins increase their secretory activity. In addition to these actions, estrogens are responsible for the growth and pigmentation of the nipples and areola and for the proliferation of the ductal systems in breast tissue during puberty. The estrogens also have an anabolic effect on other tissues, but not to the degree that androgens produce. They also increase total body protein, fat deposition and smoothness, and thickness and vascularity of the skin.

# ANALYTES

## Gonadotropins

In response to the release of GnRH from the hypothalamus, the gonadotropes of the anterior pituitary release the gonadotropins, FSH and LH. In the female, FSH is primarily responsible for the early follicular development in the ovary, whereas LH is responsible for ovulation and later development of the follicle (luteinization). In the male, FSH is primarily responsible for spermatogenesis, and LH influences the Leydig cells of the testes to produce testosterone.

Radioimmunoassay (RIA) methods are available to assess plasma levels of FSH and LH. The typical reference ranges are listed in Table 31–2.[3] These values are frequently utilized in evaluating infertility or hypogonadism. One of the most frequent uses of the LH level is in assessing ovulation. This need has led to the development of enzyme immunoassay (EIA) methods to detect urinary LH. These methods have now been modified to dipstick and membrane assays that can be utilized for home testing for LH or hCG on a daily basis in an effort to detect an LH surge and thus ovulation or pregnancy, respectively.

## Testosterone

Testosterone is synthesized by the Leydig cells of the testis of the male and small amounts may be produced by the theca cells of the ovary in the female. The main metabolites of testosterone are androsterone and dihydrotestosterone. These metabolites can be further metabolized to produce androstenediol and etiocholanolone, the 17-KS.

RIA and EIA methods for testosterone are commercially available. Heparinized plasma or serum samples can be used and are stable for approximately 1 week at refrigerator temperature or may be frozen at $-20°C$. Frozen samples are stable for approximately 6 months.

Testosterone levels are valuable in the diagnosis of hypogonadism and the presence of testicular tumors in the male as well as masculinizing tumors, usually of ovarian origin, in the female. In males, testosterone levels demonstrate a circadian pattern and peak at 7:00 A.M. They fall to their lowest levels at about 8 P.M. The reference ranges for testosterone levels are found in Table 31–3.

TABLE 31–2

**Typical Reference Ranges for Plasma FSH and LH**

|  | FSH mIU/mL | LH mIU/mL |
|---|---|---|
| Female |  |  |
| Follicular phase | 2–10 | 0–14 |
| Mid-cycle peak | 9–18 | 20–70 |
| Luteal phase | 0–9 | 0–16 |
| Postmenopause | 20–100 | 20–70 |
| Male | 2–10 | 0–9 |

FSH = follicle-stimulating hormone; LH = luteinizing hormone.

TABLE 31–3

**Reference Ranges for Plasma Testosterone**

| Males |  |
|---|---|
| Prepubertal | 10–20 ng/mL |
| Adult | 300–1000 ng/mL |
| Females |  |
| Prepubertal | 10–20 ng/mL |
| Adult | 20–75 ng/mL (higher at mid-cycle peak) |
| Pregnant | 3–4 times adult level |
| Postmenopausal | 8–35 ng/mL |

## Estradiol

Estrogens are synthesized by the ovarian granulosa cells in the female; small amounts may be produced by the adrenal cortex in the male and female, and by the testes in the male. Estradiol is the most potent of the estrogens compared to the other two estrogens, estrone and estriol.

Competitive binding RIA and EIA and enzyme-linked immunosorbent assay (ELISA) procedures are commercially available for the determination of estradiol levels. The preferred specimen is a freshly drawn, nonhemolyzed serum sample. Serum samples may be frozen at −20°C if the assay is not performed the same day it is drawn. Diurnal variations do exist (because of diurnal variations in gonadotropin levels) and so it is recommended that samples be collected at a specific time of day, especially in cases of serial blood draws.

Estradiol levels are especially useful in assessing ovarian function. Tumors of ovarian, adrenal, and testicular origin may increase levels of serum estradiol. Increased levels may also be found during pregnancy and exogenous administration of gonadotropins. Decreased levels may be found in primary and secondary ovarian failure as well as in adrenal gland malfunction. Table 31–4 lists the reference ranges for estradiol levels.

## Progesterone

Progesterone is produced mainly by the granulosa (lutein) cells of the corpus luteum in the female. It is also produced by the placenta in pregnancy and small amounts can be produced by the adrenal cortex. The main urinary metabolite is pregnanediol.

RIA, EIA, and ELISA methods are commercially available for the determination of progesterone. Serum or plasma can be utilized for the assays. Progesterone is stable for approximately 7 days at refrigerator temperatures and up to about 3 months when frozen (−20°C).

Progesterone levels have been used primarily for the evaluation of fertility in females, in particular for the detection of

ovulation and in women with luteal phase defect. Interpretation of levels must be carefully correlated with the menstrual cycle. Reference ranges are listed in Table 31–5.

## Dehydroepiandrosterone (DHEA)

DHEA is an androgen derived primarily from the adrenal gland. Therefore, measurements of DHEA and its conjugation product dehydroepiandrosterone-sulfate (DHEAS) are valuable in the assessment of adrenocortical function. RIA methods are commercially available for the determinations in nonextracted plasma. This assay has generally replaced the need for urinary 17-KS determinations in random urine samples. The assay may be performed on serum, heparinized, or EDTA plasma. The sample is stable for approximately 7 days at room temperature. The reference ranges for DHEA are 3.6 to 6.3 ng/mL for adult males and 4.4 to 6.0 ng/mL for females.

## 17-ketosteroid

The total urinary 17-KS output may be measured to assess total daily adrenal androgen production (as opposed to plasma DHEAS). Table 31–6 is a summary of the reference ranges.

TABLE 31–5

**Reference Ranges for Plasma Progesterone**

| Male | 0.12–0.3 ng/mL |
|---|---|
| Female | |
| Menstrual cycle | |
| Follicular phase | <1 ng/mL |
| Luteal phase | 5–20 ng/mL |
| Pregnancy | |
| 1st trimester | 20–50 ng/mL |
| 2nd trimester | 50–100 ng/mL |
| 3rd trimester | 100–400 ng/mL |

TABLE 31–4

**Reference Ranges for Plasma Estradiol**

| Female | |
|---|---|
| Prepubertal | 4–12 pg/mL |
| Early follicular phase | 30–100 pg/mL |
| Late follicular phase | 100–400 pg/mL |
| Luteal phase | 50–150 pg/mL |
| Postmenopausal | 5–18 pg/mL |
| Male | |
| Prepubertal | 2–8 pg/mL |
| Adult | 10–60 pg/mL |

TABLE 31–6

**Reference Ranges for Urinary 17-ketosteroid Production**

| Up to a year | <1 ng/d |
|---|---|
| 1–4 years | <2 |
| 5–8 years | <3 |
| 8–12 years | 3–10 |
| 13–16 years | 5–12 |
| Young adult male | 9–22 |
| Adult male | 8–20 |
| Adult female | 6–15 |

## CLINICAL APPLICATIONS

### Abnormalities of Testicular Function

Abnormal testicular function, either in spermatogenesis or testosterone production (or both), can be produced by a disease of the testis (primary defect) or a derangement of the pituitary (secondary defect) or hypothalamic axis (tertiary defect). The time of onset of such a defect may also determine the clinical outcome. If a testicular hypofunction begins before puberty, it may prevent the development of secondary sexual characteristics associated normally with puberty such as the deep voice, increased muscular build, and growth of axillary and facial hair. If the defect occurs after puberty, the changes are much less marked with decreased axillary and facial hair growth being the most common.

Primary hypotesticular function may be caused by an abnormal testicular development or diseases of the testes such as infection, trauma, or a tumor. Laboratory findings in this case may include increased serum gonadotropins (LH, FSH), decreased serum androgens, and urinary 17-KS. Secondary hypotesticular function may result from inadequate levels of gonadotropin (LH, FSH) production. This is usually due to a disease of the pituitary gland such as a tumor or an infection. Any of these causes may lead to male infertility, since both LH and FSH are required for androgen production and spermatogenesis, respectively.

### Male Infertility

Evaluation of male infertility includes a careful history, physical examination, and laboratory tests to assess spermatogenesis as well as the endocrine function. To assess male fertility, analysis should include sperm count and sperm motility and morphology. According to the World Health Organization (WHO) guidelines, a sperm count of <20 million/mL (oligozoospermia), a progressive motility of <50% (asthenozoospermia), and/or a proportion of <30% with normal morphology (teratozoospermia) in the ejaculate is regarded as abnormal semen.[6] Testosterone, FSH, and LH levels may be performed to provide an explanation of the semen analysis. Should these tests be inadequate in explaining the cause of the male infertility, other tests such as testis biopsy, vasograms, or testing for anti-sperm antibodies (ASA) may become necessary.[7]

The causes of male infertility are numerous and may be classified broadly as (1) pretesticular, (2) testicular, and (3) posttesticular.[8] The pretesticular causes are usually due to hypothalamic or pituitary lesions leading to the decreased production of the gonadotropins. Other common causes include hypothyroidism, Cushing's syndrome, malnutrition, and alcoholic cirrhosis. Hypothyroidism may be associated with decreased sperm counts, while the presence of pituitary Cushing's syndrome can lead to decreased testosterone levels that in turn may lead to decreased libido and impaired semen quality. Undernourishment and alcoholic cirrhosis may be valid causes of decreased gonadotropin levels and decreased testosterone production.

Primary testicular failure may be congenital or acquired. The congenital causes include failure of testicular descent (cryptorchidism) and Klinefelter's syndrome (XXY). Acquired disorders would include varicocele, tumor, orchitis or organ damage due to radiation, or chemical or drug exposure, or as a result of chemotherapy. Laboratory findings in all these conditions would result in decreased levels of testosterone and increased levels of FSH and LH. Mechanical or the functional impairment of sperm transport may also lead to infertility. Sexually transmitted diseases such as gonorrhea, which leaves scar tissues in the seminiferous tubules, may be a significant cause of sterility. Congenital defects can produce mechanical obstruction, resulting in low sperm counts or even complete absence of sperms (azoospermia). The production of ASA is clearly a contributing factor in the production of male infertility, which in some populations of subfertile men may account for as much as 10%.[7]

A primary hypertesticular function may be produced by an active testicular tumor involving especially the Leydig cells. Laboratory finding may include high serum testosterone levels, increased excretion of urinary 17-KS, and low serum LH or FSH levels. Secondary hypertesticular function may be caused by excessive gonadotropin production by the pituitary gland. The laboratory findings in this case are elevated serum levels of testosterone, LH, and FSH, and increased urinary 17-KS. The increased testosterone production has little or no clinical effect in adult males but in prepubertal males this could lead to sexual precocity and early closure of the epiphysis of long bones, producing a short stature.

### Abnormalities of Ovarian Function

Primary hypoovarian function may be due to a congenital developmental abnormality such as Turner's syndrome (with XO genotype) or to the normal age-acquired process of menopause. The major laboratory findings are decreased serum estradiol and increased FSH and LH levels (as a consequence of the lack of feedback inhibition).

Although a secondary hypoovarian function may also be caused by congenital syndromes, this is usually acquired. Some acquired examples include the development of a pituitary tumor, a postpartum necrosis of the pituitary gland (Sheehan's syndrome), infections, psychiatric disturbances, or **polycystic ovary disease** (PCOD). The most common of these is PCOD, which is characterized by hormonal alterations such as increased plasma levels of LH and androgens, lower concentrations of sex hormone-binding globulin (SHBG), and consequent higher levels of free testosterone.[9]

Tumors of the hypothalamus are rare causes of disruption of GnRH production. More common causes include stress, weight loss, exercise, and chronic illness. It must be recognized that the pituitary gland, housed in a hollow confined space in the skull (called the Turkish saddle), is the source of a number of stimulating polypeptide hormones such as TSH, CRF, ACTH, LH, and FSH. Tumor growth involving one or more cell types may lead to increased production of their respective hormones, while the growth of these cells could well suppress the normal function of adjacent cells. Thus, for example, hypersecretion of prolactin (hyperprolactinemia) due to a pituitary adenoma may result in reduced gonadotropin production leading to amenorrhea and galactorrhea and consequently infertility.[10] Hyperprolactinemia, seen in patients taking certain medications such as dopamine antagonists or in some cases of hypothyroidism, may produce the same symptoms. The laboratory findings may, therefore, be quite variable but usually include decreased serum LH and FSH, estradiol, and progesterone levels. The time of onset of the hypoovarian function is clinically important. If it begins before puberty, it results in delayed or the complete absence of menarche. If it occurs after puberty, it may result in secondary amenorrhea. Hypoovarian abnormalities usually result in **anovulation,** which is defined as the failure to produce a mature ovum for fertilization. Because ovarian function is intimately tied to the menstrual cycle, anovulation is usually accompanied by abnormal menstrual cycles as well and is a common cause of infertility. Approximately 15% of anovulatory women have hyperprolactinemia, as explained above. Therefore, laboratory investigation of the anovulatory patient may include measurement of serum prolactin levels. A TSH level may also be useful in ruling out hypothyroidism. FSH levels may be of value in distinguishing between a pituitary/hypothalamic disorder from an ovarian disorder. An ovarian disorder would yield no estradiol to provide the negative feedback mechanism necessary to control FSH levels and increased FSH levels would be expected.

## Amenorrhea

Normal menses requires a high degree of coordination among the central nervous system, the hypothalamus, the pituitary gland, and the ovaries. **Amenorrhea** is defined as the absence of menstrual discharge after puberty. Amenorrhea can be a physiologic process, such as cessation of menses during pregnancy, or it can be pathologic. The pathologic causes of amenorrhea can be classified as primary or secondary. **Primary amenorrhea** is defined as having had no previous vaginal bleeding since puberty. Signs of puberty such as breast development and appearance of pubic hair develop before menarche. In healthy females, 99% would have begun to menstruate by the age of 16. **Secondary amenorrhead** is defined as the absence of menses for 6 months or for the equivalent of three previous cycle intervals in a female who had previously menstruated on a regular basis. Even though the causes of primary and secondary amenorrhea overlap, primary amenorrhea is most frequently due to chromosomal abnormalities or structural malformations. The most common cause is Turner's syndrome (gonadal dysgenesis, 46, XO karyotype), where the ova-

ries may be replaced by fibrous tissue. About 90% of patients with Turner's syndrome never menstruate. Typically, these patients are short in stature, are sexually immature, and have a webbed neck and shield-shaped chest. Since there is no ovarian function, the major laboratory finding is increased serum FSH. Another genetic abnormality that would manifest with an increased FSH is a phenotypic female patient with a Y chromosome. The testosterone level would be expected to be in the male range and is characteristic of females with **testicular feminization.** Causes of secondary amenorrhea can be due to common occurrences such as weight loss, strenuous exercise, drugs and stress. Secondary amenorrhea due to structural abnormalities is most commonly caused by Asherman syndrome, where the endometrial lining is obliterated.[11,12] The laboratory findings include patients with normal levels of estradiol, testosterone, and progesterone but do not respond with uterine bleeding after the progesterone challenge test.

Abnormal menstrual function is a common symptom in thyroid dysfunction. In primary hypothyroidism, thyrotropin-releasing hormone (TRH), and thyroid-stimulating hormone (TSH) levels are increased. Increased TRH levels may stimulate increased prolactin production. Measurement of serum LH is valuable in the assessment of secondary amenorrhea. If the LH is high or high normal, the cause of the amenorrhea may be PCOD. These patients may be moderately overweight to obese and have a mild to moderate hirsutism. The testosterone levels will be elevated in most of these cases. If the LH and FSH levels are low, then the amenorrhea may be due to a hypothalamic or pituitary dysfunction. This dysfunction could be due to tumors, **panhypopituitarism,** or severe anorexia. Since secondary amenorrhea can be caused by many disorders, the laboratory can provide determinations so that the defective hormonal compartment can be located.

Primary ovarian hyperfunction may be due to estrogen-producing ovarian tumors (granulosa and theca cell tumors). The major laboratory findings are increased serum estradiol and decreased FSH and LH. Secondary hyperfunction is generally idiopathic. The major laboratory findings are increased serum estradiol and elevated FSH and LH. If hyperovarian function occurs prior to puberty, it results in **precocious puberty.** If it occurs after puberty, it may cause irregular uterine bleeding or postmenopausal bleeding.

## Female Infertility

Since a number of factors in the female reproductive system are required to work in synchrony to achieve pregnancy, the causes of female infertility are equally numerous, some of which have already been discussed. The causes can be traced to defects at the level of the hypothalamus, pituitary gland, the ovary, or the uterus. In addition to all the abnormalities of ovarian function that can contribute to infertility, a significant cause of infertility involves the inability of a fertilized egg to implant in an immature uterus. Luteal phase defect is a pathologic condition in which the luteal (or secretory) phase of the menstrual cycle is considerably shorter than normal (<7 days) and serum progesterone levels are inadequate to maintain pregnancy. Women with luteal phase defect usually have persistent miscarriages.[13] The major laboratory finding is reduced serum progesterone levels. Uterine leiomyomas and adenomas of smooth muscle cells are the most common tumors of the uterus. If present, they can interfere with the implantation of a fertilized ovum. Partial or total destruction of the endometrial lining of the uterus, known as Asherman's syndrome, also makes implantation impossible. Fallopian tube abnormalities usually result in decreased patency of the lumen of the oviducts. This can be caused by chronic infections, sexually transmitted diseases, as well as the estrogen-dependent endometriosis.[14]

## Precocious Puberty

**Sexual precocity** is defined as the appearance of secondary sex characteristics before the age of 8 years in girls and 9 1/2 years in boys.[15] The secondary sex characteristics in the female, pubic hair and breast development, and in the male, pubic hair, deepening of the voice, and increased muscle bulk, are produced in response to the release of the sex steroid hormones. This hormonal release eventually leads to ovulation and menstruation in girls and spermatogenesis in boys.

Sexual precocity and precocious puberty are not synonymous. Precocious puberty can be the result of two pathologic events: (1) a normal pubertal process happening at an abnormal time, and (2) an abnormal pubertal process that is independent of the integrated function of the hypothalamic-pituitary-gonadal axis. The first pathologic event is referred to as gonadotropin-dependent or true precocious puberty. The second event is referred to as gonadotropin-independent or pseudoprecocious puberty.[16,17] The most common cause of true precocious puberty is a hypothalamic hamartoma that secretes GnRH. A **hamartoma** is a condition where normal tissue is located in an abnormal location. Of course, the hamartoma is not under normal inhibitory control mechanisms and the GnRH secretion is not suppressed.

Abnormal sex steroid hormone secretion is the most common cause of **pseudoprecocious puberty.** The virilizing effect of congenital adrenal hyperplasia (CAH) or the adrenogenital syndrome are the most encountered causes of abnormal sex steroid hormone secretion. However, tumors of the gonads and adrenal gland may also lead to pseudoprecocious puberty.

Clinically, the diagnosis of precocious puberty is made primarily on the time of onset of physical signs of puberty such as the appearance of pubic hair and breast enlargement. It would appear that the laboratory would be of great value in assigning a patient to the gonadotropin-dependent or gonadotropin-independent category of precocious puberty based on the serum FSH and LH levels. However, in patients with gonadotropin-independent precocious puberty, where the sex steroid hormone levels are increased, the release of GnRH may occur because of the maturation of the hypothalamus caused by the high hormone levels. The categorization is made

by ruling out the causes of gonadotropin-independent precocious puberty by utilizing such tests as imaging studies to rule out adrenal and gonadal tumors and the measurement of steroid intermediates to rule out CAH. Once gonadotropin-independent causes have been ruled out, studies to confirm space-occupying lesions of the cranium should be performed. If this is ruled out, the diagnosis of idiopathic precocious puberty is made, which is actually the most common cause of gonadotropin-dependent precocious puberty.[13]

## DEFECTS OF ANDROGEN METABOLISM

### Hirsutism

Hirsutism is a clinical condition characterized by excessive hair growth in androgen-sensitive skin areas.[18] In women, this is may be characterized simply as male pattern hair growth. Except for rare cases of virilizing tumors or adrenal hyperplasia due to enzymatic defects, hirsutism is mainly caused by ovarian androgen overproduction (PCOD) or by peripheral hypersensitivity to normal circulating androgen levels (idiopathic hirsutism). The face, chest, abdomen, and sacral regions are commonly affected. Hirsutism is associated with normal or moderately increased levels of testosterone in the presence of normal and abnormal menstrual cycles.[19]

Laboratory testing can be extremely valuable in categorizing the cause of hirsutism. The measurement of testosterone is the test of choice in the workup of a hirsute patient. Total testosterone levels greater than 2000 ng/L suggest an adrenal or ovarian tumor. However, since free testosterone is the biologically active hormone, the free testosterone determination is the best single laboratory test to evaluate the androgen status of a patient. Because of the pulsatile release of androgens throughout the day, it has been suggested that serial pooled specimens be used for the hormone determinations.

The contributions from the adrenal glands may be assessed by measuring serum DHEAS.[20] This determination has now, for the most part, replaced the measurement of urinary 17-KS. However, it is important to note that DHEAS is water-soluble and may be excreted more easily than DHEA itself, and therefore serum levels can be underestimated. Patients with PCOD may also have elevated levels of DHEAS. In these patients, measurements of LH and FSH are helpful. In PCOD, the LH is usually increased and the FSH decreased or normal. An LH:FSH ratio of 3:1 or greater may be diagnostic of PCOD. Laboratory evaluation of levels of TSH, prolactin, and cortisol or steroid hormone precursors may prove valuable in categorizing the secondary hyperandrogenemias.

### Syndromes of Androgen Insensitivity

Androgens act through a single intracellular androgen receptor, which is encoded by a single copy gene in the X-chromosome.

Disruption of this receptor by genetic mutation results in the development of the complete androgen insensitivity syndrome (CSAI) and the female phenotype in an otherwise healthy genotypic male (46XY).[21] Affected persons suffer from androgen-regulated diseases including ambiguous genitalia, primary amenorrhea, male pseudohermaphroditism, and male infertility. The androgen resistance could be due to (1) $5\alpha$-reductase deficiency, (2) defects in the androgen receptor, or (3) receptor-positive resistance resulting from abnormalities in the postreceptor events. The deficiency of $5\alpha$-reductase results from a deficient conversion of testosterone to DHT.[22] The major laboratory findings include decreased plasma DHT levels producing elevated testosterone to DHT ratios. Levels of LH are normal or slightly increased and estrogen levels are usually within the reference range for males. The elevated testosterone level may also be explained by an increased LH level because of a defective feedback mechanism due to the androgen resistance at the hypothalamic-pituitary axis.

Patients may have defective androgen receptor function. This may range from patients who have complete testicular feminization to Reifenstein syndrome, where there is partial resistance to the infertile male syndrome.

## GONADAL FUNCTION TESTS

Invariably, the need arises for performing tests to diagnose the cause of aberrant hormone levels and determine if the defect was primary, secondary, or tertiary. The following tests may be very helpful.

### GnRH Test

GnRH controls reproduction at the tertiary level. Administration of synthetic GnRH to a patient should result in a rise in LH and FSH if the pituitary is responsive.[23] In postpubertal patients with hypogonadotropic hypogonadism, a failure of this provocative test to elevate FSH and LH is evidence of hypopituitarism.

### Clomiphene Citrate Challenge Test

Clomiphene citrate, a potent estrogen antagonist, is a mixture of the isomers enclomiphene and zuclomiphene. Administration of clomiphene citrate blocks the negative feedback action of estradiol on the hypothalamic release of GnRH in healthy women, resulting in increased LH and FSH production.[24] A failure to see this increase after clomiphene administration indicates the presence of a hypothalamic disease as the potential cause of secondary ovarian hypofunction.

### hCG Stimulation Test

Structurally, hCG is similar to LH. The hCG stimulation test exploits the fact that hCG can significantly cross react with LH. Injection of hCG mimics the effects of LH by stimulating the testis to produce testosterone.[25] The absence of this rise in serum testosterone in a patient with delayed puberty is an indication of a primary testicular defect.

## SUMMARY

Reproduction is a highly synchronized phenomenon involving the endocrine control of the gonads, which are endocrine organs in their own rights. First, there are three levels of control present in both males and females: the pulsatile release of the hypothalamic hormone GnRH represents the tertiary level. GnRH regulates the anterior pituitary gland, the secondary level that produces gonadotropins LH and FSH. The gonads (testis and ovary) respond to the gonadotropins by producing androgens and estrogens that support spermatogenesis and ovulation, respectively. The endocrine control of ovulation is a cyclic phenomenon intimately synchronized to uterine function to produce a well-prepared endometrium for implantation of a fertilized egg. Whereas ovulation stops at menopause, endocrine control of spermatogenesis is noncyclic and takes place virtually throughout the lifetime of the male.

The laboratory plays an important role not only in the diagnosis of disease states involving the reproductive systems but also in the management of infertility. Specific assay methods are now available because of the development of specific monoclonal antibodies. New procedures employing EIA techniques instead of RIA methods are quickly replacing test procedures. The ability to automate some of these procedures will increase their utility.

## REFERENCES

1. Fregly MJ, Luttage WG: *Human Endocrinology: An Interactive Text.* New York, Elsevier Science, 1982.
2. Jones RE: *Human Reproductive Biology.* 2nd ed. London, Academic Press, 1997.
3. Macklon NS, Fauser BC: Aspects of ovarian follicle development throughout life. Horm Res 52(4):161–170, 1999.
4. Nieschlag E, Simoni M, Gromoll J, et al.: Role of FSH in the regulation of spermatogenesis: clinical aspects. Clin Endocrinol 51:139–146, 1999.
5. Filicori M: The role of luteinizing hormone in folliculogenesis and ovulation induction. Fertil Steril 71:405–414, 1999.
6. World Health Organization. *Laboratory Manual for the Examination of Human Semen and Semen-cervical Mucus Interaction.* 3rd ed. New York, Cambridge University Press, 1993, pp 43–44.
7. Mazumdar S, Levine AS: Antisperm antibodies: etiology,

pathogenesis, diagnosis, and treatment. Fertil Steril 70: 799–810, 1998.

8. Hargreave T, Ghosh C: Male fertility disorders: endocrinology & metabolism. Clin North Am 27(4):765–782, 1998.

9. Franks S, Gharani N, Gilling-Smith C: Polycystic ovary syndrome: evidence for a primary disorder of ovarian steroidogenesis. J Steroid Biochem & Mol Biol 69(1–6): 269–272, 1999.

10. Biller BM: Diagnostic evaluation of hyperprolactinemia. J Reprod Med 44(12 Suppl):1095–1099, 1999.

11. Gallinelli A, Matteo ML, Volpe A, et al.: Autonomic and neuroendocrine responses to stress in patients with functional hypothalamic secondary amenorrhea. Fertil Steril 73:812–816, 2000.

12. Deligdisch L: Hormonal pathology of the endometrium. Mod Pathol 13:285–294, 2000.

13. Ogasawara M, Kajiura S, Katano K, et al.: Are serum progesterone levels predictive of recurrent miscarriage in future pregnancies? Fertil Steril 68:806–809, 1997.

14. Garrido N, Navarro J, Remohi J, et al.: Follicular hormonal environment and embryo quality in women with endometriosis. Hum Reprod Update 6(1):67–74, 2000.

15. Hines M: Abnormal sexual development and psychosexual issues. Baillieres Clin Endocrinol Metab 12:173–189, 1998.

16. Kaplowitz PB, Oberfield SE: Reexamination of the age limit for defining when puberty is precocious in girls in the United States: implications for evaluation and treatment. Drug and Therapeutics and Executive Committees of the Lawson Wilkins Pediatric Endocrine Society. Pediatrics 104(4 Pt 1):936–941, 1999.

17. Nakamoto JM: Myths and variations in normal pubertal development. West J Med 172:182–185, 2000.

18. Plouffe L Jr.: Disorders of excessive hair growth in the adolescent. Obstet Gynecol Clin North Am 27:79–99, 2000.

19. Minanni SL, Marcondes JA, Wajchenberg B, et al.: Analysis of gonadotropin pulsatility in hirsute women with normal menstrual cycles and in women with polycystic ovary syndrome. Fertil Steril 71:675–683, 1999.

20. Barth JH: Investigations in the assessment and management of patients with hirsutism. Curr Opin Obstet Gynecol 9:187–192, 1997.

21. Yong EL, Lim J, Qi W, et al.: Molecular basis of androgen receptor diseases. Ann Med 32:15–22, 2000.

22. Harris GS, Kozarich JW: Steroid 5alpha-reductase inhibitors in androgen-dependent disorders. Curr Opin Chem Biol 1:254–259, 1997.

23. Weissman A, Barash A, Shapiro H, et al.: Ovarian hyperstimulation following the sole administration of agonistic analogues of gonadotrophin releasing hormone. Hum Reprod 13:3421–3424, 1998.

24. Hannoun A, Abu Musa A, Awwad J, et al.: Clomiphene citrate challenge test: cycle to cycle variability of cycle day 10 follicle stimulating hormone level. Clin Exp Obstet Gynecol 25:155–156, 1998.

25. Tzvetkova P, Tzvetkova D, Kanchev L, et al.: hCG stimulation test for the diagnosis of androgen deficiency. Arch Androl 39:163–171, 1997.

# C H A P T E R   3 2

# Gastrointestinal and Pancreatic Function

*Claudia E. Miller*

Gastrointestinal (GI) and pancreatic disorders present with many similar clinical signs and symptoms. It is the responsibility of the physician to choose appropriate tests to diagnose the specific disorder and to initiate treatment. The laboratory, in conjunction with other health care areas, provides the answers to the diagnostic problem.

## GASTROINTESTINAL ORGANS

The organs of digestion can be divided into two groups (Figure 32–1). The first of these organ systems is the GI tract, and the second is composed of the accessory organs. The organs that comprise the GI tract include the mouth, pharynx, esophagus, stomach, small intestine, and large intestine. The GI tract has well-developed layers of smooth muscle in its walls. The churning and mixing action of the smooth muscle results in the mechanical breakdown of food. Digestive enzymes within the GI system also break down food. Several types of glands provide the GI tract with digestive enzymes and lubricating fluids that aid in the chemical breakdown of food. These glands may be simple single-celled glands located in the lining of the tract or may be part of complex organ systems located outside the GI tract entirely. These organs form a continuous tube that runs through the ventral body cavity and extends approximately 10 m from the mouth to the anus.[1]

Several important organs of the digestive system are located outside the gastrointestinal tract. The pancreas, liver, and gallbladder are important accessory organs that secrete digestive aids for the chemical breakdown of food. These organs also contain endocrine glands that secrete hormones to regulate the motor and secretory activity of the GI tract.

## Stomach

The stomach is an enlarged, specialized segment of the digestive tract located between the esophagus and small intestine. Food entering the stomach is stored and processed for absorption by the small intestine. The stomach begins the digestion of protein, mixes and physically breaks down food, and moves it along the tract. Although absorption is not a major function of the stomach, water-soluble substances are absorbed in limited quantities and some fat-soluble substances, such as ethanol, are readily and quickly absorbed.

Functionally, the stomach can be divided into four main areas called the cardiac, fundus, body, and pylorus (Figure 32–2). Each region contains distinct types of gastric glands appropriately termed **cardiac, fundic,** and **pyloric glands.** The cardiac glands are located in the cardiac zone adjacent to the esophagus. Cardiac glands produce a secretion rich in mucus. The fundic glands occupy most of the fundus and body of the stomach and are composed of parietal cells that produce hydrochloric acid and peptic or chief cells. Peptic or chief cells located in the fundic region synthesize the proenzyme pepsinogen.

The pyloric gland area of the stomach occupies a region approximately one fifth of the gastric mucosal surface area. Pyloric glands contain gastrin-producing G cells and mucus-secreting cells.

## COMPONENTS OF GASTRIC FLUID

### Hydrochloric Acid

Hydrochloric acid is secreted by parietal cells. These cells produce acid at a concentration of 150 to 160 mmol/L. The pH of gastric juice may be as low as 1.0 compared with a pH of 7.4 in blood. Parietal cells expend an enormous amount of energy to concentrate hydrogen ion. The secretion of hydrochloric acid by the gastric mucosa is continuous; however, the volume produced fluctuates considerably depending on the degree of stimulation.

### Pepsinogen

Pepsinogen is secreted by the gastric mucosa as a zymogen and converted to proteolytically active pepsin by the acid pH of the stomach. A pH below 5.0 is required for this conversion to occur. Pepsin aids in the digestion of protein by splitting peptide bonds, especially those involving aromatic amino acids such as phenylalanine, tyrosine, and leucine. The activity of pepsin is terminated when the acid gastric contents are mixed with alkaline pancreatic secretions in the small intestine.

### Gastric Lipase

Gastric juice contains a lipase that is distinct from pancreatic lipase. Gastric lipase has a broad pH optimum of pH 4.0 to 7.0. Lipolytic activity is maximal with short-chain fatty acids

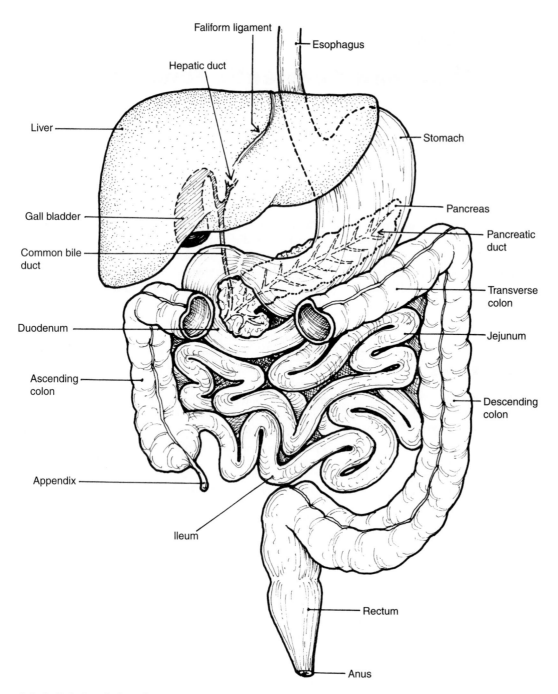

**F I G U R E   3 2 - 1**

Anatomy of the gastrointestinal tract.

as substrate. Gastric lipase may be important for digestion of short-chain triglycerides in milk.

## Mucus

The gastric mucosa is covered by a layer of mucus 1.0- to 1.5-mm thick. Mucus secretion increases following physical stimulation of the mucosa by food. The major function of the gastrointestinal mucus is to protect the mucosal epithelium from mechanical damage during the passage of food. It also provides a lubricant for the passage of food. The gastric mucus, however, does not provide an impenetrable barrier to acid since it is permeable to hydrogen ions.

## Electrolytes

The major electrolytes present in gastric juice are sodium ($Na^+$), potassium ($K^+$), chloride ($Cl^-$), and hydrogen ($H^+$). The concentration of each electrolyte in gastric juice is variable and related to the rate of secretion. In the basal state, the

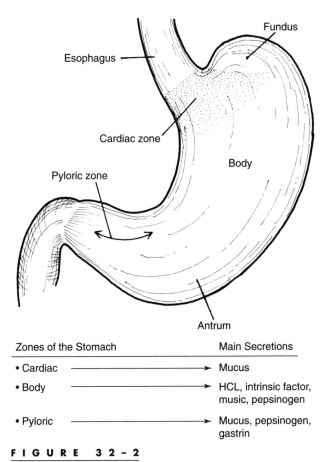

| Zones of the Stomach | Main Secretions |
|---|---|
| • Cardiac ⟶ | Mucus |
| • Body ⟶ | HCL, intrinsic factor, music, pepsinogen |
| • Pyloric ⟶ | Mucus, pepsinogen, gastrin |

**F I G U R E   3 2 - 2**

Structure of the stomach.

major electrolytes in gastric juice are sodium and chloride with small amounts of hydrogen and potassium. As the rate of secretion increases, there is a marked increase in hydrogen ion concentration with small increases in chloride and potassium concentrations. The sodium concentration decreases. At all rates of secretion, hydrogen, potassium, and chloride concentrations are greater than those in serum, whereas sodium is lower than that found in serum.

### Intrinsic Factor

Intrinsic factor produced by the parietal cells of the stomach is necessary for vitamin $B_{12}$ absorption. Achlorhydria diminishes vitamin $B_{12}$ absorption leading to pernicious anemia (see Chapter 33).

### Gastrin

Gastrin is a hormone produced and stored within the G cells located in the antral mucosa. The major physiologic effect of gastrin is the stimulation of acid secretion by the parietal cell. Acid secretion stimulated by gastrin is also accompanied by an increase in gastric blood flow and secretion of pepsinogen. Gastrin is released into interstitial fluid by various stimuli including vagal stimulation and local reflexes triggered by the presence of food in the stomach.

The major stimulus for gastrin release is amino acids. Some commonly ingested substances that also stimulate gastrin release include calcium and caffeine. Calcium, either in the gastric lumen or as increased concentrations in serum, stimulates gastrin release. Caffeine does not cause release of gastrin itself but stimulates the parietal cells directly to induce acid secretion. Release of gastrin is inhibited by acid in contact with the gastric mucosa and release is completely suppressed when the pH of the antral contents is 2.0 or lower.

## Small Intestine

Most digestion and absorption occurs in the small intestine. The functions of the small intestine include (1) the completion of digestion of food, (2) the selective absorption of nutrients and water, and (3) the passage of unabsorbed foodstuffs along the digestive tract. The function most unique to the small intestine is that of absorption. To perform this function efficiently, the small intestine contains a series of progressively finer folds that greatly increase its surface area. The mucosa is folded into transverse ridges that project into the lumen of the intestine. At the microscopic level, minute projections of the mucosa called **villi** increase the luminal surface approximately 8-fold. Each villus contains another set of projections called **microvilli** that further increase the absorptive area by a factor of about 20, so that the total absorptive area is approximately 300 square meters (3200 square feet).

The absorption of most foodstuffs is not regulated by the small intestine. It indiscriminately absorbs water, the major electrolytes, and most of the products of digestion. The absorption of calcium and iron are, however, absorbed according to the needs of the body.

## MAJOR CONSTITUENTS ABSORBED BY THE SMALL INTESTINE

### Water and Electrolytes

The intestine absorbs both exogenous fluids as well as its own secretions. The average daily volume of fluid secreted into the small intestine is approximately 12 L. If this volume were not absorbed, death from dehydration would result within 24 hours.

Water is absorbed throughout the small intestine, with most of the absorption occurring in the upper part of the tract. Absorption of water-soluble ions may occur by both active and passive transport processes. Active transport requires input of energy so that solute can be transported against an electrochemical gradient. Sodium and chloride are the major electrolytes actively transported by the small intestine, and other ions including iron, calcium, and bicarbonate are also absorbed via active transport systems.

Passive transport of ions may result from diffusion of ions down electrical or chemical concentration gradients that exist across the intestinal mucosa. Electrolytes such as lithium, iodide, bromide and potassium are absorbed by passive diffusion. Passive diffusion of solutes may also occur by a process known as **solvent drag,** which is the movement of solute in conjunction with water flow. This phenomenon accounts for the absorption of urea and other nonelectrolytes. Finally, many divalent and polyvalent ions including aluminum, barium, magnesium, and sulfate are almost completely excluded from absorption.

## Calcium

Calcium is actively absorbed against a concentration gradient throughout the small intestine and colon; however, most absorption occurs in the ileum. Calcium is bound to a specific binding protein whose synthesis is controlled by the active form of vitamin D, 1,25-dihydroxyvitamin D and the complex is absorbed through the microvillar membrane. The absorption of calcium is regulated in part by plasma calcium concentrations. As intestinal absorption of calcium rises, plasma calcium increases, which inhibits the secretion of parathyroid hormone. A reduction in parathyroid hormone production leads to decreased formation of 1,25-dihydroxyvitamin D by the kidney, which in turn leads to decreased synthesis of calcium binding protein in the intestine causing calcium absorption to cease (See Chapter 28).

## Magnesium

Magnesium is absorbed throughout the entire small intestine. Unlike calcium absorption, magnesium absorption is not vitamin D dependent. Whether magnesium can be absorbed against an electrochemical gradient or whether absorption increases in a patient with magnesium deficiency is not yet known.

## Phosphorus

Phosphorus is present in virtually all food; therefore, dietary deficiencies are rare. Phosphorus is absorbed by all segments of the small intestine by both passive and active transport processes. Absorption is increased in association with decreased dietary calcium and is augmented by the action of 1,25-dihydroxyvitamin D.

## Iron

Iron absorption is regulated by several factors including the size of the body iron stores, the rate of hematopoiesis, and bioavailability. Most iron is absorbed in the heme of hemoglobin and myoglobin. The ferrous ($Fe^{2+}$) form of inorganic iron is more rapidly absorbed compared to the ferric ($Fe^{3+}$) form. Ferrous iron binds to receptors on the brush border membrane and is absorbed by a saturable active process. The same active process also absorbs cobalt and manganese, and if any one metal is in excess, it may competitively inhibit absorption of the other.

## Vitamins

Vitamins are organic compounds that are essential for normal metabolism. Since the body cannot synthesize them, vitamins must be absorbed from dietary foodstuffs. Vitamins may be broken into two classes on the basis of their solubility in lipids or water. Lipid-soluble vitamins (A, D, E, and K) are absorbed after being solubilized within lipid micelles. Once absorbed, these vitamins are incorporated into chylomicrons and transported via the blood.

Absorption of water-soluble vitamins presents special problems. The predominant mechanism for absorption of water-soluble vitamins is probably passive diffusion except for vitamin $B_{12}$, folic acid, thiamine, and ascorbic acid, where uptake is mediated by specific transport mechanisms.

Vitamin $B_{12}$ is a large polar molecule that is absorbed following its binding with intrinsic factor. Intrinsic factor is a glycoprotein secreted by the parietal cells. The vitamin $B_{12}$–intrinsic factor complex binds to specific receptors located in the terminal portion of the ileum. The presence of calcium and magnesium, as well as an alkaline pH, is necessary for proper attachment of the $B_{12}$–intrinsic factor complex to the receptor. Any mechanism that interferes with the attachment of the vitamin $B_{12}$ intrinsic factor or with the production or secretion of intrinsic factor can lead to malabsorption of vitamin $B_{12}$.

## ACCESSORY ORGANS

### Liver and Gallbladder

The liver plays an important role in digestion because of its exocrine secretions. The biliary tract is the excretory apparatus of the liver, draining its exocrine secretions into the gastrointestinal tract (Figure 32–3). The exocrine secretion of the liver is called **bile** and is stored in the gallbladder during the fasting periods.

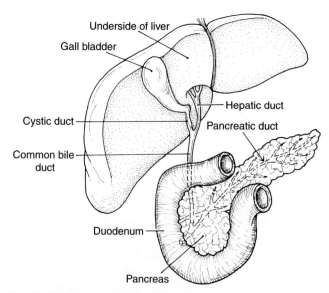

**F I G U R E    3 2 - 3**

The liver and biliary system.

The biliary tract serves as the excretory pathway for the breakdown products of hemoglobin and bilirubin. Bile also provides the main excretory pathway for toxic metabolites, cholesterol, and lipid metabolic waste products. In addition, bile is also necessary for the digestion and absorption of dietary lipids in the small intestine.

Bile acids play an essential role in the absorption of lipids. Fat that is released into the duodenum results in secretion of cholecystokinin (CCK). CCK slows gastric emptying, stimulates the pancreas to secrete lipase, as well as other digestive enzymes, and causes contraction of the gallbladder. Bile acids released into the duodenum help to emulsify fat droplets by decreasing the surface tension at the oil-water interface. This emulsification process is important in that it increases the surface area of lipids resulting in more rapid and efficient enzymatic breakdown of dietary lipids by pancreatic lipase. The concentration of bile acids in serum represents a balance between input from the intestine and clearance by the liver (see Chapter 16).

## Pancreas

The pancreas is a mixed endocrine–exocrine gland that extends transversely in the upper abdomen. The pancreas is retroperitoneal, lying behind the stomach; this location renders it inaccessible to physical examination. The head of the pancreas lies within the concavity of the duodenum on the right while its body and tail extend to the left as far as the spleen (Figure 32–4).

The pancreas is probably the most important digestive gland in the entire gastrointestinal system. Its exocrine enzyme secretions are capable of digesting all the major categories of food, while its secretion of bicarbonate is able to neutralize the acid digestive products to a pH at which the pancreatic en-

zymes can optimally function. These secretions influence the chemical composition of the duodenal contents, which in turn affects gastric secretions and gastric emptying.

The functional secretory unit of the exocrine pancreas, known as an *acinus*, consists of a roughly spherical arrangement of enzyme-secreting cells (acinar cells) arranged around a system of ductules. These networks of ductules coalesce and eventually drain into the main pancreatic duct, which in turn opens into the duodenum.

The acinar cells secrete a fluid rich in proteins, the majority of which are digestive enzymes. The nondigestive proteins present in pancreatic juice include trypsin inhibitor, a cofactor for lipase, a trace of plasma proteins, and lactoferrin, which is present in almost all exocrine secretions. Cells within the ductules and centroacinar cells produce watery secretions rich in bicarbonate and enzyme precursors or zymogens. Once secreted into the duodenum, enterokinase, an enzyme secreted by the duodenal mucosa, hydrolyzes the zymogen trypsinogen to form catalytically active trypsin. Trypsin in turn can activate the remaining pancreatic enzymes.[2] Activation of these enzymes within the duodenum, instead of within the pancreas, ensures that proteolytic autodigestion of the pancreas does not occur.

The endocrine portion of the pancreas consists of pancreatic islets called islets of Langerhans. The islets are composed of $\alpha$ and $\beta$ cells, which produce glucagon and insulin, respectively. In addition to their effects on glucose metabolism, both insulin and glucagon also influence pancreatic exocrine secretions. Insulin increases amylase synthesis and secretion by pancreatic acinar cells, and glucagon inhibits enzyme synthesis. The pancreas also produces the candidate hormone pancreatic polypeptide and contains large amounts of somatostatin that has complex effects on glucose homeostasis.

## DIGESTION

### Carbohydrates

The intestinal mucosa secretes a variety of enzymes important for the digestion of starch. Although the digestion of starch begins in the mouth by the action of salivary $\alpha$-amylase, most starch digestion takes place in the small intestine. The action of salivary and pancreatic $\alpha$-amylase yields maltose and the trisaccharide maltotriose. Amylopectin and glycogen are also hydrolyzed to maltose and oligosaccharides of glucose that are resistant to enzymatic attack. Further hydrolysis is accomplished by one or more disaccharidases located in the brush border. Lactase hydrolyzes $\beta$-galactosides exclusively, whereas isomaltase hydrolyzes the $\alpha$-1,6 glucoside bonds found in isomaltose and $\alpha$-limit dextrins. Sucrase and glucoamylase hydrolyze $\alpha$-1,4 glucoside bonds; sucrase primarily hydrolyzes sucrose and maltose, and glucoamylase hydrolyzes glucose oligosaccharides of 2 to 9 glucose residues in length (see Chapter 10).

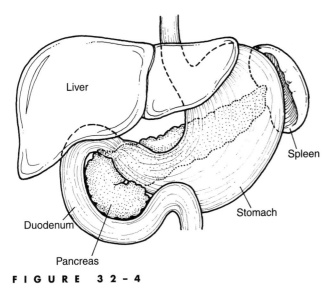

**F I G U R E   3 2 - 4**

Relation of other organs to the pancreas.

## Proteins

Protein digestion begins in the stomach with the action of pepsin and hydrochloric acid. Enterokinase is an important regulatory enzyme secreted by the intestinal mucosa. Proteolytic enzymes produced by the pancreas are secreted as inactive precursors or zymogens. Enterokinase hydrolyzes trypsinogen within the small intestine to yield the active enzyme trypsin. Trypsin in turn can readily hydrolyze many of the other inactive pancreatic enzyme precursors to yield the active enzyme. It is important that these proteolytic enzymes be secreted as inactive precursors so that autodigestion of the pancreas does not take place.

Active pancreatic enzymes—trypsin, chymotrypsin, and carboxypeptidase—act on protein to produce peptides and amino acids. These forms are easily absorbed in the ileum and jejunum (see Chapter 12).

## Fats

Dietary fat is in the form of long-chain triglycerides. Salivary lipase, which also works in the stomach, digests medium-chain triglycerides and partially digests triglycerides to form fatty acids. This process is aided by gastric lipase. However, lipid digestion takes place mainly in the intestinal lumen with the secretion of pancreatic lipase. Pancreatic lipase hydrolyzes the triglyceride molecule to monoglycerides and fatty acids.[3]

Phospholipase $A_2$ is the major pancreatic enzyme for digesting phospholipids. Cholesterol esterase digests dietary cholesterol that can only be absorbed as the free sterol (see Chapter 11).

## REGULATION OF DIGESTION BY GASTROINTESTINAL HORMONES

Many hormones help regulate gastrointestinal processes. Gastrointestinal hormones are released by endocrine cells located throughout the entire gut mucosa and control secretion, digestion, absorption, gastrointestinal motility, and release of other hormones.

Gastrointestinal hormones are released from the mucosa of the stomach and small intestine by vagal stimulation, distention by food and chemical stimulation associated with the intake of food. These hormones are initially released into the portal circulation and pass through the liver before circulating back to the digestive tract, where they exert their regulatory functions.[4]

The major gastrointestinal hormones and their important physiologic functions are given in Table 32–1.

## Cholecystokinin and Pancreozymin

Cholecystokinin (CCK) is a polypeptide containing 33 amino acids; the 8 carboxy-terminal amino acids account for all of the hormone's actions. CCK is present in mucosa cells of the duodenum and jejunum but not the ileum.

The major physiologic action of CCK is the regulation of gallbladder contraction and gastric emptying. CCK is the most potent of the gastrointestinal hormones causing gallbladder contraction. CCK also causes inhibition of gastric emptying. Since CCK has the same carboxy-terminal sequence of amino acids as gastrin, CCK also stimulates acid secretion to a small degree by competing with gastrin for the receptor sites on the hydrochloric acid (HCl)–secreting cells.

CCK is released in response to the presence of partially digested fat or partially digested proteins in the gastrointestinal tract. Carbohydrates do not affect release of CCK to any appreciable extent. The most potent stimuli for release of CCK are the essential amino acids. Increased serum calcium concentrations stimulate both gastrin and CCK release. Under normal circumstances, the effect of calcium on gastrin and CCK release is probably negligible. However, alterations in serum calcium concentrations by disease may become an important factor affecting CCK and gastrin release.

CCK has also been found in human brain, where it may function as a neurotransmitter. Release of CCK from the intestine or cerebral nerves with intake of food may function as one of the satiety signals.

## Secretin

Secretin is found throughout the entire small intestine, with the duodenum its major site of synthesis. The major stimulus for secretin release is the hydrogen ion. Below pH 4.0, release of secretin is maximal and is proportional to the amount of acid entering the duodenum. The presence of fatty acids in the gastrointestinal lumen can also cause release of secretin.

## Gastric Inhibitory Polypeptide

Gastric inhibitory polypeptide (GIP) occurs primarily in the duodenal and jejunal mucosa. GIP's *N*-terminal end has a close resemblance to glucagon and secretin. GIP was originally named because of its inhibitory effects on gastric acid secretion. However, this action has not been found to be physiologically significant. Of greater importance is the finding that GIP is much more potent in stimulating insulin release from the beta cells of the pancreas and is primarily responsible for the rapid metabolism of an oral glucose load. It has recently been called **glucose-dependent insulinotropic peptide.**

GIP release is stimulated following absorption of fat and carbohydrate; amino acids have much less of a stimulatory effect. Peak concentrations of GIP in blood occur approximately 60 minutes following the ingestion of food.

## Vasoactive Intestinal Polypeptide

Originally believed to originate from gut endocrine cells, vasoactive intestinal polypeptide (VIP) is now known to be lo-

TABLE 32-1

**Principal Actions of Major Gastrointestinal Hormones**

| HORMONE | TISSUE DISTRIBUTION | STIMULATION ACTION | INHIBITION ACTION |
|---|---|---|---|
| Secretin | Duodenum and jejunum | Pancreatic fluid and $HCO_3^-$; biliary secretion of fluid and $HCO_3^-$ | Acid secretion |
| Cholecystokinin (CCK) | Duodenum, jejunum | Gallbladder and intestinal motility; secretion of pancreatic enzymes | Gastric motility |
| Gastric inhibitory polypeptide (GIP) | Duodenum, jejunum (majority) | Insulin release; intestinal fluid and electrolyte secretion | Acid secretion; pepsin; gastrin; intestinal motility |
| Vasoactive intestinal polypeptide (VIP) | Endocrine cell and nerves of gut and central nervous system | Intestinal circular smooth muscle | None identified |
| Motilin | Upper small intestine | Small intestine and gastric motility; increase gastric emptying; increase pepsin | None identified |
| Somatostatin | Brain, hypothalamus, stomach, upper intestine, pancreas, nerve fibers | None identified | Gastric emptying; pepsin secretion; gallbladder contraction; endocrine secretion; bile; pancreatic enzymes; bicarbonate |

cated in the nerve terminals throughout the gastrointestinal tract. Particularly high concentrations are found in the wall of the gallbladder. In addition, VIP is also found in high concentration in the central nervous system, suggesting that VIP functions as a neurotransmitter, although its precise role is still unknown.

VIP is similar in structure to secretin, GIP, and glucagon. VIP-containing nerve fibers innervate gastrointestinal smooth muscle as well as exocrine pancreatic parenchyma. Following the ingestion of food, release of VIP from the nerve terminals results in relaxation of gut circular smooth muscle as well as smooth muscle in blood vessels, resulting in vasodilation. VIP also stimulates pancreatic secretion.

## Motilin

Motilin stimulates the contraction of the smooth muscles of the GI tract. In addition, it contracts the lower esophageal sphincter. It acts only in the fasting state.

## Somatostatin

The most potent inhibitor of endocrine secretions is somatostatin. It not only inhibits the release of growth hormone and thyroid-stimulating hormone but most of the gastrointestinal and pancreatic hormones as well. It also inhibits the actions of these hormones on their target tissues.

## CLINICAL APPLICATIONS

## Pathology of the Stomach

### GASTRIC CARCINOMA

Gastric cancer is the second most common fatal cancer worldwide. Dietary and genetic factors contribute to the disease. Adenocarcinoma of the stomach is usually found in the distal portion and in the prepyloric region. Usually patients have metastases before they present for examination. Therefore, the course of the disease is advanced before any treatment can be started.

Most patients with gastric carcinoma have fasting achlorhydria. They usually produce gastric acid after stimulation.

Advances in molecular oncology have improved the understanding of carcinogenesis, progression, and metastasis of gastric carcinoma. Recent studies have shown a relationship between *Helicobacter pylori* and the molecular changes from the precancerous to cancerous stage of gastric cancer. There is consideration that infection with the organism is a potential carcinogen. Chemoprevention studies are in progress.[5]

## PEPTIC ULCERS

Gastric and duodenal ulcers are grouped under the collective heading of peptic ulcer disease. Although these diseases have many features in common, their origins are quite different. One feature, however, they do share in common is the requirement for acid and pepsin. With the rare exception, a person who does not secrete acid will not develop a peptic ulcer. Ulcers form when pepsin and acid damage the mucosa and it is not able to protect and replace damaged cells.

There are environmental factors that contribute to the production of peptic ulcers. There is little evidence that consumption of any food or beverage leads to the development or persistence of ulcers. Medications such as aspirin, nonsteroidal anti-inflammatory agents, and prolonged treatment with corticosteroids have been implicated. Cigarette smoking is a risk factor. *Helicobacter pylori* is a gram-negative bacterium that causes peptic ulcer disease, gastric lymphoma, and gastric carcinoma. The organism triggers an intense leukocyte infiltration of the gastric submucosa; this is mediated by proinflammatory cytokines. Because this mechanism is common to other diseases such as cardiovascular, respiratory, neurological, autoimmune, and growth disorders, the effect of *H. pylori* on other organ systems is being studied.[6]

### Gastric Ulcers

Acid secretion in gastric ulcer disease is usually below normal. Gastric ulcers usually form because diminished gastric mucosa defenses leave the mucosa unable to withstand injury.

The decreased rate of acid secretion in gastric ulcer is due in part to the inability of the mucosa to recover acid that has been secreted and that has leaked back across the damaged mucosal barrier. In normal individuals, the gastric mucosa is relatively impermeable to $H^+$. In those cases where the mucosal barrier is damaged, $H^+$ leaks back into the mucosa. As the $H^+$ accumulates in the mucosa, the pH of the cells decreases, resulting in injury and cell death.

### Duodenal Ulcers

Patients with duodenal ulcer formation have a larger population of parietal cells than normal and as a result secrete more acid. In addition, the secretion of pepsin is about 2-fold above that seen in normal individuals as determined by measurement of plasma pepsinogen. Plasma gastrin concentrations in fasting individuals with duodenal ulcer are normal. However, the increase in gastrin response following a meal and the sensitivity to gastrin is much greater than normal.

Treatment of both duodenal and gastric ulcer disease usually consists of administering agents to neutralize secreted acids or to inhibit acid secretion. If this approach is unsatisfactory, surgical treatment such as vagotomy may be used. *H. pylori* is responsive to eradication therapy using drug regimens.

## PERNICIOUS ANEMIA

Pernicious anemia is a megaloblastic anemia with accompanying neurologic disease caused by the lack of intrinsic factor in the gastric juice. Absence of this factor prevents the absorption of vitamin $B_{12}$ (cobalamin) and folate; deficiencies result. Vitamin $B_{12}$ deficiency is suspected because of the presence of anemia, macrocytosis, and neurological symptoms. Peripheral smears show hypersegmentation of the granulocytes. Deficiencies may also be associated with clinical conditions in which anemia is absent. Additional causes of vitamin $B_{12}$ deficiency include other malabsorption problems, dietary lack (vegetarianism), bacterial overgrowth, and impaired utilization.[7]

## ZOLLINGER-ELLISON SYNDROME

The Zollinger-Ellison syndrome occurs as the result of a gastrin-secreting tumor of the pancreas or, rarely, the upper small intestine called a **gastrinoma.** Gastrinomas are usually malignant with metastasis to the lymph nodes or liver in a majority of cases.

Gastrin is released from the tumor at a high continuous rate that is not altered by intake of food. The high rate of gastrin secretion results in hypersecretion of gastric acid by the parietal cells. Most patients with a gastrinoma have peptic ulcer disease. The low duodenal pH that results causes inactivation of pancreatic enzymes, leading to maldigestion, and erodes the intestinal mucosa, producing ulceration.

When secreted in very large amounts, gastrin may inhibit the absorption of fluid and electrolytes by the intestine. The resulting large volume of fluid in the intestine, coupled with the decreased intestinal transit time, contributes to the secretory diarrhea seen in these patients. Malabsorption results.[8]

Measurement of serum gastrin concentrations in sera is extremely helpful for the diagnosis of Zollinger-Ellison syndrome. Patients with the disease usually show fasting gastrin concentrations greater than 4-fold the upper reference limit.

The evaluation of hypergastrinemia may include gastrin stimulation following intravenous calcium infusion, stimulation with protein meals, or measurement of gastrin release following infusion of secretin.

Originally, total gastrectomy to control the amount of acid secretion was the treatment for Zollinger-Ellison syndrome. New medications like histamine-receptor antagonists and antisecretory drugs have dramatically inhibited the basal and stimulated gastric acid secretion. However, surgery to resect the gastrinoma is necessary for the cure of Zollinger-Ellison syndrome.[8]

## Pathology of the Intestine

### CARCINOID SYNDROME

Carcinoid tumors are slow-growing malignancies that occur most frequently in the gastrointestinal tract and arise from the neuroendocrine cells of the gut. However, these tumors can occur at every site in the body.

These tumors produce serotonin. Serotonin is synthesized from its precursor 5-hydroxytryptophan and is metabolized to 5-hydroxyindoleacetic acid (5-HIAA). In addition to serotonin, carcinoid tumors have been found to secrete corticotropin, histamine, dopamine, prostaglandins, and kallikrein.[9]

The release of serotonin and the other vasoactive constrictors give rise to the carcinoid syndrome. Manifestations include flushing, wheezing, diarrhea, right-sided valvular heart disease, myopathy, and increased skin pigmentation. These symptoms may be paroxysmal or be triggered by agents such as alcohol, food containing tyramines (cheese, chocolate), or exercise.[10] The only method of cure for the disease is surgical excision of the tumor. Therapy is usually just supportive and cytotoxic agents are generally not helpful.

### CELIAC DISEASE (NONTROPICAL SPRUE)

Celiac disease is characterized by intolerance to wheat gliadins and related prolamines. Generalized malabsorption and small intestinal mucosal lesions characterize the disease. The intestinal villi are blunt or absent.

It is generally accepted that celiac disease is an immunologically mediated small intestine enteropathy. There is evidence of cell and humoral immunologic overstimulation. Extra-intestinal autoimmune symptoms are frequently found in celiac patients.[11]

Children are diagnosed when they present with a failure to thrive after cereals are introduced into their diet. Adults have more severe malabsorption problems than children do. When the diet eliminates all offending substances, clinical recovery is quick but intestinal histologic abnormalities change more slowly.

Undiagnosed celiac patients, or those who return to a normal diet, are exposed to a series of health risks. These include disturbance of bone calcium, reproductive and growth problems, and a possibility of increased risk of autoimmune diseases.

### COLON CANCER

Cancer of the colon accounts for approximately 20% of all cancer deaths in the United States. The main environmental risk factor is a diet high in fat and low in fiber. Such a diet has also been identified in the etiology of other gastrointestinal diseases such as diverticulosis, adenomatous polyps, and ulcerative colitis.

Colon cancer arises from adenomatous polyps that are true neoplasms. Some researchers view the development as a sequence of events from hyperplasia to the development of carcinoma. Polyps are surgically excised because of the close relationship with carcinoma. A gene (APC) has been recognized that is associated with susceptibility to colon cancer. This gene does not appear to act as a tumor suppressor gene. Instead, it is involved in DNA repair, and errors in the gene lead to instability and malignant transformation.[12]

Although colon cancer is a common malignancy, symptoms are usually vague and may include changes in bowel habits, bleeding, pain in the abdomen, weight loss, and malaise. Bleeding may be occult and initial identification can be made through occult blood–screening programs. Although the carcinoembryonic antigen (CEA) is not specific for colon cancer, it is a good tool for monitoring patients postoperatively.

### CROHN'S DISEASE

Crohn's disease, sometimes called regional or terminal ileitis, is a chronic inflammatory disorder of the intestine. It most commonly affects the ileocecal area, although it may involve virtually any part of the gastrointestinal tract. The disease has shown a dramatic increase in incidence during the past 25 years throughout the world. It usually appears in adolescents and young adults. The disease appears to have a familial occurrence. There is an increased prevalence of the disease among first-degree relatives and certain populations, especially the Ashkenazi Jews.

The etiology of the disease still remains unknown. No studies have shown any convincing evidence that the disease is caused by a specific viral or bacterial infective agent. Immunologic mechanisms as causes of Crohn's disease have also been studied since these patients have increased immunoglobulin concentrations in serum while the disease is active.

Patients with Crohn's disease frequently exhibit symptoms of diarrhea, abdominal pain, weight loss, nausea, and vomiting. Malabsorption of vitamin $B_{12}$ is also common. The high incidence of gallstones in these patients may be due to malabsorption of bile salts. Steatorrhea, which usually results from overgrowth of bacteria secondary to narrowing of the bowel, may lead to deficiencies of the fat-soluble vitamins. Patients may also be hypokalemic as the result of the severe diarrhea that occurs.

The diagnosis of Crohn's disease is usually confirmed by radiologic studies. Inflammation is discontinuous; that is, certain sections of the bowel are disease-free. Crohn's disease is often accompanied by the formation of fistulas that connect different sites in the intestinal tract with other organs. Fistulas may develop between the bowel and bladder, vagina, urethra, and skin. The risk of intestinal cancer is increased 3-fold in patients with this disease.

No curative treatment is available. Medications suppress the inflammation. Surgical resection may be necessary if the tract becomes obstructed.[13]

## LACTASE DEFICIENCY

Deficiency of the enzyme lactase, required for the conversion of lactose into glucose and galactose, occurs in much of the world's population. It can be inherited as a congenital defect or acquired in later life. Abdominal pain and distention, flatulence, and passage of loose, watery stools characterize the deficiency. Infants with congenital lactase deficiency present with profuse watery diarrhea soon after the introduction of milk. Unless the disease is quickly identified and lactose withdrawn from the diet, infants may die of dehydration.

Lactose, which remains in the intestinal lumen of patients with lactase deficiency, increases the osmotic pressure of the luminal contents. Fermentation of lactose by bacteria in the lower small intestine and colon results in the production of gas as well as lactic acid and fatty acid that also add to the osmotic effect. The osmotic retention of water in the intestinal lumen leads to diarrhea.

Absorption of disaccharides occurs on or within the brush border of the intestinal epithelial cells by specific disaccharidases. Defects for other carbohydrates due to deficiency of other brush border oligosaccharidases have also been described.

Patients with acquired lactase deficiency vary considerably in their ability to tolerate lactose. In many populations that do not normally consume milk or dairy products, lactase activity disappears from the brush border of the small intestine by 2 to 6 years of age. Northern European whites are among the few populations that are not lactase deficient in adult life. The prevalence of lactose intolerance is greater than 50% in South America, Africa, and Asia, reaching almost 100% in some Asian countries. In the United States, it is estimated that 80% of the black population and 55% of the Mexican-American population are lactase deficient.[14]

## MALABSORPTION

Malabsorption describes a number of clinical conditions in which the gastrointestinal tract inadequately absorbs one or more important nutrients. Some absorption occurs in the stomach and colon but clinically significant absorption takes place in the proximal portion of the small intestine.

Diseases of the intestinal mucosa that impair the assimilation of foodstuffs may cause malabsorption by the small bowel. Malabsorption may also occur due to maldigestion of foodstuffs. This form of malabsorption usually results from pancreatic disease such as chronic pancreatitis or fibrocystic disease of the pancreas. Malabsorption resulting from normal digestion but inadequate assimilation of foodstuffs may result from competition by bacteria or altered bacterial flora, from obstruction to the flow of lymph, from diminished mucosal surface area, or from rapid transit of small bowel contents.

Malabsorption increases with age. Slow cell turnover and continual cell renewal impact cell proliferation. Single nutrients, such as oligosaccharides and monosaccharides, bile acids, vitamin B12, carbohydrates, fats, and proteins can be malabsorbed.

Patients with malabsorption are prone to development of deficiencies of the fat-soluble vitamins A, D, E, and K. Certain conditions affecting the small bowel mucosa may also result in deficiency of water-soluble vitamins. In addition, these patients are subject to weight loss and the development of nutritional deficiencies resulting in hypoprothrombinemia, anemia, edema, ascites, and osteomalacia.

Patients with malabsorption may develop osteomalacia as the result of reduced calcium absorption. The reduced absorption of calcium has been attributed to vitamin D deficiency and also to the loss of fecal calcium complexed with fatty acids. Patients with severe forms of fat malabsorption frequently develop calcium oxalate kidney stones because of enhanced absorption of dietary oxalate.

Watery, diurnal and nocturnal, bulky, frequent stools are the hallmark of malabsorption. Steatorrhea, the presence of fat in the stool, produces a pale yellow, floating specimen. A thorough examination of the stool confirms the diagnosis of malabsorption. Other gastrointestinal features are anorexia, nausea, vomiting, abdominal distention, and excessive flatus. Abdominal pain is rare and suggests an obstruction.

Because of inadequate digestion, steatorrhea has been identified in hepatitis, extrahepatic biliary tract obstruction, biliary cirrhosis, and postgastrectomy states. Inadequate absorptive surface contributes to malabsorption due to overgrowth of bacteria in the small bowel.[15]

The site of malabsorption—intestine or pancreas—must be differentiated. The D-xylose absorption test is the most valuable tests for establishing the correct diagnosis.

Treatment of the malabsorption syndromes requires identifying the underlying cause. Antibiotic therapy is administered for malabsorption due to bacterial overgrowth. Malabsorption due to maldigestion as a result of pancreatic disease may be treated by oral supplementation with digestive enzymes.

## ULCERATIVE COLITIS

This disorder is characterized by an inflammatory reaction localized in the mucosa and submucosa of the colon. Repeated bouts of inflammation cause the bowel to become shorter, regenerating mucosa then forms polyps, and finally large portions of the colon may become necrotic. When there is severe damage to the colon, it may become filled with blood and purulent exudate.

The etiology of ulcerative colitis, like Crohn's disease, is unknown. The diseases are similar and difficult to differentiate. The major symptoms are bloody diarrhea, abdominal pain, fever, and weight loss. Laboratory findings demonstrate anemia, leukocytosis with a left shift, hypoalbuminemia, electrolyte disturbances, and elevation in sedimentation rate.[16]

Treatment of the disease involves reducing the inflammatory response and replacing the nutritional losses. Blood transfusions may be necessary. A clear liquid diet to rest the bowel and intravenous alimentation appear to be successful. Antibiotics are not used; however, corticosteroids or adenocorticotropic hormone (ACTH) are given for anti-inflammatory and immune suppression purposes.

## Pathology of the Pancreas

### CYSTIC FIBROSIS

Cystic fibrosis is a multisystem disease inherited as an autosomal recessive trait due to a defective gene carried on chromosome 7. It is seen most commonly in white populations and is rare in blacks and Asians. During the past 11 years, understanding of the physiology and genetic basis of the disease has been achieved. The cystic fibrosis gene has been cloned and its product, cystic fibrosis transmembrane conductance regulator (CFTR), has been characterized.

The defect in the cystic fibrosis gene involves the transport of chloride with a failure to excrete sodium and water; CFTR constitutes an apical chloride channel. Defective ion permeability leads to viscous epithelial secretions and obstruction in the ducts of organs such as the pancreas. The concentration of chloride, bicarbonate, and water in the pancreatic fluid is low and the acinar cells obstruct the tubules leading to destruction, fibrosis, and exocrine pancreatic insufficiency.

The resulting pancreatic insufficiency is characterized by the lack of pancreatic amylase and proteases and an increase in monosaccharide absorption. Pancreatic lipase, colipase, and phospholipase are decreased. The pancreatic dysfunction causes severe malabsorption and poor nutrition. The low level of bicarbonate in the pancreatic fluid increases the duodenal acidity. Almost all patients have chronic sinopulmonary disease. The endocrine pancreas is rarely affected.

The symptoms may range from mild to severe and onset may be present at birth or later in life. Usually the disorder is discovered between the second and twelfth month of life. Affected individuals usually present with malodorous steatorrhea and chronic pulmonary infection.

Cystic fibrosis is a systemic disease and affects many different types of exocrine glands. Pancreatic insufficiency leads to a malabsorption syndrome characterized by weakness and weight loss, steatorrhea, and deficient absorption of the fat-soluble vitamins A, D, E, and K. Deficiency of vitamin K may in turn lead to bleeding abnormalities. Patients with unexplained chronic pulmonary disease, chronic hepatobiliary disease, hypoproteinemia, edema, and failure to thrive warrant further investigation

Treatment includes pancreatic enzyme supplementation therapy. Genes for these enzymes have been cloned and acid-resistant human lipase has been commercially prepared. The gene is introduced into the hepatobiliary system or the gastrointestinal epithelium of a patient. This allows the patient to produce his own enzymes and digest nutrients.[17]

Research in cystic fibrosis includes gene therapy to correct the defective gene, protein therapy to correct the abnormal CFTR, and pharmacologic therapy to restore the chloride channels. More patients are surviving into adulthood, with the average life span being 30 years.

### ENDOCRINE TUMORS

Islet cell tumors are rare and many are nonfunctional. Endocrine tumors that are functional may occur alone or as part of the multiple endocrine neoplasia syndrome (MEN). The excess secretion of certain hormones leads to clinical syndromes.[18] Table 32–2 identifies these syndromes with clinical symptoms.

### Gastrinoma

Pancreatic gastrinoma consists of G cells that secrete gastrin, a potent stimulator of gastric acid by the stomach. G cells have

TABLE 32–2

**Pancreatic Endocrine (Islet Cell) Tumor Syndromes**

| TUMOR | HORMONE SECRETED | FORMATION SITE | SYMPTOMS | DIAGNOSIS |
|---|---|---|---|---|
| Gastrinoma | Gastrin | G cells | Zollinger-Ellison syndrome; parietal cell hyperplasia; peptic ulcers; ↑ HCl | Failure to reduce gastrin level after secretin challenge test |
| Glucagonoma | Glucagon | Alpha cells | Anemia; diabetes; rash | ↑ Glucagon |
| Insulinoma | Insulin | Beta cells | Hypoglycemia; confusion; muscle weakness; palpitations; sweating; blurred vision | Elevated insulin to glucose ratio; fasting hypoglycemia |
| Somatostatinoma | Somatostatin | Delta cells | Achlorhydria; cholelithiasis; diabetes; steatorrhea | Mass; ↑ somatostatin |
| Vipoma | Vasoactive Intestinal Peptide | Delta₁ cells | Achlorhydria; severe diarrhea; hypokalemia, acidosis; hypovolemia | Mass; severe diarrhea; ↑ vasoactive intestinal peptide |

not been demonstrated in normal pancreatic islets and electron microscopy shows that G cells resemble the gastrin-secreting cells that are normally in the duodenum. Gastrinoma causes the Zollinger-Ellison syndrome that is characterized by gastric acid hypersecretion, peptic ulceration, and elevated blood levels of gastrin.

## Glucagonoma

This rare tumor is characterized by a migratory erythematous rash, hyperglycemia, anemia, and weight loss. In addition, most patients have an 80% reduction in plasma amino acids.

## Insulinoma

Inappropriate insulin release from this beta cell tumor leads to hypoglycemia, the main clinical finding. The hypoglycemia presents as neuroglycopenia (central nervous effects due to lack of glucose to the brain) or catecholamine excess (sympathetic nervous system attempt to restore glucose). Patients are often obese because they eat to remove the hypoglycemic symptoms. These tumors, the most common of the islet cell tumors, are usually benign.

## Somatostatinoma

This delta cell pancreatic tumor is rare and presents subtle symptoms that lead to late diagnosis, usually when a mass is palpated. Somatostatinomas can occur in the pancreas or duodenum. Symptoms consist of mild diabetes, gallstones, weight loss, diarrhea, and steatorrhea.

## Vipomas

Produced in the delta$_1$ cells, vipomas cause a watery diarrhea that occurs in 100% of patients. This leads to electrolyte disturbances including hypokalemia and decreases in calcium, magnesium, and phosphorus. Achlorhydria is also present. The combination of watery diarrhea, hypokalemia, and achlorhydria is called the WDHA syndrome. The main symptom that strongly suggests the presence of a vipoma is watery diarrhea that does not abate on fasting and the absence of an osmolar gap because it is a secretory process.

## MULTIPLE ENDOCRINE NEOPLASIA

The multiple endocrine neoplasia (MEN) syndrome is characterized by the occurrence of tumors involving two or more endocrine glands within a single patient. There are two major forms of MEN: type 1, MEN1, Wermer's syndrome and type 2, MEN2, Sipple's syndrome. Each syndrome is autosomal-dominant inherited or may occur sporadically.

## MEN1 (Wermer's Syndrome)

Primary hyperparathyroidism, enteropancreatic neoplasia, pituitary neoplasia, and adrenal hyperplasia characterize MEN1. Parathyroid tumors result in hypercalcemia and are usually the first tumors to appear. Gastrinomas are the most common enteropancreatic tumors; insulinomas are the second most common. Zollinger-Ellison syndrome is the most important cause of morbidity and mortality in MEN1 patients. Prolactinomas are the most common pituitary neoplasms.

The gene causing MEN1 is localized to chromosome 11q13. Sequencing of the gene in 1997 allows for the possibility of genetic screening.

Treatment includes subtotal parathyroidectomy whenever hyperparathyroidism is diagnosed. Calcium is a stimulator of gastrin production and is believed to cause the growth of gastrinomas. In addition, patients with elevated calcium levels develop osteoporosis, peptic ulcer, and nephrolithiasis.

## MEN2 (Sipple's Syndrome)

Associated with medullary thyroid carcinoma, pheochromocytomas, and parathyroid tumors. Three variants of this syndrome are identified. The gene causing all three MEN2 variants was mapped to chromosome 10cen-10q11.2. In one variant of this syndrome, parathyroid involvement is absent and mucosal neuromas, intestinal ganglion dysfunction, and corneal abnormalities may occur. Some patients may develop tumors that are associated with both MEN1 and MEN2.[19]

## PANCREATIC CANCER

Pancreatic cancer is a virtually incurable malignancy; it is a disease that usually occurs in individuals over 60 years of age. Pathogenesis is unclear and factors such as smoking, chemical carcinogens, high-fat diet, and diabetes mellitus have been implicated.

Adenocarcinoma occurs anywhere in the pancreas, with the most frequent focus in the head. The disease is difficult to diagnose because physical signs are vague and do not appear until the cancer is advanced. Most common complaints are weight loss and an epigastric pain that radiates to the back. The 5-year survival rate is 1%; most patients die within 1 year of diagnosis.

Because of its location, carcinoma of the head of the pancreas causes early biliary obstruction and jaundice by compressing the common bile duct; biliary tract enzymes become elevated. Pancreatic adenocarcinoma usually metastasizes to the regional lymph nodes and liver. The peritoneum, adrenals, lungs, and skeletal system are other metastatic sites.[20]

There are no screening or diagnostic laboratory tests for pancreatic cancer. Monitoring for recurrence is done by measuring the fetoacinar pancreatic antigen, pancreatic cancer-associated antigen (CA-19-9), carcinoembryonic antigen (CEA), CA-50, or DU PAN-2. These are not specific tests and false positives may occur in normal patients.[21]

## PANCREATITIS

Pancreatitis is an inflammatory disorder of the exocrine pancreas that is almost always associated with acinar cell injury. As damage to the organ occurs, the endocrine portion of the gland can also be affected. Pancreatitis can be classified into acute and chronic categories. Damage to the pancreas can range from little or no acinar cell necrosis to hemorrhagic destruction of the organ. Repeated acute attacks can result in fibrosis and eventually pancreatic insufficiency.

Patients present with epigastric or upper quadrant pain that radiates to the back. Stooping over relieves the pain. Acute pancreatitis pain usually subsides within hours. Chronic pancreatitis pain lasts for a longer period and sometimes recurs as acute episodes.

## Acute Pancreatitis

This is an acute inflammatory disorder that typically presents as abdominal pain, epigastric tenderness, nausea, and vomiting. Inflammation and necrosis of the gland result in release of pancreatic enzymes into the blood. As the digestive enzymes are released, there is autodigestion of the organ. The two main triggers for this release are biliary tract disease and alcoholism (Figure 32–5).

The precise mechanism by which the pancreatic enzymes destroy the pancreas is unknown. However, the activation of trypsin is necessary. Trypsin activates pancreatic proenzymes, phospholipase $A_2$ and proelastase. Phospholipase $A_2$ attacks the phospholipids of the membranes and proelastase digests the walls of blood vessels, leading to hemorrhage. In addition, pancreatic lipase is released and causes fat necrosis.

Amylase and lipase levels are elevated in the serum and urine. Patients who recover from a bout of acute pancreatitis may show healing of the gland and restoration to its normal state as judged by its exocrine and endocrine functions and by its gross and microscopic anatomy.[22]

## Chronic Pancreatitis

This is a continuing inflammatory disease of the organ characterized by irreversible morphologic change that leads to pain and permanent loss of function (Figure 32–6). There is inflammatory change and necrosis, fibrosis, and loss of exocrine and endocrine elements. Pancreatic ducts become calcified and malabsorption results. As more and more pancreatic tissue is replaced by fibrotic tissue, the concentration of pancreatic enzymes in the serum decreases so that patients often have subnormal pancreatic enzyme activities in serum.

The most important cause of chronic pancreatitis is alcoholism. A smaller percentage of patients develop pancreatitis due to miscellaneous causes that include surgery, hypercalcemia, drugs, and hyperlipidemia. About 25% of cases are idiopathic.

Pathogenic mechanisms of how alcohol causes chronic pancreatitis are not clear. Theories include the following: (1) deposit of protein within ductules causing fibrosis, (2) pan-

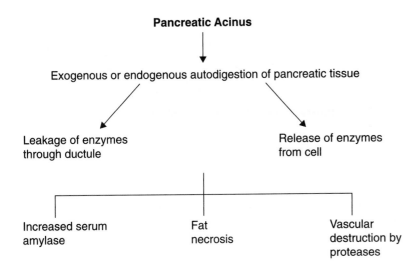

| Exogenous Causes | Endogenous Causes |
|---|---|
| Alcohol abuse | ↑ Calcium |
| Drugs | ↑ Lipids |
| Viruses | ↓ Nutrition |
| Trauma | Obstruction |

**FIGURE 32–5**

Pathogenesis of acute pancreatitis.

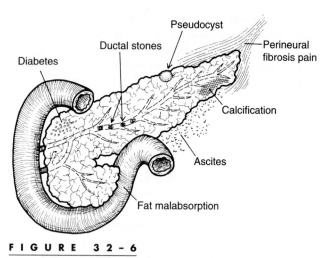

**F I G U R E   3 2 - 6**

Complications of chronic pancreatitis.

creatic lipid deposit with inflammation and fibrosis, and (3) excess free radicals attack the lipids of the membrane and lead to mast cell degeneration, platelet activation, and inflammation.[23]

Pancreatic insufficiency may occur without evidence of pancreatitis as a result of failure of release and activation of pancreatic enzymes with intestinal content.

## LABORATORY DIAGNOSIS OF DYSFUNCTION

### Diagnosis of Gastric Pathology

#### GASTRIC HYPERACIDITY AND ANACIDITY

Gastric secretions are composed of a complex mixture of hydrochloric acid, digestive enzymes, and mucus. Analysis of gastric secretions usually implies measurement of total acid output. However, detection of other components such as blood or lactic acid that are not normally found in gastric contents may be of important clinical significance. Results of gastric analysis must be interpreted carefully together with clinical and other laboratory findings.

Gastric analysis is performed for one of several reasons. The first of these is the determination of whether a patient is capable of secreting any gastric acid. The finding of anacidity is of major diagnostic importance in those patients with pernicious anemia. Measurement of the amount of acid produced may also help in the diagnosis of patients with symptoms of peptic ulcer disease. Finally, marked acidity may be helpful in diagnosing the hypersecretion characteristic of the Zollinger-Ellison syndrome.

Total gastric acid is the sum of combined and free acid. Combined acid is composed of mucoprotein, acid salts, and

organic acids; free acid refers to free HCl. Organic acids are formed when food remains in the stomach a long time and they will not be present if free HCl is available. Patients with gastric carcinoma or pyloric obstruction have elevated combined acid because of the decrease in HCl and the neutralization of HCl by the stomach contents.

For determination of basal acid output, the patient fasts overnight for 12 hours; no intake of food or liquid, smoking or physical exertion is permitted. The patient is intubated with a nasogastric tube and the tip of the tube positioned in the lowest portion of the stomach. Residual gastric fluid is first aspirated and discarded and then 4 samples are collected at 15-minute intervals (basal acid output, BAO).

Following the collection of the BAO specimens, the patient is given a gastric stimulant. Oral stimulants such as meals and alcohol do not give maximum stimulation. Gastrin or the synthetic pentagastrin, administered subcutaneously, provide maximum stimulation of acid. After stimulation, six 15-minute samples are collected (maximal acid output, MAO).

### Determination of Free HCl

The volume and pH of each sample is measured and recorded. Each specimen is titrated with 0.1 mol/L NaOH to a pH of 3.5 using Topfer's reagent (salmon pink endpoint) or a pH meter. The concentration of free HCl is calculated as follows:

$$\text{Free HCl mmol/L} = \frac{\text{mL NaOH} \times \text{Concentration of NaOH mol/L} \times 1000}{\text{Gastric specimen titrated (mL)}}$$

### Determination of Total Titratable Acidity

For total acid content, each specimen is titrated to a pH of 7.0 using a pH meter or phenol red as the indicator. Calculation is made using the above formula.

### Maximum Acid and Peak Acid Outputs

The free acid output in mmol/L is calculated in each of the first 4 poststimulation specimens; the acid outputs are averaged and the MAO is derived. The acid output per hour is calculated for all 6 poststimulation specimens; the 2 highest values are averaged, giving the peak acid output (PAO). The formula for calculating free acid for MAO and PAO is as follows:

$$\text{Free acid (mmol/h)} = \frac{\text{mmol free acid/L} \times \text{Total volume of specimen (mL)}}{1000}$$
$$\times \frac{60}{\text{Collection period of specimen (min)}}$$

## BAO/PAO Ratio

Additional diagnostic information may be obtained by using the BAO/PAO ratio as follows:

$$\frac{\text{BAO}}{\text{PAO}} \times 100 = \%\text{BAO/PAO}$$

Interpretation and reference intervals are shown in Table 32–3.

## PERNICIOUS ANEMIA

Vitamin $B_{12}$ (cobalamin) is a water-soluble vitamin that requires the presence of intrinsic factor secreted by the stomach to facilitate its absorption in the ileum. Malabsorption of vitamin $B_{12}$ may occur as a result of intrinsic factor deficiency, overgrowth of bacteria in the intestinal lumen, or resection of the terminal ileum.

In addition to the classic Schilling test, there are other approaches to the diagnosis of pernicious anemia and the accompanying deficiencies of vitamin $B_{12}$ and folate (Table 32–4).

The Schilling test is used in patients with cobalamin deficiency to document defects in absorption of the vitamin. In stage 1, vitamin $B_{12}$, labeled with radioactive cobalt, is administered orally and the percentage of ingested vitamin excreted during a 24-hour urine collection is measured. If stage 1 is abnormal, a second stage is performed 3 to 7 days later. In this procedure, radiolabeled vitamin $B_{12}$ and intrinsic factor are administered, and a 24-hour urine is collected. Individuals with pernicious anemia should have a normal excretion of the vitamin because intrinsic factor has been given.

Pernicious anemia is not the only disease that can be identified by the Schilling test. Table 32–5 gives the interpretation of Schilling results in vitamin $B_{12}$ deficient patients.[25]

## ZOLLINGER-ELLISON SYNDROME

### Gastrin

Measurement of fasting gastrin after discontinuation of medications to reduce acid output is the single best test to diagnose Zollinger-Ellison syndrome (ZES); 99% of patients will have elevated fasting gastrin levels. Pernicious anemia also demonstrates marked increases in serum gastrin concentrations. Zollinger-Ellison syndrome is characterized by gastrin-secreting non-$\beta$-islet cell tumors of the pancreas, resulting in

TABLE 32–3

**Interpretation and Reference Intervals for Gastric Acidity**

**GASTRIC RESIDUE AFTER 12-HOUR FAST**

| | |
|---|---|
| Volume | 20–100 mL (usually <50mL) |
| pH | 1.5–3.5 |
| Free acid (without stimulation) | 0–40 mmol/L |
| Free acid (after stimulation with pentagastrin) | 10–130 mmol/L |

**GASTRIC ACID SECRETION RATE**

| | |
|---|---|
| Basal acid output (BAO) | |
| Normal; gastric ulcer | Males: 0–10.5 mmol/h |
| | Females: 0–5.6 mmol/h |
| Possible duodenal ulcer | 5–15 mmol/h |
| Zollinger-Ellison syndrome | >20 mmol/h (at times, >60 mmol/h) |
| Peak acid output (PAO) | |
| Normal; gastric ulcer | Males: 12–60 mmol/h |
| | Females: 8–40 mmol/h |
| Duodenal ulcer; possible Zollinger-Ellison | Up to 60 mmol/h |
| Zollinger-Ellison syndrome | >60 mmol/h (generally not more than twice BAO) |
| BAO/PAO | |
| Normal; gastric ulcer or gastric carcinoma | <20% |
| Gastric or duodenal ulcer | 20–40% |
| Possible duodenal ulcer or Zollinger-Ellison syndrome | 40–60% |
| Zollinger-Ellison syndrome | >60% |

Modified from Burtis CA, Ashwood ER (eds): *Tietz Fundamentals of Clinical Chemistry.* 4th ed. Philadelphia, WB Saunders, 1996.

TABLE 32-4

**Laboratory Tests Used in the Diagnosis of Pernicious Anemia**

| LABORATORY TESTS | RESULTS |
|---|---|
| MCV | >100 fl (macrocytosis) |
| Peripheral blood smear | Oval macrocytes; hypersegmented neutrophils |
| Bone marrow | Megaloblastic changes |
| Serum cobalamin (vitamin B$_{12}$) | Decreased |
| Serum folate | Increased |
| Methylmalonic acid | Increased |
| Homocysteine | Increased |
| Anti-parietal cell antibodies | Present |
| Fasting serum gastrin | Increased |
| Anti-intrinsic factor antibodies | Present |
| Schilling test | Stage 1, abnormal; stage 2, normal |

MCV = mean corpuscular volume.

gastric acid hypersecretion and peptic ulceration. This syndrome can be differentiated from pernicious anemia by the fact that intragastric administration of hydrochloric acid does not change serum gastrin concentration in patients with ZES but does result in a marked decrease in gastrin in patients with pernicious anemia.

**Basal Acid Output**

The second criterion for diagnosis of ZES is elevated basal acid output (BAO). The measurement of gastric acid eliminates patients who have an elevated gastrin because of achlorhydria.

Another method to diagnose ZES is to measure gastric pH. A gastric pH of greater than 3.0 is not consistent with ZES diagnosis.

**Secretin Challenge Test**

In patients in whom gastrin and gastric acid levels do not support the diagnosis, the secretin challenge test is performed.[26,27] The previously used calcium infusion and test meal procedures are not specific and sensitive enough.

The secretin test is reliable and highly sensitive. In this test, 2 U/kg bolus of secretin is given intravenously to the fasting patient. Infused secretin normally inhibits gastrin release by the gastric mucosa. Serum gastrin levels are measured at 0, 2, 5, 10, and 15 minutes. Patients with ZES have an increase in gastrin of greater than 200 pg/mL from the basal level; this usually occurs in the 5-minute sample.[26,27]

The secretin test is useful for monitoring patients who have had a gastrinoma surgically removed. Patients with recurring ZES will have an abnormal secretin test before fasting gastrin or BAO levels become elevated.

## Diagnosis of Intestinal Pathology

### CARCINOID SYNDROME

Carcinoid tumors arise from neuroendocrine cells. They contain neurosecretory granules that are composed of a variety of hormones and biogenic amines. One of the most important of these substances is serotonin. Serotonin is synthesized from its precursor 5-hydroxytryptophan. It is subsequently metabolized to 5-hydroxyindoleacetic acid (5-HIAA), which is excreted in the urine.

In addition to serotonin, carcinoid tumors also secrete corticotropin, histamine, dopamine, neurotensin, prostaglandins, and kallikrein. It is release of these substances that causes the carcinoid syndrome.[28]

Serotonin and its metabolites are the predominant markers of this disease. Measurement of urinary 5-HIAA is the best screening test and the most reliable marker of carcinoid tu-

TABLE 32-5

**Interpretation of Schilling Results in Vitamin B$_{12}$ Deficient Patients**

| RESULTS | POSSIBLE INTERPRETATIONS |
|---|---|
| Stage 1, normal | Dietary deficiency; hypochlorhydria; partial gastrectomy; congenital deficiency |
| Stage 1, abnormal; stage 2, normal | Pernicious anemia; congenital absence of intrinsic factor; inadequate collection of urine |
| Stages 1 and 2, both abnormal | Ileal disease or resection; renal insufficiency; inadequate urine collection; bacterial overgrowth; fish tapeworm infestation; pancreatic insufficiency |

mors. Foods containing serotonin (peanuts, avocados, bananas, and chocolate) should be restricted before urine collection.

## COLON CANCER

The single most important laboratory test in the diagnosis of colon cancer is the identification of occult blood in the stool. Iron deficiency anemia is present in over half of the patients with right-sided colon involvement. Patients with left-sided sites usually are not as severely anemic because the presence of fecal blood is identified more easily. The utility of tests for the detection of blood in feces lies in the detection of hemorrhage from colon carcinoma and other occult sources of hemorrhage that may bleed intermittently.

Occult blood in the stool can be detected by chemical (guaiac), heme–porphyrin, or immunologic methods. Heme-porphyrin and immunologic methods are more expensive and more difficult to perform. Cross-reactivity with animal proteins, sample reproduction, and low specificity are additional considerations.

Most screening tests for occult blood are based on the determination of the peroxidase activity of hemoglobin. Hemoglobin and its derivatives catalyze the reaction between hydrogen peroxide and a chromogenic compound, causing the development of various shades and intensities of the particular chromogen that is used.

The major drawback of the screening methods is the choice of reagent that will detect all gastrointestinal malignancies yet be specific enough to avoid a high number of false-positive reactions. Reagents that are used differ greatly in their ability to detect peroxidase activity. Guaiac-based chemical tests remain the most popular; they are inexpensive and lend themselves to mass screening campaigns.

The guaiac method has a number of weaknesses. The ingestion of foods such as horseradish, turnips, meat, and fish that contain peroxidase activity can cause false-positive fecal peroxidase activity. Blood in the gastrointestinal tract is metabolized into its constituents that may have reduced or no peroxidase activity. Thus, hemorrhage in the upper gastrointestinal tract or an increased transit time of feces through the bowel will result in decreased peroxidase activity due to metabolism with breakdown of hemoglobin.

The determination of occult blood in the stool should be performed on at least 3 or more separate occasions with the patient on a diet free of exogenous sources of peroxidase activity.[29]

Carcinoembryonic antigen (CEA), while positive in multiple gastrointestinal diseases, should not be used as a diagnostic tool for colon cancer. However, CEA is a good monitoring test for patients who have resected malignant tumors. A rise in the CEA level may indicate recurrence of the cancer.

## LACTASE DEFICIENCY

Malabsorption of lactose may be diagnosed by an oral lactose tolerance test or measurement of hydrogen in the breath following ingestion of lactose. Although the most definitive diagnosis of lactase deficiency is histochemical examination of the brush border of the intestinal epithelium, the test is seldom performed because of its difficult and invasive nature.

The oral lactose tolerance test is probably the simplest and most direct method for diagnosis of lactase deficiency. Patients are given a 50-g oral dose of lactose and blood samples are drawn before lactose ingestion and at 15, 30, 45, 60, and 90 minutes postingestion. An increase in blood glucose concentration of at least 30 mg/dL over the fasting glucose concentration is indicative of normal lactose metabolism and absorption of the glucose end product.

Patients with less than a 20 mg/dL rise in glucose are considered lactase deficient. Patients should also be observed for signs of abdominal cramping, bloating, flatulence, and diarrhea. False-positive test results may occur in individuals with delayed gastric emptying. Therapy for lactase deficiency requires a diet that eliminates milk and foodstuffs containing lactose.

A more reliable test for the diagnosis of lactase deficiency is the measurement of breath hydrogen after the administration of lactose. Lactase-deficient patients will not absorb lactose and bacteria metabolize the disaccharide in the large bowel; large amounts of hydrogen are formed. Hydrogen passes into the circulation and is removed in the exhaled breath. The test is more difficult to perform and takes a longer time than the lactose tolerance test.[30]

## MALABSORPTION

Malabsorption of nutrients has an intestinal and luminal phase. The intestinal phase includes those processes that occur in the cells and transport channels of the organ's wall. Abnormalities of the intestinal villi, diminution of the absorptive surface, damage to the epithelial cells, and impaired transport contribute to intestinal phase malabsorption.

Luminal phase malabsorption includes interruption of the normal continuity of the stomach and duodenum (postgastrectomy), bacterial overgrowth, and deficient bile salts. In addition, because of the dependence of the intestine on pancreatic enzymes for maximum absorption, pancreatic insufficiency is another cause. In the investigation of malabsorption, it is important to distinguish between intestinal and pancreatic causes.

### $^{14}$C–Bile Acid Breath Test

This test is performed by giving the patient $^{14}$C-glycocholate orally and measuring the amount of $^{14}CO_2$ in the expired air. The test depends on bacterial cleavage of glycine from bile salts that results in production of labeled $CO_2$ in the breath. In normal patients, 90% of the compound is reabsorbed in the ileum and not metabolized. In patients with overgrowth of bacteria in the small bowel, the bacteria will deconjugate the $^{14}$C-glycocholate. A high output of $^{14}CO_2$ in the breath following oral $^{14}$C-glycocholate may be indicative of bacterial overgrowth.

## $^{14}CO_2$ Breath Test

Orally administered triglycerides containing $^{14}C$-fatty acids can be used to determine the degree to which fat is absorbed. The oxidation of $^{14}C$-fatty acids to $^{14}CO_2$ is proportional to the rate of absorption of fatty acids. Test use is limited because it takes 6 hours and involves the administration of radioactive material to the patient. In addition, the effects of other disorders of fat metabolism such as obesity and hyperlipidemia are unknown.[31]

## D-Xylose Absorption Test

The test for absorption of D-xylose is useful for the diagnosis of malabsorption. D-xylose is a pentose sugar not normally present in blood. Taken orally, D-xylose is passively absorbed in the proximal small intestine, does not rely on pancreatic secretions, and is not metabolized by the liver. Most of the absorbed D-xylose is excreted in the urine, allowing it to be used in clinical testing. The amount of D-xylose excreted into the urine over a specified time period (usually 5 hours) following ingestion is directly correlated with the amount absorbed in the GI tract.

Patients should be fasting before starting the test. A 25-g dose of D-xylose is given. After administration of the sugar, all urine voided over the next 5 hours is collected. Blood is also collected. Blood samples are usually collected at 1 hour in children and 2 hours following administration in adults. There is a difference in collection times because peak absorption is reached sooner in children when compared with adults. The amount of D-xylose present in the urine and blood is measured by a quantitative assay.

The accuracy of the D-xylose absorption test is dependent not only on the rate of absorption of D-xylose but also on the ability of the kidneys to excrete it. Patients with renal insufficiency who are unable to excrete D-xylose into the urine may be falsely classified as having malabsorption. An increased blood D-xylose concentration in the presence of a decreased urine D-xylose excretion rate would be suggestive of renal retention of D-xylose. In addition to malabsorption, low concentrations of urine and plasma D-xylose may be seen in patients with ascites, thyroid disease, vomiting, and delayed gastric emptying.

Patients given a 25-g dose of D-xylose should excrete 4 g or more of D-xylose in the urine. Patients with malabsorption due to intestinal disease absorb less D-xylose. If the D-xylose tests results are abnormal, a small bowel biopsy and aspirate for pathogens should be initiated; intestinal phase malabsorption should be suspected. If the D-xylose test results are normal, pancreatic insufficiency (luminal phase malabsorption) should be suspected.[32]

## Fecal Fat

The determination of fecal fat is performed in the evaluation of malabsorption due to pancreatic or intestinal dysfunction. The fat content of feces in normal individuals consists prima-rily of fatty acids, fatty acid salts (soaps), and neutral fats. Tests of fecal fat excretion are affected by disorders that influence digestion in the intestinal lumen as well as processes affecting absorption of fats by the mucosa. Although determination of fecal fat is useful for determining the presence of steatorrhea, it does not determine its cause.

**SCREENING TEST** An excess amount of fat in the stool is usually obvious on visual inspection. The feces are usually pale, frothy in appearance, and foul smelling. The presence of fat may be demonstrated by staining a wet preparation with an oil-soluble dye and examining it microscopically for the presence of colored fat droplets. The number of fat droplets is used to approximate the percent fat content in stool (Table 32–6). Individuals with normal fat excretion should show less than ten fat droplets in 10 high-power ($400\times$) fields on a hemocytometer.

**QUANTITATIVE MEASUREMENT** Quantitative assessment of fecal fat excretion has been classically used as the method for documenting fat excretion. In normal situations, fat excretion should not exceed 6 g per day. In malabsorption states the fat excretion increases and results in steatorrhea. Fat excretion may be normal in malabsorption states that compromise other nutrients.

Quantitative measurement requires stool collected over 3 consecutive days. For 6 days the patient consumes a diet containing approximately 100 g of fat per day.

A number of methods are available for quantitation of fecal fat. Unfortunately, many methods are nonspecific and require special equipment. The most commonly used procedure to measure fecal fat is the titration procedure of Van de Kamer. Fats are converted to soaps and then to fatty acids, which are then titrated with NaOH. The method cannot detect sterols and medium- and short-chain fatty acids.

Fecal fat determination does not define a specific cause for the malabsorption; the cause of steatorrhea might be intestinal, hepatobiliary, or pancreatic. Further tests are necessary to differentiate the cause. Pancreatic exocrine function must be almost completely lost before steatorrhea due to pancreatic insufficiency is identified.[33]

T A B L E   3 2 – 6

**Screening Test for Fecal Fat**

| AVERAGE NUMBER OF FAT DROPLETS/hpf | APPROXIMATE FAT CONTENT (%) |
|---|---|
| 10 | 5 |
| 20 | 10 |
| 30 | 15 |
| 35 | 20 |
| >40 | >30 |

## Diagnosis of Pancreatic Pathology

### CYSTIC FIBROSIS

Diagnosis of cystic fibrosis is difficult. The Cystic Fibrosis Foundation has established criteria for the diagnosis of the disease (Table 32–7).

In most cases, the diagnosis of cystic fibrosis is confirmed or excluded by the sweat test. The determination of the chloride concentration in the sweat of patients with cystic fibrosis is an extremely reliable tool for the diagnosis of the disease when performed correctly. The test should be performed when the patient is clinically stable, well hydrated, free of acute illnesses, and not receiving mineralocorticoids.

Sweat for chloride determination is collected following iontophoretic delivery of pilocarpine to the skin. Pilocarpine is a drug that stimulates sweating when introduced into the skin of the flexor surface of the forearm or thigh. A maximum amount of sweat must be collected to ensure an average sweat rate of more than 1 g/m²/min.

Although either sodium or chloride can be measured, chloride provides better discrimination between cystic fibrosis patients and unaffected individuals. A sweat chloride of greater than 60 mmol/L is consistent with the diagnosis of cystic fibrosis but the result must be related to the clinical history. In an infant under 3 months of age, a sweat chloride of greater than 40 mmol/L is highly suggestive of cystic fibrosis. The diagnosis of cystic fibrosis should not be made until an elevated sweat chloride (>60 mmol/L) is determined on two separate occasions and the criteria identified in Table 32–8 are met.

Patients with borderline results should have sweat sodium and chloride determined. Both analytes should be elevated with the chloride/sodium ratio greater than 1.0.[34,35]

Falsely decreased sweat chloride results may be obtained in patients with cystic fibrosis who are salt depleted as a result of vomiting, diarrhea, or gastric suction. False-positive test results may be seen in individuals without cystic fibrosis who have electrolyte imbalances associated with meconium ileus, hypothyroidism, congestive heart failure, and some types of renal disease that result in increased sweat chloride concentrations.

### PANCREATIC INSUFFICIENCY

Pancreatic insufficiency indicates that the exocrine function of the organ is not functional. Nutrient malabsorption is a consequence of decreasing pancreatic enzyme output. More than 90% of the secreting tissue must be destroyed before malabsorption occurs. In addition to the tests explained in this section, procedures described in the malabsorption section also can be used to diagnose pancreatic insufficiency.

The pancreas secretes many digestive enzymes. The proteolytic enzymes are secreted as the inactive precursors (zymogens). These include trypsinogen, chymotrypsinogen, proelastase, and procarboxy-peptidases A and B. Water and bicarbonate output is stimulated by secretin, a peptide hormone whose amino acid sequence is similar to glucagon. The normal bicarbonate daily

**TABLE 32–7**

**Criteria for the Diagnosis of Cystic Fibrosis**

Presence of one or more characteristic phenotypic features:
 Chronic sinopulmonary disease
 Gastrointestinal and nutritional abnormalities
  Intestinal
  Pancreatic
  Hepatic
  Failure to thrive
 Salt loss syndrome
 Male urogenital abnormalities resulting in obstructive azoospermia
OR History of cystic fibrosis in a sibling
OR Positive newborn screening
AND elevated sweat chloride on two or more occasions
OR Identification of 2 cystic fibrosis mutations
OR Abnormalities in ion transport across the nasal epithelium

output is sufficient to neutralize gastric acid production. Secretin is released whenever the pH of the duodenum falls below 4.5.

### Secretin-Cholecystokinin Test

The secretin-cholecystokinin test is a direct measurement of the exocrine ability of the pancreas. The patient's duodenum is intubated after an overnight fast. Intravenous pancreatic secretin is administered followed by cholecystokinin. Multiple specimens are collected and the volume and the amount of enzymes and bicarbonate are measured. Decreased flow and increased enzymes demonstrate obstruction of the pancreas. Other pancreatic insufficiency diseases such as cystic fibrosis, chronic pancreatitis, and calcifications have low bicarbonate and enzyme levels.[36]

### Fecal Pancreatic Enzymes

The examination of exocrine proteins in stool are used to evaluate pancreatic output and function. Fecal chymotrypsin is stable and easily measured in the laboratory. It is very sensitive for steatorrhea; however, the sensitivity decreases as the degree of pancreatic damage decreases. It is used as a monitoring test for patients diagnosed with pancreatic insufficiency.

Fecal elastase I is also stable in stool. It is proposed to be a highly sensitive and specific tubeless pancreatic function test. Like chymotrypsin, it is very sensitive for advanced pancreatic insufficiency. Sensitivity decreases in mild disease.[37]

### PABA Test

To avoid the intubation of patients suspected of pancreatic insufficiency, a tubeless noninvasive test has been introduced.

TABLE 32-8

## Conditions Associated with an Elevation in Serum Amylase

Pancreatic disease
  Pancreatitis
  Complications of pancreatitis
  Trauma
  Ductal obstruction
  Pancreatic carcinoma
  Cystic fibrosis (early)
  Excessive hormonal stimulation
Salivary disease
  Mumps
  Trauma
  Radiation
  Ductal obstruction
Gastrointestinal disease
  Perforated peptic ulcer
  Obstructed bowel
  Mesenteric infarction
  Appendicitis
  Liver disease
Gynecologic disease
  Ruptured ectopic pregnancy
  Ovarian or fallopian cysts
  Pelvic inflammatory disease
Extrapancreatic neoplasms
  Solid tumors
  Multiple myeloma
  Pheochromocytoma
Miscellaneous
  Renal failure
  Renal transplant
  Macroamylasemia
  Burns
  Acidosis
  Pregnancy
  Cerebral trauma
  Drugs
  Abdominal aortic aneurysm
  Postoperative conditions
  Anorexia, bulimia nervosa
  Idiopathic causes

Modified from Vissers RJ, Abu-Laban RB, McHugh DF: Amylase and lipase in the emergency evaluation of acute pancreatitis. J Emerg Med 17:1027–1037, 1999.

The tubeless pancreatic function test is based on the principle of decreased pancreatic function leading to increased amounts of unabsorbed food, decreased amount of pancreatic enzymes, or decreased intraluminal hydrolysis of synthetic compounds.

The patient receives N-benzoyl-L-tyrosol-p–aminobenzoic acid (BTP) and a test meal that stimulates pancreatic secretion.

BTP reacts with chymotrypsin to produce p-aminobenzoic acid (PABA). Metabolites of PABA are excreted in the urine. Lowered chymotrypsin, as found in pancreatic insufficiency, results in a decreased excretion of metabolites in the urine.[38]

## PANCREATITIS

Laboratory investigation of chronic pancreatitis centers on the tests to determine pancreatic insufficiency. In chronic pancreatitis, the exocrine function is insufficient and enzyme values are decreased. Amylase and lipase are the enzymes most frequently used in the evaluation of acute pancreatitis.[39,40] Standard treatment for exocrine pancreatic insufficiency is enteric-coated pancreatin microspheres administered at the beginning of each meal. A diet low in fat and supplemented by lipase is the treatment for steatorrhea.

### Amylase

This enzyme acts to digest starch into smaller carbohydrate groups. The two major sources of amylase are salivary glands and the pancreas; multiple other organs also produce amylase. Therefore, there are many causes of hyperamylasemia, the primary nonpancreatic reason being salivary gland involvement (Table 32–8). The lack of specificity of amylase has encouraged the measurement of isoenzymes. A new immunoinhibition assay specific for the p-form amylase (pancreatic isoenzyme) is being investigated.

Inflammation of the pancreas usually transiently elevates the level of amylase. In acute disease, amylase usually rises within 6 hours and peaks at 48 hours. It returns to normal levels within 5 to 7 days. Amylase is one of the few enzymes that are found in the urine and urinary amylase can also be measured.

The methods of amylase measurement that are most frequently used are saccharogenic, which measures the release of glucose, and chromolytic, which reacts with a polysaccharide substrate and releases a dye.

It is possible to find patients without pancreatic disease who have elevated serum amylase levels. The amylase is either bound to gamma globulins or circulates as an amylase polymer. The macroamylase molecule cannot be excreted in the urine; thus, the urine amylase levels are normal.

### Lipase

This enzyme hydrolyzes triglycerides into monoglycerides, alcohols, and fatty acids. Lipase is derived from the acinar cells of the pancreas, where it is synthesized and stored. Lipase can also be found in gastrointestinal mucosa, leukocytes, lung, and liver. Although there can be nonpancreatic causes of elevated lipase, there are not as many as those that cause hyperamylasemia (Table 32–9).

After the onset of acute pancreatitis, lipase increases within 4 hours and reaches its peak at 24 hours. It decreases within 8 to 14 days. It remains elevated longer than amylase. Lipase replaces or supplements amylase in the diagnosis of acute pancreatitis. Lipase has a higher specificity and fewer nonpancreatic causes of elevation. The development of turbidimetric

TABLE 32-9

**Conditions Associated with an Elevation in Serum Lipase[39]**

Acute pancreatitis
Chronic pancreatitis
Acute cholecystitis
Bowel obstruction or infarction
Duodenal ulceration
Pancreatic calculus
Pancreatic carcinoma
Diabetic ketoacidosis
Trauma
Idiopathic elevation

methods and the introduction of colipase have greatly enhanced the specificity of the measurement.

## Phospholipase A₂

This enzyme has been implicated in the pathogenesis of acute pancreatitis. The pathogenesis of pancreatic necrosis is still not completely understood but phospholipase $A_2$ ($PLA_2$) is liberated into the serum during an acute pancreatic attack. Previously, the proteolytic enzyme trypsin was thought to trigger autodigestion; however, PLA2 is now shown to be responsible. $PLA_2$ has been implicated in the pulmonary and renal damage that sometimes accompanies acute pancreatitis. $PLA_2$ is of diagnostic value in acute pancreatitis and can also be used in monitoring and follow-up of patients.[41]

## SUMMARY

Digestive system disorders are numerous and usually are divided into diseases of the stomach, intestine, and pancreas. Hepatic diseases are discussed in Chapter 16. The laboratory can provide assistance to the physician in the diagnosis of most of these diseases. Radiologic and surgical procedures, independently or in conjunction with the laboratory, are also used in diagnosis.

Diseases of the stomach include gastric carcinoma, peptic ulcers, Zollinger-Ellison syndrome, and pernicious anemia. Gastric acidity, gastrin, the secretin challenge test, and vitamin $B_{12}$ differentiate diagnoses.

Signs of malabsorption (steatorrhea) usually mark intestinal problems. Once a diagnosis of malabsorption has been made, it is important to determine if the site is intestinal or pancreatic. The D-xylose absorption test helps to make that decision. The secretin-cholecystokinin test may also be used. Malabsorption may result in vitamin deficiencies, osteomalacia, and carbohydrate and protein absorption abnormalities. Fecal fat, lactose tolerance, $^{14}C$-bile breath test and $^{14}CO_2$ breath test are some laboratory tests that are used in investigation.

The pancreas is both an endocrine and exocrine gland. Endocrine tumors are rare and can be difficult to diagnose. Multiple endocrine neoplasia I and II involve endocrine tumors and other diseases. Failure of exocrine functioning leads to pancreatic insufficiency as seen in chronic pancreatitis. Other exocrine pancreatic diseases include acute pancreatitis (autodigestion of the gland) and cystic fibrosis. Increased levels of amylase and lipase identify acute pancreatitis, and an abnormal sweat test is the diagnostic tool for cystic fibrosis.

## REFERENCES

1. Tortora G: *Principles of Human Anatomy.* 6th ed. New York, Harper Collins, 1992.

2. Scarpelli DG: The pancreas. In Rubin E, Farber J (eds.): *Pathology.* 2nd ed. Philadelphia, JB Lippincott, 1994, pp 788–789.

3. Wood JD: Digestion and absorption. In Rhoades RA, Tanner A (eds.): *Medical Physiology.* New York, Little Brown, 1995, pp 553–561.

4. Henderson AR, Tietz N, Rinker A: Gastric, pancreatic and intestinal function. In Burtis CA, Ashwood ER (eds.): *Tietz Fundamentals of Clinical Chemistry.* 4th ed. Philadelphia, WB Saunders, 1996, pp 595–598.

5. Chan AOO, McLuk J, Hui WM, et al: Molecular biology of gastric carcinoma: from laboratory to bedside. J Gastroenterol Hepatol 14:1150–1160, 1999.

6. Tsang KW, Lam SK: Helicobacter pylori and extradigestive diseases. J Gastroenterol Hepatol 14:844–850, 1999.

7. Snow CF: Laboratory diagnosis of vitamin $B_{12}$ and folate deficiency. Arch Intern Med 159:1289–1298, 1999.

8. Norton J: Gastrinoma: advances in localization and treatment. Surg Oncol Clin North Am 7:845–861, 1998.

9. Kulke MH, Mayer RJ: Carcinoid tumors. New Engl J Med 340:858–868, 1999.

10. Lauffer JM, Zhang T, Modlin IM: Review article: current status of gastrointestinal carcinoids. Aliment Pharmacol Ther 13:271–287, 1999.

11. Auricchio S, Troncone R, Maurano F: Coeliac disease in the year 2000. Ital J Gastroenterol Hepatol 31:773–780, 1999.

12. Da Cunha M: Genetic disorders. In Bullock BL (ed): *Pathophysiology Adaptations and Alterations in Function.* 4th ed. Philadelphia, JB Lippincott, 1996, p 79.

13. Porth CM: *Pathophysiology Concepts of Altered Health Status.* 5th ed. Philadelphia, JB Lippincott, 1998.

14. Vesa TH, Marteau P, Korpela R: Lactose intolerance. J Am Coll Nutr 19:165S–175S, 2000.

15. Bai JC: Malabsorption syndromes. Digestion 59:530–546, 1998.

16. Rubin E, Farber JL: The gastrointestinal tract. In Rubin E, Farber J (eds.): *Pathology.* 2nd ed. Philadelphia, JB Lippincott, 1994, pp 677–682.

17. Nousia-Arvanitakis S: Cystic fibrosis and the pancreas. J Clin Gastroenterol 29:138–142, 1999.

18. Metz DC: Diagnosis of non-Zollinger-Ellison syndrome, non-carcinoid syndrome, enteropancreatic neuroendocrine tumours. Ital J Gastroenterol Hepatol 31(Suppl 2): S153–S159, 1999.

19. Thakker RV: Editorial: multiple endocrine neoplasia—syndromes of the twentieth century. J Clin Endocrinol Metab 83:2617–2620, 1998.

20. Scarpelli DG: The pancreas. In Rubin E, Farber J (eds.): *Pathology.* 2nd ed. Philadelphia, JB Lippincott, 1994, pp 795–797.

21. Scarpelli DG: The pancreas. In Rubin E, Farber J (eds.): *Pathology.* 2nd ed. Philadelphia, JB Lippincott, 1994, pp 789–794.

22. Lott JA: The pancreas: function and chemical pathology. In Kaplan LA, Pesce AJ (eds.): *Clinical Chemistry Theory, Analysis, and Correlation.* 3rd ed. Chicago, Mosby, 1996, p 566.

23. Scarpelli DG: The pancreas. In Rubin E, Farber J (eds.): *Pathology.* 2nd ed. Philadelphia, JB Lippincott, 1994, pp 791–794.

24. Henderson AR, Tietz NW, Rinker AD: Gastric, pancreatic, and intestinal function. In Burtis CA, Ashwood ER (eds.): *Tietz Fundamentals of Clinical Chemistry.* 4th ed. Philadelphia, WB Saunders, 1996, pp 602–603.

25. Snow CF: Laboratory diagnosis of vitamin B12 and folate deficiency. Arch Intern Med 159:1289–1298, 1999.

26. Cadiot G, Jais P, Mignon M: Diagnosis of Zollinger-Ellison syndrome—from symptoms to biological evidence. Ital J Gastroenterol Hepatol 31(Suppl):S147–S152, 1999.

27. Norton JA: Gastrinoma advances in localization and treatment. Surg Oncol Clin North Am 7:845–861, 1998.

28. Tomassetti P: Clinical aspects of carcinoid tumours. Ital J Gastroenterol Hepatol 31(Suppl):S143–S146, 1999.

29. Simon JB: Fecal occult blood testing: clinical value and limitations. Gastroenterologist 6:66–78, 1998.

30. Shaw AD, Davies GJ: Lactose intolerance problems in diagnosis and treatment. J Clin Gastroenterol 28:208–216, 1999.

31. Henderson AR, Tietz NW, Rinker AD: Gastric, pancreatic, and intestinal function. In Burtis CA, Ashwood ER (eds.): *Tietz Fundamentals of Clinical Chemistry.* 4th ed. Philadelphia, WB Saunders, 1996, p 605.

32. Craig RM, Ehrenpreis ED: D-xylose testing. J Clin Gastroenterol 29:143–150, 1999.

33. Bai JC: Malabsorption syndromes. Digestion 59:530–546, 1998.

34. Rosenstein BJ, Cutting GR: The diagnosis of cystic fibrosis: A consensus. J Pediatr 132:589–593, 1998.

35. Rosenstein BJ: What is a cystic fibrosis diagnosis? Clin Chest Med 3:423–441, 1998.

36. Oci K, Mizushim T, Harada H, et al.: Chronic pancreatitis: functional testing. Pancreas 16:343–348, 1998.

37. Clain JE, Pearson RK: Diagnosis of chronic pancreatitis: is a gold standard necessary? Surg Clin North Am 79:829–844, 1999.

38. Oci K, Mizushim T, Harada H, et al.: Chronic pancreatitis: functional testing. Pancreas 16:343–348, 1998.

39. Vissers RJ, Abu-Laban RB, McHugh DF: Amylase and lipase in the emergency department evaluation of acute pancreatitis. J Emerg Med 17:1027–1037, 1999.

40. Layer P, Keller J: Pancreatic enzymes: secretion and luminal nutrient digestion in health and disease. J Clin Gastroenterol 28:3–10, 1999.

41. Nevalainen TJ, Hietaranta AJ, Gronroos JM: Phospholipase $A_2$ in acute pancreatitis: new biochemical and pathological aspects. Hepatogastroenterology 46:2731–2735, 1999.

CHAPTER 33

# Nutritional Status Assessment

*Sharon M. Miller and Elia Mears*

## NUTRITIONAL STATUS

Numerous simple and complex chemical reactions are required to sustain life. Nutrients provide the raw materials necessary for metabolic processes and thus for cell survival. The body is constantly in flux, with some portions being destroyed as others are being formed. Both the energy and the materials required to support cell growth and development and to maintain metabolic processes must be supplied by nutrients, preferably in a well-balanced diet. Nutrients, or nourishing substances, include carbohydrates, proteins, lipids (fats and oils), vitamins, minerals, and water.

Nutritional status is the consequence of the utilization of nutrients and directly affects the body's ability to prevent and fight disease. If nutritional status is good, the body is likely to heal wounds promptly and to fight infections or avoid infections initially because of a strong immune system. In addition, the body will be able to circulate nutrients, and route white cells and antibodies to those parts of the body in need of them. In contrast, poor nutritional status leads to deterioration of the body, its organs, and its capability to ward off infection and prevent the development of disease.

Nutritional status expresses the degree to which the physiologic needs for nutrients are met; it is a sensitive balance between nutrient intake and requirements, and it is influenced by many factors (Figure 33–1). Nutrition is an important aspect in the etiology and management of disease in our present society. Diseases such as hypertension, diabetes, osteoporosis, anemia, and vascular disease are just some of the many conditions in which nutrition is significantly involved. Appropriate assessment may detect nutritional deficiencies in the early stages of development, such that improvement may be made through nutritional intervention and support therapy may be initiated before there are serious clinical consequences.

Malnutrition is a deficiency or imbalance of one or more vital nutrients such as proteins, vitamins, minerals, or trace elements. Malnutrition is estimated to affect millions of people globally. Even in this country, it has been estimated that 30% to 50% of patients are malnourished when admitted to the hospital, and that 25% to 30% will develop malnutrition while hospitalized. Risk factors for the development of nutritional deficiencies may include age, poor food choices, low socio-economic status, chronic illness leading to loss of fluids and nutrients, hypermetabolic states, postoperative complications, and depression. Both physiologic and psychologic changes place the elderly at increased risk of suboptimal nutritional status.

Malnutrition can be characterized as developing through four stages. Stage 1 is marked by inadequate nutrient availability or imbalance as a result of a change in nutrient intake, loss, utilization by the body, or a combination of these. In stage 2 of developing malnutrition, nutrient stores become depleted. In the third stage of malnutrition, biochemical reactions or physiologic processes are affected. This state may also be called subclinical or marginal malnutrition, one which laboratory tests for specific nutrients can identify. If malnutrition is not identified and addressed at this stage, it will progress into the final stage of symptomatic malnutrition. This last stage is characterized by the presence of cellular or tissue damage due to a prolonged state of inadequate nutrient intake or excessive loss.[1]

When malnutrition is not detected and treated, there is an increase in morbidity and mortality. Patients with protein-calorie malnutrition (PCM), also known as protein-energy malnutrition (PEM), have delayed wound healing and increased susceptibility to infection, resulting in increased length of hospital stay. Of the patients identified as malnourished, few receive early or prompt nutritional support; therefore, the early identification of malnourished patients through a screening program and establishment of nutritional intervention becomes a crucial issue of quality of care.

At present, there are two approaches to nutritional assessment and monitoring. The first is the subjective approach. This method relies on medical and dietary history including recent weight loss, the ability to use the gastrointestinal (GI) tract, and functional ability. This assessment can provide a general picture of the nutritional status but does not provide detailed objective information about protein, vitamin, and mineral status. The second approach combines the subjective assessment with objective laboratory data for specific biochemical markers. These markers will often show the presence of abnormalities prior to clinical symptoms of a deficiency.

Ideally, all patients should have nutritional status assessments. The assessment process includes two phases: screening and assessment. Screening identifies patients at nutritional risk or suspected to be at risk, whereas the assessment determines

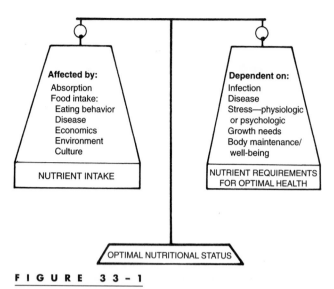

**F I G U R E   3 3 – 1**

Various factors affecting optimal nutritional status.

the nutritional status by analyzing clinical, dietary, and social history, anthropometrics (e.g., height, weight, skin folds), biochemical data, and drug-nutrient interactions. The major purpose of the assessment is to screen for nutritional risks and apply scientific techniques to determine an action plan. Conclusions drawn are used to design nutrition care plans for both inpatients and outpatients. For outpatients, nutritional evaluation should be an essential component of health promotion and disease prevention. The goals of the nutritional assessment process can be summarized as follows:

1. Identify those requiring aggressive nutrition support in order to restore or maintain nutritional status.
2. Identify appropriate medical nutrition therapies.
3. Monitor the efficiency of such therapies.

The ideal nutritional marker has the following attributes: (1) short half-life, (2) rapid response to improved nutrient intake, (3) early reflection of moderate decreased intake, (4) current nutritional status indicator, and (5) not affected by nonnutritional factor. These attributes should be applicable to the macronutrients—proteins, carbohydrates, and lipids—and to the micronutrients, vitamins and trace elements. Although the clinical laboratory can provide the physicians with information on almost all nutrients, it is commonly the patient's protein status that is used to judge his or her overall nutritional status.

## PROTEINS

### Function

Protein was the first substance recognized as a vital part of living tissue. Like fats and carbohydrates, proteins contain carbon, hydrogen, and oxygen. Proteins are unique because they

also contain about 16% nitrogen along with sulfur and sometimes other elements.

Dietary proteins are involved in the synthesis of tissue protein and other specialized metabolic functions. When the body is in a state of anabolism, proteins furnish the amino acids required to build and maintain body tissues. There are many vitamins and minerals bound to specific protein carriers for transport. Proteins, particularly albumin, also contribute to the body's homeostasis, maintaining normal osmotic relations among body fluids as shown by the appearance of edema as a result of hypoproteinemia. In addition, because of their unique structure, proteins are able to combine with acidic or basic substances to help maintain the acid-base balance required in blood and tissues.

Low-protein intakes may be tolerated by adults and children depending on the quality of protein ingested and the energy level used. To that extent, low-protein intake causes the body to compensate through an adaptation process from within and equilibrium is re-established at a lower level. Beyond a critical point, the body can no longer compensate and protein deficiency, concurrent with edema, wasting of the body tissues, and weakened immune response develops.

Protein-energy malnutrition (PEM) describes a class of clinical disorders as a result of varying degrees and combinations of protein and energy deficiency. The major forms of PEM include marasmus, in which the deficiency is primarily of energy-providing foods, kwashiorkor, characterized by protein deficiency, and marasmic kwashiorkor with deficiencies in both protein and energy.

Marasmus is a chronic condition of semi-starvation, to which the person adjusts to some extent by reduced growth. The word *marasmus* means to waste away. In its advanced stages, marasmus is characterized by muscular wasting and absence of subcutaneous fat. Victims have a "skin-and-bones" appearance since the person is slowly starving to death. It is usually associated with food shortages seen typically in wars, drought, and extreme poverty, but it may also occur in the elderly. Kwashiorkor is associated with diets high in carbohydrates in which protein intake is inadequate and of low quality. It results in extreme protein deficiency leading to hypoalbuminemia and poor immune function. Subcutaneous fat is usually preserved and muscle wasting is masked by edema. In marasmic kwashiorkor, there is a combination of symptoms of both sides. The loss of subcutaneous fat is very evident when edema is reduced in the early stages.

### Biochemical Markers for Protein Status

The synthesis of proteins can be monitored by measurement of the serum proteins listed in Tables 33–1 and 33–2. As shown, the major site of synthesis for most of the visceral proteins is the liver, one of the primary organs to be affected by protein malnutrition. The visceral proteins used as indices in the assessment of nutritional status are albumin, transferrin, retinol-binding protein, prealbumin (transthyretin), and to a lesser degree, somatomedin C and fibronectin. In addition to

T A B L E   3 3 - 1

**Serum Proteins Used in Nutrition Assessment**

| PROTEIN | HALF-LIFE | REFERENCE RANGE* | SITE(S) OF SYNTHESIS |
|---|---|---|---|
| Albumin | 21 days | 3.6–5.0 g/dL | Liver |
| Fibronectin | 15 h | 22.0–40.0 mg/dL | Endothelial cells, fibroblasts, macrophages, liver |
| Prealbumin | 2 days | 16–35 mg/dL | Liver |
| Retinol Binding Protein | 12 h | 3.0–6.0 mg/dL | Liver |
| Somatomedin C | 2–4 h | 0.10–0.40 mg/dL | Primarily liver[†] |
| Transferrin | 8 days | 200–400 mg/dL | Liver |

*May vary with age and methodology.
[†]Also in tissue to lesser extent.

their important role in nutrition assessment, these plasma proteins also play an important function as transport proteins.

## ALBUMIN

Albumin, considered the first biochemical marker of malnutrition, has been used traditionally in the assessment of hospitalized patients. Since it is an osmotic protein constituting 40% of the serum proteins, albumin has a large extravascular as well as intravascular pool. Levels less than 3.0 g/dL often are associated with malnutrition but because overhydration and dehydration affect the concentration of albumin independent of protein losses, serum albumin is an unreliable indicator of nutritional status. Owing to its long half-life, albumin is not a sensitive indicator of short-term nutrient deprivation or of the efficacy of nutrition support. However, it does help identify patients with chronic protein deficiency under conditions of adequate nonprotein calorie intake leading to marked hypoalbuminemia such as kwashiorkor. It has been established that low levels of albumin (those ≤3.5 g/dL) on admission to the hospital correlate with poor surgical outcome, poor prognosis, higher costs, and prolonged length of stay.[2] The hydration state of the patient, as well as liver or kidney disease, affect the level of albumin. Albumin is also often received by patients as part of therapy, thus making its level of little value for nutrition assessment. Age of the individual can also influence serum albumin, which declines in the elderly, most likely because of a decreased rate of albumin synthesis in the geriatric population.

## TRANSFERRIN

Transferrin is a β-globulin protein found almost completely in the intravascular space, serving as an iron-transport protein. It is the protein that binds and transports the ferric iron, and 99% of the iron in serum is bound to about one third of the transferrin pool. As a result, its synthesis is regulated by iron stores, making it an early indicator of iron deficiency. The size of the body pool of transferrin is smaller than albumin, and its half-life of 8 days makes it more likely to indicate protein depletion before albumin concentration changes.[3] However, some situations alter transferrin levels independent of nutri-

tional status. Increased levels of transferrin are associated with pregnancy, contraceptives, iron deficiency, and acute hepatitis; protein-losing states, end-stage liver disease, liver disorders, anemia, neoplastic disease, nephrotic syndrome, all cause transferrin levels to decrease.[4–6] Transferrin is, in addition, sensitive to certain antibiotics and fungicides such as aminoglycosides, tetracycline, and some of the cephalosporins.[5]

## RETINOL-BINDING PROTEIN AND PREALBUMIN

Retinol-binding protein (RBP) is a protein of low-molecular weight that functions as a carrier for retinol, the alcohol form of vitamin A. It interacts strongly with plasma transthyretin (prealbumin), circulating in plasma as a 1:1 mol/L RBP–transthyretin complex. It has been used in monitoring short-term changes in nutritional states; its usefulness as a nutritional marker is based on its short half-life (12 hours) and small body pool size. RBP concentrations tend to fall rapidly in response to protein and calorie deprivation and to respond quickly to dietary supplementation.[4–6] Although levels of prealbumin and RBP tend to parallel each other, potential problems may exist with RBP. It may have a shorter half-life than prealbumin but RBP is excreted in urine and its concentrations increase more significantly than prealbumin in patients with renal failure. In patients with chronic renal failure, plasma concentrations of RBP are increased because of its decreased catabolism by the kidney. By contrast, the catabolism of prealbumin occurs to only a small extent in the kidney, which accounts for only moderately elevated concentrations measured in advanced chronic renal insufficiency. RBP levels may also decrease in liver disease, vitamin A deficiency, acute catabolic states, postoperatively, and in hyperthyroidism.

Thyroxine-binding prealbumin serves as a transport protein for thyroxine and as a carrier protein for RBP. Prealbumin (PAB), or transthyretin, has a half-life of 2 days and a slightly larger body pool than RBP. It has a high concentration of the amino acid tryptophan, which has been shown to be a key element in the initiation of protein synthesis. In addition, PAB has one of the highest proportions of essential-to-nonessential amino acids of any protein in the body. Because of its short half-life, small pool size, tryptophan content, and

**Tests for Protein Calorie Status**

| TEST | PRINCIPLE/REQUIREMENTS | INTERPRETATION | LIMITATIONS |
|---|---|---|---|
| **VISCERAL PROTEINS** | | | |
| Albumin | Easily measured; large body pool; 60% in extravascular pool; long half-life | Decreased levels occur following protein/energy deficiency; also associated with other deficiencies | Significance confounded by liver and renal disease, pregnancy, hemodilution, and stress |
| Transferrin | Iron transport protein; smaller extravascular space than albumin; shorter half-life than albumin | Levels increased during iron deficiency and decreased by protein-energy deficiency | Significance confounded by liver disease, renal disease, pregnancy, estrogen administration, hemodilution, and stress |
| Prealbumin (transthyretin) | Transports thyroxine and carrier for RBP; short half-life | More sensitive indicator than albumin or transferrin for PCM; responds rapidly to nutritional intervention | Decreased during liver and renal disease, but to a lesser degree than albumin, and stress |
| Retinol-binding protein (RBP) | Transports retinol; filtered by glomerulus and catabolized by kidney tubule; very short half-life | Very sensitive, responds rapidly to nutritional intervention; reportedly sensitive to energy intake | Very sensitive to stress response. Also decreased in liver disease, vitamin A and zinc deficiencies; increased in chronic renal disease |
| Somatomedin C | Peptide mediator of growth hormone activity produced by the liver. Half-life few hours. Less sensitive to stress response | Decreased in chronic undernutrition; increases rapidly in nutrition support | Reduced levels seen in hypothyroidism, hypopituitarism, liver disease, estrogen usage. Costly to perform |
| **NITROGEN BALANCE** | | | |
| Urea urinary nitrogen (UUN) | Urine urea represents approximately 80% of nitrogen catabolized; requires accurate estimate of protein intake; used for TPN or tube-fed patients | Compared to actual nitrogen intake, N balance $= \dfrac{\text{protein (g)} - \text{UUN} + 4}{6.25}$ | Urine collection must be quantitative, not appropriate in renal insufficiency; inaccurate on metabolically stressed patients |
| Total urinary nitrogen (TUN) | 24-h TUN reflects to protein catabolism also requires accurate protein intake | Also compared to actual nitrogen intake, N balance $= \dfrac{\text{protein (g)} - \text{UUN} + 2}{6.25}$ | Urine collection must be quantitative; not appropriate in renal insufficiency |
| **IMMUNOLOGIC TESTS** | | | |
| Total lymphocyte count (TLC) | Calculated from the percentage of lymphocytes reported in hemogram and WBC counts | Decreased in PCM and immunocompromised patients | Decreased by viral infection chemotherapy, radiation, drugs; increased by infection and tissue necrosis |

PCM = protein-calorie malnutrition; TPN = total parenteral nutrition.

proportion of essential-to-nonessential amino acids, PAB is a better marker of visceral protein status than other proteins. PAB decreases to low levels, <10 mg/dL, with the development of severe protein calorie malnutrition and responds quickly to nutrition support with a daily increase of up to 1 mg/dL. Fluctuations in hydration status do not appear to influence its concentration to a great extent. End-stage liver disease appears to affect all protein levels in the body, but liver disease does not seem to affect PAB to the same extent or as early as it affects other visceral proteins. Patients with acute renal failure may have increased serum PAB values due to the role the kidneys play in PAB catabolism. PAB levels decrease in patients with acute phase reactions. Ingenbleek has recommended using the combined measurements of PAB and C-reactive protein, an acute phase reactant, to discriminate between the effects of an acute phase response and nutritional status in patients receiving nutritional therapy.[7] PAB measurements are useful at the initiation of nutritional therapy, as a baseline, and to monitor response to the therapy. A serum PAB concentration greater than 11 mg/dL is an entropy value that should be obtained for a patient in transition from parenteral to enteral to oral feeding. The concentration of PAB increases when more than 55% of the assessed protein and energy needs are met by the patient. If levels do not increase or if they remain below 11 mg/dL and nutritional support is being provided, the amount of nutrients, presence of disease, and/or mode of feeding must be reexamined to determine the cause. Changes in PAB have also correlated with nitrogen balance. Vanlandingham and coworkers[8] demonstrated an increase in PAB concentrations in patients with positive nitrogen balance and decreased PAB with negative nitrogen balance.

RBP and PAB have been reported to be sensitive indicators of changes in nutritional status. Carpentier and associates[9] found a definite increase in levels of RBP and prealbumin in protein-depleted, nonstressed patients receiving total parenteral nutrition. PAB was the most sensitive indicator of nutritional status in cancer patients receiving total parenteral nutrition (TPN).[10] Winkler and colleagues[11] used RBP and PAB to monitor the response to nutritional therapy during the transition of total parenteral to oral or enteral feeding. They showed a significant improvement in the concentration of the proteins during the transitional feeding period. Their data demonstrate that plasma concentrations of RBP and PAB rise at a time when other proteins, particularly transferrin and albumin, are not altered. These changes are persistent over time, and the rise in levels is maintained during the entire transitional period from TPN to oral or enteral feeding.

## SOMATOMEDIN C

Somatomedin C (SMC), also known as insulin growth factor 1, is a single-chain peptide that plays an important role in biologic growth. Its concentration is regulated by growth hormone as well as nutritional intake. Growth hormone stimulates the liver and other tissues to produce SMC. It has a proinsulin-like structure and broad anabolic properties. SMC circulates bound to carrier proteins and has a half-life of 2 to 4 hours. Studies have shown that circulating SMC levels are regulated by nutritional status, with levels particularly altered by dietary protein content. The levels fall during protein depletion and rapidly rise upon refeeding.[12] In healthy humans, SMC levels respond quickly to dietary changes in protein and calorie intake. Because of its short half-life and sensitivity to nutrient intake, SMC is a specific and sensitive marker of nutritional status. Reductions in levels occur in patients who have hypothyroidism and are receiving estrogen therapy.[4-6] However, the measurement is not easily performed in the clinical laboratory and may be too costly to justify it for routine use at this time.

## FIBRONECTIN

Fibronectin is an alpha$_2$-glycoprotein found in the lymph, blood, basement membranes, and many cell surfaces with structural functions as well as host defense functions. It serves an important role in the wound-healing process and is the major protein regulating phagocytosis. Sites of synthesis include endothelial cells, peritoneal macrophages, fibroblasts, and the liver. It is useful as a nutritional marker because it is one of the few proteins not exclusively synthesized in the liver.[13] Levels have been found to increase significantly after 1 to 4 days of adequate enteral or parenteral feeding. As with SMC, its measurement is not easy to perform, and it may be too costly to justify for routine use.

## NITROGEN BALANCE

No discussion of the serum proteins used in evaluating nutritional status is complete without the mention of nitrogen balance as one of the earlier evaluation tools. Nitrogen balance is the difference between nitrogen intake and nitrogen excretion. It is one of the most widely used indicators of protein change. In healthy humans, anabolic and catabolic rates are in equilibrium and thus the nitrogen balance is basically zero. However, during stress, trauma, or burns, nutritional intake decreases and the catabolic state increases nitrogen loss; the loss may exceed intake, leading to a negative balance. During recovery, the nitrogen balance should become positive with nutritional support. In the assessment of nitrogen balance and excretion, there are two ways of measuring urinary nitrogen losses: measuring urinary urea nitrogen and estimating total nitrogen or directly measuring total urinary nitrogen (TUN). Direct measurement is preferred and recommended, and is most significant for the unstable critically ill patient. To measure, it is essential to collect a clean, properly preserved urine sample over a 24-hour period. There is significant day-to-day variation in nitrogen excretion; therefore, multiple samples may be needed. TUN may need to be measured every other day during the initial most catabolic stage of illness and then weekly thereafter. TUN is important in the determination of the success of a nutrition plan.[14]

## TABLE 33-3

### Dietary Reference Intakes: Recommended Intakes for Individuals

Food and Nutrition Board, Institute of Medicine, National Academies[†]

| LIFE STAGE GROUP | CALCIUM (mg/d) | PHOSPHORUS (mg/d) | MAGNESIUM (mg/d) | VITAMIN D (µg/d)[a,b] | FLUORIDE (mg/d) | THIAMIN (mg/d) | RIBOFLAVIN (mg/d) | NIACIN (mg/d)[c] | VITAMIN B6 (mg/d) | FOLATE (µg/d)[d] | VITAMIN B12 (µg/d) | PANTOTHENIC ACID (mg/d) | BIOTIN (µg/d) | CHOLINE[e] (mg/d) | VITAMIN C (mg/d) | VITAMIN E[f] (mg/d) | SELENIUM (µg/d) |
|---|---|---|---|---|---|---|---|---|---|---|---|---|---|---|---|---|---|
| Infants | | | | | | | | | | | | | | | | | |
| 0–6 mo | 210* | 100* | 30* | 5* | 0.01* | 0.2* | 0.3* | 2* | 0.1* | 65* | 0.4* | 1.7* | 5* | 125* | 40* | 4* | 15* |
| 7–12 mo | 270* | 275* | 75* | 5* | 0.5* | 0.3* | 0.4* | 4* | 0.3* | 80* | 0.5* | 1.8* | 6* | 150* | 50* | 6* | 20* |
| Children | | | | | | | | | | | | | | | | | |
| 1–3 y | 500* | 460 | 80 | 5* | 0.7* | 0.5 | 0.5 | 6 | 0.5 | 150 | 0.9 | 2* | 8* | 200* | 15 | 6 | 20 |
| 4–8 y | 800* | 500 | 130 | 5* | 1* | 0.6 | 0.6 | 8 | 0.6 | 200 | 1.2 | 3* | 12* | 250* | 25 | 7 | 30 |
| Males | | | | | | | | | | | | | | | | | |
| 9–13 y | 1,300* | 1,250 | 240 | 5* | 2* | 0.9 | 0.9 | 12 | 1.0 | 300 | 1.8 | 4* | 20* | 375* | 45 | 11 | 40 |
| 14–18 y | 1,300* | 1,250 | 410 | 5* | 3* | 1.2 | 1.3 | 16 | 1.3 | 400 | 2.4 | 5* | 25* | 550* | 75 | 15 | 55 |
| 19–30 y | 1,000* | 700 | 400 | 5* | 4* | 1.2 | 1.3 | 16 | 1.3 | 400 | 2.4 | 5* | 30* | 550* | 90 | 15 | 55 |
| 31–50 y | 1,000* | 700 | 420 | 5* | 4* | 1.2 | 1.3 | 16 | 1.3 | 400 | 2.4 | 5* | 30* | 550* | 90 | 15 | 55 |
| 51–70 y | 1,200* | 700 | 420 | 10* | 4* | 1.2 | 1.3 | 16 | 1.7 | 400 | 2.4[g] | 5* | 30* | 550* | 90 | 15 | 55 |
| >70 y | 1,200* | 700 | 420 | 15* | 4* | 1.2 | 1.3 | 16 | 1.7 | 400 | 2.4[g] | 5* | 30* | 550* | 90 | 15 | 55 |
| Females | | | | | | | | | | | | | | | | | |
| 9–13 y | 1,300* | 1,250 | 240 | 5* | 2* | 0.9 | 0.9 | 12 | 1.0 | 300 | 1.8 | 4* | 20* | 375* | 45 | 11 | 40 |
| 14–18 y | 1,300* | 1,250 | 360 | 5* | 3* | 1.0 | 1.0 | 14 | 1.2 | 400[h] | 2.4 | 5* | 25* | 400* | 65 | 15 | 55 |
| 19–30 y | 1,000* | 700 | 310 | 5* | 3* | 1.1 | 1.1 | 14 | 1.3 | 400[h] | 2.4 | 5* | 30* | 425* | 75 | 15 | 55 |
| 31–50 y | 1,000* | 700 | 320 | 5* | 3* | 1.1 | 1.1 | 14 | 1.3 | 400[h] | 2.4 | 5* | 30* | 425* | 75 | 15 | 55 |
| 51–70 y | 1,200* | 700 | 320 | 10* | 3* | 1.1 | 1.1 | 14 | 1.5 | 400 | 2.4[g] | 5* | 30* | 425* | 75 | 15 | 55 |
| >70 y | 1,200* | 700 | 320 | 15* | 3* | 1.1 | 1.1 | 14 | 1.5 | 400 | 2.4[g] | 5* | 30* | 425* | 75 | 15 | 55 |
| Pregnancy | | | | | | | | | | | | | | | | | |
| ≤18 y | 1,300* | 1,250 | 400 | 5* | 3* | 1.4 | 1.4 | 18 | 1.9 | 600[i] | 2.6 | 6* | 30* | 450* | 80 | 15 | 60 |
| 19–30 y | 1,000* | 700 | 350 | 5* | 3* | 1.4 | 1.4 | 18 | 1.9 | 600[i] | 2.6 | 6* | 30* | 450* | 85 | 15 | 60 |
| 31–50 y | 1,000* | 700 | 360 | 5* | 3* | 1.4 | 1.4 | 18 | 1.9 | 600[i] | 2.6 | 6* | 30* | 450* | 85 | 15 | 60 |

| Lactation | | | | | | | | | | | | | | | | |
|---|---|---|---|---|---|---|---|---|---|---|---|---|---|---|---|---|
| ≤18 y | 1,300* | 1,250 | 360 | 5* | 3* | 1.4 | 1.6 | 17 | 2.0 | 500 | 2.8 | 7* | 35* | 550* | 115 | 19 | 70 |
| 19–30 y | 1,000* | 700 | 310 | 5* | 3* | 1.4 | 1.6 | 17 | 2.0 | 500 | 2.8 | 7* | 35* | 550* | 120 | 19 | 70 |
| 31–50 y | 1,000* | 700 | 320 | 5* | 3* | 1.4 | 1.6 | 17 | 2.0 | 500 | 2.8 | 7* | 35* | 550* | 120 | 19 | 70 |

**NOTE:** This table presents Recommended Dietary Allowances (RDAs) in bold type and Adequate intakes (AIs) in ordinary type followed by an asterisk (*). RDAs and AIs may both be used as goals for individual intake. RDAs are set to meet the needs of almost all (97% to 98%) of individuals in a group. For healthy breastfed infants, the AI is the mean intake. The AI for other life-stage and gender groups is believed to cover needs of all individuals in the group, but lack of data or uncertainty in the data prevent being able to specify with confidence the percentage of individuals covered by this intake.

[a] As cholecalciferol, 1 μg cholecalciferol = 40 IU vitamin D.

[b] In the absence of adequate exposure to sunlight.

[c] As niacin equivalents (NE). 1 mg of niacin = 60 mg of tryptophan; 0–6 months = preformed niacin (not NE).

[d] As dietary folate equivalents (DFE). 1 DFE = 1 μg food folate = 0.6 μg of folic acid from fortified food or as a supplement consumed with food = 0.5 μg of a supplement taken on an empty stomach.

[e] Although AIs have been set for choline, there are few data to assess whether a dietary supply of choline is needed at all stages of the life cycle, and it may be that the choline requirement can be met by endogenous synthesis at some of these stages.

[f] As α-tocopherol. α-Tocopherol includes $RRR$-α-tocopherol, the only form of α-tocopherol that occurs naturally in foods, and the 2R-stereoisomeric forms of α-tocopherol ($RRR$-, $RSR$-, $RRS$-, and $RSS$-α-tocopherol) that occur in fortified foods and supplements. It does not include the 2S-stereoisomeric forms of α-tocopherol ($SRR$-, $SSR$-, $SRS$-, and $SSS$-α-tocopherol), also found in fortified foods and supplements.

[g] Because 10 to 30 percent of older people may malabsorb food-bound $B_{12}$, it is advisable for those older than 50 years to meet their RDA mainly by consuming foods fortified with $B_{12}$ or a supplement containing $B_{12}$.

[h] In view of evidence linking folate intake with neural tube defects in the fetus, it is recommended that all women capable of becoming pregnant consume 400 μg from supplements or fortified foods in addition to intake of food folate from a varied diet.

[i] It is assumed that women will continue consuming 400 μg from supplements or fortified food until their pregnancy is confirmed and they enter prenatal care, which ordinarily occurs after the end of the periconceptional period—the critical time for formation of the neural tube.

[†] Reprinted with permission from *Dietary Reference Intakes: Applications in Dietary Assessment.* Copyright 2000 by the National Academy of Sciences. Courtesy of the National Academy Press, Washington, D.C.)

## C-REACTIVE PROTEIN

C-reactive protein (CRP) is an acute-phase protein (reactant), which increases dramatically under conditions of sepsis, infection, and inflammation. CRP rises in concentration 4 to 6 hours before other acute-phase reactants respond. During this period, synthesis rates of CRP as well as other acute phase proteins increase, whereas prealbumin and albumin decrease. Additionally, a significant negative nitrogen balance usually occurs secondary to the greater protein catabolism. When the anabolic process once again predominates, the rate of synthesis of CRP decreases. At this point, short half-life proteins such as prealbumin, fibronectin, and SMC begin to be synthesized from the available substrates and become useful nutritional markers once again. Therefore, during this hypermetabolic phase, monitoring the CRP value is important until the condition improves. Then the use of shorter half-life proteins once again defines the nutritional status of the patient.

## LYMPHOCYTE COUNT

Lymphocyte count is also a marker of nutritional deprivation. Total lymphocyte count (TLC) is a quick and inexpensive test that may be a useful indicator of nutritional status and outcome. In protein calorie malnutrition, the lymphocyte count is often below $2.5 \times 10^9$/L. Blackburn and colleagues have suggested that a count of 0.8 to $1.2 \times 10^9$/L indicates a moderate nutritional deficit and a value below $0.8 \times 10^9$/L represents a severe nutritional deficit. Marked lymphopenia in the absence of other primary causes such as immunodeficiency or viral infection may suggest the presence of malnutrition.[15]

## VITAMINS AND MINERAL STATUS

### Functions and Intake Recommendations

Vitamins are essential organic molecules that may be supplied by the diet or, in some instances, synthesized by the body or its intestinal microflora. Vitamins perform a variety of biochemical functions. Members of the B family enhance the activity of selected enzymes by serving as precursors or components of coenzymes or prosthetic groups. Vitamins C and E and provitamin A carotenoids (e.g., beta carotene) are antioxidants that protect cells from damage by scavenging free radicals. A vitamin D metabolite, i.e., 1,25-dihydroxyvitamin D, functions as a calcium and phosphate-regulating hormone. A form of vitamin A is part of the visual pigment rhodopsin.

Biochemical assessment of vitamin status may **directly** measure the concentration of the vitamin, its precursor or its metabolites in body fluids and tissues. Tests of this type provide a "snapshot" or static indication of vitamin status. In functional assays, the vitamin level is quantitated **indirectly** by evaluating enzymatic activity or a physiologic response in which the vitamin is necessary. Direct methods give information only on the level of the vitamin in the body pool from which the specimen was obtained. Functional assays reflect the extent to which the concentration of vitamin present throughout the body is able to support the demands of metabolism; this promotes a more dynamic interpretation of vitamin status. Usually the determination of vitamin status is conducted only as part of a detailed assessment of a patient and is prompted by information obtained from clinical and dietary history. For example, risk of certain inherited metabolic disorders, the presence of certain chronic diseases, long-term use of selected drugs, evidence of malnutrition, or concern about the effectiveness of nutritional therapy will prompt the physician to order laboratory tests of vitamin status. This may be changing as emphasis continues to shift toward prevention of disease and dysfunction and the improvement of overall health.[16] Wellness testing is increasingly of interest to members of the baby boomer generation who wish to avoid many of the degenerative disorders associated with aging.[17] Populations at greatest risk for vitamin deficiency are pregnant women, infants and children, and the elderly. While consumption of megadoses of vitamins is a growing popular practice, it has the potential for serious negative health consequences. Vitamin intoxication, although less common than deficiency, can produce irreversible pathologic changes and requires prompt identification. Vitamins share a designation as essential micronutrients but they do not possess a common chemical structure. For convenience, they are segregated into two categories, water-soluble and fat-soluble vitamins. The water-soluble vitamins are soluble in aqueous environments such as the cytoplasm and extracellular fluids, are cleared by the kidneys, and excreted in the urine. In contrast to fat-soluble vitamins, most water-soluble vitamins are retained in the body for only short periods. Despite the ease with which they are usually disposed of, under certain circumstances water-soluble vitamins can reach levels at which they cause adverse effects. Because they are stored in the liver and adipose tissue, fat-soluble vitamins are more likely to accumulate to harmful levels than are water-soluble vitamins. In either undernutrition or malnutrition, deficiencies of both the water- and fat-soluble vitamins are common.

In 2000, the Food and Nutrition Board of the Institute of Medicine, National Academy of Sciences, announced a new, more inclusive system of providing quantitative recommendations for nutrient intake (Table 33–3).[18] Recommended dietary allowances (RDAs) identify the average daily dietary intake sufficient to meet the nutritional requirements of about 98% of healthy people in a specific age and gender grouping. While retaining the RDA additional reference, values were identified as part of the dietary reference intakes (DRIs) including estimated average requirement (EAR), adequate intake (AI), and tolerable upper intake level (UL). An EAR is the amount of a nutrient that is believed to meet the requirements of 50% of the healthy individuals in a specified age and gender group. RDAs are set higher than EARs. The DRI RDA is arbitrarily set at 2 standard deviations (SDs) above the EAR (RDA = EAR + 2 SD$_{EAR}$). If a standard deviation cannot be calculated, a 10% coefficient of variation is usually assumed and the RDA is calculated to be equal to 1.2 times the value of the EAR (RDA = 1.2 × EAR). If there is insufficient data to suggest an EAR and subsequent RDA, an AI is identified. Adequate intake is an intake based on observed or experimentally determined approximations of nutrient intake by a group of healthy people (Table 33–4). The UL is the maximum intake unlikely to cause an adverse reaction. ULs have been established for many, but not all, nutrients because of insufficient data. For example, ULs cannot yet be established for thiamin, riboflavin, vitamin B$_{12}$, pantothenic acid, or biotin.[19] This approach emphasizes the important role of nutrients in maintaining health and reducing the risk of chronic diseases and developmental disorders—not just the traditional goal of preventing deficiency diseases. As recently as January, 2001, the Institute of Medicine of the National Academy of Science released a report recommending quantitative reference intake for vitamin A, vitamin K, boron, chromium, copper, iodine, iron, manganese, molybdenum, nickel, vanadium, and zinc.

Although it may be convenient to think of vitamin status in absolute terms—normal, deficient, or excessive—in reality, a physiologic continuum exists from overt deficiency through intoxication. Somewhere in the mid-portion of the vitamin status continuum typically lies the concentration that is required to support the metabolism in a healthy individual, responding to conventional physiologic stress. Vitamin intake requirements are influenced by situations that provide physiologic challenges such as pregnancy, pathologic conditions, or age-influenced amendments in vitamin processing. An individual's vitamin intake that is necessary to achieve an appropriate vitamin level will fluctuate over time as circumstances change. Failure of the vitamin level to be adjusted in response to changing needs leads to incomplete metabolic compensation and vitamin status will degrade, progressing gradually through various states of inappropriateness. When vitamin

### TABLE 33–4

**Dietary Reference Intakes: Tolerable Upper Intake Levels (UL$^a$)**

Food and Nutrition Board, Institute of Medicine, National Academies†

| LIFE STAGE GROUP | CALCIUM (g/d) | PHOSPHORUS (g/d) | MAGNESIUM (mg/d)$^b$ | VITAMIN D (μg/d) | FLUORIDE (mg/d) | NIACIN (mg/d)$^c$ | VITAMIN B$_6$ (mg/d) | FOLATE (μg/d)$^c$ | CHOLINE (g/d) | VITAMIN C (mg/d) | VITAMIN E (mg/d)$^d$ | SELENIUM (μg/d) |
|---|---|---|---|---|---|---|---|---|---|---|---|---|
| Infants | | | | | | | | | | | | |
| 0–6 mo | ND$^e$ | ND | ND | 25 | 0.7 | ND | ND | ND | ND | ND | ND | 45 |
| 7–12 mo | ND | ND | ND | 25 | 0.9 | ND | ND | ND | ND | ND | ND | 60 |
| Children | | | | | | | | | | | | |
| 1–3 y | 2.5 | 3 | 65 | 50 | 1.3 | 10 | 30 | 300 | 1.0 | 400 | 200 | 90 |
| 4–8 y | 2.5 | 3 | 110 | 50 | 2.2 | 15 | 40 | 400 | 1.0 | 650 | 300 | 150 |
| Males, Females | | | | | | | | | | | | |
| 9–13 y | 2.5 | 4 | 350 | 50 | 10 | 20 | 60 | 600 | 2.0 | 1,200 | 600 | 280 |
| 14–18 y | 2.5 | 4 | 350 | 50 | 10 | 30 | 80 | 800 | 3.0 | 1,800 | 800 | 400 |
| 19–70 y | 2.5 | 4 | 350 | 50 | 10 | 35 | 100 | 1,000 | 3.5 | 2,000 | 1,000 | 400 |
| <70 y | 2.5 | 3 | 350 | 50 | 10 | 35 | 100 | 1,000 | 3.5 | 2,000 | 1,000 | 400 |
| Pregnancy | | | | | | | | | | | | |
| ≤18 y | 2.5 | 3.5 | 350 | 50 | 10 | 30 | 80 | 800 | 3.0 | 1,800 | 800 | 400 |
| 19–50 y | 2.5 | 3.5 | 350 | 50 | 10 | 35 | 100 | 1,000 | 3.5 | 2,000 | 1,000 | 400 |
| Lactation | | | | | | | | | | | | |
| ≤18 y | 2.5 | 4 | 350 | 50 | 10 | 30 | 80 | 800 | 3.0 | 1,800 | 800 | 400 |
| 19–50 y | 2.5 | 4 | 350 | 50 | 10 | 35 | 100 | 1,000 | 3.5 | 2,000 | 1,000 | 400 |

$^a$UL = The maximum level of daily nutrient intake that is likely to pose no risk of adverse effects. Unless otherwise specified, the UL represents total intake from food, water, and supplements. Owing to lack of suitable data, ULs could not be established for thiamin, riboflavin, vitamin B$_{12}$, pantothenic acid, biotin, or any carotenoids. In the absence of ULs, extra caution may be warranted in consuming levels above recommended intakes.

$^b$The ULs for magnesium represent intake from a pharmacological agent only and do not include intake from food and water.

$^c$The ULs for niacin, folate, and vitamin E apply to synthetic forms obtained from supplements, fortified foods, or a combination of the two.

$^d$As α-tocopherol; applies to any form of supplemental α-tocopherol.

$^e$ND = Not determinable due to lack of data of adverse effects in this age group and concern with regard to lack of ability to handle excess amounts. Source of intake should be from food only to prevent high levels of intake.

†Reprinted with permission from *Dietary Reference Intakes: Applications in Dietary Assessment.* Copyright 2000 by the National Academy of Sciences. Courtesy of the National Academy Press, Washington, D.C.

needs are unmet, but before overt symptoms of deficiency (or intoxication) appear, the individual's metabolism may continue to perform but in a suboptimal manner. Even less than overt disruptions have adverse health consequences. It is in this stage of imbalance that laboratory findings are especially valuable because they permit detection of a problem and intervention to correct it before micronutrient stores are influenced, biochemical processes adversely affected, and evidence of cellular changes or tissue damage appears. In special situations, the body's intake of vitamin may need to exceed the RDA to achieve optimal physiologic responsiveness in new or modified circumstances. Therapeutic vitamin usage in amounts that substantially exceed the RDA may be required to restore homeostasis or strengthen the body's ability to effectively deal with extraordinarily stressful conditions. Only by this means may it be possible to restore optimal physiologic function and improve patient outcomes.

## Water-Soluble Vitamins

### ASCORBIC ACID

Ascorbic acid (vitamin C) functions as a potent reducing agent and can donate one or two of its electrons to an acceptor molecule (Figure 33–2). A number of enzymes require vitamin C for maximum activity. Eight enzymes depend specifically on vitamin C as an electron donor or reducing agent, including 3 that participate in formation of the structural protein collagen, 2 that participate in formation of the activated acyl transport molecule carnitine, and 1 each catalyzing biosynthesis of the neurotransmitter, norepinephrine; amidation of peptide hormones; and metabolism of the amino acid tyrosine.[20] Other activities which vitamin C promotes but is not absolutely essential for include metabolism of cholesterol to bile acids, steroid metabolism in the adrenals, histamine synthesis, hepatic metabolism of aromatic drugs and carcinogens, leukocyte function, and nonheme iron absorption in the small intestine. Vitamin C also functions as a reducing agent or antioxidant in nonenzymatic reactions. It can, for example, donate electrons to a free radical, thereby "scavenging" or eliminating it. Free radicals are generally highly reactive and transient, although they do vary in degree of reactivity and duration of existence. A free radical's ability to damage cellular constituents is due to the presence of an unpaired electron in its outer orbital—a very unstable condition. A reaction sequence is initiated in which the free radical extracts an electron from a neighboring macromolecule (i.e., protein, nucleic acid, lipid, or carbohydrate), thereby restoring its own electronic configuration to a stable form. The newly created free radical continues the chain reaction by extracting an electron from another molecule and, in a domino effect, new free radicals continue to be generated. Antioxidants like vitamins C and E and beta carotene

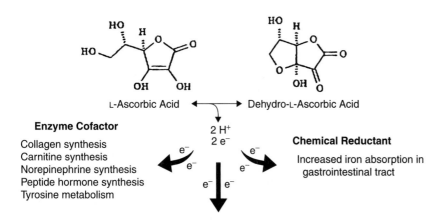

**FIGURE 33-2**

Actions of vitamin C. Oxidation of vitamin C (L-ascorbic acid) sequentially releases two donor electrons that become available for biochemical reactions observed in vivo and/or in vitro. Up and down arrows mean an increase or decrease in level. (From: Levine M et al.: Criteria and recommendations for vitamin C intake. JAMA 281:1415, 1999.)

prevent or disrupt the repeated production of free radicals. For example, vitamin C reduces aqueous free radicals. In the process, ascorbic acid loses an electron, becoming a relatively stable and only weakly reactive ascorbyl radical, and protects other substrates from oxidative damage.[21] Damage caused by free radicals as well as other reactive oxygen and nitrogen species that are not radicals has been linked to degenerative changes seen in chronic diseases including arthritis, cardiovascular disease, Alzheimer's disease, and diabetes, as well as to DNA mutations that may give rise to cancer and to the aging process itself.[22] As a free radical scavenger ascorbic acid, along with vitamin E, may suppress the oxidative modification of low-density lipoproteins (LDLs) by preventing lipid peroxidation, thus reducing the risk of atherogenesis.[23] Impaired vascular function is part of the clinical expression of atherosclerosis. Low plasma levels of vitamin C have been associated with hypertension.[24] Ascorbic acid treatment (500 mg/d) may have a sustained beneficial effect on coronary artery disease (CAD) by improving endothelium-mediated vasodilation.[25] Vitamin C provides protection against oxidative damage to DNA.[26] In the GI tract, vitamin C may act as a reducing agent to prevent the formation of potentially carcinogenic compounds such as nitrosamines.[27] Some evidence suggests that ascorbic acid may optimize the immune response by enhancing leukocyte functions. Cataract development may be delayed by optimizing vitamin C status, thus protecting the lens protein crystallin from oxidative damage. Damaged proteins aggregate and precipitate, causing the lens of the eye to become cloudy.[21]

Ascorbic acid deficiency is known as scurvy. It is characterized by hemorrhagic disorders including petechiae and swollen, bleeding gums, as well as impaired wound healing and anemia. Abnormally low plasma levels of ascorbic acid may precede scorbutic symptoms. In addition to deficient intake of ascorbic acid, blood levels are decreased by chronic inflammatory diseases and acute and chronic infections. The RDA for ascorbic acid was raised in 2000 to 75 mg/d and 90 mg/d for adult women and men, respectively. Cigarette smoking decreases the serum concentration of vitamin C and increases the risk of cancer and cardiovascular disease.[28] Because smokers experience increased oxidative stress and metabolic turnover of vitamin C, their recommended intake was increased by an additional 35 mg/d.[29] Generally, high intakes of ascorbic acid are associated with few adverse reactions. A tolerable upper intake level (UL) of 2000 mg/d has been established based on avoiding the adverse effect of osmotic diarrhea. Individuals with hemochromatosis, glucose-6-phosphate dehydrogenase (G-6-PD) deficiency, or those at risk for formation of certain types of kidney stones should avoid consuming large amounts of the vitamin. At high levels of intake, absorption efficiency declines and any circulating excesses are rapidly cleared by the kidney. Routine urinalysis on a specimen that contains a high concentration of vitamin C may be difficult because of interference from ascorbic acid if a peroxidase-redox indicator system is part of the reagent stick tests for glucose or hemoglobin. Ascorbic acid nutriture is most commonly assayed by measur-ing plasma levels of the vitamin, although urine and leukocyte concentrations can also be measured. Two methods are commonly used, an assay employing colorimetric detection after reaction of the vitamin with dinitrophenylhydrazine or an assay using high-performance liquid chromatography (HPLC) with electrochemical detection.

The serum reference range for vitamin C is 0.4 to 0.6 mg/dL, and deficiency is <0.2 mg/dL.

## B VITAMINS

**Thiamin (B₁)** functions as a coenzyme in energy metabolism, particularly carbohydrate metabolism. The coenzyme, thiamin pyrophosphate (TPP), is required for the activity of transketolase in the pentose phosphate pathway (also known as the hexose monophosphate shunt). Thiamin pyrophosphate can be phosphorylated to thiamin triphosphate (TTP), which is believed to play a key role in nerve conduction. Thiamin is rapidly absorbed from foods in the small intestine. It is excreted in the urine. The clinical condition associated with the chronic deficiency of thiamin is called beriberi. It is most often found in underdeveloped countries of the world and is characterized by symptoms involving the nervous (dry beriberi) and cardiovascular systems (wet beriberi). In the United States, thiamin deficiency is most frequently observed among chronic alcoholics with accompanying malnutrition. Decreased intake, impaired absorption, and increased requirements all appear to play a role in the development of thiamin deficiency in alcoholics. Extreme thiamin deficiency may lead to nerve degeneration and development of Wernicke's encephalopathy, Korsakoff's psychosis, or a combined disorder. Thiamin requirements are elevated in individuals on high carbohydrate diets. Patients at risk of developing a thiamin deficiency include individuals fed intravenously for prolonged periods, renal patients on long-term hemodialysis, and those with chronic febrile infections. Because of reports that there is a significant correlation between thiamin status and neuropsychologic function, a clinician may request laboratory evaluation of thiamin status in an elderly patient experiencing depression or a sleep disorder before prescribing sedative hypnotics. Excess thiamin is easily cleared by the kidneys and there is no evidence of thiamin toxicity by oral administration. High-dose therapy with thiamin has been effective in the treatment of certain inborn errors of metabolism, including one form of maple syrup urine disease (branched-chain ketoaciduria).[30] Lactic acidosis arising from an inherited disorder of the enzyme pyruvate dehydrogenase is responsive to treatment with thiamin. The EAR for thiamin is 1.0 mg/d for men and 0.9 mg/d for women. The RDA of thiamin for an adult male is 1.2 mg/d and for an adult female, 1.1 mg/d. For pregnant women, the RDA is 1.4 mg/d and for lactating women, 1.5 mg/d.

The concentration of thiamin in serum or urine can be measured manually by the fluorometric thiochrome method or by using HPLC. However, neither serum nor urine concentrations are as prognostic as is the measurement of erythrocyte transketolase (ETK) activity. The enzymatic assay of

ETK activity provides a functional measurement of thiamin. The sensitivity of the ETK activity assay can be further improved by measuring the enzyme activity before and after addition of TPP. The presence of TPP ensures optimal enzyme activity. If the increase in activity after addition of TPP is >25%, thiamin deficiency is present.

The reference ranges for thiamin are as follows:

Serum, 0.21–0.43 $\mu$g/dL
Urine, >100 $\mu$g/24 h
ETK activity increase with TPP
   Adequate, 0% to 14%
   Marginal deficiency, 15% to 24%
   Deficiency, >25%

**Riboflavin (B$_2$)** functions primarily as a component of two coenzymes, flavin mononucleotide (FMN) and flavin adenine dinucleotide (FAD). These two coenzymes catalyze a variety of oxidation-reduction reactions including those involved in the electron-transport chain, lipid metabolism, sterol biosynthesis, and the intermediary metabolism of amino acids, purines, and pyrimidines. Riboflavin is also necessary for the conversion of vitamin B$_6$ into its active coenzyme form. Dietary riboflavin is absorbed in the small intestine and transported in the blood bound to albumin. Riboflavin, along with a variety of oxidation products, is excreted in the urine. Consumption of excessive amounts of the vitamin can impart an orange color to a specimen. Riboflavin deficiency commonly occurs along with other nutrient deficiencies. Conditions such as alcoholism and starvation, which lead to deficiency of the B vitamins in general, also cause riboflavin deficiency. Chronic diarrhea and malabsorption syndromes can produce riboflavin deficiency. Riboflavin metabolism is altered in thyroid disease and vitamin excretion is enhanced in diabetes mellitus. Certain drugs antagonize the action or metabolism of riboflavin, including psychoactive drugs and tricyclic antidepressants. The possibility exists that a newborn being treated for hyperbilirubinemia by phototherapy may develop a deficiency because of riboflavin's photosensitivity.[31] Recent evidence suggests that plasma riboflavin is an independent determinant of plasma total homocysteine (tHcy) concentration. Intracellular tHcy is either converted to cysteine via the vitamin B$_6$-dependent transsulfuration pathway or remethylated to form the amino acid methionine. Two additional B vitamins are required for the successful enzyme-catalyzed remethylation. Vitamin B$_{12}$ is needed as the coenzyme, methylcobalamin, and folate in the physiologically active form of 5-methyltetrahydrofolate serves as a methyl donor.[32] Because riboflavin is the precursor of FMN and FAD, which serve as prosthetic groups for the flavoenzymes involved in the metabolism of vitamin B$_6$, folate and vitamin B$_{12}$, riboflavin status may influence homocysteine metabolism, affect plasma tHcy concentration and thus alter the risk of cardiovascular disease.[33] The DRI RDA of riboflavin for male adults is 1.3 mg/d; for female adults, it is 1.1 mg/d; for children, 0.5 to 0.6 mg/d, and for pregnant and lactating women, 1.4 and 1.6 mg/d, respectively. There is no increase in recommended intake for either men or women over the age of 50.

The concentration of riboflavin in serum or urine can be measured using HPLC with quantitation by fluorometry. However, neither blood nor urine levels of riboflavin are as sensitive indicators of riboflavin status as is the stimulation of erythrocyte glutathione (GSH) reductase activity by the coenzyme FAD. Erythrocyte glutathione reductase (EGR) has an absolute requirement for FAD and its activity is a reflection of the bioavailability of riboflavin. The enzyme activity is measured spectrophotometrically before and after addition of FAD.

The reference ranges for riboflavin are as follows:

Serum, 4 to 24 $\mu$g/dL
Urine, >120 $\mu$g/24 h
GSH reductase increase with FAD
   Adequate, 0% to 20%
   Marginal deficiency, 20% to 40%
   Deficiency, >40%

**Niacin** is a water-soluble vitamin whose requirement in humans is met in part by the conversion of the diet-derived amino acid tryptophan to niacin. Niacin is the generic term used for both nicotinic acid and nicotinamide. Niacin functions as a component of the two coenzymes NAD and NADP, which are necessary for many metabolic processes, including tissue respiration, fatty acid and steroid syntheses, and glycolysis. Nicotinic acid is a component of glucose tolerance factor, an organochromium complex that potentiates insulin response. Niacin is absorbed in the small intestine and excess is excreted in the form of metabolites in the urine.

The clinical syndrome resulting from niacin deficiency is called pellagra. This deficiency syndrome is associated with diets providing very low levels of niacin and tryptophan. Corn protein is low in tryptophan. A diet composed primarily of cornmeal will not provide adequate amounts of the precursor amino acid and the risk for poor niacin status is increased. Niacin deficiency may also be seen in alcoholism, carcinoid syndrome, and Hartnup disease. Pharmacologic doses (3 to 9 g/d) of nicotinic acid are given therapeutically to decrease serum cholesterol and triglyceride levels. In today's cost-conscious health care environment, its use offers an inexpensive alternative to the use of high-cost prescription medications. After only 1 month, total cholesterol has been reported to fall by 20% to 25% and triglycerides by 25% to 45%. An increase in HDL-cholesterol and reduction of Lp(a), a variant of LDL, have also been reported. Although toxicity of niacin is low, large doses of nicotinic acid have been reported to cause "niacin hepatitis," gout, and impaired glucose tolerance. There have also been isolated reports of macular edema associated with consumption of high dosages.[34] Not surprisingly it is essential that liver enzyme concentrations be monitored during nicotinic acid therapy. Ingestion of large amounts of nicotinic acid can trigger release of the vasodilator histamine, causing flushing of the skin and itching. The RDA of niacin for an adult male is 16 mg/d and for an adult female 14 mg/d. For pregnant women the recommended dietary intake is 18 mg/d; for lactating women, 17 mg/d, and for children, 6 to 8 mg/d. No increased intake is believed necessary with aging.

Neither blood nor urinary niacin levels are of value in assessing niacin nutritional status. The primary metabolites of nicotinamide are N-methylnicotinamide (NMN) and N-methyl-2-pyridone-5-carboxamide (2-py). Nicotinic acid is metabolized to N-methylnicotinic acid. Niacin status may be assessed by measuring the concentration of metabolites in the urine using HPLC methods.

**Pyridoxine (B$_6$)** is the collective name given to three related compounds or vitamers: pyridoxine, pyridoxal, and pyridoxamine. These compounds are converted in the liver, erythrocytes, and other tissues to pyridoxal phosphate (PLP) and pyridoxamine phosphate (PMP), which serve primarily as coenzymes in transamination reactions. PLP also functions in the metabolism of amino acids and lipids. The enzyme that catalyzes the phosphorylation reaction requires zinc for activation. Zinc status, therefore, influences B$_6$ metabolism. Vitamin B$_6$ plays an essential role in maintaining the functional integrity of the brain. Limited evidence suggests that doses of 50 to 100 mg/d may be beneficial in reducing overall premenstrual symptoms and in relieving depression associated with PMS.[35] High doses of B$_6$ are purported to reduce the pain of carpal tunnel syndrome. It is also required for the formation of δ-aminolevulinic acid, an intermediate in porphyrin synthesis, as well as maintenance of immune responsiveness and endocrine metabolism. Along with vitamin B$_{12}$ and folate, vitamin B$_6$ is required in the metabolism of the atherogenic amino acid homocysteine. Elevated levels of plasma homocysteine appear to be an independent risk factor for the development of occlusive vascular disease and for venous thrombosis.[36] Hyperhomocysteinemia is also associated with neural tube defects and complications of pregnancy.[37] Vitamin B$_6$ is readily absorbed from the intestinal tract and is excreted in the urine in the form of metabolites such as 4-pyridoxic acid (4-PA).

Vitamin B$_6$ deficiency rarely occurs alone and is most commonly seen in individuals deficient in several B vitamins. Those particularly at risk for deficiency are uremic patients, patients with liver disease, absorption syndromes or malignancies, and chronic alcoholics. High intake of protein increases the requirement for vitamin B$_6$. Therefore, a high-protein diet may cause a rapid onset of deficiency if the increased requirements are not met. Pregnancy and use of estrogen-containing oral contraceptives also cause decreased vitamin B$_6$. Pyridoxine deficiency has been reported to cause convulsions, dermatitis, and a form of sideroblastic anemia. In what may be evidence of a rebound phenomenon, newborns whose mothers had consumed moderately high amounts of pyridoxine during pregnancy experienced seizures when their serum B$_6$ levels normalized at birth.[38] Genetically determined disorders responsive to megavitamin therapy with B$_6$ include homocystinuria, cysthioninuria, xanthurenic acidurias, hyperoxalurias and infantile convulsions.[30] Vitamin B$_6$ has very low

toxicity but long-term high doses may cause severe sensory neuropathy and ataxia. Daily intakes of 500 mg have been associated with neurotoxicity. The DRI RDA of vitamin B$_6$ for adult men and women is 1.3 mg/d; 0.5 mg/d for children; 1.9 mg/d for pregnant women, and 2.0 for women who are breastfeeding. For men and women over 50 years of age the DRI RDAs are 1.7 mg/d and 1.5 mg/d, respectively. Tolerable upper intake for B$_6$ is 100 mg/d for adults including pregnant and lactating women aged 19 and older. With pregnancy in women 18 or younger, the UL is 80 mg/d.[18]

Blood plasma contains several forms of vitamin B$_6$ but the most important is PLP. Plasma PLP concentration can be quantitated using a radioenzymatic method or by HPLC. As with thiamin and riboflavin, a functional assay is often best for determining vitamin status. The functional assay for vitamin B$_6$ involves measuring the enzyme activity of erythrocyte aspartate aminotransferase (AST) before and after stimulation with PLP.

The reference ranges for pyridoxine are as follows:

Whole blood
    Adequate, 30 to 80 ng/mL
    Deficiency, <5 ng/mL
AST activity increases with PLP
    Adequate, >50%
    Deficiency, <50%

**Biotin** serves as a cofactor for the activation of four carboxylases that are essential in fatty acid synthesis, gluconeogenesis, and the breakdown of branched-chain amino acids. The enzyme that covalently links biotin to a lysine residue in the inactive apocarboxylase to form the active holoenzyme is holocarboxylase synthetase (HCS). Dietary biotin exists free or in protein-bound form as biocytin, the lysyl derivative of biotin. During digestion, biocytin and biotinyl peptides along with free biotin are liberated by proteolytic enzymes. The enzyme biotinidase catalyzes the release of free biotin from biocytin and biotinyl peptides. When biotinidase is deficient or absent, biotin cannot be liberated from ingested food nor be recovered from the carboxylases to which it is attached. Biotin reclamation in the body is an important mechanism for maintaining adequate vitamin availability. Deficiency of the biotin-liberating enzyme can secondarily create a biotin deficiency. Free biotin is absorbed in the small intestine. Biocytin not metabolized by biotinidase is excreted in the urine. Biotin is also synthesized by bacteria in the colon but not in sufficient amounts to maintain a normal biotin status. It is excreted in the urine and feces.

In humans, biotin deficiency can be produced by ingestion of large amounts of avidin, a glycoprotein found in raw egg white. Avidin irreversibly binds biotin and prevents its absorption. Impaired uptake of biotin may occur in gastrointestinal disorders such as achlorhydria or chronic inflammatory bowel disease. Biotin deficiency has also been noted in patients receiving long-term parenteral nutrition without biotin supplementation.[39] Biotin deficiency also occurs in infants and children with genetic defects of carboxylase and biotinidase enzymes. There are two types of multiple carboxylase deficiency (MCD). In the neonatal form, presenting symptoms usually include vomiting, lethargy, and hypotonia. The neonatal disorder is due to a deficiency in the enzyme holocarboxylase synthetase. Biotinidase deficiency is the primary defect in most children with late-onset MCD. Many of the symptoms of biotinidase deficiency mimic those found in epilepsy and cerebral palsy. Late-onset or juvenile form manifestations include seizures, hypotonia, hearing loss, skin rash, conjunctivitis, hair loss, ataxia, and developmental delay. Newborn screening for biotinidase deficiency permits prompt therapeutic intervention before irreparable tissue damage occurs. Biochemical findings linked to deficiency of the vitamin include organic aciduria, hyperammonemia, and ketolactic acidosis. No intoxication from biotin has been described. Large oral doses ($\geq$10 mg/d) of biotin are routinely given to treat biotin-dependent inborn errors of metabolism.[40] The DRI RDA set for biotin is 30 $\mu$g/d for adult men and women, 8 to 12 $\mu$g/d for children, 30 $\mu$g/d for pregnant women, and 35 $\mu$g/d for women who are breastfeeding.

Biotin and biotin metabolites in body fluids can be measured by using HPLC to separate the compounds, followed by quantitation of the fractions using a sequential, solid-phase avidin-binding assay.[41] Levels of biotin are rarely measured in the clinical setting; state public health laboratories are more common sites for this kind of testing.[42] Use of tandem mass spectrometry (MS/MS) offers increased test sensitivity and specificity and allows large numbers of samples to be run quickly. This methodology permits multiple screenings on a single specimen of dried blood collected on filter paper and thus lends itself to screening of newborns for a variety of inherited metabolic disorders, including those producing biotin deficiency. A microbiologic method has been employed in research settings but the assay does not detect most biotin metabolites. Biotinidase activity may be assessed directly or indirectly with measurements of the enzyme itself, plasma and urinary concentrations of biotin and its metabolites, or the levels of organic acids whose metabolism is dependent on the activity of biotin-requiring carboxylases. It must be noted that not all biotinidase-deficient individuals develop organic aciduria. Serum biotinidase activity can be measured easily and inexpensively by a quantitative colorimetric procedure or by fluorometry. Affected infants and children have 0% to 10% of normal adult activity. Levels between 10% to 30% of mean normal activity levels are considered partial biotinidase deficiency.[43] Radioassays for measuring biotinidase activity have proven to be sensitive tests, an especially important consideration when assaying limited-quantity neonatal serum.

The reference ranges for biotin are as follows:

Plasma
    Adequate, 0.82 to 2.87 nmol/L
    Deficiency, <1.02 nmol/L

**Cobalamin (B$_{12}$)** are terms used interchangeably to refer to a large group of cobalt-containing compounds. Technically,

B$_{12}$ refers specifically to cyanocobalamin. Cobalamin (Cbl) is synthesized by microorganisms, and only animal products (including meat, milk, and eggs) provide an adequate dietary source of the vitamin. In the stomach, gastric acid and the proteolytic enzyme pepsin release vitamin B$_{12}$ from the dietary proteins to which it is bound. If production of gastric acid is diminished, vitamin liberation from proteins will be reduced. R proteins, collectively known as haptocorrins, are found in most body fluids including saliva and gastric juice. Free cobalamin is bound by R proteins and the complex enters the small intestine. Pancreatic proteases catalyze the release of the cobalamin. Intestinal absorption of the free vitamin B$_{12}$ occurs in the ileum and is mediated by a unique binding glycoprotein called intrinsic factor (IF). IF is secreted by parietal cells of the gastric mucosa. If very large amounts of cobalamin are ingested, intestinal uptake can occur by passive diffusion as well as IF-mediated absorption. Newly absorbed vitamin B$_{12}$ is transported to tissues primarily bound to transcobalamin (TC) II, one of a group of carrier globulins. Coenzyme forms of vitamin B$_{12}$ are methylcobalamin and adenosylcobalamin. B$_{12}$ functions in oxidative degradation of amino acids and in lipid and carbohydrate metabolism. Conversion of methylmalonyl-coenzyme A (CoA) to succinyl-CoA (a TCA cycle intermediate) requires adenosyl-Cbl (Ado-Cbl) as a coenzyme. This reaction is part of the pathway for the breakdown of certain amino acids and odd-chain fatty acids. Succinyl-CoA is further metabolized through the tricarboxylic acid (TCA) cycle. In B$_{12}$ deficiency, methylmalonyl-CoA conversion to succinyl-CoA is blocked and methylmalonic acid (MMA) will accumulate in the blood and urine (Figure 33–3).

As mentioned earlier in this chapter, several vitamins participate in the reactions associated with methionine and homocysteine metabolism. Methionine is considered to be a glucogenic amino acid since its catabolism yields an intermediate of the TCA cycle, succinyl CoA, which can be used to form glucose. Because of this, cobalamin deficiency will affect carbohydrate metabolism. An inadequate amount of methionine linked to a deficiency of vitamin B$_{12}$ decreases the availability of S-adenosylmethionine (SAM). S-adenosylmethionine is required for a large number of methylation reactions including those essential to myelin maintenance. This may be the basis for the neurologic lesions associated with deficiency of B$_{12}$. Serum levels of MMA and tHcy are sensitive biomarkers of Cbl deficiency. An individual whose serum cobalamin is less than 150 pmol/L, plasma tHcy greater than 20 $\mu$mol/L, and plasma MMA exceeding 0.41 $\mu$mol/L would easily be classified as cobalamin-deficient. Some patients, however, may have increased concentration of only one metabolite, usually MMA. Elevated concentrations of metabolites precede the appearance of hematologic abnormalities and reduction of serum Cbl concentration. Increases in tHcy are strongly associated with higher risk of vascular disease.[44]

Cobalamin, unlike most water-soluble vitamins, is retained in the body for long periods. It is stored, primarily in the form of adenosylcobalamin, in the liver. Smaller amounts

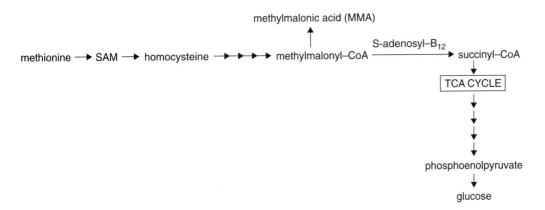

**FIGURE 33-3**

Methionine metabolism.

are stored in other tissues including muscle, bone, kidneys, heart, brain, and spleen. Despite severe malabsorption, it may take 2 to 5 years (even as long as 20 years) for an individual to deplete these stores and develop a deficiency.[45] Excess vitamin $B_{12}$ is excreted in the urine.

The most common cause of $B_{12}$ deficiency is malabsorption of the vitamin. In most individuals, Cbl absorption is impaired due to pernicious anemia, atrophic gastritis, or hypochlorhydria. In older adults, protein-bound vitamin $B_{12}$ malabsorption is linked to reduced activity of the proteolytic enzyme pepsin and a reduction in gastric acid secretion. Although these changes interfere with release of cobalamin from dietary protein, there is no change in the ability to absorb free and synthetic vitamin $B_{12}$. In pernicious (megaloblastic) anemia (PA), $B_{12}$ deficiency arises because of lack or dysfunction of intrinsic factor, which prevents absorption of vitamin $B_{12}$ in any form, protein-bound or free.[46] Autoantibodies to gastric parietal cells and to IF are detectable in serum of patients with PA. Pernicious anemia primarily affects individuals over 60 years of age. Vitamin $B_{12}$ deficiency can also occur as a result of dietary deficiency (e.g., strict vegetarians or vegans); as a result of loss of ingested vitamin $B_{12}$ (e.g., fish tapeworm infestation); as a consequence of various malabsorption diseases (e.g., sprue and celiac disease); or from surgical removal or bypass of IF–synthesizing gastric tissue (e.g., partial gastrectomy or gastric bypass). A decrease in serum Cbl levels has been reported after 3 to 4 years of treatment with certain antiulcer medications that block the formation of gastric acid.[47] Low vitamin $B_{12}$ levels often occur in folate deficiency. On examination of blood smears, observation of neutrophil hypersegmentation or megaloblastic anemia should prompt biochemical evaluation of cobalamin status. High folate intake can mask hematologic evidence of cobalamin deficiency but does not prevent the progression of neurologic lesions, including spinal cord damage. In the older adult, hematologic evidence of Cbl deficiency may never develop and only neuropsychiatric manifestations of deficiency are noted (see Figure 33–4). Toxicity

of vitamin $B_{12}$ has not been reported. The dietary reference intake RDA of vitamin $B_{12}$ is 2.4 $\mu$g/d for adult men and women, 2.6 $\mu$g/d for pregnant women, and 2.8 $\mu$g/d for lactating women. For children, 0.9 to 1.2 $\mu$g/d of cobalamin is recommended. It has been suggested that individuals aged 51 years and older should consume supplements or foods fortified with non-protein–bound vitamin $B_{12}$. This recommendation is based upon the observation that 10% to 30% of older adults do not absorb food-bound forms of the vitamin (Figure 33–5).[18]

In a research setting, determination of vitamin $B_{12}$ concentration may be by a microbiologic assay using *Lactobacillus leichmannii* or *Euglena gracilis*. A thorough evaluation of vitamin $B_{12}$ nutriture calls for measurement of serum cobalamin, methylmalonic acid, and homocysteine concentrations. In a clinical laboratory, a competitive protein-binding radioassay that is highly specific for cobalamin is routinely used to assess serum $B_{12}$. The binding protein may be purified hog intrinsic factor or a mixture of IF and R proteins. Release of the vitamin from the binding protein must occur before quantitation and can be accomplished by heat denaturation (boiling) or inactivation at alkaline pH (no-boil). Vitamin $B_{12}$ deficiency can be determined by measuring MMA in urine or assessing its serum levels by gas chromatography/mass spectrometry (GC/MS) methods. Urine concentration of MMA is about 40 times greater than the serum concentration and is usually expressed as a ratio of MMA to creatinine. Plasma tHcy concentration can be measured using HPLC and fluorescent detection.[48] Electron tandem mass spectrometry, a new technology, may make determinations of both tHcy and MMA more attractive by lowering reagent and labor costs and shortening assay time.[49]

The reference ranges for vitamin $B_{12}$ are as follows:

Serum
    Adequate, 110 to 800 pg/mL
    Borderline, 100 to 300 pg/mL
    Deficiency, <100 pg/mL

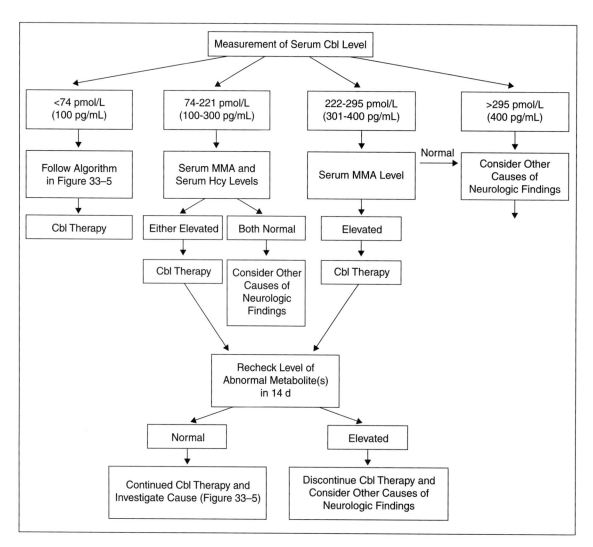

**FIGURE 33-4**

Evaluation of neurologic symptoms and signs suggestive of possible cobalamin (Cbl) deficiency in patients with normal complete blood cell counts. MMA denotes methylmalonic acid, Hcy, homocysteine. (From: Snow CF: Laboratory diagnosis of vitamin $B_{12}$ and folate deficiency: A guide for the primary care physician. Arch Intern Med 159:1289, 1999.)

The reference range for methylmalonic acid is:

Plasma, >0.41 μmol/L

The reference ranges for homocysteine are as follows:

Total homocysteine
    Plasma, 5 to 15 μmol/L (desirable <10)
Hyperhomocysteinemia[50]
    Moderate, 15 to 30 μmol/L
    Intermediate, 30 to 100 μmol/L
    Severe, >100 μmol/L

**Folate** is the generic term used for compounds that are derived from folic acid or pteroylglutamic acid (PGA). Most folates in food are polyglutamates. Folates play critical roles in cell division and protein synthesis. Enzymes requiring folic acid as a coenzyme catalyze the reactions of one-carbon metabolism. Reactions for which folate is required include serine and glycine metabolism, histidine metabolism, thymidylate synthesis, methionine synthesis, and purine synthesis. Metabolic actions of cobalamin and folate are interdependent. For example, folate is critical for synthesis of SAM, which serves as a methyl donor for over 100 biochemical reactions.[49] The hematologic changes that result from deficiency of either vitamin are indistinguishable. Folate polyglutamates in the diet are hydrolyzed to monoglutamates by conjugases in the small intestine and are quickly absorbed. In uptake and transport across the intestine, folate is reduced to tetrahydrofolate and methylated or formylated. Body stores of folate are relatively

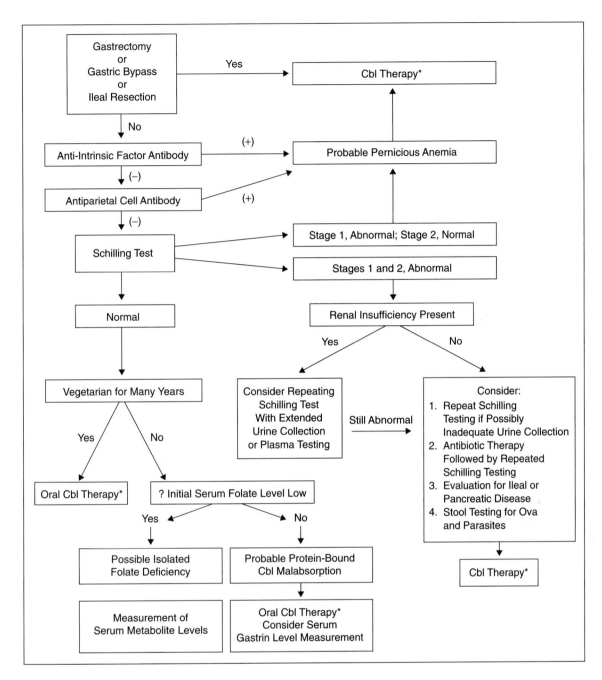

**FIGURE  33-5**

Approach to the patient with hematologic abnormalities and a serum cobalamin (Cbl)
level less than 74 pmol/L (100 pg/mL). *Patient's complete blood count should be
monitored until hematologic abnormalities are corrected. (From: Snow CF: Laboratory
diagnosis of vitamin $B_{12}$ and folate deficiency: A guide for the primary care
physician. Arch Intern Med 159:1289, 1999.)

small. RBC folate levels that reflect tissue stores of the vitamin
are much higher than serum levels; even slight hemolysis will
falsely elevate serum folate. Serum folate, which is principally
methyltetrahydrofolate, registers short-term dietary effects. Excess vitamin is excreted in the urine and feces. Large quantities of folate are synthesized by intestinal microflora.

Compromised folate status may be found in a variety of
clinical conditions including megaloblastic anemia, alcoholism, malabsorption syndromes, carcinomas, liver disease,
chronic hemodialysis, and hemolytic and sideroblastic anemias. Although hematologic changes are typically associated
with folate deficiency, neuropsychiatric manifestations such as
depression and dementia have also been noted. Maternal use
of drugs that antagonize the metabolism of folate increase the

risk of fetal defects of the brain and spinal cord, heart, urinary tract, and mouth. Many of the anticonvulsant drugs (e.g., phenytoin, phenobarbital) used to treat epilepsy lead to development of folate deficiency. Methotrexate, an especially potent folate antagonist, is used not only as a cancer chemotherapeutic agent but also in the treatment of rheumatoid arthritis and psoriasis. Several other drugs have been shown to adversely affect folate levels including sulfasalazine, used to treat inflammatory bowel disease; cholestyramine, used to treat elevated cholesterol levels; and isoniazid and cycloserine for tuberculosis therapy. Oral contraceptive steroid use is associated with lowered folate concentrations in both serum and erythrocytes. Because it may take as long as 4 months for folate status to normalize, a woman who stops using oral contraceptives in hopes of becoming pregnant may not be able to optimize her folate concentration before conception. Folate is needed very early in embryogenesis for the formation of the brain and spinal cord. All women capable of having children, whether they plan to become pregnant or not, should consume at least 400 $\mu$g daily of synthetic folic acid from food and/or supplements, in addition to eating a diet rich in leafy, dark green vegetables, legumes, and citrus fruits. This will substantially reduce the risk of fetal neural tube defects and may also lower the risk of a Down syndrome pregnancy.[51] A recent survey reported that about 30% of people in the United States and 33% of women of reproductive age took a supplement that contained folic acid in the month preceding the survey.[52] Poor folate status has been associated with an increased risk of colon cancer in several epidemiologic studies.[53] Increased risk of heart disease associated with elevated tHcy levels is related to folate status as well as availability of vitamins $B_{12}$ and $B_6$.[54] There are no known cases of folate intoxication; however folate supplementation at high levels can mask a vitamin $B_{12}$ deficiency. The DRI RDA of folate for adult men and women is 400 $\mu$g/d, 150 to 200 $\mu$g/d for children, 600 $\mu$g/d for pregnant women, and 500 $\mu$g/d for lactating women.

The reference method for serum folate determination is a microbiologic assay employing *Lactobacillus casei*. In the clinical laboratory, a competitive protein-binding radioassay for folate in serum and erythrocytes is routinely performed. The binder protein often utilized is $\beta$-lactoglobulin, a milk folate binder. Folate must be released from the binding protein by alkaline conditions or chemical reagents before it can be quantitated. In the development of folate deficiency, serum levels fall first, followed by a decrease in erythrocyte folate levels and the ultimate hematologic manifestations. It is often helpful to measure both serum and erythrocyte levels since serum levels indicate circulating folate and erythrocyte levels better approximate tissue stores.

The reference ranges for folate are as follows:

  Serum, 3 to 16 ng/mL
  Erythrocyte
    Adequate, 150 to 630 ng/mL
    Borderline, 150 to 250 ng/mL
    Deficient stores, <150 ng/mL

**Pantothenic acid** is a member of the B complex of vitamins. However, assessment of pantothenic acid status is rarely performed and deficiency is seen only in severe malnutrition. As a constituent of coenzyme A (CoA), the vitamin is essential in the production of energy from fats, carbohydrates, and proteins. Pantothenic acid also functions as part of the acyl carrier protein (ACP) that is part of the fatty acid synthetase complex and is involved in acetylation reactions that may protect cell proteins from degradation.

## Fat-Soluble Vitamins

### VITAMIN A

Vitamin A designates a group of compounds essential for vision, cellular differentiation, growth, reproduction, and immune system function. Naturally occurring compounds with vitamin A activity are retinol, retinal (retinaldehyde), and retinoic acid. The involvement of vitamin A in cell differentiation is the basis for its links to cancer. Fruits and vegetables contain carotenoids, some of which are precursors to retinol. When beta carotene is cleaved, it forms retinol and retinoic acid. Pro-vitamin A carotenes (i.e., beta carotene) provide over half of the retinol requirement in the American diet. Retinol and carotene are absorbed from the small intestine into the circulation via the lymphatic system as retinyl esters in chylomicrons. The retinyl esters are rapidly taken up and stored by the liver, at which point they are attached to retinol-binding protein (RBP). After secretion into the circulation, the vitamin A–RBP complex is further joined to prealbumin and is released into the blood.

Vitamin A deficiency is most common among young children living in nonindustrialized countries of the world, although poor inner-city children may also be deficient. The most common origin of poor vitamin status is insufficient dietary intake. Vitamin A has been called the "anti-infection" vitamin; it appears to be important in maintaining T lymphocyte functions and for antibody response to bacterial, parasitic, and viral infections. Increased risk of complications and death from measles among children with a poor vitamin A status is well known. Deficiency may also occur as a result of chronic fat malabsorption. An early sign of vitamin A deficiency is poor dark adaptation or night blindness.[55] Other causes of abnormal dark adaptation include zinc and protein deficiencies. Prolonged deficiency may lead to corneal ulceration and eventually to total blindness. Low levels of vitamin A are found in diseases that impair small intestinal function or liver function. Subclinical vitamin deficiency occurs among patients with Crohn's disease, alcoholic cirrhosis, a history of small intestine bypass surgery, and pancreatic insufficiency. When ingested in high doses, either chronically or acutely, vitamin A causes toxic symptoms or teratogenic effects. Isotretinoin (13-cis-retinoic acid) used in acne treatment has proven to be teratogenic, and if ingested during the first trimester of pregnancy, increases the rate of spontaneous abortion. Signs and symptoms of intoxication include nausea, fatigue, hair coarsening and loss, drying and scaling of the skin, and bone pain. Limited human data suggest that skeletal changes associated with hypervitaminosis A include increased resorption and decreased bone formation. Epidemiologic studies indicate that skeletal damage may occur with intake of amounts of vitamin A that can easily be obtained from the diet and supplements. The possibility has been raised that subclinical hypervitaminosis A may be a common contributor to the development of osteoporosis.[56] Excessive intake of vitamin A can lead ultimately to liver damage and can increase the risk of certain birth defects. High doses of vitamin A may be obtained from ingestion of excess vitamin supplements or large amounts of fish liver (e.g., cod liver) oils, which are rich in vitamin A. The tolerable upper intake level (UL) of vitamin A for an adult is 3000 $\mu$g/d. Carotenoids, on the other hand, are not known to be toxic. This is due to a reduced efficiency of carotene absorption at high doses and limited conversion to vitamin A. Vitamin A activity is expressed as retinol equivalents. One retinol equivalent (RE) is equal to 1 $\mu$g all-*trans*-retinol or 3.33 IUs or 12 $\mu$g beta carotene. The DRI RDA of vitamin A for an adult male is 900 $\mu$g/d and for an adult female, 700 $\mu$g/d. Older literature may report vitamin A activity in international units. Because there is insufficient data on which to base a recommendation, no RDAs have been set for beta carotene or other carotenoids. Beta carotene has many functions such as quenching singlet oxygen and scavenging free radicals. The interest in beta carotene's potential as a protective agent against cancer and heart disease stem from its function as an antioxidant. However, in two important studies (ATBC[57] and CARET),[58] beta carotene was found to have adverse effects, including increases in lung cancer incidence and deaths from cardiovascular disease and total deaths, rather than beneficial effects. More work is clearly needed before any recommendations on intake are developed.

Measurement of retinol is the most common means of assessing vitamin A status in the clinical setting. Retinol may be assayed using a direct fluorometric method or by HPLC. Toxicity is best assessed by measuring retinyl ester levels in serum rather than retinol. Measurement of the various forms of vitamin A (retinol, retinyl esters) is accomplished using HPLC methods.

The reference rangs for retinol are as follows:

Plasma, 300 to 800 $\mu$g/L
Severe deficiency, <100 $\mu$g/L

## VITAMIN D

Vitamin D refers to a group of related compounds. Vitamin D is essential for development and maintenance of skeletal integrity and for calcium and phosphate homeostasis. Exposure to UV light (sunlight) triggers synthesis of cholecalciferol (vitamin $D_3$) from 7-dehydrocholesterol in the skin. Increased levels of melanin in the skin raise the length of time that skin must be exposed to UV light for cutaneous synthesis of vita-

min D. Persons with very dark skin pigmentation may require as much as a 6 times longer exposure to sunlight to synthesize the same amount of vitamin D as a person with light skin.[59] Enzyme-catalyzed hydroxylation of vitamin $D_3$ takes place in the liver to form 25-hydroxyvitamin $D_3$ (25-OH $D_3$), which is also known as calcidiol. An additional hydroxylation occurs in the kidney to form 1,25-dihydroxyvitamin $D_3$ (1,25(OH)$_2D_3$) or calcitriol. The concentration of calcitriol is tightly regulated and varies in response to changes in concentrations of parathyrin (PTH), calcium, phosphate, estrogen, and possibly other hormones. Subscripts are often used to identify the origin of the vitamin and its metabolites. Vitamin $D_3$ is of animal origin. The form of the vitamin found in plants is ergocalciferol or vitamin $D_2$. Vitamin D in foods occurs as cholecalciferol or ergocalciferol. The most active metabolite of vitamin D is 1,25(OH)$_2D_3$, a potent calcium and phosphate mobilizing hormone. It stimulates intestinal absorption of calcium and phosphate for bone growth and metabolism and, together with PTH, promotes the mobilization of calcium and phosphate from bone and modifies renal excretion of calcium and phosphorus. Vitamin D is absorbed in the small intestine and requires bile salts for uptake. The vitamin is stored in the liver and excreted in the bile.

Vitamin D deficiency is characterized by inadequate mineralization of the bone. In infants and children, severe deficiency impairs the body's ability to absorb calcium, causing poor bone development and a deformation of the skeleton called nutritional rickets. Children whose diet is low in vitamin D or who have little exposure to sunlight (UV) are at high risk for rickets. The Industrial Revolution with the widespread use of child labor and urban air pollution made rickets common among young people in the late 1890s. Infants Hospital in Boston reported that 80% of infants younger than 2 years old showed physical evidence of rickets. In the early years of the 20th century, better understanding of the importance of dietary and environmental factors (exposure to ultraviolet light/sunlight) in the prevention of nutritional rickets helped virtually eliminate this crippling disease in the United States.[60] Recent reports suggest that there is a reemergence of nutritional rickets throughout this country due to an increase in breastfeeding of infants who do not receive supplemental vitamins.[61] The biochemical indicators of rickets, including serum levels of calcidiol, alkaline phosphatase, parathyrin, and calcium, respond quickly to vitamin D supplementation. In adults, hypovitaminosis D leads to undermineralization of bone matrix, resulting in excessive bone loss and osteomalacia. Low levels of vitamin D are reported with small bowel disease, chronic renal failure, hepatobiliary disease, pancreatic insufficiency, hypoparathyroidism, and use of anticonvulsant drugs. Renal rickets can develop in patients on hemodialysis because of the inability of failing kidneys to synthesize calcitriol from calcidiol. Inadequate exposure to sunlight and avoidance of dairy products that are fortified with vitamin D contribute to poor vitamin D status among the elderly. Vitamin D is potentially toxic, especially in children. The effects of excessive vitamin D intake include hypercalcemia and hypercalciuria, which can lead to calcium deposits in soft tissue and irreversible renal and cardiac damage and hypercalciuria. Elevated levels of vitamin D are present in hyperparathyroidism, hypophosphatemia, and during pregnancy. The RDA of vitamin D for adults is 5 μg/d (200 IU), for children, 10 μg/d, for breastfed infants, 5 to 8 μg/d, and 10 μg/d for pregnant and lactating women. For older women (postmenopausal) and men, studies suggest the need for even greater intake of vitamin D, along with calcium, to reduce the risk of osteoporosis. In osteoporosis, decreased bone mass markedly increases fracture risk. The annual medical costs of osteoporosis are projected to reach almost $50 billion by the year 2040. If this comes to pass, osteoporosis will cost more than most other age-related chronic diseases including stroke, cancer, or diabetes. Although the public tends to associate osteoporosis with aging, bone loss prevention is essential at all ages. Excessive exercise and eating disorders may place young women and men at increased risk of osteoporotic fracture.[62] In addition to their role in bone health, metabolites of vitamin D may be involved in differentiation and proliferation of cells in the immune system, the epidermis, and perhaps in the inhibition of growth of certain cancer cells. For people 51 to 70 years of age, 10 μg/d (400 IU) is suggested, and for those 71 years of age and older, 15μg/d (600 IU). A compelling case can be made for an even higher requirement for vitamin D, as much as 800 to 1000 IUs daily by probably all older adults to increase serum 25-OH D$_3$ levels and minimize any seasonal variation in concentration. Although excessive intake can cause hypercalcemia and metastatic calcifications, these complications do not seem to appear unless daily intake exceeds 2400 IUs. The UL has been set conservatively at 50 μg/d (2000 IUs).[63]

The two forms of vitamin D most commonly measured in the clinical laboratory are 25-OH D$_3$ and 1,25(OH)$_2$D$_3$. The 25-OH D$_3$ is the major circulating form of vitamin D and its measurement is the best indicator of vitamin D nutritional status as well as vitamin D intoxication. Reference ranges vary with season and geographic location. The most metabolically active form of vitamin D [1,25(OH)$_2$D$_3$] is a reflection of the body calcium homeostasis. Serum levels of calcitriol are a poor indicator of vitamin D status because of tight hormonal control. It is often useful to measure PTH and calcium levels in conjunction with 1,25(OH)$_2$D$_3$. These levels are useful in diagnosing primary hyperparathyroidism, in diagnosing different types of rickets, in monitoring patients with chronic renal failure, and in assessing compliance with 1,25(OH)$_2$D$_3$ therapy. Laboratory methods for assaying vitamin D metabolites must be very sensitive because of the low circulating concentrations of the vitamin. Quantitation may be performed using radioassay methods or HPLC in conjunction with competitive protein binding.

The reference ranges for vitamin D are as follows:

25-OH D$_3$, 14 to 42 ng/mL
1,25(OH)$_2$D$_3$, 15 to 45 pg/mL

## VITAMIN E

Vitamin E functions in the body as a powerful antioxidant; it is a primary free radical scavenger in membranes. The most important compounds exhibiting the biologic activity of vitamin E are the tocopherols. Alpha-tocopherol is the most biologically active and widely distributed form of vitamin E. It is alpha-tocopherol that is most often measured in the laboratory. As a fat-soluble antioxidant, vitamin E can prevent peroxidation of polyunsaturated fatty acids (PUFAs) in cell membranes. The vitamin is critical for maintenance of cell membrane integrity and many functions that occur at the cell membrane level including drug metabolism, heme biosynthesis, mitochondrial electron transport, and neuromuscular function. In addition, vitamin E increases the resistance of LDL to oxidative modification and thereby reduces the risk of atherogenesis.[64] Other micronutrients including selenium, ascorbic acid (vitamin C), and perhaps, beta carotene and other carotenoids may also help protect against oxidative damage. There also may be an intracellular, antiatherogenic effect of alpha-tocopherol (1200 IU/d for 8 weeks) in monocytes that decreases their ability to release harmful reactive oxygen species.[65] Absorption of dietary vitamin E is most efficient in the jejunum, where it is attached to lipoproteins and transported via the lymphatics. As an individual's lipoprotein level varies, so will vitamin E status. Vitamin E is stored in the liver and in a variety of tissues with high lipid content; it is excreted largely in the feces.

Vitamin E deficiency commonly occurs in two groups of individuals: premature, very low birth weight infants and patients who do not absorb fat normally. In patients receiving parenteral nutrition, vitamin E and selenium nutriture may be compromised and biochemical monitoring for deficiency is suggested. Evidence of peroxidative stress and diminished plasma antioxidant defenses have been reported in patients receiving parenteral nutrition.[66] Signs of deficiency include increased platelet aggregation, increased fragility of erythrocytes that can lead to hemolytic anemia reproductive failure, muscular atrophy and wasting, and neurological defects. Some, but not all, studies have suggested that low levels of vitamin E are related to increased risk of lung cancer. In healthy elderly, supplementation with 800 mg of alpha-tocopherol for 1 month improved immune responsiveness by increasing delayed-type hypersensitivity (DTH) response, increasing production of interleukin-2, enhancing proliferation of T lymphocytes in response to certain mitogens, and decreasing prostaglandin E2 synthesis and overall lipid peroxidation. An immunostimulatory effect by 200 mg/d of vitamin E consumed for 235 days has been linked to a 65% increase in DTH, a 6-fold increase in antibody titer to hepatitis B and a significant increase in antibody titer to tetanus vaccine among healthy elderly.[67] Supplemental vitamin E intake of at least 100 IU/d for at least 2 years may reduce the risk of coronary artery disease.[68,69] Megavitamin therapy has been useful in treating patients with peripheral vascular disease. Intermittent claudication improved after 12 to 18 months of vitamin E therapy. In patients with moderately severe Alzheimer's disease, alpha-tocopherol (2000 IU/d) appears to slow nerve damage. The brain has a high metabolic requirement for oxygen and a high concentration of polyunsaturated fatty acids. These two factors increase tissue vulnerability to lipid peroxidation. Vitamin E acting as an antioxidant may protect the nerve tissue from free radical damage, thereby impeding neurodegenerative processes. The American Psychiatric Association has approved the use of vitamin E supplements to delay progress of Alzheimer's disease. Vitamin E status is an important determinant of cardiovascular disease risk. Recently, there has been speculation that the protective effect of vitamin E on memory and cognition may be due at least in part to the protection it provides against vascular disease.[70] Pharmacologic doses of vitamin E seldom produce toxic effects but may significantly impair the absorption of vitamins D and K. The DRI RDA of vitamin E for adult men and women is 15 mg/d. This is equivalent to 22 IUs of natural source vitamin E or 33 IUs of the synthetic form.[19]

Vitamin E is easily quantitated in serum or plasma using HPLC methods. The erythrocyte fragility test based on the percentage of RBCs hemolyzed after exposure to $H_2O_2$ (>20% is considered to reflect vitamin E deficiency) is subject to too many variables to be an acceptable assessment method.

The reference ranges for vitamin E are as follows:

Serum alpha-tocopherol
    Adequate, >7 mg/L
    Low, 5 to 7 mg/dL
    Deficiency, <5 mg/dL

## VITAMIN K

Vitamin K is the name for a group of compounds all of which are essential for the formation of prothrombin (factor II) and several other coagulation proteins, including factors VII, IX, and X, and proteins C, S, and Z. The vitamin is necessary to convert the precursor forms to the functional forms of these coagulation proteins. This transformation occurs in the liver. Phylloquinone, found in dark-green, leafy vegetables, is the primary dietary source of vitamin K. Patients with cystic fibrosis are at risk of vitamin K deficiency due to pancreatic insufficiency and/or hepatobiliary disease.[71] Dietary vitamin K is absorbed primarily in the terminal ileum and possibly in the colon. Intestinal bacteria synthesize a form of vitamin K (menaquinones) but probably only provide a small portion of the daily human requirement.[72] Vitamin K is stored briefly in the liver and then distributed widely among body tissues. Especially for a fat-soluble vitamin, the body pool of vitamin K is quite small (less than the pool for vitamin $B_{12}$) and it turns over rapidly. A metabolite of vitamin K is excreted in the urine.

Traditionally, vitamin K has been viewed as necessary for hemostasis and the major sign of vitamin K deficiency is defective clotting of the blood. Evidence is accumulating that suggests it also has important roles in the production of many other proteins. Vitamin K plays an important role in bone metabolism and the maintenance of skeletal integrity. Though not confirmed by all studies, serum vitamin K levels have been associated positively with bone mineral density. Low serum concentrations of vitamin K have been reported in patients with osteoporotic fractures of the spine and hip.[73-75] The effect of vitamin K on bone appears to be in its role as a cofactor for carboxylation of glutamic acid residues to form γ-carboxyglutamic acid (Gla) residues in vitamin K-dependent proteins. The γ-carboxyglutamic acid residues serve as calcium-binding sites in the protein. A vitamin-K dependent bone protein, osteocalcin, has been found to be a very sensitive marker of vitamin K nutritional status. Osteocalcin, the most abundant noncollagenous protein in mature bone matrix, is produced by osteoblasts and its circulating level has been used as a marker of bone formation. The calciotropic hormone $1,25(OH)_2D_3$ promotes synthesis of osteocalcin, which may act by influencing bone mineralization. Recent studies suggest that fracture risk is associated with depressed or undercarboxylation of osteocalcin. A deficiency of vitamin K in patients with cystic fibrosis may adversely affect skeletal growth. Vitamin K metabolism or action and bone remodeling are reported to be altered in response to short- and long-term exposure to microgravity conditions during space flight. Dietary deficiency in adults is rare. However, vitamin K deficiency can occur in individuals with malabsorption syndrome and liver disease. High doses of vitamins A and E may antagonize the action of vitamin K. Broad-spectrum antibiotic (e.g., neomycin) therapy may cause vitamin K deficiency by destroying much of the naturally occurring, vitamin K–synthesizing intestinal microflora. Patients receiving total parenteral nutrition are also at increased risk of deficiency. In the case of anticoagulant therapy with vitamin K antagonists such as coumarin, prothrombin, and factors VII, IX, and X are synthesized but are nonfunctional. An apparent vitamin K deficiency, leading to hemorrhagic predisposition, may be observed when drugs such as warfarin, one of the coumarin-based oral anticoagulants, are used in the treatment of thromboembolic disease. Even when minidose warfarin (1 mg/d) is administered to healthy individuals, the percentage of undercarboxylated osteocalcin increases by about 170% after a week of treatment.[76] Breast milk is low in vitamin K, the neonatal liver is immature with respect to prothrombin synthesis, and the infant gut is sterile during the first few days of life. Not surprisingly breastfed infants are at greater risk for hemorrhagic disease of the newborn than formula-fed infants.[77] A single intramuscular dose of 1 mg of phylloquinone is administered at birth to protect against vitamin K–deficiency bleeding. Maternal supplementation with 5 mg/d of phylloquinone during the first 3 months of nursing improves the vitamin K status of infants who are exclusively breastfed. Natural forms of vitamin K such as phylloquinone have not been reported to cause toxic effects even in large doses. However, ingestion of large amounts of vitamin K–containing foods can diminish the effectiveness of oral anticoagulants. Administration of menadione, a synthetic analog of vitamin K, to neonates must be avoided because it will trigger toxic reactions including hemolytic anemia, hyperbilirubinemia, kernicterus, brain damage, and death. An UL cannot yet be established for vitamin K because of insufficient available data. The adequate intake (AI) for vitamin K has been increased for adult males to 120 μg/d and for adult females to 90 μg/d.

Although procedurally difficult, it is possible to measure phylloquinone (and menaquinone) levels directly by HPLC with fluorometric detection but its concentration reflects only recent dietary intake. Serum total osteocalcin (OC) and the percentage of undercarboxylated osteocalcin (%ucOC) are more sensitive measures of vitamin K status than the traditional blood coagulation tests. Assessment procedures use differences in binding of undercarboxylated and fully carboxylated osteocalcin to the salts, barium sulfate, or hydroxyapatite. Technical difficulties have raised questions about test reliability.[78,79] Methods employed include barium-sulfate–binding RIA and hydroxyapatite-binding RIA. The plasma concentration of undercarboxylated or incompletely γ-carboxylated clotting factors such as prothrombin (II), also known as PIVKA-II (proteins induced by vitamin K absence or antagonism) is also responsive to depletion and repletion with phylloquinone and can be measured by immunoassay.[80] Assessment of urinary excretion of γ-carboxyglutamic acid (Gla) in a 24-hour period can be useful in evaluating vitamin nutriture. Urinary Gla can be determined by derivitization, followed by HPLC with fluorometric detection. Vitamin K compounds are not routinely quantitated in the clinical laboratory due to the difficulty of the methods. Therefore, prothrombin time (PT) is used as a functional indicator of vitamin K status. However, prolonged prothrombin time is a late indicator of vitamin K deficiency and the test is not sufficiently sensitive for use in monitoring patient response to nutritional support therapy.

The reference range is 11.6 to 13.6 seconds (varies with method used); with deficiency, there is a prolonged PT.

The DRI RDAs, AIs, and ULs of the vitamins discussed in the preceding section are summarized in Tables 33–3, 33–4, and 33–5.

## TRACE AND ULTRATRACE ELEMENTS

Minerals are inorganic elements that constitute a very small portion of the body weight (only about 4%) but are essential for many vital processes. These inorganic elements are often tightly complexed with proteins to form a functioning unit, for example hemoglobin, thyroxine, and the metalloenzymes.

Minerals are often divided into two groups. The **major minerals** or macroelements are present in quantities greater than 5 g in the body and are required at levels of intake of at least 100 mg/d.[19] Examples are calcium, phosphorus, potassium, sodium, chloride, magnesium, and sulfur. The major minerals are nutritionally important, but are discussed in Chapters 21 and 28. The microelements are usually considered as two groups: trace elements and ultratrace elements. Trace elements include iron, zinc, manganese, copper, and fluorine. Ultratrace elements include selenium, molybdenum, iodine, chromium, boron, and cobalt. Nickel, vanadium, arsenic, and silicon are also elements that may be essential or beneficial to humans. The **trace elements** are those minerals present in quantities less than 5 g in the body and required in amounts

**Recommended Dietary Allowances (RDA) or Adequate Intake (AI) of Vitamins for Adults**

| WATER-SOLUBLE VITAMINS | | FAT-SOLUBLE VITAMINS | |
|---|---|---|---|
| Ascorbic acid (C) | *M: 90 mg/d<br>F: 75 mg/d | Retinol (A) | M: 900 μg/d<br>F: 700 μg/d |
| Thiamine (B₁) | M: 1.2 mg/d<br>F: 1.1 mg/d | Vitamin D | M: 5 μg/d<br>F: 5 μg/d |
| Riboflavin (B₂) | M: 1.3 mg/d<br>F: 1.1 mg/d | Tocopherol (E) | M: 15 mg/d<br>F: 15 mg/d |
| Pyridoxine (B₆) | M: 1.3 mg/d<br>F: 1.3 mg/d | Vitamin K* | M: 120 μg/d<br>F: 90 μg/d |
| Cobalamin (B₁₂) | M: 2.4 mg/d<br>F: 2.4 mg/d | | |
| Folate | M: 400 μg/d<br>F: 400 μg/d | | |
| Niacin | M: 16 mg/d<br>F: 14 mg/d | | |
| Biotin | M: 30 μg/d<br>F: 30 μg/d | | |

M = male; F = female.

*AI (adequate intake) for vitamin K. Note: The AI is not equivalent to an RDA.

## TABLE 33-6

**Clinical Manifestations Associated with Deficiency of Ultratrace Elements**

| ULTRATRACE ELEMENT | CLINICAL MANIFESTATION |
|---|---|
| Chromium | Impaired glucose tolerance |
| | Hyperinsulinemia |
| | Reactive hypoglycemia |
| | Hyperglycemia and glycosuria |
| | Hyperlipidemia |
| Vanadium | Influences glucose metabolism |
| | Mimics action of insulin |
| Molybdenum | Mental retardation |
| | Neuropsychiatric symptoms |
| Nickel | No definitive manifestations described |
| Cobalt | No definitive manifestations described |
| Tin | No definitive manifestations described |

ranging from 1 to 100 mg/d. Despite their small amounts, these trace elements are crucial to sustaining life. **Ultratrace elements** are also important but they are required in very small amounts (e.g., <1 mg/d). In a variety of pathologic conditions, circulating levels of trace elements may be altered (Table 33–6). The trace and ultratrace elements believed to be essential for life are listed in Table 33–7. The RDA has been established for iron, iodine, selenium, zinc, copper, and molybdenum. An RDA range has been recommended for fluoride and manganese. These 8 inorganic nutrients are discussed in some detail below. Dietary intakes for many of the remaining minerals have not been determined. Therefore, chromium, cobalt, nickel, silicon, tin, and vanadium will receive limited discussion. In a variety

## TABLE 33-7

**Essential Trace and Ultratrace Elements**

Chromium
Cobalt
Copper
Fluoride
Iodine
Iron
Manganese
Molybdenum
Nickel
Selenium
Silicon
Tin
Vanadium
Zinc

of pathologic conditions, circulating levels of trace and ultratrace elements may be altered (Table 33–8).

## Analytical Methods

A variety of analytical techniques have proved useful in the separation, identification, and quantitation of chemical compounds including trace and ultratrace elements. Because these elements are present in biologic specimens in such small amounts, an analytical method's limit of detection is a critical factor in evaluating its utility for these micronutrient assays.

## Trace Elements

### IRON

Iron is perhaps the most well known trace element. It is available in the diet in two forms: heme and nonheme iron. As a constituent of hemoglobin, myoglobin, the cytochromes of the electron transport chain and a number of enzymes, it functions in the important roles of oxygen delivery to tissues and energy transformation. Iron is absorbed by the intestinal mucosa. The individual's iron status influences absorption efficiency so that physiologic needs are met but excessive intake is avoided. Generally heme iron, which is found in meat, is better absorbed than nonheme iron, which is found mainly in plant material. If an individual is not deficient in iron, about 5% or less of ingested nonheme iron is absorbed, whereas 20% to 30% of heme iron is absorbed. In iron deficiency absorption may increase to more than 50% of ingested nonheme iron if the deficiency is severe.[81] Dietary factors such as tannic acid in tea and phytates in cereals and bran can inhibit iron uptake. Ascorbic acid (vitamin C) promotes the uptake of nonheme iron. Approximately 70% of the iron in the body is found in red blood cells as part of the hemoglobin molecule. Another 5% is in the form of myoglobin in the muscles. About 20% of iron is stored intracellularly in the proteins ferritin and hemosiderin. Ferritin is the primary iron storage form in the liver, spleen, and bone marrow. In iron overload, hemosiderin deposits are increased substantially. The remaining 5% of the body's iron is found as a component of oxidative enzymes. Circulating iron is bound to the transport protein, transferrin. Under normal conditions, only a very small amount of iron is lost from the body. Even in healthy individuals, minute amounts of blood and sloughed mucosal cells from the GI tract pass out of the body in the feces. Some iron is lost in the urine and by desquamation of surface cells of the skin.[82] Iron is also lost through menstruation and by chronic or acute hemorrhage.

Worldwide iron deficiency is one of the most common nutritional problems. Infants, children, young women, and the elderly are at greatest risk of inadequate intake. Pica, a craving for unusual nonfoods (starch, dirt, clay, ice) or crunchy or salty foods, has been associated with iron deficient anemia. Iron deficiency ultimately results in anemia due to impaired hemoglobin synthesis. Three stages of iron deficiency have been iden-

**Factors Affecting Concentration of Selected Trace and Ultratrace Elements**

| ANALYTE | FACTORS AFFECTING CONCENTRATION |
|---|---|
| Chromium (S) | ↓ Diabetic children, pregnancy |
| Copper (S) | ↑ Pregnancy, estrogen, birth control pills, infection, inflammation |
| | ↓ Wilson's disease, Menkes's syndrome, protein malnutrition, cystic fibrosis |
| Iron (S) | ↑ Hemochromatosis, acute leukemia, acute hepatitis, thalassemia, excessive Fe therapy |
| | ↓ Iron deficiency anemia, infection, hypothyroidism, kwashiorkor |
| Manganese (S, P, WB) | ↑ Industrial exposure, myocardial infarction, acute hepatitis |
| | ↓ Seizure disorders, phenylketonuria |
| Molybdenum (S, P, WB) | |
| Selenium (S, P, WB) | ↑ Industrial toxicity |
| | ↓ Cardiomyopathy (Keshan disease), GI cancer, pregnancy, cirrhosis, hepatitis |
| Zinc (P) | ↑ Coronary heart disease, arteriosclerosis |
| | ↓ Estrogens, oral contraceptives, acute infections, acrodermatitis enteropathica, leukemias, pregnancy |

S = serum; P = plasma; WB = whole blood; ↑ = increased; ↓ = decreased.

Adapted from Milne DB: Laboratory assessment of trace element and mineral status. In Bogden JD, Klevay LM (eds.): *Clinical Nutrition of the Essential Trace Elements and Minerals: The Guide for Health Professionals*. Totowa, NJ, Humana Press Inc., 2000.

tified.[83] The first is a depletion of iron stores. The second stage of iron deficiency is characterized by iron deficient erythropoiesis and the third stage is the development of iron deficiency anemia. Iron deficiency can be caused by a decrease in dietary intake, accelerated losses, or a block in the mobilization of stored iron. A block in iron mobilization is caused by many chronic diseases and the resulting deficiency is often referred to as anemia of chronic disease. Long-term use of certain medications such as nonsteroidal anti-inflammatory drugs (NSAIDs) increase the risk of GI ulceration and development of iron deficient anemia. Toxicity resulting from iron in foods has never been reported. However, excess iron ingested as ferrous sulfate or other supplemental forms can be extremely toxic. Even one 0.3 mg tablet of ferrous sulfate may increase the serum iron concentration by 300 to 500 $\mu$g/dL.[84] In the United States alone, over 2000 cases of iron poisoning are reported per year. Most of these cases are children who have ingested iron supplements formulated for adults.[85] Iron toxicity can also occur as a result of the iron-loading disorder hemochromatosis. Hemochromatosis is the result of a genetic defect that leads to enhanced iron absorption. Multiple transfusions can also produce chronic iron overload. In iron overload, the accumulation of excess iron in the body can cause extensive organ damage leading to a variety of disorders, including heart disease, liver disease, and cancer.[86] The pathology of iron overload may be from the catalytic role of iron in reactions that generate highly damaging free radicals. The DRI RDA of iron for adult men and postmenopausal women is 8 mg/d, 27 mg/d for pregnant women, and for premenopausal women, 18 mg/d. The adult tolerable upper intake level (UL) for iron has recently been reduced from 75 mg/d to 45 mg/d.

There are many laboratory tests available for assessing iron status. The definitive test is the examination of a bone marrow aspirate. A smear of the marrow is stained with Perls' stain (Prussian blue), which is specific for iron. The particles of stained iron, as well as the number of sideroblasts, are counted and will be decreased in iron deficiency. Although it is a definitive test, the bone marrow examination is not routinely performed because of its highly invasive nature and the great discomfort afforded the patient. It is used when all other diagnostic procedures have been exhausted.

Serum ferritin assay is the test of choice for assessing iron stores (see Chapter 21). Ferritin is quantitated by a variety of methods including radioimmunoassay (RIA), enzyme immunoassay (EIA), immunoradiometric assay (IRMA), and immunofluorometric assay. Reference values vary considerably with the method of assay.

Serum iron concentration, total iron-binding capacity (TIBC) and transferrin saturation are widely used to assess iron status. TIBC is the maximum amount of iron that plasma transferrin can bind. Serum iron is determined by measuring the amount of iron bound to transferrin. Circulating iron is best evaluated by calculating the transferrin (Tf) saturation. The Tf saturation is highly sensitive to recent dietary iron intake. Normally, transferrin is about one third saturated with iron; in deficiency, Tf saturation drops to <15% and iron supply becomes limiting for tissue needs and erythropoiesis requirements. Following measurement of serum iron and TIBC, the transferrin saturation is expressed as a percentage:

$$\frac{\text{Serum iron}}{\text{TIBC}} \times 100 = \% \text{ Transferrin saturation}$$

Serum iron and TIBC are most often quantitated using colorimetric methods. However, both may also be assayed using atomic absorption spectrophotometry (AAS) or by an electrochemical method.

Several hematology tests are used in assessing iron status. Since the ultimate effect of iron deficiency is impaired heme synthesis, tests such as hemoglobin concentration, hematocrit, and red blood cell indices (i.e., mean cell volume [MCV] and mean cell hemoglobin [MCH]) are indicators of late-stage iron deficiency. Iron deficiency anemia is suggested by hemoglobin concentration <12 g/dL for women and 14 g/dL for men. Hematocrits of <37% and 40% for women and men, respectively, are typical of iron deficiency anemia.[87] These measurements are most often performed in a hematology laboratory using an automated hematology instrument.

Finally, the zinc protoporphyrin/heme (ZPP/H) ratio is a functional test for iron status. In the absence of sufficient iron for erythropoiesis, zinc is inserted into the protoporphyrin ring structure of heme. Zinc protoporphyrin accumulates in developing red cells. The ZPP/H ratio, a very sensitive indicator of relative iron deficient erythropoiesis, becomes abnormal very early in the development of iron deficiency. The ZPP/H ratio is easily determined in a sample of whole blood using an instrument called an hematofluorometer.

The reference range for ferritin in men is 20 to 250 ng/mL and in women 20 to 200 ng/mL. Iron deficiency is present at <10 ng/mL and iron overload at >220 ng/mL.

The Tf saturation in men is 20% to 50% and in women, 15% to 50%. Iron deficiency is present at <15%.

The reference range for ZPP/H is <80 $\mu$mol ZPP/mol heme and is increased in iron deficiency.

## IODINE

Iodine is an essential constituent of the thyroid hormones, thyroxine ($T_4$) and triiodothyronine ($T_3$). The storage form of the thyroid hormones in the thyroid gland is the iodine-containing glycoprotein thyroglobulin. Thyroglobulin contains 90% of the total iodine in the gland. Proteolytic enzymes break down thyroglobulin and $T_4$ and $T_3$ are released into the circulation. The pituitary hormone thyroid-stimulating hormone (TSH) controls thyroid secretion. As the blood level of $T_4$ falls, TSH secretion is increased. The iodine in $T_4$ accounts for >80% of all serum iodine. The most abundant thyroid hormone is thyroxine but $T_3$ is the most active thyroid hormone. Deficiency of selenium impairs the conversion of $T_4$ to $T_3$.[88] These hormones regulate the basal metabolic rate of the body. As a result of this function, iodine is important to the growth and development of the body tissues, especially the nervous system. It is essential for normal fetal development. Good sources of iodine include seafood and iodized salt. Water from very deep wells can also be a good source of iodine. Iodine is rapidly absorbed from the GI tract and transported to the thyroid gland for synthesis into thyroid hormones. The main excretory route for iodine is via the urine.

An enlargement of the thyroid gland, known as a goiter, is the most easily recognized evidence of iodine deficiency. Thyroid tissue growth occurs in response to TSH. In severe iodine deficiency, TSH is increased significantly. A major outcome of fetal iodine deficiency is the condition of cretinism, which is characterized by mental deficiency, deaf mutism, and sometimes dwarfism. States require screening of newborns for congenital hypothyroidism, which is the most common cause of infant mental retardation. Blood from heelsticks of newborns is collected on to filter paper, dried, and typically sent to a laboratory for testing. The potential toxic effects of dietary iodine are not clear but there seems to be a wide margin of safety for iodine consumption. Normal diets supply <2000 $\mu$g of iodine a day but intake >2 mg/d reportedly causes no adverse effects. Iodine-induced hyperthyroidism rarely has been reported linked to food (iodized salt) supplementation efforts. The RDA of iodine for adults is 150 $\mu$g/d.

The assessment of iodine nutriture is best accomplished by evaluation of thyroid function tests. Determination of TSH and $T_4$, as well as $T_3$, is readily accomplished by automated immunoassay methods.

## SELENIUM

Selenium is a cofactor of two important enzymes: the antioxidant enzyme glutathione peroxidase, and the thyroid hormone–converting enzyme thyroxine deiodinase. Glutathione peroxidase, an oxidant defense enzyme, protects against the damaging effects of peroxides that are produced when fats are oxidized. The role of selenium as an antioxidant is closely related to two other micronutrients, vitamins E and C. The selenoprotein thyroxine deiodinase catalyzes the conversion of thyroxine ($T_4$) into triiodothyronine ($T_3$). In addition to its actions as part of selenium-dependent enzymes, selenium is thought to have a role in the enhancement of immunocompetence and the production of anticarcinogenic metabolites. The mineral is required for testosterone biosynthesis and formation and development of normal spermatozoa.[89] Normally, selenium is consumed as part of protein and a person consuming diets low in protein may become selenium deficient. Selenium is absorbed in the GI tract. The absorption depends on the solubility of selenium and the amount of sulfur present. The control of selenium excretion in man is not clearly understood; however the main route of excretion is urine.

Three disorders are linked to selenium deficiency: Keshin disease, Kashin-Beck disease, and hypothyroid cretinism.[90] Selenium deficiency predisposes children and women of childbearing age to a cardiomyopathy called Keshan disease, which can lead to congestive heart failure. A significant inverse relationship has been reported between plasma selenium concentration and risk of coronary heart disease.[91] Kashin-Beck disease is an osteoarthropathy of the hands and fingers, elbows, knees, and ankles in children and adolescents. The third disorder, hypothyroid cretinism, is characterized by thyroid injury, decreased $T_3$ production, and mental and growth retardation. Populations at risk for selenium deficiency include those living in areas with low selenium content in the soil used for growing foods, those who are malnourished in general, those with catabolic diseases, and those with inflammatory bowel disease. Individuals with phenylketonuria (PKU) or milder hyperphenylalaninemias (HPAs) who are consuming protein-restricted diets are at risk of selenium deficiency. Deficiency of the selenium cofactor may lead to hypothyroidism in the elderly.[92] Low selenium levels may be observed in a variety of pathologic conditions including colon, gastric, pancreatic and prostate cancers, and cirrhosis. Some epidemiologic and intervention studies suggest an important role for selenium in cancer prevention.[93] A recently initiated study, the Selenium and Vitamin E Cancer Prevention Trial (SELECT), will follow older men in the United States and Canada for a least 7 years to see if taking selenium and/or vitamin supplements has any affect in prostate cancer prevention. Marginal deficiency has been associated with a significantly greater incidence of adverse mood states such as depression, anxiety, hostility, and confusion.[94] Selenium toxicity has been reported resulting from excessive dietary intakes as well as from industrial exposure. Symptoms of selenosis (selenium toxicity) include loss of hair, weakened fingernails, and garlic odor on the breath. The RDA of selenium for both males and females is 55 $\mu$g/d. The upper intake level has been set at 400 $\mu$g/d.[29]

Although it may be measured in serum, plasma, RBCs, whole blood, urine, and hair, selenium levels in whole blood are the most common means of assessing selenium nutritional status.[94,95] To avoid contamination, samples must be collected in metal-free containers. In cases of toxicity, measurement of urinary excretion of selenium may be helpful. Whole-blood selenium is quantitated by AAS or with a fluorometric method; urine samples are analyzed using AAS. The activity of plasma gluthathione peroxidase reflects recent changes in selenium intake. A useful functional index for selenium status is the measurement of glutathione peroxidase activity in erythrocytes. This test, using a UV method, is apt to be run in research settings and is not routinely available in a clinical laboratory.

The reference ranges and toxicity level are as follows:

Whole blood, 58 to 234 $\mu$g/L
Serum, 50 to 140 $\mu$g/L
Urine, 7 to 160 $\mu$g/L
Toxicity, >400 $\mu$g/L

## ZINC

The formation of collagen is dependent on the trace element zinc. Zinc is also a component of insulin, is involved in its storage and release and apparently serves to increase the duration of insulin action after it is injected. Furthermore, zinc is required by at least 70, perhaps over 200, enzymes involved in metabolic activities such as the release of carbon dioxide from tissues to the lungs, synthesis of protein, DNA, and RNA and carbohydrate metabolism. DNA and RNA polymerase activity is dependent on zinc. Zinc functions in cell division and

growth, spermatogenesis, ova formation, pituitary and adrenal gland function, in night vision, in immune defenses, in taste acuity, and in the wound-healing process. Zinc is primarily absorbed in the jejunum and circulates bound to albumin, macroglobulin, and transferrin. In severe hypoalbuminemia, total plasma zinc levels may be low. The major route of excretion from the body is in pancreatic and intestinal secretions but some zinc (400 to 600 $\mu$g or about 5% of total daily zinc) is excreted in the urine and a small amount is lost in sweat.

Zinc deficiency is often associated with diets low in animal protein but high in dietary fiber, which binds zinc, rendering it unable to be absorbed. Febrile diseases and trauma cause zinc to be redistributed from the circulation to the liver, causing an apparent zinc deficiency. Infections cause increased loss of zinc through urinary excretion. In burn patients, the cutaneous loss of zinc is greatly elevated and may lead to zinc deficiency. Therapeutic doses of oral zinc can cause nausea and GI disturbances. Because zinc competes with copper for absorption and transport, zinc supplements can cause a copper-deficiency–induced anemia.[87] A number of diseases predispose a patient to developing zinc deficiency, including alcoholism, inflammatory bowel disease, celiac disease, short bowel syndrome, cystic fibrosis, nephrotic syndrome, hemolytic anemia, and anorexia nervosa. Treatment with anabolic or metal-chelating drugs can cause zinc deficiency. The most commonly recognized signs of zinc deficiency are hair loss and skin lesions. These cutaneous changes seen in zinc deficiency vary widely between patients. The inherited disorder acrodermatitis enteropathica is also a manifestation of zinc deficiency.[96] Owing to the necessity of zinc for collagen formation, poor wound healing is another symptom of zinc deficiency. Individuals with diabetes have been observed to have altered zinc status, including low serum levels of zinc. Correction of zinc deficiency in patients with type 1 diabetes has led to reduced lipid peroxidation. This may be related to the protection of insulin from free radical damage by zinc.[97] Ingestion of zinc lozenges has been claimed to be useful in the treatment of colds by significantly reducing the severity and average duration of cold symptoms. However, study results have been contradictory and it may be that timing of therapy initiation, dosage, and absorption factors are crucial to the final outcomes.[98,99] Chronic ingestion of high doses of zinc supplements may lead to toxicity. Poisoning can also be caused by drinking from galvanized vessels and from inhalation of the fumes of zinc salts. The RDA of zinc for an adult male is 11 mg/d and for an adult female, 8 mg/d.

Zinc levels in blood and urine are easily measured in the laboratory by AAS methods. Serum or plasma are the most common specimens analyzed for nutritional assessment purposes. Urine values are helpful in toxicity studies. The serum concentration of zinc is subject to circadian variations that peak at 0900 and 1800 hours.[100] Zinc levels also decrease postprandially. Therefore, it is best to assay zinc levels from a morning sample after fasting. As with all trace elements, care must be taken to collect samples in metal-free containers and use metal-free glassware or plastic during all steps of analysis.

The reference ranges for zinc are as follows:

Serum/plasma
    Adequate, 70 to 150 $\mu$g/dL
    Deficiency, <70 $\mu$g/dL
Urine
    Adequate, 150 to 1200 $\mu$g/24 h
    Toxicity, >1200 $\mu$g/24 h

## COPPER

Copper, along with iron, is involved in the synthesis of hemoglobin. Copper functions in the formation of collagen and the maintenance of the myelin sheath surrounding nerve fibers. It also is involved in skeletal development, in the function of the immune system, in the formation of melanin for pigmentation, and as a component of the enzyme superoxide dismutase. Reduced availability of copper may thus impair the body's antioxidant defenses. Copper is primarily absorbed in the stomach and duodenum. It circulates bound to albumin and as part of an acute phase protein called ceruloplasmin, which is also important in iron metabolism. Recent studies suggest that about 60% to 70% of plasma copper is bound to ceruloplasmin.[101] The main route of excretion is in the feces.

Copper deficiency occurs in a variety of conditions. Patients with shortened bowels are at risk for copper deficiency, as are infants fed only cow's milk. Menkes' disease, a rare genetic disease, results in impaired copper utilization and therefore severe deficiency. Clinical manifestations include mental retardation, kinky hair, scurvylike bone defects, and generalized arterial disease. Menkes' disease is also known as "kinky hair" syndrome or "steely hair" disease. Copper absorption may be impaired in patients with small bowel disease and in those with high intakes of competing trace elements such as zinc and cadmium. Signs of deficiency include hypochromic anemia, neutropenia, and demineralization of bone. Copper toxicity can occur as a result of ingestion of copper-contaminated solutions such as acidic foods or liquids processed or stored in copper vessels or brass containers, use of copper intrauterine devices (IUDs), or exposure to copper fungicides. Wilson's disease, a genetic disorder, causes toxic copper accumulation, particularly in the liver, kidney, brain, and eyes. Corneal pigmentation in the form of so-called Kayser-Fleischer rings indicates copper deposition in the central nervous system. Early recognition of Wilson's disease is important so that prompt treatment can stop its progression. Although the pathogenic mechanism is unknown, it appears that there is a defect in energy metabolism in Wilson's disease. It has been suggested that free radical formation and oxidative damage, probably due to the accumulation of copper in the mitochondria, are involved.[102] Toxicity from dietary sources is extremely rare. The RDA has recently been established for copper as 900 $\mu$g/d for adult men and women.

At present, there is no laboratory test to adequately assess copper nutriture. Inductively coupled plasma–mass spectrometry (ICP-MS) has proved a powerful tool for trace-element detection in urine, serum, plasma, whole blood, and tissues. More than one element can be detected at the same time. The technique can be used to determine the concentration of many substances including iron, zinc, cobalt, and copper. Serum copper levels are quantitated by AAS and inductively coupled plasma–mass spectrometry methods, but circulating copper concentration is not a valid index of copper status. Ceruloplasmin, the protein-copper complex, has been suggested as an indicator for copper status. However, ceruloplasmin is strongly influenced by hormonal changes and inflammation, which limits its usefulness as an indicator. Copper and ceruloplasmin increase with use of oral contraceptives, in pregnancy and in malignancy. Current research is showing the activity of copper-containing enzymes such as erythrocyte superoxide dismutase and cytochrome oxidase in platelets or leukocytes to be a better indicator of metabolically active copper stores. Improved methods for determining activity of these enzymes in tissues and blood cells will provide a means of reliably assessing copper status. These assays, however, are not routinely available.[101]

The reference ranges for copper are as follows:

Serum
    Males, 70 to 140 $\mu$g/dL
    Females, 80 to 155 $\mu$g/dL
    Adults over age 60 years
        Males, 85 to 170 $\mu$g/L
        Females, 85 to 190 $\mu$g/L
    Pregnant females, 120 to 300 $\mu$g/dL
    Blacks, 8% to 12% higher
    Wilson's disease, 40 to 60 $\mu$g/dL
Urine, 3 to 35 $\mu$g/24 h
    Wilson's disease, >100 $\mu$g/24 h

## FLUORINE (FLUORIDE)

The trace element fluorine, as fluoride, has the primary function of maintaining dental health. Fluoride is deposited in the enamel portion of teeth and acts by enhancing the ability of the teeth to withstand the acid formed by cavity-causing bacteria. It has also been suggested that fluoride may play a role in protecting adult bone structure and in the treatment of osteoporosis. The main route of excretion is in urine.

Fluoride deficiency in humans leads to increased susceptibility to dental caries. In laboratory animals, deficiency has resulted in anemia and impaired growth and reproduction. Fluoride is toxic when consumed in excess. Chronic toxicity, known as fluorosis, affects bone health, kidney function, and possibly muscle and nerve function. The estimated safe and adequate daily intake of fluoride is 1.5 to 4.0 mg/d with primary sources being fluoridated water and fluoride toothpaste and mouth rinses. Beverages such as bottled water and commercially prepared foods processed with fluoridated water also supply fluoride to the diet.

TABLE 33-9

**Laboratory Assessment and Indices for Monitoring Selected Ultratrace Elements**

| ULTRATRACE ELEMENT | SPECIMEN | REFERENCE RANGE | TOXIC LEVEL | ASSAY METHOD |
|---|---|---|---|---|
| Chromium | Whole blood | 2–10 ng/mL | >100 ng/mL | AAS |
| | Serum, plasma | 0.1–2 ng/mL | >5 ng/mL | |
| | Urine (24 h) | <8 μg/24 h | >100 μg/24 h | |
| | Urine (random) | <0.5–6 ng/mL | >30 μg/g creatinine | |
| Cobalt | Whole blood | 0.5–3.9 ng/mL | Not established | ICP-MS |
| | Serum, plasma | 0.1–0.4 ng/mL | | |
| | Urine (24 h) | <2 μg/24 h | Not established | AAS |
| | Urine (random) | <2 ng/mL | Not established | AAS |
| Fluorine (fluoride) | Serum | 0.01–0.2 μg/mL | >8.0 mg/L | ISE |
| | Urine | 0.2–3.2 μg/mL | | |
| Nickel | Whole blood | 4–28 ng/mL | >100 ng/mL | AAS |
| | Serum | 1.5–4 ng/mL | >10 ng/mL | |
| | Urine (24 hrs) | <6.4 μg/24 h | Not established | |
| | Urine (random) | <5 ng/mL | >10 ng/mL | |

AAS = atomic absorption spectrometry; ICP-MS = inductively coupled plasma–mass spectrometry; ISE = ion-specific electrode.

Adapted from Leiken JB, Davis A, Tharratt RS, Dickey JH. Selected topics related to occupational exposures. Disease-a-Month 46(9), 2000.

Fluoride is not measured clinically as part of nutritional assessment. However, techniques such as ion-selective potentiometry and gas-liquid chromatography are available to measure fluoride in plasma and urine (Table 33–9). Measurement of fluoride is usually reserved for monitoring fluoride treatment or cases of toxicity.

The reference ranges for fluoride are as follows:

Plasma or serum, 0.01 to 0.2 μg/mL
Urine, 0.2 to 3.2 μg/mL
Toxicity, >8.0 mg/L

## MANGANESE

Manganese functions in activating a wide variety of enzymes including decarboxylases, hydrolases, kinases, and transferases. It functions biochemically in oxidative phosphorylation, fatty-acid metabolism and synthesis of proteins, cholesterol, and mucopolysaccharides. Manganese is absorbed in the small intestine. It may be bound to alpha$_2$-macroglobulin for transport in the portal circulation to the liver. If oxidized, it may be transported from the liver by transferrin. Iron competes with manganese for common binding sites during absorption. It is excreted primarily via the bile in the feces.

Women with osteoporosis have been reported to have lowered plasma manganese levels, but manganese deficiency has not been observed in free-living human populations. However, deficiency has been observed in institutionalized, malnourished individuals. Signs of deficiency include poor reproductive function, growth retardation, abnormal formation of bone,

and impaired glucose tolerance. Because the liver maintains manganese homeostasis, any disorder that interrupts enterohepatic circulation poses a risk of manganese deficiency. Toxicity has only been observed in workers exposed to high concentrations of manganese dust or fumes. Toxicity has not been observed as a consequence of dietary intake. The recently established AI for manganese is 2.3 mg/d for adult men and 1.8 mg/d for adult women.

Progress in the field of manganese nutrition has been thwarted by the lack of a practical method for assessing manganese status. Manganese can be quantitated in the blood and urine by AAS methods. However, consistent differences in manganese levels of repleted versus depleted subjects have not been observed.

## Ultratrace Elements

### MOLYBDENUM

Molybdenum is a constituent of the metalloenzymes aldehyde oxidase, sulfite oxidase, and xanthine oxidase, which are involved in the metabolism of nucleic acids to uric acid. Molybdenum is absorbed rapidly in the GI tract and transported to the liver. Its primary route of excretion is the urine (90%), with a lesser amount (10%) removed in the bile.[103]

The RDA for molybdenum has recently been set at 45 μg/d for men and women. The requirement for molybdenum is so low that it is easily furnished in the typical American diet. Molybdenum deficiency due to dietary restriction occurs only very rarely. It has been reported in patients receiving parenteral methionine therapy. Biochemical evidence of deficiency includes abnormal sulfur metabolism and uric acid production; clinical presentation includes mental disturbance and ultimately coma (See Table 33–6). Chronic exposure to high environmental concentrations of molybdenum produces loss of appetite, lethargy, diarrhea, and anemia; uric acid concentrations in both serum and urine are elevated.

Molybdenum is not routinely assayed in the clinical laboratory. However, it can be quantitated in blood and urine by AAS methods. However, the limit of quantitation of AAS is too high to evaluate deficiency. The requisite sensitivity can be achieved if neutron activation analysis is used. This technique is not readily available. Increased plasma methionine and decreased urinary uric acid are characteristic laboratory findings in molybdenum deficiency.

## CHROMIUM

Chromium is part of the organic compound called glucose tolerance factor (GTF). Because of its function as part of GTF, chromium is important in maintaining normal glucose metabolism.[104] By potentiating the action of insulin, chromium increases glucose uptake by cells and promotes intracellular car-

bohydrate and lipid metabolism. Chromium is absorbed intestinally and excreted in urine.

Deficient chromium intake is believed to be an aggravating factor in the development of impaired glucose tolerance and type 2 diabetes. Chromium supplementation appears to achieve beneficial responses in subjects with demonstrated glucose intolerance.[105] Supplemental chromium for women with gestational diabetes has been reported to improve glucose tolerance and decrease hyperinsulinemia. Reversal of uncontrolled, steroid-induced diabetes has also been described.[106] Chromium deficiency has also been reported in protein calorie malnutrition and some cases of coronary artery disease. Toxicity due to dietary chromium has not been reported. However, chronic exposure of workers to dust containing chromate has been linked with an increased incidence of bronchial cancer. Studies of chromium nutrition are scarce; therefore, it is difficult to establish a recommended intake. The recently set AI for young men is 35 $\mu$g/d and 25 $\mu$g/d for young women.

Because of lack of methods to diagnose chromium status, it is rarely measured in the laboratory. In the research setting, chromium lends itself to measurement by AAS techniques (See Table 33–9).

TABLE 33–10

**Adult Reference Ranges for Biochemical Markers of Micronutrient Status Commonly Assayed in the Clinical Laboratory**

| TEST | SPECIMEN | REFERENCE RANGE |
|---|---|---|
| **Vitamin status** | | |
| Ascorbic acid (C) | Serum | 0.4–0.6 mg/dL |
| Cobalamin (B$_{12}$) | Serum | 110–800 pg/mL |
| Folate | Serum | 3–16 ng/mL |
| | RBC | 130–630 ng/mL |
| Retinol (A) | Serum | 300–800 $\mu$g/L |
| 25-OH D$_3$ | Serum | 14–42 ng/mL |
| 1,25(OH)$_2$D$_3$ | Serum | 15–45 pg/mL |
| Tocopherol (E) | Serum | 5–7 mg/L |
| **Trace/ultratrace element status** | | |
| Ferritin | Serum | M: 20–250 ng/mL |
| | | F: 20–200 ng/mL |
| Transferrin saturation | Serum | M: 20–50% |
| | | F: 15–50% |
| | Whole blood | <80 $\mu$mol/mol |
| Zinc protoporphyrin/heme ratio | Whole blood | 58–243 $\mu$g/dL |
| | Urine | 7–160 $\mu$g/L |
| Selenium | Serum | 70–150 $\mu$g/dL |
| | Urine | 150–1200 $\mu$g/d |
| Zinc | Serum | M: 70–140 $\mu$g/dL |
| | Urine | F: 80–155 $\mu$g/dL |
| Copper | | 3–35 $\mu$g/24 h |

M = male; F = female.

## COBALT

The only known nutritional function of **cobalt** is as an integral component of vitamin $B_{12}$ (cobalamin). It is abundant in the diet and is absorbed from the GI tract. In humans, there are no reports of cobalt deficiency leading to vitamin $B_{12}$ deficiency. There is no evidence that cobalt in the human diet is limited; therefore, no RDA is necessary. Assay methods for cobalt include both AAS and ICP-MS (See Table 33–9).

## NICKEL

Studies have shown nickel to be important for growth, reproduction, hematopoiesis, and iron and zinc metabolism. Nickel is absorbed in the small intestine and excreted in urine. Low levels of nickel may occur in patients with cirrhosis or chronic uremia. Toxicity has not been reported from dietary intake, although toxicity due to industrial exposure has been observed. The requirement for nickel in humans is very low. A safe and adequate intake is probably in the range of 35 to 500 μg/d. The most reliable means of evaluating nickel status is the measurement of serum and urine nickel concentration. Although rarely performed, nickel may be quantitated by AAS techniques (See Table 33–9).

## SILICON

Silicon is apparently involved in the normal growth of bone. Silicon deficiency leads to structural abnormalities of the long bones and skull as well as impaired connective tissue formation.

## TIN

Investigations suggest that stunted growth and impaired reproduction may be linked to diets very low in tin and vanadium. The site of action for tin is in fatty tissue, where it is believed to be involved in oxidation-reduction reactions. This, however, is speculation. There are no reports of clinical conditions arising from tin deficiency in humans.

## VANADIUM

Vanadium influences various aspects of glucose metabolism including uptake by cells, oxidation, and synthesis of glycogen. It appears to mimic the effect of insulin.[107] See Table 33–6. Most ingested vanadium is not absorbed and passes out of the body in the feces. Absorbed vanadium is eliminated by renal excretion. The human requirement for vanadium is not established, but it has been estimated to be between 10 and 25 μg/d. A typical American diet probably supplies 10 to 60 μg daily. Reported levels of vanadium in healthy adults are:[87]

Plasma or serum, 0.02 to 10 ng/mL
Urine, 0 to 10 μg/24 h
Hair, 0.01 to 2.2 μg/g

Nutritional requirements for these trace elements are extremely low and are easily met by levels naturally occurring in food and water. The biochemical markers of protein, carbohydrate, lipid, vitamin, and trace element status discussed in this chapter are summarized in Table 33–10.

## SUMMARY

Nutritional assessment encompasses myriad methods to define the nutritional status of an individual. The common goal of these methods is to identify the patient with altered nutritional status that might lead to adverse clinical events. Objective evaluation of nutritional status is essential for identifying patients at risk for malnutrition, for delivering appropriate nutritional care, and for monitoring progress of nutritional therapy. As the benefits of nutritional therapy are more widely recognized, the demand for nutritional assessment will increase.

The incidence of malnutrition, especially among hospitalized populations, has been well established and the adverse effects of even marginal malnutrition are beginning to be recognized. The RDAs for the essential nutrients have been carefully defined in an effort to avoid the occurrence of malnutrition. However, regardless of these efforts, and as a result of numerous social and economic factors, many segments of the population remain at risk for development of nutrient deficiencies. Marginal malnutrition and single nutrient deficiencies may be difficult to diagnose prior to the advanced stages of clinical symptoms. However, specific biochemical changes are often present before the manifestation of symptoms and improved laboratory procedures aid in the identification of malnutrition well before symptoms or tissue damage appear.

There are several components of a complete nutritional assessment. Dietary, physical, and anthropometric data as well as biochemical data are all important factors in determining the nutritional status of an individual. These four types of measurements are employed collectively to obtain the most complete and accurate picture of an individual's nutritional status. Presymptomatic malnutrition can be diagnosed with specific and sensitive assays. The clinical laboratory's importance in nutritional assessment lies in the ability to objectively measure the levels of both macronutrients and micronutrients.

### REFERENCES

1. Labbe R, Veldee M: Nutrition in the clinical laboratory. Clin Lab Med 13:314, 1993.
2. Mullen JL, Buzby GP, Walman MT, et al.: Prediction of operative morbidity and mortality by preoperative nutritional assessment. Surg Forum 30:80, 1979.
3. Ingenbleek Y, Van Den Schrieck HG, DeNayer P, et al.: Albumin, transferrin and thyroxine-binding prealbumin/retinol-binding protein (TBPA-RBP) complex in assessment of malnutrition. Clin Chim Acta 63:61, 1975.
4. Gibson R: *Principles of Nutritional Assessment.* New York, Oxford University Press, 1990.

5. Spiekerman M: Proteins used in nutritional assessment. Clin Lab Med 13:353, 1993.

6. Charney P: Nutrition assessment in the 90's: Where are we now? Nutr Clin Pract 10:131, 1995.

7. Ingenbleek Y: Usefulness of prealbumin as nutritional indicator. In Allen RC, Bienvenu J, Laurent P, Suskind RM (eds.): *Marker Proteins in Inflammation.* New York, Walter de Gruyter, 1982, p 37.

8. Vanlandingham S, Spiekerman M, Newmark SR: P realbumin: A parameter of visceral protein levels during albumin infusion. J Parenter Enter Nutr 6:230, 1982.

9. Carpentier YA, Barthel J, Bruyns J: Plasma protein concentration in nutritional assessment. Proc Nutr Soc 4: 405, 1982.

10. Bourry J, Milano G, Caldani C, et al.: Assessment of nutritional proteins during parenteral nutrition of cancer patients. Ann Clin Lab Sci 12:158, 1982.

11. Winkler MF, Gerrior S, Pomp A, et al.: Use of retinol-binding protein and prealbumin as indicators of the response to nutrition therapy. J Am Diet Assoc 89:684, 1989.

12. Clemmons DR, Underwood LE, Dickerson RN, et al.: Use of plasma somatomedin-C/insulin-like growth factor 1 measurements to monitor the response to nutritional repletion in malnourished patients. Am J Clin Nutr 41:191, 1985.

13. Mosher DF: Physiology of fibronectin. Ann Rev Med 35:561, 1984.

14. Konstantinides FN: Nitrogen balance studies in clinical nutrition. Clin Pract 7:231, 1992.

15. Blackburn GL, Bistrian BR, Maini BS, et al.: Nutritional and metabolic assessment of the hospitalized patient. Parenter Enter Nutr 1:11, 1977.

16. Statland BE: Vitamins and minerals: Passing fads or keys to health. MLO 25(12):21, 1993.

17. Auxter S: Testing the "wellness" of baby boomers. Clin Lab News 24(7):29, 1998.

18. Yates AA, Schlicker SA, Suitor CW: Dietary reference intakes: The new basis for recommendations for calcium and related nutrients, B vitamins and choline. J Am Diet Assoc 98:699, 1998.

19. Monsen ER: Dietary reference intakes for the antioxidant nutrients: Vitamin C, vitamin E, selenium, and carotenoids. J Am Diet Assoc 100:637, 2000.

20. Levine M, Rumsey SC, Daruwala R, et al.: Criteria and recommendations for vitamin C intake. JAMA 281: 1415, 1999.

21. Carr AC, Frei B: Toward a new recommended dietary allowance for vitamin C based on antioxidant and health effects in humans. Am J Clin Nutr 69:1086, 1999.

22. Miller SM: Antioxidants and aging. MLO 29(9):42, 1997.

23. Bankson D, Kestin M, Rifai N: Role of free radicals in cancer and atherosclerosis. Clin Lab Med 13:463, 1993.

24. Ness AR, Khaw KT, Bingham S, Day NE: Vitamin C status and blood pressure. J Hypertens 14:503,1996.

25. Gokce N, Keaney JF, Frei B, Holbrook M, et al.: Long-term ascorbic acid administration reverses endothelial vasomotor dysfunction in patients with coronary artery disease. Circulation 99:3234, 1999.

26. Noroozi M, Angerson WJ, Lean MEJ: Effects of flavonoids and vitamin C on oxidative DNA damage to human lymphocytes. Am J Clin Nutr 67:1210, 1998.

27. Correa P: Human gastric carcinogenesis. Cancer Res 52:6735, 1992.

28. Loria CM, Klag MJ, Caulfield LE, Whelton PK: Vitamin C status and mortality in U.S. adults. Am J Clin Nutr 72:139, 2000.

29. National Academy of Science, Food and Nutrition Board, Institute of Medicine: *Dietary Reference Intakes for Vitamin C, Vitamin E, Selenium, and Carotenoids.* Washington, DC, National Academy Press, 2000.

30. Dashman T, Sansaricq C: Nutrition in the management of inborn errors of metabolism. Clin Lab Med 13:407, 1993.

31. Lockitch G, Halstead AC: Pediatric nutrition. In Soldin SJ, Rifai N, Hicks JMB (eds.): *Biochemical Basis of Pediatric Disease.* 2nd ed. Washington, DC, AACC Press, 1995, p 19.

32. Jacobsen DW: Homocysteine and vitamins in cardiovascular disease. Clin Chem 44:1833, 1998.

33. Hustad S, Ueland PM, Vollset SE, Zhang Y, et al.: Riboflavin as a determinant of plasma total homocysteine: Effect modification by the methylenetetrahydrofolate reductase C677T polymorphism. Clin Chem 46:1065, 2000.

34. Callanan D, Blodi BA, Martin DF: Macular edema associated with nicotinic acid (niacin). JAMA 279:1702, 1998.

35. Wyatt KM, Dimmock PW, Jones PW, O'Brien S: Efficacy of vitamin B-6 in the treatment of premenstrual syndrome: Systematic review. BMJ 318:1375, 1999.

36. Refsum H, Ueland PM, Nygard O, Vollset SE: Homocysteine and cardiovascular disease. Annu Rev Med 49:31, 1998.

37. Ray JG, Laskin CA: Folic acid and homocyst(e)ine metabolic defects and the risk of placental abruption, pre-eclampsia and spontaneous pregnancy loss: A systematic review. Placenta 20:519, 1999.

38. South M: Neonatal seizures after use of pyridoxine in pregnancy. Lancet 353:1940, 1999.

39. Innis SM, Allardyce DB: Possible biotin deficiency in adults receiving long-term total parenteral nutrition. Am J Clin Nutr 37:185, 1983.

40. Zempleni J, Mock DM: Bioavailability of biotin given orally to humans in pharmacologic doses. Am J Clin Nutr 69:506, 1999.

41. Zempleni J, Mock DM: Advanced analysis of biotin metabolites in body fluids allows a more accurate mea-

surement of biotin bioavailability and metabolism in humans. J Nutr 129:494S, 1999.

42. Baranoski CLN, Miller SM: Biotinidase deficiency: The screening of newborns. Part 2. ADVANCE for Administrators of the Laboratory 8(9):22, 1999.

43. Wolf B: Disorders of biotin metabolism. In Scriver CR, Beaudet AL, Sly WS, Valle D (eds.): *The Metabolic and Molecular Basis of Inherited Disease.* 7th ed. New York, McGraw-Hill, 1995, p 3151.

44. Williams RH, Maggiore JA: Hyperhomocysteinemia. Pathogenesis, clinical significance, laboratory assessment, and treatment. Lab Med 30:468, 1999.

45. Snow CF: Laboratory diagnosis of vitamin B₁₂ and folate deficiency. Arch Intern Med 159:1289, 1999.

46. Ho C, Kauwell GPA, Bailey LB: Practitioners' guide to meeting the vitamin B-12 recommended dietary allowance for people aged 51 years and older. J Am Diet Assoc 99:725, 1999.

47. Koop H: Metabolic consequences of long-term inhibition of acid secretion by omeprazole. Aliment Pharmacol Ther 6:399, 1992.

48. Ueland PM, Refsum H, Stabler SP, Malinow MR, et al.: Total homocysteine in plasma or serum: Methods and clinical applications. Clin Chem 29:1764, 1993.

49. Klee GG: Cobalamin and folate evaluation: Measurement of methylmalonic acid and homocysteine vs vitamin B₁₂ and folates. Clin Chem 46:1277, 2000.

50. Williams RH, Maggiore JA: Hyperhomocysteinemia. Pathogenesis, clinical significance, laboratory assessment, and treatment. Lab Med 30(7):468, 1999.

51. Miller SM: Preventing and detecting neural tube defects. MLO 31(5):32, 1999.

52. Balluz LS, Kieszak SM, Philen RM, Mulinare J: Vitamin and mineral supplement use in the United States. Arch Fam Med 9:258, 2000.

53. Weir DG, Scott JM: Colonic mucosal folate concentrations and their association with colorectal cancer. Am J Clin Nutr 68:763, 1998.

54. McCully KS: Homocysteine, folate, vitamin B₆, and cardiovascular disease. JAMA 279:392, 1998.

55. Russell R: The vitamin A spectrum: From deficiency to toxicity. Am J Clin Nutr 71:878, 2000.

56. Binkley N, Krueger D: Hypervitaminosis A and bone. Nutr Rev 58(5):138, 2000.

57. Alpha-Tocopherol, Beta-Carotene Cancer Prevention Study Group: The effect of vitamin E and beta-carotene on the incidence of lung cancer and other cancers in male smokers. N Engl J Med 330:1029, 1994.

58. Omenn GS, Goodman GE, Thornquist M, Balmes J, et al.: Risk factors for lung cancer and for intervention effects in CARET, the beta-carotene and retinol efficacy trial. J Natl Cancer Inst 88:1550, 1996.

59. Fitzpatrick S, Sheard NF, Clark NG, Ritter ML: Vitamin D-deficient rickets: A multifactorial disease. Nutr Rev 58(7):218, 2000.

60. Welch TR, Bergstrom WH, Tsang RC: Vitamin D-deficient rickets: The reemergence of a once-conquered disease. J Pediatr 137:143, 2000.

61. Kreiter SR, Schwartz RP, Kirkman HN Jr, et al.: Nutritional rickets in African American breast-fed infants. J Pediatr 137:153, 2000.

62. Miller PD: Management of osteoporosis. Dis Mon 45(2):24, 1999.

63. Utiger RD: The need for more vitamin D. N Engl J Med 338:828, 1998.

64. Jialal I, Devaraj S: Low-density lipoprotein oxidation, antioxidants, and atherosclerosis: A clinical biochemistry perspective. Clin Chem 42:498, 1996.

65. Devaraj S, Li D, Jialal I: The effects of alpha tocopherol supplementation on monocyte function. Decreased lipid oxidation, interleukin 1β secretion, and monocyte adhesion to endothelium. J Clin Invest 98:756, 1996.

66. Jonas CR, Ziegler TR: Nutrition support and antioxidant defenses: A cause for concern. Am J Clin Nutr 68:765, 1998.

67. Meydani SN, Meydani M, Blumberg JB, et al.: Vitamin E supplementation and in vivo immune response in healthy elderly subjects. A randomized controlled trial. JAMA 227:1380, 1997.

68. Rimm E, Stampfer M, Ascherio A, et al.: Vitamin E consumption and risk of coronary heart disease in men. N Engl J Med 328:1450, 1993.

69. Stampfer M, Hennekens C, Manson J, et al.: Vitamin E consumption and the risk of coronary disease in women. N Engl J Med 328:1444, 1993.

70. Miller JW: Vitamin E and memory: Is it vascular protection? Nutr Rev 58(4):109, 2000.

71. Rashid M, Durie P, Andrew M, Kalnins D, et al.: Prevalence of vitamin K deficiency in cystic fibrosis. Am J Clin Nutr 70:378, 1999.

72. Booth SL, Suttie JW: Dietary intake and adequacy of vitamin K. J Nutr 128:785, 1998.

73. Weber P: The role of vitamins in the prevention of osteoporosis—A brief status report. Int J Vitam Nutr Res 69(3):194, 1999.

74. Feskanich D, Weber P, Willett WC, Rockett H, et al.: Vitamin K intake and hip fracture in women: A prospective study. Am J Clin Nutr 69:74, 1999.

75. Booth SL, Tucker KL, Chen H, Hannan MT, et al.: Dietary vitamin K intakes are associated with hip fractures but not with bone mineral density in elderly men and women. Am J Clin Nutr 71:1201, 2000.

76. Sokoll LJ, O'Brien ME, Camilo ME, Sadowski JA: Undercarboxylated osteocalcin and development of a method to determine vitamin K status. Clin Chem 8(Part 1):1121, 1995.

77. Greer FR, Marshall SP, Foley AL, Suttie JW: Improving the vitamin K status of breastfeeding infants with maternal vitamin K supplements. Pediatrics 99:88, 1997.

78. Booth SL: Warfarin use and fracture risk. Nutr Rev 58(1):20, 2000.

79. Gundberg CM, Nieman SD, Abrams S, Rosen H: Vitamin K status and bone health: An analysis of methods for determination of undercarboxylated osteocalcin. J Clin Endocrinol Metab 83:3258, 1998.

80. Sokoll LJ, Sadowski JA: Comparison of biochemical indexes for assessing vitamin K nutritional status in a healthy adult population. Am J Clin Nutr 63:566, 1996.

81. Yip R, Mehra M: Individual functional roles of metal ions in vivo. Iron. In Berthon G (ed.): *Handbook of Metal-Ligand Interactions in Biological Fluids. Bioinorganic Medicine.* Vol. I. New York, Marcel Dekker, 1995, p 207.

82. Monsen E: The ironies of iron. Am J Clin Nutr 69:831, 1999.

83. Dallman PR, Siimes MA, Stekel A: Iron deficiency in infancy and childhood. Am J Clin Nutr 33:86, 1980.

84. Fairbanks VF, Klee GG: Biochemical aspects of hematology. In Burtis CA (ed.): *Tietz Textbook of Clinical Chemistry.* 3rd ed. Philadelphia, WB Saunders, 1999, p 1702.

85. National Research Council: Iron. *A Report of the Subcommittee on Iron, Committee on Medical and Biologic Effects of Environmental Pollutants, Division of Medical Sciences, Assembly of Life Sciences.* Washington DC, National Academy Press, 1986.

86. de Valk B, Marx JJM: Iron, atherosclerosis, and ischemic heart disease. Arch Intern Med 159:1542, 1999.

87. Groff JL, Gropper SS: *Advanced Nutrition and Human Metabolism.* 3rd ed. Belmont, CA, Wadsworth, 2000, p 402.

88. Arthur J: Interrelationships between selenium deficiency, iodine deficiency, and thyroid hormones. Am J Clin Nutr 57:253S, 1993.

89. Rayman MP: The importance of selenium to human health. Lancet 356:233, 2000.

90. Utiger RD: Kashin-Beck disease—Expanding the spectrum of iodine-deficiency disorders. N Engl J Med 339:1156, 1998.

91. Mikkelsen SL, Bottner RK, Paoli C: Selenium and other plasma element concentrations in coronary heart disease. Lab Med 23(2):122, 1992.

92. Chan S, Gerson B, Subramaniam S: The role of copper, molybdenum, selenium, and zinc in nutrition and health. Clin Lab Med 18(4):673, 1998.

93. Ip C: Lessons from basic research in selenium and cancer prevention. J Nutr 128:1845, 1998.

94. Lockitch G: Trace elements in pediatrics. J Int Fed Clin Chem 9(2):46, 1996.

95. Ash O: Trace elements: When essential nutrients become poisonous. Lab Med 26(4):266, 1995.

96. Ulmer DD: Trace elements. N Engl J Med 297(6):318, 1977.

97. Anderson RA: Role of dietary factors: Micronutrients. Nutr Rev 58 (II):S10, 2000.

98. Jackson J, Peterson C, Lesho A: A meta-analysis of zinc salt lozenges and the common cold. Arch Intern Med 157:2372, 1997.

99. Prasad AS, Fitzgerald JT, Bao B, Beck FWJ, Chandrasekar PH: Duration of symptoms and plasma cytokine levels in patients with the common cold treated with zinc acetate. Ann Intern Med 2000 133:245, 2000.

100. Guillard O, Pirious A, Gombert J, Reiss D: Diurnal variation of zinc, copper and magnesium in the serum of normal fasting adults. Biomed 31:193, 1979.

101. Milne D: Assessment of copper nutritional status. Clin Chem 40:1479, 1994.

102. Gu M, Cooper JM, Butler P, Walker AP, Mistry PK, et al.: Oxidative-phosphorylation defects in liver of patients with Wilson's diseased. Lancet 356:469, 2000.

103. Chan S, Gerson B, Subramaniam S: The role of copper, molybdenum, selenium, and zinc in nutrition and health. Clin Lab Med 18(4):673, 1998.

104. Vincent JB: Quest for the molecular mechanism of chromium action and its relationship to diabetes. Nutr Rev 58(3):(I)67, 2000.

105. Anderson RA: Chromium, glucose intolerance and diabetes. J Am Coll Nutr 17:548, 1998.

106. Ravina A, Slezak L, Mirsky N, et al.: Reversal of corticosteroid-induced diabetes with supplemental chromium. Diabet Med 16:164, 1999.

# CHAPTER 34

# Point-of-Care Testing

*Jean D. Holter*

Point-of-care testing (POCT) is also called near-patient testing. It is generally any analytical laboratory testing of a patient specimen that occurs near the location of the patient and outside the main clinical laboratory of the hospital. Most analytical tests performed in a point-of-care setting are classified as waivered by the Clinical Laboratory Improvement Act '88 (CLIA '88). This type of testing is classified as waivered because it typically does not pose a significant risk to the patient.[1]

The purpose of developing a point-of-care laboratory is to provide the physician with the results in a timely manner when a decision needs to be made concerning care for the patient. Situations in which point-of-care test results are needed would be in the emergency department, the operating room, and the intensive and critical care units. A timely result may also be justified in other areas of the hospital, but the emphasis should be on immediate results that benefit the patient and not for the sake of convenience. The major concern of the physicians that has led to the establishment of a POCT laboratory is the turnaround time, which is the time from the physician's request to the time the actual laboratory result is reported.

In the outpatient/ambulatory care setting, it is important that the physician obtain laboratory test results as soon as possible. This situation may be better served by a satellite laboratory rather than a POCT laboratory. For the hospitalized patient, the emphasis is on medical management and the reduction of the length of stay for the patient. The question then is, does POCT reduce the length of stay and improve the medical management of the patient?

The characteristics of most POCT systems are that they are self-contained and portable. The system should require minimal training of personnel to operate the instruments and minimal maintenance to maintain the system. The longer the reagents are stable at room temperature, the less chance of reagent problems during testing. A system that generates a printout of the results and can be interfaced to a laboratory computer would be advantageous.

## THE POCT LABORATORY

### Variables

Many POCT laboratories are developed because of the turnaround time in relation to the main laboratory testing. Turnaround time in the main laboratory can be affected by preanalytical variables, analytical variables, and postanalytical variables. The preanalytical variables include the time from the physician request, to the drawing of the blood specimen, and the delivery of the sample to the laboratory. POCT laboratories decrease many of the prenalytical variables because the personnel are in that particular area and can obtain the sample and analyze it as soon as the sample is obtained. If the sample is being collected by the main laboratory personnel, the laboratory needs to be notified, the phlebotomist needs to obtain the sample, and the sample needs to be delivered to the laboratory. There could be delays depending on the responsibilities and the location of the phlebotomist at the time of the physician's request. POCT reduces the time involved in the preanalytical area. The use of a pneumatic tube system that connects the laboratory to each area of the hospital and outpatient areas has assisted in reducing the preanalytical time for specimen transport to the main laboratory. This may be the solution rather than POCT.

Most samples for POCT testing are obtained via a fingerstick. This sample can be contaminated with interstitial fluids if the specimen is not collected properly, which results in a preanalytical error.

For the analytical time, the delay in the main laboratory is related to the number of other requests being performed. If the laboratorian has 10 urgent requests to be analyzed, they are analyzed in the order received in the laboratory since the laboratorian has no knowledge that a particular patient has a more critical condition than another patient. The actual analysis time of the sample is not very different between that performed in the POCT and the main laboratory because similar methodologies are utilized.

The postanalytical variables are related to the reporting of the patient result. A POCT laboratorian can deliver the result directly to the physician in minutes after completing the analysis. In the main laboratory, depending on the system used, the report may need to be telephoned to the physician, the floor, or the nurse. The result may need to be entered onto a log sheet that is transferred to a report or manually entered into a computer. If the procedure and the laboratory are computerized, the result may need to be verified by the technologist before the result is sent to the unit requesting the test. Since the laboratory is servicing all areas of the hospital, there may be a delay in the results being completed and the physician knowing the result. If the result is computerized and sent to the requesting unit, then it is the responsibility of someone on that unit to check for the result.

## Personnel

If the POCT is classified as waived by CLIA '88, then anyone can perform the tests. POCT is generally performed by non-laboratorians or nonmedical technologists. The personnel must be trained in the procedure and complete competencies related to test performance annually. The personnel performing POCT testing must have a knowledge of the procedure so that they can interpret the results as being valid or not. Many of the problems with the test results relate to the technique of the personnel performing the test. An inaccurate technique may lead to inaccurate results.

## Need for POCT

The administration of the institution must decide if a POCT laboratory is required. The underlying basis for this is that patient care will be improved. POCT testing should be of high quality so that results are similar to those of the main laboratory. This quality and reliability is especially important so that the physician has results that are a continuous evaluation for patient care. A study correlating the results between the two laboratories will be required.

Another factor to be considered is the cost of the POCT. Usually, POCT costs are higher than the cost in the main laboratory. The point-of-care instrumentation is less expensive than the instrumentation in the main laboratory, but the cost of reagents and consumables is typically higher than those of the main laboratory. The main laboratory is able to batch tests, which results in lower consumable costs.

The instruments for the POCT laboratory will need to be calibrated on a periodic basis (usually every 24 hours) and quality control samples will need to be analyzed at predetermined intervals. For some POCT instruments, the quality control testing may be performed every 24 hours or every time a patient test is analyzed. These quality control samples need to be evaluated before the patient test result is completed and released. In addition, the quality control samples must be analyzed and evaluated on a monthly basis.

Other factors that influence the POCT laboratory are the competency of the personnel available to perform the tests requested. In the final evaluation, does patient care benefit by having the laboratory tests performed in a POCT laboratory? Will these results improve patient care and outcomes?

Can the problem be corrected without the expense of a POCT laboratory? Is this something that a pneumatic tube system can correct? Or is there some other inadequacy in the current testing system in the main laboratory? If the turnaround time for the test can be improved without the use of a POCT laboratory, then the POCT laboratory is not warranted.

Another variable is the cost of personnel to perform the test. Who will be performing the tests? In some hospitals, the laboratory is responsible for performing the POCT. This can

be expensive if a technologist is paid to be available to perform the tests and has no other responsibilities. Once this person is given other responsibilities, the turnaround times may be adversely affected. If the nursing personnel are performing the test, then time may be taken away from patient care. Although it may not take much time to perform the test, say about 10 minutes to run controls and the sample, and the nurse performs 10 tests each shift, that is 100 minutes that the nurse is not available for direct patient care during a particular shift.

The instrument will also require periodic maintenance. Is a maintenance contract needed for the instrument? How often is maintenance required? How long does it take to perform the maintenance?

Space needs to be dedicated to the storage of reagents and the instruments when they are not in use. This can mean the addition of a refrigerator or other storage space. In addition to space for reagents and the instruments, there needs to be some mechanism for the disposal of biological materials. Depending on the location of the POCT, this may or may not be a problem.

There will also need to be someone responsible for the ordering of supplies and validating that the new reagents are comparable to the reagents in use. A new reagent must be evaluated before patient samples can be analyzed. This is accomplished through calibration and quality control procedures.

## EVALUATION

There needs to be some evaluation of the current system in the main laboratory and the possibility of the establishment of a POCT laboratory. This evaluation is best done with a committee composed of physicians that desire POCT, laboratory personnel, nursing staff, and any other personnel that would be involved in the use of a POCT laboratory.

The evaluation of the tests and equipment is time consuming. The choice of the instrument, the correlation of results, calculating the costs, and the training of personnel can be time consuming as well as costly. Other evaluations require the establishing of control ranges, proficiency testing, the verification of reference ranges, and the reporting of the results.

The first step is to decide what is required. Search the market to determine what tests and instruments are available. A chart comparing the desired parameters and what is available in the market by system or instrument aids the committee in determining if a system meets all or any of the required needs. It is beneficial to visit a similar facility that has the system to see what their experience has been, both good and bad. Once the instrument or system decision has been made, there needs to be a system of correlation of results with the main laboratory and the training of the personnel that will perform the tests. The ideal situation is one in which an instrument can be trial tested in the institution before being purchased. Once the system has been chosen and delivered, the system for calibration and quality control needs to be established. Policies will need to be defined and a procedures manual developed. During this period, an evaluation of the staffing requirements needs to be performed.

## Training Program

There will need to be a training program developed for all the personnel that will perform the tests. If nonlaboratorians will be performing the testing, the need for quality control and quality assurance will need to be emphasized. Nonlaboratory personnel usually do not understand the importance of quality control and calibration. The maintenance and the quality control may be viewed as unnecessary and time consuming and the value of troubleshooting may not be apparent. Some personnel will feel that if it gives a result on the patient sample, then there is no problem with the instrument.

The personnel must understand the principle of the procedure and the implications of the results obtained. If not, they will not be able to determine the adequate function of the system.

Proper patient identification and sample collection are other areas that need to be emphasized during the training sessions. All of this training must be documented for accreditation purposes.

Many systems have the capabilities to "lockout" unauthorized personnel. If someone has not been through a training course or has not demonstrated annual competencies, they would not be able to perform the testing. The training programs need to be available every time new personnel are hired so that they are trained to perform the POCT and become a functional part of the team.

The last area for training deals with how the results are reported. The results need to be documented. A minimum of documentation includes the patient's name, hospital number, date, time, test being performed, the person performing the test, and the result. There needs to be a permanent record of these results. Some hospitals enter the results into the laboratory computer system, while other hospitals use a manual method. Whichever method is utilized, there needs to be some mechanism to produce the bill related to performing the test. If no bill is produced, then the tests are being performed for free, and none of the costs associated with the testing can be recovered.

## Clinical Laboratory Improvement Act

There are many federal and state regulations involved with laboratory testing. The Clinical Laboratory Improvement Act (CLIA '88) administered through the Health Care Financing Administration (HCFA) is the major regulatory issue relating to laboratories unless the state requirements concerning laboratories are more stringent. CLIA subjects all clinical laboratories to the same quality standards and is considered "site neutral" regardless of where the testing is performed.[2] Each institution must obtain a CLIA certificate in order to perform laboratory testing. It is the decision of the institution whether the POCT laboratory will be included in the main laboratory certificate or if the POCT laboratory will have a separate certificate. CLIA requires that proficiency testing and quality control be performed, even for waived testing in an institutional setting where higher categories of testing are performed.

The CLIA waived tests[3] are simple laboratory tests and procedures that include the following:

1. tests are approved by the Food and Drug Administration (FDA) for home testing
2. simple and accurate methodologies where the likelihood of erroneous results are negligible
3. poses no risk of harm to the patient if the test is performed incorrectly
4. automated or self-contained
5. no manipulation of the sample before analyzing
6. provides a direct readout of the results

Table 34–1 is a list of tests that are currently in the waivered category. These tests are classified[3] based on the following:

1. uses direct unprocessed specimens
2. contains fail-safe mechanisms by giving no results when results are outside of the reportable range or the system has a malfunction
3. contains instructions written at the seventh grade level of comprehension.

## College of American Pathologists Requirements

The College of American Pathologists (CAP) inspects many clinical laboratories and has defined a POCT laboratory as any laboratory that does not require permanent dedicated space and exists outside the main laboratory. This includes handheld devices and instruments that are transported to the patient area for testing (CAP Checklist Section 30). The CAP checklist for POCT does not include satellite laboratories that have dedicated space. CAP does not categorize the tests; CLIA does. If the main laboratory personnel are responsible for the POCT, then the main laboratory checklist includes the POCT laboratory inspection. If not, each POCT site must complete a checklist in order to be CAP accredited.

The CAP accreditation for POCT requires the following:

1. proficiency tests and review of results
2. quality control program with weekly review
3. specimen and patient identification integrity maintained with an assessing system
4. system to detect and correct clerical errors and unexpected results
5. review of results no later than the next routine working shift
6. procedure manual to include principle, clinical significance, specimen type, reagents, calibration, quality control, procedure steps, calculations, reference ranges, and interpretation
7. system for reporting results with reference ranges

TABLE 34-1

**List of Current Waivered CLIA Tests (4/2001)**

- Dipstick or tablet reagent urinalysis
- Fecal occult blood
- Ovulation test by visual color
- Urine pregnancy test by visual color
- Erythrocyte sedimentation rate (ESR)—nonautomated
- Hemoglobin by copper sulfate—nonautomated
- Hemoglobin—HemoCue, HemoSite meter
- Blood glucose, FDA-approved monitoring devices, home use
- Glucose—HemoCue
- Spun hematocrit
- Hematocrit—Wampole STAR-CRIT, Micro Diagnostics
- Cholesterol—ChemTrak AccuMeter, Advanced Care, Accu-Check. ENA.C.T, Lifestream Technologies, LDX, Polymer Technology Systems
- Urine albumin—Boehringer Mannheim Chemstrip Micral, Roche
- Ketones, blood—Polymer Technology Systems
- *Helicobacter pylori*—Quick Vue, Delata West, GI Supply HP-FAST, Abbott Signify, Becton Dickinson Link 2, Applied Biotech, Quidel, Princeton BioMeditech, Trinity BioTech
- One-step Strep A Test—Quick Vue, Binax NOW, Wyntek Diagnostics OSOM, Applied Biotech SureStrep A, LifeSign LLC
- pH—color comparison
- Gastric occult blood—SmithKline Gastrooccult
- Antbodies to *H. pylori*—SmithKline
- LXN fructosamine test
- Prothrombin time—CoaguCheck PST
- Coagulation Factors II, V, VII, X—Avosure PT
- Glycosylated hemoglobin—Bayer DCA 2000
- Mononucleosis—Mono-Plus WB-Wampole, Genzyme, Wyntek Diagnostics, Princeton BioMeditech, Quidel, Applied Biotech
- Alcohol–Saliva—STC Diagnostics QED
- Nicotine, urine—Dynagen
- Urine bladder tumor—Bion Diagnostics
- Catalase—Diatech Diagnostics Uriscreen
- Urine drugs—Pamtech
- Influenza, types A and B—Quidel Quick Vue

8. critical values and notification of physician
9. upper and lower limits of test analysis
10. documentation of person performing the test
11. verification of reagent performance and reagent labels with appropriate dates and proper storage
12. calibration and standards documented and verified after changing reagents, quality control failure, and after main-

tenance and service that follows manufacturer recommendations
13. control material at more than one concentration analyzed for each test daily
14. evidence for corrective action based on control values
15. maintenance records
16. physician (preferably a pathologist) or doctoral scientist responsible for the testing
17. personnel trained and competencies
18. compliance with safety requirements.

Laboratory testing can be performed in the main laboratory or in a POCT laboratory. The main concern of all of the regulatory agencies is the quality of testing, and that the testing benefits the patient and ultimately results in better care for the patient or a reduction in the time that a patient stays in the hospital.

## POCT TESTING AND INSTRUMENTATION

### Instruments

Most of the instruments utilized for POCT use whole blood for analysis and have disposable reagent unit-dose devices.[5] These instruments typically have a low throughput but a rapid response time. The following are examples of instruments: (1) the Abbott Vision is a centrifugal analyzer that can utilize whole blood,[5] and (2) the Clinistat uses a slide similar to the Ektachem by Johnson & Johnson that has individual slides for each test.[5] The most popular POCT instrument is the i-STAT Analyzer. This is a portable handheld analyzer that contains the calibrator and the reagents in a prepackaged cartridge.

### POC Tests

Many tests may be performed as POCT but not all of them meet the requirement of better patient management. The most common POCT is the bedside glucose test for the management of patients with diabetes. Other tests commonly performed are urinalysis and coagulation testing.

The area that justifies a POCT laboratory is the emergency department. The tests performed depend on the population that the emergency department serves. Tests that are categorized as emergency can offer a definitive diagnosis and lead to specific therapy.[6] These tests are blood glucose, hemoglobin and hematocrit, and arterial pH and blood gases.[6] Additional POCT such as electrolytes do not appear to be justified in the emergency department situation.[7] Many hospitals have a satellite laboratory that offers a variety of tests for the emergency department and reduces the turnaround time associated with the testing. Other tests that may be beneficial to patient care would be cardiac profiles. These would best be completed in a satellite laboratory rather than a POCT.

A parathyroid hormone (PTH) assay that is available during parathyroid hormone surgery as a POCT has been demonstrated to be invaluable at hospitals that offer this service.[8] The PTH is utilized to confirm the complete removal of the PTH secreting glands during the surgery. This has increased the success rate of this surgery and decreased the amount of time a patient is in the operating room. Hospitals that utilize this testing have the test performed by personnel from the main laboratory. The instrument is kept on a cart and is taken to the surgical area to analyze the PTH POCT. This requires that there is always a trained technologist available to perform the test. A major time commitment on the part of the laboratory personnel is required, but this is justified through the decreased time in the operating room, which yields a direct patient care benefit.

## BILLING

### Medicare

Medicare expects any area of the hospital performing laboratory testing to follow the same guidelines and requirements. The test must have a Current Procedural Terminology (CPT) code and the laboratory revenue center code.[9] These codes indicate the test methodology and the hospital cost center. The other medicare requirement is the Advanced Beneficiary Notice, where the patient must sign for the requested test and be billed for the test if Medicare determines that the test is not medically necessary.[9]

### Advances

Advances in POCT are related to the technology of the testing where there is bar code capabilities for patient identification and bar code links to the hospital computer system.[10] Employee identification can also be included in the bar code system, eliminating the need for manual entry. This bar code can be linked to competency ratings and the lockout feature activated if this information is not current. Bar coding of reagents and controls can also eliminate the testing of a sample when the control has not been analyzed or a different lot number of reagents is utilized. Being able to directly link the POCT device to the hospital or laboratory computer eliminates the problems associated with the documentation of the test result as a permanent record.

## SUMMARY

Point-of-care testing is any testing performed outside the main clinical laboratory and may or may not be performed by laboratory personnel. To develop a POCT laboratory, there must be a demonstrated benefit to the patient that is not met by having the test performed in the main laboratory. A POCT laboratory cannot be established solely for convenience. The preanalytical and postanalytical variables are decreased with a POCT.

To have a successful POCT laboratory, the equipment, personnel, and the benefits must be evaluated. This process may be very time consuming. Regulations affecting POCT are CLIA and CAP. POCT can be billed under Medicare with the CPT code and laboratory revenue center codes.

POCT testing has been successful in various situations, including the emergency department and the operating room. Before beginning POCT, the laboratory personnel may want to examine the current situation to determine whether any improvements can be made in the current system.

### REFERENCES

1. Bishop M, Duben-Englekirk J, Fody E (eds.): *Clinical Chemistry: Principles, Procedure, Correlations.* 4th ed. Philadelphia, Lippincott Williams & Wilkins, 2000, p 142.
2. Kaplan LA, Pesce AJ (eds.): *Clinical Chemistry Theory, Analysis, Correlation.* 3rd ed. St. Louis, MO, Mosby, 1996.
3. http/www.phppo.cdc.gov/clia/docs/hsq225p.html, p2,12.
4. http/www.phppo.cdc.gov/clia/docs/hsq225p.html, p5.
5. Burtis C, Ashwood E (eds.): *Tietz Textbook of Clinical Chemistry.* 2nd ed. Philadelphia, WB Saunders, 1994, pp 366–368.
6. Betlej TM, Maturen A: The emergency department and the clinical laboratory. Clin Lab News 25(8):12–16, 1999.
7. Sainato D: POCT in the emergency department: Opportunities are increasing, but not all applications work. Clin Lab News 25(4):12–13, 1999.
8. Remaley A, Woods J, Glickman J: Point-of-care testing of parathyroid hormone during the surgical treatment of hyperparathyroidism. MLO 31:21–27, 1999.
9. Sainato D: POCT vs. Central lab testing: When it comes to medicare billing, HCFA says it's all the same. Clin Lab News 25(4)15, 1999.
10. Seiler J: Trends in point-of-care testing. Adv Med Lab Professionals 11(19):26–29, 1999.

# CHAPTER 35

# Laboratory Assessment of Psychiatric Disorders

*Jane Adrian*

## SUPPORTING THE PSYCHIATRIC DIAGNOSIS AND PLAN OF TREATMENT

The clinical laboratory may play a role in the assessment of psychiatric disorders at three levels. The first is to assist in ruling out that the individual has an organic cause for the presenting complaint. The second is, at present, a very limited role in identifying biologic abnormalities characteristic of psychiatric disorders. The third category of the clinical laboratory's participation is in monitoring medications and therapy. Each role and the related disorders are discussed in this chapter.

The *Diagnostic and Statistical Manual of Mental Disorders* (DSM IV-R)[1] is published by the American Psychiatric Association in a effort to provide common language and a methodical approach to the diagnosis of mental disorders. The DSM IV-R supplements and expands the *International Classification of Diseases* (ICD),[2] "Chapter 5, Mental and Behavioral Disorders." This chapter underscores that the distinctions between general medical conditions and mental disorders are purely for the convenience of this discussion. In other words, the term *illness* refers to both mental disorders *and* general medical conditions. Just as mental disorders are related to physical or biologic conditions, general medical conditions are related to behavioral or psychosocial issues.

The clinical laboratorian has a role to play in removing the boundary that has developed between "mental" and "physical" disorders. The professional's selection of language is imperative in this regard. Since these diagnoses reflect a condition or set of symptoms, they do not describe the individual. Therefore, rather than referring to the "schizophrenic," choose to say the individual with schizophrenia. Rather than referring to the person as an alcoholic, say the individual presents with alcohol dependence.

The DSM IV-R defines a **mental disorder** as

> . . . a clinically significant behavioral or psychological syndrome or pattern that occurs in an individual and that is associated with present distress (e.g., a painful symptom) or disability (i.e., impairment in one or more important areas of functioning) or with a significantly increased risk

of suffering death, pain, disability, or an important loss of freedom.[1]

The definition excludes culturally sanctioned events, conflicts between individuals, conflicts between the individual and society, and deviant behavior unless these present as a frank symptom contributing to the dysfunction of the individual. The mental disorder "must currently be considered a manifestation of a behavioral, psychological or biological dysfunction in the individual."[1]

Although grouped together in the past, today psychiatric diagnoses are divided into those relating to developmental disabilities or mental retardation and those relating to mental illness. Just as individuals with a medical diagnosis of anemia may experience psychiatric problems as well, individuals whose condition is diagnosed as mental retardation may also exhibit symptoms of mental illness, such as depression in addition to anemia. Mental illnesses are grouped as psychoses in ICD-9 and DSM IV-R codes 290 to 299 and codes 300-316. The three broad categories of disorders are organic psychotic conditions; other psychoses; and neurotic, personality, and other nonpsychotic mental disorders. Examples of the differentiation may be reviewed in Table 35–1.

Individuals who are developmentally disabled are classified under mental retardation in ICD-9 and DSM IV-R codes 317-319. The level of retardation is designated as mild, moderate, severe, or profound.

When working with other professionals in the area of abnormal psychology, it may be useful to realize that there are two somewhat opposing schools of thought in the diagnosis and treatment of these conditions: the medical model and the behavioral model. The medical model focuses on symptoms, diagnoses, etiologies, prescribed treatments, and prognosis; the behavior model focuses on observable behavior. The behavior model presupposes that mental disorders are the result of learned conditioning. Treatment plans include heavy components of conditioning. Although these two points of view need not be mutually exclusive, the clinical laboratory scientist can expect rather deep differences of opinion with regard to approaches to the diagnosis and treatment of these conditions. In tandem, the two models represent powerful options for the treatment of mental disorders.

T A B L E   3 5 – 1

**Differential Categories of Mental Illness According to the *Diagnostic and Statistical Manual of Mental Disorders* and *International Classification of Diseases***

| CATEGORY | EXAMPLES |
|---|---|
| Organic psychotic conditions (290–294) | Dementia, such as senile and arteriosclerotic; Alcohol and/or drug psychosis; Transient organic psychotic conditions such as delirium, delusions, hallucinations, or anxiety; Chronic organic psychotic conditions such as amnesia, Alzheimer disease, cerebral lipidosis, epilepsy, Huntington's chorea. |
| Other psychoses (295–299) | Schizophrenia, mania, manic depression, bipolar affective, paranoia, delusions |
| Neurotic, personality and other nonpsychotic mental disorders (300–316) | Anxiety, hysteria, multiple personality, dissociative disorder, compulsive personality disorder, antisocial disorder, narcissism, avoidance, passive-aggressive, sexual deviation. Includes the physiologic malfunction arising from mental factors such as psychogenic paralysis, dysuria, dysmenorrhea, or stammering, etc. |

## MEDICAL CONDITIONS UNDERLYING PSYCHIATRIC DIAGNOSIS AND TREATMENT

The clinical laboratory plays a pivotal role in assisting the clinician in uncovering or ruling out an organic cause for an individual's illness. For example, the individual who may present with fatigue and pica with ice chips may in fact display a hematologic picture consistent with iron deficiency anemia instead of a psychosis.

Broad and generalized laboratory screenings seldom yield diagnostic information that justifies the expense. However, an example of laboratory tests from which to select a screening battery to rule out underlying medical conditions may include a combination of those in Table 35–2.[3]

These test batteries include basic chemistry and hematologic screening tests to evaluate renal and hepatic function and to exclude underlying anemia as well as other possible challenges to homeostasis. Neuroendocrine tests with abnormal results of thyroid function tests and cortisol determinations may represent sources of underlying depression. Although not generally included in screening batteries at this time, other hormone abnormalities are often associated with mental illness. Some of these include prolactin (an anterior pituitary hormone), growth hormone, gonadotrophin-releasing hormone, and somatostatin. Sex hormones such as estrogen, testosterone, follicle-stimulating hormone, and luteinizing hormone have been linked to behavior disorders. Seasonal affective disorder has been linked to abnormal levels of melatonin.[4] The implication of tests to determine levels of catecholamines in psychiatric disorder are addressed later in this chapter.

The list, in addition to the routine hematology and chemical screens, includes some of the tests related to endocrine function and laboratory support in ruling out sexually transmitted disease, the use of illicit drugs, and the misuse of prescription medication that also play a role in determining possible underlying causes of psychiatric episodes. The toxicologic tools may extend to the determination of heavy metals and even nonspecific tests suggesting inflammation or underlying protein abnormalities.

The diagnosis of Wilson's disease or hepatolenticular degeneration is an example of a condition that may present with neurological and psychological symptoms that is caused by an organic deficiency. Wilson's disease is an inherited disorder of copper metabolism. An individual with suspected Wilson's disease may develop, among other symptoms, inappropriate behavior, disrupted coordination, personality change, cognitive impairment, anxiety, and depression. The diagnosis is made through the clinical laboratory confirmation of decreased ceruloplasmin. Ceruloplasmin is an $\alpha_2$-globulin containing copper. In Wilson's disease, the body fails to incorporate copper into apoceruloplasmin; increased levels of plasma and tissue-free copper result. The tissues at particular risk are the liver and brain. Note that abnormal levels of ceruloplasmin can indicate other conditions. Low ceruloplasmin implicates Menkes's kinky hair syndrome, protein loss indicative of nephrotic syndromes, malabsorption, and advanced liver disease. High ceruloplasmin implicates neoplasia, inflammatory responses, and pregnancy in addition to copper intoxication. Consequently, copper levels in serum and urine must be determined in order to rule out Wilson's disease. In summary, laboratory studies to confirm a diagnosis of Wilson's disease will demonstrate decreased ceruloplasmin, decreased serum copper, increased 24-hour urine copper excretion, increased copper in the liver, and abnormal

**TABLE 35–2**

**Laboratory Screening Tests to Rule Out Some Underlying Organic Disorders**

Complete blood count (CBC)
Serum electrolytes
Stools for occult blood
Renal function tests
  Blood urea nitrogen
  Creatinine
  Urinalysis
Hepatic function tests
  Aspartate aminotransferase (AST)
  Alanine aminotransferase (ALT)
  Bilirubin, total and direct
  Gamma-glutamyltransferase
  Alkaline phosphatase
Lipid profile tests
  Cholesterol
  High-density lipoprotein
  Low-density lipoprotein
  Triglycerides
Nutritional assessment
  Total protein
  Albumin
  Prealbumin
  Calcium
Metabolic assessment
  Glucose
  Iron
  $B_{12}$
  Folate
Basal endocrine tests
  Thyroid function tests
    Thyroid-stimulating hormone
    Free $T_4$ (Thyroxine)
    Total $T_3$
    Cortisol
Infectious disease (in individuals determined at risk)
  Syphilis—*Treponema pallidum* (RPR or VDRL, Venereal Disease Research Laboratory)
  Hepatitis
  Human immunodeficiency virus
  Lyme disease
Toxicology (in individuals determined at risk)
  Alcohol
  Heavy metals
    Mercury
    Copper
    Lead
Nonspecific test suggestive of inflammation or underlying protein abnormalities
  Erythrocyte sedimentation rate
  C-reactive protein
  Myoglobin

liver function tests. This is an example of an organic origin of a disease that may present with primarily psychiatric symptoms.

Another view of this same category of assessment involves high levels of zinc. Some authors suggest that excessive therapeutic zinc may block the intestinal absorption of copper. This may be characterized by laboratory findings consistent with decreased copper such as hypochromic microcytic anemia with leukopenia, generalized neutropenia, and zero ceruloplasmin. However, in this case, the specific therapy would initiate with a decrease in zinc supplement.

A selection of the laboratory tests listed in Table 35–2 will undoubtedly be a part of any series of diagnostic tools that also may include an electrocardiogram, an electroencephalogram, computed tomography or magnetic resonance imaging, or possible radiographs. The clinical history and interview remain the most powerful diagnostic tool available to the clinician.

## SCREENING FOR THE BIOCHEMICAL BASIS OF PSYCHIATRIC DISORDERS

Scientists continue to search for specific biochemical markers diagnostic of specific psychiatric disorders. A number of neurotransmitters have been identified, and it is believed that several different disturbances involving the neurotransmitters may result in psychoses. Researchers realize that the psychiatric disturbance may be due to the

- decreased or increased synthesis of the neurotransmitter
- decreased or increased storage of the neurotransmitter
- increased or decreased numbers of receptors
- changes in concentrations of enzymes responsible for reuptake of the particular neurotransmitter.

At the present time, however, note that any actual laboratory measurement of blood or urine neurotransmitters such as the catecholamines (dopamine, norepinephrine, and epinephrine) or serotonin are *not* used to confirm that diagnoses of psychoses. Instead, the metabolites of these neurotransmitters may be used to confirm and to monitor related tumors. Specifically, the use of homovanillic acid, a major terminal metabolite of the dopamine pathway and vanillylmandelic acid, the major terminal metabolite of the norepinephrine pathway, are used to diagnose and monitor neuroblastoma, ganglioneuroma, and pheochromocytoma. These are discussed in detail elsewhere in this text.

It is thought that compromised serotonin metabolism resulting in reduced cerebrospinal fluid (CSF) levels of 5-hydroxyindole acetic acid (5-HIAA) may result in anxiety, depression, outward and self-directed aggression, and suicide. Indeed, serotonin-potentiating drugs such as clomipramine, trazadone, and fluoxetine have been used successfully to reduce these behaviors. Some researches have further observed that the ratio of CSF 5-HIAA to dopamine (HVA) levels is low in individuals with a diagnosis of schizophrenia; moreover, this ratio increased after treatment. Some further studies suggest a possible relationship between a diagnosis of attention deficit hyperactivity disorder (ADHD) and increased levels of CSF HVA stemming from dopaminergic dysfunction. However, at this time, no measure of serotonin levels or its metabolites is correlated with a psychiatric diagnosis. Today, blood serotonin levels are used practically to track carcinoid syndromes.

Decreased CSF levels of 5-HIAA have been associated with self- and other-directed aggression and may predict aggression. Studies suggest a possible relationship between a diagnosis of ADHD and levels of increased levels of CSF HVA stemming from dopaminergic dysfunction.

Monoamine oxidase (MAO) and neuropeptides such as catechol-O-methyltransferase, dopamine $\beta$-hydroxylase (low levels associated with undersocialized conduct disorders), and adenylate cyclase in the CSF are currently performed in the context of research to study psychiatric disorders. Indices of central monoaminergic activity have been of most interest. Examples of these metabolites of interest include: serotonin (5-hydroxyindole acetic acid, 5-HIAA), dopamine (HVA), and noradrenaline (3-methoxy-4-hydroxyphenylglycol).[5]

Increased levels of central neuropeptides have been implicated in obsessive-compulsive disorders. This finding has been linked to the role of the central neuropeptides to arousal and conditioned behaviors. Increased CSF levels of corticotropin-releasing hormone, vasopression, and oxytocin have been implicated with symptoms suggesting obsessive-compulsive disorder, anxiety, and depression. These observations remain theoretical and have yet to influence clinical practice.

These once purported biologic markers to aid in the diagnosis of psychiatric disorders have failed the test of time:

- dexamethasone suppression test
- thyrotropin-releasing hormone stimulation test
- corticotropin-releasing hormone stimulation test
- fenfluramine challenge

The dexamethasone suppression test challenges the individual with 1 mg of dexamethasone, a synthetic steroid that suppresses adrenocorticotropin (ACTH) secretion, which further results normally in decreased cortisol level. An abnormal result is documented by a nonsuppression of cortisol after the dexamethasone challenge. This test was initially touted as a marker of depression. However, studies have proved many false positives, and the test has been discarded as a predictor of depression. Test results neither mirror prognosis nor aid in the selection of medication for mental disorders.

Today, the test is used to distinguish among causes of elevated cortisol levels. If the cortisol level is successfully suppressed, then the feedback mechanism is intact and the clinician may rule out Cushing's syndrome.

The thyrotropin-releasing hormone stimulation test, considered diagnostic when a thyroid-stimulating hormone level is decreased below baseline after a challenge with thyrotropin, was thought to indicate depression. Time has proved this test

more useful in differentiating pituitary failure from hypothalamic hypothyroidism.

The corticotropin-releasing hormone stimulation test is another neuroendocrine challenge test. Normally, the corticotropin-releasing hormone is released by the hypothalamus and further acts on the pituitary to cause a release of adrenocorticotropin. Decreased ACTH postchallenge may be indicative of depression.

In the research setting, fenfluramine-induced prolactin has been used to demonstrate psychopathology associated with mood disorders. Specifically, fenfluramine induces presynaptic release of serotonin, which in turn stimulates cortisol and prolactin release.[6] In summary, the results of these tests remain associative, lack sensitivity, specificity, and reliability as diagnostic tools of psychiatric illness.

It may be more significant to point out that a number of endocrine-associated disorders do exhibit psychiatric manifestations. For example, depression often precedes a diagnosis of diabetes mellitus or hypothyroid. In fact, a long list of symptoms, including, but not limited to anxiety, depression, mental retardation, dementia, restlessness, and psychosis, have been linked to abnormal thyroid function tests.

## MONITORING THERAPEUTIC TREATMENT

Although not a major player in the screening or confirmation of specific psychosis, the clinical laboratory has a significant role in monitoring the therapeutic levels of some medications, and perhaps more importantly, in protecting the safety of the individual through monitoring for adverse events related to medications. Current and emerging medications for mental disorders have wrought miracles in the world of psychotherapy. Individuals once confined to institutions housing thousands can now successfully live meaningful lives in their communities. Moreover, understanding of the mechanism of mental disorders may be attributed more to observing the success or failure of the medication than any specific test that the clinical laboratory has had to offer.

Most of these medications, however, affect not only the neurological system, but may also alter the function of the bone marrow, the liver, the kidneys, or impair electrolyte balance. For this reason, baseline values for organ functions before initiating treatment is imperative.

The clinical laboratory supports the therapeutic monitoring of some of these medications such as carbamazepine, valproic acid, phenytoin, phenobarbital, and primadone when used for seizure control, for example. The pharmacokinetics of therapeutic drug monitoring, such as absorption, distribution, metabolism and elimination, dose responses, half-life, steady state, therapeutic ranges, drug-to-drug interactions, and monitoring schedules are addressed elsewhere in this text. The clinical laboratory scientist must become aware that when these medications are used "off label," the published therapeutic values for effective seizure control may not apply.

**TABLE 35-3**

### Classes of Medications and Typical Monitoring for Adverse Effects

| CLASS OF MEDICATION | RECOMMENDED MONITORS |
|---|---|
| Benzodiazepines (diazepam, alprazolam, chlordiazepoxide) | Liver function tests |
| Antipsychotics (chlorpromazine, haloperidol, clozapine) | Hematologic monitoring for leukopenia, agranulocytosis, anemia, liver function tests |
| Tricyclics and tetracyclics (imipramine, desipramine, nortriptyline) | Electrocardiogram |
| Monoamine oxidase inhibitors (moclobemide, phenelzine, tranylcypromine) | Blood pressure |
| Lithium | Thyroid function tests, electrolytes for hyponatremia, renal function, leukocytosis, electrocardiogram |
| Antiseizure medications | Differs per medication—liver function tests, renal function tests, complete blood counts, electrocardiograms, electrolytes |

For example, valproate has been successful in controlling seizure disorder. It has been also used to treat manic episodes in bipolar disorder, especially in cases that have become refractory to lithium therapy. In addition, valproate is increasingly used as a mood stabilizer. Note, however, that the therapeutic range for this medication has been established for controlling seizure disorders. Therapeutic ranges for these additional uses have yet to be confirmed.

As useful as valproate has proved to be, the clinical laboratory is key to monitoring associated adverse events, which are evidenced through hematologic, hepatic, and renal studies. In some individuals, the platelet counts may decrease and the red cells become macrocytic. The change in platelet numbers appears to be dose related. When the dose of the valproate is reduced, the number of platelets rebounds.[7]

There are many new medications for psychiatric disorders that do not require therapeutic monitoring of levels because plasma levels do not correlate with clinical response. However, as in the preceding example with valproate, the potential adverse events associated with the use of the medication must be systematically monitored through laboratory tests. Examples of the class of medications and typical recommendations for monitors for adverse effects are seen in Table 35-3.

## SUMMARY

The clinical laboratory may play a significant role in the medical assessment of individuals presenting with possible psychosis and in monitoring potentially adverse effects of medications. However, for the moment, the clinical laboratory has yet to find a useful role in assisting the clinician in diagnosing mental illness. The clinical history and presenting behavior remains the most important tool in differentiating the diagnosis of individuals with psychiatric disorders.

## REFERENCES

1. American Psychiatric Association. *Diagnostic and Statistical Manual of Mental Disorders.* 4th ed. Washington, DC, American Psychiatric Press, Inc., 2000.

2. *International Classification of Diseases.* 9th Revision. Los Angeles, CA, Practice Management Information Corporation, 2000.

3. Morihisa JM, Rosse RB, Cross CD: Laboratory and other diagnostic tests in psychiatry. In Hales RH, Yudofsky SC (eds.): *Synopsis of Psychiatry.* Washington, DC, American Psychiatric Press, 1996, p 274.

4. Kaplan HI, Sadock BJ: *Synopsis of Psychiatry: Behavioral Sciences/Clinical Psychiatry.* Philadelphia, Lippincott Williams & Wilkins, 1994.

5. Zametkin AJ: Laboratory and diagnostic testing in child and adolescent psychiatry: A review of the past 10 years. J Am Acad Child Adolesc Psychiatry 37:5, 1998.

6. Cleare AJ, Murray RM, O'Keane V: Do noradrenergic reuptake inhibitors affect serotonergic function in depression? Psychopharmacology 134:4, 1997.

7. Trannel TJ, Ahmed I, Boebert D: Occurrence of thrombocytopenia in psychiatric patients taking valproate. Am J Psychiatry 157:1, 2001.

# CHAPTER 36

# Biochemical Assessment During Pregnancy

*George B. Kudolo*

## BIOCHEMICAL CHANGES

Significant biochemical, physiologic, and metabolic changes accompany the transition from an ordinary menstrual cycle, lasting approximately 4 weeks, to pregnancy (the condition of carrying a developing baby), which may last 40 to 42 weeks. Pregnancy begins with the implantation of a fertilized egg in a well-prepared endometrial layer of the uterus (conception) during the luteal phase of the menstrual cycle. This leads to the postponement of menstruation for that cycle. The delay and subsequent absence of menstruation is therefore the earliest physiologic indication of pregnancy, even before biochemical confirmatory urinary or blood tests provide definitive results. The dating of the pregnancy and the expected date of delivery may thus be estimated on the basis of the last menstrual period (LMP).

To meet the increasing demands of the developing baby, whose biochemical and metabolic needs are also constantly changing, the mother undergoes significant physiologic changes. Almost every organ function in the mother is modified, and many biochemical and metabolic indices found in the maternal circulation may vary considerably when compared with values in the nonpregnant female. The hormonal profile of the mother is also considerably different from the nonpregnant state as the mother physiologically adapts to the presence of the developing baby. In fact, three distinct endocrine systems can be identified during pregnancy: the maternal and fetal endocrine systems and the placenta. Unlike the maternal and the fetal systems, however, the placenta is an endocrine system that does not possess its own stores of precursors for hormone synthesis. Instead, the placenta obtains its precursors from both the maternal and fetal systems. Increased uterine blood flow and placental plasma membrane permeability during pregnancy ensure that the placenta is well perfused with both maternal and fetal blood supply. Therefore biochemical tests of the maternal blood may reveal the health of the fetoplacental unit and thereby the well-being of the developing baby.

Some of the analytes found in the maternal circulation may be unique only to the period of pregnancy. Others are common to all females, only the values may now be altered because of the pregnancy. The biochemical compounds that are found in the maternal circulation during pregnancy may therefore be derived from any of the three sources and can be used as markers for assessing the maternal and fetoplacental well-being. Three distinct body fluids are routinely available to the clinical chemistry laboratory for the measurements of analytes for the management of pregnancy: maternal blood and urine as well as **amniotic fluid,** a major component of the intrauterine environment. An understanding of the synthesis and metabolism of the various biochemical compounds in these body fluids is important for accurate interpretation of the results of analytical measurements.

## Maternal Changes

The hallmark of the luteal (or secretory) phase of the menstrual cycle is progesterone, which supports endometrial preparation for implantation of the zygote. The ovarian corpus luteum is the main source of progesterone production at this time. A maximal progesterone concentration of 10 to 20 ng/mL may be reached in approximately 4 to 7 days after ovulation, and its supportive role extends well into the early stages of pregnancy. This important function of the corpus luteum is sustained by increasing plasma levels of human chorionic gonadotropin (hCG) from the developing embryo up to about 50 days into the pregnancy (Table 36–1). Early studies in which the corpus luteum was removed after day 50 of pregnancy confirmed that the placenta takes over from the corpora lutea as the major source of progesterone production with no deleterious effect on the development of the baby.[1]

Estradiol levels, which in a normal menstrual cycle peak during the follicular phase, continue to increase throughout pregnancy producing a wide range of metabolic effects. Estradiol is the predominant estrogen present in the nonpregnant female but the predominant estrogen found during pregnancy is estriol, which is synthesized primarily by the placenta using precursors from both the maternal and fetal adrenal sources (Figure 36–1). Note that the maternal liver conjugates a substantial amount of the circulating estriol to produce the water-soluble estriol glucuronide, which is then excreted in the maternal urine. Therefore, plasma estriol is not a true reflection

TABLE 36-1

### Reference Levels of Serum Human Chorionic Gonadotropin (hCG) Hormone During Pregnancy

| WEEK FROM THE LAST MENSTRUAL PERIOD | AMOUNT OF hCG (mU/mL)* |
|---|---|
| 3 | 5–50† |
| 4 | 3–426 |
| 5 | 19–7,340 |
| 6 | 1,080–56,500 |
| 7–8 | 7,650–229,000 |
| 9–12 | 25,700–288,000 |
| 13–16 | 13,300–254,000 |
| 17–24 | 4,060–165,400 |
| 25–40 | 3,640–117,000 |

*Serum samples assayed using antiserum raised against the β-subunit of hCG.

†hCG levels <5 mU/mL indicates the absence of pregnancy.

of the endogenous placental estriol synthesis. Measurement of this analyte is, however, important for assessment of the fetoplacental unit, as explained later in the chapter.

Table 36–2 summarizes the important changes in hormone synthesis during pregnancy. In the pituitary gland, the increasing estrogen levels lead to the suppression of the activity of the gonadotropes, follicle-stimulating hormone (FSH) and luteinizing hormone (LH) producing cells, through a negative feedback effect but increased activity of the prolactin-producing cells. This gives rise to increased prolactin synthe-

sis with plasma concentration rising over 10 times the levels found in the nonpregnant state.[1] Although no significant increase in thyroid-stimulating hormone (TSH) is demonstrable during pregnancy, total thyroxine ($T_4$) and triiodothyronine ($T_3$) is increased over 50%; this is due essentially to estrogen-dependent increase in the synthesis of thyroxine-binding globulin (TBG). This may be doubled by the end of the first trimester and may remain elevated throughout pregnancy. The increased TBG level in turn leads to increased $T_4$ production, which may be mistaken for hyperthyroidism since 99.9% of $T_4$ is bound to TBG. Estimation of the free $T_4/T_3$ and free $T_4$ index ($FT_4I$) in most pregnancies clearly confirms a euthyroid state. The maternal liver is stimulated to produce several other transport proteins such as ceruloplasmin, transferrin, and transcortin during pregnancy. Parathyroid hormone (PTH) levels are increased over 30% during the course of a normal pregnancy, with no appreciable changes in the levels of calcitonin. To ensure adequate absorption of calcium, which is needed by the developing baby, 1,25 dihydroxyvitamin $D_3$ levels are usually elevated.

The function of the maternal adrenal glands is important during pregnancy. Although an increased maternal adrenal androgen production (androstenedione and dehydroepiandrosterone) may play an important part in the development of such pathological conditions as ambiguous genitalia in the baby, it is clear that this anomaly is usually caused by genetic defects in the fetal adrenal function rather than the mother's androgen level. Instead, these androgens may be transferred to the placenta for the synthesis of estriol (Figure 36–1). Only very small changes can be seen in the maternal serum levels of pituitary adrenocorticotropic hormone (ACTH) during pregnancy, and yet plasma cortisol levels may be significantly in-

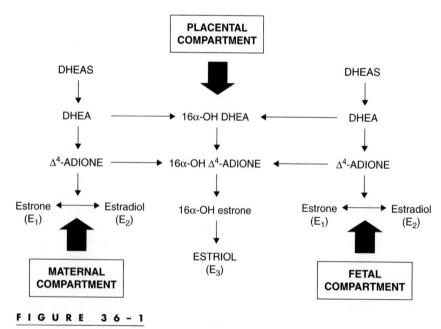

FIGURE 36-1

Sources of estrogens during pregnancy.

TABLE  36-2

**The Effects of Pregnancy on Selected Hormones**

| ORGAN | STAGE OF PREGNANCY | |
|---|---|---|
| | BEFORE | AT TERM |
| Pituitary gland | | |
| FSH (mU/mL) | 2–15 | <2 |
| LH (mU/mL) | 5–25 | <2 |
| PRL (ng/mL) | 5–25 | 100–300 |
| GH (ng/mL) | <5 | <7 |
| TSH (μU/mL) | <5 | <5 |
| ACTH (pg/mL) | 7.8–120 | 12–60 |
| Ovary | | |
| Estradiol (ng/mL) | 0.07–0.3 | 5–25 |
| Progesterone (ng/mL) | 1–25 | 70–250 |
| Thyroid and | | |
| parathyroid glands | | |
| $T_4$ (μg/dL) | 5–12 | 7–18 |
| $T_3$ (ng/dL) | 50–250 | 120–280 |
| PTH (μEq/mL) | 20–60 | 20–120 |
| Calcitonin (pg/mL) | 50–350 | 40–450 |
| Adrenal gland | | |
| Cortisol (μg/dL) | 5–25 | 10–40 |
| Aldosterone (μg/dL) | 2–10 | 40–150 |

creased during pregnancy. This increase may be caused by (1) reduced metabolic cortisol clearance during pregnancy, or (2) the fact that cortisol is transported in the peripheral circulation bound to its specific binding protein transcortin (corticosteroid-binding globulin, CBG), which is increased during pregnancy.

It has long been known that during pregnancy maternal fasting plasma glucose levels decline from the mid-80 mg/dL to mid-70 mg/dL. At night, the maternal blood glucose levels fall as the developing baby draws glucose from the maternal circulation. In normal pregnancy, postprandial blood glucose peaks rarely exceed 130 mg/dL at 1 hour and 120 mg/dL at 2 hours.[2] Deviations from this may necessitate evaluating the expectant mother for the presence of gestational diabetes mellitus. As described later, development of this metabolic derangement has serious consequences for both mother and child during pregnancy.

Maternal plasma volume may increase by 45% to 50% during pregnancy and a dilutional effect may explain some of the decreases in many of the values of the routine laboratory tests.[3] The increase observed in some test values may actually be an underestimation (Table 36–3). Greater increases of plasma volume have been observed with heavier infants and twins, whereas smaller volume increases have been associated with preeclampsia.[4] Figure 36–2 is a schematic summary of the interrelationships between maternal blood specimens and

other body fluids that are routinely available for biochemical tests during pregnancy. Because the amniotic fluid is derived from both the maternal blood and fetal sources (including excreted urine and desquamated epithelial cells), it is an excellent specimen for examination of the fetoplacental unit and for screening for genetic diseases. The volume of amniotic fluid increases with gestation (about 30 mL at 10 weeks to about 1 L at 38 weeks). The volume of the amniotic fluid may itself provide clues about the pregnancy. For example, **oligohydramnios,** a condition with less than 400 mL of amniotic fluid, may be indicative of reduced placental blood flow.[5]

Normal pregnancy is characterized by a decrease in mean arterial pressure accompanied by an increase in cardiac output. Maternal renal plasma flow is increased, with as much as a 45% increase in creatinine clearance during pregnancy.[1,6] Therefore, biochemical compounds in the blood are quickly filtered into the urine and serum levels of several analytes may become artificially decreased. For example, serum urea nitrogen and creatinine are decreased during pregnancy. Maternal urine is therefore an excellent specimen for biochemical tests. Additionally, unlike the blood collected by venipuncture and amniotic fluid collected by amniocentesis, urine collection is relatively simple and noninvasive.

Pregnancy is also a state of hypercoagulability because of the increased concentration of coagulation factors, decreased levels of coagulation inhibitors (e.g., antithrombin III, protein C, and protein S) and decreased fibrinolytic capacity.[7–9] Protein S levels seem to significantly decrease throughout pregnancy, whereas protein C and antithrombin III levels remain normal. There is also increased platelet activation during pregnancy, thus creating a state of not only hypercoagulability, but also of hypersensitivity of the blood platelets.[9] This markedly increases the risk for venous thromboembolism.

## Fetal Changes

One of the most important events that takes place during fetal development is sexual differentiation. The developing individual is described as an embryo during the first 8 weeks of life. Thereafter, the preferred term *fetus* is used.[10] The most important period of pregnancy is undoubtedly between 4 and 8 weeks of embryonic life when the development of the major internal and external organs begins. Undifferentiated sex organs, capable of developing into either sex depending on or even in spite of the fetal genotype, become visible after week 5. By the 7th week, the embryo has two sets of reproductive tracts: the **müllerian ducts** may develop into the female reproductive tract and the **wolffian ducts** may develop into the male reproductive system. In a fetus with an XY genotype, a decision is made to retain the male reproductive system because of the presence of the SRY gene found on the Y chromosome.[10] Two testicular secretions are released when the testes become functional: (1) testosterone, synthesized by the interstitial or **Leydig cells;** and (2) **müllerian inhibitory factor** (MIF), synthesized by the **Sertoli cells.** In response to signals

TABLE 36-3

**Biochemical Findings During Pregnancy**

| ELECTROLYTES (SERUM) | | ENZYMES (SERUM) | |
|---|---|---|---|
| Sodium | ↓ | Lactate dehydrogenase | ⇒ |
| Potassium | ↓ | Aspartate aminotransferase | ⇒ |
| Chloride | ↓ to ⇒ | Alanine aminotransferase | ⇒ |
| Bicarbonate | ↓ | Creatine kinase | ↓ |
| Calcium | ↓ | Triacylglycerol acylhydrolase (lipase, LPS) | ↑ |
| Magnesium | ↓ | Cholinesterase | ↓ |
| Phosphorus | ↓ | Leucine aminopeptidase | ↑ |
| Osmolality | ↓ | α-Amylase (AMS) | ⇒ |
| | | Alkaline phosphatase | ↑ |
| | | Acid phosphatase | ⇒ |

| PROTEINS (SERUM) | | LIPIDS (SERUM) | |
|---|---|---|---|
| Total protein | ↓ | Triglycerides | ↑ |
| Albumin | ↓ | Cholesterol | ↑ |
| $\alpha_1$-Globulins | ↑ | Phospholipids | ↑ |
| $\alpha_2$-Globulins | ↑ | Free Fatty Acids | ↑ |
| $\beta$-Globulins | ↑ | HDL | ↑ |
| $\gamma$-Globulins | ↓ | | |

| NONPROTEIN NITROGENS (SERUM) | | VITAMINS (SERUM) | |
|---|---|---|---|
| Urea nitrogen | ↓ | Folate | ↓ |
| Creatinine | ↓ | $B_{12}$ | ↓ |
| Uric Acid | ↓ to ⇒ at term | C | ↓ |
| | | $B_6$ | ↓ |

↑ = increased; ↓ = decreased; ⇒ = unaltered.

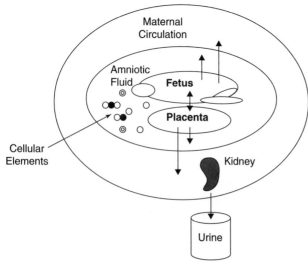

**FIGURE 36-2**

A schematic representation of the source of the body fluids used for the biochemical analysis during pregnancy.

from the SRY gene, MIF is released, which leads to the degeneration of the female reproductive tract. Together with MIF, testosterone supports the development of the vas deferens and related internal structures of the male reproductive tract.

In the fetus with an XX genotype, the development of female structures does not depend on functional ovarian function. The development of both internal and external genitalia begins by default when the genetic signals from the SRY gene are not received by the 12th week of gestation. The regression of the male wolffian ducts is completed by the end of the first trimester, but ovarian development continues throughout pregnancy. During the first trimester, the fetal pituitary gland is not fully functional and so placental hCG, which cross-reacts with LH, most likely stimulates testosterone production by the Leydig cells in the fetal testes. By the second trimester, the pituitary gland matures and gonadotropins (LH and FSH), growth hormone (GH), TSH, and ACTH are released. The gonadotropin secretions stimulate ovarian oocyte maturation, which continues throughout pregnancy so that by the end of gestation, each ovary in a female child contains approximately

$0.8-1.0 \times 10^6$ eggs. Maturation of the follicles, however, does not commence until puberty. The fetal hypothalamic-pituitary axis is matured by the third trimester and is now able to control fetal hormone synthesis using the feedback system.

The fetal adrenal gland produces the androgens dehydroepiandrosterone (DHEA) and androstenedione. In the fetal liver, the conjugated form, dehydroepiandrosterone sulfate (DHEAS), is converted to $16\alpha$-OH DHEAS and transported into the placenta as a precursor for estriol synthesis (see Figure 36–1). The fetal liver is the predominant blood-forming organ, a role that is taken over by the bone marrow after the 5th month of gestation. The metabolic function of the liver does not reach full maturity until about 1 month after birth even in full-term babies. Therefore, hepatic metabolism of substances such as excess bilirubin may become inefficient. This explains why every newborn baby may develop physiologic jaundice because of its inability to process excess bilirubin produced by excessive destruction of the red blood cells.[11,12] The fetal liver (as well as the yolk sac and the gastrointestinal tract) is, however, capable of synthesizing alpha-fetoprotein (AFP),[6] a glycoprotein with chemical and physical similarity to albumin. Within the fetal circulation, AFP levels peak (200 to 400 mg/dL) between the 12th and 15th week of gestation. The peak levels also coincide with the period of organogenesis in the fetus, and so malformations at this time, such as neural tube defects, may facilitate the leakage of AFP into the amniotic fluid. After the 16th week, the levels of AFP decline progressively throughout gestation so that at birth, AFP levels found in cord blood are usually less than 5 mg/dL and serum levels are <50 ng/mL at 1 year. Adult AFP levels are usually <30 ng/mL. AFP from fetal sources leaks into the maternal circulation with increasing age of gestation; peak levels are found between weeks 34 and 36.

Like the liver, several fetal organs do not reach full maturity at term, but many of them are nevertheless compatible with life. In these cases, no tests are necessary to verify the maturity of these organs before delivery in threatened pregnancies. Maturity of the fetal lung, on the other hand, determines the ability of the baby to breathe on its own after birth. Lung maturity must be completed before birth, and tests are available to assess lung maturity in cases where the pregnancy is threatened or the mother must undergo an elective cesarean delivery before term.

## Placental Endocrine Changes

Placentation begins between weeks 6 and 8 of gestation and is usually complete by the 12th week.[13] The placenta is the predominant source of the protein hormone hCG and human placental lactogen (hPL), progesterone and estriol utilizing precursors from both fetal and maternal sources. The quantity of these products, which is usually proportional to the placental mass, is secreted predominantly into the maternal circulation. Only minute quantities reach the fetal circulation. The syncytiotrophoblastic cells in the placental villi also produce enzymes such as alkaline phosphatase (ALP), which migrates into the

maternal circulation. The placental alkaline phosphatase (PALP) is an isoenzyme that is quite distinct from other forms of ALP found in other tissues in the body. PALP is resistant to heat (65°C for 30 minutes) and urea (3M urea for 18 minutes) but is inhibited by 5 mM L-phenylalanine. These characteristics allow the laboratory to identify the actual source of the enzyme. In fact, it is identical to the Regan isoenzyme, which is a carcinoembryonic antigen (CEA). Many other compounds, such as oxytocinase, cystine aminopeptidase, and leucine aminopeptidase (LAP), are produced by the placenta but assays for these enzymes are not performed routinely in the clinical laboratory.

The placenta plays a unique role not only in the development of the fetus but also in the general health of the mother. It has been suggested that reduced placental perfusion is the convergence point for the development of several pathogenic processes such as eclampsia during pregnancy.[14] Reduced placental perfusion may lead to reduced supply of oxygen and nutrients and restricted intrauterine growth and therefore low birth weight.

## ANALYTES

### Human Chorionic Gonadotropin

Human chorionic gonadotropin (hCG) is a glycoprotein that is synthesized by the syncytiotrophoblast cells of the placental villi. As shown in Table 36–1, serum hCG levels rise with increasing age of gestation, with peak levels of about 100,000 mU/mL found around the 14th week (after the last menstrual period, LMP). Thereafter, serum hCG levels begin to fall, until when at term, only 15,000 mU/mL may be found.[1] Such high levels are obviously above the renal threshold; therefore, serum hCG is filtered intact into the urine. Thus both urine and serum specimens may be used for the measurement of hCG. Structurally, the molecule is a dimer consisting of alpha ($\alpha$) and beta ($\beta$) glycoprotein subunits. The $\alpha$-subunit is identical in several protein hormones such as LH, FSH, and TSH. Dissociation of the subunits leads to loss of biological activity. Because the $\beta$-subunit of hCG is unique and dissimilar to the other hormones, antibodies raised to it can be used for specific measurement of hCG. The physiologic functions of hCG are (1) to support the secretion of progesterone by the corpus luteum until the placenta can produce enough hormone, (2) to promote steroidogenesis by the fetoplacental unit, and (3) to promote gonadal development in the fetus.

There is significant cross-reaction between hCG and LH because of their structural similarity. Therefore, the most important requirement for the measurement of hCG during pregnancy is the use of an antiserum with specific recognition for the $\beta$-subunit. Both urine and serum specimens may be used. However, urine specimens are used primarily in qualitative assays. There are several commercial kits for urine hCG measurements. The choice of tests may depend on the stage of pregnancy and the extent of hydration (i.e., urine output) since test sensitivity is often a problem. To assure the sensitivity of the assays, the urine sample may be concentrated, which is usually accomplished by restricting fluid intake and collecting the first voided morning specimen. The qualitative urine assays may not become positive until 8 to 14 days after the first missed menstrual period.[11] Sensitivity of the test may also depend on the underlying principle. The basic underlying principle used in the rapid qualitative pregnancy test is an agglutination inhibition reaction using either a slide test or a test tube matrix. In the slide test format, an hCG antiserum is first added to a urine specimen followed by the addition of hCG-coated latex particles. An agglutination reaction (hCG antigen–anti-hCG antiserum reaction) may be prevented only by a sufficiently high concentration of urinary hCG (positive test = pregnancy). In the absence of high urinary hCG, the hCG antiserum interacts preferentially with the hCG-coated latex particles to form an agglutination reaction within 2 minutes (negative test). The test tube format of this test is based on the same principle, except that the hCG-coated latex particles are replaced by erythrocytes. Another difference is that the agglutination reaction may take about 2 hours to develop. The slide tests are less sensitive than the tube tests. False-positive reactions may occur in about 5% of the cases and may be caused by the presence of proteins, pituitary gonadotropin LH, erythrocytes, leukocytes, and bacteria as well as certain drug metabolites. False-negative reactions also occur mainly because of the lack of sensitivity, since concentrations less than 1000 mU/mL may be undetectable (i.e., before day 8 since the LMP). Accuracy of these qualitative tests is about 94%. Because of the ease and speed of performing these tests, the urinary pregnancy test is a valuable home screening for the presence of pregnancy.

Serum samples are used for a more sensitive and accurate measurement of hCG using immunoassay techniques based on antisera raised against the $\beta$-subunit of hCG. The high sensitivity of the immunoassay techniques (about 200-fold more sensitive than urine qualitative tests and quantitative serum tests using antiserum against the intact hCG) may allow the detection of pregnancy as early as day 8 of gestation. Several variations of the immunoassay techniques are now available, including radioimmunoassay (RIA), enzyme immunoassays (EIA), and solid-phase, double-antibody sandwich, enzyme-linked immunoadsorbent (ELISA) assays. Gross hemolysis, turbidity, or lipemia of a serum sample may cause false-positive reactions.

The determination of pregnancy is only one clinical application for the measurement of hCG. Consistently low levels of hCG may be useful in diagnosing ectopic pregnancies. Another application in which serum hCG levels may be of benefit is in patients with gestational trophoblastic neoplasms or other hCG-producing tumors. After the tumor has been removed or treated, an increase in hCG levels may indicate recurrence of the tumor.

## Human Placental Lactogen

Human placental lactogen (hPL), also known as human chorionic somatomammotropin (hCS), is a polypeptide produced by the syncytiotrophoblastic cells in the placenta. Structurally, hPL shares similarity with both human growth hormone (hGH) and PRL. It has been suggested that the actions of hPL include (1) stimulation of the corpus luteum to produce estrogen and progesterone, (2) stimulation of the development of the mammary glands during pregnancy without causing milk secretion, and (3) somatotropic actions similar to those caused by GH. It is believed that hPL is one of the factors that contributes to carbohydrate metabolism changes during pregnancy.[15] The transport mechanism of hPL into the amniotic cavity is still unclear. Its concentration in the amniotic fluid is about 15 to 20 times lower than those found in the maternal circulation. Levels of hPL increase throughout the gestation period and correlate with placental weight.[15] Therefore, serum levels may reflect the integrity of the fetoplacental unit. The measurement of hPL is used to assess placental function during pregnancy, confirm the diagnosis of uterine cysts or tumors, and confirm diagnosis and monitor treatment of tumors outside the uterus that secrete human placental lactogen. Values are decreased with toxemia, molar pregnancy (hydatidiform mole), choriocarcinoma, and placental insufficiency. Increased hPL may be associated with multiple pregnancies, diabetes, and Rh incompatibility. The method of choice for the determination of hPL involves RIA techniques. A number of commercial kits are available. Serum is the specimen of choice and must be frozen immediately if there is a delay in measurement.

The measurement of human placental lactogen levels may be of some value in high-risk pregnancies, but there is not enough evidence to evaluate the use of hPL tests in routine care during pregnancy. Table 36–4 lists levels of human placental lactogen.

## Estriol

Estrogen synthesis in the woman is significantly altered during pregnancy, with the placenta rather than the ovary be-

**T A B L E   3 6 – 4**

**Reference Levels of Human Placental Lactogen (hPL) During Pregnancy**

| WEEK OF PREGNANCY | hPL (μg/mL) |
|---|---|
| 22 | 1.0–3.8 |
| 26 | 1.5–4.5 |
| 30 | 2.8–5.8 |
| 34 | 3.4–6.9 |
| 38 | 3.6–8.2 |
| 42 | 3.0–8.0 |

coming the major biosynthetic site. Estriol, rather than estradiol, becomes the major estrogen with milligram quantities being produced by the placenta using precursors derived from both maternal and fetal adrenal glands. The fetal adrenal gland produces dehydroepiandrosterone sulfate (DHEAS) and androstenedione. In the fetal liver, DHEAS is first hydroxylated to 16$\alpha$-OH DHEAS and subsequently converted to 16$\alpha$-OH androstenedione in the placenta. Just as the conversion of androgens, testosterone, and androstenedione to estrogens in the ovary is catalyzed by the aromatase enzyme system (19-hydroylase, 19-oxidase and 10,19-desmolase), the androgen 16$\alpha$-OH androstenedione is converted to estriol in the presence of the aromatase enzyme system. Placental estriol arrives at the maternal surface in a free state but is rapidly conjugated by the maternal liver to produce the water-soluble sulfate and glucuronide conjugates, which are excreted in the maternal urine. No unconjugated estriol is found in the maternal urine. Only about 14% of plasma estriol exists in the unconjugated form. Figure 36–1 summarizes the interrelationship between the maternal and fetal systems for providing precursors to the placenta for the production of estriol in the pregnant female.

Plasma (and urine) estriol levels may be used to assess the ability of the fetal adrenals to supply adequate amounts of androgens to the placenta and the ability of the placenta to process the precursors into estriol. These functions may be dependent on the fetal weight, fetal adrenal status, placental size, and the presence or deficiency of specific placental enzymes. The excretion of estriol in the urine is dependent not only on placental estriol synthesis but also on the mother's ability to conjugate the estriol in the liver and excrete the conjugated compound in the urine. Urinary and plasma estriol can therefore be used to predict problems that may affect these different parameters during pregnancy. Since the fetoplacental size increases with pregnancy, the levels of estriol rise as pregnancy progresses. Monitoring estriol levels in high-risk pregnancies as an assessment of the fetoplacental unit is particularly important. For example, if the estriol level drops 40% to 45% below the established mean of previous measurements, it may be an early indicator of fetoplacental distress. Proper interpretation of such tests may, however, be affected by several factors including the efficiency of maternal hepatic and renal functions. This may affect the amount of conjugated estriol excreted in the urine and the amount of estriol that is recirculated in the serum.[16] If the maternal liver cannot conjugate the estriol, free levels of estriol might increase in the plasma and free estriol may appear in the urine. If there is a maternal renal disease that significantly decreases the glomerular filtration rate, it may lead to decreased urinary estriol excretion and increased plasma estriol levels. By itself, however, there appears to be no beneficial effects of estriol measurement on fetal outcome.[17] It is most useful when used in combination with hCG and AFP.

Estriol determinations can be performed on urine (random or 24-hour collections), plasma, or serum. Unconjugated estriol assays are performed using serum. The specimens are stable at 4 to 10°C. Several manufacturers (including Amerlex-M, Eastman Kodak, Rochester, NY, and Diagnostic Systems Laboratories, Webster, TX) now have kits, all employing the RIA technique capable of measuring either the unconjugated or total estriol (which includes the conjugated form). A hydrolysis step is usually required in the procedure to measure unconjugated estriol.

## Alpha-fetoprotein

The most common diagnostic use of AFP levels is for the screening of maternal serum for the detection of open neural tube defects (spina bifida or anencephaly) or as a preliminary screen for Down syndrome.[18,19] Clearly, with an open spinal column or head, more AFP may leak out. High maternal serum AFP may suggest that the baby has one of these problems. For approximately 3.5% to 4% of women who have AFP values above 2.0 multiples of the mean, a repeat sample is recommended if the pregnancy is not too far advanced. About half of those with repeat testing will have a normal second value and may require no further testing. A second elevated AFP level may warrant examination with a fetal sonogram to confirm gestational age and also rule out multiple pregnancy. For women whose gestational age is confirmed and there is only one fetus, recalculation of the AFP is not necessary, and these patients are customarily offered amniocentesis for amniotic fluid AFP. Low maternal serum AFP levels may be an indication for the triple marker screen for Down syndrome risk assessment. However, should the triple screen results indicate an abnormality, the test may not be repeated, since a second normal value has not been shown to modify the initial risk. Instead, it is customary to recalculate the gestational age on the first sample for clarification purposes.

The results of maternal serum AFP concentration are usually expressed in relationship to the multiple of the median (MOM) for an appropriate gestational age. Interpretation is difficult and should be made in connection with maternal weight, age, race, and presence of diseases such as insulin-dependent (type 1) diabetes mellitus.[20,21] The following formula is used to adjust MOM for maternal weight.

$$\text{Expected MOM} = 10^{0.2658 - 0.00188 \text{ (maternal weight in pounds)}}$$

Even though maternal age per se does not affect the AFP synthesis, the risk of many chromosomal abnormalities increases with maternal age. The maternal weight correlates directly with maternal circulatory volume. By adjusting MOM for maternal weight, maternal serum AFP may be more accurately interpreted.[21]

The concentrations of maternal serum AFP are approximately 10% higher in black women than in white, Hispanic, or Oriental women.[22] Therefore, the MOM should be decreased by 10% in black women before interpretation.

Mothers with type 1 diabetes mellitus have 20% to 40% lower levels of serum AFP than those without the disorder.

The MOM should be corrected by dividing by an appropriate factor (0.7).[22] Increased serum AFP is found in several other diseases such as alcoholic liver disease and chronic active hepatitis. In fact, in adults with hepatocellular carcinoma, serum AFP may be as high as 3000 ng/mL.[23]

AFP is most commonly measured using RIA or EIA techniques including the microparticle enzyme immunoassay technique (Abbott Laboratories). Maternal serum or amniotic fluid can be utilized as specimens and the AFP is very stable even at ambient temperatures.

## Bilirubin

The analysis of bilirubin pigments in amniotic fluid during pregnancy can be a valuable tool to the clinician in evaluating the status of an infant that may or may not be affected by fetal-maternal incompatibility. This may be assessed using either the Liley or Queenan charts.[24] Even though the term *bilirubin* is used, these pigments should probably be described as bilirubinoid because of their molecular complexity. The procedure for the measurement of the bilirubinoid pigments in amniotic fluid ($\Delta A_{450}$) is discussed in greater detail in Chapter 16. Unconjugated bilirubin peaks at 450 nm on a spectral scan of amniotic fluid. The degree of elevation of this peak has been correlated with the severity of erythroblastosis fetalis.

The amniotic fluid is obtained through a procedure known as **amniocentesis.** Amniocentesis is performed by the introduction of a needle through the maternal abdominal and uterine walls into the amniotic cavity. Approximately 10 mL of fluid are withdrawn. The procedure may be done as early as 22 weeks' gestation if there is a previous history of hemolytic disease of the newborn or serologic evidence of incompatibility.

## Surfactant Phospholipids

The lung is the last organ to mature in the developing fetus. The lung is primarily a fluid-filled organ during pregnancy and has to quickly adapt to breathing in a gaseous environment within minutes of birth. A defect in lung maturation may make this transition a difficult or even impossible one. Both proper anatomic and functional maturation of the lung are required before birth. Pulmonary surfactants reduce the surface tension between fluid lining and the air in the lungs. The pulmonary surfactant is a complex chemical mixture of lipids, proteins, and less than 5% carbohydrates.[6] The predominant lipids are phosphatidylcholine (PC) (lecithin), phosphatidylglycerol (PG), and phosphatidylinositol (PI). Amniotic fluid sphingomyelin is present in relatively small quantities (~2%), and even though it may be derived from sources other than the lungs, it is frequently used in assays because it serves as an internal standard against the more specific phospholipids being measured. These chemical compounds are produced by specialized alveolar cells called type II granular pneumocytes and packaged into storage granules called the *lamellar bodies.* As pregnancy progresses and the fetus begins to breathe, pulmonary fluids escape out of the respiratory tract into the amniotic fluid. The measurement of surfactant phospholipids in amniotic fluid has become an important diagnostic tool in the evaluation of fetal lung maturity and thus the prevention of respiratory distress syndrome (RDS).[25]

Several methods are available for evaluating fetal lung maturity that exploit either the chemical or physical properties of the surfactants.[26] In general, amniotic fluid is harvested during amniocentesis being careful not to contaminate the specimens with blood, meconium, or vaginal secretions (if specimen was collected vaginally after the rupture of the membranes). These contaminants interfere with most test procedures. The most commonly used measurement of the chemical constituents of the surfactant in amniotic fluid is the lecithin/sphingomyelin (L/S) ratio because the concentration of lecithin relative to sphingomyelin increases with gestation.[6] A peak in L/S is reached between 34 and 36 weeks of gestation that coincides with fetal lung maturity. An L/S ratio $\geq 2$ is indicative of fetal maturity in a normal pregnancy and $\geq 3$ for mothers with diabetes. This is a semiquantitative test that employs the thin-layer chromatography technique. A minimum of 3 mL of amniotic fluid are required for the test. The amniotic fluid must be centrifuged to remove all cellular elements because the organic (acetone) phospholipid extracts may be artifactually increased by plasma membrane phospholipids.

Determination of either PG or PI as percentage of total phospholipid content of the amniotic fluid improves the diagnostic accuracy of the L/S ratio. By running a two-dimensional thin-layer chromatography of a cold acetone phospholipid extract of the amniotic fluid, the percentage of PG or PI can be estimated. A PG level >3% of the total phospholipid extract is indicative of fetal lung maturity.

The amniotic fluid supernatant should be assayed or stored at refrigerator temperature or frozen. Phospholipid levels decrease at room temperature. If stored, the specimen should be mixed gently before analysis since the phospholipids settle to the bottom during storage.

Procedures that exploit the physical properties of the pulmonary surfactants are also available.[26–28] The most common of these is the foam stability index (FSI), which is based on the principle that more surfactant activity is required to support a stable foam formation when the amniotic fluid is mixed with increasing concentration of ethanol. A set of 6 test tubes is set up containing varying amounts of 95% ethanol (0.55, 0.51, 0.49, 0.47, 0.45, and 0.43 mL) and 0.5 mL of amniotic fluid added. The final concentrations correspond to 0.50, 0.48, 0.47, 0.46, 0.45, and 0.44, respectively. The tubes are shaken vigorously for 30 seconds before examination for a stable ring of bubbles. The highest concentration of ethanol that supports a stable foam is the FSI and a value of $\geq 0.47$ is indicative of fetal lung maturity.

## CLINICAL APPLICATIONS

### Respiratory Distress Syndrome

Respiratory distress syndrome (RDS) is the most common disturbance found in babies born prematurely (before 37 weeks and with birth weight <2500 g). Also called hyaline membrane disease, RDS is a lung disorder that is caused by insufficient synthesis of pulmonary surfactant. As a result, exchange of oxygen and carbon dioxide in the lungs' alveolar sacs during breathing is inefficient and incomplete. The disease causes difficulty in breathing and gradually leads to collapse of the lungs. The reduced oxygenation of the organs in the rest of the body may result in heart failure, kidney failure, intestinal disease, bleeding into the brain, chronic lung disease, cerebral palsy, and later in life, learning disorders.

Nearly all babies born before 32 weeks of pregnancy will develop RDS, and about 25% of these very premature babies will die of RDS and associated problems.[26] Fetal lung maturity tests therefore offer the physician the opportunity to assess whether medical care can best be given in utero if the lungs are not matured yet or in the nursery if fetal maturity can be verified. Instances when fetal lung maturity testing may be required include anticipated early delivery because of medical or obstetrical mishaps, premature rupture of the fetal membranes, or in mothers who may have to undergo a repeat cesarean delivery.

### Down Syndrome and Spina Bifida

Down syndrome (trisomy 21) occurs in 0.99 per 1000 births, with the risk of incidence increasing with the maternal age. About 10% to 20% of the infants die in the first year, predominantly from cardiovascular defects. Trisomy 18 is a more severe chromosomal abnormality, with an incidence rate of about 1 in 8000 births. Two thirds of cases diagnosed before birth are aborted before delivery.[29] Before the introduction of biochemical serum markers, most Down syndrome babies were not discovered before birth. Genetic screening (amniocentesis at 16 to 18 weeks of gestation) of mothers who are 35 years and older at the time of delivery has been helpful in detecting some of these babies but it has been estimated that about 80% of these babies were also born to mothers who were younger than 35 years old. During the early part of the 1980s, it was discovered that there was an association between low maternal serum AFP levels and increased risk of Down syndrome.[30,31] Subsequently, it was established that maternal serum hCG, unconjugated estriol, and AFP were also associated with Down syndrome.[18–20] Indeed, using the triple markers (AFP, hCG, and unconjugated estriol) increased the detection rate to about 60%, compared to about 25% when AFP was used alone. The triple-marker screen also reduced the false-positive rate considerably to less than 7%. The triple-marker screen is used as a screening tool to detect fetuses with neural tube defects (e.g., anencephaly, spina bifida), ventral wall defects, and several cytogenetic trisomies. This triple-marker screen with a mid-trimester risk cutoff level of 1:190 (most laboratories use a conservative cutoff level of 1:250) is the most efficient for optimizing the detection rate and minimizing the false-positive rate. The cutoff level, calculated using the median values for AFP, hCG, and unconjugated estriol and the maternal age, is determined using a computer program, such as the Alpha program (Logical Medical Systems, London).

The use of the triple-marker screening test is particularly useful for women younger than 35 years of age who would, under normal circumstances, not be considered for amniocentesis. Pregnant women with advancing maternal age or with family or pregnancy history of problems of these genetic abnormalities definitely benefit from undergoing these tests. The results have the best predictive value if the serum samples are collected between 15 and 18 weeks of gestation.

### Erythroblastosis Fetalis

Erythroblastosis fetalis is also known as the hemolytic disease of the newborn. It is a disease of the fetus caused by an incompatibility between fetal and maternal red blood cells.[32] Fetal erythrocytes may cross the placenta in small numbers during pregnancy or in larger numbers at birth due to fetal-maternal hemorrhage. When an Rh(D)-negative mother is first exposed to Rh-positive fetal cells, she is sensitized to the D antigen. In subsequent pregnancies, further stimulation with D positive fetal cells may cause production of anti-D, which can cross the placenta and attack the Rh-positive fetal cells. This results in the destruction of fetal erythrocytes. Clinical manifestation of the RhD hemolytic disease may range from an asymptomatic mild anemia to hydrops fetalis or stillbirth associated with severe anemia and jaundice. The jaundice is due to an extra bilirubin burden on the fetal liver. Since the excretory function of the liver does not reach full maturity until about 4 weeks after birth even in full-term babies, there is inadequate hepatic conjugation of the excess bilirubin. Therefore, relatively large quantities of unconjugated bilirubin remain in the fetal circulation. Unconjugated bilirubin is toxic to the brain, where it preferentially accumulates leading to the condition known as **kernicterus.** Babies who survive this disease are known to be mentally retarded. Historically, the best known blood incompatibility involves the Rh blood group system, but other blood systems may be involved. For example, hemolytic disease of the newborn due to anti-S antibodies has been reported.[33] The anemia produced as a result of excessive loss of the erythrocytes also stimulates hematopoiesis in the fetal bone marrow, spleen, and liver. Increased hematopoiesis in the liver may lead to destruction of the fetal liver cells, which may in turn lead to decreased protein synthesis. The result may be a reduction in oncotic pressure, producing edema or hydrops in the fetus.[34]

The degree of fetal erythrocyte destruction can be monitored by determining the bilirubinoid level in the amniotic fluid using the $\Delta A_{450}$ spectrophotometric procedure. Generally, 10 mL of amniotic fluid are required and must be stored in the dark, where it is stable for 30 days at room temperature or up to 9 months when stored at 4°C. Proper interpretation of the results takes into account the gestational age.

## Gestational Diabetes Mellitus

**Gestational diabetes mellitus** (GDM) is defined as any degree of glucose intolerance with onset or first recognition during the pregnancy.[35] This definition of GDM does not rule out that the disease could well have started before the pregnancy or concurrently with conception. Even though in most instances the disease may disappear after pregnancy, it is also possible that the disease may persist after delivery of the baby. In the United States, approximately 135,000 pregnancies are complicated by GDM annually (~1 out of 20 pregnancies). The incidence rate may, however, range from 1% to 15% depending on the ethnicity of the community being sampled: Native-American, Hispanic-American and African-American populations generally have higher incidence rates of diabetes than the white population.[36,37]

Women with advanced maternal age, marked obesity, personal history of GDM, glycosuria, or a strong family history (first-degree relative) of diabetes are at great risk of GDM and so must undergo glucose testing at the earliest convenience or at the first prenatal visit. Retesting is recommended between 24 and 28 weeks of gestation.[38] The current criteria for diagnosis of diabetes (a fasting plasma glucose >126 mg/dL or a random plasma glucose >200 mg/dL) when confirmed on a subsequent occasion meets the threshold for the diagnosis of diabetes in pregnancy and may require no further testing. If the results are not definitive and the woman is in a high-risk group for GDM, it is the recommendation of the American Diabetes Association that the 75-g or 100-g oral glucose tolerance test (OGTT) be performed.[39] Table 36–5 summarizes the diagnostic criteria during the tests. Two or more of the plasma glucose concentrations must be met or exceeded for a positive diagnosis of GDM.

T A B L E   3 6 – 5

**Diagnosis of Gestational Diabetes Mellitus with 75-g or 100-g Oral Glucose Tolerance Test**

| LOAD TIME | 75-g GLUCOSE LOAD (mg/dL) | 100-g GLUCOSE LOAD (mg/dL) |
|---|---|---|
| Fasting | 95 | 95 |
| 1 h | 180 | 180 |
| 2 h | 155 | 155 |
| 3 h | — | 140 |

Women with GDM are at increased risk of development of type 2 diabetes mellitus after pregnancy since risk factors such as obesity promote insulin resistance even in the nonpregnant state. The same problems known to occur in infants born to women with preexisting diabetes such as neonatal hypoglycemia, jaundice, and respiratory distress syndrome are also found in GDM. In a population-based study of Magee et al,[38] women with GDM had a significantly higher likelihood of experiencing any of 33 possible perinatal morbidities. The offsprings of women with GDM have increased risks of developing diabetes later in life, but the most common complication of GDM is **macrosomia,** which is loosely defined as birth weight in excess of 8.5 to 9 lb (4000 to 4500 g).[39,40] Macrosomia is found in 15% to 45% of diabetic pregnancies. Large for the gestational age is diagnosed when infants are at or above the 90th, 95th, or in some instances, 97.5th percentile for gestational age after adjustment for such variables as gender and birth order.[41] Mounting evidence shows that macrosomic newborns of diabetic mothers experience excessive rates of neonatal morbidity compared with normal birthweight neonates.[42]

Several studies have confirmed that insulin plays a significant role in the development of macrosomia. Apparently, as a result of hyperglycemic episodes in the maternal circulation, fetal hyperinsulinemia is created that promotes storage of excess nutrients.[42] In fact, fetal hyperinsulinemic episodes lasting only 1 to 2 hours may produce detrimental effects.

Evaluation of the mother early in the pregnancy for detecting hyperglycemia may help to keep the mother in metabolic control through insulin treatment and adjustment of caloric intake. Oral hypoglycemic agents are not recommended during pregnancy. Maternal surveillance can easily be accomplished by measurement of blood glucose and glycated hemoglobin (Hb $A_{1c}$) levels. Urine glucose is also helpful since it is noninvasive. Fetal insulin and C-peptide can be measured by sampling the amniotic fluid. In the long run, control of maternal blood glucose levels will be a benefit to both mother and baby.

## HELLP Syndrome

Pregnancy-induced hypertension, especially eclampsia, affects 7% to 10% of all pregnancies and contributes substantially to both maternal and fetal mortality and morbidity.[43] The classic findings in severe preeclampsia are hypertension, with systolic blood pressure >160 mm Hg or diastolic blood pressure >110 mm Hg, proteinuria >5 g/24 h, oliguria <400 mL/24 h, cerebral or visual disturbances, and/or pulmonary edema or cyanosis. Approximately 10% of patients with severe preeclampsia develop a serious variant of preeclampsia known as HELLP syndrome. First coined by Weinstein in 1982, HELLP is an acronym for h̲emolysis, e̲levated l̲iver function, and l̲ow p̲latelet count.[44] Pregnancies complicated by this syndrome are associated with poor maternal and perinatal outcome. Reported maternal mortality ranges from 0% to 24%. In addition, the mothers are at increased risk for developing several diseases including pulmonary edema, adult respiratory distress syndrome (ARDS), disseminated intravascular coagulopathy (DIC), ruptured liver hematomas, and acute renal failure.[45–48]

## SUMMARY

The first major change accompanying pregnancy is the endocrine modification of the luteal phase of the menstrual cycle leading to a postponement of menstruation. Significant biochemical, physiologic, and metabolic changes accompany the transition from an ordinary menstrual cycle to pregnancy. To meet the increasing demands of the developing baby whose biochemical and metabolic needs are also constantly changing, the mother undergoes significant physiologic changes, some of which predispose her and the baby to serious health consequences. Almost every organ function in the mother is modified and many biochemical and metabolic indices found in the maternal circulation may vary considerably when compared with values in the nonpregnant female. Increased maternal uterine blood flow and placental plasma membrane permeability during pregnancy allow adequate perfusion of the placental beds for exchange of oxygen and nutrients to the fetus and the surrounding amniotic fluid, a major component of the intrauterine environment. Three distinctive body fluids (maternal blood and urine and the amniotic fluid) are available to the laboratory for the measurements of several analytes that the clinician may use to monitor the well-being of the mother and baby. Some of the analytes found in the maternal circulation (e.g., hCG and AFP) or amniotic fluid may be unique only to the period of pregnancy and therefore may be used to assess the progress of the pregnancy or for the screening of birth defects. Clearly, the laboratory plays a significant role in the care and management of both normal and abnormal pregnancies.

## REFERENCES

1. Greene MF, Fencl DM, Tulchinsky D: Biochemical aspects of pregnancy. In Tietz NW (ed.): *Textbook of Clinical Chemistry.* 1st ed. Philadelphia, WB Saunders, 1986, p 1745.
2. Coustan DR: Gestational diabetes. In *Diabetes and Digestive Disease.* 2nd ed. Bethesda, MD, National Institutes of Health, NIH publication No. 95–1468, 1995, p 703.
3. Chapman A, Abraham WT, Zamudio S, et al.: Temporal relationships between hormonal and hemodynamic changes in early human pregnancy. Kidney Int 54:2056, 1998.
4. Moore TR: Fetal growth in diabetic pregnancy. Clin Obstet Gynecol 40:771, 1997.
5. Magann EF, Isler CM, Chauhan SP, Martin JN Jr.: Am-

6. Ashwood ER: Clinical chemistry of pregnancy. In Burtis CA, Ashwood ER (eds.): *Tietz Textbook of Clinical Chemistry.* 2nd ed. Philadelphia, WB Saunders, 1994, p 2107.
7. Faught W, Garner P, Jones G, et al.: Changes in protein C and protein S levels in normal pregnancy. Am J Obstet Gynecol 172:147, 1995.
8. Bremme K, Ostund E, Almqvist I, et al.: Enhanced thrombin generation and fibrinolytic activity in normal pregnancy and the puerperium. Obstet Gynecol 80:132, 1992.
9. Bonnar J: Haemostasis and coagulation disorders in pregnancy. In Bloom AL, Thomas DP (eds.): *Haemostasis and Thrombosis.* 2nd ed. Edinburgh, Churchill Livingstone, 1987, p 570.
10. Haqq CM, King C, Ukiyama E, Falsafi S, et al.: Molecular basis of mammalian sexual determination: activation of mullerian inhibiting substance gene expression by SRY. Science 266:1494, 1994.
11. Grupp-Phelan J, Taylor JA, Liu LL, Davis RL: Early newborn hospital discharge and readmission for mild and severe jaundice. Arch Pediatr Adolesc Med 153:1283, 1999.
12. Moyer VA, Ahn C, Sneed S: Accuracy of clinical judgment in neonatal jaundice. Arch Pediatr Adolesc Med 154:391, 2000.
13. Trudinger B: Fetal-placental circulation and placentation in normal and hypertensive pregnancies. In Jacobsen H, Striker G, Klahr S (eds.): *The Principles and Practice of Neurology.* 2nd ed. St. Louis, MO, Mosby, 1995, p 431.
14. Pijnenborg R: Uterine haemodynamics as a possible driving force for endovascular trophoblast migration in the placental bed. Med Hypotheses 55:114, 2000.
15. Cao X, Qin W, He Z: Changes of carbohydrate metabolism in normal pregnancy and its relationship with placental lactogen concentrations. Chin J Obstet Gynecol 33:80, 1998.
16. Doche C, Bartoli M, Mercier S, et al.: Prenatal screening for Down syndrome: preanalytical precautions. Prenat Diagn 20:684, 2000.
17. Neilson JP, Cloherty LJ: Hormonal placental function tests for fetal assessment in high risk pregnancies. Cochrane Database of Systematic Reviews [computer file] (2):CD000108, 2000.
18. Kellner LH, Weiss RR, Weiner Z, et al.: Fetus-placenta-newborn: The advantages of using triple-marker screening for chromosomal abnormalities. Am J Obstet Gynecol 172:831, 1995.
19. Cate S, Ball S: Multiple marker screening for Down syndrome—whom should we screen? J Am Bd Fam Pract 12:367, 1999.
20. Knight GJ, Palomaki GE, Haddow JE: Use of maternal

serum alpha-fetoprotein measurement to screen for Down syndrome. Clin Obstet Gynecol 31:306, 1988.

21. Kramer RL, Yaron Y, O'Brien JE, et al.: Effect of adjustment of maternal serum alpha-fetoprotein levels in insulin-dependent diabetes mellitus. Am J Med Genet 75:176, 1998.

22. O'Brien JE, Dvorin E, Drugan A, et al.: Race-ethnicity-specific variation in multiple-marker biochemical screening: Alpha-fetoprotein, hCG, and estriol. Obstet Gynecol 89:355, 1997.

23. Gambarin-Gelwan M, Wolf DC, Shapiro R, et al.: Sensitivity of commonly available screening tests in detecting hepatocellular carcinoma in cirrhotic patients undergoing liver transplantation. Am J Gastroenterol 95:1535, 2000.

24. Scott F, Chan FY: Assessment of the clinical usefulness of the 'Queenan' chart versus the 'Liley' chart in predicting severity of rhesus iso-immunization. Prenat Diagn 18:1143, 1998.

25. Barrington KJ, Finer NN: Recent advances. Care of near term infants with respiratory failure. BMJ 315:1215, 1997.

26. McElrath TF, Norwitz ER, Robinson JN, et al.: Differences in TDx fetal lung maturity assay values between twin and singleton gestations. Am J Obstet Gynecol 182:1110, 2000.

27. Piazze JJ, Anceschi MM, Maranghi, et al.: The biophysical/biochemical test. A new marker of fetal lung maturity in borderline cases. J Reprod Med 44:611, 1999.

28. Kucuk M: Tap test, shake test and phosphatidylglycerol in the assessment of fetal pulmonary maturity. Int J Gynaecol Obstet 60:9, 1998.

29. Hook EB, Cross PK, Schreimemachers DM: Chromosomal abnormality rates at amniocentesis and in liveborn infants. JAMA 249:2034, 1983.

30. Merkatz IR, Nitowski HM, Macri JN, Johnson WE: An association between low maternal serum alpha-fetoprotein and fetal chromosomal abnormalities. Am J Obstet Gynecol 148:886, 1984.

31. Hershey DW, Crandall BF, Scroff PS: Maternal serum alpha-fetoprotein screening of fetal trisomies. Am J Obstet Gynecol 153:224, 1985.

32. Urbaniak SJ, Greiss MA: RhD haemolytic disease of the fetus and the newborn. Blood Rev 14:44, 2000.

33. Parsh BS. Hemolytic disease of the newborn due to anti S antibodies. J Natl Med Assoc 92:91, 2000.

34. Wy CA, Sajous CH, Loberiza F, Weiss MG: Outcome of infants with a diagnosis of hydrops fetalis in the 1990s. Am J Perinat 16:561, 1999.

35. Schwartz ML, Ray WN, Lubarsky SL: The diagnosis and classification of gestational diabetes: Is it time to change our tune? Am J Obstet Gynecol 180:1560, 1999.

36. Dooley SL, Metzger BE, Cho NH: Gestational diabetes mellitus: Influence of race on disease prevalence and perinatal outcomes in a US population. Diabetes Care 40(Suppl 2):25, 1991.

37. Harris MI, Hadden WC, Knowler WC, Bennett PH: Prevalence of diabetes and impaired glucose tolerance and plasma glucose levels in US population aged 20–74 yr. Diabetes 36:523, 1987.

38. Magee MS, Walden CE, Benedetti TJ, Knopp RH: Influence of diagnostic criteria on the incidence of gestational diabetes and perinatal morbidity. JAMA 269:609, 1993.

39. American Diabetes Association: Clinical practice recommendations 2000. Diabetes Care 23:S77, 2000.

40. Sacks DA: Fetal macrosomia and gestational diabetes: What's the problem? Obstet Gynecol 81:775, 1993.

41. Grassi AE, Giuliano MA: The neonate with macrosomia. Clin Obstet Gynecol 43(2):340, 2000.

42. Schwartz R, Gruppuso PA, Petzol K, et al.: Hyperinsulinemia and macrosomia in the fetus of the diabetic mother. Diabetes Care 17:640, 1994.

43. Xiong X, Mayes D, Demianczuk N, et al.: Impact of pregnancy-induced hypertension on fetal growth. Am J Obstet Gynecol 180:207, 1999.

44. Weinstein L: Syndrome of hemolysis, elevated liver enzymes, and low platelet count: A severe consequence of hypertension in pregnancy. Am J Obstet Gynecol 142:159, 1982.

45. Osmers RGW, Schütz E, Diedrich F, et al.: Increased serum levels of hyaluronic acid in pregnancies complicated by preeclampsia or hemolysis, elevated liver enzymes, and low platelets syndrome. Am J Obstet Gynecol 178:341, 1998.

46. Van Dam PA, Reiner M, Baekelandt M, et al.: Disseminated intravascular coagulation and the syndrome of hemolysis, elevated liver enzymes, and low platelets in severe preeclampsia. Obstet Gynecol 73:97, 1989.

47. Martin JN Jr., Rinehart BK, May WL, et al.: The spectrum of severe preeclampsia: comparative analysis by HELLP (hemolysis, elevated liver enzyme levels, and low platelet count) syndrome classification. Am J Obstet Gynecol 180:1373, 1999.

48. Sibai BM, Ramadan MK: Acute renal failure in pregnancies complicated by hemolysis, elevated liver enzymes, and low platelets. Am J Obstet Gynecol 168:1682, 1993.

# CHAPTER 37

# Neonatal and Pediatric Laboratory Assessment

*Eileen Carreiro-Lewandowski*

## DEVELOPMENTAL DIFFERENCES

The pediatric population includes neonates, infants, children, and young adults up until the age of 18. Beginning at birth, the infant rapidly adapts from life inside the placenta to the extrauterine environment, undergoing many systemic changes throughout childhood until the completion of growth at the end of adolescence. These stages are often marked in a chronological manner, matched with an expected range of relative physiologic developments beginning with gestational age as a fetus. Environmental, socioeconomic, and genetic factors also play an important role in determining pediatric wellness or disease at any stage of development, making interpretation of laboratory data relative to established reference ranges particularly critical. Therefore, the associated reference ranges need to reflect the maturation changes in this population as well as any variation caused by the different methods and laboratory instruments utilized in test performance, including those used in point-of-care testing. Regardless of the population served, laboratories need to establish or verify published and manufacturer's reference ranges. At this time, several good references addressing establishment of reference ranges for the pediatric population include the National Committee for Clinical Laboratory Standards (NCCLS) C28-A[1] and two texts entitled *The Biochemical Basis of Pediatric Disease*[2] and *Pediatric Reference Ranges*.[3]

Although the biochemical, physiologic, and metabolic processes may be similar in both the pediatric and adult population, the developmental differences that have an impact on all organ systems vary considerably. Members of the pediatric population should not be considered as "miniature" adults. Assuming birth occurs at the proper gestational age and development, also known as full term (approximately 40 weeks' gestation), the age groups associated with each stage may be defined as: the newborn or neonate, birth to 1 month; the infant, 1 month to 1 year; early childhood, 1 year through 4 years; middle childhood, 5 years through 10 years; and adolescence, 11 years through the 17th year.[4] The term *perinatal* refers to the period preceding, during, or immediately after birth and may be used in association with the term *neonatal*. Preterm refers to the infant born prematurely, before 38 weeks

of gestation or weighing less than 5 to 5.5 lb.[5] A comparison of changes in body composition with growth and aging (Figure 37–1) illustrates the differences in minerals, proteins, fat, and water at different stages. It is quickly apparent that any analyte confined to or associated with these compartments would need to be assessed in reference to the compartment at various stages of development and maturation.[6] For most analytes, the same pathologic processes causing values to be outside a reference range in the adult population would have the same impact on those analytes in the pediatric population, provided the values are interpreted within the proper context. There are unique circumstances that arise in the pediatric and neonatal population and these topics are briefly discussed in this chapter.

## PERINATAL PHYSIOLOGY

### Respiratory System

Perinatal physiology reveals that the fetus, immersed in amniotic fluid, must make the transition from total dependency on the placenta for gas exchange, nutrition, and excretion to an independent air-breathing organism.[7] Failure to successfully make the transition results in some type of neonatal disorder. While in utero, the placenta provides the exchange of $CO_2$ for $O_2$ in the fetus. The fetal lungs and alveoli are fairly developed by 25 weeks but are filled with amniotic fluid rather than air. Fetal breathing movements, present at this time, push the amniotic fluid from the fetal alveoli up through the tracheobronchial tree for gas exchange. At this stage of development, surface tension in the fetal lungs is not an issue, but once born, the alveoli fill with air, causing very high surface tensions to exist between the alveoli and chest cavity linings. Pulmonary surfactant material is needed to keep the alveoli from collapsing (atelectasis). The surfactant material is composed of a mixture of phospholipids including phosphatidylcholine (also known as lecithin), phosphatidylglycerol, phosphatidylinositol, sphingomyelin, and three surface-active proteins. By 34 to 35 weeks' gestation, enough surfactant, housed in bundles called *lamellar bodies*, is usually produced to prevent atelectasis.

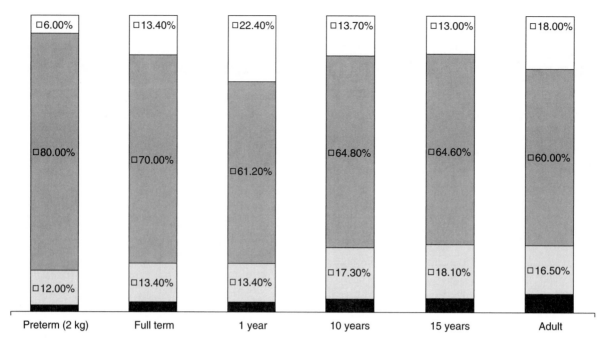

Body composition with growth.

Inadequate surfactant, usually associated with immaturity, is a primary defect in respiratory distress syndrome (RDS). Laboratory testing for fetal lung maturity involves several approaches that detect the amount of various substances including a ratio of lecithin to sphingomyelin (L/S ratio), the level of one or more of the phospholipids, and/or the number of lamellar bodies,[8,9] and others.

## Circulation and Hematopoiesis

Circulation in the fetus is actually opposite to that in the newborn.[10] Because the placenta is the source of oxygenated fetal blood, not the fetal lungs, the fetal circulation basically bypasses the lungs, allowing the oxygen rich blood to easily move into the fetal head and thoracic area. The pulmonary artery has a much higher relative resistance than does the right ventricle and blood flows from the right ventricle to the aorta via a fetal ductus in the heart and out to systemic circulation. There also exists a difference in pressures between the right and left atrium. Left atrial pressure is low because little blood is returned from the lungs, but the right atrial pressure remains high because of the large volume of blood returning from the placenta. This causes a flap of the foramen ovale to remain open and further support the shunting of blood from the right to the left with an increase in relative blood flow. Normally, this flap closes shortly after birth as the pressure in the lungs markedly increases when air is inhaled. The $PO_2$ of systemic fetal blood is very low at about 25 mm Hg. The high percentage of fetal hemoglobin present (70%), and its high affinity for oxygen coupled with the increased blood flow associ-

ated with the systemic fetal circulation, ensures that the fetal tissues are adequately oxygenated. After birth, systemic resistance increases above the pulmonary resistance caused by air breathing. The increased $PO_2$ (95 to 98 mmHg) plus cord clamping at birth causes the umbilical arteries to constrict, resulting in reduced blood flow (and therefore pressure) to the right atrium, whereas left atrial pressure increases. The blood flow now reverses, creating left-to-right adult-like shunting of the blood through the fetal ductus, which then closes in about 24 hours after birth. The closing of the ductus further aids the left-to-right direction of blood flow through the heart.

At birth, the abrupt increase in $PO_2$ also causes erythropoietin levels to fall so that the amount of hemoglobin decreases from about 16 g/dL at birth to approximately 12g/dL at 3 months. This drop in hemoglobin constitutes a type of physiologic anemia. During this period, the reduced $O_2$ tension signals the production of erythropoietin and bone marrow production of red blood cells. In utero, erythrocyte production is heavily dependent on the liver and spleen and less on the bone marrow. As the infant grows, changes in the marrow cause some of the red (hematopoietic) marrow to begin being replaced by yellow (fatty) marrow, resulting in less dependence on the liver and spleen as sites of red cell production. In addition, the lifespan of red cells in infants is decreased to ~60 to 80 days rather than the children and adult red cell lifespan of 120 days. Red blood cell turnover in premature infants is even more rapid, where the lifespan may be as short as 20 to 30 days.[7] These cells are metabolically more active, resulting in increased glucose consumption for glycolysis. Another change in blood cellular components is a "shift to the left" (increased numbers of immature erythrocytes and leukocytes, particularly neutrophils and lymphocytes) that usually disappears by 3 months of age. Collectively, there is a decreased efficiency of the reticuloendothelial system at birth.

## Immunity

The newborn's immune system is immature at birth. Most of the antibody present is from IgG that crosses the placenta because IgM, IgA, IgE, and complement do not. The fetus produces trace amounts of IgM and IgG by the 30th week but because of the antigen-free environment of the fetus, only trace amounts are produced in utero. After 22 weeks' gestation, placental transfer of IgG increases reaching maternal levels, or slightly higher, at birth. Levels in premature infants are decreased relative to their gestational age. After birth, catabolism of maternal IgG occurs, and since it only has a half-life of approximately 25 days, results in a physiologic hypogammaglobulinemia. The hypogammaglobulinemia begins to resolve at about 6 months of age as the infant's production of immunoglobulins increases to sufficient levels. Transfer of maternal IgG and immune factors via breast milk helps compensate for the newborn's immature immune system. In addition, newborns have a reduced antibody response to many antigens including those in vaccines. By 1 year, the IgG levels approximate 70% of adult levels. IgM reaches adult immunoglobulin levels at 1 year, IgG by 8 years, and IgA by the 11th year.[12] Lymphocytic cytotoxic activity at birth, including natural killer cells, B and T cells, is considerably lower than seen in adult lymphocytes. At 12 hours after birth, neutrophil and monocyte phagocytosis is normal in healthy infants but chemotaxis is decreased. This ultimately contributes to the overall poor immunity of healthy full-term newborns, and premature neonates have an even less effective defense system.

## Gastrointestinal and Liver

A newborn's gastrointestinal tract, while fully developed, is functionally immature because the processes of digestion and elimination have been aided by the placenta. At birth, the entire intestine is filled with a substance called *meconium*, which consists of intestinal gland secretions and some amniotic fluid that appears as a dark brownish-green substance. In healthy newborns, meconium is passed, usually within 24 to 48 hours after birth. Following an infant's first feeding and meconium defecation, normal bowel movements occur and normal flora in the gut begin to be present. A newborn has slower bowel motility than an older child. The gastric pH at birth is fairly neutral and then falls to a more acidic pH of about 3. The pH does not stabilize until 3 years of age as the gastric mucosa develops. Gastric emptying is slower than adults until about 6 months of age. Both of these factors have an impact on drug absorption.

Liver adaptation to the extrauterine environment may take several days, even in a full-term healthy infant. Full understanding of liver function and bilirubin metabolism, breakdown of hemoglobin from red blood cells (see Chapter 16), is helpful in assessing the differences between the pediatric and adult liver functions. The fetal liver is relatively immature because the placenta aids in the conjugation and excretion of toxic substances, including fetal bilirubin. Approximately 50% of healthy, full-term newborns display an unconjugated hyperbilirubinemia at 24 to 48 hours that generally resolves by day 7 and is often referred to as physiologic jaundice. This usually transient condition is due to low concentrations of the liver enzymes responsible for bilirubin conjugation, namely glucuronyl transferases. Hemolysis, associated with the trauma of birth, can also contribute to the increased bilirubin. Because of decreased bowel motility in the newborn, use of the enterohepatic pathway for bilirubin excretion may be increased. Additionally, a newborn's small intestine contains some residual $\beta$-glucuronidase, an enzyme capable of deconjugating bilirubin glucuronide, forming even more unconjugated bilirubin utilizing this pathway. Early feedings (within 4 hours) increase bowel motility and decrease the level of bilirubin and hyperbilirubinemia.[13] The newborn also lacks the intestinal bacteria responsible for oxidizing bilirubin to urobilinogen, resulting in unchanged conjugated bilirubin excretion to appear in the newborn stool and responsible for the characteristic yellow-green stool. Infants born to mothers with diabetes may be prone to hyperbilirubinemia because of initial feeding difficulties. Formula-fed infants have lower values than those infants who are breast fed.[14,15] Increased bilirubin in immature infants may persist for a longer time, sometimes as long as 14 days. Increased bilirubin before 24 hours, conjugated bilirubinemia, or a hyperbilirubinemia that lasts longer than expected are reasons for concern and further evaluation. Neonatal metabolism of other substances, such as drugs, is generally slower, but many other factors such as drug administration, elimination, drug distribution, and plasma protein binding all influence the drug half-life, which is considered later in this chapter.

## Renal

Kidney function in the newborn is generally deficient and greatly depends on gestational age. The glomerular filtration rate (GFR) and tubular secretions functionally mature during the first 2 years of life. Neonatal GFR is about 30% of the adult rate. The effective renal blood flow during the first 48 hours is approximately 34 to 99 mL/min/1.73m$^2$. It increases to a range of 54 to 166 mL/min/1.73m$^2$ within 2 to 3 weeks after birth and attains and surpasses adult levels of about 600 mL/min/1.73m$^2$ by age 1 to 2 years. The newborn's concentrating ability is about 25% lower than an adult's, and reabsorption of sodium appears to be less efficient than in an older infant or child, primarily because of the limited concentrating ability of the kidneys. The infant's kidneys are also less able to excrete hydrogen ions, which may lead to an acidotic state.

Inherited disorders of the kidney may include cystinuria and Fanconi's syndrome. In hereditary Fanconi's syndrome, renal tubular defects cause impaired reabsorption of glucose, amino acids, bicarbonate, uric acid, water, potassium, and phosphate.[16] The clinical features of proximal tubular acidosis, hypophosphatemia, hypokalemia, polyuria, and polydipsia usually appear in infancy. Growth retardation and failure-to-thrive syndrome may also be present. Fanconi's syndrome may be acquired and is often associated with cystinuria.[17]

## Prematurity

As was previously defined, a premature infant is one born before 37 weeks' gestation or weighing less than 5.0 lb. These are generalized criteria and may differ from one facility or reference text to another. A small-for-gestational-age infant, even when postterm, may exhibit the same organ system immaturity of an infant that is born at an earlier gestational age. Regardless, a neonate classified by either criterion, usually has less body fat and a high surface-area-to-body-mass ratio, resulting in very poor body temperature control. Even full-term infants are prone to hypothermia. Hypothermia causes increased metabolic demands. Consequently, there may be an increased utilization of $O_2$ and glucose that may lead to tissue hypoxia and/or an overproduction of organic acids that may, in turn, contribute to metabolic acidosis. The renal function in the premature neonate is impaired since the concentrating and diluting ability of the kidneys is less than that of a full-term infant. This also means that the kidneys are unable to properly excrete organic acids, further adding to the metabolic acidosis. In an attempt to minimize the hypothermia, most infants are immediately placed on a warmed surface or in a warm incubator. However, care must be taken to minimize dehydration that can lead to electrolyte derangement. Insufficient surfactant can cause respiratory problems, particularly RDS. The immature liver is less likely to adequately control bilirubin and the diminished sucking and swallowing reflexes in a premature infant may hinder oral and nasogastric tube feedings, further contributing to the bilirubin burden. The immature immune system makes a premature infant more susceptible to infection, and the added interventions (i.e., increased handling, indwelling catheters, IVs, venipuncture, and endotracheal tubes) by medical staff may increase the risk of nosocomial infections.

## Postmaturity

An infant delivered beyond 42 weeks' gestation is considered by many as postmature.[18] The major concern is the ability of the placenta to remain intact as the fetus continues its dependence on the mother. Postmature infants may be larger for their gestational age, causing concern for trauma during the birthing process. Infants born to women with diabetes are at greatest risk for postmaturity. Their larger size is attributed to high levels of available glucose during gestation. They are at an increased risk for hypoglycemia, RDS, and hyperbilirubinemia. The RDS risk is largely caused by a delay in moth-

ers with diabetes having poor glycemic control during the pregnancy to produce adequate levels of surfactant at birth. The hyperbilirubinemia may be caused by either an increase in hematocrit, any trauma experienced during birth, difficulty with oral feeding, or any combination of these.

## LABORATORY ASSESSMENT IN THE PEDIATRIC POPULATION

### Acid-Base and RDS

Premature infants are particularly susceptible to RDS, also known as *hyaline membrane disease*, which often develops immediately or within a few hours after birth. In severe RDS, the atelectasis progressively worsens, causing retention of $PCO_2$ and an associated respiratory acidosis. Since the atelectasis also causes poor oxygenation of that area of the lung, hypoxemia results, anaerobic metabolism ensues, and a metabolic acidosis develops. Blood gas results (low pH, increased $PCO_2$, and low $PO_2$) are useful in assessing the extent of RDS.

Laboratory evaluation of RDS may start with amniocentesis. Amniocentesis provides a means to collect and analyze amniotic fluid. Because amniotic fluid is in communication with fetal alveoli, assessment of the amount of lecithin to sphingomyelin (surfactant phospholipids), expressed as the L/S ratio, is a valuable tool to determine if the fetus is ready for extrauterine survival or the degree of risk of RDS. An L/S ratio greater than 2, which occurs at about 34 weeks' gestation, indicates about a 5% chance of RDS.[21] Another test, demonstration of the presence of phosphatidylglycerol, which is excreted at about 36 weeks' gestation, may better predict fetal lung maturity, but this remains somewhat controversial.[22] In addition to amniocentesis, the L/S ratio and phosphatidylglycerol value from maternal vaginal pools or neonatal endotracheal or gastric aspirates taken immediately after birth, along with radiographic information, can assist in the assessment of fetal lung maturity.

Tests for assessing fetal lung maturity, or the likelihood of RDS, in amniotic fluid include analysis using thin-layer chromatography to determine the L/S ratio and/or the level of phosphatidylglycerol (PG) or phosphatidylinositol (PI), either separately or simultaneously. These tests are rather laborious and time consuming. Unless the laboratory performs them often, more rapid tests (<2 hours) for RDS assessment are often employed. Included in this category are the foam stability index (evaluates bubble stability), lamellar body (packages of surfactant material) counts using automated cell counters,[23] or immunoassays, such as fluorescent polarization or semiquantitative slide tests, used alone or in combination.

### Electrolyte and Water Metabolism

Insensible water loss in neonates due to increased skin permeability to water, the relative high surface-area-to-body-mass ratio, increased respiratory and metabolic rates, positioning under phototherapy light, and placement on a warmer or in a warm environment can quickly cause dehydration. As seen in Figure 37–1, both premature and full-term infants have higher body water volumes that will quickly cause marked changes with relatively little water loss by volume. Dehydration, usually due to diarrhea, is a major cause of morbidity and mortality in infants worldwide. Overhydration can be serious in ill pediatric patients with cerebral edema, impaired renal or circulatory function, or immature organ systems. There is less room for error when replacement therapy is given.

Hypernatremia (serum sodium > 150 mmol/L), like in the adult (Chapter 21), results from water loss in excess of sodium loss, increased sodium intake, or a combination of both. Dehydration is a major concern as previously discussed, but in addition to the newborn risks, diarrhea, high fever, and/or vomiting can also contribute to significant water loss. In the case of increased sodium intake, the serum sodium value may actually be within the expected reference range or even decreased if edema is present or if water has shifted to the extracellular compartment to offset the sodium increase (dilutional hyponatremia). Hyponatremia can also result if salt loss is greater than water loss, usually via the kidneys or GI tract as may be the case with conditions associated with vomiting or diarrhea. Assessment of solute status using a serum and/or urine osmolality, urine specific gravity, BUN, creatinine, hemoglobin, hematocrit, and total protein or albumin may be helpful.

Changes in potassium are caused by the same conditions that would cause these changes in an adult, except for the higher risk from dehydration discussed previously. Rate of replacement therapy for infants depends on the severity of the dehydration but generally occurs over a 48-hour period.

Chloride values generally reflect changes in sodium and bicarbonate values. A sweat chloride determination is used to evaluate for cystic fibrosis. The sample is obtained either by iontophoresis collection or use of a surface electrode. In a patient having a family history of cystic fibrosis or an infant demonstrating complications associated with the disease, the diagnosis is confirmed if the sweat chloride value is greater than 60 mmol/L.[24] These complications include meconium passage problems, or infants with malabsorption, those who fail to appropriately gain weight, or who have pulmonary or pancreatic problems.

Hypocalcemia can be classified as early-onset (within the first few hours of life) or late-onset (occurring after 3 days) when the total serum calcium value is <8 mg/dL in full-term infants, <7 mg/dL in a preterm infant, or an ionized calcium <3.0 mg/dL. Early-onset is associated with a transient hypoparathyroidism, especially in preterm infants because of abrupt cessation of ionized calcium coming from the mother or a poor renal phosphate response to parathyroid hormone (PTH). A delayed adaptation to their own ionized calcium levels is seen in infants born to mothers with greater than normal ionized calcium levels present in the maternal blood, as seen in diabetes or hyperparathyroidism. Late-onset hypo-

calcemia is rare and usually associated with bottle-fed infants consuming formula very high in phosphate (cow's milk) or in DiGeorge syndrome (hypoplasia of the thymus and parathyroids), where the infant itself has hypoparathyroidism. Hypomagnesemia, while rare, may be associated with low calcium and should be suspected when treatment of hypocalcemia has not rectified the clinical situation and seizures continue to occur.

Phosphate levels in neonates and children are higher, 50% and 30%, respectively, than those in adults because of increased requirements for growth. Growth hormone causes increases in blood phosphate by probable alterations in its excretion, causing transient hyperphosphatemia seen in early infancy and periodically throughout childhood, most notably in children 5 years and younger.[25] Abnormal elevations in neonates may be caused by sudden increases in phosphate intake, particularly those bottle-fed with cow's milk. Hypophosphatemia occurs in rickets, an X-linked dominant trait, or more rarely, acquired rickets associated with benign mesenchymal tumors or vitamin D deficiency. Rickets results in soft bones and is linked with frequent bone fractures and retarded growth. The hallmark biochemical change in this disease is the low phosphate.[26] As calcium levels fall, PTH production is stimulated, thereby restoring the calcium levels but at the expense of phosphate, which is excreted to very low levels. Once below a critical threshold, bone mineralization fails to occur properly. Phosphate levels in defining hypophosphatemia in neonates differ depending on the type of feedings; neonates fed breast milk have lower values than those fed with formula. A greater incidence of vitamin D deficiency has been detected in breast-fed African-American neonates whose mothers did not take vitamin D supplements.

## Hyperbilirubinemia

A serum total bilirubin concentration >10 mg/dL in preterm newborns or >15 mg/dL in full-term newborns and/or an elevated bilirubin that occurs within 24 hours of birth constitutes hyperbilirubinemia and should be investigated.[27] Increased bilirubin levels may be due to increased erythrocyte destruction, conjugation problems, or decreased excretion of bilirubin but most often involves physiologic jaundice in newborns. The mechanisms surrounding physiologic jaundice have been discussed earlier in this chapter. Table 37–1 lists major causes of neonatal hyperbilirubinemia. In newborns, jaundice is evident at total bilirubin levels of 4 to 5 mg/dL. The increased bilirubin consists of unconjugated (indirect) bilirubin. Recall that unconjugated bilirubin is bound to albumin as it is transported to the liver for conjugation. Any circumstances that allow for decreased bilirubin binding by albumin (i.e., low albumin levels, competition for binding sites by other compounds such as hydrogen ions, or certain drugs, or when very high unconjugated bilirubin is present overwhelming the amount of albumin present) will cause "free" bilirubin to exist. If the free bilirubin crosses the blood–brain barrier, as might happen with prematurity, it causes a condition known as

T A B L E   3 7 - 1

**Predominant Changes in Selected Causes of Neonatal Hyperbilirubinemia**

**UNCONJUGATED**

Physiologic jaundice
Respiratory distress syndrome (RDS)
Erythroblastosis fetalis (fetal-maternal blood group/
   type incompatibility)
Hemolysis
   Inherited (G6PD deficiency pyruvate kinase
      deficiency, thalassemia, spherocytosis)
   Acquired
Polycythemia
Increased enterohepatic circulation (delayed
   feeding, infant of diabetic mother)
Hypothyroidism

**CONJUGATED**

Cholestasis/liver disease
Biliary atresia
Inherited disorders (galactosemia, cystic fibrosis,
   Niemann-Pick type C, fructose intolerance,
   alpha₁-antitrypsin deficiency)
Defects in bile acid synthesis
Sepsis
Intrauterine infections

kernicterus, which can result in motor dysfunction and mental retardation. There is no cure and there is no cut-off bilirubin level above which kernicterus can be accurately predicted. Treatment of the physiologic jaundice of the newborn consists of reducing the amount of unconjugated bilirubin, including early feeding for proper intestinal motility, phototherapy causing bilirubin degradation, and in severe cases, exchange transfusions via an umbilical vein catheter.

Other causes, besides physiologic jaundice–associated hyperbilirubinemia, must be investigated in newborns when the condition persists or does not begin to resolve using traditional treatment. A condition known as breast milk jaundice may be considered when all other causes of jaundice have been ruled out. The mechanism is not well understood, but interruption of breastfeeding for several days with substitution of formula use seems to resolve the jaundice. Bilirubin levels can become quite elevated. If a further reduction of bilirubin levels is necessary, phototherapy and exchange transfusion is undertaken. Other causes for increased unconjugated bilirubin include hemolytic disorders, Gilbert's syndrome (an apparent clinically insignificant mild increase in unconjugated bilirubin often detected in young adults and after a prolonged fasting period), and Crigler-Najjar syndrome (an autosomal inherited disorder having two forms that affects glucuronosyltransferase activity).

Type I Crigler-Najjar is the most severe and patients usually die of kernicterus within the first year of life. The milder form, type II, causes less severe hyperbilirubinemia since the glucuronosyltransferase activity is diminished but not to a degree that causes neurological damage. Type II can be treated with phenobarbital, which induces the enzyme activity of the partially deficient glucuronosyltransferase.

Conjugated types of hyperbilirubinemia in the pediatric population have similar origins to those associated with the adult population. Besides those, several inherited disorders may need to be evaluated. Dubin-Johnson syndrome is a rare autosomal recessive disorder involving impaired excretion of bilirubin, causing a mild elevated bilirubin and highly pigmented liver. Rotor's syndrome is similar to Dubin-Johnson, except there is no liver pigmentation. Both are benign disorders.

## Carbohydrates

Hypoglycemia (glucose level <40mg/dL in the full-term newborn or <30 mg/dL in the preterm newborn) usually occurs because of deficient glycogen stores. Hypoglycemia can lead to neurological impairment, and therefore requires prompt treatment. Glycogen stores can quickly be depleted in any hypermetabolic situation (i.e., RDS), hypoxic states, or in preterm or low-birth weight infants whose stores are deficient at the time of birth. Infants born to mothers with diabetes are often hypoglycemic because they are accustomed to a state of hyperinsulinism associated with an increased supply of glucose from the mother. The sudden cessation of available glucose at birth causes a rapid fall in the infant's glucose within hours. This same phenomenon may also occur if an intravenous infusion of glucose and water is abruptly stopped.

Glycogen storage diseases (Chapter 10), associated with defective glycogen-related enzymes, may result in hypoglycemia not corrected with ordinary measures. Von Gierke's type IA, IB, IC, ID, Pompe's disease (type II), Forbes/Cori's (type III), Andersen's disease (type IV), and Hers' disease (type VI) all manifest themselves in the newborn period or early childhood.

Galactosemia (inborn error of metabolism) ultimately results in a lack of conversion of galactose (mostly found in lactose and dairy products) to glucose with an accumulation of galactose in the blood. The infant appears normal at birth but becomes anorexic and jaundiced after consuming breast milk or lactose-containing formula. Vomiting, poor growth, hepatomegaly, septicemia, and a renal Fanconi's syndrome can develop. Galactosemia is also associated with cataract development in the affected child. Fructose intolerance results in hypoglycemia and is treated by removing fructose or sucrose from the diet.

Hyperglycemia in neonates is less frequently encountered. However, low birth weight or preterm infants if given intravenous glucose too rapidly may become hyperglycemic, resulting in osmotic diuresis and a dehydration that may be life threatening. Transient neonatal diabetes mellitus usually resolves itself in a few days, but if accompanied by severe hyperosmolality, may result in neurological damage.

## Enzymes

Enzyme levels (Chapter 15) mimic those found in the adult population for a given disorder. Elevated alkaline phosphatase (ALP) levels are associated with periods of rapid bone growth. The expected levels in children younger than 10 years old are almost four times that of adult levels. Peak activity in males is higher and occurs later than that of females, but occurs during puberty for both males and females. Female levels decrease sooner than males to adult levels, approximately 15 and 20 years, respectively.

Elevations in creatine kinase (CK) and each of its isoenzymes (CK-MM, MB, BB) have been reported in both healthy as well as ill neonates.[28] Immediately after birth, the levels of all three CK isoenzymes rise to a maximum in 5 to 8 hours. The mechanism of action is thought to be due to skeletal muscle trauma to the infant during birth. Mode of delivery appears to affect the level of isoenzyme elevation. Infants delivered by cesarean section tend to have lower levels of CK-MM and CK-MB. Elevations can persist for up to 10 days, and some authors have emphasized the relationship of elevated CK-BB in neonates with an asphyxia event in utero or poor obstetric outcome as measured by low Apgar scores.

Although widespread immunization programs have eradicated many childhood diseases, mumps and mononucleosis can have profound effects on serum enzymes, notably amylase, lipase, and lactate dehydrogenase.

## Proteins

As with other analytes, reference values for protein levels need to be ascertained for corresponding age and expected amounts of body proteins. However, the disorders that affect protein levels in adults would affect the pediatric population in a similar manner.

Wilson's disease is an inherited disorder that interrupts normal copper deposition because of a deficiency of ceruloplasmin, the copper-carrying protein. The copper concentration of affected individuals is 20 times greater than that of unaffected individuals. However, elevated levels of copper are seen in almost all newborns up to about 3 months of age, so diagnosis is unreliable before 6 months of age.[29] Clinical manifestations are rarely seen before 5 years of age. Wilson's disease may begin with neurological problems or present as hepatitis, but it is progressive. This disease is often fatal by the age of 30 years unless continual lifelong treatment is instituted.[30]

Aminoacidurias (see Chapter 13) are a result of inherited disorders that affect enzymes in amino acid metabolism. A list of aminoacidurias often included in newborn metabolic screening may be found in Table 37–2.

One protein of special note is alpha$_1$-antitrypsin. Deficiency of this protein, in the pediatric population, clinically manifests itself as liver disease such as neonatal hepatitis or cholestasis in the first few months of life. It can also appear as emphysema in young adults. The gene for alpha$_1$-antitrypsin is on chromosome 14 and the over 70 alleles can result in normal, reduced, or zero levels of this protease inhibitor. PiZZ is the most serious combination causing up to 25% of those affected to eventually develop cirrhosis and portal hypertension and die before the age of 12 years.[31]

## Nonprotein Nitrogen

Cord values of urea nitrogen are much higher than those seen in the adult population. Premature infants and newborns have a wider reference range for this analyte than do adults. Creatinine values are lower as would be expected because of the immaturity of the kidneys and smaller muscle mass as compared to adults.

It should be recalled that liver abnormalities that interfere with the proper formation of urea from ammonia might cause elevations in ammonia levels. One disorder that is associated with the pediatric population is Reye's syndrome.

TABLE 37–2

**New England Newborn Screening Program, June 2000**

| METABOLIC | ENDOCRINE | HEMOGLOBINOPATHIES | INFECTIONS |
|---|---|---|---|
| Analysis of amino acids, biotinidase enzyme, trypsinogen, and acylcarnitine | T$_4$<br>17-OHP | Hemoglobin phenotypes | Toxoplasmosis |
| Disorders detected: | | | |
|   Galactosemia | Hypothyroidism | Sickle cell | |
|   PKU | Adrenal hyperplasia | | |
|   Maple syrup urine disease | | | |
|   MCAD (medium-chain acyl-CoA<br>    dehydrogenase) | | | |
|   Cystic fibrosis | | | |
|   Homocystinuria | | | |
|   Biotinidase enzyme deficiency | | | |

The etiology of Reye's syndrome remains unclear; however, it is associated with a viral-like syndrome plus ingestion of aspirin that results in an encephalopathy and fatty infiltration of the liver. It occurs most often in children ages 6 to 12 years of age. The most characteristic aspect of the disease is a marked increase in ammonia levels. Increases in transaminases (AST and ALT), LD, and ALP are also noted. Because of the widespread public awareness of the disease and its association with aspirin, few pediatric aged individuals are given any aspirin products, and the incidence of the disease has dramatically decreased.[32]

## Thyroid

Congenital hypothyroidism occurs with an approximate frequency of 1 in 4000 births in the United States. Thyroid hormone levels change rapidly during the first few days and weeks of life. At or within 30 minutes after birth, thyroid-stimulating hormone (TSH), also called thyrotropin, is at its highest levels. Levels gradually fall to reach those of adults by about 4 weeks after birth. Thyroxine ($T_4$) peaks at about 24 hours and then drops. It is important to assess the level of thyroid hormones in the neonate because cretinism, a condition causing mental retardation from low thyroid hormone levels, is a preventable condition. Screening programs exist in all developed countries in the world. The most frequently used screening test employs filter-paper spots filled with blood, usually obtained by a heelstick. This sample is eluted from the paper and evaluated for $T_4$ levels. If the $T_4$ level is found to be outside a certain percentile value, a TSH level is determined using a different spot on the same filter-paper collection. Many agencies automatically do the TSH level first, followed by a $T_4$ level.

## Lipids

At birth, plasma cholesterol concentrations are about 66 mg/dL and equally distributed between low-density lipoproteins (LDL) and high-density lipoproteins (HDL) with a trace amount taken up by very low-density lipoproteins (VLDL). Triglyceride levels are approximately 36 mg/dL. The values rise during the first few months of life to a total cholesterol value of about 155 mg/dL, LDL cholesterol averaging 90 mg/dL, and HDL levels of about 53 mg/dL and remain unchanged until after puberty.

Coronary heart disease (CHD) manifests itself clinically by the third or fourth decade but it is widely accepted that the process begins very early in life. Although little CHD is present in the pediatric population, studies have shown a direct relationship between early lipid values and those found later in life. Evaluating lipids at an early age, particularly for those who have a family history of increased risk of CHD or elevated lipids and treating as needed, may prevent or delay the development of this disease.

The National Cholesterol Education Panel (NCEP)[33] and American Academy of Pediatrics[34] have made several recommendations concerning the screening and associated cutoff levels for this population. A desirable level in children and adolescents of total cholesterol is <170 mg/dL, and for LDL cholesterol, the desirable level is <110 mg/dL. High levels for these two constituents are ≥200 mg/dL and ≥130 mg/dL, respectively. Low HDL cholesterol values are <35 mg/dL in this population. Recommended screening should begin after 2 years of age, whenever the infant has a parent with a total cholesterol level >240 mg/dL, or a family history (mother, father, grandparent, aunt, uncle) of documented CHD, myocardial infarction, cerebrovascular disease, or sudden cardiac death. Criticism regarding these criteria for screening have emerged since parental self-reporting of cholesterol levels may miss as many as 90% of children with total cholesterol values above the 75th percentile by population.[35] A risk assessment flow chart, Figure 37–2, recommended by the NCEP Expert Panel on Blood Cholesterol in Children and Adults, attempts to address interventions (diet, drug therapy) in those individuals found outside of the levels indicated.

One lipid disorder that may be expressed in the pediatric population is familial hypercholesterolemia (FH). FH, an inherited disorder, causes a defect in the LDL receptor gene that is expressed as an increased LDL and total cholesterol, both present at birth. It can be inherited as either a homozygous or heterozygous trait. The levels of LDL cholesterol are 2 to 3 times higher in the heterozygous population and 4 to 6 times higher in the homozygous population than the levels found in the normal population. Because of the increased cholesterol, these patients have cholesterol deposits in skin, tendons, and arteries. Homozygous FH patients usually develop cutaneous xanthomas by age 4 and have juvenile atherosclerosis and marked hypercholesterolemia. Heterozygotes are more difficult to detect at an early age because the deposition changes do not often occur until later in life but xanthomas are usually present by the end of the second decade. For a more complete discussion of lipid abnormalities, see Chapter 11.

## Drug Monitoring

Review of perinatal physiology makes it apparent that the rate of drug absorption, protein-binding, liver metabolism, and excretion can be quite different from that found in adults, especially in preterm and younger children. While the mechanisms are the same, see Chapter 23, the efficiency of these mechanisms is not. This means that the dosage (in mg/kg), bioavailability, half-life, and associated laboratory values (i.e., therapeutic range, peak and trough levels) should reflect these differences. Many drugs have a plasma half-life 2 to 3 times longer in newborns than in adults, and because of the greater amount of body water, the dose of water-soluble drugs may need decreasing. After the age of 1 year, the elimination and liver processing of some drugs surpass that of adults and dosages need to be adjusted accordingly. Alternate or unexpected

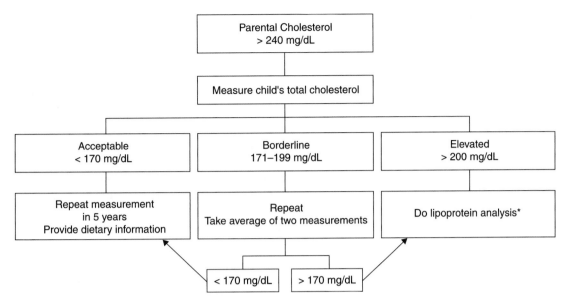

**FIGURE 37-2**

Pediatric lipid testing. *First step in child with positive family (parent, aunt, uncle, grandparent) history of premature (less than 55 years) cardiovascular disease.

sources of drugs, such as breast milk or via the skin through diapers (i.e., dyes, antibacterials), may alter drug metabolism or cause toxicity and should be considered. Patient compliance can be at issue even for a routine 10-day course of antibiotics (noncompliance estimated at 71% by day 6),[36] and it is expected that more complex regimens that do not have direct apparent benefit may be even higher. Parents may not completely understand their role and the importance of strict adherence to the medication directions. Adolescent patients may assume responsibility for their medication administration but suffer from the same issues as their parents. Chronically ill adolescents may need additional support in accepting behaviors that are in their best interest and eliminating those that are contraindicated by their illness.

## Metabolic Screening

Inborn errors of metabolism represent a large group of inherited disorders caused by enzyme deficiency in a particular metabolic pathway. These include the aminoacidurias (i.e., PKU), lysosomal storage disease (i.e., Gaucher's and Tay-Sachs), cystic fibrosis, plus any enzyme involved in the urea cycle (i.e., citrullinemia), carbohydrate metabolism (i.e., glycogen storage diseases, glucose-6-phosphate dehydrogenase-G6PD), lipid disorders (i.e., medium-chain acyl-CoA dehydrogenase-MCAD, which is suspected but not confirmed as a possible cause or precipitating factor in sudden infant death syndrome)[37] or other enzyme abnormalities resulting in erythrocyte defects (i.e., hereditary spherocytosis, sickle cell disease, thalassemias, porphyrias) or platelet and coagulation defects (i.e., hemophilia, thrombocytopenias). Since some of these disorders are very rare,

not all are screened for at birth. Clinical and family history, such as known disease in a primary family member, including aunts, uncles, and grandparents, or an unexplained death (sudden infant death) in a sibling, or inclusion in a high-risk group (i.e., Ashkenazi Jews for Gaucher's or Tay-Sachs disease or males from Mediterranean areas for G6PD deficiency) often determines the necessity of screening for some individuals. Newborn screening programs concentrate on those tests that can identify the most frequently occurring inherited disorders that can be readily cured or effects diminished (i.e., PKU, screening for hypothyroidism) in the area population and performed in a cost-effective, rapid manner, with test methods having few false positives and no false negatives. In the United States, screening programs are often dictated and performed by local public health laboratories or their approved designated laboratories. Table 37-2 lists those tests currently (June 2000) performed as part of the routine New England Newborn Screening Program[38] with follow-up testing on any tests considered abnormal.

Infants suffering from a metabolic disorder that is not readily apparent or suspected often demonstrate a failure to thrive, or gain weight, or do not grow or develop as expected. Symptoms that occur after feeding has begun, such as projectile vomiting, lethargy, seizures, nonspecific liver disease, renal disease, cataracts, apparent sepsis, particularly in severe or chronic response to common problems or hematologic abnormalities, may indicate a metabolic disorder once more common causes have been ruled out. In older children, evidence of skeletal abnormalities, growth maturation aberrations, severe behavioral changes, loss of motor skills, difficulty walking, opthalmic abnormalities, hypoglycemia, hepatic problems, or metabolic acidosis may hallmark a need to investigate the

TABLE 37-3

### Odors Associated with Metabolic Disease

| DISORDER | ODOR |
|---|---|
| Maple syrup urine disease | Maple syrup (urine) |
| Isovaleric acidemia | Sweaty socks |
| Phenylketonuria (PKU) | Musty, damp |
| Hawkinsuria | Chlorine, bleach, swimming pool |
| Trimethylaminuria | Ammonia, fishy |
| Tyrosinemia (hypermethioninemia) | Cabbage, rancid butter |
| Diabetes | Fruity, acetone |

presence of underlying genetic disease. Some metabolic disorders are associated with certain odors in patients or their urine (Table 37–3).[39]

Congenital disorders (present at birth) affecting any major organ system (e.g., heart, kidneys, lung, brain, eye, neuromuscular) or chromosome abnormalities (e.g., Down's, Turner's) are investigated based on clinical presentation and will not be discussed here. Some congenital disorders, depending on the severity, do represent a high risk for infants whenever a major organ function is compromised, whereas others, such as Duchenne's muscular dystrophy, cystic fibrosis, or Marfan's syndrome, may not present until the adolescent years or even later. Diagnosis of these genetic disorders has advanced largely due to DNA technology.

## SUMMARY

Interpretation of neonatal and pediatric laboratory values must be evaluated in light of the maturation and development of the child. Special consideration is given to neonates because of their need to quickly transition from intrauterine to the extrauterine environment. Depending on the gestational age, preterm infants are at greater risk to develop complications. These include RDS, hyperbilirubinemia that may lead to kernicterus, suffer increased risk of infection or electrolyte and metabolic derangements associated with hypothermia and dehydration. Drug levels in the pediatric population are affected by variances in drug absorption, protein binding, volume of distribution, metabolism, especially liver mechanisms, and alterations in excretion.

Abnormal laboratory values in the pediatric population are often caused by the same disease conditions and circumstances that affect the adult population; however, these biochemical changes must be recognized within the scope of reference ranges that are age and developmentally appropriate. Some inherited disorders are readily apparent within the first few days or months of life; others do not express themselves until later in childhood or even later in life. Newborn metabolic screening tests are designed to detect the most prevalent disorders for which medical intervention can positively impact the patient outcome. In the United States, PKU and thyroid testing are among the most common disorders screened for at birth, usually in centralized state laboratories.

## REFERENCES

1. National Committee for Clinical Laboratory Standards (NCCLS) C28-A: How to define, determine, and utilize reference intervals in the clinical laboratory. Villanova, PA, NCCLS, 1995.
2. Soldin SJ, Rifai N, Hicks JM (eds.): *The Biochemical Basis of Pediatric Disease.* Washington DC, American Association for Clinical Chemistry Press, 1992.
3. Soldin SJ, Brugnara C, Hicks JM (eds.): *Pediatric Reference Ranges.* 3rd ed. Washington DC, American Association for Clinical Chemistry Press, 1999.
4. Beers MH (ed): *The Merck Manual.* Westpoint, PA, Merck & Co., 1999.
5. Thomas CL (ed.): *Taber's Cyclopedic Medical Dictionary.* Philadelphia, FA Davis Co., 1999.
6. Walker WA, Watkins JB (eds.): *Nutrition in Pediatrics.* Ontario, Canada, Dekker, 1996.
7. Bergman RE, Kleigman RM (eds.): *Nelson's Textbook of Pediatrics.* 15th ed. Philadelphia, WB Saunders, 1995.
8. Ashwood ER, Palmer SE, Lenke RR: Rapid fetal lung maturity testing: Commercial versus NBD-phosphatidylcholine assay. Obstet Gynecol 81:1048–1053, 1992.
9. Ashwood ER: Standards of laboratory practice: Evaluation of fetal lung maturity. Clin Chem 43:1–4, 1997.
10. McChance K, Huether SE (eds.): *Pathophysiology: The Biologic Basis for Disease in Adults and Children.* 3rd ed. St. Louis, MO, Mosby-Yearbook, 1998.
11. Fyler DC (ed.): *Nada's Pediatric Cardiology.* Philadelphia, Hanley & Belfus, 1992.
12. Splawski JB, Jelinek DM, Lipsky PE: Delineation of the functional capacity of human neonatal lymphocytes. J Clin Invest 87:545, 1992.
13. Suchy FJ (ed.): *Liver Disease in Children.* St. Louis, MO, Mosby, 1994.
14. Alpay F, Saricic SU, Tosuncuk, HD: The value of first-day bilirubin measurement in predicting the development of significant hyperbilirubinemia in healthy term newborns. Pediatrics 106:E16, 2000.
15. Clemons RM: Neonatal jaundice and diet. Arch Pediatr Adolesc Med 153:184–8, 1999.
16. Gregory M, Schwartz GJ: Diagnosis and treatment of renal tubular disorders. Sem Nephrol 18:317–329, 1998.
17. Toth-Heyden P, Drukker A, Guinard JP: The stressed neonatal kidney: From pathology to clinical management of neonatal vasomotor nephropathy. Pediatr Nephrol 14:227–239, 2000.

18. Haymond, MW: Hypoglycemia in infants and children. Endocrinol Metab Clin North Am 18:211–252, 1989.

19. Green A, Morgan I: *Neonatology and Clinical Biochemistry.* London, ACB Venture Publications, 1993.

20. Burtis CA, Ashwood ER (eds.): *Tietz Textbook of Clinical Chemistry.* 3rd ed. Philadelphia, WB Saunders, 1999.

21. Sher G, Statland BE, Knutzen VK: Diagnostic reliability of the lecithin/sphingomyelin ratio assay and the quantitation foam stability index test: Results of a comparative study. J Reprod Med 27:51–55, 1982.

22. Ashwood ER: Standards of laboratory practice: Evaluation of fetal lung maturity. Clin Chem 43:1–4, 1997.

23. Delance CR, Bowie LJ, Dohnal JC, et al.: Amniotic fluid lamellar body count: A rapid and reliable fetal lung maturity test. Obstet Gynecol 86:235–239, 1995.

24. Rosenstein BJ, Zeitlin PL: Cystic fibrosis. Lancet 351: 277–282, 1998.

25. Crofton PM: What is the cause of benign transient hyperphosphatemia: A study of 35 cases. Clin Chem 34: 335–40, 1988.

26. Aiken CG, Sherwood RA, Lenney W: Role of plasma phosphate measurements in detecting rickets of prematurity and in monitoring treatment. Ann Clin Biochem 30 (Pt 5): 469–475, 1993.

27. Kelley DA: Jaundice in the neonate. Med Interne 22: 461–464, 1994.

28. Quivers ES, Murphy NJ, Soldin SJ: The effect of gestational age, birth weight and disease on troponin I and creatine kinase MB in the first year of life. Clin Biochem 32:419–421, 1999.

29. Stremmel W: Wilson disease: Clinical presentation, treatment and survival. Ann Intern Med 115:720–726, 1991.

30. Thomas GR, Forbes JR, Roberts EA, et al.: The Wilson disease gene: Spectrum of mutations and their consequences. Nature Genet 9:210–217, 1995.

31. Lomas DA, Evans DL, Finch JT: The mechanism of Z alpha-1-antitrypsin accumulation in the liver. Nature 357:605–607, 1992.

32. Casteels-van Daele M, Van Geet C, Wouters K, et al.: The changing pattern of Reye's syndrome: 1982–1990. Arch Dis Child 76:79, 1997.

33. National Cholesterol Education Program: Report of the Expert Panel on Blood Cholesterol Levels in Children and Adolescents. US Department of Health and Human Services, Bethesda, MD, NIH publication No. 91-2732, 1991.

34. American Academy of Pediatrics Committee on Nutrition: Indication for cholesterol testing in children. Pediatrics 83:141–142, 1989.

35. Lauer RM, Clarke WR: Use of cholesterol measurements in childhood for the prediction of adult hypercholesterolemia: The Muscatine study. JAMA 264:3034–3038, 1990.

36. Beers MH, (ed): *The Merck Manual.* Westpoint, Merck & Co., 1999.

37. Daneman D: Disorders of carbohydrate metabolism in infants and children. In Soldin SJ, Rifai N, Hicks JM (eds.): *The Biochemical Basis of Pediatric Disease.* Washington DC, American Association for Clinical Chemistry Press, 1992; p 295.

38. Massachusetts Institute of Public Health, Jamaica Plains, Massachusetts. New England (MA, RI, NH, VT) Newborn Screening Program, 2000.

39. Bishop M, Duben-Engelkirk JL, Fody E (eds.): *Clinical Chemistry: Principles, Procedures, Correlations.* 4th ed. Philadelphia, Lippincott Williams & Wilkins, 2000.

40. Ashwood, A: Standards of laboratory practice: Evaluation of fetal lung maturity. Clin Chem 43:211–214, 1997.

41. Piper JM, Xenakis EM, Langer O: Delayed appearance of pulmonary maturation markers is associated with poor glucose control in diabetic pregnancies. J Matern Fetal Med 7:148–153, 1998.

42. Delgado JC, Greene MF, Winkelman JW, et al.: Comparison of disaturated phosphatidylcholine and fetal lung maturity surfactant/albumin ratio in diabetic and nondiabetic pregnancies. Am J Clin Pathol 113:151–153, 2000.

43. Dubin SB: Assessment of fetal lung maturity. Practice parameter. Am J Clin Pathol 110:723–732, 1998.

44. Aranda JV: Pharmacologic effects of theophylline in the newborn. J Allergy Clin Immunol 78 (4 Pt 2):773–80, 1986.

# CHAPTER 38

# Geriatric Laboratory Assessment

*Sharon M. Miller*

## THE 'NEW' ELDERLY

Across all ethnic and racial groups, the elderly are the fastest growing segment of society. In current usage, the terms **elderly, seniors,** and **older adults** are used interchangeably to identify individuals aged 65 years or older. During the 20th century, the number of individuals over the age of 65 increased by a factor of 11, and the number of those younger than 65 has increased by only 3-fold[1] (Figure 38–1). About 13% of all Americans (or 1 in 8) is elderly. In 1998, 34.4 million Americans were over the age of 65.[2] Beginning in 2011, the baby boomer generation (individuals born between 1946 and 1961) will begin to enter the ranks of the elderly. By 2030, seniors will increase in number to an estimated 70 million, one half of whom will be 75 years of age or older. By the year 2050, according to the U.S. Census Bureau projections, 80 million (or 1 in 5) Americans could be elderly. The "oldest-old," or those aged 85 and older, are the fastest growing segment of the population. Currently, there are over 4 million Americans over the age of 85. They constitute 10% of the elderly and just over 1% of the total population. With the influx of the survivors of the baby boomer generation, as many as 19 million Americans could occupy this chronologic niche in 2050. If that occurs, the oldest old would make up almost one quarter of the elderly and 5% of all Americans. Although the number of centenarians is difficult to determine reliably, there may currently be as many as 70,000 persons 100 years of age or older. This group has more than doubled since 1980. By 2005, the number is predicted to double again, and by 2050, this age group could include as many as 1 million persons.[3] By the middle of this century, we may no longer be able to consider ourselves a nation of the young. Perhaps as soon as 2025, there may be twice as many elderly as there are adolescents and children.[1]

Although there are racial differences, overall life expectancy at birth is about 76 years. The elderly population is becoming more racially and ethnically diverse. In 1998, minorities constituted about 16% of seniors; in 2030 they will make up about 25% of the group. Between 1989 and 2030, the white, non-Hispanic portion of the population 65 years of age and older will increase by 79%. In this same period, older

minorities will increase by 220%.[2] There are also gender differences in life expectancy. Among seniors, women outnumber men at all ages. Elderly women outnumber elderly men by about 3 to 2 (20.2 million to 14.2 million). About 4 in 5 centenarians are women.[1] Almost 90% of women born in 1990 are expected to live to age 65, and more than 50% will live to be 85. The average age of menopause onset is 51 years. In 1997, more than 8 million women in the United States turned 50. Today's woman may spend one third of her life in the postmenopausal years. With the loss of estrogen production at or around menopause, there are physical changes and potential increased risk for certain chronic conditions such as osteoporosis.[4] Clearly, health concerns of older adults are becoming predominately problems of elderly women. The increasing number of older adults will have a profound effect on our economy, culture, and health care.

Aging is a dynamic biologic continuum and there is great variability in the age of onset, rate, and course of both structural and functional changes. Not all tissues age at the same pace. The establishment of laboratory reference values in the elderly is complicated by a multitude of factors including the presence of subclinical undiagnosed disorders, polypharmacy, differential decline in physiologic functions among individuals, and the effects of diet and exercise. With increasing age, the probability of having more than one chronic disorder or disease increases. Elderly women are more likely than elderly men to have two or more chronic conditions (referred to as comorbidity). Five of the six leading causes of death among older Americans are chronic diseases (Figure 38–2). Among the most common chronic conditions affecting the elderly are arthritis, hypertension and heart disease, and disorders that limit communications such as hearing loss, cataracts, and visual disorders such as macular degeneration.[1] With the exception of hearing loss, women have higher rates for all chronic diseases than men.[5] Approximately 18% of elderly have diabetes mellitus. Persons with diabetes typically have higher blood pressure and are more likely to die from heart disease and stroke than individuals without the disease.[6] Over the age of 50, about one half of all women and one fourth of all men have diseases of the bone that increase fracture risk and the likelihood of permanent disability.[7] The major causes of death for those persons age 65 and over are heart disease, cancer, and

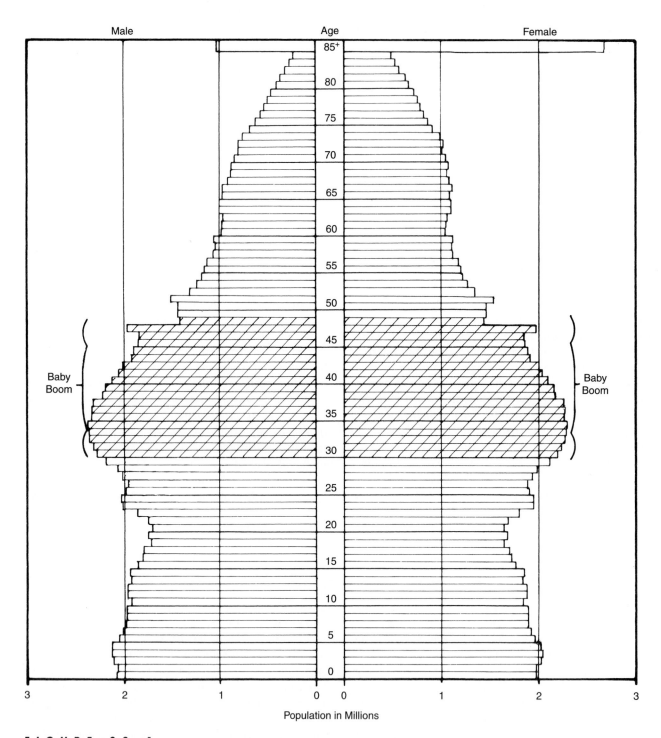

**FIGURE 38-1**

Population by age and sex, July 1, 1994 (From U.S. Census Bureau; "65+ in the United States," published April 1996; census.gov/prod/1/pop/p23-190/ p23190-e.pdf)

stroke. Chronic obstructive pulmonary disease as well as pneumonia and influenza are also among the leading causes of morbidity in the elderly.[1]

As the population ages, more of our health care resources will need to be directed toward the promotion of health, not just disease prevention, and to the early detection and monitoring of changes associated with chronic and degenerative disorders. Laboratorians will need to be familiar with the health problems most common among the elderly and be able to interpret laboratory data in the context of age- and medication-

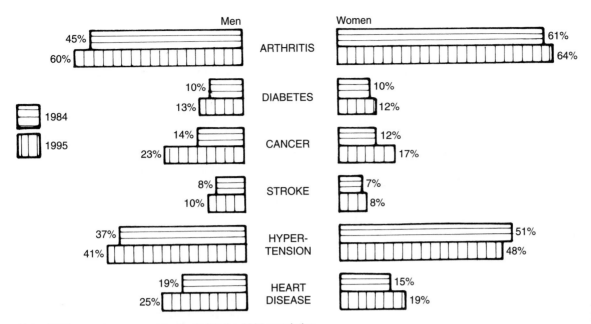

Note: 1984 percentages are age-adjusted to the 1995 population.
Reference population: These data refer to the civilian noninstitutional population.
Source: Supplement on Aging and Second Supplement on Aging.

**FIGURE 38-2**

Percentage of persons age 70 or older who reported having selected chronic
conditions, by sex, 1984 and 1995. (From Federal Interagency Forum on Aging—
Related Statistics; "Older Americans 2000: Key Indicators of Well Being, Chronic
Health Conditions," published March 1999; agingstats.gov/chafrtbook2000)

related variations as well as classic pathologic changes. But what
changes in anatomy and physiologic function are linked specifically to aging? As a consequence of well-documented age-
related physiologic changes, what alterations in analyte concentrations are predictable? Can we establish geriatric reference
ranges for analytes on the basis of data collected from elderly
subjects, presumed "healthy" because they are asymptomatic?
Chronologic grouping is convenient but, in isolation, not necessarily meaningful in risk assessment given the great diversity
of environmental factors to which individuals are exposed over
the lifespan. The physiologic and functional status of two 30-
year-old individuals is more likely to be similar than that of
two 80-year-old individuals. It seems reasonable to suspect that
many older adults have at least one subclinical or undiagnosed
disorder or disease. After all, an individual with type 2 diabetes may have his condition undiagnosed for as long as 10
years and during that time be presumed to be healthy. In reality, microvascular and macrovascular changes are taking place
that increase the risk for long-term complications, including
nephropathy, neuropathy, retinopathy, and cardiovascular disease. Before we consider the significance of biochemical
changes presenting in an older adult and the utility of establishing geriatric reference ranges, we need to better understand
the process of aging.

## THEORIES OF AGING

Aging results from highly complex interactions of the individual and the environment. Is it an unalterable natural process, or is it susceptible to control or delay through human intervention? Currently, there are two broad, but overlapping,
collections of theories that attempt to explain the origins and
mechanics of aging. In stochastic theories, the accumulation
of random "errors" or cellular damage over time is viewed as
leading to impaired cellular function, inability to maintain homeostasis (aging), and death. Nonstochastic theories emphasize that genetic "programming" is the determinant of cellular
aging. Also included among nonstochastic theories is the concept of intrinsic pacemakers of the aging process. Certain organs or organ systems such as the immune and neuroendocrine
systems may be susceptible to programmed senescence. Immune senescence is probably a result of both deterioration and
loss of regulation of the aging immune system. The following
observations support the immune impairment theory of aging: (1) decreased lymphocyte responsiveness to mitogens and
antigens, (2) increased incidence of neoplasia and autoimmunity, and (3) increased susceptibility to infection.[8-10] The

critical change in the aging immune system may be a diminished proliferative response. Involution of the thymus, which begins at puberty, could explain a reduction in T-lymphocyte numbers that some researchers have reported occurs with aging. While there may not be an absolute decrease in the number of T lymphocytes, there does seem to be a redistribution in numbers of cells among the various subsets of T cells. Qualitative changes in both T- and B-lymphocyte function may contribute to declining immune status with aging.[10] Reduction in cytokine secretion, especially of interleukin-2 (IL-2), is noted along with a reduction in the density of IL-2 receptors on cell membranes. IL-2 stimulates the proliferation and differentiation of T cells. One particular immune function that diminishes with age is the ability to remove lymphocytes that cross-react to self-antigens.[11] Changes in humoral immunity often arise secondary to changes in T-cell function. Blood levels of immunoglobulins G and A are increased in very old, healthy elderly, whereas IgM levels are mildly reduced.[12,13] A decrease in antibody production in response to immunization (vaccination failure) is noted with lower peak serum values and an accelerated decay of antibody titer over time. Although there is a diminished capacity for immune response to "new" antigens, there is an increase in circulating autoantibodies. Increased incidence of malignancies in older adults may be linked to a decrement in immune surveillance. Although aging is associated with compromised immune system performance in many seniors, some elderly have an immune system as vigorous as that of a young adult.[14] The neuroendocrine aging theory emphasizes changes in the hypothalamic-pituitary gland target-organ relationship over time, leading to various neuroendocrine deficiencies.[15] Production of growth hormone (GH) by the pituitary gland declines by 14% per decade, beginning in the 30s. The result is a lower serum level of GH and insulinlike growth factor I (IGF-I), also known as somatomedin C, a GH-hormone regulated substance that mediates many of the effects of GH.[16] Many of the physiologic and metabolic changes that are observed in normal aging are opposite to the effects of GH and suggest that these changes are from falling GH concentration. For example, GH decreases body fat and cholesterol and increases lean body mass, muscle strength, aerobic capacity, and bone density. Normal aging is associated with increases in total body fat and increasing circulating levels of cholesterol and triglycerides and decreases in lean body mass, muscle strength, aerobic capacity, and bone mineral density.

Genetic control theories of lifespan focus attention on the finite number of times "normal" cells seem to be able to divide.[3] For example, a cell might be able to divide successfully 50 times before it ultimately enters a nondividing state called **replicative senescence.** After that, the cell may become damaged or genetically altered. Removal of such terminally differentiated, damaged, or dysfunctional cells occurs by means of "cellular suicide" or apoptosis, a term derived from the Greek meaning "to drop out." **Apoptosis,** the rapid and controlled destruction of a cell, is initiated following the activation of cer-

tain cell-death proteins by any one of several signals. The process of apoptosis facilitates tissue remodeling.[17] An internal "biological clock" of some sort appears to preset a cell's maximum lifespan. The basis for a biological clock may be the telomeres, nucleic acid sequences extending from the ends of chromosomes. With each round of DNA replication, telomeres are shortened. When the telomeres are finally lost, the cell stops dividing and becomes senescent. The enzyme telomerase, found only in cancer and germ cells, appears to repair and replace the end-protecting telomeres, thereby resetting the biological clock that controls the cell's lifespan.[15,18] Telomere shortening may not be the direct signal for stopping the cell cycle. Loss of the telomeres, the physical ends of the chromosomes, may lead to breaks in the DNA. Cells respond to DNA damage by increasing their production of the tumor suppressor gene product, p53, an inhibitor of cell division and potent inducer of apoptosis. Increasing levels of p53 protein induce synthesis of a cell-cycle inhibitor, p21, which causes irreversible arrest of growth during the early stages of cell differentiation.[19] New research suggests that p21 not only inhibits cell-cycle progression but it also up-regulates multiple genes that have been implicated in age-related diseases including atherosclerosis, Alzheimer's disease, amyloidosis, and arthritis. It may become possible to fight age-related diseases by targeting their common link—p21.[20]

Stochastic or injury-based theories of aging are based on the belief that random events over time can cause sufficient macromolecular abnormalities and somatic damage to impair cell function (aging) and trigger cell death. Two currently popular theories of this type are (1) posttranslational macromolecular modification (e.g., cross-linking or glycation), and (2) free radical damage/oxidative stress.[3,8,21] Over time, posttranslational modification of both structural and functional proteins may occur. Molecular modifications may arise from chemical alterations to or conformational changes of the proteins. Such modifications have been found to involve the stability, structural integrity, and functional properties of these proteins. As a rule, such changes lead to a reduction or loss of biologic activity.[22] Cross-linking of the structural proteins collagen and elastin in arterial walls would increase vessel rigidity. Reduction of the vessels' ability to relax to accommodate changes in blood pressure would contribute to development of hypertension. Reduced enzyme activity and alteration of surface membrane receptors may arise from damage to protein tertiary structure. Impaired binding of hormones by altered cell membrane receptors could be the basis for increased occurrence of certain endocrine disorders among seniors. Peripheral tissue resistance to insulin and the resulting impairment of glucose homeostasis may be due to this phenomenon. The most common chemical causes of these age-related protein modifications are glycation and oxidation. Glucose reacts nonenzymatically with an amino group of a protein to form a glycated product. Reaction depends on the glucose concentration and the length of time the protein is in contact with the sugar. This process is initially reversible, although even temporary glycation can alter protein structure and function. With time, additional irreversible changes occur to produce an advanced glycation end product (AGE). AGEs contribute to many of the pathophysiologic changes that accompany long-standing diabetes. AGEs can occur not only on long-lived structural proteins such as collagen, elastin, myelin, and the ocular lens protein crystallin, but also on short-lived proteins, on lipids, and on nucleic acids. It is common for AGE-modified molecules to cross-link with or trap other molecules. For example, AGE-collagen can trap so-called "innocent bystander" soluble molecules on the connective tissue matrix (Figure 38–3). It has been proposed that low-density lipoprotein (LDL) immobilization on long-lived glycated proteins of vessel walls promotes the accumulation of lipids in fibrous plaques. This might be the basis for the relationship between hyperglycemia and increased risk of macrovascular disease.[23] In addition, this model has been used to explain the thickening of the renal basement membrane by the trapping of immunoglobulins and albumin by AGE-collagen. Tissue damage,

complement activation, and increased recognition and uptake of modified proteins by macrophages would follow.

Another explanation of why we age is the free radical theory. Free radicals are atoms or molecules that have one or more unpaired electrons in its outer shell. These chemical species are continually being produced endogenously as byproducts of metabolism. They are also produced by activated phagocytes during the inflammatory response. Exogenous sources of free radicals include drugs, pesticides, ozone, UV-light, and other forms of radiation as well as air pollutants including cigarette smoke.[24] Some of the most important and potent oxygen-derived reactants generated include the superoxide anion radical, the hydroxyl radical, hydrogen peroxide, and singlet molecular oxygen. In singlet molecular oxygen ($^1O_2$) the outermost electron is excited by light to an orbital higher than that which it normally occupies. Like free radicals, singlet oxygen can damage cells and tissues. In vivo sources of singlet oxygen include photochemical reactions and reactions of ozone with selected biologic molecules. Several reactive nitrogen species,

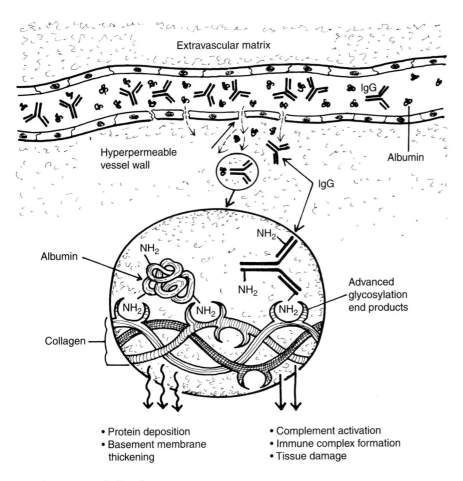

**FIGURE 38-3**

Trapping of "innocent bystander" molecules by advanced glycosylation end products (age) of collagen. (From Vlassara H, Brownlee M, et al.: Nonenzymatic glycosylation: Role in the pathogenesis of diabetic complications. Clin Chem 32(10B):B38, 1986.)

T A B L E   3 8 - 1

**Free Radicals and Reactive Oxygen Species**

| RADICALS | | NONRADICAL SPECIES | |
|---|---|---|---|
| HO• | Hydroxyl radical | $^1O_2$ | Singlet oxygen |
| RO• | Alkoxyl radical | $ONOO^-$ | Peroxynitrite |
| ROO• | Peroxyl radical | $H_2O_2$ | Hydrogen |
| NO• | Nitric oxide | | peroxide |
| | radical | | |
| $O_2^{\overline{\bullet}}$ | Superoxide | | |
| | anion radical | | |

among them nitric oxide and peroxynitrite, are also produced (Table 38–1). Because they carry an unpaired electron, free radicals, although short-lived, are typically reactive and can oxidize nucleic acids, proteins, lipids, or carbohydrates. An estimated 10,000 oxidative "hits" are sustained daily by the DNA in every human cell. Oxidation can alter the structure and function of the target molecule.[25] Detrimental outcomes include deactivation of cell enzymes, cross-linkage and aggregation of proteins, alteration or misreading of DNA, lipid peroxidation, and depolymerization of cell polysaccharides. Free radical oxidation of low-density lipoproteins (LDLs) is thought to be an important contributor to the development of atherosclerosis.[26] Free radicals routinely create more free radicals and reactive oxygen species (ROS), thereby triggering long sequences or chain reactions of destructive activity. The accumulation of irreversible oxidative damage to cells and tissues could be the basis for the changes we associate with normal aging. Free radical damage to immune cell membrane lipids may impair the ability of immune cells to respond normally to challenge. Free radicals and reactive oxygen species are implicated in many disorders common among the elderly including cardiovascular disease, arthritis, cancer, cataracts, and neurodegenerative diseases such as Alzheimer's.[27–29]

Lens proteins have a very slow rate of turnover. Over time, they are especially vulnerable to accumulated oxidative damage such as cross-linkages. If they are altered, lens proteins aggregate and precipitate and the lens' transparency to light is reduced. This is suggested as the basis for lens opacification, i.e., cataract development, which is very common among seniors. Neurodegenerative diseases linked to oxidative stress are Parkinson's disease and Alzheimer's disease.[28] Oxidative stress is generally considered to be a substantial excess of free radicals and ROS in comparison to available antioxidants in the body. An array of antioxidant defenses help prevent free radical formation or limit their damaging effects. Free radical scavengers in cells include enzymes such as superoxide dismutase, glutathione reductase, catalase, and peroxidase. Plasma proteins complex with or sequester transition metals (e.g., transferrin/iron, ceruloplasmin/copper). This prevents the metals' participation in the generation of free radicals. Dietary antioxidants such as

vitamins C and E and beta-carotene are also part of the body's defenses. Their presence in adequate amounts helps protect cells from oxidant damage. For example, vitamin E is the most effective lipid-soluble antioxidant in cell membranes. It is present in notably high concentrations in immune cell membranes whose high polyunsaturated fatty acid (PUFA) content puts them at high risk of oxidative damage.[30–32] Although still in its infancy, there is substantial interest in and research on measurement of clinical markers of oxidative stress to assess the progress of various pathophysiologic conditions as well as aging. Markers of tissue injury caused by oxidative stress or antioxidant depletion include lipid-oxidative products such as the short-chain serum aldehyde, malondialdehyde (MDA), and breath pentane. The thiobarbituric acid reactive substances (TBARS) assay measures lipid-peroxidation markers such as MDA. There is no consensus on the utility of these assays in assessing the aging process or the risk of mortality.

## BIOCHEMICAL CHANGES

To varying degrees, the following changes are associated with the aging process: (1) atrophy of tissues and organs, (2) progressive decline in physiologic responsiveness, especially under stress, (3) increased susceptibility to most malignancies, (4) increased vulnerability to trauma, infections, and immune system disruptions, and (5) decreased capacity to adequately oxygenate tissues.[8] Age-associated alterations in function that place the elderly at increased risk of serious clinical problems usually produce biochemical changes detectable by the laboratorian. Establishment of clinical chemistry reference ranges specifically for seniors has been proposed for a number of analytes (Table 38–2). However, the magnitude, and often even the direction, of analyte change reported in various clinical studies of the elderly is highly variable.[33] This is not unexpected, given that the majority of clinical studies are cross-sectional rather than longitudinal, and that data are often reported as mean values and intragroup variability is high among the elderly. It is also likely that in healthy elderly, biochemical evidence of functional decline appears only under stress. It has often been commented that the elderly are more heterogeneous than any other chronologically defined group. An extensive study of reference intervals in the "fit" elderly considered over 15,000 measurements of 47 analytes obtained from 236 individuals ages 60 to 90; 22 individuals from 91 to 99 years of age and 69 individuals 100 years or older.[34] Although differences from the reference values determined on younger adults were noted, these variations were mild or moderate. This study as well as review of the literature suggests that only a few laboratory values can be identified as changing in response to aging itself. Many clinicians accept that the greatest benefit derived from laboratory data comes from monitoring a specific individual's test values over time. More information is likely to be obtained by comparing changes from personal baseline

TABLE 38-2

**Laboratory Values That Do and Do Not Change with Age (65 years or older unless otherwise specified)**

| CATEGORY | VALUES THAT DO NOT CHANGE | VALUES THAT CHANGE | DEGREE OR TYPE OF CHANGE |
|---|---|---|---|
| Chemistry | Serum bilirubin<br>AST<br>ALT<br>GGTP | Alkaline phosphatase | Increases 0%–20% for men and 0%–37% for women between ages 30 and 80 y |
| | | Serum albumin | Slight decrease |
| | | Serum magnesium | Decreases 15% between ages 30 and 80 y |
| | | Uric acid | Slight increase |
| Lipids | | Total cholesterol | Increases 30–40 mg/dL by age 55 in women and age 60 in men. |
| | | HDL cholesterol | Increases 30% in men and decreases 30% in women between ages 30 and 80 y |
| | | Triglycerides | Increases 30% in men and 50% in women between ages 30 and 80 y |
| Blood Glucose | | Fasting blood glucose | Increases 2 mg/dL per decade after age 30 |
| | | 1-h postprandial blood glucose | Increases 10 mg/dL per decade after age 30 |
| | | 2-h postprandial blood glucose | Increases up to 100 mg/dL plus age in years after 40 |
| Pulmonary arterial blood gas | pH<br>PaCO$_2$ | PaO$_2$ | Decreases 25% between ages 30 and 80 y |
| Renal function | Serum creatinine | Creatinine clearance | Decreases 10 mL/min/1.73 m$^3$ per decade |
| Thyroid function | T$_4$ | T$_3$ | Possible slight decrease |
| | | TSH | Possible slight decrease |
| Hematology | Hematocrit<br>Hemoglobin | Leukocyte count | Slight decrease |
| | Red blood cell indices | ESR | Rises (upper limit, 40 mm/h in men and 45 mm/h in women) |
| | Platelet count | Vitamin B$_{12}$ | Slight decrease |

ALT = alanine aminotransferase; AST = aspartate aminotransferase; ESR = erythrocyte sedimentation rate; GGTP = gamma-glutamyl transpeptidase; HDL = high-density lipoprotein; TSH = thyrotropin; T$_4$ = thyroxine; T$_3$ = triiodothyronine. (From Brigden ML, Heathcote JC: Problems in interpreting laboratory tests. What do unexpected results mean? Postgrad Med 107(7):145, 2000.)

values throughout adult life than in referring to generalized "geriatric reference ranges." Still, there is merit in identifying laboratory values that seem to be most susceptible to change with aging.

Increases are generally, though not universally, observed among healthy elderly for only a few analytes: BUN, uric acid, alkaline phosphatase (women), lactate dehydrogenase, fasting blood glucose, postprandial glucose, glycated hemoglobin,

fructosamine, total cholesterol, and triglycerides. Because of reduced skeletal mass, serum creatinine is likely to remain unchanged during aging despite reduction in creatinine clearance. Decreased values are commonly reported for growth hormone, triiodothyronine, albumin, total protein, creatinine clearance, hemoglobin, iron, folate, and vitamin B$_{12}$. Although the decline in serum albumin is small and may be due to dietary rather than physiologic changes, the consequence of its decline is that reference ranges for substances bound to albumin may be altered even though the unbound fraction remains constant.[13,34,35]

Effects of preanalytical variables such as patient position (sitting versus lying), level of exercise, dietary practices, drug, caffeine or alcohol ingestion, smoking, time of day of specimen collection, and duration of tourniquet application may be especially important when assessing the significance of laboratory findings from seniors. For example, the elderly are often identified as a supine population, engaging in only minimal physical activity. This lifestyle impacts selected analytes. There is about a 10% increase in total protein when an individual moves from lying down to a standing position. Levels of protein-bound analytes will therefore be affected by the nondisease variable of posture. A postural change can produce a 15% variation in total cholesterol and high-density lipoprotein (HDL) cholesterol determinations. Physical activity also influences laboratory results. Vigorous exercise shortly before blood collection can produce a 6% increase in total cholesterol level.[35] Elevations of serum enzymes such as creatine kinase (CK) are observed 5 to 15 hours after exercise when an individual, although healthy, is out of condition. Use of diuretics is common among elderly for the treatment of hypertension. Long-term diuretic use impairs glucose tolerance in some individuals. Diuretic therapy increases serum uric acid by 1 to 1.5 mg/dL and may precipitate or aggravate gout in some patients. Thiazide-like diuretics deplete the body's magnesium and potassium.[36,37] Table 38–3 summarizes the effects of selected drugs on laboratory results.

Aging is a complex phenomenon involving biochemical and physiologic adjustments. The aging of specific systems within the individual depends on the interactions of inheritance, hormonal and immunologic regulation, and environmental stressors such as diet, exercise, drug use, and infection. It is essential to keep this diversity in mind when biochemical measures of physiologic function are examined. Physiologic changes associated with the normal aging process may affect susceptibility to disease, the way in which a disorder is manifested, and the body's ability to reestablish homeostasis. A key feature of physiologic aging is the inability to maintain homeostasis under stress. In the absence of stress, age-related changes in physiology, although measurable, are often not clinically significant. Differentiating between pathologic conditions and age-associated deterioration of function in the older adult may be especially difficult. In seniors, disease presentation is often atypical.[38] Nonspecific complaints are common and so-called classic symptoms, seen in younger persons, are absent. Because of this, delay in diagnosis often occurs. Pneumonia, thyroid disorders, pulmonary embolism, and myocardial infarction are only a few of the clinical conditions that often present nonspecifically in the elderly (Table 38–4). Among older adults, the most common undetected diseases

TABLE 38–3

**Selected in vivo Drug Interaction**

**AGENTS ASSOCIATED WITH DECREASED SERUM ALBUMIN**

| | | | |
|---|---|---|---|
| Acetaminophen | Cathartics | Niacin | |
| Anticonvulsants | Estrogens | | |

**AGENTS ASSOCIATED WITH INCREASED BUN**

| | | | |
|---|---|---|---|
| Acetaminophen | Diazepam | Indomethacin | Penicillin |
| Allopurinol | Hydralazine | Levodopa | Propranolol |
| Thiazides | Salicylates | Tetracyclines | Streptokinase |

**AGENTS ASSOCIATED WITH INCREASED SERUM CREATININE**

| | | | |
|---|---|---|---|
| Acetaminophen | Alkaline antacids | Minoxidil | Thiazides |
| Barbiturates | Penicillin | Streptokinase | |

**AGENTS ASSOCIATED WITH INCREASED SERUM URIC ACID**

| | | | |
|---|---|---|---|
| Antineoplastic agents | Ethanol | Levodopa | Niacin |
| Prednisone | Salicylates | Thiazides | |

**AGENTS ASSOCIATED WITH INCREASED SERUM ALKALINE PHOSPHATASE**

| | | | |
|---|---|---|---|
| Acetaminophen | Barbiturates | Diazepam | Niacin |
| Allopurinol | Colchicine | Estrogens | Propranolol |
| Anticonvulsants | Coumarin derivatives | Gold | Thiazides |

TABLE 38-4

**Diseases Likely to Present Nonspecifically
In The Elderly**

Pneumonia
Tuberculosis
Myocardial infarction
Pulmonary embolism
Hypothyroidism
Hyperthyroidism
Alcoholism

are anemia, bacteriuria, hyperlipidemia, diabetes, bleeding colonic lesions, hypothyroidism, and electrolyte disturbances.

Age-related changes in weight and body composition occur. Total body water is decreased from approximately 60% at age 25 to 50% at age 70.[36] Studies have consistently demonstrated clinically important losses of fat-free mass (FFM) with age in both men and women. This phenomenon is known as **sarcopenia.**[39] Over an individual's lifetime, there is a decrease in lean body mass of about 15% due to atrophy of skeletal muscle and viscera. Between the ages of 30 and 70, FFM declines by as much as 40%.[39] Even within lean tissue such as muscle, fat content increases with aging. As a result, the total volume available for the distribution of water-soluble drugs and nutrients diminishes. As women age, they tend to gain weight. Although lean body mass decreases slightly, there is a greater increase in percent body fat. Men tend to maintain a stable body weight as they grow older, with a decrease in lean body mass offset by an equivalent increase in body fat. Increase in body fat expands the body's storage capacity for lipid-soluble drugs and nutrients and increases the potential for toxic accumulation of these substances. Secretion of GH by the pituitary falls by about one third between the ages of 25 and 65 years. At least in part, the decrease in lean body mass, expansion of adipose tissue, and thinning of skin that occurs with aging can be traced to diminished secretion of this hormone.[16] Aging is associated with an increasingly more central deposition of fat in both men and women.[39] In men, this change in fat distribution progresses slowly with aging; in women, the central accumulation of fat may begin only after menopause. The longer a woman is postmenopausal, the higher her proportion of body fat to fat-free mass. Whether use of hormone replacement therapy (HRT) influences menopause-related changes in body weight is unclear. Both men and women show a gradual weight loss as they progress from "young-old" to "old-old."

## Renal Function

Changes in the urinary tract are among the most readily identified as being age-related for any organ system. Major functions of the kidney include (1) glomerular filtration, (2) fluid and elec-

trolyte homeostasis, (3) acid-base homeostasis, (4) blood pressure regulation, (5) calcium and phosphorus metabolism, and (6) erythropoiesis. Renal function alterations with aging are well-documented.[36] As the kidneys age, organ size decreases, glomerular sclerosis increases, renal tubular changes occur, and renal blood flow is altered. Between the ages of 30 and 80, renal mass declines by 20 to 25%.[36,40] Tissue loss is mainly cortical and involves both glomeruli and tubules. As the kidney ages, there is a steady increase in the number of sclerotic glomeruli. In the renal tubules, the length and volume of the proximal convoluted portion, in particular, decrease. Basement membrane thickening is reported more often in the tubules than in the glomeruli. Renal vascular changes occur and blood flow to many glomeruli is reduced or cut off.

Linked at least in part to anatomic changes are numerous functional abnormalities. Under normal physiologic conditions, the aging kidney may be capable of maintaining homeostasis. However, in response to stress (disease, medications, environmental factors), older individuals show decreased adaptive capacity. Reduction in GFR is the single most important physiologic change observed in the aging kidney.[36] Glomerular function declines with age as the number of functioning glomeruli is reduced and renal blood is diminished. After the age of 40, the GFR rate, as estimated by creatinine clearance, declines on average by 0.8 and 1.0 mL/min per 1.73 $M^2$ or by approximately 1% per year in the absence of any overt clinical disease (Figure 38–4).[41,42] However, not all healthy elderly show a decrease in GFR. In the Baltimore Longitudinal Study of Aging, which followed over 1000 healthy individuals for up to 30 years, about 30% of participants showed no decline at all in creatinine clearance, in some instances for as long as 25 years.[36] Measurement of serum creatinine concentration is a convenient means of estimating renal function. Serum creatinine, derived from metabolism of muscle creatine, is removed from the blood by urinary excretion, primarily filtration. Its concentration in the blood is therefore an approximate index of glomerular filtration. In young adults, there is an excellent inverse correlation between plasma creatinine and GFR. In these individuals, a single plasma creatinine value is a reasonable indicator of GFR. Loss of lean body (muscle) mass with aging means that less creatinine will be produced. Despite the usual decline in GFR with age, serum creatinine concentration is unlikely to change with age and could remain between 0.8 and 1.0 mg/dL throughout life. Because of this, serum creatinine values may be misleading (Figure 38–5). A serum creatinine concentration considered to reflect an acceptable GFR in a young adult might be evidence of renal insufficiency in an older individual. Use of the Cockcroft and Gault formula permits rapid calculation of creatinine clearance from the plasma or serum creatinine level, taking into account the patient's age, weight, and gender. But, while it is useful, it tends to overestimate creatinine clearance, especially in the very old.[36]

$$\text{Creatinine clearance in males (mL/min)} = \frac{(140 - \text{Age in years}) \times \text{Weight (kg)}}{72 \times \text{Serum creatinine (mg/dL)}}$$

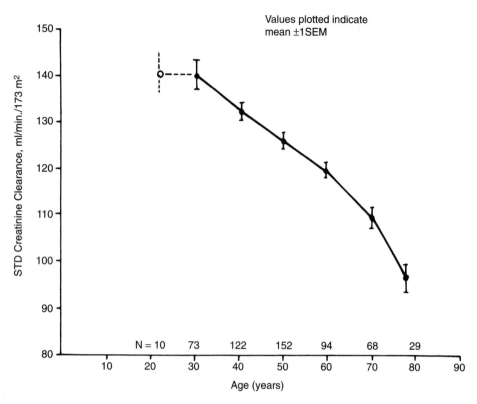

**F I G U R E   3 8 - 4**

The effect of age on creatinine clearance in men. (From Rowe JW: Renal system. In Rowe JW, Besdine RW (eds.): *Geriatric Medicine*. 2nd ed. Boston, Little, Brown, 1988.)

Since creatinine clearance is approximately 15% less in females, this value must be multiplied by 0.85 to obtain the corrected value for women.

Assessment of kidney function by quantitation of blood urea nitrogen (BUN) may also be unreliable in the elderly. Urea formation is related to protein intake. BUN levels tend to increase with age as renal function is compromised but reduction in protein intake, a common dietary problem in older adults, may offset any increase due to diminished glomerular filtration.

Alterations in renal tubular functions contribute to difficulties in fluid, electrolyte, and acid-base homeostasis among the elderly. Diminished ability to conserve water and concentrate urine is common among seniors. In healthy young adults, urine osmolality can reach 1200 mOsm/kg during maximum renal water conservation. The maximum urinary osmolality achieved in an 80-year-old may be only 400 to 500 mOsm/kg.[36] Further reduction in urinary concentrating ability often is due to conditions or medications common to the elderly such as urinary tract infection or obstruction, malnutrition, or the use of diuretics. Inability to regulate water balance may be due to an age-related reduction in renal responsiveness to antidiuretic hormone (ADH).[36] Thus, the older individual is less able to cope with either dehydration or water load. Delayed sodium conservation response, narrowed limits for potassium homeo-

stasis, increased renal threshold for glucose and altered excretion of acid are also common findings among seniors.

Increased blood pressure is not a normal part of aging; many individuals do not demonstrate a rise in blood pressure with increasing age. Atherosclerotic changes, decreased vascular elasticity, inappropriate sodium intake and/or retention, and progressive loss of nephrons contribute to increased peripheral vascular resistance and blood pressure elevation with age. Hypertension significantly increases the risk of mortality and as many as two thirds of seniors are hypertensive. End-stage renal disease (ESRD) is a condition closely related to high blood pressure. Physical conditioning, which improves the aerobic capacity of older adults by increasing both cardiac output and oxygen use, also appears to lessen the vascular stiffening associated with aging. Salt sensitivity of arterial pressure regulation increases with aging and chronic consumption of a high salt diet might contribute to arterial stiffening and increased systolic pressure. The single most potent, common, and treatable risk factor for cardiovascular disease in women is hypertension.[38,43,44] Diastolic pressure rises with age but should stabilize or decrease slightly after age 60. Systolic pressure continues to increase after age 55 until age 70 or 80 but should not exceed 160 mm Hg. A higher percentage of men than women have high blood pressure (HBP) until age 55; from ages 55 to 74, the percentage of women is somewhat

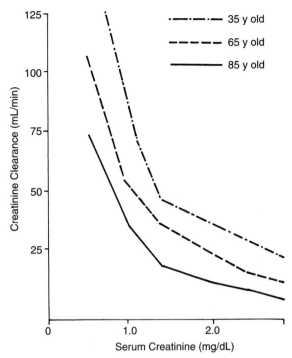

**FIGURE 38-5**

Relationship of age and serum creatinine concentration to creatinine clearance (Cockroft and Gault calculation) in a 50-kg male. (From Meyer RB: Renal function in aging. J Amer Geriatr Soc 37:794, 1989.)

higher. From age 75 upward, a higher percentage of women have HBP than men.[45] The Framingham Study data link high rates of cardiovascular disease and stroke with systolic hypertension in the elderly.[44] Isolated systolic hypertension is defined as systolic blood pressure 140 mm Hg or greater and diastolic blood pressure less than 90 mm Hg. Over 30% of persons older than 75 have resting isolated systolic blood pressures greater than 160 mm Hg (Figure 38–6). An increase in systolic blood pressure from 140 to 185 mm Hg in a 70-year-old nearly doubles the probability of a cardiovascular event.[44] More elderly blacks are hypertensive than are elderly whites.[45]

Magnesium and potassium affect vascular resistance and imbalances can give rise to hypertension. Among the elderly, deficiencies of these two electrolytes are common. Magnesium is important in controlling arterial tone and stimulating the release of the vasodilator prostaglandin (PGI$_2$). Deficiency of magnesium plays a key role in regulating plasma potassium concentration. Hypomagnesemia can lead to hypokalemia by promoting loss of potassium, which in the urine and feces. Total body potassium declines with age, probably due to loss of muscle mass and excessive renal loss of potassium, which is especially common in elderly patients taking thiazide and loop diuretics. Potassium, the major intracellular cation, is involved in energy metabolism, membrane transport, and maintenance of the potential difference across cell membranes. Potassium also exerts a blood-pressure lowering effect. Even in healthy elderly, routine assessment of serum potassium is advisable. Both

hyperkalemic and hypokalemia can be deadly because there is interference with the ability of cells to depolarize and repolarize normally. Changes in the excitability of nerve and muscle cells are evident.[40] Hypokalemia is characterized by muscle weakness, paralysis, and cardiac conduction defects. Maintenance of the body's potassium balance depends on the effectiveness of renal excretion. Loss of renal mass with aging limits the amount of potassium that can be transported in a given time. Reduced tubular responsiveness to aldosterone also limits the effectiveness of potassium excretion. Elderly patients are therefore at increased risk of hyperkalemia, especially in response to a potassium-load (potassium supplement or a salt-substitute rich in potassium chloride) or drugs that interfere with potassium excretion (potassium-sparing diuretics such as spironolactone).[36] Severe hyperkalemia can lead to peripheral vascular collapse and cardiac arrest. Seniors are more likely to become dehydrated and experience hypotension in response to diuretics, acute febrile illnesses, or in situations where salt and water limitations exist. Older adults often show a sluggish response to a sodium load, making it difficult for them to manage conditions of sodium excess. Similarly, response to sodium deprivation is slowed. Even healthy seniors may take twice as long as young adults to reduce sodium excretion and restore equilibrium when they are placed on low-salt diets. Acid-base

Prevalence of Hypertension (>160/95 mm Hg) in U.S.

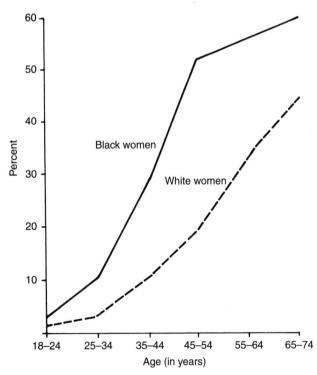

**FIGURE 38-6**

Prevalence of hypertension (>160/95 mm Hg) in the United States. (From Byyny RL, Speroff L: *A Clinical Guide for the Care of Older Women.* 2nd ed. Baltimore, Williams & Wilkins, 1996.)

disturbances are common in the elderly. Under stress, older adults experience a greater difficulty in maintaining a normal acid-base equilibrium. Diminished acid excretory ability has been linked to decreased tubular secretion of ammonia, which buffers about one half of the acid excreted.[36]

Loss of renal mass with aging may have consequences beyond those readily associated with kidney function. Anemia is a common finding in older adults, although it is most often associated with a number of chronic diseases.[35] Hemoglobin tends to decrease with age in men over 60, although in women, values do not decline until the mid-80s. More than a deficiency of micronutrients such as iron, folate, or cobalamin in elderly may be responsible for the decline in hemoglobin and hematocrit. It has been suggested that ineffective erythropoiesis due to declining erythropoietin (EPO) release as renal tissue is lost reduces the body's ability to stimulate red blood cell formation in response to reduction in tissue oxygenation. The anemia of chronic renal failure is due to decreased EPO production. A possible defect in EPO production has also been suggested as a main cause of anemia in chronic rheumatic disorders. In the elderly, there is a decline in red blood cell mass indicated by within reference range, but not elevated, hematocrit values in spite of a reduction in total body water. Whatever its origin, anemia of any degree demands a clinical follow-up. Skeletal integrity may be adversely affected by the loss of renal tissue. Synthesis of the potent calciotropic hormone 1,25-dihydroxyvitamin $D_3$ occurs only in the renal cortex. Impaired vitamin D status, leading to disruption of calcium metabolism and loss of bone density, may arise from progressive loss of renal tissue with aging.

Age-related decline in renal function places seniors at increased risk of drug toxicity. Polypharmacy, the consumption of multiple drugs simultaneously, often for extended periods, is common practice among the elderly. These patients receive 30% of all prescription drugs and 40% of all over-the-counter medications.[40] Total body water decrease and total body fat increase with age reduce the volume for distribution of water-soluble drugs and increase the volume of distribution for lipid-soluble drugs. As renal function declines, drugs accumulate in the tissues at levels in excess of the therapeutic dose. Aminoglycosides, lithium, digoxin, procainamide, and cimetidine are prescribed for medical conditions commonly found in seniors. These medications have potentially toxic effects and their prolonged retention due to impaired renal function poses a serious risk. Therapeutic monitoring is essential to guide dose adjustments. The adverse cumulative effect of polypharmacy and reduced renal excretion is exemplified by the inhibition of metabolism of the anticoagulant warfarin by the ulcer medication cimetidine.[46] A number of other age-related changes in physiology influence the body's handling of drugs as can be seen in Table 38–5.

Changes in lower urinary tract functions create major health problems for the elderly. These age-related changes can increase vulnerability of older adults to urinary incontinence. Incontinence reportedly affects 10 million adults in the United States, including an estimated 30% of community-dwelling

## TABLE 3 8 – 5

### Age-Related Changes That Influence Drug Handling

Gastric pH increased
Gastric emptying impaired
Visceral blood flow reduced
Gastrointestinal motility reduced
Gastrointestinal absorptive surface reduced and thinned
Lean body mass reduced
Total body fat relatively increased (until advanced age)
Metabolically active tissue decreased
Total body water decreased
Plasma albumin concentration reduced
Liver mass reduced
Hepatic microsomal enzyme activity reduced
Regional blood flow from liver and kidney redistributed
Glomerular filtration rate reduced
Renal tubular function impaired

Modified from Swift CG: Drug therapy. In Pathy MSJ, Finucane P (eds.): *Geriatric Medicine. Problems and Practices.* London, Springer-Verlag, 1989, pp 299–311.

elderly and 50% to 70% of those living in nursing homes.[47] Women are twice as likely as men to suffer from incontinence. Significant causes of reversible urinary incontinence include drugs, delirium, and infection. Four types of incontinence have been identified. Stress incontinence is most commonly encountered in women who have given birth to many children. Control of bladder function is adversely affected by weakened supporting pelvic muscles, resulting from multiple pregnancies, and compromise or loss of urethral sphincter integrity permits leakage when intraabdominal pressure is raised, as occurs in coughing, sneezing, or lifting heavy objects. In overflow incontinence, the bladder cannot empty normally and becomes overdistended. Causes include medications, obstructive problems in women, and prostate hypertrophy in men. Urge incontinence is due to uninhibited bladder contractions in response to an urge to void. Causes include lesions of the central nervous system and local irritating factors such as urinary tract infections. Functional incontinence occurs when the lower urinary tract function is intact but cognitive impairment and immobility affect urination. Urinary tract infections are very common in older adults and most individuals are asymptomatic. In men and women aged 65 and older, the prevalence of bacteriuria is 10% and 20%, respectively. Most older persons with bacteriuria are asymptomatic. Urinary incontinence in seniors appears to be unrelated to the presence or absence of asymptomatic bacteriuria.[48]

Laboratory assessment of patients with incontinence usually includes a urinalysis, creatinine clearance, and postvoid residual urine volume. Other tests suggested are urine culture, blood glucose (polyuria may be associated with diabetes mellitus), and urinary cytology.

## Glucose Homeostasis

The appearance of hyperglycemia with advancing age is well documented. The ability of the body to maintain glucose homeostasis after a glucose challenge is progressively impaired. Glucose tolerance declines with age even in the absence of overt diabetes, which is usually type 2. The prevalence of diabetes in men and women in the U.S. population, based on the National Health and Nutrition Examination Survey, 1988–1994 (NHANES III) and using American Diabetes Association (ADA) criteria, is shown in Figure 38–7. Total prevalence of diabetes increases from 1% to 2% in young adults to 18% to 20% of those aged 60 to 74 years. From age 75 upward, incidence rates of diagnosed and undiagnosed diabetes plateau. After age 65, prevalence rates are higher for men than women. A confirmed fasting plasma glucose (FPG) value greater than or equal to 126 (mg/dL) indicates a diagnosis of diabetes mellitus (DM).[49] New diagnostic criteria for diabetes call for the recognition of an intermediate group of individuals whose glucose levels are not so high that they meet the criteria for diabetes but whose levels are too high to be considered "normal." The terms impaired glucose tolerance (IGT) and impaired fasting glucose (IFG) refer to a metabolic situation that is between normal glucose homeostasis and diabetes. IGT and IFG are not clinical entities themselves but indicate risk for future diabetes and cardiovascular disease. Under new ADA guidelines, patients with either IFG or IGT merit a diagnosis of prediabetes. Both are associated with the insulin resistance syndrome also known as syndrome X. An FPG less than 110 mg/dL is considered to be the upper limit of normal, partly because a value greater than this is associated with a progressively greater risk of developing microvascular and macrovascular complications. IFG is defined as a FPG $\geq$ 110 mg/dL but less than 126 mg/dL. Rates of IFG increase with age. Prevalence is higher for men than women in all racial and ethnic groups. When an oral glucose tolerance test (OGTT) is conducted, a confirmed plasma glucose value >200 mg/dL 2 hours after ingestion of a solution containing 75 g of anhydrous glucose dissolved in water supports a diagnosis of diabetes. A laboratory designation of impaired glucose tolerance (IGT) is applied to an individual in whom a fasting plasma glucose is <126 mg/dL and who, in response to an OGTT, has a 2-hour value $\geq$140 but <200 mg/dL.[50] Figure 38–7 shows the prevalence of diabetes, both diagnosed and undiagnosed, by gender and age. Table 38–6 shows the percentage of undiagnosed diabetes and IFG in the population as a function of age, gender, and race and ethnic origin.

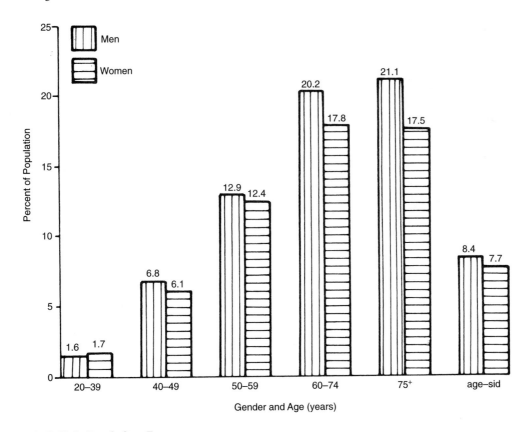

**F I G U R E   3 8 - 7**

Prevalence of diabetes in men and women in the U.S. population age $\geq$20 years, based on NHANES III. (From Harris MI, Flegal KM, Cowie CC, et al.: Prevalence of diabetes, impaired fasting glucose, and impaired glucose tolerance in U.S. adults. Third National Health and Nutrition Examination Survey, 1988–1994. Diabetes Care 21:518, 1998.)

TABLE  38-6

**Percentage of the U.S. Population ≥20 Years of Age with Undiagnosed Diabetes and Impaired Fasting Glucose Based on NHANES III (1988–1994) and 1997 American Diabetes Association Fasting Plasma Glucose Diagnostic Criteria**

| RACE/SEX | AGE (YEARS) | | | | | | |
|---|---|---|---|---|---|---|---|
| | 20–39 | 40–49 | 50–59 | 60–74 | ≥75 | ≥20 | ≥20* |
| **Undiagnosed diabetes** | | | | | | | |
| All races† | | | | | | | |
| Both sexes | 0.6 | 2.5 | 4.6 | 6.2 | 5.7 | 2.7 | 2.8 |
| Men | 0.5 | 3.6 | 3.3 | 8.4 | 7.3 | 3.0 | 3.1 |
| Women | 0.6 | 1.6 | 5.8 | 4.5 | 4.7 | 2.4 | 2.5 |
| Non-Hispanic White | | | | | | | |
| Both sexes | 0.4 | 2.1 | 4.0 | 6.0 | 4.9 | 2.5 | 2.5 |
| Men | 0.4 | 2.9 | 3.5 | 8.2 | 6.0 | 2.9 | 2.9 |
| Women | 0.4 | 1.3 | 4.4 | 4.3 | 4.3 | 2.1 | 2.0 |
| Non-Hispanic Black | | | | | | | |
| Both sexes | 1.4 | 3.9 | 6.1 | 7.7 | 4.9 | 3.4 | 3.6 |
| Men | 1.1 | 4.3 | 3.0 | 6.6 | 0.0 | 2.6 | 2.7 |
| Women | 1.7 | 3.7 | 8.5 | 8.5 | 7.6 | 4.0 | 4.5 |
| Mexican-American | | | | | | | |
| Both sexes | 1.5 | 5.9 | 10.0 | 4.9 | 8.0 | 3.4 | 4.5 |
| Men | 1.5 | 6.8 | 12.9 | 6.3 | 10.1 | 3.8 | 5.4 |
| Women | 1.5 | 4.9 | 7.5 | 3.5 | 6.2 | 3.0 | 3.6 |
| **Impaired fasting glucose** | | | | | | | |
| All races† | | | | | | | |
| Both sexes | 2.8 | 7.1 | 8.0 | 14.0 | 14.1 | 6.9 | 6.9 |
| Men | 4.5 | 10.1 | 9.2 | 16.2 | 17.9 | 8.7 | 8.8 |
| Women | 1.2 | 4.3 | 6.8 | 12.3 | 11.9 | 5.2 | 5.0 |
| Non-Hispanic White | | | | | | | |
| Both sexes | 2.7 | 6.7 | 7.7 | 13.9 | 13.7 | 6.9 | 6.8 |
| Men | 4.8 | 10.2 | 9.1 | 15.6 | 18.4 | 9.0 | 8.9 |
| Women | 0.8 | 3.2 | 6.4 | 12.5 | 11.0 | 5.0 | 4.6 |
| Non-Hispanic Black | | | | | | | |
| Both sexes | 2.8 | 7.0 | 10.0 | 12.1 | 15.7 | 6.2 | 7.0 |
| Men | 3.3 | 6.7 | 9.3 | 15.4 | 18.7 | 6.7 | 7.7 |
| Women | 2.5 | 7.2 | 10.5 | 9.8 | 14.1 | 5.2 | 6.4 |
| Mexican-American | | | | | | | |
| Both sexes | 4.4 | 11.8 | 8.6 | 17.1 | 14.7 | 7.3 | 8.9 |
| Men | 5.7 | 15.6 | 8.6 | 24.5 | 18.3 | 9.3 | 11.6 |
| Women | 2.9 | 7.9 | 8.6 | 10.1 | 11.9 | 5.2 | 6.3 |

Undiagnosed diabetes is defined as fasting plasma glucose ≥126 mg/dl; impaired fasting glucose is defined as fasting plasma 110–125 mg/dl.

*Values are age- and sex-standardized.

†Values include those of racial and ethnic groups not listed separately.

(From Harris MI, Flegal KM, Cowie CC, et al.: Prevalence of diabetes, impaired fasting glucose and impaired glucose tolerance in U.S. adults. Third National Health and Nutrition Examination Survey, 1988–1994. Diabetes Care 21(4):518, 1998.)

Over 6 million Americans aged 65 years or older have diabetes: 18.4% of all people in this age group.[51] Minorities are at increased risk for diabetes. Diabetes is the sixth leading cause of death among Hispanics and the number 4 cause of death among women and elderly Hispanics. One quarter of blacks between 65 and 74 years of age have diabetes.[52] Some degree of deterioration in glucose tolerance is estimated to be present in more than 60% of individuals over age 60.[53]

A multitude of factors contribute to glucose intolerance in people of all ages. Especially problematic among seniors are:

obesity (more than 40% above ideal body weight), decreased physical activity, loss of lean body mass, poor dietary habits, and alterations in insulin action. Although modest elevation of blood glucose may be the "norm" among older adults, it is important to keep in mind that normality does not imply harmlessness. The prevalence of disorders of glucose metabolism can be expected to increase as our population becomes increasingly more overweight, sedentary, racially and ethnically diverse, and elderly.

Individuals with IGT do not necessarily progress to overt diabetes. They are, however, at increased risk of cardiovascular disease including coronary heart disease, hypertension, and arterial disease. Complications specific for diabetes such as retinopathy, nephropathy, and neuropathy are rarely observed. In view of similarities in structural and functional changes, diabetes has been suggested as an example of accelerated aging.[22,23]

Laboratory assessment of glycemic control is essential among seniors. With age, it appears that the body's ability to efficiently dispose of glucose is compromised. Fasting blood glucose levels increase from 1 to 2 mg/dL per decade over the age of 30.[35] A more marked increase of as much as 5 mg/dL/decade has been suggested by some studies. Although the reference range in men is higher than women at all ages, the difference is not judged to be sufficient to require a gender-specific reference range. At menopause, fasting glucose levels increase but oral contraceptives, used by both pre and post-menopausal women, can also elevate plasma glucose. Fasting glucose levels are less influenced by age than specimens taken at random during the day. In 1- to 2-hour postprandial specimens, average glucose increases of 4 mg/dL per decade after age 40 are noted, with elevations as high as 8 to 15 mg/dL per decade reported.[54]

Because of the increased renal threshold for glucose and decreased GFR, interpretation of the urine glucose test becomes problematic. As noted previously, the absence of glycosuria does not exclude a diagnosis of diabetes or impaired glucose tolerance. Renal glycosuria identified in a young adult may become less pronounced as the individual ages.

Insulin secretion in response to a glucose challenge is altered with age.[15,54] The average increase in postglucose loading specimens is about 10 mg/dL at 1 hour and 5 mg/dL at 2 hours per decade past 35 years of age. In seniors, the size of the loading dose has less effect on the blood glucose levels than it does in young adults. Normally, mean glucose levels in the OGTT are higher in the afternoon and evening than in morning tests, but this diurnal variation is blunted in seniors. The OGTT curve can be subdivided into three phases. In phase 1, occurring within about 1 hour after loading, the slope of the curves for both young and old adults are similar. This suggests that intestinal absorption of glucose is not impaired with age. Phase 2, the time required to reach peak glucose levels, varies significantly with age. Maximum glucose levels are attained in young adults in about one-half hour. In seniors, peak values are not reached for 60 to 75 minutes postloading. This portion of the OGTT curve reflects the critical period of age-dependent deteriorated glycemic control. During this period,

rising glucose and insulin levels do not trigger peripheral uptake due to tissue insensitivity to the hormone. Insulin resistance is more commonly encountered in older subjects. In the third phase of the curve, glucose enters the cells and is metabolized. Although the rate of restoration is similar in all adults, the absolute length of time required to return to preload levels is longer in the elderly.

Hyperglycemia, even if mild, is not a benign condition. Plasma osmolality is increased as serum glucose levels rise. Because of the delayed or diminished ability of aging kidneys to promptly excrete excessive amounts of glucose, there is an increase in the risk for hyperosmolar nonketotic coma in the elderly. In response to the high osmolality of the extracellular fluid, water moves out of those cells in which glucose entry is insulin dependent. In these tissues, intracellular dehydration results. However, in insulin-independent tissue such as the brain, glucose enters the cells. In response, water will shift into these cells and swelling of brain tissue from intracellular edema occurs. Shock and coma follow with patient mortality ranging from 30% to 50%. This syndrome of life-threatening hyperosmolality caused by marked hyperglycemia is almost exclusively observed in older adults. Insulin levels may be sufficient to prevent ketosis but not hyperglycemia. Biochemical findings associated with hyperosmolar nonketotic coma include: plasma glucose >600 mg/dL; serum osmolality >330 mOsm/kg; absent or minimal serum ketones; arterial blood pH >7.3; serum bicarbonate >20 mmol/L, and negative or small urine ketones.

Diabetes appears to accelerate the aging process. A person with diabetes may appear physiologically to be 10 years older than their chronologic age.[55] As discussed earlier in the section on theories of aging, hyperglycemia is responsible for reversible and irreversible changes to a variety of proteins. Any protein, whether long or short-lived, is susceptible to glycation. Proteins with relatively short half-life such as serum proteins (i.e. albumin) and hemoglobin can exhibit altered reactivities and conformation changes related to reversible glycation from mild long-term hyperglycemia. Assessment of glycemic control over time in a patient is possible by measuring serum glycated proteins (i.e., serum fructosamine) and glycated hemoglobin. Even in seniors whose OGTT results are within reference range, glycated hemoglobin levels that reflect glycemic control over the previous 2 to 3 months are reported to be elevated. Healthy young adults have approximately 5% to 7% HbA$_{1C}$; among healthy seniors over 70, 9% of hemoglobin is glycated. On average each 1% change in glycated hemoglobin represents a 25 to 35 mg/dL change in plasma glucose. Varying serum protein levels in the elderly do not appear to diminish the usefulness of the fructosamine assay as long as the albumin concentration is greater than 3 g/dL.

Postprandial serum insulin levels are increased in older adults. In women, insulin levels are higher at all times during the OGTT. Hyperinsulinemia or an underlying insulin-resistant state may contribute to the development of atherosclerosis, hypertension, and/or increased risk of coronary heart disease (CHD).[56] Hypertension develops in about one half of diabetics, about 50% of persons with type 2 diabetes have dyslipidemia and about 80% are obese. Hypertension is significantly linked to elevated insulin levels. Increased insulin levels are also associated with elevated triglycerides and reduced high-density lipoprotein (HDL) cholesterol. It has been suggested that an insulin-androgen association is the basis for the difference in response of nondiabetic men and women to glucose and insulin within the normal range. Altered glucose homeostasis with aging has been attributed to insulin deficiency (either relative or absolute) and/or decreased sensitivity of target tissues to the hormone and less efficient insulin-induced suppression of hepatic glucose output. Distribution of the increased body fat that occurs with aging is important. Metabolic changes arising from fat redistribution and accumulation in a centralized location (trunk and internal organs) contributes to increasing difficulty in postprandial glucose disposal. The importance of central fat distribution in the elderly is an area of current study. Two proteins are currently being examined for a possible role in altered glucose metabolism. Amylin, a small polypeptide cosecreted with insulin, has been proposed as a mediator of insulin resistance. Leptin, a hormone secreted from fat cells, regulates appetite and modulated insulin action. The clinical value of measuring these plasma analytes is unclear.[57] Reduced numbers of peripheral cell receptors for insulin as adipose tissue replaces muscle, impaired binding of the hormone by cell membrane receptors, and increasing occurrence of postreceptor or intracellular defects would effectively increase tissue resistance to insulin.[58] Difficulty in the conversion of proinsulin to insulin could lead to relative hyperproinsulinemia. Several recent studies have demonstrated that type 2 DM and IGT are characterized by relative hyperproinsulinemia.

## Lipids

The coronary risk factors that in general apply to middle-aged adults also apply to the elderly.[43] The Framingham Heart Study played a key role in identifying coronary heart disease (CHD) risk factors.[59] The study, begun in 1948, is an ongoing observational study of the population of Framingham, Massachusetts. It is credited with uncovering some of the basic risk factors for cardiovascular disease including cigarette smoking, hypertension, high serum total cholesterol and various cholesterol fractions, low levels of HDL cholesterol, and diabetes mellitus. Other risk factors include obesity, physical inactivity, hypertriglyceridemia, small low-density lipoprotein (LDL) particles, increased lipoprotein (a), abnormalities in several coagulation factors, and family history of premature CHD. The significance of elevated serum homocysteine as an independent causative risk factor for cardiovascular disease continues to be a topic of much study and debate.[60,61] Numerous studies suggest it may play a role in atherogenic and thrombogenic disease. Autooxidation of homocysteine produces potent reactive oxygen species and free radicals, including superoxide anion and hydroxyl radicals in addition to hydrogen peroxide. The

resulting endothelial damage caused by these oxidants may play a role in atherothrombotic disease (Figure 38–8).[62] Total homocysteine (tHcy) concentrations are partly determined by folate, vitamin $B_{12}$, and vitamin $B_6$ status.[63] Advancing age is also included as a risk factor because cardiovascular diseases, such as hypertension and coronary atherosclerosis, exhibit an exponential increase in incidence and prevalence in older people (Figure 38–9).

In 1997, CHD accounted for almost one half of deaths among all seniors, male and female.[64] In view of this, many cross-sectional studies of the elderly have been criticized since the elderly assessed could be viewed as "survivors" and not representative of the larger group of seniors. Even longitudinal studies may be difficult to interpret given the recent changes in diet and exercise that have come to characterize the lifestyle of many older adults in our society. Plasma total cholesterol and triglycerides increase with advancing age. During the premenopausal period, women tend to have lower total cholesterol than men. Of even greater clinical significance, is the higher values for HDL cholesterol for women. Between the ages of 50 and 60, women show a distinct increase in total cholesterol, coincidental with declining estrogen production at menopause. Of interest is the recent Heart and Estrogen/Progestin Replacement Study (HERS) that has raised questions about the cardiovascular benefit of hormone replacement therapy in women with CHD.[65]

Among seniors ages 65 to 74, about 22% of men and 41% of women have total cholesterol levels of 240 mg/dL or higher.[66] Median cholesterol levels have been reported to increase by as much as 40 mg/dL between the ages of 60 and 79.[12] After age 75, declines in median serum cholesterol level have been noted and attributed to survivor bias. Increased total serum cholesterol and LDL-cholesterol are risk factors for CHD in both men and women. However, Framingham Study data indicate that women have a lower absolute risk for CHD compared with men up to age 75.[59] However, cardiovascular disease is still the number one cause of death among both men and women.

Epidemiologic studies of cholesterol and CHD risk in the elderly have suggested that elevated serum cholesterol poses a lesser risk for CHD among elderly men, although it remains significantly associated with CHD in older women. Findings from epidemiological studies must be viewed with caution and the duration of long-term follow-up of participants considered. Other ongoing, prospective epidemiologic studies of CHD and stroke among men of Japanese ancestry living in Hawaii suggest that the serum cholesterol level is an independent predictor of CHD, even among men over the age of 65 years. These investigations continue to link hypercholesterolemia with CHD in elderly as well as middle-aged men.[67] Based on Framingham data, there was a slight increase in mean high-density lipoprotein levels between 60 and 80 years of age. However, low-density lipoprotein (LDL) levels dropped by almost 9%.[68] In the Honolulu group, mean high-density lipoproteins also increased slightly but LDL levels changed by

**What Happens to Homocysteine**

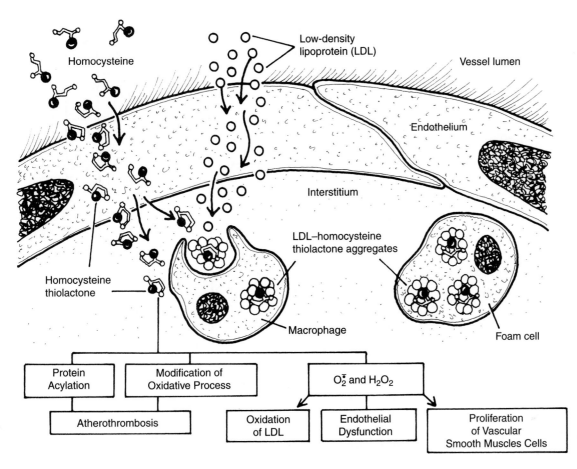

**F I G U R E    3 8 - 8**

What happens to homocysteine. (From Welch GN, Upchurch GR Jr, Loscalzo J: Homocysteine, oxidative stress and vascular disease. Hosp Pract 32(6):81, 1997.)

only about 1% over the same age range. Plasma triglycerides increase markedly with aging. In men, the increase is significant by as early as 40 years with values reaching a plateau between age 50 and 60 and even declining with advancing age. In women, levels increase significantly between 50 and 60 and plateau or decline in later years. The decrease in lipoprotein lipase activity reported with aging may account in part for changes in plasma triglyceride levels. The relationship of hypertriglyceridemia to CHD in the general population still remains controversial. However, Framingham data support hypertriglyceridemia in women, especially postmenopause, as an independent and highly significant risk factor for CHD.

## Blood Gases

Arterial blood gas (ABG) measurements are useful in determining a patient's acid-base balance, evaluating efficiency of the respiratory tract and monitoring respiratory therapy. Even in healthy young adults, pulmonary function begins to decline

after about the mid-30s.[3,35,38] This decline is linked to cumulative, adverse changes throughout the respiratory system including decreased lung elasticity, loss of alveolar surface area for gas exchange, and chest wall stiffness. Arterial oxygen pressure decreases by about 25% between the ages of 30 and 80. When interpreting blood gas results the $PaO_2$ of a 75-year-old should typically be 75 mm Hg or greater.[35]

A suggested correction[35] for the patient's age is:

$$PaO_2 \text{ (mm Hg)} = 100.1 - (0.325 \times \text{age in years})$$

No consensus exists as to whether aging results in $CO_2$ retention with a resultant change in $PCO_2$ and pH. It has been reported that carbon dioxide pressure ($PCO_2$) increases by about 2% for every 10 years after age 50. An increase in bicarbonate ion concentration is also noted with aging and would compensate for the increase in $PCO_2$ and maintain pH within reference range.[12]

Estimated Prevalence of Cardiovascular Disease
in Americans Age 20 and Older by Age and Gender
United States 1988–1994

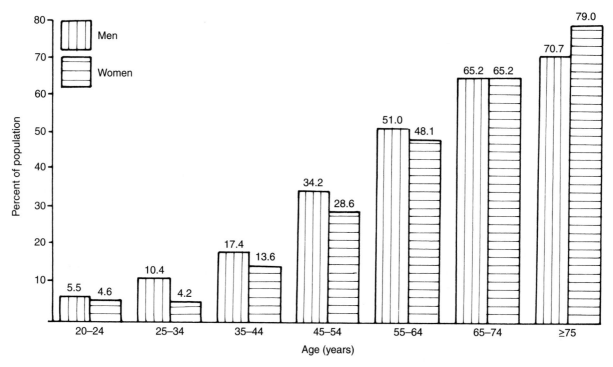

Source: NHANES III (1988–94), CDC/NCHS and the American Heart Association

**F I G U R E    3 8 - 9**

Estimated prevalence of cardiovascular diseases in Americans 20 years and older,
by age and sex–United States 1988–1994. (From American Heart Association.
*2000 Heart and Stroke Statistical Update.* Dallas, TX, American Heart Association,
1999.)

Common causes of acid-base disturbances in the elderly include pneumonia, chronic obstructive pulmonary disease (COPD), tuberculosis, pulmonary emboli, and congestive heart failure.[37] Increased frequency of these conditions along with less effective and less consistent compensatory response patterns are noted in seniors. Pneumonia often goes unrecognized in older adults because of atypical presentation.[69] The classic features of fever, cough, chest pain, and sputum production are frequently not observed. More often the patient complains of being tired and weak, has little appetite but no cough. Pneumonia in seniors is most often bacterial in origin and is the leading cause of death due to infectious disease. The most common pathogen is *Streptococcus pneumoniae*. However, in about one third of all cases of pneumonia in patients over the age of 70, the causative agents are gram-negative bacilli. Incidence of pulmonary tuberculosis (TB) is highest among elderly populations regardless of gender, race, or ethnicity. In 1992, seniors accounted for just under one quarter of all TB cases. Among residents in long-term care facilities, the TB case rate is especially high.[70] The umbrella term COPD describes conditions in which there is a progressive development of air-

flow limitation. The lungs lose elasticity, alveolar ducts and bronchi enlarge, and the number of alveoli decrease, especially at the base of the lung.[38] Because of these changes complete pulmonary function cannot be restored. Included in this group of disorders is chronic bronchitis and emphysema.[71] Evidence is accumulating that oxidative stress, especially from the free radicals in cigarette smoke, plays an important role in COPD.[72] Nearly 16 million individuals have COPD, which is now the fourth leading cause of death in the United States and the only common cause of death whose incidence is increasing. Among seniors, frequent causes of sudden deterioration in already impaired airflow include (1) respiratory infection, (2) myocardial infarction, (3) sedatives, (4) air pollution, and (5) systemic illness, including sepsis or other organ system failure.

## Hepatic Function

Ultrasound studies show a decrease in liver volume with age. Hepatic blood flow also declines.[73] A decline in hepatocyte perfusion may account for changes in the liver's clearance of specific high extraction drugs. Most medications are taken orally and are absorbed in the small intestine. Some drugs are removed or extracted from the portal circulation and undergo significant presystemic metabolism in the liver. This immediate processing is called the *first-pass effect*. If hepatic metabolic activity declines, there will be a reduction in the first-pass effect and an increase in the bioavailability of these high extraction drugs. In the elderly, elevated bioactive or free drug levels of such potent medications as methyldopa, propranolol, verapamil, desipramine, meperidine, and lidocaine are linked to reduced first-pass clearance.[74]

Hepatic detoxification occurs by two groups of metabolic processes: (1) microsomal oxidation, reduction, or hydrolysis and (2) conjugation with glucuronic acid, sulfate, glycine, and other groups. Activity of the microsomal or phase I enzymes whose action results in the production of more polar and often inactive water-soluble metabolites seems to decrease with aging. Prolonged elimination of some benzodiazepines, tricyclic antidepressants, theophylline, and several nonsteroidal anti-inflammatory drugs (NSAIDs) is the result of age-related reduction in hepatic metabolism.[46,74] Specifically, changes in phase I enzyme activity reduce metabolism of antipyrine, diazepam, imipramine, amitriptyline, and phenytoin.[26] Cumulative effects of psychoactive drugs (including benzodiazepines), caused by impaired metabolism and delayed elimination, are often associated with falls producing hip fractures in the elderly.[46] Activities of conjugation or phase II enzymes whose actions produce such water-soluble drug derivatives as glucuronides for renal excretion do not appear to change with age. Increased prevalence of drug-induced hepatotoxicity in seniors is probably due to a combination of factors including polypharmacy, decline in the phase I hepatic drug-metabolizing enzymes, hepatic blood flow, and liver mass. Altered plasma protein binding and smaller distribution volume also may contribute to hepatotoxicity. Although the specific cause is not clear, antituberculosis medications (isoniazid, rifampin and pyrazinamide) are more likely to cause liver damage in older patients.[73]

The liver of the older adult is less able to initiate enzyme-catalyzed metabolic transformations in response to nutritional imbalances or deficiencies. Glycogen reserves are diminished and the capacity for gluconeogenesis is reduced. Modest decline in serum albumin levels has been reported in elderly but only rarely do levels fall below reference range unless there is accompanying malnutrition or disease. The liver is the principal site of alcohol metabolism. Superoxide radicals formed in the hepatic breakdown of ethanol are especially damaging to an already aging organ.

Bile production is a major function of the liver. Constituents of bile include water, bile acids or salts and bile pigments (primarily bilirubin), cholesterol, and various inorganic salts. Precipitation of material present in the bile produces stone.[75] In the United States, gallstones are formed predominantly of cholesterol. It has been suggested that increased cholelithiasis in the elderly is due to supersaturation of the bile

as a result of increased hepatic secretion of cholesterol.[76] At the same time, there is decreased synthesis of mucus and bile acids. Gallstones affect 15% to 20% of adults of all ages and 30% to 50% of seniors by age 75. Between the ages of 80 and 89 years, gallstones were identified in 22% of men and 38% of women. Over the age of 90, the prevalence increases to 31% in men. At all ages, gallstones are almost twice as likely to occur in women. Most gallstones are asymptomatic. Bilirubin levels remain unchanged in healthy elderly.

## Enzymes

Attempts have been made to discern a pattern to enzyme changes reportedly associated with the normal aging process. Contradictory findings from various studies have made interpretation and correlation of results exceedingly difficult.[77] It appears that overall the activity and synthesis of hepatic enzymes is not substantially affected by aging. Alterations in enzyme levels and kinetic properties as well as shifts in isoenzyme patterns have been suggested on the basis of various animal models. Substantial data exist on changes in lactate dehydrogenase (LD), aspartate transaminase (AST), alanine transaminase (ALT), alkaline phosphatase (ALP), and creatine kinase (CK) and its isoenzymes. Whether these findings are due to normal aging, underlying pathologic changes, and/or occur in response to drug use is not always clear. Alteration in muscle mass, hepatic synthesis, and renal function all contribute to changing enzyme levels. For example, serum gamma-glutamyltransferase (GGT) from the liver is elevated in seniors. The increase may be due to enzyme induction by certain drugs, including ethanol. Anticonvulsants can produce a marked increase in serum GGT. Induction of hepatic enzymes by antiepileptic drugs such as phenobarbital and phenytoin has been reported in elderly men.[78] Although LD levels have been reported to show a moderate increase with aging, overall the findings do not support a need for adjustment of the reference range for this enzyme. Serum AST is 10% higher in adult men of all ages in comparison to adult women. Most studies reveal an age-related increase of the enzyme in women but the degree of elevation is unclear. Levels in elderly women have been reported to exceed those of young women by as much as 25% to 50%. Men aged 70 or older have average serum AST values that are 10% higher than those of young adult men. The liver is the richest source of ALT. The ALT levels in elderly men are 10% to 15% higher than those in elderly women. In women, ALT levels tend to remain fairly constant with aging but men show an age-related decrease of the enzyme. It is unclear whether this pattern is related to changing hepatic physiology or is linked to differential exposure to alcohol and other hepatotoxins. Serum ALP is a critical analyte in geriatric chemistry. The two most common sources of elevated ALP are liver and bone. As a product of osteoblastic synthesis, bone-specific alkaline phosphatase is a biochemical marker of bone formation.[79] New immunoassays are available to differentiate bone and liver forms of the enzyme. Both sex and age influence serum ALP levels. In young adults, ALP levels are 10% to 15% higher in men. In the elderly, sex differences in enzymes disappear due to a marked, age-related progressive elevation of ALP in women. It has been suggested that the significant rise in serum ALP seen at menopause may be related to the accelerated loss of bone as estrogen levels drop. Overall, there is a rise in ALP levels with aging. In older women, menopause induced a 50% increase in bone-specific ALP.[79] Elderly men have serum ALP levels somewhat less than 10% higher than those in young adults. It has been suggested that separate reference intervals for ALP be established for seniors, particularly for older women. In the elderly, ALP activity is induced by antiepileptic drugs at least at the same level as in younger subjects.

Total serum CK activity and the MB isoenzyme are routinely used in the diagnosis of acute myocardial infarction (AMI). An AMI presentation is often atypical among seniors when compared to younger patients. Among the elderly, a feeling of weakness, difficulty in breathing, and fainting are often reported. If chest pain is present, its pattern of distribution is often atypical. EKG changes are less likely to be significant. Because of these differences in presentation, AMI is not considered during the first 24 hours after symptom onset in as high as 50% of elderly patients. Laboratory tests show an elevated serum CK-MB with a normal total CK twice as often among patients age 70 or older as in younger adults. Reduced muscle mass in seniors leads to a progressive decline in CK levels with aging. Because of this, total CK levels may remain within the reference range despite the occurrence of an AMI in an elderly patient, particularly one who is small and sedentary. However, CK-MB, which is found mainly in the heart, will constitute a greater percentage of total CK values postinfarct even in the elderly. Serum amylase levels increase slightly in healthy seniors over 60, approaching the upper limits found in young adults.[80] Increased serum amylase level is attributed in part to the enzyme's retention in the body as renal function declines.

## Proteins

Albumin is the main protein synthesized in the liver. Serum concentrations depend on hepatic synthesis, degradation in peripheral tissues, and intravascular and extravascular distribution in extracellular fluids. The functions of serum albumin include maintaining the body's osmotic pressure, acting as a temporary amino acid storage site, and binding and transporting a variety of molecules including nutrients, metabolites, hormones, and drugs to peripheral tissues. Total serum protein concentrations change very little with age in the absence of significant disease, trauma, or malnutrition. Reduced protein levels due to protein-energy malnutrition (PEM) (a condition resulting from regularly consuming insufficient amounts of energy foods and too little protein) occur in all individuals,

irrespective of age. However, even in well-nourished elderly, a slight decline in serum albumin is noted.[81] Although the magnitude of the decrease varies considerably among studies, between the ages of 30 and 80, serum albumin decreases by 10% to 15%; a decline of a little over 0.5 g/L per decade has been reported recently.[80,82,83] Low serum albumin concentrations have been found to be significantly associated with reduced muscle mass (sarcopenia) in relatively healthy, well-nourished men and women. Sixty percent of total body albumin is extravascular in muscle and skin and serum albumin exchanges with this pool. The mechanism underlying the relationship of the somatic protein reserves and serum albumin is not known. If albumin is decreased, a greater percentage of highly protein bound drugs will exist in the body as the free or bioactive form. For elderly patients, clinicians must lower drug dosage of phenytoin, warfarin, salicylates, sulfonamides, thyroxine, and tricyclic antidepressants to achieve a given free-drug level because at least 90% of each of these medications is bound to serum proteins. Albumin also binds between 50% and 90% of protein-bound calcium. The age-related decline in serum albumin contributes to the decline in total calcium observed in the elderly. Modest elevation of serum calcium can occur in the hyperalbuminemia of dehydration, a common phenomenon in seniors. To improve diagnostic usefulness, serum total calcium levels should be corrected for changes in albumin above or below 4 g/dL. A commonly applied simple formula used to obtain albumin-adjusted calcium is:

$$Ca\ adj(mg/dL) = Ca\ total(mg/dL) - Albumin\ (g/dL) + 4.0$$

Circadian and seasonal variations in total plasma proteins, not exclusively related to circadian rhythms in blood volume, have been noted in healthy young and elderly subjects.[84] The 24-hour mean concentrations of plasma proteins showed larger seasonal variation in elderly groups (7 to 8 g/L) than in young men (2 to 5 g/L). Seasonal changes in plasma proteins were more marked in the elderly. The seasonal peak occurred in October and the seasonal trough in the period March to June. The yearly mean (±SEM) of plasma proteins was 67.4 ± 1.3 g/L in elderly men, approximately 4 g/L less than in the young men (71.7 ± 0.5 g/L). Especially in older adults, such changes in plasma proteins may significantly affect drug binding and transportation.[74]

## Thyroid Function

Reports on age-related changes in structure and function of the thyroid gland conflict. Increased nodularity and fibrosis of the gland are generally agreed upon. Marked changes in thyroid hormone levels do not accompany aging unless there is some underlying disorder or coexisting nutritional problem.[85] Incidence of both hypothyroidism and hyperthyroidism rises in the elderly.[15,86] Diagnosis of thyroid dysfunction in the elderly is often delayed since many of the clinical manifestations may be nonspecific, atypical, or the metabolic and behavioral changes misinterpreted as part of the "normal aging process."[15]

Among the elderly, subclinical hypothyroidism is common, especially in women.[87] As high as 4% of elderly men and 8% of women may be hypothyroid.[85] Dry, flaky, inelastic skin; sparse, dry hair; frequent constipation; forgetfulness and inattentiveness are not uncommon even with normal thyroid function. Such nonspecific complaints as fatigue, sensitivity to cold, weakness, and lethargy would be more likely to suggest a diagnosis of hypothyroidism to the clinician if they were reported by a young, rather than older, adult. Elderly patients are more likely than younger patients to present with central nervous system symptoms, including loss of hearing, sensations of numbness, prickling or tingling, psychiatric manifestations, and coma or cardiovascular abnormalities. Particularly in older persons, there is increased risk of angina and congestive heart failure. Electrocardiographic changes and elevated levels of AST, LD, and CK are also observed. Older individuals with hypothyroidism experience a weight loss rather than a weight gain as seen in young adults. Diagnosis depends on detecting a raised serum TSH. Thyroid therapy is common in the elderly. The overall prevalence of thyroid hormone use in older adults has been reported to be 7%. Inappropriate thyroid treatment is particularly hazardous in the elderly since it may worsen manifestations of coronary heart disease.

The occurrence of hyperthyroidism also increases with age and may exist in 7% to 12% of seniors.[85] One quarter to one third of all cases of hyperthyroidism occur in persons over age 60.[15] Excessive $T_3$ and/or $T_4$ production by a thyroid nodule may cause thyrotoxicosis in the elderly. The anatomic changes of fibrosis and atrophy associated with glandular aging make nodule detection by palpation difficult. The most common sign of hyperthyroidism in seniors is weight loss; dramatic wasting of muscle and weakness is often noted. Cardiovascular symptoms are common, including atrial fibrillation, congestive heart failure, angina, and pulmonary edema. Hyperthyroidism as it presents among seniors has been referred to as "apathetic thyrotoxicosis," since common features include patient confusion, depression, and lack of animation. Even subclinical hyperthyroidism may result in accelerated bone turnover and increased risk of osteoporosis.[88]

Thyroid uptake of iodine may be reduced in older adults and changes in hormone biosynthesis have been reported. Serum $T_3$ concentrations decline slightly with age; TSH has been reported to fluctuate minimally. Some authors report slight increase, others a small decrease. In healthy elderly, thyroxine levels ($T_4$) remain essentially constant.[35] It has been suggested that low $T_3$ concentrations in seniors are due to a reduction in hormone binding by thyroxine-binding globulin (TBG) but this has not been confirmed. Thyroid gland responsiveness to endogenous or administered TSH does not appear to differ significantly between young and old adults.[85]

With increasing age, TSH response to thyrotropin-releasing hormone (TRH) is reportedly lessened in men but not women.[85] Difficulty in correctly diagnosing thyroid disease in seniors on the basis of clinical presentation underscores the importance of laboratory test interpretation. Screening for thyroid abnormalities should be an integral part of health care for seniors, particularly women. The single best test to exclude thyroid disease is TSH measurement.[89] An abnormal thyroid function test should never be attributed simply to growing older.

A summary of commonly reported changes in circulating hormonal levels seen with aging is found in Table 38–7.

TABLE 38–7

**Commonly Reported Changes in Circulating Hormonal Levels Seen With Aging**

| HORMONE | CHANGE |
| --- | --- |
| Pituitary related | |
| Growth hormone | ↓ |
| Prolactin | N |
| Somatomedin C | ↓ |
| Arginine vasopressin | ↑ |
| Thyroid | |
| Thyroxine ($T_4$) | N |
| Triiodothyronine ($T_3$) | ↓ |
| Adrenal | |
| Cortisol | N |
| Dehydroepiandrosterone | ↓ |
| Aldosterone | ↓ |
| Renin | ↓ |
| Norepinephrine | ↑ |
| Epinephrine | N or ↑ |
| Pancreatic | |
| Insulin | ↑ |
| Gonadal | |
| Estrogen (females) | ↓ |
| Testosterone (males) | ↓ |
| Luteinizing hormone | ↑ |
| Follicle-stimulating hormone | ↑ |
| Calcium regulatory | |
| Parathyrin (PTH) | ↑ or N |
| Calcitonin | N |
| 25-OH-vitamin D | ↓ |
| 1,25-dihydroxyvitamin D | ↓ |

N = no change; ↓ = decrease; ↑ = increase.
Modified from Morley JE, Korenman SG: Aging. In Bagdade JD, et al. (eds.): *The Year Book of Endocrinology.* Chicago, Year Book Medical Publishers, 1987, p 107.

## NUTRITION IN AGING

Nutritional problems are common among seniors (see Chapter 33).[90] The prevalence of undernutrition and malnutrition increases with advancing age. A wide range of factors have important effects on the nutritional status of the elderly. These factors fall into three major categories: (1) physiologic changes, (2) age-associated pathologic conditions, and (3) environmental aspects including physical, biologic, psychologic, and cultural-socioeconomic variables.[91] Decreased food consumption as physical activity declines, limited dietary choices linked to limited income, fewer opportunities for shopping due to physical disability, and greater incidence of diseases that alter the body's metabolic requirements are contributing factors to the development of suboptimal or inadequate nutriture in older adults.[92] To age successfully, that is to maintain high levels of mental and physical function, to minimize the risk for disability or disease, and to sustain interest in and derive pleasure from activities of living, including social contact with family and friends, requires an optimal nutritional status.[93]

How the body is able to respond to the multitude of stressors to which it is subjected daily or over extended periods depends in part on the adequacy of nutrition. More than 80% of older adults have chronic diseases that may be affected by diet.[94] Shifts in nutrient intake, requirements, and metabolism have been reported among institutionalized seniors and those living independently in the community. Even in healthy older adults, a variety of changes in physiology and metabolism have been recognized that affect nutritional needs. In an evaluation of the Elderly Nutrition Program of the Older Americans Act, 67% to 88% of participants were identified as being at moderate to high nutritional risk.[92] Significant numbers of seniors have marginal or inadequate intake of various nutrients including thiamin, riboflavin, niacin, vitamins $B_6$, $B_{12}$, folic acid, D, C, calcium, iron, zinc, and protein.[95] The need for geriatric recommended dietary allowances (RDAs) for specific nutrients is strongly advocated.[96,97]

Many of the physiologic changes that occur during aging have already been discussed earlier in this chapter. There are other functional alterations that affect eating behaviors. Seniors often experience a loss of appetite. Sense of taste changes with aging and the sense of smell becomes less acute. Many drugs adversely affect appetite, taste, and smell. Not surprisingly, less food is likely to be eaten if little sensory pleasure is derived from the activity. Poor dentition, decreased production of saliva, and difficulty in chewing and swallowing also affect ingestion. Alterations in the structure and function of the gastrointestinal tract may limit nutrient uptake. Lactase deficiency, particularly common in elderly Blacks and Asians, causes carbohydrate maldigestion. These are only a few of the factors that contribute to poor nutritional status in older adults.[91]

Dietary energy is mainly provided by the macronutrients—protein, carbohydrate, and fat. According to data from the third National Health and Nutrition Examination Survey (NHANES), as women age their energy intake declines from about 1600 kilocalories/day between the ages of 60 and 69; to 1400 kcal/day between 70 and 79 years of age; to 1300 kcal/day at 80 years or older. Men show a similar decline in energy intake from 2100 kcal/day between 60 and 69; to about 1900 kcal/day from 70 to 79, and 1800 kcal/day from 80 years and upwards.[98] Fewer than 1,000 kcal/day are consumed by 15% to 20% of those over age 60. Diets that fall below about 1200 kcal/day often provide inadequate amounts of protein, calcium, iron, and vitamins.

In a typical American diet, about 15% of energy comes from proteins. However, protein requirements may actually be higher in elderly than in younger adults. Proteins are essential nutritionally because of their constituent amino acids, which the body uses to synthesize its own proteins and nitrogen-containing molecules. Foods high in protein may be too expensive for many seniors and consumption of dietary carbohydrates and fat, less expensive sources of calories, may be increased. Without adequate dietary protein, normal metabolism cannot be sustained.

Among seniors, protein-energy malnutrition (PEM) is the most common form of malnutrition. In PEM, the body loses energy stores and protein mass. As the body is depleted of glycogen, fat and protein, body weight falls and protein-related cellular functions are diminished. Both skeletal muscle and visceral proteins are lost if the energy deficit becomes more severe and protein breakdown occurs. Virtually every organ is affected including the brain, heart, lungs, liver, and kidneys.[99] As the visceral protein pool is reduced, hepatic protein synthesis declines and there is a decrease in serum transport proteins, fluid and electrolyte imbalances arise, and susceptibility to infection increases. In nutritionally depleted individuals, wounds heal slowly and immune responsiveness is weakened. PEM can originate directly from inadequate food intake or secondarily due to inadequate nutrient absorption or utilization, increased nutritional requirements, or increased loss of nutrients.[100]

Protein-energy undernutrition as well as malnutrition (PEM) compromises the health of seniors. As long as they remain free of infection, injury, or other stress, malnourished seniors may be able to function adequately. The additional nutritional demands arising from trauma, surgery, inflammation, or sepsis may be impossible to meet without dietary supplements or nutritional support. Up to 60% of elderly patients are protein-energy undernourished at the time of admission or acquire nutritional deficits during hospitalization. This deterioration of nutritional status substantially increases the risk for complications and death. A discussion of laboratory assessment of nutritional status may be found in Chapter 33 of this text. To what extent vitamin and trace mineral requirements change with aging in the absence of stress, malabsorption, or disease remains controversial.

## VITAMIN STATUS

Older adults are becoming increasingly more aware of the financial as well as personal benefits of staying well and living independently for as long as possible. Consumption of vitamins and mineral supplements is viewed by the public as one means of forestalling functional deterioration and physical disability associated with aging and as a protection in medical concerns ranging in severity from colds to heart disease and cancer. Use of dietary supplements is widespread, with at least 40% of the U. S. population taking vitamins regularly. Among individuals 60 years of age and older, over 50% of women and 40% of men consume a supplement.[101] Among more affluent seniors, this percentage increases to almost 70%. Micronutrient and drug handling tends to alter with age because of factors such as changes in body composition, impairment of renal function, and reduction of hepatic clearance. Assessment of vitamin status needs to play a key role in preventive medicine, particularly in high-risk groups such as seniors. Overdosing, as well as underdosing, by those using supplements has potential health effects. A sampling of the wide variety of signs and symptoms that may be associated with nutritional imbalance in older adults is presented in Table 38–8. Many of the age-related functional changes already discussed affect vitamin status. The importance of drug–nutrient interaction cannot be overstated. Drugs and vitamins frequently interact with the outcome being a vitamin deficiency due to nonavailability rather than dietary inadequacy. Deficiencies of B vitamins are produced with greater frequency by this type of interaction than deficiencies of other water-soluble vitamins. Age-associated decline in renal function leads to prolonged retention of water-soluble vitamins, thereby placing the individual at increased risk of developing adverse side effects from their ingestion. Increase in adipose tissue and decrease in lean body mass may expand the storage potential for fat-soluble vitamins, which can then accumulate to toxic levels. In both instances, substantial increase in vitamin intake may have serious consequences.

In addition to overt micronutrient deficiencies, many elderly are at risk for subclinical or marginal deficiencies of vitamins and trace elements. Frequently cited as likely to be present at less than optimal levels are vitamins $B_{12}$, $B_6$, D, C, folate, and thiamin, as well as zinc and selenium.

Vitamin C levels in whole blood, plasma, and white blood cells decline with aging. Women's plasma levels of vitamin C are higher than men's on the same controlled diet. This raises the possibility that men are at greater risk of developing a vitamin C deficiency even though they consume the RDA. Drug-induced deficiency of the vitamin has been reported among cigarette smokers and users of oral contraceptive steroids. Aspirin and barbiturates promote urinary excretion of ascorbic acid, thereby reducing body levels. Low levels of vitamin C can lead to joint pain, easy bruising, fatigue, and impaired cognition. Such problems may be inappropriately dismissed as simply a natural consequence of aging. Questions have been raised by researchers as to the real incidence and prevalence of hypovitaminosis C. Evidence suggests that a large proportion of the elderly have suboptimal vitamin C levels.[102] Although direct evidence is limited, low vitamin C status may increase the risk of mortality from cardiovascular disease and cancer.[103] It has been suggested that subclinical deficiency of vitamin C is the basis for the loss of tissue repair ability, diminished connective tissue integrity, and delayed wound healing seen in older adults. Functioning as a potent reducing agent, vitamin C is a specific electron donor for 8 enzymes. Reactions for which adequate amounts of vitamin C is pivotal include syntheses of collagen, carnitine, norepinephrine, tyrosine metabolism, and activation of a variety of hormones and releasing factors including calcitonin, releasing factors for growth hormone, corticotropin and thyrotropin.[104] Vitamin C also increases iron absorption in the gastrointestinal (GI) tract. It seems likely that the anticarcinogenic function of vitamin C is tied to its antioxidant properties in the aqueous phase of the cell, where it is a powerful scavenger of several reactive oxygen metabolites and free radicals. Vitamin C may play a role in the prevention of atherogenesis and cardiovascular disease by inhibition of metal-catalyzed LDL oxidation or by improving vasodilation and vascular reactivity by decreasing interactions of nitric oxide with oxidants.[105,106] High levels of vitamin C are thought to decrease the risk of cataracts by protecting lens protein from oxidation. Other roles for the vitamin include enhancement of immunologic response and the lowering of cholesterol levels in some individuals. Regeneration of oxidized vitamin E by vitamin C has also been proposed. One preliminary study has even linked daily use of vitamin C and E supplements to a delay in the progression of Parkinson's disease by virtue of their effective reduction or elimination of free radicals in brain tissue.[107]

Most vitamins function as cofactors in enzyme catalyzed reactions. The B complex vitamins thiamin, riboflavin, $B_6$, $B_{12}$, and folate are critical for the synthesis of neurotransmitters including norepinephrine, dopamine, serotonin, gamma amino butyric acid (GABA), and acetylcholine. In addition, thiamin, riboflavin, folate, and vitamin $B_{12}$ function as coenzymes in the methylation pathways that synthesize 5-methyltetrahydrofolate and S-adenosylmethionine, both of which have notable antidepressive activity. Significant correlation between thiamin status and neuropsychologic function, indicated by cognitive performance and brain electrophysiology, has been reported.[108] Folate and $B_{12}$ status have been linked to cognitive function including reasoning ability, judgment, and memory.[109] Collectively, these observations suggest a central role for B vitamins in the development and treatment of disorders of affective and cognitive function encountered in many older adults.[110] Marginal or subclinical vitamin deficiencies could alter brain function and adversely affect the activities of daily

TABLE 38-8

**Symptoms and Signs of Nutritional Deficiencies in the Elderly**

**Protein-energy malnutrition**
  Low body weight
  Diminished subcutaneous fat
  Pallor and fatigue
  Temporal wasting
  Dermatitis
  Impaired immunity with increased risk of infection
  Hypoproteinemia and edema
**Vitamin deficiency**
  B$_1$
    Anorexia
    Malaise
    Weakness of legs
    Pins and needles (burning feet syndrome)
    Sluggish or absent reflexes
    Palpitations
    Heart failure
    Encephalopathy
  B$_2$
    Cheilosis
    Angular stomatitis
    Misty vision with burning sensation in the eyes
    Orogenital syndrome
    Excessive hair loss
  B$_6$
    Depression and mood changes
    Irritability and forgetfulness
    Peripheral neuropathy
    Altered reflexes
    Spinal ataxia
    Anemia
    Easily fatigued
  Folate
    Anorexia
    Depression, memory loss
    Paranoia
    Megaloblastic anemia
  C
    Loss of energy
    Spontaneous bruising
    Arthralgia
    Gingivitis
    Bleeding gums

**Vitamin deficiency** (continued)
  D
    Bone pains
    Unsteady gait
    Spontaneous fractures
    Accelerated loss of vertical height
    Loss of mobility
    Muscle weakness and aches
  A
    Poor night vision
    Dermatitis
  B$_{12}$
    Megaloblastic anemia
    Glossitis
    Cognitive impairment
    Dementia
    Peripheral neuropathy
**Mineral deficiency**
  Calcium, phosphorous
    Aches and pains
    Osteoporosis
    Repeated fractures
  Zinc
    Loss of taste and sense of smell
    Excessive hair loss
    Prostatism
    Impaired night vision
    Poor wound healing
    Anorexia
  Iodine
    Goiter
  Fluoride
    Dental caries
  Copper
    Hypochromic, microcytic anemia
    Neutropenia
    Bony abnormalities
  Chromium
    Glucose intolerance
  Selenium
    Cardiomyopathy
    Myositis
    Hemolytic anemia

Adapted from Gupta KL, Dworkin B, Gambert SR. Manifestations of common nutritional disorders in the elderly. Geriatrics 43:87–97, 1988.

living. Individuals in whom mild deficiencies of B vitamins have been identified complain of lack of appetite and weight loss, poor coordination, tiredness, irritability, forgetfulness, depression, and sleep disturbances. It has been suggested that evaluation of thiamin status is highly desirable when depres-

sion and sleep disorders occur in the elderly before the physician prescribes sedative hypnotics.[111]

Vitamin B$_6$ (pyridoxine) functions in a wide variety of reactions related to amino acid and protein metabolism. Serum levels of the metabolically active coenzyme form of the vitamin, pyridoxal 5'-phosphate, decrease with age throughout adult life. Dietary patterns and medication usage may be the cause of the hypovitaminosis. The elderly are at increased risk of $B_6$ deficiency; several studies indicate that 50% of seniors consume only three quarters or less of the RDA for this vitamin. Drugs that interact with vitamin $B_6$ include isoniazid, cycloserine, L-dopa, penicillamine, and theophylline.[112,113] Vitamin $B_6$ deficiency impairs interleukin-2 (IL-2) production and lymphocyte proliferation in older adults.[14] In instances of overt deficiency, personality changes, loss of sense of responsibility, and clinical depression have been reported. Also noted has been the decrement of both humoral and cell-mediated immunity as evidenced by reduced DNA synthesis in lymphocytes in response to T and B cell mitogens.[114,115] A recent study demonstrated that vitamin $B_6$ deficiency decreases the total number of peripheral lymphocytes, mitogenic responses of T and B cells, and IL-2 production in healthy older adults. Immunocompetence can be improved by supplementation. Lymphocyte proliferation responses increased in elderly subjects following 8 weeks of supplementation with 50 mg/day of vitamin $B_6$.[14] However, prolonged ingestion of megadoses

of vitamin $B_6$ can lead to peripheral neuropathy with loss of muscle coordination and severe sensory dysfunction. Based upon findings from the Nurses' Health Study, an ongoing prospective study of women aged 30 to 55 at the time of enrollment in 1976, women can benefit from increased intake of vitamins $B_6$ and folate from both diet and supplements. Women with the highest intake of vitamin $B_6$ and folate seem to be about 50% less likely to develop heart disease when compared to women with the lowest intakes of the vitamins.[116] Low intakes of both of these B vitamins have been linked to elevated blood homocysteine levels, a cause of arterial occlusion.

DNA synthesis and cell division are dependent on the availability of vitamin $B_{12}$, also referred to as cobalamin. Vitamin $B_{12}$ is involved in two types of reactions as a coenzyme (Figure 38–10). A $B_{12}$-containing enzyme catalyzes the removal of a methyl group from 5-methyltetrahydrofolate and its delivery to homocysteine. By this reaction, homocysteine is converted to methionine and tetrahydrofolate (THF) is regenerated. If a person is deficient in cobalamin much of their folate is "trapped" as methyltetrahydrofolate, a metabolically

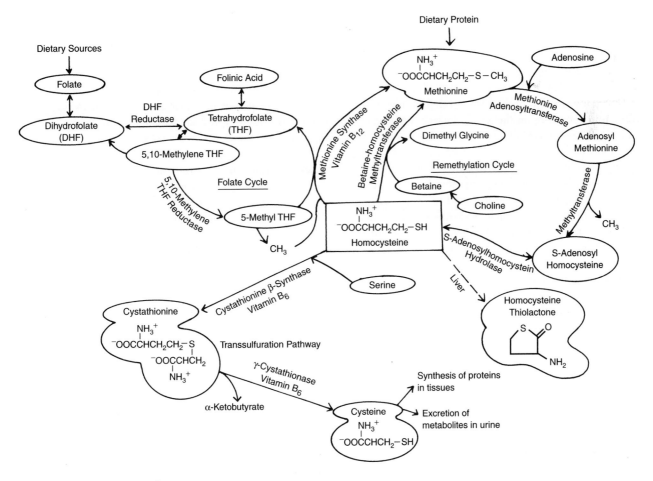

**FIGURE  38-10**

Methionine cycle and homocysteine metabolism. (Modified from Solomon BP, Duda CT: Homocysteine determinations in plasmas. Current Separations 17:3, 1998.)

inactive form as far as nucleotide synthesis is concerned. The "folate trap" explains why the hematologic evidence of B$_{12}$ deficiency is morphologically indistinguishable from a folate deficiency. Vitamin B$_{12}$ is also involved in rearrangement reactions such as the conversion of methylmalonyl CoA to succinyl CoA, which is the point of entry for some of the carbon atoms of the amino acids (methionine, isoleucine, threonine, and valine) into the tricarboxylic acid (TCA) cycle. Meat, dairy products, and fortified breakfast cereals are dietary sources of the vitamin. With advancing age, serum levels of B$_{12}$ decline. Deficiency of the vitamin has been reported in 10% to 20% of U.S. seniors.[117] Projections suggest that 2 to 5 million Americans over the age of 60 have subnormal cobalamin concentrations.[118] Depending on the technique used, the lower limit of the reference range for serum B$_{12}$ varies.[119] Usually the threshold for defining risk of vitamin deficiency is set at about 148 pmol/L (200 pg/mL).[95] In healthy elderly, rates of gastric acid secretion remain essentially unchanged with advancing age.[120] However, disease and/or use of certain medications can influence gastric secretions and thereby alter bioavailability of vitamin B$_{12}$. The two major gastric disorders of cobalamin assimilation are pernicious anemia and food-cobalamin malabsorption.[121] Loss of immune self-tolerance among seniors may permit the development of autoantibodies to gastric parietal cells or intrinsic factor. Pernicious anemia (PA) is an autoimmune disorder in which antibodies to intrinsic factor (IF) and gastric parietal cells are produced followed by destruction of gastric tissue. Decreased gastric secretions reduce the availability of IF for formation of the IF-B$_{12}$ complex, thus reducing cobalamin absorption in the small intestine. PA accounts for only a small percentage of all instances of low cobalamin levels in the elderly. The prevalence of untreated PA among the elderly is estimated to be 2% to 3%.[121] Loss or destruction of parietal cells whether from gastric atrophy, gastrectomy, or gastric bypass decreases gastric acid production and impairs release of B$_{12}$ from dietary protein. Gastritis may arise from chronic infection by the bacterium, *Helicobacter pylori.* Infection with *H. pylori* increases with aging from about 10% in young adults to over 60% in individuals 50 years of age or greater. By age 75, 80% of Americans are seropositive.[122] Gastritis due to *H. pylori* may progress to atrophic gastritis with hypochlorhydria or achlorhydria. Atrophic gastritis affects the availability of protein-bound cobalamin in 10% to 40% of adults over the age of 60, depending on the diagnostic criteria applied and the population studied.[123,124] General malabsorption due to ileal disease or resection or to pancreatic insufficiency may also compromise cobalamin uptake.

B$_{12}$ deficiency may also arise due to drug–nutrient interaction. Chronic use of medications that suppress gastric acidity or in other ways adversely affect cobalamin levels is common with older patients. Included among these drugs are cholestyramine, metformin, cimetadine, potassium chloride, neomycin, and the anti-rheumatoid drug, colchicine.[119,124] Ethanol interferes with vitamin absorption. Estimates of alcohol abuse or dependency vary from 2% to 10% of individu-

als over the age of 60.[125] Among elderly admitted to nursing homes and general hospital wards, 15% to 20% have been found to be alcohol dependent. Classic presentation of vitamin B$_{12}$ deficiency includes both hematologic and neurologic manifestations. In the elderly the only indication of deficiency may be neuropsychiatric abnormalities; macrocytosis (MCV > 100 fl) and/or megaloblastic anemia may never develop.[119] In the absence of hematologic evidence of cobalamin deficiency, serum levels of methylmalonic acid (MMA) and serum total homocysteine (tHcy) may be evaluated. Serum levels of these metabolites have proved to be highly sensitive indicators of tissue deficiency of cobalamin. A recent study suggests that plasma tHcy is a better marker of cobalamin and folate tissue status than serum MMA.[126] Renal insufficiency can cause elevation of serum levels of both metabolites, but the increase is modest compared to that observed in cobalamin deficiency.[119] References ranges for MMA and tHcy vary greatly among laboratories. This variability may be due to several factors including the assay methodology, differences in sample collection, and perhaps the selection of reference individuals. Some researchers recommend a plasma total homocysteine reference interval of 5.8 to 11.9 $\mu$mol/L for subjects over 60 years of age and 0.06 to 0.25 $\mu$mol/L for methylmalonic acid.[127]

Cobalamin deficiency is indicated by serum values for these analytes greater than the upper threshold of the reference range. Symptoms of deficiency (serum cobalamin levels <148 pmol/L) in the elderly may include sensory and memory impairment, loss of coordination and abnormalities of gait, and mood or personality changes. Some evidence suggests a role for the vitamin in bone metabolism. If correct, the decline in cobalamin levels with aging may contribute to the development of osteopenia among seniors. Data from a recent prospective epidemiologic study suggest a relationship between serum vitamin B$_{12}$ concentrations and risk of breast cancer among postmenopausal women.[128] Excluding cancers of the skin, breast cancer is the most common cancer in women. Only lung cancer causes more deaths in women.[129] Breast cancer incidence increases with age. There appear to be three categories of determinants of breast cancer risk: heredity, hormonal and reproductive factors, and environmental factors. Although the precise mechanism is still not clear, B$_{12}$ depletion may enhance carcinogenesis. One potential mechanism is an increase in DNA strand breakage. A folate trap produced by a cobalamin deficiency decreases thymidine and purine synthesis and may enable uracil, rather than thymidine, to be incorporated into DNA. Removal of the uracil by a repair enzyme causes a temporary break in the DNA. In a study of healthy elderly men or young adults, increased chromosome breakage correlated with a deficiency of B$_{12}$ (or folate) or with elevated levels of homocysteine.[128] The new recommended intake of vitamin B$_{12}$ for adults has been increased from the 1989 RDA of 2.0 $\mu$g/day to 2.4 $\mu$g/day. In addition, because B$_{12}$ is more readily absorbed when it is not protein-bound, individuals over the age of 50 are encouraged to obtain most of their vitamin from supplements or fortified foods.[124] Cobalamin deficiency with an elevated serum MMA is more prevalent among elderly white than black women. However, elevated serum tHcy and folate deficiency are more common in elderly black than white women.[130]

Folate deficiency (RBC folate <140 ng/mL or plasma folate <3 ng/mL) has been one of the most common vitamin deficiencies, occurring in about 10% of the U.S. population. Limited evidence suggests that nearly one half of low-income (mainly Blacks) elderly are deficient in the vitamin.[131] This may be changing since the Food and Drug Administration approved the addition of folic acid (the synthetic form of the vitamin) to cereals and flour products as of January 1, 1998. Fortified foods include most enriched breads, flours, corn meal, rice, noodles, macaroni, and grain products.[132] Low-income elderly are more likely to develop folate deficiency than are more affluent seniors. Up to 60% of older adults at the lower end of the socioeconomic scale are deficient in folate as compared with 6% of those with high income. Dietary sources of folate, the naturally occurring form of the vitamin, include leafy dark-green vegetables, dried beans and peas, and citrus fruits and juices. Food selection is influenced directly by income as well as seasonal availability. Fresh fruits and vegetables may be prohibitively expensive for seniors on a fixed income. Adding to the potential for folate deficit is that the vitamin is heat sensitive and it is inactivated by prolonged cooking.

Folate coenzymes are involved in numerous reactions including nucleic acid synthesis, methionine regeneration, and in the transfer of one-carbon units required for normal metabolism.[133] Intake of the vitamin may be adequate if the elderly individual is unstressed. However, in circumstances where need is increased, e.g., acute leukemia, drug-induced or autoimmune hemolytic anemia, metastatic cancer, multiple myeloma, or hemodialysis, dietary intake may be inadequate. In addition, drugs such as phenytoin, cycloserine, and various chemotherapeutic agents, e.g., methotrexate, can induce a folate deficiency. The effects of folic acid are blocked by the antibiotic trimethoprim and the high-pressure medication triamterene. Widespread use of antacids and cimetidine among the elderly may pose a threat to the pH-sensitive folate-transporting system by elevating intestinal pH. As pointed out earlier, the metabolism of folate and vitamin B$_{12}$ are intimately connected. Clinical presentation of a deficiency includes megaloblastic anemia and some mental dysfunction such as memory loss and confusion. Folate also appears to play an important role in preventing depression. Patients with megaloblastic anemia commonly suffer from depression, which may progress to dementia and peripheral neuropathy. Low or deficient serum or RBC folate levels (plasma folate ≤2.5 ng/ml and RBC folate <200 ng/ml) have been found in 15% to 38% of patients diagnosed with depression. There seems to be a direct relationship between folate deficiency and the emergence or severity of depressive illness.[134] Administration of folate (50 mg/day) without any antidepressants to elderly depressed patients resulted in improvement within 6 weeks. But caution is needed. Excessive intake of folate may exacerbate depression. Folate supplementation (15 mg/day) has

been reported to improve treatment with antidepressants, MOA-inhibitors, and lithium in folate-deficient patients. A recent longitudinal study of a small sample of elderly Catholic nuns indicated a strong relationship of low serum folate and cerebral atrophy associated with Alzheimer's disease.[109] Epidemiologic studies have suggested that a diminished folate status is associated with an increased risk of colon, esophageal, and cervical cancer.[131,135] Colorectal cancer is the second most common cause of cancer-related death in both men and women. Folate deficiency causes massive incorporation of uracil into human DNA and chromosomes breaks. It has been suggested that folate deficiency produces DNA strand breaks in the p53 tumor suppressor gene and site-specific protooncogene DNA hypomethylation. Perhaps hypomethylation of DNA "switches on" certain genes, whereas methylation would keep them turned off.[136] Folate also plays a role in the pathogenesis of cardiovascular disease.

The hormonal form of vitamin D, calcitriol (1,25-dihydroxyvitamin D$_3$), is essential for maintenance of the body's calcium balance. The precursor of this potent calciotropic hormone is provitamin D$_3$, 7-dehydrocholesterol, found in the skin and converted by ultraviolet light to previtamin D$_3$. Not only does skin thickness decrease with age, there is also an age-dependent decrease in the epidermal concentration of provitamin D$_3$.[137] Young adults possess at least twice the capacity to form previtamin D$_3$ as do older adults (Figure 38–11).

Previtamin D$_3$ transforms to vitamin D$_3$ and following two hydroxylation reactions (first in the liver and second in the kidneys) 1,25-dihydroxyvitamin D$_3$ is formed. The hepatic hydroxylase reaction results in the synthesis of 25-hydroxyvitamin D$_3$, also known as calcidiol. Vitamin D deficiency in seniors may arise due to deprivation of sunlight (homebound

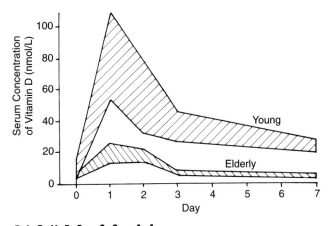

**FIGURE 38–11**

Circulating concentrations of vitamin D in response to a whole-body exposure to one minimal erythemal dose in healthy young and elderly subjects. (From Holick MF: Environmental factors that influence the cutaneous production of vitamin D. Am J Clin Nutr 61(Suppl): 638S, 1995.)

or institutionalized elderly being especially at risk), avoidance of dairy products due to lactase deficiency or low income or intestinal malabsorption and recently increasing use of sunscreens in older adults who have developed skin cancer.[138] The possibility has recently been raised that obesity-associated vitamin D insufficiency may be due to decreased bioavailability of vitamin D from both endogenous and exogenous sources because it is deposited in body fat compartments. If vitamin D levels are low, there will be a decrease in absorption of dietary calcium and the extracellular calcium concentration will decline. Increased secretion of the parathyroid hormone, parathyrin, helps offset the developing hypocalcemia by promoting the release of calcium from bone. Reduced hepatic and renal mass accompanied by diminished hydroxylase activity also contribute to the elderly having lower serum levels of both $25\text{-OH-D}_3$ and $1,25\text{-}(OH)_2D_3$. Serum concentration of $25\text{-OH-D}_3$ is the best clinical evidence of vitamin D status. The level of 25-dihydroxyvitamin $D_3$ in the elderly may be only one half that in young adults, thereby leading to a 1,25-dihydroxyvitamin $D_3$ deficiency. Calcitriol acts on the major target organs, bone, kidney, and the gastrointestinal tract to promote uptake and retention of calcium. Animal models suggest that with aging there is a reduction in number of intestinal and skeletal receptors for calcitriol. Serum calcium levels and bone integrity are dependent on the adequacy of vitamin D nutriture.[139] 1,25-dihydroxyvitamin $D_3$ may play a role in regulation of osteoblast function. During bone matrix formation, osteoblasts synthesize the protein osteocalcin that functions as a binding factor for calcium. By stimulating osteocalcin synthesis, vitamin D may be a necessary component of the vitamin K-dependent carboxylation process in bone. Among the elderly increased risk of osteoporosis and hip and other fractures has been traced to secondary hyperparathyroidism brought on by vitamin D deficiency.[140] Optimum vitamin D status confers a variety of benefits beyond that of promoting bone health. Low levels of the vitamin have been linked to increased risk of certain cancers (skin, colon, breast, and prostate), because $1,25\text{-}(OH)_2D_3$ is a potent inhibitor of cell proliferation and inducer of cell maturation. A possible role for calcitriol in the immune response has been proposed in which the vitamin alters T and B cell function and macrophage activity thereby suppressing autoimmunity.

Acting as an enzyme cofactor, vitamin K mediates the postranslational gamma carboxylation of protein-bound glutamic acid residues. It is in this way involved in the synthesis of several blood coagulation factors and the bone matrix protein, osteocalcin. Osteocalcin is thought to act as a regulator of bone mineralization. Age-related changes in vitamin K nutriture or metabolism are suggested by increased sensitivity to warfarin among healthy elderly with no known liver damage. Possible explanations include an increase in the free fraction of the drug due to declining serum albumin levels, altered binding affinity of vitamin K to the clotting factor synthesizing system, or depletion of vitamin K stores with age. High serum concentration of <u>under</u> carboxylated osteocalcin (ucOC) and low serum concentrations of vitamin K are associated with in-

creased risk of hip fracture in elderly men and women. Some, but not all, studies suggest a low vitamin K intake is associated with lowered bone mineral density. Some studies indicate that vitamin K decreases urinary calcium excretion.[141,142]

Vitamin E (alpha-tocopherol) acting as a free radical and peroxide scavenger in the lipid phase of the cell protects cell members from oxidative damage. Normal neurologic structure and function as well as red blood cell integrity and platelet aggregation require adequate supplies of vitamin E. Although plasma levels of vitamin E are not altered with age, platelet levels reportedly decline in healthy elderly. Supplementation with vitamin E has been shown to improve immune responsiveness in healthy elderly.[30,143] Enhanced cell-mediated immunity has been demonstrated by (1) increased delayed-type hypersensitivity (DTH) response, (2) increased IL-2 production, (3) increased T cell proliferation in response to certain mitogens, and (4) decreased synthesis of $PGE_2$ and plasma lipid peroxides.[30] By virtue of its function as an antioxidant, vitamin E seems to delay the progression (if not the development) of Alzheimer's disease.[144] Vitamin E has several potentially protective effects on the cardiovascular system. Studies suggest that the vitamin protects against the oxidation of LDL and decreases the deposition of atherogenic oxidized LDL in arterial walls, inhibits platelet aggregation and adhesion, prevents smooth muscle proliferation, and preserves normal coronary dilation.[32,145]

## REFERENCE RANGES

Establishing reference intervals for the elderly poses a challenge for the laboratorian. The purpose of a reference range or reference interval is to provide a reference point to which the patient's result can be compared to make a medical decision.[146] But there is little evidence that aging, in the absence of some underlying subclinical pathology, alters the reference range of many analytes.[147] The National Committee for Clinical Laboratory Standards (NCCLS) provides detailed guidance on how to define and determine reference intervals in the clinical laboratory.[146] But even when these guidelines are followed, establishing an appropriate reference interval can be tricky. Most clinical studies are cross-sectional and among the elderly only the survivors are available for study at advanced age. On the other hand, the presence of subclinical disorders or deficiencies in seniors may contaminate the data collection and skew the results. For example, the determination of plasma total homocysteine is becoming a more important diagnostic test. Increased assessment of this analyte is based on the evidence that hyperhomocysteinemia is a significant risk factor for cardiovascular disease. Methyltetrahydrofolate and vitamin $B_{12}$ are coenzymes in homocysteine metabolism, and if folate or cobalamin status is inadequate, homocysteine concentration will rise. Unfortunately, a high percentage of elderly are not obtaining sufficient folic acid and/or $B_{12}$ to keep their homocysteine levels low. How then do you establish a reference range

T A B L E    3 8 - 9

**Modifiable Aspects of Aging**

| AGING MARKER | LIFESTYLE ADJUSTMENT(S) REQUIRED |
|---|---|
| Cardiac reserve | Exercise, nonsmoking |
| Glucose tolerance | Weight control, exercise, diet |
| Memory | Training, practice |
| Osteoporosis | Weight-bearing exercise, diet |
| Physical endurance | Exercise, weight control |
| Physical strength | Exercise |
| Pulmonary reserve | Exercise, nonsmoking |
| Serum cholesterol | Diet, weight control, exercise |
| Systolic blood pressure | Salt limitation, weight control, exercise |

Adapted from Aiken LR: *Aging: An Introduction to Gerontology.* Thousand Oaks, CA, Sage Publications, 1995.

for homocysteine? Since the implementation of fortification of cereals and flour products with folic acid began in 1998, early reports are encouraging that improved folate status is lowering homocysteine levels. What now becomes of the previously established reference range for total homocysteine? Initial assumptions that homocysteine levels increased as a result of "normal" aging have been overturned. Perhaps we will discover that more analyte concentration changes in seniors are attributable to diet, body weight, and exercise (Table 38–9). Successful strategies to maintain mental and physical function in old age incorporate the use of hormones, improved nutrition, weight control, selected vitamin supplementation, and regular exercise.[3]

As seniors become more conscious of the importance of following an active healthy lifestyle whether they are 65, 75, or 85 years old, we may begin to see laboratory values for the fit elderly much like those characteristic of middle-aged healthy adults. Declining levels of sex hormones impact selected analytes but hormone replacement therapy is available. Postmenopausal women are at increased risk of osteoporosis but clinicians now know that osteoporosis and the associated alterations in calcium metabolism that once seemed virtually an inevitability of advanced age are both preventable and treatable. As our understanding of which changes are inevitable and which are preventable is refined, we may see less need for geriatric reference intervals. With elderly patients, perhaps emphasis should be placed on critical values or medical decision limits rather than population-based geriatric reference intervals. For example, the National Cholesterol Education Program (NCEP) has established risk-associated lipid limits. Although an older patient's serum total cholesterol might be within a "healthy geriatric reference interval," clinical intervention would be appropriate based on scientific and medical knowledge that a such total cholesterol concentration places the senior at increased risk of cardiovascular disease. An abnormal laboratory finding in an older patient may simply be

that—an abnormal result suggesting a clinical disorder and warranting further testing. Perhaps the most useful laboratory information is that of the individual acquired throughout their adult life. Comparison of a person's cholesterol level at age 70 to that at age 50 might be more enlightening for the clinician than reliance on a geriatric reference range.

## CLINICAL APPLICATIONS

Unless we make substantial progress in the prevention, early detection and treatment of disorders that cause the greatest disability and produce the greatest need for long-term care, the aging of our population will have catastrophic consequences for our health care system. Laboratory data can be especially helpful to the physician with respect to two age-dependent, costly to manage conditions among the elderly: dementia and hip fracture.

### Dementia

The American Psychiatric Association defines dementia as a syndrome of acquired and persistent impairment in cognitive and intellectual functioning.[148] The prevalence of dementia increases rapidly with advancing age (Figure 38–12).

A wide variety of underlying disorders can affect the integrity of the central nervous system and cause dementia. Among the conditions are neurogenerative disorders, vascular injuries, infections, drug-induced or metabolic disruptions, and trauma. Alzheimer's disease (AD) is a progressive, degenerative disease of the brain and the most common cause of

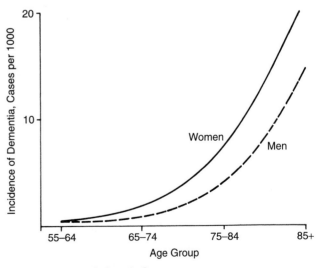

**F I G U R E    3 8 - 1 2**

Estimated incidence of dementia in older individuals as a function of age. (From Birge SJ, Morrow-Howell N, Proctor EK: Hip fracture. In Perry HM, III (ed.): *The Aging Skeleton, Clinics in Geriatric Medicine.* Philadelphia, WB Saunders, 1994.)

dementia among seniors in the United States[149]; the second most common cause of dementia in seniors is vascular dementia. Common features of dementia include short-term memory loss, impaired judgment, diminished problem-solving abilities, and attention problems. Behavioral problems include personality changes and sleep disturbances. Forgetfulness severe enough to interfere with the daily activities of living is a frequent early sign of AD. The devastating consequences of Alzheimer's disease are well-known to the general public. The greatest risk for Alzheimer's is age. Alzheimer's disease afflicts almost 4 million Americans; between 6% and 10% of the population over the age of 65 and more than 50% of those over 85 years of age.[150,151] Alzheimer's cases double for every 5 years of age between 65 and 85 (Figure 38–13). The occurrence of dementia among elderly nursing home residents is even more common. Half of all residents in long-term care facilities suffer from AD or a related disorder.[149] By the middle of the century, or perhaps earlier, it is possible that 14 million Americans will be diagnosed with AD. National annual costs of caring for AD patients are estimated conservatively at $125 billion. Appearance of abnormalities called **neurofibrillary tangles** and deposition of senile plaques in the cerebral cortex are associated with neuronal cell destruction.

Risk factors for AD include age and family history. Four specific mutations contribute to AD. Defective genes located on chromosomes 1, 14, 19, and 21 seem to be involved in the accumulation of a protein fragment called **amyloid beta protein.** $\beta$-Amyloid deposits in the brain are a contributing, but not the sole, factor involved in the pathogenesis of Alzheimer's disease. Spontaneous generation of free radicals and ROS by $\beta$-amyloid causes damage to cell membrane lipids and proteins. $\beta$-Amyloid also generates radicals through interaction with iron and zinc, both of which are increased in the brain of subjects with AD.[28] Antioxidants, such as vitamin E which inhibits lipid peroxidation, appear to reduce $\beta$-amyloid-

induced neuron death.[152] At the present time, there is no routine biochemical test that can be used to diagnose Alzheimer's disease. AD can only be definitely diagnosed at autopsy.

Unlike Alzheimer's, acquired cognitive disorders can be traced to metabolic, toxic, infectious, or neoplastic origins and may be reversible (Table 38–10).

Clinical studies have reported the percentage of all dementias that are potentially reversible as ranging from a low of 5% to a high of 30%, depending on the population examined.[151] Numerous drugs, selected vitamin deficiencies, heavy metal intoxication, and intracranial infections are among the possible causes of dementing disorders. Endocrinopathies of the parathyroid and thyroid and deficiency states of thiamin, cobalamin, folate, and possibly vitamin C are frequently encountered among older adults and may be associated with cognitive impairment. A recent study of healthy elderly over 60 years of age reported numerous correlations between electroencephalographic (EEG) indices of neuropsychologic function and indicators of thiamin, riboflavin, and iron status. There is growing evidence that patients with affective disorders have vitamin $B_{12}$, $B_6$, and folate deficiencies and those with psychotic depression have lower $B_{12}$ levels. Both affective and cognitive function improve with selected B vitamin supplementation. Recommendations on laboratory test performance for the differential diagnosis of dementing diseases include a complete blood count, differential, erythrocyte sedimentation rate, electrolyte panel, blood urea nitrogen, creatinine, blood glucose, calcium and phosphorus levels, hepatic function tests, thyroid function (TSH), triglycerides and cholesterol, vitamin $B_{12}$ and folate levels, urinalysis (which may include 24-hour urinary free cortisol, urine heavy metals, and drug screening), syphilis serology, and perhaps HIV antibody testing. Arterial blood gases, serum protein electrophoresis, and an electrocardiogram may also provide useful information in selected situations. Cerebrospinal fluid analysis is appropriate to exclude

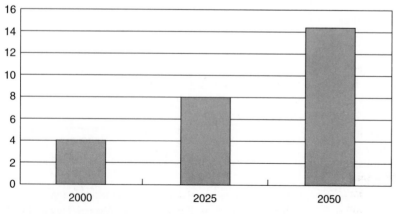

**Projection of Americans Affected with Alzheimer's Disease (in millions)**

**FIGURE  38-13**

Americans with Alzheimer's disease (Statistics courtesy of the Alzheimer's Association)

TABLE 38-10

**Potentially Reversible Etiologies of Dementia**

**Metabolic, Toxic, or Systemic**
 Vitamin deficiencies
  $B_{12}$ (pernicious anemia)
  Thiamin ($B_1$) (Wernicke's encephalopathy)
  Nicotinic acid (pellagra)
 Dehydration
 Renal failure
 Hepatic failure
 Pulmonary failure
 Endocrine failure
  Hyperthyroid and hypothyroid
  Adrenal insufficiency and Cushing's syndrome
  Hypoparathyroidism and hyperparathyroidism
 Drugs
  Alcohol
  Psychotropic agents
  Neuroleptics
  Antidepressants
  Anxiolytics/sedatives/hypnotics
  Stimulants
 Antiparkinsonian agents
  Anticholinergics
  Amantadine
  Levodopa (L-dopa)
  Bromocriptine
 Antihistamines
 Cardiovascular agents
 Hypoglycemic agents
 Anticonvulsants
 Analgesics
 Other
  Cimetidine
  Metoclopramide
  Corticosteroids
  Carbon monoxide
  Antimicrobials
  Organophosphates
 Heavy metal poisoning (lead, mercury, thallium, manganese)

**Chronic infections**
 Neurosyphilis
 TB, fungal, and protozoal
 Whipple's disease
 Sarcoidosis
**Immunologic**
 Granulomatous angiitis
 Limbic encephalitis
**Other intracranial disease**
 Subdural hematoma
 Neoplasm
 Normal pressure hydrocephalus
 Seizures
**Psychiatric "pseudodementia"**
**Miscellaneous**
 Sensory deprivation/intensive care unit psychosis
 Fecal impaction

causes of chronic meningeal inflammation.[149] These tests may detect the presence of coexisting medical conditions such as urinary tract infections, hypothyroidism, or evidence of side effects from medications. In such instances, treatment of the previously unsuspected medical problem frequently reduces the disability associated with the dementing disorder.

## Hip Fracture

Injury is among the leading causes of death in persons over 65 and most of these fatal injuries are fall-related. Nonfatal in-

juries include serious soft-tissue damage as well as broken bones. Twenty-eight million Americans, predominately older men and women, have disorders that affect their skeletal integrity. Approximately 10 million have osteoporosis, and conservatively, another 20 million have osteopenia or low bone mass, both conditions placing them at increased risk of fracture. Among postmenopausal women, 30% to 50% have osteoporosis. Approximately 50% of all Americans over the age of 75 have osteoporosis.[153] It has been estimated that as many as 1.5 million fractures annually are the result of osteoporosis. These fractures include 700,000 vertebral fractures, 240,000 wrist fractures, and 250,000 hip fractures.[154,155] Total direct costs associated with these fractures was $17 billion in 2001 (approximately $49 million daily). One third of the elderly fall each year and 90% of hip fractures occur as a result of a fall, although some occur spontaneously.[156] Hip fracture, the most severe osteoporotic fracture, is likely to cause serious functional impairment, reduced quality of life, and institutionalization. The prevalence and cost of osteoporosis continues to rise as the elderly population grows. Unless there is a dramatic change in lifestyle that improves Americans' overall calcium balance, by the middle of this century the projected annual cost of hip fractures alone could be a staggering $240 billion[157] (Figure 38–14). In addition to these costs, fractures cause pain, deformity, loss of independence and even increased risk of death.[154] The risk of hip fracture increases exponentially with age. Hip fracture rates are highest in whites and lowest in blacks. By age 70, 40% of women will suffer a hip fracture.[153] In white women over the age of 85, the incidence of hip fracture is about 3% annually. A woman's lifetime risk of hip fracture alone is equal to the combined risk of developing breast, uterine, and ovarian cancer. Mortality 6 months after hip fracture is 10% to 20% and one half of survivors never walk again without assistance.[156]

Genetic, environmental, hormonal, and nutritional factors are all determinants of peak bone mass and the retention of skeletal integrity over time. Serum concentrations of all metabolites of vitamin D are likely to decline with advancing age. As a result, calcium uptake from the GI tract is reduced. The importance of estrogen (and testosterone) in maintaining adult bone mass is known. Orchiectomy for prostate cancer is frequently followed by severe osteoporosis.[158] Cessation of estrogen at menopause leads to accelerated bone loss (Figure 38–15). Cumulatively, these events are reflected in reduced skeletal integrity.

Bone strength depends upon architecture as well as composition.[159] Changes in bone turnover, mass, and mineraliza-

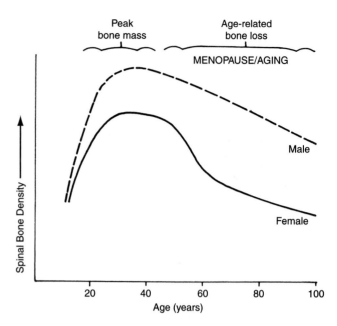

**F I G U R E   3 8 - 1 5**

Bone mass as a function of age and gender. (From Hough S: Fast and slow bone losers: Relevance to the management of osteoporosis. Drugs and Aging 12(Suppl 1):1, 1998.)

tion can increase risk of osteomalacia and osteoporosis among seniors, both men and women[160] (Table 38–11).

In Europe and the United States, between 30 and 40% of elderly hip fracture patients are deficient in vitamin D. A lack of vitamin D suppresses bone remodeling, disrupting the linkage between bone formation, and resorption.[154] Osteoporosis is now defined by the World Health Organization as a disease of fracture risk determined by comparison of an individual's bone mineral density (BMD) measurements to that of a young, healthy reference group. Low bone mass, or osteopenia, is defined as a BMD between 1.0 and 2.5 SD below the mean for the reference group. Osteoporosis is defined as a BMD that is greater than 2.5 SD below the mean.[161]

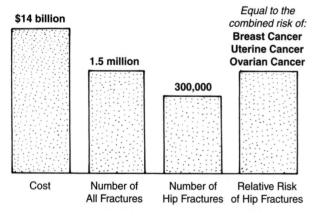

**F I G U R E   3 8 - 1 4**

Annual disease burden of osteoporosis in the United States (From the National Osteoporosis Foundation and Older Women's League)

T A B L E   3 8 – 1 1

**Osteoporosis Risk Factors**

Female sex
White or Asian race
Positive family history
Age
Early menopause/menstrual history
Diet low in calcium
Smoking
Excessive alcohol or caffeine intake
Sedentary lifestyle
Medications, disease

Osteoporosis is both preventable and treatable.[162] Early identification by the laboratory of individuals whose calcium homeostasis is impaired should prompt BMD assessment and aggressive treatment by the clinician to prevent or retard skeletal deterioration. Measurement of biochemical markers in the urine and serum can provide information about significant changes in bone remodeling within 3 to 6 months after therapy initiation. Other factors that place an individual at increased risk of injury from falls can be identified at least partially by laboratory evaluation include dementia, postural hypotension, and biochemical deficiencies that affect neurologic and musculoskeletal function and thus impair balance and gait.

## SUMMARY

The percentage of the population identified as elderly is increasing at an astonishing rate. The challenge that this presents, now and in the future, to our health care delivery system and resources is unprecedented. To keep older adults healthy and living in the community for the maximum length of time will require expanded knowledge of functional and structural changes associated with aging. The greatest challenge for those studying the elderly is the ability to differentiate parameters that change because of physiologic and biochemical alterations that occur with passage of time from those changes that may be attributed to disease processes and medication effects. Perhaps establishment of geriatric reference ranges for healthy elderly is beneficial for a few selected analytes. The greater challenge remains to clarify the clinical significance of biochemical changes seen in the aging process. Laboratory findings can be especially useful to the clinician both in identifying seniors who are at increased risk of various age-associated disorders and as a basis for action to optimize metabolism and maximize physiologic function. The contribution of laboratory assessment in supporting successful aging, in increasing longevity, and in maintaining the highest possible quality of life for the longest period cannot be overestimated. We must better understand the nature of the modifiable factors that will permit individuals to continue to function effectively with increasing age. It is time to replace society's negative image of aging with a new optimistic positive view, and laboratory data can help clinicians in the development and implementation of strategies to improve the health and increase the vigor of seniors.

## REFERENCES

1. U.S. Bureau of the Census: Statistical brief. Sixty-five plus in the United States. Available at: http://www.census.gov/socdemo/www/agebrief.html. Accessed August 6, 2000.
2. AARP 1999: A profile of older Americans. Available at: http://www.aoa.dhhs.gov/stats/profile/default/htm. Accessed August 6, 2000.
3. Howard RB, Hoel D: Grow old along with me. Postgrad Med 102(4):216, 1997.
4. Greendale GA, Lee NP, Arriola ER: The menopause. Lancet 353:571, 1999.
5. Houston DK, Johnson MJ, Nozza RJ, et al.: Age-related hearing loss, vitamin B-12, and folate in elderly women. Am J Clin Nutr 69:564, 1999.
6. National Diabetes Fact Sheet: Available at: http://www.cdc.gov/diabetes/pubs/facts98.htm. Accessed February 16, 2000.
7. Christensen RH: The basics of bone metabolism. Clin Lab News 24(5):10, 1998.
8. Knight JA: *Free Radicals, Antioxidants, Aging, and Disease.* Washington, DC, AACC Press, 1999.
9. Chandra RK: Graying of the immune system. JAMA 277:1398, 1997.
10. Cearlock D, Laude-Flaws M: Stress, immune function, and the older adult. MLO 29(10):36, 1997.
11. Blechman MB, Gelb AM: Aging and gastrointestinal physiology. Clin Geriatr Med 15(3):429, 1999.
12. Gorman L: Aging: Laboratory testing and theories. Clin Lab Sci 8:24, 1995.
13. Lesourd BM, Mazari L, Ferry M: The role of nutrition in immunity in the aged. Nutr Rev 56(Suppl II):S113, 1998.
14. Heurser MD, Adler WH: Immunological aspects of aging and malnutrition. Clin Geriatr Med 13(4):697, 1997.
15. Knight J: *Laboratory Medicine and the Aging Process.* Chicago, American Society of Clinical Pathologists, 1996.
16. Lieberman SA, Hofman AR: The somatopause. Should growth hormone deficiency in older people be treated? Clin Geriatr Med 19(4):6671, 1997.
17. McKenney CA, Romzer MR, Ziemba SE: Apoptosis—When cells die. Lab Med 30(12):791, 1999.
18. Bodnar AG, Ouellette M, Frolkis M, Holt SE, et al.: Extension of life-span by introduction of telomerase into normal human cells. Science 279(5349):349, 1998.
19. Wynford-Thomas D: Cellular senescence and cancer. J Pathol 187:100, 1999.
20. Chang B-D, Watanabe K, Broude EV, et al.: Effects of p21^Waf1/Cip1/Sdi1 on cellular gene expression: Implications for carcinogenesis, senescence, and age-related diseases. Proc Natl Acad Sci 97:4291, 2000.
21. Vijg J: Understanding the biology of aging: The key to prevention and therapy. J Am Geriatr Soc 43:426, 1995.
22. Gafni A: Structural modifications of proteins during aging. J Am Geriatr Soc 45:871, 1997.
23. Vlassara H: Recent progress in advanced glycation end products and diabetic complications. Diabetes 46(Suppl 2):S19, 1997.

24. Miller SM: Antioxidants and aging. MLO 29(9):42, 1997.

25. Ames BN, Shigenaga MK, Hagen TM: Oxidants, antioxidants and the degenerative diseases of aging. Proc Natl Acad Sci USA 90:7915, 1993.

26. Mylonas C. Kouretas D: Lipid peroxidation and tissue damage. A review. In vivo 13:295, 1999.

27. Halliwell B: Antioxidants and human disease: A general introduction. Nutr Rev 55(Suppl II):S44, 1997.

28. Markesbery WR: The role of oxidative stress in Alzheimer disease. Arch Neurol 56(12):1449, 1999. Available at: http://archneur.ama-assn.org/issues/v56n12/full/nmr8390.html. Accessed August 6, 2000.

29. Oldham KM, Bowen PE: Oxidative stress in critical care: Is antioxidant supplementation beneficial? J Am Diet Assoc 98:1001, 1998.

30. Meydani SN, Beharaka AA: Recent developments in vitamin E and immune response. Nutr Rev 56(Suppl II):S49, 1998.

31. Sies H, Stahl W: Vitamins E and C, β-carotene, and other carotenoids as antioxidants. Am J Clin Nutr 62(Suppl):1315S, 1995.

32. Emmert DH, Kirchner JT: The role of vitamin E in the prevention of heart disease. Arch Fam Med 8:537, 1999.

33. Faulkner WR, Meites S: Geriatric Clinical Chemistry: Reference Values. Washington, DC, AACC Press, 1994.

34. Tietz NW, Shuey DF, Wekstein DR: Laboratory values in fit aging individuals—sexagenarians through centenarians. Clin Chem 38:1167, 1992.

35. Brigden ML, Heathcote JC: Problems in interpreting laboratory tests. What do unexpected results mean? Postgrad Med 107(7):145, 2000.

36. Beck LH: Changes in renal function with aging. Clin Geriatr Med 14(2):199, 1998.

37. Sica DA: Renal disease, electrolyte abnormalities, and acid-base imbalance in the elderly. Clin Geriatr Med 10(1):197, 1994.

38. Andresen GP: Assessing the older patient. RN 61(3):37, 1998.

39. Schwartz RS: Obesity in the elderly, in Bray GA, Bouchard C (eds.): Handbook of Obesity. New York, Marcel Dekker, 1998, p 103.

40. Hassan A: Renal disease in the elderly. Postgrad Med 100(6):44, 1996.

41. Lubran MM: Renal function in the elderly. Ann Clin Lab Sci 25(2):122, 1995.

42. Anderson S: Effects of aging on the renal glomerulus. Am J Med 80:435, 1986.

43. Liebson PR, Amsterdam EA: Prevention of coronary heart disease. Part II. Secondary prevention, detection of subclinical disease, and emerging risk factors. Dis Mon 46(1):1, 2000.

44. Byyny RL, Speroff L: A Clinical Guide for the Care of Older Women. 2nd ed. Baltimore, Williams & Wilkins, 1996.

45. American Heart Association: High blood pressure. Available at: http:www//americanheart.org/statistics/06hghbld.html. Accessed August 9, 2000.

46. Montamat SC, Cusack BJ, Vestal RE: Management of drug therapy in the elderly. N Engl J Med 321:303, 1989.

47. Busby-Whitehead J, Johnson TM: Urinary incontinence. Clin Geriatr Med 14(2):285, 1998.

48. Wood CA, Abrutyn E: Urinary tract infections in older adults. Clin Geriatr Med 14(2):267, 1998.

49. Harris MI, Flegal KM, Cowie CC, Eberhardt MS, et al.: Prevalence of diabetes, impaired fasting glucose, and impaired glucose tolerance in U.S. adults. Third National Health and Nutrition Examination Survey, 1988–1994. Diabetes Care 21:518, 1998.

50. The Expert Committee on the Diagnosis and Classification of Diabetes Mellitus: Report of the Expert Committee on the Diagnosis and Classification of Diabetes Mellitus. Diabetes Care 20:1183, 1997.

51. National Diabetes Fact Sheet: Available at: http://www.cdc.gov/diabetes/pubs/facts98.htm. Accessed May 23, 2000.

52. Miller SM, Lefevre MA:. Changes, challenges of diabetes. ADVANCE for Administrators of the Laboratory 9(9):50,2000.

53. Gilden JL: Nutrition and the older diabetic. Clin Geriatr Med 15(2):371, 1999.

54. Perry HM: The endocrinology of aging. Clin Chem 45(8):1369, 1999.

55. Morley JE: An overview of diabetes mellitus in older persons. Clin Geriatr Med 15(2):211, 1999.

56. Burchfiel CM, Sharp DS, Curb JD, Rodriguez BL et al.: Hyperinsulinemia and cardiovascular disease in elderly men. The Honolulu Heart Program. Arterioscler Thromb Vasc Biol 18:450, 1998.

57. Ceddia RB, William Jr. WN, Lima FB, et al.: Pivotal role of leptin in insulin effects. Braz J Med Biol Res 31:715, 1998.

58. Kotz CM, Billington CJ, Levine AS: Obesity and aging. Clin Geriatr Med 15(2):391, 1999.

59. Grundy SM, Balady GJ, Criqui MH, Fletcher G, et al.: Primary prevention of coronary heart disease: Guidance from Framingham. Circulation 97:1876, 1998.

60. Refsum H, Ueland PM, Nygard O, Vollset SE: Homocysteine and cardiovascular disease [Review]. Annu Rev Med 49:31, 1998.

61. Folsom AR, Nieto FJ, McGovern PG, Tsai M, et al.: Prospective study of coronary heart disease incidence in relation to fasting total homocysteine, related genetic polymorphisms, and B vitamins. The Atherosclerosis Risk in Communities (ARIC) Study. Circulation 98:204, 1998.

62. Welch GN, Loscalzo J: Homocysteine and athero-thrombosis. N Engl J Med 338:1042, 1998.

63. Jacobsen DW: Homocysteine and vitamins in cardiovascular disease. Clin Chem 44(8B):1833, 1998

64. American Heart Association: Coronary heart disease and angina pectoris. Available at: http://www.americanheart.org/statistics/04cornry.html. Accessed August 9, 2000.

65. Hulley S, Grady D, Bush T, et. al.: For the Heart and Estrogen/Progestin Replacement Study (HERS) Research Group. Randomized trail of estrogen plus progestin for secondary prevention of coronary heart disease in postmenopausal women. JAMA 280:605, 1998.

66. American Heart Association: Older Americans and cardiovascular diseases. Available at: http://www.americanheart.org/statistics/biostats/biool.htm. Accessed August 9, 2000.

67. Benfante R, Reed D: Is elevated serum cholesterol level a risk factor for coronary heart disease in the elderly? JAMA 263:393, 1990.

68. Kannel WB: Nutritional contributors to cardiovascular disease in the elderly. J Am Geriatr Soc 34:27, 1986.

69. Aldin CM, Gilmer DF: Immunity, disease processes, and optimal aging. In Cavanaugh JC, Whitbourne SK (eds.): Gerontology: An Interdisciplinary Approach. New York, Oxford University Press, 1999, p 123.

70. McDermott LJ, Mehta JB, Duff AK: Tuberculosis. Part 1. Dis Mon 43(3):115, 1997.

71. Barnes PJ: Chronic obstructive pulmonary disease. JAMA 343:269, 2000.

72. Marangon K, Herbeth B, Lecomte E, et al.: Diet, antioxidant status, and smoking habits in French men. Am J Clin Nutr 67:231, 1998.

73. Varanasi RV, Varanasi SC, Howell CD: Liver diseases. Clin Geriatr Med 15(3):559, 1999.

74. Annesley TM: Special considerations for geriatric therapeutic drug monitoring. Clin Chem 35:1337–1341, 1989.

75. Simon JA, Hudes ES: Serum ascorbic acid and gallbladder disease prevalence among US adults. Arch Intern Med 160:931, 2000.

76. Affronti J: Biliary disease in the elderly patient. Clin Geriatr Med 15(3):571, 1999.

77. Griffiths JC: Enzyme changes in healthy older individuals. In Faulkner WR, Meites S (eds.): Geriatric Clinical Chemistry Reference Values. Washington, DC, AACC Press, 1994; p. 117.

78. Cho C, Flynn RJ: Hepatic enzyme induction by antiepileptic drugs in the elderly male. Lab Med 21(12):823, 1990.

79. Gundberg CM: Biochemical markers of bone formation. Clin Lab Med 20(3):489, 2000.

80. Shamburek RD, Farrar JT: Disorders of the digestive system in the elderly. N Engl J Med 322:438, 1990.

81. Baumgartner RN, Koehler KM, Romero L, Garry PJ: Serum albumin is associated with skeletal muscle in elderly men and women. Am J Clin Nutr 64:552, 1996.

82. Annesley T: Pharmacokinetic changes in the elderly. Clin Lab Sci 3(2):100–102, 1990.

83. Williamson JS, Wyandt CM: What the pharmacist should know about food and drug interactions. Hosp Pharm Report 12(4):43, 1998.

84. Touitou Y, Touitou C, Bogdan A, et al.: Differences between young and elderly subjects in seasonal and circadian variations of total plasma proteins and blood volume as reflected by hemoglobin, hematocrit, and erythrocyte counts. Clin Chem 32(5):801, 1986.

85. Mooradian AD: Normal age-related changes in thyroid hormone economy. Clin Geriatr Med 11(2):159, 1995.

86. Perry III HM: The endocrinology of aging. Clin Chem 45:8(B):1369, 1999.

87. Sawin CT: Subclinical hypothyroidism in older persons. Clin Geriatr Med 11(2):231, 1995.

88. Gambert SR: Hyperthyroidism in the elderly. Clin Geriatr Med 11(2):181, 1995.

89. Feldkamp CS: Thyroid testing algorithms. Clin Lab News 23(10):6, 1997.

90. Miller SM: Successful aging in America. Part 1, Nutrition, the elderly, and the laboratory. MLO 29(3):22, 1997.

91. Gariballa SE, Sinclair AJ: Nutrition, aging and ill health. Br J Nutr 80:7, 1998.

92. American Dietetic Association: Position of the American Dietetic Association: Nutrition, aging and the continuum of care. J Am Diet Assoc 96(10):1048, 1996.

93. Rowe JW, Kahn RL: Successful Aging. New York, Dell, 1998.

94. Anon: An apple a day keeps old age away. Drug Ther Perspect 14(5):5, 1999.

95. Haller J: The vitamin status and its adequacy in the elderly: An international overview. Int J Vitam Nutr Res 69(3):160, 1999.

96. Blumberg J: Nutrient requirements of the healthy elderly—Should there be specific RDAs? Nutr Rev 52(8) Suppl II:S15, 1994.

97. Lachance P, Langseth L: The RDA concept: Time for a change? Nutr Rec 52(8):(I)266, 1994.

98. McDowell MA, Briefel RR, Alaimo K, et al.: Energy and Macronutrient Intakes of Persons Ages 2 Months and Over in the United States: Third National Health and Nutrition Examination Survey, Phase 1, 1988–91. Washington, DC: National Center for Health Statistics, Centers for Disease Control and Prevention, U.S. Department of Health and Human Services, Publication no. 255, 1994.

99. Gallagher S, Miller S: Nutrition, the older adult, and the laboratory. ADVANCE for Administrators of the Laboratory 6(1):45, 1997.

100. Hill JO, Kriketos AD, Peters JC.: Disturbances of energy balance, In Stipanuk MH (ed.): *Biochemical and Physiological Aspects of Human Nutrition.* Philadelphia, WB Saunders, 2000, p 439.

101. Balluz LS, Kieszak SM, Philen RM, Mulinare J: Vitamin and mineral supplement use in the United States. Results from the Third National Health and Nutrition Examination Survey. Arch Fam Med 9:258, 2000.

102. Carr AC, Frei B:Toward a new recommended dietary allowance for vitamin C based on antioxidant and health effects in humans. Am J Clin Nutr 69:1086, 1999.

103. Loria CM, Klag MJ, Caulfield LE, Whelton PK: Vitamin C status and mortality in U.S. adults. Am J Clin Nutr 72:139, 2000.

104. Levine M, Rumsey SC, Darurvala R, Park JB, et al.: Criteria and recommendations for vitamin C intake. JAMA 281:1415, 1999.

105. Padayatty SJ, Levine M: Vitamin C and myocardial infarction: The heart of the matter. Am J Clin Nutr 71: 1027, 2000

106. Halliwell B: Ascorbic acid: Hype, hoax or healer. Am J Clin Nutr 65:1891, 1997.

107. Van Pelt D: Vitamins may help fight Parkinson's disease. Insight 4:56, 1988.

108. Tucker DM, Penland JG, Sandstead HH, et al.: Nutrition status and brain function. Am J Clin Nutr 52:93, 1990.

109. Snowden DA, Tully CL, Smith CD, Riley KP, Markesbery WR: Serum folate and the severity of atrophy of the neocortex in Alzheimer disease: Findings from the Nun Study. Am J Clin Nutr 71:993, 2000.

110. Bell IR, Edman JS, Morrow FD, et al.: B complex vitamin patterns in geriatric and young adult inpatients with major depression. J Am Geriatr Soc 39(3):252, 1991.

111. Smidt LJ, Cremin FM, Grivetti LE, et al.: Influence of thiamin supplementation on the health and general well-being of an elderly Irish population with marginal thiamin deficiency. J Gerontol Med Sci 46(1):M16, 1991.

112. Leklem J: Vitamin B$_6$, in: Machlin LJ (ed.): *Handbook of Vitamins.* 2nd ed. New York, Marcel Dekker, 1991, p 341.

113. Bartel PR, Ubbink JB, Delport R, et al.: Vitamin B-6 supplementation and theophylline-related effects in humans. Am J Clin Nutr 60:93, 1994.

114. Meydani SN, Ribaya-Mercado JD, Russell RM, et al.: Vitamin B$_6$ impairs interleukin 2 production and lymphocyte proliferation in elderly adults. Am J Clin Nutr 53:1275, 1991.

115. Talbott MC, Miller LT, Kerkvliet NI: Pyridoxine supplementation: Effect on lymphocyte responses in elderly persons. Am J Clin Nutr 46:659, 1987.

116. Rimm E, Willett W, Hu F, et al.: Folate and vitamin B$_6$ from diet and supplements in relation to risk of coronary heart disease among women. JAMA 279:359, 1998.

117. Stabler SP, Lindenbaum J, Allen RH: Vitamin B-12 deficiency in the elderly: Current dilemmas. Am J Clin Nutr 66:741, 1997.

118. Carmel R: Cobalamin, the stomach, and aging. Am J Clin Nutr 66:750, 1997.

119. Snow CF: Laboratory diagnosis of vitamin B$_{12}$ and folate deficiency. Arch Intern Med 159:1289, 1999.

120. Feldman M: The mature stomach. Still pumping out acid? JAMA 278:681, 1997.

121. Carmel R: Prevalence of undiagnosed pernicious anemia in the elderly. Arch Intern Med 156:1097, 1996.

122. Borum ML: Peptic-ulcer disease in elderly. Clin Geriatr Med 15(3):457, 1999.

123. Hurwitz A, Brady DA, Schaal E, Samloff IM, et al.: Gastric acidity in older adults. JAMA 278:659, 1997.

124. Tucker KL, Rich S, Rosenberg I, Jacques P, et al.: Plasma vitamin B-12 concentrations relate to intake source in Framingham Offspring Study. Am J Clin Nutr 71:514, 2000.

125. Gallo JJ, Fulmer T, Paveza GJ, Reichel W: *Handbook of Geriatric Assessment.* 3rd ed, Gaithersburg, MD, Aspen Publications, 2000.

126. Nilsson K, Gustafson L, Hultberg B: The plasma homocysteine concentration is better than that of serum methylmalonic acid as a marker for sociopsychological performance in a psychogeriatric population. Clin Chem 46(5):691, 2000.

127. Rasmussen K, Moller J, Lynbak M, et al.: Age- and gender-specific reference intervals for total homocysteine and methylmalonic acid in plasma before and after vitamin supplementation. Clin Chem 42(4):630, 1996.

128. Wu K, Helzlsouer KJ, Comstock GW, et al.: A prospective study on folate, B$_{12}$, and pyridoxal 5'-phosphate (B$_6$) and breast cancer. Cancer Epidemiol Biomarkers Prev 8:209, 1999.

129. Landis SH, Murray T, Bolden S, et al.: Cancer statistics, 1999. CA Cancer J Clin 49:8, 1999.

130. Stabler SP, Allen RH, Fried LP, Pahor M, et al.: Racial differences in prevalence of cobalamin and folate deficiencies in disabled elderly women. Am J Clin Nutr 70(5):911, 1999.

131. Blount BC, Mack MM, Wehr CM, MacGregor JT, et al.: Folate deficiency causes uracil misincorporation into human DNA and chromosome breakage: Implications for cancer and neuronal damage. Proc Natl Acad Sci USA 94:329095, 1997.

132. Food and Drug Administration: Food standards: amendment of standards of identity for enriched grain products to require addition of folic acid. Final rule. Fed Regist 61:8781, 1996.

133. Bailey LB, Gregory III JF: Folate metabolism and requirements. J Nutr 129:779, 1999.

134. Alpert JE, Fava M: Nutrition and depression: The role of folate. Nutr Rev 55(5):145, 1997.

135. Kim Y-I: Folate and carcinogenesis: Evidence, mechanisms, and implications. J Nutr Biochem 10:66, 1999

136. Weir DG, Scott JM: Colonic mucosal folate concentrations and their association with colorectal cancer. Am J Clin Nutr 68:763, 1998.

137. Holick MF: Vitamin D: The underappreciated D-lightful hormone that is important for skeletal and cellular health. Current Opinion in Endocrinology and Diabetes 9:87–98, 2002.

138. Holick MF: McCollum Award Lecture, 1994: Vitamin D-new horizons for the 21st century. Am J Clin Nutr 60:619, 1994.

139. Dawson-Hughes B: Calcium and vitamin D nutritional needs of elderly. J Nutr 126:1165S, 1996.

140. Utiger RD: The need for more vitamin D. N Engl J Med 338(12):828, 1998.

141. Feskanich D, Weber P, Willett WC, Rockett H, et al.: Vitamin K intake and hip fractures in women: A prospective study. Am J Clin Nutr 69:74, 1999.

142. Booth SL, Tucker KL, Chen H, Hannan MT, et al.: Dietary vitamin K intakes are associated with hip fracture but not with bone mineral density in elderly men and women. Am J Clin Nutr, 71:1201, 2000.

143. Pallast EG, Schouten EG, deWaart FG, Fonk HC: Effect of 50- and 100-mg vitamin E supplements on cellular immune function in noninstitutionalized elderly persons. Am J Clin Nutr 69(6):1273, 1999.

144. Grundman M: Vitamin E and Alzheimer disease: The basis for additional clinical trails. Am J Clin Nutr 71(2)(Suppl):630S, 2000.

145. Spencer AP, Carson DS, Crouch MA. Vitamin E and coronary artery disease. Arch Intern Med 159: 1313, 1999

146. National Committee for Clinical Laboratory Standards. *How to Define and Determine Reference Intervals in the Clinical Laboratory*, 2nd ed., Wayne, PA, NCCLS, 2000.

147. Knight J: Laboratory issues regarding geriatric patients. Lab Med 28(7):458, 1997.

148. American Psychiatric Association: *Diagnostic and Statistical Manual of Mental Disorders*, 4th ed., Washington DC, American Psychiatric Press, 1994.

149. Mezey MD, Mitty EL, Bottrell MM, Ramsey GC, Fisher T: Advance directives. Older adults with dementia. Clin in Geriatr Med 16(2):255, 2000.

150. Shuster JL: Palliative care for advanced dementia. Clin Geriatr Med 16(2):373, 2000.

151. Fletcher K, Damgaard P: Alzheimer's disease: Present & future issues. ADVANCE for Administrators of the Laboratory 8(1): 59, 1999.

152. Sano M, Ernesto C, Thomas RG, Klauber MR, et al.: A controlled trial of selegiline, alpha-tocopheral, or both as treatment for Alzheimer's disease. N Engl J Med 336:1216, 1997.

153. Kohlmeier L: Osteoporosis: Risk factors, screening and treatment. *Proceedings from the 50th Annual Meeting of the American Academy of Family Physicians Scientific Assembly.* September 16–20, 1998.

154. Falk R, Dagenais RJ: Osteoporosis. Can a future epidemic be prevented? ADVANCE for Administrators of the Laboratory 6(8):46, 1997.

155. Black DM, Cooper C: Epidemiology of fractures and assessment of fracture risk. Clin Lab Med 20(3):439, 2000.

156. Greenspan SL: A 73-year-old woman with osteoporosis. JAMA 281(16):1531, 1999.

157. Stauffer ME: Osteoporosis and metabolic bone disease. Forward. Clin Lab Med 20(3):xi, 2000.

158. De La Rosette JJMCH, D'Ancona FCH, Debruyne FMJ: Current status of thermotherapy of the prostate. J Urology 157(2):Abstracts, 1997.

159. Rosen CJ: Pathophysiology of osteoporosis. Clin Lab Med 20(3):455, 2000.

160. Odell WD, Health III H: Osteoporosis: Pathophysiology, prevention, diagnosis, and treatment. Dis Mon 39(11):789, 1993.

161. Falk RA, Miller SM: Clinical evaluation, management of osteoporosis. ADVANCE for Administrators of the Laboratory 8(5):57, 1999.

162. *Physician's Guide to Prevention and Treatment of Osteoporosis.* Washington, DC, National Osteoporosis Foundation, 1998.

# Index

Note: Page numbers followed by *t* and *f* indicate tables and figures, respectively.

Relative centrifugal force (RCF), 13
  nomogram for, 13, 14f
Renal arteries, 361
Renal blood flow (RBF), 361–362, 362f
  neonatal, 639
Renal calculi, 379, 396
Renal corpuscle. *See* Glomerulus
Renal cortex, 355, 356f
Renal disease, 391–395
Renal failure, 391–392
  acute, 391–392
  chronic, 392
    and hypocalcemia, 516
    plasma alkaline phosphatase levels in,
      282t
  and ketoacidosis, 433
Renal hilus, 355, 361
Renal medulla, 355, 356f
Renal osteodystrophy, 516
Renal pelvis, 355, 356f
Renal pyramids, 355, 356f
Renal replacement therapy, 396
Renal transplantation, 397
Renal tubule(s), 360–361, 361f
  function of, assessment of, 214, 384–387
Renin, 362, 403
  circulating levels of, age-related changes
    in, 669t
  secretion of, 370, 403
  as tumor marker, 328t, 331
Renin-angiotensin-aldosterone system, 403,
  404f
Renin-angiotensin system, 370–371
Replicative senescence, 652
Reproductive system
  female, 539–544, 541f
  male, 537–539, 538f, 539f
Resolution, of digital display, 143
Respiration, 424–426
Respiratory acidosis, 432t, 434
Respiratory alkalosis, 432t, 434
Respiratory disorders, 431, 434
Respiratory distress syndrome, 633
  acid-base status in, 640
  laboratory evaluation in, 640
  pathophysiology of, 633, 638
  in postmature infant, 640
  in premature infant, 640
Respiratory system, perinatal physiology of,
  637–638
Response, drug producing, 441
Restriction endonuclease, 114
  in identification of base sequences in
    DNA, 268–269, 269f
Restriction fragment length polymorphisms
  (RFLPs), 114–115
Retention jaundice, 298–299
Reticular dysgenesis, 252
Retinal, 596
Retinoic acid, 596

Retinol, 596
Retinol-binding protein (RBP), 596
  analysis of, 212
    procedures for, 581–583, 582t
  function of, 212
  half-life of, 581
Retinyl esters, 596
Retrovirus, 254
Reverse cholesterol transport, 186, 186f
Reverse osmosis, 11
Reverse transcriptase, 119
Reverse translation, 112
Reverse triiodothyronine (rT₃), 500
Reye's syndrome, 306, 643–644
  serum AST and ALT in, 280, 281t
  serum creatine kinase (CK) and CK
    isoenzymes in, 279t
RhD hemolytic disease, 633
Rheumatic fever, acute, effector mechanism
  in, 241t
Rheumatoid arthritis, 249–250
  antinuclear antibodies in, 242, 244t, 250
  effector mechanism in, 241t
  HLA association in, 240t
  target antigen in, 240t
Riboflavin. *See* Vitamin B₂
Ribonuclease, as tumor marker, 326t,
  326–327
Ribonucleoprotein, antibodies to, 242–243
Ribosomal RNA (rRNA), 95, 97, 97f
  assays for, specimen collection and
    handling for, 98
Ribosome(s), 97
Rickets, 516, 597–598, 641
RNA polymerase, 97, 97f, 119
  type I, antibody to, 243
RNA (ribonucleic acid), 95
  antibodies to, 243, 244t
  assays for, specimen collection and
    handling for, 98
  structure of, 95, 96f
Robotics, 131–132
Rohypnol, 469
Rotor's syndrome, 304, 642
Rouleaux, in multiple myeloma, 217
R proteins, 592
RS-61443, for immunosuppression, 397
RS-232 interface standard, 150, 150f
Rubella, congenital, and diabetes mellitus,
  161

## S

Safety, 27–39. *See also* Chemical safety;
  Fire safety
  employee training in, 29
  information on, resources for, 39
  in laboratory
    manager for, 38
    program for, 38

Safety (*Cont.*)
  practices promoting, 27–29
  regulations concerning, 27
Safety equipment, for laboratory, 38
Salicylates
  abuse and overdose of, 466, 467t, 468
    and ketoacidosis, 433
    and Reye's syndrome, 306
    serum levels of, quantitation of, 468
    toxicology of, 456t
Salicylic acid, formulation of, 443
Saliva, for drug screening, 471
Salkowski reaction, 190
Sandhoff's disorder, 198
Sarcoidosis, hypercalcemia in, 517
Sarcomas, 323
Sarcopenia, 657
Schilling test, for pernicious anemia
    diagnosis, 571, 572t
Scintillation, 101
Scleroderma
  antinuclear antibodies in, 244t, 248, 248t
  target antigen in, 240t
Screen, computer. *See* Monitor
Scurvy, 589
SDS PAGE, 210
SDy/x, calculation of, 71
Secobarbital, abuse and overdose of, 467t,
  468
Secondary active tubular transport, 366
Second messenger, 480, 485
Secretin, 562, 563t
Secretin challenge test, 572
Secretin-cholecystokinin test, 575
Secretory endometrium, 543
Secretory phase of menstrual cycle, 542
Sedative/hypnotics, abuse and overdose of,
  466, 468
Selective (discretionary) analysis, definition
  of, 131
Selective IgA deficiency, 251, 253
Selective IgG deficiency, 251, 253
Selenium, 603–604
  analytical procedures for, 603
  deficiency of, 603
    signs and symptoms of, in elderly, 672t
  factors affecting concentration of, 601t
  functions of, 603
  recommended dietary allowance for, 584t
  reference ranges for, 604
  toxicity of, 603
  upper intake level for, 587t
Self-tolerance, 239–240
Semen, 537
  composition of, 539t
Seminiferous tubule, 537, 538f
Senescence, replicative, 652
Sensitivity
  of diagnostic test, 72
  of radioimmunoassay, 102

Vitamin B$_{12}$ (*Cont.*)
  deficiency of, 593
    and affective disorders, 678
    approach to patient with hematologic
      abnormalities and, 593,
      595*f*
    and carcinogenesis, 674
    in elderly, 672*t*, 673–674
    evaluation of neurologic symptoms of,
      593, 594*f*
    in elderly, 655, 655*t*
  functions of, 592–593, 671, 673*f*,
    673–674
  malabsorption of, 564, 571, 593
  recommended dietary allowance for, 584*t*,
    600*t*, 674
  reference ranges for, 594–595
  storage of, 290
Vitamin C, 187, 588–589
  analytical procedures for, 589
  deficiency of, 589
    in elderly, 671, 672*t*
  functions of, 587–588
  recommended dietary allowance for, 584*t*,
    600*t*
  reference ranges for, 589
  upper intake level for, 587*t*
Vitamin D, 597–598
  analytical procedures for, 598
  and calcium levels, 512–513, 513*t*
  deficiency of, 515–516, 597–598
    in elderly, 672*t*, 675–676, 680
    in pediatric patient, 641
  formation of, 675, 675*f*
  functions of, 597
  recommended dietary allowance for, 584*t*,
    588*t*
  reference ranges for, 598
  storage of, 290
  toxicity of, 517, 598
  upper intake level for, 587*t*
Vitamin E, 187, 654
  analytical procedures for, 599
  deficiency of, 598–599
  functions of, 598, 676
  recommended dietary allowance for, 584*t*,
    588t
  reference ranges for, 599
  storage of, 290
  supplementation of, in elderly, 676
  upper intake level for, 587*t*
Vitamin intoxication, 586
Vitamin K, 599–600
  analytical procedures for, 600
  deficiency of, 599–600
  in elderly, 676
  functions of, 599, 676
  recommended dietary allowance for,
    588*t*
  reference ranges for, 600
  storage of, 290

Vitamin status, assessment of, 586
  direct, 586
  indirect, 586
VITROS analyzer, 136–137
Vitros clinical chemistry slides for bilirubin,
  293*f*, 293–294, 294*f*
V$_{max}$, 264–265
Volatiles
  identification of, 459
  quantitation of, 459
  toxicology of, 456*t*, 457–460
Volume of distribution, 445
von Gierke's disease, 167–168, 168*t*, 642
VP AFFIRM, 116*f*, 116–117

# W

Waldenström's macroglobulinemia, 217
Waste disposal, 28
Water
  absorption of, 559–560
  daily requirement of, 363
  deionization of, 11
  distillation of, 11
  filtration of, 11
  impurities in, 10
  metabolism of, assessment of, in neonates
    and children, 640–641
  purification of, methods for, 11
  purity of, specifications for, 10, 10*t*
  reabsorption of, antidiuretic hormone
    and, 384, 402
  reagent grade
    NCCLS standards for, 10, 10*t*
    quality control for, 11
    uses of, 11
  total body, 401
Water deprivation test, 485, 487
Waterhouse-Friderichsen syndrome, 527
Water-insoluble bilirubin, 288
Water of hydration, 22
Water-soluble bilirubin, 288
Water-soluble vitamins, 586, 587–596
  recommended dietary allowances for,
    588*t*
Watson-Schwartz test, 350–351
Weber-Christian disease, 251
Weighing, of substances, 11
  balances for, 11–12
Weight
  age-related changes in, 657
  definition of, 11
Wermer's syndrome, 568
Westgard multirule system, 55–61
Westgard QC website, 55
Wet beriberi, 590
White blood cells (WBCs), in urine, 389,
  390
Wide area network (WAN), 147
Wilson's disease, 301–302, 604–605, 643
  diagnosis of, 214, 301

Wilson's disease (*Cont.*)
  differential diagnosis of, 301
  etiology of, 301
  laboratory diagnosis of, 301–302, 620–621
  pathophysiology of, 214
  prevalence of, 301
  psychiatric symptoms in, 301, 620–621
  treatment of, 302
Wiskott-Aldrich syndrome, 251, 253
Wolffian ducts, 627, 628
Wolframs syndrome, and diabetes mellitus,
  161
Workstations, 145–146
WT1, 337

# X

Xanthine oxidase, 606
XENIX, 146
Xenotransplantation, 317
X-linked hyper IgM syndrome, 251, 253
X-linked lymphoproliferative disease, 251,
  253
X rays, 37, 81, 82*f*
D-Xylose absorption test, 574

# Y

Yeast, in urine, 390
Y intercept, 70–71
  error identified by, 72*t*

# Z

Zero-order kinetics, 445
Zimmerman reaction for determination of
  17-ketogenic steroids, 524, 525*f*
Zinc, 604
  analytical procedures for, 604
  deficiency of, 604
    signs and symptoms of, 604
      in elderly, 672*t*
  excess of, laboratory diagnosis of, 621
  factors affecting concentration of, 602*t*
  functions of, 604
  reference ranges for, 604
  toxicity of, 604
Zinc protoporphyrin, 343, 348, 462–464,
  463*f*, 463–464
  analytical procedures for, 352
Zinc protoporphyrin/heme ratio (ZPP/H),
  602
Zip™ disks, 142, 143
Zollinger-Ellison syndrome (ZES), 330,
  564–565
  diagnosis of, 571–572
Zona fasciculata, 521, 522*f*
Zona glomerulosa, 521, 522*f*
Zona reticularis, 521, 522*f*
Zone electrophoresis, 209
Zwitterion, 203